Pediatric Dosage Handbook

2nd Edition 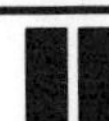 1993-94

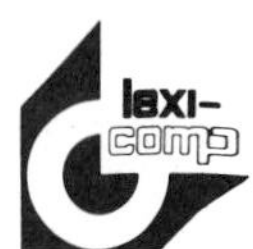

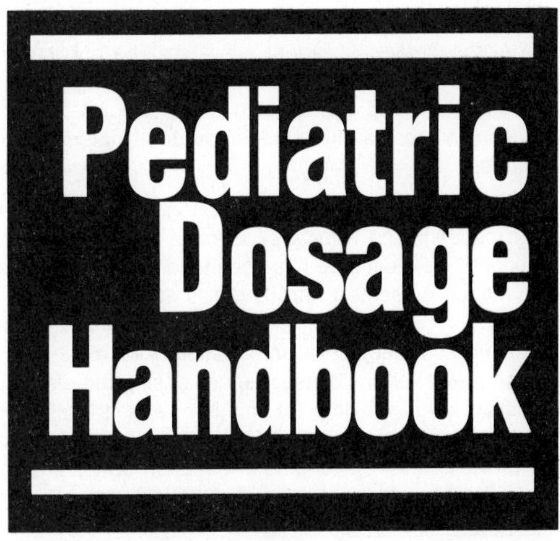

2nd Edition  *1993-94*

Carol K. Taketomo, PharmD
Pharmacy Manager
Children's Hospital of Los Angeles
Los Angeles, California

Jane Hurlburt Hodding, PharmD
Supervisor, Children's Pharmacy
Memorial Miller Children's Hospital
Long Beach, California

Donna M. Kraus, PharmD
Assistant Professor of Pharmacy Practice
Departments of Pharmacy Practice and Pediatrics
Clinical Pharmacist
Pediatric Intensive Care Unit
University of Illinois at Chicago
Chicago, Illinois

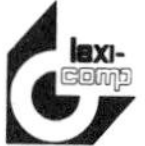

LEXI-COMP, INC
Hudson (Cleveland/Akron)

NOTICE

This handbook is intended to serve the user as a handy reference and not as a complete drug information resource. It does not include information on every therapeutic agent available. The publication covers 541 commonly used drugs and is specifically designed to present important aspects of drug data in a more concise format than is typically found in medical literature or product material supplied by manufacturers.

The nature of drug information is that it is constantly evolving because of ongoing research and clinical experience and is often subject to interpretation. While great care has been taken to ensure the accuracy of the information presented, the reader is advised that the authors, editors, reviewers, contributors, and publishers cannot be responsible for the continued currency of the information or for any errors or omissions in this book or for any consequences arising therefrom. Because of the dynamic nature of drug information, readers are advised that decisions regarding drug therapy must be based on the independent judgment of the clinician, changing information about a drug (eg, as reflected in the literature and manufacturer's most current product information), and changing medical practices. The editors are not responsible for any inaccuracy of quotation or for any false or misleading implication that may arise due to the text or formulas as used or due to the quotation of revisions no longer official.

The editors, authors, and contributors have written this book in their private capacities. No official support or endorsement by any federal or state agency or pharmaceutical company is intended or inferred.

If you have any suggestions or questions
regarding any information presented in this handbook,
please contact our drug information pharmacist at

1-800-837-LEXI

This manual was produced using the FormuLex™ Program —
A complete publishing service of Lexi-Comp Inc.

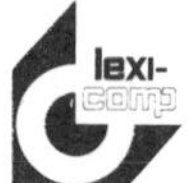

Lexi-Comp Inc.
1100 Terex Road
Hudson, Ohio 44236-3771
(216) 650-6506

ISBN 0-916589-09-9

TABLE OF CONTENTS

RAPID DRUG FINDER SERIES EDITORIAL ADVISORY PANEL

ABOUT THE AUTHORS

Carol K. Taketomo, PharmD

Dr Taketomo received her doctorate from the University of Southern California School of Pharmacy. Subsequently, she completed a clinical pharmacy residency at the University of California Medical Center in San Diego. With over 16 years of clinical experience at one of the largest pediatric teaching hospitals in the nation, she is an acknowledged expert in the practical aspects of pediatric drug distribution and clinical pharmacy practice.

In her current capacity as Pharmacy Manager at Children's Hospital of Los Angeles, Dr Taketomo plays an active role in the education and training of the medical, pharmacy, and nursing staff. She coordinates the Pharmacy Department's quality assurance and drug use evaluation programs; maintains the hospital's strict formulary program; and is the editor of the housestaff manual. Her particular interests are strategies to influence physician prescribing patterns and methods to decrease medication errors in the pediatric setting. She has been the author of numerous publications, and is an active presenter at professional meetings. She currently holds an appointment with the University of Southern California School of Pharmacy.

Dr Taketomo is a member of the American Pharmaceutical Association (APhA), American Society of Hospital Pharmacists (ASHP), California Society of Hospital Pharmacists (CSHP), and Southern California Pediatric Pharmacy Group.

Jane Hurlburt Hodding, PharmD

Dr Hodding earned a doctorate and completed her pharmacy residency at the University of California School of Pharmacy in San Francisco. She has held teaching positions as Assistant Clinical Professor of Pharmacy at UCSF as well as Assistant Clinical Professor of Pharmacy Practice at the University of Southern California in Los Angeles. Currently, Dr Hodding is the Supervisor of Children's Pharmacy at Memorial Miller Children's Hospital in Long Beach, California.

Throughout her 16 years of pediatric pharmacy practice, Dr Hodding has actively pursued methods to improve neonatal intensive care, pediatric intensive care, and parenteral nutrition. She has published numerous articles covering neonatal medication administration and aminoglycoside and theophylline clearance in premature infants.

Dr Hodding is a member of the American Pharmaceutical Association (APhA), American Society of Hospital Pharmacists (ASHP), California Society of Hospital Pharmacists, and Southern California Pediatric Pharmacy Group. She is frequently an invited speaker on the topics of Monitoring Drug Therapy in the NICU, Fluid and Electrolyte Therapy in Children, Drug Therapy Considerations in Children, and Parenteral Nutrition in the Premature Infant.

Donna M. Kraus, PharmD

Dr Kraus has 16 years of active pharmacy experience dealing as an educator and working pharmacist. She has dealt with the clinical problems of determining appropriate pediatric dosages and pharmacotherapy. Her research areas include pediatric drug dosing, developmental pharmacokinetics and pharmacodynamics.

After earning her doctorate degree at the University of Illinois, Dr Kraus completed a postdoctoral pediatric specialty residency at the University of Texas Health Science Center in San Antonio. She has, for the past 10 years, served as a Pediatric Intensive Care Clinical Pharmacist and currently also holds the appointment of Assistant Professor of Pharmacy Practice in both the Departments of Pharmacy Practice and Pediatrics at the University of Illinois in Chicago.

Dr Kraus has been an active member of numerous professional associations including the American Pharmaceutical Association (APhA), American Society of Hospital Pharmacists (ASHP), Illinois Pharmacists Association (IPhA), American College of Clinical Pharmacy (ACCP), and the Illinois College of Clinical Pharmacy (ICCP).

Dr Kraus has been a continual contributor of articles and information to enhance the practice of pediatric pharmacy and is the APhA designated author for this handbook.

PREFACE

This second edition of the *Pediatric Dosage Handbook* is designed to be a practical and convenient guide to the dosing and usage of medications in children. The pediatric population is a dynamic group, with major changes in pharmacokinetics and pharmacodynamics taking place throughout infancy and childhood. Therefore, the need for the evaluation and establishment of medication dosing regimens in children of different ages is great.

Special considerations must be taken into account when dosing medications in pediatric patients. Unfortunately, due to a lack of appropriate studies, most medications commonly used in children do not have FDA approved labeling for use in pediatric patients. Only 30% of drugs used in children in a 1988 survey carried FDA approval in their labeling. Seventy-five percent of medications listed in the *1990 Physicians Desk Reference* carry some type of precaution or disclaimer statement for use in children.[1] The recently proposed FDA labeling changes, which would require expanded information in the Pediatric Use section of the package insert for all prescription drugs, would help to increase dissemination of pediatric drug information. Most commonly used pharmacy references, however, do not include information regarding pediatric dosing, drug administration, or special pediatric concerns. It is, therefore, not surprising that in order to obtain pediatric dosing information, oftentimes the pediatric clinician is faced with extensive literature searches to arrive at a logical dose.

This handbook was developed with the intent to serve as a compilation of recommended pediatric doses found in the literature and to provide relevant clinical information regarding the use of drugs in children. This 2nd edition incorporates additions and revisions in format which we hope the user will find beneficial. Drug monographs have been updated and revised and 20 new medications have been added. The Pharmacodynamics and Pharmacokinetics fields have been reformatted for easier and quicker access to information. Adverse reactions are now arranged according to organ system. Three new fields of information have been added to the drug monographs and include:

> **Administration** which incorporates the guidelines for the proper administration of parenteral medications;
> **Monitoring Parameters** which lists laboratory tests and patient parameters to assess for the efficacy and toxicity of drug therapy; and
> **Extemporaneous Preparations** which lists formulations for oral liquid dosage forms with appropriate references.

For dosing information, when both milligram and milligram per kilogram doses are listed, the milligram per kilogram dosing method is preferred. When ranges of doses are listed, initiate therapy at the lower end of the range and titrate the dose accordingly. References are listed at the end of drug monographs to support doses listed when little dosing information exists. Additional clinical drug information which is relevant to the practice of pediatric pharmacotherapy is also included within each monograph and in the appendices. The appendix section has also been expanded and reorganized to be more "user friendly."

We hope this 2nd edition continues to be a valuable and practical source of clinical drug information for the pediatric health care professional. We welcome comments to further improve future editions.

---

[1] Food and Drug Letter, Washington Business Information, Inc. November 23, 1990.

ACKNOWLEDGMENTS

This handbook exists in its present form as a result of the concerted efforts of many individuals. The publisher and president of Lexi-Comp Inc, Robert D. Kerscher and the director of special projects, Laura C. Lawson, American Pharmaceutical Association (APhA) deserve much of the credit for bringing the concept of such a book to fruition.

Other members of the Lexi-Comp staff whose contributions were invaluable and whose patience with the editors' enumerable drafts, revisions, deletions, additions, and enhancements was inexhaustible include: Leonard L. Lance, RPh, pharmacy editor; Diane Harbart, MT (ASCP), medical editor; Lynn Coppinger, director of product development; Barbara F. Kerscher, production manager; Jeanne Eads, Beth Daulbaugh, Lisa Leukart, and Julie White, assistant production managers; Alexandra Hart, composition specialist; Jil Neuman, Julie Kelley, and Jackie Mizer, production assistants; Jeff J. Zaccagnini, Brian B. Vossler, and Jerry M. Reeves, sales managers; Edmund A. Harbart, vice-president, custom publishing division; and Jack L. Stones, vice-president, reference publishing division. The complex computer programming required for the typesetting of the book was provided by Dennis P. Smithers, Jay L. Katzen, Dale E. Jablonski, and David C. Marcus, system analysts, under the direction of Thury L. O'Connor, vice-president.

Other APhA staff members whose contributions were important are James P. Caro, senior director, Programming and Publications and James V. McGinnis, manager of art and production. A special thanks goes to Chris Lomax, PharmD, director of pharmacy, Children's Hospital, Los Angeles, who played a significant role in bringing APhA and Lexi-Comp together.

In addition, sincere appreciation to Vaughn W. Floutz, PhD who served as editorial consultant and contributor.

Much of the material contained in the book was a result of pediatric pharmacy contributors throughout the United States and Canada. Lexi-Comp has assisted many pediatric medical institutions to develop hospital-specific formulary manuals that contains clinical drug information as well as dosing. Working with these pediatric clinical pharmacists, pediatric hospital pharmacy and therapeutics committees, and hospital drug information centers, Lexi-Comp has developed an evolutionary drug database that reflects the practice of pediatric pharmacy in these major pediatric institutions.

Dr Taketomo would like to thank Robert Taketomo, PharmD, MBA and Chris Lomax, PharmD for their professional guidance and continued support, and the pharmacy staff at Childrens Hospital Los Angeles for their assistance.

In addition, the authors wish to thank their families, friends, and colleagues who supported them in their efforts to complete this handbook.

HOW TO USE THE PEDIATRIC DOSAGE HANDBOOK

The *Pediatric Dosage Handbook, 2nd Edition* is divided into four sections.

The first section is a compilation of introductory text pertinent to the use of this book.

The drug information section of the handbook, in which all drugs are listed alphabetically, details information pertinent to each drug. Extensive cross-referencing is provided by brand name and synonyms.

The third section is an invaluable appendix section with charts, tables, nomograms, and guidelines.

The last section of this handbook is an index listing drugs in their unique therapeutic category.

Alphabetical Listing of Drugs

Drug information is presented in a consistent format and provides the following:

Generic Name	U.S. adopted name
Pronunciation Guide	
Related Information	Cross-reference to other pertinent drug information found in the Appendix
Brand Names	Common trade names
Synonyms	Other names or accepted abbreviations for the generic drug
Therapeutic Class	Systematic classification of medications
Use	Information pertaining to appropriate indications or use of the drug
Restrictions	DEA classification for federally scheduled controlled substances
Pregnancy Risk Factor	Five categories established by the FDA to indicate the potential of a systemically absorbed drug for causing birth defects
Contraindications	Information pertaining to inappropriate use of the drug
Warnings	Hazardous conditions related to use of the drug
Precautions	Disease states or patient populations in which the drug should be cautiously used
Adverse Reactions	Side effects are grouped by body system
Drug Interactions Stability	Comments and/or considerations are offered when appropriate
Mechanism of Action	How the drug works in the body to elicit a response
Pharmacodynamics	Dose-response relationships including onset of action, time of peak action, and duration of action
Pharmacokinetics	Drug movement through the body over time. Pharmacokinetics deals with absorption, distribution, metabolism, half-life, bioavailability, protein binding, and elimination of drugs. Pharmacokinetic parameters help predict drug concentration and dosage requirements.

Usual Dosage	The amount of the drug to be typically given or taken during therapy
Administration	Information regarding the recommended final concentrations and rates for administration of the drug are listed when appropriate.
Monitoring Parameters	Laboratory tests and patient physical parameters that should be monitored for safety and efficacy of drug therapy are listed when appropriate.
References Levels	Therapeutic and toxic serum concentrations listed when appropriate
Test Interactions	Listing of assay interferences when relevant; (S) = Serum; (U) = Urine
Patient Information Nursing Implications Additional Information	Comments and/or considerations are offered when appropriate
Dosage Forms	Information with regard to form, strength, and availability of the drug
Extemporaneous Preparations	Directions for preparing liquid formulations from solid drug products. May include stability information and references (listed when appropriate).
References	Bibliographic information referring to specific pediatric literature findings, especially doses

Appendix

The appendix offers a compilation of tables, guidelines, and conversion information which can often be helpful when considering patient care. This section is broken down into various sections for ease of use.

Therapeutic Category & Key Word Index

This index provides a useful listing by an easy-to-use therapeutic classification system.

DEFINITION OF AGE GROUP TERMINOLOGY

Information in this handbook is listed according to specific age or by age group. The following are definitions of age groups and age-related terminologies. These definitions should be used unless otherwise specified in the monograph.

Gestational age (GA)	The time from conception until birth. More specifically, gestational age is defined as the number of weeks from the first day of the mother's last menstrual period (LMP) until the birth of the baby. Gestational age at birth is assessed by the date of the LMP and by physical exam (Dubowitz score).
Postnatal age (PNA)	Chronological age since birth
Postconceptional age (PCA)	Age since conception. Gestational age plus postnatal age (PCA = GA + PNA)
Neonate	0-4 weeks of age
Premature neonate	Neonate born at <37 weeks gestation
Full-term neonate	Neonate born at 37-42 weeks (average ≈40 weeks) gestation
Infant	1 month to 1 year of age
Child/Children	1-12 years of age
Adolescent	12-18 years of age
Adult	>18 years of age

FDA PREGNANCY CATEGORIES

Throughout this book there is a field labeled Pregnancy Risk Factor (PRF) and the letter A, B, C, D or X immediately following which signifies a category. The FDA has established these five categories to indicate the potential of a systemically absorbed drug for causing birth defects. The key differentiation among the categories rests upon the reliability of documentation and the risk:benefit ratio. Pregnancy Category X is particularly notable in that if any data exists that may implicate a drug as a teratogen and the risk:benefit ratio is clearly negative, the drug is contraindicated during pregnancy.

These categories are summarized as follows:

A Controlled studies in pregnant women fail to demonstrate a risk to the fetus in the first trimester with no evidence of risk in later trimesters. The possibility of fetal harm appears remote.

B Either animal-reproduction studies have not demonstrated a fetal risk but there are no controlled studies in pregnant women, or animal-reproduction studies have shown an adverse effect (other than a decrease in fertility) that was not confirmed in controlled studies in women in the first trimester and there is no evidence of a risk in later trimesters.

C Either studies in animals have revealed adverse effects on the fetus (teratogenic or embryocidal effects or other) and there are no controlled studies in women, or studies in women and animals are not available. Drugs should be given only if the potential benefits justify the potential risk to the fetus.

D There is positive evidence of human fetal risk, but the benefits from use in pregnant women may be acceptable despite the risk (eg, if the drug is needed in a life-threatening situation or for a serious disease for which safer drugs cannot be used or are ineffective).

X Studies in animals or human beings have demonstrated fetal abnormalities or there is evidence of fetal risk based on human experience, or both, and the risk of the use of the drug in pregnant women clearly outweighs any possible benefit. The drug is contraindicated in women who are or may become pregnant.

SAFE WRITING

Health professionals and their support personnel frequently produce handwritten copies of information they see in print; therefore, such information is subjected to even greater possibilities for error or misinterpretation on the part of others. Thus, particular care must be given to how drug names and strengths are expressed when creating written healthcare documents.

The following are a few examples of safe writing rules suggested by the Institute for Safe Medication Practices, Inc.*

1. There should be a space between a number and its units as it is easier to read. There should be no periods after the abbreviations mg or mL.

Correct	Incorrect
10 mg	10mg
100 mg	100mg

2. Never place a decimal and a zero after a whole number (2 mg is correct and 2.0 mg is incorrect). If the decimal point is not seen because it falls on a line or because individuals are working from copies where the decimal point is not seen, this causes a tenfold overdose.

3. Just the opposite is true for numbers less than one. Always place a zero before a naked decimal (0.5 mL is correct, .5 mL is **in**correct).

4. Never abbreviate the word unit. The handwritten U or u, looks like a 0 (zero), and may cause a tenfold overdose error to be made.

5. Q.D. is not a safe abbreviation for once daily, as when the Q is followed by a sloppy dot, it looks like QID which means four times daily.

6. O.D. is not a safe abbreviation for once daily, as it is properly interpreted as meaning "right eye" and has caused liquid medications such as saturated solution of potassium iodide and lugol's solution to be administered incorrectly. There is no safe abbreviation for once daily. It must be written out in full.

7. Do not use chemical names such as 6-mercaptopurine or 6-thioguanine, as 6 fold overdoses have been given when these were not recognized as chemical names. The proper names of these drugs are mercaptopurine or thioguanine.

8. Do not abbreviate drug names (5FC, 6MP, 5-ASA, MTX, HCTZ CPZ, PBZ, etc) as they are misinterpreted and cause error.

9. Do not use the apothecary system or symbols.

10. When writing an outpatient prescription, write a complete prescription. A complete prescription can prevent the prescriber, the pharmacist, and/or the patient from making a

*From "Safe Writing" by Davis NM, PharmD and Cohen MR, MS, Lecturers and Consultants for Safe Medication Practices, 1143 Wright Drive, Huntingdon Valley, PA 19006. Phone: (215) 947-7566.

mistake and can eliminate the need for further clarification. The legible prescriptions should contain:

a. patient's full name
b. for pediatric or geriatric patients: their age (or weight where applicable)
c. drug name, dosage form and strength; if a drug is new or rarely prescribed, print this information
d. number or amount to be dispensed
e. complete instructions for the patient, including the purpose of the medication
f. when there are recognized contraindications for a prescribed drug, indicate to the pharmacist that you are aware of this fact (ie, when prescribing a potassium salt for a patient receiving an ACE inhibitor, write "K serum leveling being monitored")

SELECTED REFERENCES

AMA Drug Evaluations Subscription, American Medical Association, Department of Drugs, Division of Drugs and Toxicology, Winter, 1993.

Drug Interaction Facts, St Louis, MO: J.B. Lippincott Co (Facts and Comparisons Division), 1993.

Facts and Comparisons, St Louis, MO: J.B. Lippincott Co (Facts and Comparisons Division), 1993.

Feigin RD and Cherry JD, *Textbook of Pediatric Infectious Diseases,*3rd ed, Philadelphia, PA: WB Saunders Company, 1992.

Handbook on Extemporaneous Formulations, Bethesda, MD: American Society of Hospital Pharmacists, 1987.

Handbook of Nonprescription Drugs, 9th ed, Washington, DC: American Pharmaceutical Association, 1990.

Jacobs DS, Kasten Jr BL, DeMott WR, et al, *Laboratory Test Handbook with Key Word Index*, 2nd ed, Hudson, OH: Lexi-Comp Inc, 1990.

Levin D, *Essentials of Pediatric Intensive Care*, 1st ed, St Louis, MO: Quality Medical Publishing, Inc, 1990.

McEvoy GK and Litvak K, *AHFS Drug Information*, Bethesda, MD: American Society of Hospital Pharmacists, 1993.

Nahata MC and Hipple TF, *Pediatric Drug Formulations,* Harvey Whitney Books Company, 1st ed, 1990.

Nelson JD, *1993-1994 Pocketbook of Pediatric Antimicrobial Therapy*, 10th ed, Baltimore, MD: Williams & Wilkins, 1993.

Phelps SJ and Cochran EB, *Guidelines for Administration of Intravenous Medications to Pediatric Patients,* 4th ed, Bethesda, MD:American Society of Hospital Pharmacists, 1993.

Physician's Desk Reference, 47th ed, Oradell, NJ: Medical Economics Books, 1993.

Pizzo PA and Poplack DG, *Principles and Practice of Pediatric Oncology*, 2nd ed, Philadelphia, PA: JB Lippincott Company.

Radde IC and MacLead SM, *Pediatric Pharmacology and Therapeutics*, St Louis, MO: Mosby, 1993.

Report of the Committee on Infectious Diseases, American Academy of Pediatrics, 22nd ed, 1991.

Rogers MC, *Textbook of Pediatric Intensive Care*, 2nd ed, Baltimore, MD: Williams & Wilkins, 1992.

Rudolph AM, *Rudolph's Pediatrics*, 19th ed, Norwalk, CT: Appleton & Lange, 1991.

Trissel L, *Handbook of Injectable Drugs*, 7th ed, Bethesda, MD: American Society of Hospital Pharmacists, 1992.

United States Pharmacopeia Dispensing Information (USP DI), 13th ed, Rockville, MD: United States Pharmacopeial Convention, Inc, 1993.

Yaffe SJ and Aranda JV, *Pediatric Pharmacology: Therapeutic Principles in Practice,* Philadelphia, PA: WB Saunders Company, 1992.

ALPHABETICAL LISTING OF DRUGS

A-ase *see* Asparaginase *on page 60*

Abbokinase® *see* Urokinase *on page 590*

Accutane® *see* Isotretinoin *on page 325*

Acephen® [OTC] *see* Acetaminophen *on this page*

Aceta® [OTC] *see* Acetaminophen *on this page*

Acetaminophen (a seet a min' oh fen)

Related Information

OTC Cold Preparations, Pediatric *on page 723-726*

Overdose and Toxicology Information *on page 696-700*

Brand Names Acephen® [OTC]; Aceta® [OTC]; Anacin-3® [OTC]; Apacet® [OTC]; Banesin® [OTC]; Dapa® [OTC]; Datril® [OTC]; Dorcol® [OTC]; Feverall™ [OTC]; Genapap® [OTC]; Halenol® [OTC]; Myapap® Drops [OTC]; Neopap® [OTC]; Panadol® [OTC]; Tempra® [OTC]; Tylenol® [OTC]

Synonyms APAP; N-Acetyl-P-Aminophenol; Paracetamol

Therapeutic Category Analgesic, Non-Narcotic; Antipyretic

Use Treatment of mild to moderate pain and fever; does not have antirheumatic effects

Pregnancy Risk Factor B

Contraindications Hypersensitivity to acetaminophen, G-6-PD deficiency

Warnings May cause severe hepatic toxicity with overdose

Adverse Reactions

Dermatologic: Rash

Renal & genitourinary: Renal injury with chronic use

Miscellaneous: Hypersensitivity reactions (rare)

Mechanism of Action Inhibits the synthesis of prostaglandins in the central nervous system and peripherally blocks pain impulse generation; produces antipyresis from inhibition of hypothalamic heat regulating center

Pharmacokinetics

Protein binding: 20% to 50%

Metabolism: At normal therapeutic dosages the parent compound is metabolized in the liver to sulfate and glucuronide metabolites, while a small amount is metabolized by microsomal mixed function oxidases to a highly reactive intermediate (N-acetyl-imidoquinone) which is conjugated with glutathione and inactivated; at toxic doses (as little as 4 g in a single day) glutathione can become depleted, and conjugation becomes insufficient to meet the metabolic demand causing an increase in N-acetyl-imidoquinone concentration, which is thought to cause hepatic cell necrosis.

Half-life:

Neonates: 2-5 hours

Adults: 1-3 hours

Peak serum concentrations: Occur 10-60 minutes after normal oral doses, but may be delayed in acute overdoses

Usual Dosage Oral, rectal:

Children: 10-15 mg/kg/dose every 4-6 hours as needed; do **not** exceed 5 doses in 24 hours; alternatively, the following doses may be used. See table.

Acetaminophen

Age	Dosage (mg)	Age	Dosage (mg)
0–3 mo	40	4–5 y	240
4–11 mo	80	6–8 y	320
1–2 y	120	9–10 y	400
2–3 y	160	11 y	480

Adults: 325-650 mg every 4-6 hours or 1000 mg 3-4 times/day; do **not** exceed 4 g/day

Reference Range Toxic concentration with probable hepatotoxicity: >200 µg/mL at 4 hours or 50 µg/mL at 12 hours

Dosage Forms

Caplet: 160 mg, 325 mg, 500 mg
Drops: 48 mg/mL (15 mL); 60 mg/0.6 mL (15 mL)
Elixir: 120 mg/5 mL, 160 mg/5 mL, 167 mg/5 mL, 325 mg/5 mL
Liquid, oral: 160 mg/5 mL
Suppository, rectal: 120 mg, 125 mg, 325 mg, 650 mg
Suspension: 100 mg/mL, 160 mg/mL
Tablet: 325 mg, 500 mg, 650 mg
Tablet, chewable: 80 mg, 160 mg

Acetaminophen and Codeine Phosphate

(a seet a min' oh fen and koe' deen)

Related Information

Overdose and Toxicology Information *on page 696-700*

Brand Names Capital® and Codeine; CodAphen®; Phenaphen® With Codeine; Tylenol® With Codeine

Synonyms Codeine Phosphate and Acetaminophen

Therapeutic Category Analgesic, Narcotic

Use Relief of mild to moderate pain

Restrictions C-III; C-IV

Pregnancy Risk Factor C

Contraindications Hypersensitivity to acetaminophen or codeine phosphate

Warnings Tablets contain metabisulfite which may cause allergic reactions

Precautions Use with caution in patients with hypersensitivity reactions to other phenanthrene derivative opioid agonists (morphine, hydrocodone, hydromorphone, levorphanol, oxycodone, oxymorphone) or respiratory disease or compromise

Adverse Reactions

Cardiovascular: Palpitations, hypotension, bradycardia, peripheral vasodilation
Central nervous system: CNS depression, dizziness, drowsiness, sedation
Dermatologic: Pruritus
Endocrine & metabolic: Antidiuretic hormone release
Gastrointestinal: Nausea, vomiting, constipation, biliary tract spasm
Ocular: Miosis
Renal & genitourinary: Urinary retention
Respiratory: Respiratory depression
Miscellaneous: Histamine release, increased intracranial pressure, physical and psychological dependence

Drug Interactions CNS depressants, phenothiazines, tricyclic antidepressants may potentiate the adverse effects of codeine

Usual Dosage Oral (doses should be titrated to appropriate analgesic effect):

Children: Analgesic: 0.5-1 mg codeine/kg/dose every 4-6 hours
- 3-6 years: 5 mL 3-4 times/day as needed
- 7-12 years: 10 mL 3-4 times/day as needed
- >12 years: 15 mL every 4 hours as needed

Adults: 1-2 tablets every 4 hours with a maximum of 12 tablets/24 hours

Dosage Forms

Capsule:
- #2: Acetaminophen 325 mg and codeine phosphate 15 mg
- #3: Acetaminophen 325 mg and codeine phosphate 30 mg
- #4: Acetaminophen 325 mg and codeine phosphate 60 mg

Elixir: Acetaminophen 120 mg and codeine phosphate 12 mg per 5 mL with alcohol 7% (C-IV)

Suspension, oral, alcohol free: Acetaminophen 120 mg and codeine phosphate 12 mg per 5 mL (C-IV)

Tablet: Acetaminophen 500 mg and codeine phosphate 30 mg; acetaminophen 650 mg and codeine phosphate 30 mg

Tablet:
- #1: Acetaminophen 300 mg and codeine phosphate 7.5 mg
- #2: Acetaminophen 300 mg and codeine phosphate 15 mg
- #3: Acetaminophen 300 mg and codeine phosphate 30 mg
- #4: Acetaminophen 300 mg and codeine phosphate 60 mg

Acetaminophen and Hydrocodone *see* Hydrocodone and Acetaminophen *on page 292*

Acetaminophen and Oxycodone Hydrochloride *see* Oxycodone Hydrochloride and Acetaminophen *on page 427*

Acetazolamide (a set a zole' a mide)

Brand Names AK-Zol®; Dazamide®; Diamox®

Therapeutic Category Carbonic Anhydrase Inhibitor; Diuretic, Carbonic Anhydrase Inhibitor

Use Treatment of glaucoma by lowering intraocular pressure; a diuretic; adjunct treatment of refractory seizure and acute altitude sickness

Pregnancy Risk Factor C

Contraindications Hypersensitivity to acetazolamide or other sulfonamides; patients with hepatic disease or insufficiency; decreased serum sodium and/or potassium; adrenocortical insufficiency; hyperchloremic acidosis; or severe renal disease

Warnings I.M. administration is painful because of the alkaline pH of the drug

Precautions Use with caution in patients with respiratory acidosis, diabetes mellitus, and gout

Adverse Reactions

Cardiovascular: Cyanosis

Central nervous system: Paresthesias, muscle weakness, drowsiness, fatigue, vertigo, fever

Dermatologic: Rash

Endocrine & metabolic: Hypokalemia, hyperchloremic metabolic acidosis

Gastrointestinal: GI irritation, anorexia, nausea, vomiting, dry mouth, melena

Hematologic: Bone marrow suppression

Hepatic: Hepatic insufficiency

Ocular: Myopia

Renal & genitourinary: Dysuria, renal calculi

Respiratory: Hyperpnea

Drug Interactions Increases lithium excretion; may decrease the rate of excretion of other drugs such as procainamide, quinidine, and tricyclic antidepressants; may increase the excretion of salicylates and phenobarbital; may inactivate methenamine in the urine

Stability After reconstitution, acetazolamide injection is stable for 1 week when stored under refrigeration

Mechanism of Action Competitive, reversible inhibition of the enzyme carbonic anhydrase resulting in ↑ renal excretion of sodium, potassium, bicarbonate, and water and ↓ formation of aqueous humor

Pharmacodynamics

Onset of action: Varies between 2 minutes with the I.V. form to 2 hours with the extended release capsule

Peak effect:

- Capsule: 3-6 hours
- Tablet: 1-4 hours
- I.V.: 15 minutes

Duration:

- Capsule: 18-24 hours
- Tablet: 8-12 hours
- I.V.: 4-5 hours

Pharmacokinetics

Distribution: Distributes into erythrocytes, kidneys, and breast milk; crosses the blood-brain barrier and the placenta; a milk/plasma ratio of 0.25 has been reported

Half-life: 2.4-5.8 hours

Elimination: 70% to 100% of an I.V. or tablet dose and 47% of an extended release capsule is excreted unchanged in the urine within 24 hours

Usual Dosage

Children:

- Glaucoma:
  - Oral: 8-30 mg/kg/day or 300-900 mg/m^2/day divided every 8 hours
  - I.M., I.V.: 20-40 mg/kg/day divided every 6 hours, not to exceed 1 g/day
- Edema: Oral, I.M., I.V.: 5 mg/kg or 150 mg/m^2 once daily
- Epilepsy: Oral: 8-30 mg/kg/day in 1-4 divided doses, not to exceed 1 g/day

Adults:
  Glaucoma:
    Oral: 250 mg 1-4 times/day or 500 mg sustained release capsule twice daily
    I.M., I.V.: 250-500 mg, may repeat in 2-4 hours
  Edema: Oral, I.M., I.V.: 250-375 mg once daily
  Epilepsy: Oral: 8-30 mg/kg/day in 1-4 divided doses, not to exceed 1 g/day
  Altitude sickness: Oral: 250 mg every 8-12 hours or 500 mg extended release capsules every 12-24 hours; therapy should begin 24-48 hours before and continued during ascent and for at least 48 hours after arrival at the high altitude

Dosing interval in renal impairment: Children and Adults:
  Cl_{cr} 10-50 mL/minute: Administer every 12 hours
  Cl_{cr} <10 mL/minute: Avoid use

Administration Reconstitute with at least 5 mL sterile water to provide an I.V. solution containing not more than 100 mg/mL; maximum concentration: 100 mg/mL; maximum rate of I.V. infusion: 500 mg/minute

Monitoring Parameters Serum electrolytes, periodic hematologic determinations

Test Interactions May cause false-positive results for urinary protein with Albustix®, Labstix®, Albutest®, Bumintest®

Patient Information Do not crush or chew long-acting capsule; take with food

Nursing Implications Tablet may be crushed and suspended in cherry or chocolate syrup to disguise the bitter taste of the drug

Additional Information Sodium content of 500 mg: 2.049 mEq

Extended release capsules are indicated only for use for the adjunctive treatment of open-angle or secondary glaucoma and the prevention of high altitude sickness

Dosage Forms

Capsule, sustained release: 500 mg
Injection: 500 mg/5 mL
Tablet: 125 mg, 250 mg

Extemporaneous Preparation(s) Tablets may be crushed and suspended in cherry, chocolate, raspberry, or other highly flavored carbohydrate syrup to a maximum concentration of 100 mg/mL; suspensions are stable for 7 days; stability data for compounding a 25 mg/mL oral suspension from crushed tablets is available in the following reference.

Alexander KS, Haribhakti RP, and Parker GA, "Stability of Acetazolamide in Suspension Compound From Tablets," *Am J Hosp Pharm*, 1991, 48(6):1241-4.

Acetoxymethylprogesterone *see* Medroxyprogesterone Acetate *on page 359*

Acetylcholine Chloride (a se teel koe' leen)

Brand Names Miochol®

Therapeutic Category Cholinergic Agent, Ophthalmic; Ophthalmic Agent, Miotic

Use To produce complete miosis in cataract surgery, keratoplasty, iridectomy and other anterior segment surgery where rapid miosis is required

Pregnancy Risk Factor C

Contraindications Hypersensitivity to acetylcholine chloride; acute iritis and acute inflammatory disease of the anterior chamber

Warnings Open under aseptic conditions only

Adverse Reactions

Cardiovascular: Transient bradycardia and hypotension
Ocular: Iris atrophy, temporary lens opacities (attributed to osmotic effect of 5% mannitol present in preparation)

Stability Prepare solution immediately before use

Mechanism of Action Causes contraction of the sphincter muscles of the iris, resulting in miosis and contraction of the ciliary muscle, leading to accommodation

Pharmacodynamics

Onset of action: Miosis occurs promptly
Duration: ~10-20 minutes

(Continued)

Acetylcholine Chloride *(Continued)*

Usual Dosage Adults: 0.5-2 mL of 1% injection (5-20 mg) instilled into anterior chamber before or after securing one or more sutures

Dosage Forms Powder, intraocular: 20 mg

Acetylcysteine (a se teel sis' tay een)

Brand Names Mucomyst®; Mucosol®

Synonyms *N*-Acetylcysteine; *N*-Acetyl-L-cysteine

Therapeutic Category Antidote, Acetaminophen; Mucolytic Agent

Use Adjunctive therapy in patients with abnormal or viscid mucous secretions in acute and chronic bronchopulmonary diseases, pulmonary complications of surgery and cystic fibrosis; diagnostic bronchial studies; antidote for acute acetaminophen toxicity

Pregnancy Risk Factor B

Contraindications Known hypersensitivity to acetylcysteine

Warnings Since increased bronchial secretions may develop after inhalation, percussion, postural drainage and suctioning should follow

Precautions If bronchospasm occurs, administer a bronchodilator; discontinue acetylcysteine if bronchospasm progresses

Adverse Reactions

Dermatologic: Generalized urticaria

Gastrointestinal: Stomatitis, nausea, vomiting, hemoptysis

Hepatic: Mild increases in liver function tests have occurred after oral therapy

Respiratory: Bronchospasm, rhinorrhea

Stability Store opened vials in the refrigerator; use within 96 hours

Mechanism of Action Exerts mucolytic action through its free sulfhydryl group which opens up the disulfide bonds in the mucoproteins thus lowering the viscosity. The exact mechanism of action in acetaminophen toxicity is unknown. It may act by maintaining or restoring glutathione levels or by acting as an alternative substrate for conjugation with the toxic metabolite.

Pharmacodynamics

Onset of action: Upon inhalation, mucus liquefaction occurs maximally within 5-10 minutes

Duration of mucus liquefaction: More than 1 hour

Pharmacokinetics

Half-life:

- Reduced acetylkcysteine: 2 hours
- Total acetylcysteine: 5.5

Usual Dosage

Acetaminophen poisoning: Children and Adults: Oral: 140 mg/kg; followed by 17 doses of 70 mg/kg every 4 hours; repeat dose if emesis occurs within 1 hour of administration; therapy should continue until all doses are administered even though the acetaminophen plasma level has dropped below the toxic range

Inhalation: Acetylcysteine 10% and 20% solution (Mucomyst®) (dilute 20% solution with sodium chloride or sterile water for inhalation); 10% solution may be used undiluted

- Infants: 1-2 mL of 20% solution or 2-4 mL 10% solution until nebulized given 3-4 times/day
- Children: 3-5 mL of 20% solution or 6-10 mL of 10% solution until nebulized given 3-4 times/day
- Adolescents: 5-10 mL of 10% to 20% solution until nebulized given 3-4 times/day
- **Note:** Patients should receive an aerosolized bronchodilator 10-15 minutes prior to acetylcysteine

Meconium ileus equivalent: Children and Adults: 100-300 mL of 4% to 10% solution by irrigation or orally

Monitoring Parameters Determine acetaminophen level as soon as possible, but no sooner than 4 hours after ingestion (to ensure peak levels have been obtained); liver function tests (when used in acetaminophen overdose)

Patient Information Clear airway by coughing deeply before aerosol treatment

Nursing Implications Assess patient for nausea, vomiting, and skin rash following oral administration for treatment of acetaminophen poisoning; intermittent aerosol treatments are commonly given when patient arises, before meals, and just before retiring at bedtime

Additional Information For treatment of acetaminophen overdosage, administer orally as a 5% solution; dilute the 20% solution 1:3 with a cola, orange juice or other soft drink; use within 1 hour of preparation

Dosage Forms Solution, as sodium: 10% (4 mL, 10 mL, 30 mL); 20% (4 mL, 10 mL, 30 mL, 100 mL)

References

Dart RC and Rumack BH, "Acetaminophen Hepatotoxicity After Prolonged Ingestion," (letter to the editor), *Pediatrics*, 1993, 91:1021-2.

Acetylsalicylic Acid *see* Aspirin *on page 61*

Achromycin® *see* Tetracycline Hydrochloride *on page 552*

Achromycin® V *see* Tetracycline Hydrochloride *on page 552*

Aciclovir *see* Acyclovir *on this page*

Acid Mantle® [OTC] *see* Aluminum Acetate *on page 33*

Acidulated Phosphate Fluoride *see* Fluoride *on page 255*

ACT *see* Dactinomycin *on page 169*

ACT® [OTC] *see* Fluoride *on page 255*

Actagen® [OTC] *see* Triprolidine and Pseudoephedrine *on page 586*

ACTH *see* Corticotropin *on page 153*

Acthar® *see* Corticotropin *on page 153*

Actidose-Aqua® [OTC] *see* Charcoal *on page 121*

Actidose® With Sorbitol [OTC] *see* Charcoal *on page 121*

Actifed® [OTC] *see* Triprolidine and Pseudoephedrine *on page 586*

Actinomycin D *see* Dactinomycin *on page 169*

Activated Carbon *see* Charcoal *on page 121*

Activated Charcoal *see* Charcoal *on page 121*

Activated Dimethicone *see* Simethicone *on page 524*

Activated Ergosterol *see* Ergocalciferol *on page 224*

Activated Methylpolysiloxane *see* Simethicone *on page 524*

ACV *see* Acyclovir *on this page*

Acycloguanosine *see* Acyclovir *on this page*

Acyclovir (ay sye' kloe ver)

Brand Names Zovirax®

Synonyms Aciclovir; ACV; Acycloguanosine

Therapeutic Category Antiviral Agent, Oral; Antiviral Agent, Parenteral; Antiviral Agent, Topical

Use Treatment of initial and prophylaxis of recurrent mucosal and cutaneous herpes simplex (HSV-1 and HSV-2) infections; herpes simplex encephalitis; herpes zoster infections; varicella-zoster infections in healthy, nonpregnant persons >13 years, children >12 months who have a chronic skin or lung disorder or are receiving long-term aspirin therapy, and immunocompromised patients

Pregnancy Risk Factor C

Contraindications Hypersensitivity to acyclovir

Precautions Use with caution in patients with renal disease, dehydration, underlying neurologic disease, and in patients with hypoxia, hepatic or electrolyte abnormalities; dosage should be reduced in patients with renal impairment

Adverse Reactions

Central nervous system: Headache, lethargy, tremulousness, delirium, coma, dizziness, seizures, pain, insomnia

Dermatologic: Skin rash

Gastrointestinal: Nausea, vomiting

(Continued)

Acyclovir *(Continued)*

Hematologic: Bone marrow depression
Hepatic: Elevation of liver enzymes
Local: Phlebitis at injection site, local pain and stinging with topical use
Renal & genitourinary: Nephrotoxicity
Respiratory: Sore throat
Miscellaneous: Diaphoresis

Drug Interactions Zidovudine; probenecid (decreases renal clearance of acyclovir)

Stability Acyclovir is incompatible with blood products and protein-containing solutions; reconstituted 50 mg/mL solution should be used within 12 hours; do not refrigerate reconstituted solutions as they may precipitate

Mechanism of Action Inhibits DNA synthesis and viral replication by competing with deoxyguanosine triphosphate for viral DNA polymerase and being incorporated into viral DNA

Pharmacokinetics

Absorption: Oral: 15% to 30%; food does not appear to affect its absorption
Distribution: Widely distributed throughout the body including brain, kidney, lungs, liver, spleen, muscle, uterus, vagina, and the CSF
Protein binding: <30%
Half-life, terminal phase:
- Neonates: 4 hours
- Children 1-12 years: 2-3 hours
- Adults: 2-3.5 hours (with normal renal function)

Peak serum levels: Oral: Within 1.5-2 hours
Elimination: Primary route is the kidney with 30% to 90% of a dose excreted unchanged in the urine, following a small amount of hepatic metabolism; requires dosage adjustment with renal impairment; hemodialysis removes ~60% of a dose while removal by peritoneal dialysis is to a much lesser extent

Usual Dosage

Neonates: HSV infection: I.V.: 1500 mg/m^2/day divided every 8 hours or 30 mg/kg/day divided every 8 hours for 10-14 days

Children: Oral:
- Herpes zoster in immunocompromised patients: 250-600 mg/m^2/dose 4-5 times/day
- Varicella zoster (chickenpox): 20 mg/kg/dose (maximum: 800 mg/dose) 4 times/day for 5 days; begin treatment at the earliest sign or symptom

Adults: Oral:
- Genital herpes infection: 200 mg every 4 hours while awake (5 times/day)
  - Prophylaxis: 200 mg 3-4 times/day or 400 mg twice daily
- Herpes zoster in immunocompromised patients: 800 mg every 4 hours (5 times/day) for 7-10 days
  - Prophylaxis: 400 mg 5 times/day
- Varicella zoster: 20 mg/kg/dose (maximum: 800 mg/dose) 4 times/day for 5 days; begin treatment at the earliest sign or symptom

Children and Adults:
- I.V. (dosage for obese patients should be based on ideal body weight):
  - Mucocutaneous HSV infection: 750 mg/m^2/day divided every 8 hours **or** 15 mg/kg/day divided every 8 hours for 7 days
  - HSV encephalitis: 1500 mg/m^2/day divided every 8 hours **or** 30 mg/kg/day divided every 8 hours for 10 days (or up to 14-21 days)
  - Varicella-zoster virus infection: 1500 mg/m^2/day divided every 8 hours **or** 30 mg/kg/day divided every 8 hours for 7 days
  - Herpes zoster in immunocompromised patients: 7.5 mg/kg/dose every 8 hours
- Topical: Apply ½" ribbon of ointment for a 4" square surface area every 3 hours (6 times/day) for 7 days
- I.V.: Prophylaxis of bone marrow transplant recipients:
  - Autologous patients who are HSV seropositive: 150 mg/m^2/dose every 12 hours; with clinical symptoms of herpes simplex: 150 mg/m^2/dose every 8 hours
  - Autologous patients who are CMV seropositive: 500 mg/m^2/dose every 8 hours; for clinically symptomatic CMV infection, consider replacing acyclovir with ganciclovir

Dosing interval in renal impairment for children ≥6 months and adults:

Oral:

200 mg 5 times/day: Cl_{cr} <10 mL/minute: Administer every 12 hours

800 mg 5 times/day: Cl_{cr} 10-25 mL/minute: Administer every 8 hours; Cl_{cr} <10 mL/minute: Administer every 12 hours

I.V.:

Cl_{cr} 25-50 mL/minute: Administer every 12 hours

Cl_{cr} 10-25 mL/minute: Administer every 24 hours

Cl_{cr} <10 mL/minute: 50% decrease in dose, administer every 24 hours

Administration Reconstitute vial for injection with paraben-free sterile water; administer by slow I.V. infusion over at least 1 hour at a final concentration not to exceed 7 mg/mL; in patients who require fluid restriction, a concentration of up to 10 mg/mL has been infused; concentration >10 mg/mL increases the risk of phlebitis

Monitoring Parameters Urinalysis, BUN, serum creatinine, liver enzymes, CBC

Nursing Implications Maintain adequate hydration and urine output the first 2 hours after I.V. infusion to decrease the risk of nephrotoxicity

Additional Information Sodium content of 1 g: 4.2 mEq

Dosage Forms

Capsule: 200 mg

Injection: 50 mg/mL (10 mL, 20 mL)

Ointment, topical: 5% (15 g)

Suspension, oral: 200 mg/5 mL

Tablet: 800 mg

References

Balfour HH Jr, Kelly JM, Suarez CS, et al, "Acyclovir Treatment of Varicella in Otherwise Healthy Children," *J Pediatr*, 1990, 116(4):633-9.

Dellamonica P, Carles M, Lokiec F, et al, "Preventing Recurrent Varicella and Herpes Zoster With Oral Acyclovir in HIV-Seropositive Patients," *Clin Pharm*, 1991, 10(4):301-2.

Dunkle LM, Arvin AM, Whitley RJ, et al, "A Controlled Trial of Acyclovir for Chickenpox in Normal Children," *N Engl J Med*, 1991, 325(22):1539-44.

Englund JA, Fletcher CV, and Balfour HH Jr, "Acyclovir Therapy in Neonates," *J Pediatr*, 1991, 119(1 Pt 1):129-35.

Meyers JD, Reed EC, Shepp DH, et al, "Acyclovir for Prevention of Cytomegalovirus Infection and Disease After Allogenic Marrow Transplantation," *N Engl J Med*, 1988, 318(2):70-5.

Novelli VM, Marshall WC, Yeo J, et al, "High-Dose Oral Acyclovir for Children at Risk of Disseminated Herpes Virus Infections," *J Infect Dis*, 1985, 151(2):372.

Adalat® *see* Nifedipine *on page 413*

Adamantanamine Hydrochloride *see* Amantadine Hydrochloride *on page 34*

Adapin® *see* Doxepin Hydrochloride *on page 207*

Adenine Arabinoside *see* Vidarabine *on page 599*

Adenocard® *see* Adenosine *on this page*

Adenosine (a den' oh seen)

Brand Names Adenocard®

Synonyms 9-Beta-D-ribofuranosyladenine

Therapeutic Category Antiarrhythmic Agent, Miscellaneous

Use Treatment of paroxysmal supraventricular tachycardia (PSVT); orphan drug for treatment of brain tumors in conjunction with BCNU

Pregnancy Risk Factor C

Contraindications Known hypersensitivity to adenosine, second and third degree A-V block or sick-sinus syndrome unless pacemaker placed

Warnings Heart block, including transient asystole may occur as well as other arrhythmias; if arrhythmia is not due to re-entry pathway through A-V node or sinus node (ie, atrial fibrillation, flutter, or tachycardia or ventricular tachycardia), adenosine will not terminate the arrhythmia but can produce transient ventriculoatrial or A-V block; possible mutagenic effects

Precautions Possible bronchoconstriction in asthmatics; use with caution in patients with underlying dysfunction of sinus or A-V node; initial adenosine dose should be significantly decreased in patients receiving dipyridamole

(Continued)

Adenosine *(Continued)*

Adverse Reactions

Cardiovascular: Flushing, arrhythmias, minimal hemodynamic disturbances, chest pain, bradycardia, heart block

Central nervous system: Irritability, headaches, lightheadedness

Gastrointestinal: Nausea

Respiratory: Dyspnea

Drug Interactions Dipyridamole potentiates effects of adenosine; methylxanthines antagonize effects; carbamazepine may increase heart block

Stability Do **not** refrigerate, precipitation may occur; no preservatives, discard unused portion

Mechanism of Action Slows conduction time through the A-V node, interrupting the re-entry pathways through the A-V node, restoring normal sinus rhythm

Pharmacokinetics

Clinical effects occur rapidly and are very brief

Metabolism: Metabolized in blood and tissue → inosine → adenosine monophosphate (AMP) and hypoxanthine → xanthine → uric acid

Half-life: <10 seconds, thus adverse effects are usually rapidly self limiting

Usual Dosage Rapid I.V. (**Note:** Higher doses may be needed for administration via peripheral vs central vein):

Children: PALS dose for treatment of SVT: 0.1 mg/kg; if not effective, give 0.2 mg/kg; maximum single dose: 12 mg

Alternatively: Initial dose: 0.05 mg/kg; if not effective within 2 minutes, increase dose in 0.05 mg/kg increments every 2 minutes to a maximum dose of 0.25 mg/kg or until termination of PSVT; median dose required: 0.15 mg/kg; do not exceed 12 mg/dose

Adults: 6 mg, if not effective within 1-2 minutes, 12 mg may be given; may repeat 12 mg bolus if needed

Administration For rapid bolus I.V. use only, give over 1-2 seconds; administer at I.V. site closest to patient; follow each bolus with normal saline flush

Monitoring Parameters Continuous EKG, heart rate, blood pressure, respirations

Nursing Implications Be alert for possible exacerbation of asthma in asthmatic patients

Additional Information Short action an advantage; not effective in atrial flutter, atrial fibrillation, or ventricular tachycardia

Dosage Forms Injection, preservative free: 3 mg/mL (2 mL)

References

Emergency Cardiac Care Committee and Subcommittees, American Heart Association, "Guidelines for Cardiopulmonary Resuscitation and Emergency Cardiac Care, III: Adult Advanced Cardiac Life Support" and "VI: Pediatric Advanced Life Support," *JAMA*, 1992, 268(16):2199-241 and 2262-75.

Till J, Shinebourne EA, Rigby ML, et al, "Efficacy and Safety in the Treatment of Supraventricular Tachycardia in Infants and Children," *Br Heart J*, 1989, 62(3):204-11.

Zeigler V, "Adenosine in the Pediatric Population: Nursing Implications," *Pediatr Nurs*, 1991, 17(6):600-2.

ADH *see* Vasopressin *on page 595*

Adlone® *see* Methylprednisolone *on page 379*

ADR *see* Doxorubicin Hydrochloride *on page 208*

Adrenalin® *see* Epinephrine *on page 220*

Adrenaline *see* Epinephrine *on page 220*

Adrenocorticotropic Hormone *see* Corticotropin *on page 153*

Adriamycin PFS™ *see* Doxorubicin Hydrochloride *on page 208*

Adriamycin RDF™ *see* Doxorubicin Hydrochloride *on page 208*

Adrucil® *see* Fluorouracil *on page 257*

Adsorbent Charcoal *see* Charcoal *on page 121*

Adsorbocarpine® *see* Pilocarpine *on page 459*

Adsorbonac® [OTC] Ophthalmic *see* Sodium Chloride *on page 527*

Advil® [OTC] *see* Ibuprofen *on page 300*

AeroBid® *see* Flunisolide *on page 253*

Aerolate® *see* Theophylline *on page 554*

Aerolate III® *see* Theophylline *on page 554*

Aerolate JR® *see* Theophylline *on page 554*

Aerolate SR® S *see* Theophylline *on page 554*

Aeroseb-Dex® *see* Dexamethasone *on page 178*

Aeroseb-HC® *see* Hydrocortisone *on page 293*

Aerosporin® *see* Polymyxin B Sulfate *on page 466*

Afrin® Nasal Solution [OTC] *see* Oxymetazoline Hydrochloride *on page 429*

Afrinol® [OTC] *see* Pseudoephedrine *on page 497*

Aftate® [OTC] *see* Tolnaftate *on page 573*

Agoral® Plain [OTC] *see* Mineral Oil *on page 390*

AHF *see* Antihemophilic Factor, Human *on page 55*

AHG *see* Antihemophilic Factor, Human *on page 55*

A-hydroCort® *see* Hydrocortisone *on page 293*

Akarpine® *see* Pilocarpine *on page 459*

AK-Chlor® *see* Chloramphenicol *on page 124*

AK-Con® *see* Naphazoline Hydrochloride *on page 403*

AK-Dex® *see* Dexamethasone *on page 178*

AK-Dilate® Ophthalmic Solution *see* Phenylephrine Hydrochloride *on page 453*

AK-Homatropine® *see* Homatropine Hydrobromide *on page 287*

AK-Mycin® *see* Erythromycin *on page 226*

AK-Nefrin® Ophthalmic Solution *see* Phenylephrine Hydrochloride *on page 453*

Akne-Mycin® *see* Erythromycin *on page 226*

AK-Pentolate® *see* Cyclopentolate Hydrochloride *on page 161*

AK-Poly-Bac® *see* Bacitracin and Polymyxin B Sulfate *on page 74*

AK-Pred® *see* Prednisolone *on page 476*

AK-Spore H.C.® *see* Neomycin, (Bacitracin) Polymyxin B and Hydrocortisone *on page 406*

AK-Sulf® *see* Sulfacetamide Sodium *on page 539*

AK-Taine® *see* Proparacaine Hydrochloride *on page 490*

AK-Tracin® *see* Bacitracin *on page 73*

AK-Trol® *see* Dexamethasone, Neomycin and Polymyxin B *on page 180*

AK-Zol® *see* Acetazolamide *on page 18*

Ala-Tet® *see* Tetracycline Hydrochloride *on page 552*

Albalon® Liquifilm® *see* Naphazoline Hydrochloride *on page 403*

Albuminar® *see* Albumin Human *on this page*

Albumin Human (al byoo' min)

Related Information

CPR Pediatric Drug Dosages *on page 614*

Brand Names Albuminar®; Albutein®; Buminate®; Plasbumin®

Synonyms Normal Human Serum Albumin; Normal Serum Albumin (Human); Salt Poor Albumin

(Continued)

Albumin Human *(Continued)*

Therapeutic Category Blood Product Derivative; Plasma Volume Expander

Use Plasma volume expansion and maintenance of cardiac output in the treatment of certain types of shock or impending shock; hypoproteinemia

Pregnancy Risk Factor C

Contraindications Patients with severe anemia or cardiac failure; known hypersensitivity to albumin; avoid 25% concentration in preterm infants due to risk of IVH

Precautions Rapid infusion of albumin solutions may cause vascular overload. Do not administer albumin to burn patients for the first 24 hours after the burn (capillary exudation of albumin will occur)

Adverse Reactions

Cardiovascular: Precipitation of congestive heart failure or pulmonary edema, hypertension, tachycardia, hypervolemia, hypotension due to hypersensitivity

Central nervous system: Fever, chills

Dermatologic: Rash

Gastrointestinal: Nausea, vomiting

Stability Use within 4 hours after opening vial, do not use if turbid or contains a deposit

Mechanism of Action Provides increase in intravascular oncotic pressure and causes mobilization of fluids from interstitial into intravascular space

Pharmacodynamics Duration of volume expansion: ~24 hours

Pharmacokinetics Half-life: 21 days

Usual Dosage 5% should be used in hypovolemic or intravascularly depleted patients; 25% should be used in patients with fluid or sodium restrictions. Dose depends on condition of patient. I.V.:

Children:

Hypoproteinemia: 0.5-1 g/kg/dose; infuse over 2-4 hours; may repeat every 1-2 days

Hypovolemia: 0.5-1 g/kg/dose; may repeat as needed; maximum dose: 6 g/kg/day

Adults: 25 g; no more than 250 g should be administered within 48 hours

Administration I.V. after initial volume replacement:

5%: Do not exceed 2-4 mL/minute

25%: Do not exceed 1 mL/minute

Monitoring Parameters Observe for signs of hypervolemia, pulmonary edema, and cardiac failure

Nursing Implications Albumin administration must be completed within 6 hours after entering container, provided that administration is begun within 4 hours of entering the container; use 5 micron filter or larger, do **not** give through 0.22 micron filter

Additional Information Albumin contains 130-160 mEq of sodium per liter; osmolarity: 5% albumin = 300 mOsm/L; 25% albumin = 1500 mOsm/L

Dosage Forms Injection: 5% (50 mL, 250 mL, 500 mL, 1000 mL); 25% (10 mL, 20 mL, 50 mL, 100 mL)

Albutein® *see* Albumin Human *on previous page*

Albuterol (al byoo' ter ole)

Brand Names Proventil®; Ventolin®

Synonyms Salbutamol

Therapeutic Category Beta-2-Adrenergic Agonist Agent; Bronchodilator; Sympathomimetic

Use Used as a bronchodilator in reversible airway obstruction due to asthma or COPD

Pregnancy Risk Factor C

Contraindications Hypersensitivity to albuterol or any component or adrenergic amine

Precautions Use with caution in patients with hyperthyroidism, diabetes mellitus; cardiovascular disorders including coronary insufficiency or hypertension; excessive or prolonged use can lead to tolerance

Adverse Reactions

Cardiovascular: Tachycardia, palpitations, peripheral vasodilatation

Central nervous system: Tremor, nervousness, CNS stimulation; hyperactivity and insomnia occur more frequently in younger children than adults

Endocrine & metabolic: Hypokalemia
Gastrointestinal: GI upset
Respiratory: Irritation of oropharynx

Drug Interactions Action of albuterol is antagonized by beta-adrenergic blocking agents such as propranolol; cardiovascular effects are potentiated in patients also receiving MAO inhibitors or tricyclic antidepressants; concomitant administration of sympathomimetics may result in enhanced cardiovascular effects

Mechanism of Action Relaxes bronchial smooth muscle by action on $beta_2$ receptors with little effect on heart rate

Pharmacodynamics

Nebulization/oral inhalation:
- Peak bronchodilation: Within 0.5-2 hours nebulization
- Duration: 2-5 hours

Oral:
- Peak bronchodilatation: 2-3 hours
- Duration: 4-6 hours

Extended release tablets: Duration: Up to 12 hours

Pharmacokinetics

Metabolism: Metabolized by the liver to an inactive sulfate

Half-life:
- Oral: 2.7-5 hours
- Inhalation: 3.8 hours

Elimination: 30% appears in the urine as unchanged drug

Usual Dosage

Oral:
- 2-6 years: 0.1-0.2 mg/kg/dose 3 times/day; maximum dose not to exceed 4 mg 3 times/day
- 6-12 years: 2 mg/dose 3-4 times/day; maximum dose not to exceed 24 mg/day (divided doses)
- >12 years: 2-4 mg/dose 3-4 times/day; maximum dose not to exceed 8 mg 4 times/day

Inhalation MDI: 90 μg/spray:
- <12 years: 1-2 inhalations 4 times/day using a tube spacer
- ≥12 years: 1-2 inhalations every 4-6 hours

Inhalation: Nebulization: 0.01-0.05 mL/kg of 0.5% solution every 4-6 hours; intensive care patients may require more frequent administration; minimum dose: 0.1 mL; maximum dose: 1 mL diluted in 1-2 mL normal saline

Oral inhalation (Rotahaler®): Children >4 years and Adults: 200-400 μg every 4-6 hours

Monitoring Parameters Serum potassium, heart rate, respiratory rate; arterial or capillary blood gases (if patient's condition warrants)

Patient Information Do not exceed recommended dosage; rinse mouth with water following each inhalation to help with dry throat and mouth

Nursing Implications Before using, the inhaler must be shaken well

Dosage Forms

Aerosol, oral: 90 μg/spray (17 g)
Capsules, for inhalation (Rotacaps®): 200 μg
Inhalation: 0.083% (3 mL); 0.5% (20 mL)
Syrup, as sulfate, alcohol and sugar free (strawberry flavor): 2 mg/5 mL (480 mL)
Tablet, as sulfate: 2 mg, 4 mg
Tablet, extended release: 4 mg

References

O'Callaghan C, Milner AD, and Swarbrick A, "Nebulized Salbutamol Does Have a Protective Effect on Airways in Children Under One Year Old," *Arch Dis Child*, 1988, 63(5):479-83.

Rachelefsky GS and Siegel SC, "Asthma in Infants and Children - Treatment of Childhood Asthma: Part II," *J Allergy Clin Immunol*, 1985, 76(3):409-25.

Schuh S, Parkin P, Rajan A, et al, "High- Versus Low-Dose, Frequently Administered, Nebulized Albuterol in Children With Severe, Acute Asthma," *Pediatrics*, 1989, 83(4):513-8.

Schuh S, Reider MJ, Canny G, et al, "Nebulized Albuterol in Acute Childhood Asthma: Comparison of Two Doses," *Pediatrics*, 1990, 86(4):509-13.

Alcaine® *see* Proparacaine Hydrochloride *on page 490*

Alconefrin® Nasal Solution [OTC] *see* Phenylephrine Hydrochloride *on page 453*

Aldactone® *see* Spironolactone *on page 533*

Aldomet® *see* Methyldopa *on page 376*

Alfenta® *see* Alfentanil Hydrochloride *on this page*

Alfentanil Hydrochloride (al fen' ta nill)

Related Information

Narcotic Analgesics Comparison Chart *on page 721-722*

Overdose and Toxicology Information *on page 696-700*

Brand Names Alfenta®

Therapeutic Category Analgesic, Narcotic; General Anesthetic

Use Analgesia; analgesia adjunct; anesthetic agent

Restrictions C-II

Pregnancy Risk Factor C

Contraindications Hypersensitivity to alfentanil hydrochloride; increased intracranial pressure; severe respiratory depression

Warnings Rapid I.V. infusion may result in skeletal muscle and chest wall rigidity → impaired ventilation → respiratory distress/arrest; inject slowly over 3-5 minutes; nondepolarizing skeletal muscle relaxant may be required

Precautions Use with caution in patients with bradycardia

Adverse Reactions

Cardiovascular: Bradycardia, peripheral vasodilation, hypotension, increased intracranial pressure

Central nervous system: Drowsiness, dizziness, sedation, CNS depression

Endocrine & metabolic: Antidiuretic hormone release

Gastrointestinal: Nausea, vomiting, constipation

Ocular: Miosis

Renal & genitourinary: Biliary or urinary tract spasm

Respiratory: Respiratory depression

Miscellaneous: Physical and psychological dependence with prolonged use

Drug Interactions CNS depressants, phenothiazines, tricyclic antidepressants may potentiate the adverse effects of opiate agonists

Mechanism of Action Binds with stereospecific receptors at many sites within the CNS, increases pain threshold, alters pain reception, inhibits ascending pain pathways

Pharmacodynamics

Onset: Within 5 minutes

Duration: <15-20 minutes

Pharmacokinetics

Distribution: V_{dB}:

- Newborns, premature: 1 L/kg
- Children: 0.163-0.48 L/kg
- Adults: 0.46 L/kg

Protein binding:

- Neonates: 67%
- Adults: 88% to 92%
- Bound to $alpha_1$ acid glycoprotein

Half-life, elimination:

- Newborns, premature: 320-525 minutes
- Children: 40-60 minutes
- Adults: 83-97 minutes

Elimination: Hepatic metabolism

Usual Dosage Doses should be titrated to appropriate effects; wide range of doses is dependent upon desired degree of analgesia/anesthesia

Children <12 years: Dose not established

Adults: Use lean body weight for patients who weigh >20% over IBW; see table.

Monitoring Parameters Respiratory rate, blood pressure, heart rate, neurological status (for degree of analgesia/anesthesia)

Additional Information Alfentanil may produce more hypotension compared to fentanyl, therefore, be sure to administer slowly and ensure patient has adequate hydration

Alfentanil

Indication	Approximate Duration of Anesthesia (min)	Induction Period (Initial Dose) (μg/kg)	Maintenance Period (Increments/ Infusion)	Total Dose (μg/kg)	Effects
Incremental injection	≤30	8–20	3–5 μg/kg or 0.5–1 μg/kg/min	8–40	Spontaneously breathing or assisted ventilation when required.
	30–60	20–50	5–15 μg/kg	Up to 75	Assisted or controlled ventilation required. Attenuation of response to laryngoscopy and intubation.
Continuous infusion	>45	50–75	0.5–3.0 μg/kg/min average infusion rate 1–1.5 μg/kg/min	Dependent on duration of procedure	Assisted or controlled ventilation required. Some attenuation of response to intubation and incision, with intraoperative stability.
Anesthetic induction	>45	130–245	0.5–1.5 μg/kg/min or general anesthetic	Dependent on duration of procedure	Assisted or controlled ventilation required. Administer slowly (over three minutes). Concentration of inhalation agents reduced by 30–50% for initial hour.

Dosage Forms Injection, preservative free: 500 μg/mL (2 mL, 5 mL, 10 mL, 20 mL)

References

Davis PJ, Killian A, Stiller RL, et al, "Pharmacokinetics of Alfentanil in Newborn Premature Infants and Older Children," *Dev Pharmacol Ther*, 1989, 13(1):21-7.

Marlow N, Weindling AM, Van Peer A, et al, "Alfentanil Pharmacokinetics in Preterm Infants," *Arch Dis Child*, 1990, 65(4 Spec No):349-51.

Meistelman C, Saint-Maurice C, Lepaul M, et al, "A Comparison of Alfentanil Pharmacokinetics in Children and Adults," *Anesthesiology*, 1987, 66(1):13-6.

Alglucerase

Brand Names Ceredase®

Synonyms Glucocerebrosidase

Therapeutic Category Enzyme, Glucocerebrosidase

Use Long-term enzyme replacement in patients with confirmed Type I Gaucher's disease who exhibit one or more of the following conditions: Moderate to severe anemia; thrombocytopenia and bleeding tendencies; bone disease; hepatomegaly or splenomegaly

Pregnancy Risk Factor C

Adverse Reactions

Central nervous system: Fever, chills

Gastrointestinal: Abdominal discomfort, nausea, and vomiting

Local: Discomfort, burning, and swelling at the site of injection

Drug Interactions No information available at this time

Mechanism of Action Glucocerebrosidase is an enzyme prepared from human placental tissue. Gaucher's disease is an inherited metabolic disorder caused by the defective activity of beta-glucosidase and the resultant accumulation of glucosyl ceramide laden macrophages in the liver, bone, and spleen. The disease affects an estimated 10,000-15,000 people in the United States, primarily of Eastern European Jewish descent, with up to 5,000 being symptomatic and requiring treatment. Alglucerase acts by replacing the missing enzyme associated with Gaucher's disease.

Pharmacodynamics Onset of significant improvement in symptoms:

Hepatosplenomegaly and hematologic abnormalities: Occurs within 6 months

(Continued)

Alglucerase *(Continued)*

Improvement in bone mineralization: Noted at 80-104 weeks of therapy

Pharmacokinetics Half-life, elimination: ~4-20 minutes

Usual Dosage Usually administered as a 20-60 units/kg I.V. infusion over 1-2 hours, usually repeated every 2 weeks; it has been given as frequently as every other day or as infrequently as every 4 weeks

Administration Dilute to a final volume of 100 mL or less of normal saline and infuse I.V. over 1-2 hours; an in-line filter should be used; do not shake solution as it denatures the enzyme

Monitoring Parameters CBC, platelets, liver function tests

Dosage Forms Injection: 10 units/mL (5 mL); 80 units/mL (5 mL)

References

Barton NW, Brady RO, Dambrosia JM, et al, "Replacement Therapy for Inherited Enzyme Deficiency - Macrophage-targeted Glucocerebrosidase for Gaucher's Disease," *N Engl J Med*, 1991, 324(21):1464-70.

Alkaban-AQ® *see* Vinblastine Sulfate *on page 601*

Alka-Mints® [OTC] *see* Calcium Carbonate *on page 94*

Alkeran® *see* Melphalan *on page 360*

Aller-Chlor® [OTC] *see* Chlorpheniramine Maleate *on page 128*

Allerest® 12 Hours Nasal Solution [OTC] *see* Oxymetazoline Hydrochloride *on page 429*

Allerest® Eye Drops [OTC] *see* Naphazoline Hydrochloride *on page 403*

Allerfrin® [OTC] *see* Triprolidine and Pseudoephedrine *on page 586*

Allergan® Ear Drops *see* Antipyrine and Benzocaine *on page 56*

AllerMax® [OTC] *see* Diphenhydramine Hydrochloride *on page 195*

Allerphed [OTC] *see* Triprolidine and Pseudoephedrine *on page 586*

Allopurinol (al oh pure' i nole)

Brand Names Zyloprim®

Therapeutic Category Uric Acid Lowering Agent

Use Prevention of attack of gouty arthritis and nephropathy; also used to treat secondary hyperuricemia which may occur during treatment of tumors or leukemia; to prevent recurrent calcium oxalate calculi

Pregnancy Risk Factor C

Contraindications Hypersensitivity to allopurinol

Precautions Reduce dosage in renal impairment; discontinue drug at the first sign of rash

Adverse Reactions

Central nervous system: Drowsiness, fever, neuritis

Dermatologic: Pruritic maculopapular rash, exfoliative dermatitis

Gastrointestinal: GI irritation

Hematologic: Leukocytosis, leukopenia, thrombocytopenia, eosinophilia, bone marrow suppression

Hepatic: Hepatitis

Ocular: Cataracts

Renal & genitourinary: Renal impairment

Drug Interactions Inhibits metabolism of azathioprine and mercaptopurine; use with ampicillin or amoxicillin may increase the incidence of skin rash; chlorpropamide, thiazides, trimethoprim/sulfamethoxazole, ethacrynic acid

Mechanism of Action Decreases the production of uric acid by inhibiting the action of xanthine oxidase, an enzyme that converts hypoxanthine to xanthine and xanthine to uric acid

Pharmacodynamics Decrease in serum uric acid occurs in 1-2 days with a nadir achieved in 1-3 weeks

Pharmacokinetics

Absorption: Oral: ~80% absorbed from the GI tract

Distribution: Distributes into breast milk
Protein binding: <1%
Metabolism: ~75% of the drug is metabolized to active metabolites, chiefly oxypurinol
Half-life:
Parent: 1-3 hours
Oxypurinol metabolite: 18-30 hours in patients with normal renal function
Peak serum levels: Within 2-6 hours
Allopurinol and oxypurinol are dialyzable

Usual Dosage Oral:
Children: 10 mg/kg/day in 2-3 divided doses or 200-300 mg/m^2/day in 2-4 divided doses; maximum dose: 800 mg/day
Alternative:
<6 years: 150 mg/day in 3 divided doses
6-10 years: 300 mg/day in 2-3 divided doses

Children >10 years and Adults (daily doses >300 mg should be administered in divided doses):
Myeloproliferative neoplastic disorders: 600-800 mg/day in 2-3 divided doses for prevention of acute uric acid nephropathy for 2-3 days starting 1-2 days before chemotherapy
Gout:
Mild: 200-300 mg/day
Severe: 400-600 mg/day

Dosing adjustment in renal impairment:
Cl_{cr} >50 mL/minute: No dosage change
Cl_{cr} 10-50 mL/minute: Reduce dosage to 50% of recommended
Cl_{cr} <10 mL/minute: Reduce dosage to 30% of recommended

Monitoring Parameters CBC, liver function tests, renal function, serum uric acid

Patient Information Report any skin rash, painful urination, blood in urine, irritation of the eyes, or swelling of lips or mouth

Nursing Implications Give after meals with plenty of fluid

Dosage Forms Tablet: 100 mg, 300 mg

Extemporaneous Preparation(s) Crush tablets to make a 5 mg/mL suspension in simple syrup; stable 14 days under refrigeration.

Nahata MC and Hipple TF, *Pediatric Drug Formulations*, 1st ed, Harvey Whitney Books Co, 1990.

References

Bennett WM, Aronoff GR, Golper TA, et al, *Drug Prescribing in Renal Failure*, Philadelphia, PA: American College of Physicians, 1987.

Krakoff IH and Murphey ML, "Hyperuricemia in Neoplastics Disease in Children: Prevention With Allopurinol, A Xanthine Oxidase Inhibitor" *Pediatrics*, 1968, 41(1 Pt 1):52-6.

Alphamul® [OTC] *see* Castor Oil *on page 109*

AlphaNine® *see* Factor IX Complex (Human) *on page 239*

Alphatrex® *see* Betamethasone *on page 81*

Alprazolam (al pray' zoe lam)

Related Information
Overdose and Toxicology Information *on page 696-700*

Brand Names Xanax®

Therapeutic Category Antianxiety Agent; Benzodiazepine

Use Treatment of anxiety; adjunct in the treatment of depression; management of panic attacks

Restrictions C-IV

Pregnancy Risk Factor D

Contraindications Hypersensitivity to alprazolam or any component; there may be a cross-sensitivity with other benzodiazepines; severe uncontrolled pain, narrow angle glaucoma, severe respiratory depression, pre-existing CNS depression; not to be used in pregnancy or lactation

Warnings Withdrawal symptoms including seizures have occurred 18 hours to 3 days after abrupt discontinuation; when discontinuing therapy, decrease daily dose by no more than 0.5 mg every 3 days; reduce dose in patients with significant hepatic disease

(Continued)

Alprazolam *(Continued)*

Precautions Safety has not been established in children <18 years of age

Adverse Reactions

Central nervous system: Drowsiness, dizziness, confusion, sedation, ataxia, headache

Gastrointestinal: Dry mouth, constipation, diarrhea, nausea, vomiting

Ocular: Blurred vision

Miscellaneous: Physical and psychological dependence with prolonged use

Drug Interactions Cimetidine may ↓ and enzyme inducers may ↑ metabolism of alprazolam; CNS depressants may enhance CNS effects

Mechanism of Action Binds at stereospecific receptors at several sites within the central nervous system, including the limbic system, reticular formation; effects may be mediated through GABA

Pharmacokinetics

Absorption: Oral: Rapidly and well absorbed

Distribution: 0.9-1.2 L/kg; distributes into breast milk

Protein binding: 80%

Metabolism: Extensive in the liver; major metabolite is inactive

Half-life: 12-15 hours

Peak serum levels: Within 1-2 hours

Elimination: Excretion of metabolites and parent compound in the urine

Usual Dosage Oral:

Children <18 years: Dose not established; investigationally in children 7-16 years of age (n=13), initial doses of 0.005 mg/kg or 0.125 mg/dose were given 3 times/day for situational anxiety and increments of 0.125-0.25 mg were used to ↑ doses to maximum of 0.02 mg/kg/dose or 0.06 mg/kg/day; a range of 0.375-3 mg/day was needed

Adults: 0.25-0.5 mg 2-3 times/day, titrate dose upward; maximum: 4 mg/day

Nursing Implications Give with food; assist with ambulation during beginning of therapy; allow patient to rise slowly to avoid fainting

Dosage Forms Tablet: 0.25 mg, 0.5 mg, 1 mg, 2 mg

References

Bernstein GA, Garfinkel BD, and Borchardt CM, "Comparative Studies of Pharmacotherapy for School Refusal," *J Am Acad Child Adolesc Psychiatry*, 1990, 29(5):773-81.

Pfefferbaum B, Overall JE, Boren HA, et al, "Alprazolam in the Treatment of Anticipatory and Acute Situational Anxiety in Children With Cancer," *J Am Acad Child Adolesc Psychiatry*, 1987, 26(4):532-5.

Simeon JG and Ferguson HB, "Alprazolam Effects in Children With Anxiety Disorders," *Can J Psychiatry*, 1987, 32(7):570-4.

Alprostadil (al pross' ta dil)

Brand Names Prostin VR Pediatric®

Synonyms PGE_1; Prostaglandin E_1

Therapeutic Category Prostaglandin

Use Temporary maintenance of patency of ductus arteriosus in neonates with ductal-dependent congenital heart disease until surgery can be performed. These defects include cyanotic (ie, pulmonary atresia, pulmonary stenosis, tricuspid atresia, Fallot's tetralogy, transposition of the great vessels) and acyanotic (ie, interruption of aortic arch, coarctation of aorta, hypoplastic left ventricle) heart disease.

Pregnancy Risk Factor X

Contraindications Respiratory distress syndrome or persistent fetal circulation

Warnings Apnea occurs in 10% to 12% of neonates with congenital heart defects especially in those weighing <2 kg at birth and usually appears during the first hour of drug infusion

Adverse Reactions

Cardiovascular: Systemic hypotension, flushing, bradycardia, rhythm disturbances

Central nervous system: Seizure-like activity, fever

Endocrine & metabolic: Cortical proliferation of long bones has been seen with long-term infusions

Gastrointestinal: Diarrhea

Hematologic: Inhibition of platelet aggregation

Respiratory: Respiratory depression, apnea

Stability Compatible in D_5W, $D_{10}W$, and saline solutions; refrigerate ampuls at 2°C to 8°C

Mechanism of Action Causes vasodilation by means of direct effect on vascular and ductus arteriosus smooth muscle

Pharmacokinetics

Metabolism: ~70% to 80% is metabolized by oxidation during a single pass through the lungs (metabolite 13,14 dihydro-PGE_1 is active)

Half-life: 5-10 minutes; since the half-life is so short, the drug must be administered by continuous infusion

Elimination: Metabolites are excreted in urine

Usual Dosage Infants: 0.05-0.1 μg/kg/minute; with therapeutic response, rate is reduced to lowest effective dosage; with unsatisfactory dose, rate is increased gradually; maintenance: 0.01-0.4 μg/kg/minute

PGE_1 is usually given at an infusion rate of 0.1 μg/kg/minute; but it is often possible to reduce the dosage to ½ or even $^1/_{10}$ without losing the therapeutic effect. The mixing schedule is shown in the table.

Add 1 Ampul (500 μg) to:	Concentration (μg/mL)	Infusion Rate	
		mL/min/kg Needed to Infuse 0.1 μg/kg/min	mL/kg/24 h
250 mL	2	0.05	72
100 mL	5	0.02	28.8
50 mL	10	0.01	14.4
25 mL	20	0.005	7.2

Administration I.V. continuous infusion into a large vein or alternatively through an umbilical artery catheter placed at the ductal opening; maximum concentration listed (per package insert) for I.V. infusion: 20 μg/mL

Monitoring Parameters Arterial pressure, respiratory rate, heart rate, temperature, pO_2

Nursing Implications Prepare fresh solution every 24 hours; if hypotension or pyrexia occurs, the infusion rate should be reduced until symptoms subside; apnea or bradycardia requires drug discontinuation with cautious reinstitution at a lower dose

Additional Information Therapeutic response is indicated by an increase in systemic blood pressure and pH in those with restricted systemic blood flow and acidosis, or by an increase in oxygenation (pO_2) in those with restricted pulmonary blood flow; response usually evident within 30 minutes. Alprostadil has also been used investigationally for the treatment of pulmonary hypertension in infants and children with congenital heart defects with left-to-right shunts. Alprostadil was administered via continuous infusion into the right pulmonary artery.

Dosage Forms Injection: 500 μg/mL (1 mL)

References

Weesner KM, "Hemodynamic Effects of Prostaglandin E_1 in Patients With Congenital Heart Disease and Pulmonary Hypertension," *Cathet Cardiovasc Diagn*, 1991, 24(1):10-5.

Aluminum Acetate

Brand Names Acid Mantle® [OTC]; Bluboro® [OTC]; Boropak®; Domeboro® [OTC]; Pedi-Boro® [OTC]

Synonyms Burow's Solution

Therapeutic Category Topical Skin Product

Use Astringent wet dressing for relief of inflammatory conditions of the skin and to reduce weeping that may occur in dermatitis; treatment of superficial infections of the external auditory canal; reduce edema and crusting associated with moist ear canals; used prophylactically against swimmer's ear

Pregnancy Risk Factor C

Contraindications Use with topical collagenase

(Continued)

Aluminum Acetate *(Continued)*

Precautions Do not use plastic or other impervious material to prevent evaporation

Adverse Reactions Local: Irritation

Usual Dosage Children and Adults:

Topical: Soak the affected area in the solution 2-4 times/day for 15-30 minutes or apply wet dressing soaked in the solution 2-4 times/day for 30-minute treatment periods; rewet dressing with solution every few minutes to keep it moist

Otic: Instill 4-6 drops every 2-3 hours initially, then every 4-6 hours until itching or burning subsides

Patient Information Keep away from eyes, external use only

Nursing Implications One tablet dissolved in a pint of water makes a modified Burow's solution equivalent to a 1:40 dilution, 2 tablets: 1:20 dilution, 4 tablets: 1:10 dilution

Dosage Forms

Powder, to make topical solution: 1 packet/pint of water = 1:40 solution
Solution, otic: Aluminum acetate 1:10 with acetic acid 2% (60 mL)
Tablet: 1 tablet/pint = 1:40 dilution

Aluminum Sucrose Sulfate, Basic *see* Sucralfate *on page 538*

Alupent® *see* Metaproterenol Sulfate *on page 367*

Amantadine Hydrochloride (a man' ta deen)

Brand Names Symadine®; Symmetrel®

Synonyms Adamantanamine Hydrochloride

Therapeutic Category Antiviral Agent, Oral

Use Symptomatic and adjunct treatment of parkinsonism; also used in prophylaxis and treatment of influenza A viral infection

Pregnancy Risk Factor C

Contraindications Hypersensitivity to amantadine hydrochloride or any component

Precautions Use with caution in patients with liver disease, epilepsy, history of recurrent eczematoid dermatitis, uncontrolled psychosis, and in those receiving CNS stimulant drugs; modify dosage in patients with renal impairment and in patients with active seizure disorders

Adverse Reactions

Cardiovascular: Orthostatic hypotension, edema
Central nervous system: Dizziness, confusion, headache, insomnia, difficulty in concentrating, anxiety, restlessness, irritability, hallucinations
Gastrointestinal: Nausea, vomiting, dry mouth
Renal & genitourinary: Urinary retention
Miscellaneous: Livedo reticularis

Drug Interactions Additive anticholinergic effects in patients receiving drugs with anticholinergic activity; additive CNS stimulant effect with CNS stimulants

Mechanism of Action As an antiviral, blocks the uncoating of influenza A virus preventing penetration of virus into host and inhibits M_2 protein in the assembly of progeny virions; antiparkinsonian activity may be due to its blocking the reuptake of dopamine into presynaptic neurons and causing direct stimulation of postsynaptic receptors

Pharmacokinetics

Absorption: Well absorbed from the GI tract
Half-life, patients with normal renal function: 10-28 hours
Peak serum levels: 1-4 hours
Elimination: 80% to 90% excreted unchanged in the urine by glomerular filtration and tubular secretion
0% to 5% removed by hemodialysis

Usual Dosage Oral:

Children:

1-8 years: 5-9 mg/kg/day in 2 divided doses; maximum: 200 mg/day
9-12 years: 100-200 mg/day in 2 divided doses

Note: After first influenza A virus vaccine dose, amantadine prophylaxis may be administered for up to 6 weeks or until 2 weeks after the second dose of vaccine; administer a 10-day course of therapy following exposure

Adults:

Parkinson's disease: 100 mg twice daily

Influenza A viral infection: 200 mg/day in 1-2 divided doses

Prophylaxis: Minimum 10-day course of therapy following exposure or continue for 2-3 weeks after influenza A virus vaccine is given

Dosing interval in renal impairment:

Cl_{cr} 30-50 mL/minute: Administer 100 mg/day

Cl_{cr} 15-29 mL/minute: Administer 100 mg every other day

Cl_{cr} <15 mL/minute: Administer 200 mg every 7 days

Monitoring Parameters Renal function

Patient Information May impair ability to perform activities requiring mental alertness or coordination; do not abruptly discontinue therapy, may precipitate a parkinsonian crisis

Nursing Implications If insomnia occurs, the last daily dose should be taken several hours before retiring

Dosage Forms

Capsule: 100 mg

Syrup: 50 mg/5 mL

References

Strong DK, Eisenstat DD, Bryson SM, et al, "Amantadine Neurotoxicity in a Pediatric Patient With Renal Insufficiency," *DICP*, 1991, 25(11):1175-7.

Amcort® *see* Triamcinolone *on page 579*

Amen® *see* Medroxyprogesterone Acetate *on page 359*

Americaine® [OTC] *see* Benzocaine *on page 77*

A-methaPred® *see* Methylprednisolone *on page 379*

Amethocaine Hydrochloride *see* Tetracaine Hydrochloride *on page 551*

Amethopterin *see* Methotrexate *on page 374*

Amicar® *see* Aminocaproic Acid *on next page*

Amikacin Sulfate (am i kay' sin)

Related Information

Blood Level Sampling Time Guidelines *on page 694-695*

Medications Compatible With PN Solutions *on page 649-650*

Overdose and Toxicology Information *on page 696-700*

Brand Names Amikin®

Therapeutic Category Antibiotic, Aminoglycoside

Use Treatment of documented gram-negative enteric infection resistant to gentamicin and tobramycin; documented infection of mycobacterial organisms susceptible to amikacin

Pregnancy Risk Factor C

Contraindications Hypersensitivity to amikacin sulfate or any component; cross sensitivity may exist with other aminoglycosides

Warnings Aminoglycosides are associated with significant nephrotoxicity or ototoxicity; the ototoxicity is directly proportional to the amount of drug given and the duration of treatment; tinnitus or vertigo are indications of vestibular injury and impending bilateral irreversible deafness; renal damage is usually reversible

Precautions Use with caution in neonates due to renal immaturity that results in a prolonged half-life; patients with pre-existing renal impairment, auditory or vestibular impairment, hypocalcemia, myasthenia gravis, and in conditions which depress neuromuscular transmission; dose and/or frequency of administration must be modified in patients with renal impairment

Adverse Reactions

Dermatologic: Rash

Musculoskeletal: Neuromuscular blockade

Otic: Ototoxicity

Renal & genitourinary: Nephrotoxicity

Drug Interactions Penicillins and cephalosporins; loop diuretics may potentiate the ototoxicity of the aminoglycosides; neuromuscular blocking agents and general anesthetics may potentiate neuromuscular blockade

(Continued)

Amikacin Sulfate *(Continued)*

Mechanism of Action Inhibits protein synthesis in susceptible bacteria by binding to ribosomal subunits

Pharmacokinetics

Distribution: Primarily distributed into extracellular fluid (highly hydrophilic); poor penetration into the blood-brain barrier even when meninges are inflamed; V_d is increased in neonates and patients with edema, ascites, fluid overload; V_d is decreased in patients with dehydration; crosses the placenta

Half-life:

- Infants:
  - Low birth weight, 1-3 days of age: 7-9 hours
  - Full term >7 days: 4-5 hours
- Children: 1.6-2.5 hours
- Adults: 2-3 hours
- Anuria: 28-86 hours; half-life and clearance are dependent on renal function

Peak serum levels:

- I.M.: Within 45-120 minutes
- I.V.: Within 30 minutes following a 30-minute infusion

Elimination: 94% to 98% is excreted unchanged in the urine via glomerular filtration within 24 hours

Dialyzable (50% to 100%)

Usual Dosage I.M., I.V. (dosage should be based on an estimate of ideal body weight)

Neonates:

- 0-4 weeks, <1200 g: 7.5 mg/kg/dose every 18-24 hours
- Postnatal age ≤7 days:
  - 1200-2000 g: 7.5 mg/kg/dose every 12-18 hours
  - >2000 g: 10 mg/kg/dose every 12 hours
- Postnatal age >7 days:
  - 1200-2000 g: 7.5 mg/kg/dose every 8-12 hours
  - >2000 g: 10 mg/kg/dose every 8 hours

Infants and Children: 15-22.5 mg/kg/day divided every 8 hours

Adults: 15 mg/kg/day divided every 8-12 hours

Dosing interval in renal impairment: Loading dose: 5-7.5 mg/kg; subsequent dosages and frequency of administration are best determined by measurement of serum levels and assessment of renal insufficiency

Some patients may require larger or more frequent doses if serum levels document the need (ie, cystic fibrosis or febrile granulocytopenic patients)

Administration Administer by intermittent I.V. infusion over 30 minutes at a final concentration not to exceed 5 mg amikacin/mL

Monitoring Parameters Urinalysis, urine output, BUN, serum creatinine, peak and trough serum amikacin concentrations; be alert to ototoxicity

Reference Range Peak: 20-30 μg/mL; Trough: <10 μg/mL

Patient Information Report loss of hearing, ringing or roaring in the ears, or feeling of fullness in head

Nursing Implications Drug levels should be obtained after the third dose; peak serum levels should be drawn 30 minutes after the end of a 30-minute infusion; trough levels are drawn within 30 minutes before the next dose; provide optimal patient hydration

Dosage Forms Injection: 50 mg/mL (2 mL); 250 mg/mL (2 mL, 4 mL)

References

Vogelstein B, Kowarski AA, and Lietman PS, "The Pharmacokinetics of Amikacin in Children," *J Pediatr*, 1977, 91(2):333.

Amikin® *see* Amikacin Sulfate *on previous page*

2-Amino-6-mercaptopurine *see* Thioguanine *on page 560*

Aminobenzylpenicillin *see* Ampicillin *on page 48*

Aminocaproic Acid (a mee noe ka proe' ik)

Brand Names Amicar®

Therapeutic Category Hemostatic Agent

Use Treatment of excessive bleeding resulting from systemic hyperfibrinolysis and urinary fibrinolysis

Pregnancy Risk Factor C

Contraindications Disseminated intravascular coagulation; hematuria of upper urinary tract

Warnings Aminocaproic acid may accumulate in patients with decreased renal function

Precautions Use with caution in patients with cardiac, renal or hepatic disease

Adverse Reactions

Cardiovascular: Hypotension, bradycardia and arrhythmias (following rapid I.V. administration), nasal congestion

Central nervous system: Dizziness, headache, tinnitus, malaise

Dermatologic: Rash

Gastrointestinal: GI irritation

Musculoskeletal: Myopathy, acute rhabdomyolysis

Drug Interactions Oral contraceptives and estrogens

Mechanism of Action Competitively inhibits activation of plasminogen thereby reducing fibrinolysin, without inhibiting lysis of clot

Pharmacodynamics

Peak effects: Within 2 hours after oral administration

Therapeutic effects: Within 1-72 hours after the dose

Pharmacokinetics

Distribution: Widely distributes through intravascular and extravascular compartments

Metabolism: Hepatic metabolism is minimal

Half-life: 1-2 hours

Elimination: 40% to 60% excreted as unchanged drug in the urine within 12 hours

Usual Dosage

Children: Oral, I.V.:

Loading: 100-200 mg/kg; maintenance: 100 mg/kg/dose every 6 hours; maximum daily dose: 30 g **or** I.V. loading dose: 100 mg/kg or 3 g/m^2 followed by a continuous infusion of 33.3 mg/kg/hour or 1 g/m^2/hour; total dosage should not exceed 18 g/m^2/day

Traumatic hyphema: 100 mg/kg/dose every 4 hours (maximum: 5 g/dose; maximum daily dose: 30 g/day)

Adults:

Oral: For the treatment of acute bleeding syndromes due to elevated fibrinolytic activity, give 5 g during first hour, followed by 1-1.25 g/hour for about 8 hours or until bleeding stops; daily dose should not exceed 30 g

I.V.: Give 4-5 g during first hour followed by continuous infusion at the rate of 1-1.25 g/hour, continue for 8 hours or until bleeding stops

Administration Maximum concentration for I.V. dilution: 20 mg/mL; administer single doses over at least 1 hour

Monitoring Parameters Fibrinogen, fibrin split products, serum creatinine kinase (long-term therapy)

Nursing Implications Rapid I.V. injection (IVP) should be avoided since hypotension, bradycardia, and arrhythmias may result

Dosage Forms

Injection: 250 mg/mL (20 mL, 96 mL, 100 mL)

Syrup (raspberry flavor): 1.25 g/5 mL (480 mL)

Tablet: 500 mg

References

McGetrick JJ, Jampol LM, Goldberg MP, et al, "Aminocaproic Acid Decreases Secondary Hemorrhage After Traumatic Hyphema," *Arch Ophthalmol*, 1983, 101(7):1031-3.

Aminophyllin™ *see* Aminophylline *on this page*

Aminophylline (am in off' i lin)

Related Information

Medications Compatible With PN Solutions *on page 649-650*

Overdose and Toxicology Information *on page 696-700*

Brand Names Aminophyllin™; Phyllocontin®; Truphylline®

Synonyms Theophylline Ethylenediamine

(Continued)

Aminophylline *(Continued)*

Therapeutic Category Bronchodilator

Use As a bronchodilator in reversible airway obstruction due to asthma or COPD; for neonatal idiopathic apnea/bradycardia spells

Pregnancy Risk Factor C

Contraindications Uncontrolled arrhythmias

Warnings Some commercial products may contain sulfites which may produce hypersensitivity reactions in sensitive individuals

Adverse Reactions See Theophylline monograph

Drug Interactions See Theophylline monograph

Mechanism of Action See Theophylline monograph

Pharmacokinetics Aminophylline is the ethylenediamine salt of theophylline, pharmacokinetic parameters are those of **theophylline**

Absorption: Oral absorption depends upon the dosage form

Distribution: V_d: 0.45 L/kg; distributes into breast milk (approximates serum concentration); crosses the placenta.

Patient Group	Approximate Half-Life (h)
Neonates	
Premature	30
Normal newborn	24
Infants	
4-52 weeks	4-30
Children/Adolescents	
1-9 years	2-10 (4 avg)
9-16 years	4-16
Adults	
Nonsmoker	4-16 (8.7 avg)
Smoker	4.4
Cardiac compromised, liver failure	20-30

Dosage Form	Time to Peak
Liquid	30 min
Uncoated tablet	2 h
Enteric coated tablet	5 h
Chewable tablet	1-1.5 h
Extended release	4-7 h
Intravenous	<30 min

Fraction available: 80% (eg, 100 mg aminophylline = 80 mg theophylline)

Half-life is highly variable and dependent upon age, liver function, cardiac function, lung disease, and smoking history (see table)

Metabolism: Metabolized in the liver by demethylation and oxidation; in neonates a small portion of theophylline is metabolized to caffeine

Elimination: 10% excreted in the urine as metabolites; neonates excreted a greater percentage in the urine (up to 50%)

Usual Dosage All dosages based upon **aminophylline**

Neonates:

Apnea of prematurity:

Loading dose: 5 mg/kg

Maintenance: Initial: 5 mg/kg/day every 12 hours; increased dosages may be indicated as liver metabolism matures (usually >30 days of life); monitor serum levels to determine appropriate dosages

Theophylline levels should be initially drawn after 3 days of therapy; repeat levels are indicated 3 days after each increase in dosage or weekly if on a stabilized dosage

Treatment of acute bronchospasm:

Loading dose (in patients not currently receiving aminophylline or theophylline): 6 mg/kg (based on aminophylline) given I.V. over 20-30 minutes

Approximate I.V. maintenance dosages are based upon **continuous infusions**; bolus dosing (often used in children <6 months of age) may be determined by multiplying the hourly infusion rate by 24 hours and dividing by the desired number of doses/day (usually in 3-4 doses/day)

6 weeks to 6 months: 0.5 mg/kg/hour

6 months to 1 year: 0.6-0.7 mg/kg/hour

1-9 years: 1-1.2 mg/kg/hour

9-12 years and young adult smokers: 0.9 mg/kg/hour

12-16 years: 0.7 mg/kg/hour

Adults (healthy, nonsmoking): 0.7 mg/kg/hour

Older patients and patients with cor pulmonale patients with congestive heart failure or liver failure: 0.25 mg/kg/hour

Oral dose: See Theophylline, (consider mg theophylline available when using aminophylline products)

Dosage should be adjusted according to serum level measurements during the first 12- to 24-hour period. Avoid using suppositories due to erratic, unreliable absorption. See table.

Guidelines for Drawing Theophylline Serum Levels

Dosage Form	Time to Draw Level
I.V. bolus	30 min after end of 30 min infusion
I.V. continuous infusion	12–24 h after initiation of infusion
P.O. liquid, fast-release tab	Peak: 1 h post a dose after at least 1 day of therapy Trough: Just before a dose after at least 1 day of therapy
P.O. slow-release product	Peak: 4 h post a dose after at least 1 day of therapy Trough: Just before a dose after at least 1 day of therapy

Administration Dilute with I.V. fluid to a concentration of 1 mg/mL and infuse over 20-30 minutes; maximum concentration: 25 mg/mL; maximum rate of infusion: 0.36 mg/kg/minute, and no greater than 25 mg/minute

Monitoring Parameters Serum theophylline levels, heart rate, respiratory rate, number and severity of apnea spells (when used for apnea of prematurity); arterial or capillary blood gases (if applicable)

Reference Range Therapeutic level: For asthma 10-20 µg/mL; for neonatal apnea 6-13 µg/mL (serum levels are reduced for neonatal apnea due to decreased binding of theophylline to fetal albumin resulting in a greater amount of free "active" theophylline)

Dosage Forms

Injection: 25 mg/mL (10 mL, 20 mL) - 250 mg (equivalent to 197 mg theophylline) per 10 mL; 500 mg (equivalent to 394 mg theophylline) per 20 mL

Liquid, oral:105 mg (equivalent to 90 mg theophylline) per 5 mL (240 mL)

Suppository, rectal: 250 mg (equivalent to 198 mg theophylline) - 500 mg (equivalent to 395 mg theophylline)

Tablet: 100 mg (equivalent to 79 mg theophylline) - 200 mg (equivalent to 158 mg theophylline)

Tablet, sustained release: 225 mg (equivalent to 178 mg theophylline)

Amiodarone Hydrochloride (a mee' oh da rone)

Brand Names Cordarone®

Therapeutic Category Antiarrhythmic Agent, Class III

Use Management of resistant, life-threatening ventricular arrhythmias unresponsive to conventional therapy with less toxic agents; has also been used for treatment of supraventricular arrhythmias unresponsive to conventional therapy

Pregnancy Risk Factor C

Contraindications Hypersensitivity to amiodarone; severe sinus node dysfunction, marked sinus bradycardia; second and third degree A-V block; bradycardia-induced syncope, except if pacemaker is placed; thyroid disease

(Continued)

Amiodarone Hydrochloride *(Continued)*

Warnings Not considered first-line antiarrhythmic due to high incidence of toxicity; 75% of patients experience adverse effects with large doses; discontinuation is required in 5% to 20% of patients; reserve for use in life-threatening arrhythmias refractory to other therapy

Precautions Avoid during pregnancy and while breast feeding (fetal/neonatal goiters, hypothyroidism, and possible cerebral damage may occur)

Adverse Reactions

Cardiovascular: Atropine resistant bradycardia, heart block, sinus arrest, myocardial depression, congestive heart failure, paroxysmal ventricular tachycardia, hypotension

Central nervous system (20% to 40% incidence): Lack of coordination, fatigue, malaise, tremor, abnormal gait, ataxia, paresthesia, dizziness, headache, insomnia, nightmares

Dermatologic: Slate blue discoloration of skin, photosensitivity, rash

Endocrine & metabolic: Hypothyroidism (or less commonly hyperthyroidism), hyperglycemia, ↑ triglycerides

Gastrointestinal: Nausea, vomiting, anorexia, constipation

Hematologic: Coagulation abnormalities, thrombocytopenia

Hepatic: ↑ liver enzymes, severe hepatic toxicity (potentially fatal), ↑ bilirubin, ↑ serum ammonia

Ocular: Corneal microdeposits, photophobia

Respiratory (potentially fatal): Interstitial pneumonitis, hypersensitivity pneumonitis, pulmonary fibrosis; may present with cough, fever, dyspnea, malaise, chest x-ray changes

Drug Interactions Amiodarone may increase plasma concentrations of digoxin and cardiac glycosides, flecainide, procainamide, quinidine, warfarin, and phenytoin resulting in toxicities; combined use with beta blockers, digitalis or calcium channel blockers may result in bradycardia, sinus arrest; use with class I antiarrhythmics → ventricular arrhythmias; amiodarone + general anesthetics may result in bradycardia, hypotension, heart block; cholestyramine may possibly ↓ amiodarone serum levels.

Mechanism of Action A class III antiarrhythmic agent which inhibits adrenergic stimulation, prolongs the action potential and refractory period in myocardial tissue; decreases A-V conduction and sinus node function

Pharmacodynamics

Onset of effect: 3 days to 3 weeks after starting therapy

Maximum effect: 1 week to 5 months

Duration of effects after discontinuation of therapy: 7-50 days

Mean onset of effect and duration after discontinuation may be shorter in children vs adults

Pharmacokinetics

Distribution: V_d: 66 L/kg (range: 18-148 L/kg); crosses placenta; distributes to breast milk in concentrations higher than maternal plasma concentrations

Protein binding: 96%

Metabolism: Metabolized in liver, major metabolite N-desethylamiodarone (active)

Bioavailability: ~50% (range: 20% to 80%)

Half-life (oral chronic therapy): 40-55 days (range: 26-107 days); half-life is shortened in children vs adults

Elimination: Via biliary excretion; possible enterohepatic recirculation; <1% excreted unchanged in urine

Nondialyzable

Usual Dosage

Children <1 year of age should be dosed as calculated by body surface area.

Children: Loading dose: 10-15 mg/kg/day or 600-800 mg/1.73 m^2/day for 4-14 days or until adequate control of arrhythmia or prominent adverse effects occur (this loading dose may be given in 1-2 divided doses/day); dosage should then be reduced to 5 mg/kg/day or 200-400 mg/1.73 m^2/day given once daily for several weeks; if arrhythmia does not recur reduce to lowest effective dosage possible; usual daily minimal dose: 2.5 mg/kg; maintenance doses may be given for 5 of 7 days/week.

Adults: Ventricular arrhythmias: 800-1600 mg/day in 1-2 doses for 1-3 weeks, then 600-800 mg/day in 1-2 doses for one month; maintenance:

400 mg/day; lower doses are recommended for supraventricular arrhythmias.

Monitoring Parameters Heart rate and rhythm, EKG, pulmonary function tests, thyroid function tests, liver enzymes

Reference Range Therapeutic: 0.5-2.5 mg/L (SI: 1-4 μmol/L) (parent); desethyl metabolite (active) is present in equal concentration to parent drug

Test Interactions Thyroid function tests: Amiodarone partially inhibits the peripheral conversion of thyroxine (T_4) to tri-iodothyronine (T_3); serum T_4 and reverse tri-iodothyronine (RT_3) concentrations may be increased and serum T_3 may be decreased; most patients remain clinically euthyroid, however, clinical hypothyroidism or hyperthyroidism may occur

Nursing Implications Administer with food; avoid exposure of patient to sunlight; use sunscreen, sunglasses; intoxication with amiodarone necessitates EKG monitoring; bradycardia may be atropine resistant, I.V. isoproterenol or cardiac pacemaker may be required; hypotension, heart block and QT prolongation may also be seen; patients should be monitored for several days following ingestion due to long half-life

Dosage Forms Tablet: 200 mg

References

Coumel P and Fidelle J, "Amiodarone in the Treatment of Cardiac Arrhythmias in Children: One Hundred Thirty-five Cases," *Am Heart J*, 1980, 100(6 Pt 2):1063-9.

Garson A Jr, Gillette PC, McVey P, et al, "Amiodarone Treatment of Critical Arrhythmias in Children and Young Adults," *J Am Coll Cardiol*, 1984, 4(4):749-55.

Shahar E, Barzilay Z, Frand M, et al, "Amiodarone in Control of Sustained Tachyarrhythmias in Children With Wolff-Parkinson-White Syndrome," *Pediatrics*, 1983, 72(6):813-6.

Amitone® [OTC] *see* Calcium Carbonate *on page 94*

Amitriptyline Hydrochloride (a mee trip' ti leen)

Related Information

Overdose and Toxicology Information *on page 696-700*

Brand Names Elavil®; Endep®; Enovil®

Therapeutic Category Antidepressant, Tricyclic

Use Treatment of various forms of depression, often in conjunction with psychotherapy; analgesic for certain chronic and neuropathic pain

Pregnancy Risk Factor D

Contraindications Hypersensitivity to amitriptyline (cross-sensitivity with other tricyclics may occur); narrow-angle glaucoma; patients receiving MAOI within past 14 days

Warnings Do not discontinue abruptly in patients receiving high doses chronically

Precautions Use with caution in patients with cardiac conduction disturbances, cardiovascular disease, seizure disorders, history of urinary retention, hyperthyroidism or those receiving thyroid hormone replacement

Adverse Reactions Anticholinergic effects may be pronounced; moderate to marked sedation can occur (tolerance to these effects usually occurs)

Cardiovascular: Postural hypotension, arrhythmias, tachycardia, sudden death

Central nervous system: Sedation, weakness, fatigue, tremor, anxiety, confusion, insomnia, impaired cognitive function, seizures, extrapyramidal symptoms are possible

Dermatologic: Photosensitivity

Endocrine & metabolic: Rarely SIADH

Gastrointestinal: Dry mouth, constipation, ↓ lower esophageal sphincter tone, GE reflux, ↑ appetite and weight gain

Hematologic: Rarely agranulocytosis, leukopenia, eosinophilia

Hepatic: ↑ liver enzymes, cholestatic jaundice

Ocular: Blurred vision, ↑ intraocular pressure

Renal & genitourinary: Urinary retention

Miscellaneous: Allergic reactions

Drug Interactions Amitriptyline may ↓ the effects of guanethidine and may ↑ the effects of other CNS depressants, adrenergic agents (epinephrine, isoproterenol), anticholinergic agents and warfarin. With MAO inhibitors, hy-

(Continued)

Amitriptyline Hydrochloride *(Continued)*

perpyrexia, tachycardia, hypertension, confusion, seizures, and death have been reported. Cimetidine and methylphenidate may ↓ the metabolism and phenobarbital may ↑ the metabolism of amitriptyline; with clonidine → hypertensive crisis

Stability Protect injection and Elavil® 10 mg tablets from light

Mechanism of Action Increases the synaptic concentration of serotonin and/or norepinephrine in the central nervous system by inhibition of their reuptake by the presynaptic neuronal membrane

Pharmacodynamics Onset of action: Therapeutic antidepressant effects begin in 7-21 days maximum effects may not occur for ≥2 weeks

Pharmacokinetics

Distribution: Crosses placenta; enters breast milk

Metabolism: Metabolized in the liver to nortriptyline (active), hydroxy derivatives and conjugated derivatives

Half-life, adults: 9-25 hours (15-hour average)

Peak serum levels: Within 4 hours

Elimination: Renal excretion of 18% as unchanged drug; small amounts eliminated in feces by bile

Usual Dosage

Chronic pain management: Children: Oral: Initial: 0.1 mg/kg at bedtime, may advance as tolerated over 2-3 weeks to 0.5-2 mg/kg at bedtime

Depressive disorders: Oral:

- Children: Investigationally initial doses of 1 mg/kg/day given in 3 divided doses with increases to 1.5 mg/kg/day have been reported in a small number of children (n=9)
- Adolescents: Initial: 25-50 mg/day; may give in divided doses; ↑ gradually to 100 mg/day in divided doses

Adults:

- Oral: 30-100 mg/day single dose at bedtime or in divided doses; dose may be gradually increased up to 300 mg/day; once symptoms are controlled, ↓ gradually to lowest effective dose
- I.M.: 20-30 mg 4 times/day

Monitoring Parameters Heart rate, blood pressure

Reference Range Therapeutic: Amitriptyline plus nortriptyline (active metabolite) 100-250 ng/mL (SI: 360-900 nmol/L); nortriptyline 50-150 ng/mL (SI: 190-570 nmol/L). Toxic: >0.5 μg/mL (500 ng/mL)

Nursing Implications Do not administer I.V.

Dosage Forms

Injection: 10 mg/mL (10 mL)

Tablet: 10 mg, 25 mg, 50 mg, 75 mg, 100 mg, 150 mg

References

Kashani JH, Shekim WO, and Reid JC, "Amitriptyline in Children With Major Depressive Disorder: A Double-Blind Crossover Pilot Study," *J Am Acad Child Psychiatry*, 1984, 23(3):348-51.

Ammonium Chloride

Therapeutic Category Diuretic, Miscellaneous; Metabolic Alkalosis Agent; Urinary Acidifying Agent

Use Diuretic or systemic and urinary acidifying agent; treatment of hypochloremic states

Pregnancy Risk Factor B

Contraindications Severe hepatic and renal dysfunction; patients with primary respiratory acidosis

Adverse Reactions

Cardiovascular: Bradycardia

Central nervous system: Mental confusion, coma, headache

Dermatologic: Rash

Endocrine & metabolic: Metabolic acidosis secondary to hyperchloremia

Gastrointestinal: GI irritation

Local: Pain at site of injection

Respiratory: Hyperventilation

Mechanism of Action Its dissociation to ammonium and chloride ions increases acidity by increasing free hydrogen ion concentration which combines with bicarbonate ion to form CO_2 and water; the net result is the replacement of bicarbonate ions by chloride ions

Pharmacokinetics

Absorption: Absorbed rapidly from the GI tract with absorption being complete in 3-6 hours

Metabolism: Metabolized in the liver

Elimination: Excreted in the urine

Usual Dosage The following equations represent different methods of chloride or alkalosis correction utilizing either the serum HCO_3^-, the serum Cl^- or the base excess

Correction of refractory hypochloremic metabolic alkalosis: Dose mEq = 0.5 (L/kg) x wt (kg) x [serum HCO_3^--24] mEq/L; give $\frac{1}{2}$ to $\frac{2}{3}$ of the calculated dose, then re-evaluate

Correction of hypochloremia: mEq NH_4Cl = 0.2 L/kg x wt x [103 - serum Cl^-] mEq/L, give $\frac{1}{2}$ to $\frac{2}{3}$ of calculated dose, then re-evaluate

Correction of alkalosis via base excess method: mEq NH_4Cl = 0.3 L/kg x wt (kg) x base excess (mEq/L), give $\frac{1}{2}$ to $\frac{2}{3}$ of calculated dose, then re-evaluate

Children: Oral, I.V.: 75 mg/kg/day in 4 divided doses for urinary acidification; maximum daily dose: 6 g

Adults:

Oral: 2-3 g every 6 hours; maximum daily dose: 12 g

I.V.: 1.5 g/dose every 6 hours

Administration Dilute to 0.2 mEq/mL and infuse I.V. over 3 hours; maximum concentration: 0.4 mEq/mL; maximum rate of infusion: 1 mEq/kg/hour

Monitoring Parameters Serum electrolytes, serum ammonia

Patient Information Take oral dose after meals

Nursing Implications Rapid I.V. injection may increase the likelihood of ammonia toxicity

Dosage Forms

Injection: 5 mEq/mL (20 mL)

Tablet: 500 mg

Tablet, enteric coated: 500 mg

Amonidrin® [OTC] *see* Guaifenesin *on page 278*

Amoxapine (a mox' a peen)

Related Information

Overdose and Toxicology Information *on page 696-700*

Brand Names Asendin®

Therapeutic Category Antidepressant, Tricyclic

Use Treatment of neurotic and endogenous depression and mixed symptoms of anxiety and depression

Pregnancy Risk Factor C

Contraindications Hypersensitivity to amoxapine; cross-sensitivity with other tricyclics may occur; narrow-angle glaucoma; patients receiving MAO inhibitors within past 14 days

Warnings Do not discontinue abruptly in patients receiving high doses chronically

Precautions Use with caution in patients with seizures, cardiac conduction disturbances, cardiovascular diseases, urinary retention, hyperthyroidism, or those receiving thyroid replacement

Adverse Reactions Cardiac toxicities and risk of seizure are usually greater than anticholinergic effects

Cardiovascular: Hypotension, arrhythmias

Central nervous system: Tardive dyskinesia, drowsiness, dizziness, nervousness, insomnia, neuroleptic malignant syndrome, seizures, fever, extrapyramidal effects

Dermatologic: Rash

Endocrine & metabolic: Amenorrhea, galactorrhea

Gastrointestinal: Dry mouth, constipation

Hematologic: Leukopenia

Ocular: Blurred vision

Drug Interactions May possibly ↓ effects of clonidine and guanethidine; may ↑ effects of central nervous system depressants, adrenergic agents, anticholinergic agents; with monamine oxidase inhibitors, hyperpyrexia,

(Continued)

Amoxapine *(Continued)*

tachycardia, hypertension, seizures and death may occur; similar interactions as with other tricyclics may occur

Mechanism of Action Reduces the reuptake of serotonin and norepinephrine and blocks the response of dopamine receptors to dopamine

Pharmacodynamics Onset of action: Antidepressant effects usually occur after 1-2 weeks

Pharmacokinetics

Absorption: Oral: Well absorbed
Distribution: V_d: 0.9-1.2 L/kg; distributes into breast milk
Protein binding: 80%
Metabolism: Extensive in the liver; 8-hydroxy metabolite is active
Half-life:
- Parent drug: 11-16 hours
- Active metabolite (8-hydroxy): 30 hours

Peak serum levels: Within 1-2 hours
Elimination: Excretion of metabolites and parent compound in the urine

Usual Dosage Once symptoms are controlled, decrease gradually to lowest effective dose. Oral:

Children: Not established in children <16 years of age

Adolescents: Initial: 25-50 mg/day; ↑ gradually to 100 mg/day; may give as divided doses or as a single dose at bedtime

Adults: Initial: 25 mg 2-3 times/day, if tolerated, dosage may be increased to 100 mg 2-3 times/day; may be given in a single bedtime dose when dosage <300 mg/day
- Maximum daily dose:
  - Outpatient: 400 mg
  - Inpatient: 600 mg

Monitoring Parameters Blood pressure, heart rate and rhythm

Reference Range Therapeutic: Amoxapine 20-100 ng/mL (SI: 64-319 nmol/L); 8-OH amoxapine 150-400 ng/mL (SI: 478-1275 nmol/L); both 200-500 ng/mL (SI: 637-1594 nmol/L)

Dosage Forms Tablet: 25 mg, 50 mg, 100 mg, 150 mg

Amoxicillin (a mox i sill' in)

Related Information

Endocarditis Prophylaxis *on page 659*

Brand Names Amoxil®; Biomox®; Polymox®; Trimox®; Wymox®

Synonyms Amoxycillin; *p*-Hydroxyampicillin

Therapeutic Category Antibiotic, Penicillin

Use Infections caused by susceptible organisms involving the respiratory tract, otitis media, sinusitis, skin, and urinary tract; prophylaxis of bacterial endocarditis; spectrum similar to ampicillin except amoxicillin is less active against *Shigella* and *Enterobacter*

Pregnancy Risk Factor B

Contraindications Hypersensitivity to amoxicillin, penicillin, or any component

Warnings High percentage of patients with infectious mononucleosis have developed rash during therapy with amoxicillin

Precautions In patients with renal dysfunction, doses and/or frequency of administration should be modified in response to the degree of renal impairment

Adverse Reactions

Central nervous system: Fever
Dermatologic: Rash
Gastrointestinal: Diarrhea
Miscellaneous: Superinfection

Drug Interactions Probenecid, allopurinol

Stability Suspensions are stable for 14 days at room temperature or if refrigerated; refrigeration is preferred

Mechanism of Action Interferes with bacterial cell wall synthesis during active multiplication, causing cell wall death and resultant bactericidal activity against susceptible bacteria

Pharmacokinetics

Absorption: Rapid and nearly complete; food does not interfere with absorption

Distribution: Distributes into liver, lungs, prostate, muscle, middle ear effusions, maxillary sinus secretions, bile, and into ascitic and synovial fluids
Protein binding: 17% to 20%; lower in neonates
Metabolism: Partial
Peak levels:
Capsule: Within 2 hours
Suspension: 1 hour
Half-life:
Neonates, full-term: 3.7 hours
Infants and Children: 1-2 hours
Adults with normal renal function: 0.7-1.4 hours
Patients with Cl_{cr} <10 mL/minute: 7-21 hours
Elimination: Renal excretion (80% as unchanged drug)
Moderately dialyzable (20% to 50%); ~30% removed by 3-hour hemodialysis

Usual Dosage Oral:
Children: 20-50 mg/kg/day in divided doses every 8 hours
Uncomplicated gonorrhea: ≥2 years: 50 mg/kg plus probenecid 25 mg/kg in a single dose; do not use this regimen in children <2 years of age, probenecid is contraindicated in this age group
Subacute bacterial endocarditis prophylaxis: 50 mg/kg 1 hour before procedure and 25 mg/kg 6 hours later, not to exceed adult dose

Adults: 250-500 mg every 8 hours; maximum dose: 2-3 g/day
Uncomplicated gonorrhea: 3 g plus probenecid 1 g in a single dose
Endocarditis prophylaxis: 3 g 1 hour before procedure and 1.5 g 6 hours later

Dosing interval in renal impairment: Cl_{cr} <10 mL/minute: Administer every 12-24 hours

Monitoring Parameters With prolonged therapy, monitor renal, hepatic, and hematologic function periodically; assess patient at beginning and throughout therapy for infection; observe for signs and symptoms of anaphylaxis

Patient Information May be administered with meals

Dosage Forms
Capsule: 250 mg, 500 mg
Drops, oral: 50 mg/mL (15 mL, 30 mL)
Suspension, oral: 125 mg/5 mL (5 mL, 80 mL, 100 mL, 150 mL, 200 mL); 250 mg/5 mL (5 mL, 80 mL, 100 mL, 150 mL, 200 mL)
Tablet, chewable: 125 mg, 250 mg

References

Dajani AS, Bisno AL, Chung KJ, et al, "Prevention of Bacterial Endocarditis Recommendations by the American Heart Association," *JAMA*, 1990, 264(22):2919-22.

Amoxicillin and Clavulanate Potassium *see* Amoxicillin and Clavulanic Acid *on this page*

Amoxicillin and Clavulanic Acid

Brand Names Augmentin®

Synonyms Amoxicillin and Clavulanate Potassium

Therapeutic Category Antibiotic, Penicillin

Use Infections caused by susceptible organisms involving the lower respiratory tract, otitis media, sinusitis, skin and skin structure, and urinary tract; spectrum same as amoxicillin in addition to beta-lactamase producing *B. catarrhalis*, *H. influenzae*, *N. gonorrhoeae*, and *S. aureus* (not MRSA)

Pregnancy Risk Factor B

Contraindications Known hypersensitivity to amoxicillin, clavulanic acid, or penicillin; concomitant use of disulfiram

Warnings High percentage of patients with infectious mononucleosis have developed rash during therapy with amoxicillin

Precautions In patients with renal dysfunction, doses and/or frequency of administration should be modified in response to the degree of renal impairment

Adverse Reactions
Central nervous system: Headache

(Continued)

Amoxicillin and Clavulanic Acid *(Continued)*

Dermatologic: Rash, urticaria

Gastrointestinal: Nausea, vomiting, pseudomembranous colitis; incidence of diarrhea (9%) is higher than with amoxicillin alone

Miscellaneous: Vaginal candidiasis

Drug Interactions Probenecid, allopurinol, disulfiram

Stability Reconstituted oral suspension should be kept in refrigerator; discard unused suspension after 10 days

Mechanism of Action Clavulanic acid binds and inhibits beta-lactamases that inactivate amoxicillin resulting in amoxicillin having an expanded spectrum of activity

Pharmacokinetics

Absorption: Both amoxicillin and clavulanate are well absorbed

Metabolism: Clavulanic acid: Metabolized in the liver

Half-life of both agents in adults with normal renal function: ~1 hour; amoxicillin pharmacokinetics are not affected by clavulanic acid

Peak levels: Within 2 hours

Elimination: Amoxicillin: Excreted primarily unchanged in the urine

Usual Dosage Oral:

Children <40 kg: 20-40 mg (amoxicillin component)/kg/day in divided doses every 8 hours

Adults: 250-500 mg every 8 hours; maximum dose: 2 g/day

Dosing interval in renal impairment:

- Cl_{cr} 15-30 mL/minute: Administer every 12-18 hours
- Cl_{cr} 5-15 mL/minute: Administer every 24-36 hours
- Cl_{cr} <5 mL/minute: Administer every 48 hours

Monitoring Parameters With prolonged therapy, monitor renal, hepatic, and hematologic function periodically

Test Interactions May interfere with urinary glucose determinations using Clinitest®

Patient Information Adverse GI effects may occur less frequently if given with food

Additional Information Potassium content: 0.16 mEq of potassium per 31.25 mg of clavulanic acid; since both the '250' and '500' tablets contain the same amount of clavulanic acid, two '250' tablets are not equivalent to one '500' tablet

Dosage Forms

Suspension, oral (banana flavor):

- 125: Amoxicillin trihydrate 125 mg and clavulanic acid 31.25 mg per 5 mL (75 mL, 150 mL)
- 250: Amoxicillin trihydrate 250 mg and clavulanic acid 62.5 mg per 5 mL (75 mL, 150 mL)

Tablet:

- 250: Amoxicillin trihydrate 250 mg and clavulanic acid 125 mg
- 500: Amoxicillin trihydrate 500 mg and clavulanic acid 125 mg

Tablet, chewable:

- 125: Amoxicillin trihydrate 125 mg and clavulanic acid 31.25 mg
- 250: Amoxicillin trihydrate 250 mg and clavulanic acid 62.5 mg

References

Arguedas AG, Zaleska M, Stutman HR, et al, "Comparative Trial of Cefprozil vs Amoxicillin Clavulanate Potassium in the Treatment of Children With Acute Otitis Media With Effusion," *Pediatr Infect Dis J*, 1991, 10(5):375-80.

Gan VN, Kusmiesz H, Shelton S, et al, "Comparative Evaluation of Loracarbef and Amoxicillin-Clavulanate for Acute Otitis Media," *Antimicrob Agents Chemother*, 1991, 35(5):967-71.

Thoene DE and Johnson CE, "Pharmacotherapy of Otitis Media," *Pharmacotherapy*, 1991, 11(3):212-21.

Amoxil® *see* Amoxicillin *on page 44*

Amoxycillin *see* Amoxicillin *on page 44*

Amphojel® [OTC] *see* Antacid Preparations *on page 53*

Amphotericin B (am foe ter' i sin)

Brand Names Fungizone®

Therapeutic Category Antifungal Agent, Systemic; Antifungal Agent, Topical

Use Treatment of severe systemic infections and meningitis caused by susceptible fungi such as *Candida* species, *Histoplasma capsulatum*, *Cryptococcus neoformans*, *Aspergillus* species, *Blastomyces dermatitidis*, *Torulopsis glabrata*, and *Coccidioides immitis*; fungal peritonitis; irrigant for bladder fungal infections; and topically for cutaneous and mucocutaneous candidal infections

Pregnancy Risk Factor B

Contraindications Hypersensitivity to amphotericin or any component

Warnings I.V. amphotericin is used primarily for the treatment of patients with progressive and potentially fatal fungal infections; not to be used for common clinically inapparent forms of fungal disease

Precautions Due to the nephrotoxic potential of amphotericin, other nephrotoxic drugs should be avoided

Adverse Reactions

Cardiovascular: Hypotension, hypertension, cardiac arrhythmias, flushing
Central nervous system: Fever, delirium, headache, chills
Endocrine & metabolic: Hypokalemia, hypomagnesemia
Gastrointestinal: Anorexia, nausea, vomiting
Hematologic: Anemia, leukopenia, thrombocytopenia
Local: Phlebitis
Renal & genitourinary: Renal tubular acidosis, renal failure (oliguria, azotemia, ↑ serum creatinine)

Adverse effects due to intrathecal amphotericin:
- Central nervous system: Headache, paresthesia, pain along lumbar nerves, arachnoiditis
- Gastrointestinal: Nausea, vomiting
- Ocular: Vision changes
- Renal & genitourinary: Urinary retention

Drug Interactions Nephrotoxic drugs → toxic effects may be additive; corticosteroids may ↑ potassium depletion caused by amphotericin; may predispose patients receiving cardiac glycosides or skeletal muscle relaxants to toxicity secondary to hypokalemia

Stability Reconstitute only with sterile water without preservatives, not bacteriostatic water; benzyl alcohol, sodium chloride, or other electrolyte solutions may cause precipitation; can be diluted in D_5W, $D_{10}W$, up to $D_{20}W$; for I.V. infusion, an in-line filter (>1 micron mean pore diameter) may be used; short-term exposure (<24 hours) to light during I.V. infusion does **not** appreciably affect potency

Mechanism of Action Binds to ergosterol altering cell membrane permeability in susceptible fungi and causing leakage of cell components with subsequent cell death

Pharmacokinetics

Distribution: Minimal amounts enter the aqueous humor, bile, amniotic fluid, pericardial fluid, pleural fluid, and synovial fluid; poor CSF penetration
Protein binding: 90%
Half-life: Increased in small neonates and young infants
- Initial: 15-48 hours
- Terminal phase: 15 days

Poorly dialyzed

Usual Dosage Minimum dilution for amphotericin B infusions: 0.1 mg/mL

Infants and Children:
- Test dose: I.V.: 0.1 mg/kg/dose to a maximum of 1 mg; infuse over 30-60 minutes
- Initial therapeutic dose (if the test dose is tolerated): 0.25 mg/kg
- The daily dose can then be gradually increased, usually in 0.25 mg/kg increments on each subsequent day until the desired daily dose is reached; in critically ill patients, more rapid dosage acceleration (up to 0.5 mg/kg increments on each subsequent day) may be warranted
- Maintenance dose: 0.25-1 mg/kg/day given once daily; infuse over 2-6 hours; once therapy has been established, amphotericin B can be administered on an every-other-day basis at 1-1.5 mg/kg/dose
- I.T.: 25-100 μg every 48-72 hours; increase to 500 μg as tolerated

Adults:
- Test dose: I.V.: 1 mg infused over 20-30 minutes
- Initial therapeutic dose (if the test dose is tolerated): 0.25 mg/kg

(Continued)

Amphotericin B *(Continued)*

The daily dose can then be gradually increased, usually in 0.25 mg/kg increments on each subsequent day until the desired daily dose is reached

Maintenance dose: I.V.: 0.25-1 mg/kg/day once daily, infuse over 2-6 hours; or 1-1.5 mg/kg/dose every other day; do not exceed 1.5 mg/kg/day

I.T.: 100 μg every 48-72 hours; increase to 500 μg as tolerated

Children and Adults:

Bladder irrigation: 5-15 mg amphotericin/100 mL of sterile water irrigation solution at 100-300 mL/day. Fluid is instilled into the bladder; the catheter is clamped for 60-120 minutes and the bladder drained. Perform irrigation 3-4 times/day for 2-5 days.

Dialysate: 1-4 mg/L of peritoneal dialysis fluid either with or without low-dose I.V. amphotericin B therapy

Topical: Apply to affected areas 2-4 times/day

Administration Amphotericin is administered by I.V. infusion over 2-6 hours at a final concentration not to exceed 0.1 mg/mL. In patients unable to tolerate a large fluid volume, amphotericin B 0.25 mg/mL in D_5W given through a central venous catheter is the highest concentration reported to have been administered.

Monitoring Parameters BUN and serum creatinine levels should be determined every other day while therapy is increased and at least weekly thereafter; serum potassium and magnesium should be monitored closely; monitor electrolytes, liver function, hematocrit, CBC regularly; monitor input and output; monitor for signs of hypokalemia (muscle weakness, cramping, drowsiness, EKG changes, etc); blood pressure, temperature

Patient Information Amphotericin cream may slightly discolor skin and stain clothing; personal hygiene is very important to help reduce the spread and recurrence of lesions; avoid covering topical applications with occlusive bandages; most skin lesions require 1-3 weeks of therapy

Nursing Implications Cardiovascular collapse has been reported after rapid amphotericin injection; may premedicate patients who experience mild adverse reactions with acetaminophen and diphenhydramine 30 minutes prior to the amphotericin infusion. Meperidine may help to reduce rigors.

Additional Information Reversing sodium depletion may prevent amphotericin B-induced nephrotoxicity. Dosage adjustments are not necessary with renal impairment. If decreased renal function is due to amphotericin, the daily dose can be decreased by 50% or the dose can be given every other day.

Dosage Forms

Cream: 3% (20 g)

Powder for injection, lyophilized: 50 mg

Lotion: 3% (30 mL)

Ointment, topical: 3% (20 g)

References

The Ad Hoc Advisory Panel on Peritonitis Management. "Continuous Ambulatory Peritoneal Dialysis (CAPD) Peritonitis Treatment Recommendations: 1989 Update," *Perit Dial Int*, 1989, 9(4):247-56.

Benson JM and Nahata MC, "Pharmacokinetics of Amphotericin B in Children," *Antimicrob Agents Chemother*, 1989, 33(11):1989-93.

Gallis HA, Drew RH, and Pickard WW, "Amphotericin B: 30 Years of Clinical Experience," *Rev Infect Dis*, 1990, 12(2):308-29.

Kintzel PE and Smith GH, "Practical Guidelines for Preparing and Administering Amphotericin B," *Am J Hosp Pharm*, 1992, 49(5):1156-64.

Koren G, Lau A, Klein J, et al, "Pharmacokinetics and Adverse Effects of Amphotericin B in Infants and Children," *J Pediatr*, 1988, 113(3):559-63.

Ampicillin (am pi sill' in)

Related Information

Endocarditis Prophylaxis *on page 659*

Brand Names Marcillin®; Omnipen®; Omnipen®-N; Polycillin®; Polycillin-N®; Principen®; Totacillin®; Totacillin®-N

Synonyms Aminobenzylpenicillin

Therapeutic Category Antibiotic, Penicillin

Use Treatment of susceptible bacterial infections caused by streptococci, pneumococci, nonpenicillinase-producing staphylococci, *Listeria*, meningococci; some strains of *H. influenzae*, *Salmonella*, *Shigella*, *E. coli*, *Enterobacter*, and *Klebsiella*.

Pregnancy Risk Factor B

Contraindications Known hypersensitivity to ampicillin (penicillins)

Warnings High percentage of patients with infectious mononucleosis have developed rash during therapy with ampicillin

Precautions Dosage adjustment may be necessary when Cl_{cr} <10-15 mL/minute

Adverse Reactions

- Central nervous system: Seizures
- Dermatologic: Rash
- Gastrointestinal: Diarrhea, nausea, vomiting, glossitis, colitis
- Hematologic: Eosinophilia, hemolytic anemia, thrombocytopenia, neutropenia
- Renal & genitourinary: Interstitial nephritis
- Miscellaneous: Drug fever

Drug Interactions Aminoglycosides, probenecid, chloroquine

Stability Oral suspension stable for 14 days under refrigeration; reconstituted solutions for I.M. or direct I.V. should be used within one hour; solutions for I.V. infusion will be inactivated by dextrose at room temperature; if dextrose containing solutions are to be used as a diluent, the resultant solution will only be stable for 2 hours vs 8 hours in solutions containing the 0.9% sodium chloride injection

Mechanism of Action Interferes with bacterial cell wall synthesis during active multiplication, causing cell wall death and resultant bactericidal activity against susceptible bacteria

Pharmacokinetics

- Absorption: Oral: 50%
- Distribution: Distributes into bile; penetration into CSF occurs with inflamed meninges only
- Protein binding:
  - Neonates: 10%
  - Adults: 15% to 18%
- Half-life:
  - Neonates:
    - 2-7 days: 4 hours
    - 8-14 days: 2.8 hours
    - 15-30 days: 1.7 hours
  - Children and Adults: 1-1.8 hours
  - Anuric patients: 8-20 hours
- Time to peak serum concentration: Within 1-2 hours following oral administration
- Elimination: ~90% of the drug is excreted unchanged in the urine within 24 hours
- ~40% is removed by hemodialysis

Usual Dosage

- Neonates: I.M., I.V.:
  - Postnatal age ≤7 days:
    - ≤2000 g: 50 mg/kg/day divided every 12 hours; meningitis: 100 mg/kg/day divided every 12 hours
    - >2000 g: 75 mg/kg/day divided every 8 hours; meningitis: 150 mg/kg/day divided every 8 hours
  - Postnatal age >7 days:
    - <1200 g: 50 mg/kg/day divided every 12 hours; meningitis: 100 mg/kg/day divided every 12 hours
    - 1200-2000 g: 75 mg/kg/day divided every 8 hours; meningitis: 150 mg/kg/day divided every 8 hours
    - >2000 g: 100 mg/kg/day divided every 6 hours; meningitis: 200 mg/kg/day divided every 6 hours
- Infants and Children: I.M., I.V.: 100-200 mg/kg/day divided every 4-6 hours; meningitis: 200-400 mg/kg/day divided every 4-6 hours; maximum dose: 12 g/day
- Adults: I.M., I.V.: 500 mg to 3 g every 4-6 hours
- Children: Oral: 50-100 mg/kg/day divided every 6 hours; maximum dose: 2-3 g/day

(Continued)

Ampicillin *(Continued)*

Adults: Oral: 250-500 mg every 6 hours

Adult dosing interval in renal impairment:
Cl_{cr} 10-30 mL/minute: Administer every 6-12 hours
Cl_{cr} <10 mL/minutes: Administer every 12 hours

Administration Ampicillin can be administered IVP over 3-5 minutes at a rate not to exceed 100 mg/minute or I.V. intermittent infusion over 15-30 minutes; final concentration for I.V. administration should not exceed 100 mg/mL (IVP) or 30 mg/mL (I.V. intermittent infusion)

Monitoring Parameters With prolonged therapy monitor renal, hepatic, and hematologic function periodically

Test Interactions False-positive urinary glucose (Benedict's solution, Clinitest®); + Coombs' [direct]

Patient Information Food decreases rate and extent of absorption; take on an empty stomach

Nursing Implications Ampicillin and gentamicin should not be mixed in the same I.V. tubing or administered concurrently

Additional Information Appearance of a rash should be carefully evaluated to differentiate a nonallergic ampicillin rash from a hypersensitivity reaction. Ampicillin rash occurs in 5% to 10% of children receiving ampicillin and is a generalized dull red, maculopapular rash, generally appearing 3-14 days after the start of therapy. It normally begins on the trunk and spreads over most of the body. It may be most intense at pressure areas, elbows, and knees. Incidence of ampicillin rash is higher in patients with viral infections, *Salmonella* infections, lymphocytic leukemia, or patients with hyperuricemia who are receiving allopurinol

Sodium content of suspension (250 mg/5 mL, 5 mL): 10 mg (0.4 mEq)
Sodium content of 1 g: 66.7 mg (3 mEq)

Dosage Forms
Capsule, as anhydrous: 250 mg, 500 mg
Capsule, as trihydrate: 250 mg, 500 mg
Powder for injection, as sodium: 125 mg, 250 mg, 500 mg, 1 g, 2 g, 10 g
Powder for oral suspension, as trihydrate: 125 mg/5 mL (5 mL unit dose, 80 mL, 100 mL, 150 mL, 200 mL); 250 mg/5 mL (5 mL unit dose, 80 mL, 100 mL, 150 mL, 200 mL); 500 mg/5 mL (5 mL unit dose, 100 mL)
Powder for oral suspension, drops, as trihydrate: 100 mg/mL (20 mL)

References

Brown RD, Campoli-Richards DM, "Antimicrobial Therapy in Neonates, Infants, and Children," *Clin Pharmacokinet*, 1989, 17(Suppl 1):105-15.

Ampicillin and Sulbactam

Brand Names Unasyn®

Synonyms Sulbactam and Ampicillin

Therapeutic Category Antibiotic, Penicillin

Use Treatment of susceptible bacterial infections involved with skin and skin structure, intra-abdominal infections, gynecological infections; spectrum is that of ampicillin plus organisms producing beta-lactamases such as *S. aureus*, *H. influenzae*, *E. coli*, *Klebsiella*, *Acinetobacter*, *Enterobacter* and anaerobes

Pregnancy Risk Factor B

Contraindications Hypersensitivity to ampicillin, sulbactam or any component, or penicillins

Warnings Should not be administered to patients with mononucleosis; not FDA approved for children <12 years of age

Precautions Modify dosage in patients with renal impairment

Adverse Reactions
Cardiovascular: Chest pain
Central nervous system: Fatigue, malaise, headache, chills
Dermatologic: Rash (2%); itching
Gastrointestinal: Diarrhea (3%); nausea, vomiting, candidiasis, flatulence, enterocolitis, pseudomembranous colitis
Hematologic: ↓ WBC, neutrophils, platelets, hemoglobin, and hematocrit
Hepatic: ↑ liver enzymes
Local: Pain at injection site (I.M.: 16%, I.V.: 3%); thrombophlebitis (3%)
Renal & genitourinary: Dysuria, ↑ BUN and creatinine

Miscellaneous: Hairy tongue, hypersensitivity reactions

Drug Interactions Probenecid (↓ elimination of ampicillin and sulbactam); allopurinol

Stability Ampicillin/sulbactam infusion solution is stable for 8 hours in 0.9% sodium chloride injection at room temperature; incompatible when mixed with aminoglycosides

Mechanism of Action The addition of sulbactam, a beta-lactamase inhibitor, to ampicillin extends the spectrum of ampicillin to include beta-lactamase producing organisms; ampicillin acts by inhibiting bacterial cell wall synthesis during the stage of active multiplication

Pharmacokinetics

Distribution: Distributed into bile, blister and tissue fluids; poor penetration into CSF with uninflamed meninges; higher concentrations attained with inflamed meninges

Protein binding:

- Ampicillin: 28%
- Sulbactam: 38%

Half-life: Ampicillin and sulbactam are similar: 1-1.8 hours and 1-1.3 hours, respectively in patients with normal renal function

Elimination: ~75% to 85% of both drugs are excreted unchanged in the urine within 8 hours following administration

Usual Dosage Unasyn® (ampicillin/sulbactam) is a combination product; each 3 g vial contains 2 g of ampicillin and 1 g of sulbactam. Sulbactam has very little antibacterial activity by itself, but effectively extends the spectrum of ampicillin to include beta-lactamase producing strains that are resistant to ampicillin alone; therefore, dosage recommendations for Unasyn® are based on the **ampicillin** component.

I.M., I.V.:

- Children: 100-200 mg ampicillin/kg/day divided every 6 hours; maximum dose: 8 g ampicillin/day
- Adults: 1-2 g ampicillin every 6-8 hours; maximum dose: 8 g ampicillin/day

Dosing interval in renal impairment:

- Cl_{cr} 15-29 mL/minute: Administer every 12 hours
- Cl_{cr} 5-14 mL/minute: Administer every 24 hours

Administration Can be administered by slow I.V. injection over 10-15 minutes at a final concentration for administration not to exceed 45 mg Unasyn® (30 mg ampicillin and 15 mg sulbactam)/mL

Monitoring Parameters With prolonged therapy monitor hematologic, renal, and hepatic function

Test Interactions False-positive urinary glucose levels (Benedict's solution, Clinitest®)

Additional Information Sodium content of 1.5 g (1 g ampicillin plus 0.5 g sulbactam): 5 mEq

Dosage Forms Powder for injection: 1.5 g = ampicillin sodium 1 g and sulbactam sodium 0.5 g; 3 g = ampicillin sodium 2 g and sulbactam sodium 1 g

References

Dajani AS, "Sulbactam/Ampicillin in Pediatric Infections," *Drugs*, 1988, 35(Suppl 7):35-8.

Goldfarb J, Aronoff SC, Jaffé A, et al, "Sultamicillin in the Treatment of Superficial Skin and Soft Tissue Infections in Children," *Antimicrob Agents Chemother*, 1987, 31(4):663-4.

Kulhanjian J, Dunphy MG, Hamstra S, et al, "Randomized Comparative Study of Ampicillin/Sulbactam vs Ceftriaxone for Treatment of Soft Tissue and Skeletal Infections in Children," *Pediatr Infect Dis J*, 1989, 8(9):605-10.

Syriopoulou V, Bitsi M, Theodoridis C, et al, "Clinical Efficacy of Sulbactam/Ampicillin in Pediatric Infections Caused by Ampicillin-Resistant or Penicillin-Resistant Organisms," *Rev Infect Dis*, 1986, 8(Suppl 5):S630-3.

Amrinone Lactate (am' ri none)

Brand Names Inocor®

Therapeutic Category Adrenergic Agonist Agent

Use Treatment of low cardiac output states (sepsis, congestive heart failure); adjunctive therapy of pulmonary hypertension

(Continued)

Amrinone Lactate *(Continued)*

Pregnancy Risk Factor C

Contraindications Hypersensitivity to amrinone lactate or sulfites (contains sodium metabisulfite)

Precautions Monitor for hypotension, thrombocytopenia, hepatotoxicity, and GI effects; monitor fluids and electrolytes. Diuresis may result from improvement in cardiac output and may require dosage reduction of diuretics.

Adverse Reactions

Cardiovascular: Hypotension (1.3% incidence), ventricular and supraventricular arrhythmias (3% incidence); may be related to infusion rate

Gastrointestinal: Nausea, vomiting, abdominal pain, anorexia

Hematologic: Thrombocytopenia (2.4% incidence), may be dose related

Hepatic: Hepatotoxicity (0.2% incidence), discontinue amrinone if significant ↑ in liver enzymes with symptoms of idiosyncratic hypersensitivity reaction (ie, eosinophilia) occurs

Stability Do not directly dilute with dextrose-containing solutions, chemical interaction occurs; may be administered I.V. into running dextrose infusions. Furosemide forms a precipitate when injected in I.V. lines containing amrinone.

Mechanism of Action Inhibits myocardial cyclic adenosine monophosphate (cAMP) phosphodiesterase activity and increases cellular levels of cAMP resulting in a positive inotropic effect; also possesses systemic and pulmonary vasodilator effects

Pharmacodynamics

Onset of action: I.V.: Within 2-5 minutes

Peak effect: Within 10 minutes

Duration: Dose dependent with low doses lasting ~30 minutes and higher doses lasting ~2 hours

Pharmacokinetics

Distribution: V_d:

- Neonates: 1.8 L/kg
- Infants: 1.6 L/kg
- Adults: 1.2 L/kg

Protein binding: 10% to 49%

Metabolism: Metabolized in the liver

Half-life:

- Neonates, 1-2 weeks of-age: 22.2 hours
- Infants 6-38 weeks of age: 6.8 hours; negative correlation of age with half-life in infants 4-38 weeks of age
- Adults, normal volunteers: 3.6 hours
- Adults with CHF: 5.8 hours

Elimination: Excreted (60% to 90% as metabolites) in the urine within 24 hours

Usual Dosage Note: Dose should not exceed 10 mg/kg/24 hours

Neonates: 0.75 mg/kg I.V. bolus over 2-3 minutes followed by maintenance infusion 3-5 μg/kg/minute; I.V. bolus may need to be repeated in 30 minutes; see Additional Information

Children: 0.75 mg/kg I.V. bolus over 2-3 minutes followed by maintenance infusion 5-10 μg/kg/minute; I.V. bolus may need to be repeated in 30 minutes

Adults: 0.75 mg/kg I.V. bolus over 2-3 minutes followed by maintenance infusion of 5-10 μg/kg/minute

Administration May be administered undiluted for I.V. bolus doses. For continuous infusion: Dilute with 0.45% or 0.9% sodium chloride to final concentration of 1-3 mg/mL use within 24 hours

Monitoring Parameters Blood pressure, heart rate, platelet count, liver enzymes

Nursing Implications Do **not** "Y" furosemide IVP into amrinone solutions

Additional Information Preliminary pharmacokinetic studies estimate total initial bolus doses of 3-4.5 mg/kg given in divided doses in neonates and infants to obtain serum concentrations similar to therapeutic adult levels. The actual use of these higher doses has been reported in a very small number of infants (n=7). Further studies are needed to define pediatric dosing guidelines.

Dosage Forms Injection: 5 mg/mL (20 mL)

References

Lawless S, Burckart G, Diven W, et al, "Amrinone in Neonates and Infants After Cardiac Surgery," *Crit Care Med*, 1989, 17(8):751-4.

Lawless ST, Zaritsky A, and Miles MV, "The Acute Pharmacokinetics and Pharmacodynamics of Amrinone in Pediatric Patients," *J Clin Pharmacol*, 1991, 31(9):800-3.

Anacin® [OTC] *see* Aspirin *on page 61*

Anacin-3® [OTC] *see* Acetaminophen *on page 16*

Anaprox® *see* Naproxen *on page 404*

Anbesol® Maximum Strength [OTC] *see* Benzocaine *on page 77*

Ancef® *see* Cefazolin Sodium *on page 110*

Ancobon® *see* Flucytosine *on page 249*

Andro® *see* Testosterone *on page 550*

Andro-Cyp® *see* Testosterone *on page 550*

Andro-L.A.® *see* Testosterone *on page 550*

Andronate® *see* Testosterone *on page 550*

Andropository® *see* Testosterone *on page 550*

Anectine® Chloride *see* Succinylcholine Chloride *on page 537*

Anectine® Flo-Pack® *see* Succinylcholine Chloride *on page 537*

Anergan® *see* Promethazine Hydrochloride *on page 488*

Anestacon® *see* Lidocaine Hydrochloride *on page 342*

Aneurine Hydrochloride *see* Thiamine Hydrochloride *on page 559*

Anexia® *see* Hydrocodone and Acetaminophen *on page 292*

Ansaid® *see* Flurbiprofen Sodium *on page 261*

Ansamycin *see* Rifabutin *on page 513*

Antacid Preparations

Brand Names Amphojel® [OTC]; Basaljel® [OTC]; Gaviscon® [OTC]; Maalox® [OTC]; Maalox® Plus Extra Strength [OTC]; Mylanta® [OTC]; Mylanta®-II [OTC]; Riopan® [OTC]; Tums® [OTC]

Use Relief of stomach upset associated with hyperacidity; prevention of stress ulcer bleeding; treatment of duodenal ulcer and gastroesophageal reflux disease. Aluminum hydroxide is also used to reduce phosphate absorption in hyperphosphatemia; calcium carbonate is used to treat calcium deficiency and magnesium oxide is used to treat hypomagnesemia.

Warnings Use aluminum-containing antacids with caution in patients with gastric outlet obstruction, in patients with uremia who are not receiving dialysis and in patients who have an upper GI hemorrhage; use magnesium-containing products with caution in patients with renal impairment

Adverse Reactions

Sodium-containing antacids:
Cardiovascular: Fluid retention

Aluminum-containing antacids:
Central nervous system: Dementia, encephalopathy, seizures, confusion, coma
Endocrine & metabolic: Osteomalacia, hypophosphatemia
Gastrointestinal: Constipation

Calcium-containing antacids:
Endocrine & metabolic: Milk-alkali syndrome

Magnesium-containing antacids:
Gastrointestinal: Laxative effects, diarrhea

Mechanism of Action Neutralize gastric acidity increasing gastric pH; inhibits proteolytic activity of pepsin when gastric pH is increased >4

Usual Dosage Oral:

Peptic ulcer disease:
Children: 5-15 mL/dose every 3-6 hours or 1-3 hours after meals and at bedtime

(Continued)

Antacid Preparations *(Continued)*

Adults: 15-45 mL every 3-6 hours or 1-3 hours after meals and at bedtime

Prophylaxis against GI bleeding:
- Neonates: 1 mL/kg every 4 hours as needed
- Infants: 2-5 mL/dose every 1-2 hours, titrate to gastric pH >5
- Children: 5-15 mL/dose every 1-2 hours, titrate to gastric pH >5
- Adults: 30-60 mL every 1-2 hours, titrate to gastric pH >5

Hyperphosphatemia:
- Children: Use $Al(OH)_3$ or aluminum carbonate gel product only. 50-150 mg/kg/day (as aluminum hydroxide gel) divided every 4-6 hours; titrate to normal serum phosphorus level
- Adults: 500-1800 μg of $Al(OH)_3$ 3-6 times/day between meals and at bedtime

Antacid Preparations

Generic/Therapeutic Groupings Brand Names	$Al(OH)_3$*	$Mg(OH)_2$*	$CaCO_3$*	Other Content	Sodium† (mg)	ANC‡ (mEq)	How Supplied
Aluminum carbonate gel (basic)							
Basaljel®	400			Simethicone, saccharin, sorbitol	2.9	12	Suspension
	500				2.8	12	Capsule
	500				2.8	13	Tablet
Aluminum hydroxide gel							
Amphojel®	320			Saccharin, sorbitol	< 2.3	10	Suspension
	300				1.8	8	Tablet
	600				2.9	16	
Aluminum/magnesium hydroxide							
Maalox®	225	200		Saccharin, sorbitol	1.4	13.3	Suspension
	200				0.7	9.7	Tablet/chewable
Maalox® Plus Extra Strength	500	450		Simethicone 25 mg saccharin, sorbitol (sugar-free)	1.2	29	Suspension
Aluminum hydroxide/magnesium carbonate							
Gaviscon®	31.7			Magnesium carbonate 412 mg, sodium alginate, EDTA, saccharin, sorbitol	13	3–4	Suspension
Aluminum hydroxide/magnesium trisilicate							
Gaviscon®	80			Magnesium trisilicate 20 mg, alginic acid, sodium bicarbonate	19	0.5	Tablet/chewable
Calcium carbonate							
Tums®			500		≤ 2	10	Tablet/chewable
Calcium carbonate suspension			1250		< 5		Suspension

* Liquids in mg per 5 mL; capsules and tablets in mg.
† mg of sodium per tablet, capsule, or 5 mL of liquid (23 mg = 1 mEq sodium)
‡ Acid neutralizing capacity per tablet, capsule, or 5 mL of liquid.

Monitoring Parameters GI complaints, stool frequency

Patient Information Antacids may impair or increase absorption of many drugs, do not take oral medications within 1-2 hours of an antacid dose unless specifically instructed to do so

Dosage Forms See table.

Antidigoxin Fab Fragments *see* Digoxin Immune Fab *on page 191*

Antidiuretic Hormone *see* Vasopressin *on page 595*

Antihemophilic Factor, Human (an tee hee moe fill' ik)

Brand Names Hemofil® M; Humate-P®; Kōate®-HP; Kōate®-HS; KoGENate®; Monoclate-P®; Profilate® OSD

Synonyms AHF; AHG; Factor VIII

Therapeutic Category Antihemophilic Agent; Blood Product Derivative

Use Management of hemophilia A in patients whom a deficiency in factor VIII has been demonstrated

Pregnancy Risk Factor C

Contraindications Hypersensitivity to mouse protein (Monoclate-P®; Hemofil® M, Method M, Monoclonal Purified; and Antihemophilic Factor (Human), Method M, Monoclonal Purified contain trace amounts of mouse protein)

Precautions Antihemophilic factor is prepared from pooled plasma and even with heat treated or other viral attenuated processes, the risk of viral transmission (ie, viral hepatitis, HIV) is not totally eradicated. Progressive anemia and hemolysis may occur in individuals with blood groups A, B, and AB who receive large or frequent doses due to trace amounts of blood group A and B isohemagglutinins.

Adverse Reactions

Cardiovascular: Flushing, tachycardia

Central nervous system: Paresthesia, headache

Gastrointestinal: Nausea, vomiting

Miscellaneous: Allergic vasomotor reactions, tightness in neck or chest

Stability Dried concentrate should be refrigerated, but may be stored at room temperature for up to 6 months depending upon specific product; if refrigerated, the dried concentrate and diluent should be warmed to room temperature before reconstitution; gently agitate or rotate vial after adding diluent, do not shake vigorously; do **not** refrigerate after reconstitution, precipitation may occur; administer within three hours after reconstitution; Method M, monoclonal purified products should be administered within 1 hour after reconstitution

Mechanism of Action A protein in normal plasma which is necessary for clot formation and maintenance of hemostasis; activates factor X in conjunction with activated factor IX; activated factor X converts prothrombin to thrombin, which converts fibrinogen to fibrin and with factor XIII forms a stable clot

Pharmacokinetics

Distribution: Does not readily cross the placenta

Half-life: 4-24 hours with a mean of 12 hours (biphasic)

Usual Dosage I.V. (individualize dosage based on coagulation studies performed prior to and during treatment at regular intervals):

Hospitalized patients: 20-50 units/kg/dose; may be higher for special circumstances. Dose can be given every 12-24 hours and more frequently in special circumstances.

Formula to approximate percentage increase in plasma antihemophilic factor: Units required = body weight (kg) x 0.5 x desired increase factor VIII (% of normal)

Administration I.V. administration only; maximum rate of administration is product dependent: Monoclate-P® 2 mL/minute; Humate-P® 4 mL/minute; administration of other products should not exceed 10 mL/minute; use filter needle to draw product into syringe; reduce rate of administration or temporarily discontinue if patient becomes tachycardiac

Monitoring Parameters Heart rate before and during I.V. administration; plasma antihemophilic factor levels prior to and during treatment

(Continued)

Antihemophilic Factor, Human *(Continued)*

Reference Range Plasma antihemophilic factor level: Desired: Approximately 30% of normal for effective hemostasis in patients with hemorrhage; approximately 5% to 10% of normal for hemarthrosis; approximately 30% to 50% of normal to prevent hemorrhage for minor surgical procedures; approximately 80% to 100% of normal for major surgical procedures (give dose 1 hour prior to OR); approximately 30% to 60% of normal may be required for at least 10-14 days postoperatively.

Dosage Forms Injection: Single-dose vials with varied units; 10 mL, 20 mL, 30 mL

Antilirium® *see* Physostigmine Salicylate *on page 457*

Antiminth® [OTC] *see* Pyrantel Pamoate *on page 499*

Antipyrine and Benzocaine (an tee pye' reen)

Brand Names Allergan® Ear Drops; Auralgan®; Auroto®; Otocalm® Ear

Synonyms Benzocaine and Antipyrine

Therapeutic Category Otic Agent, Analgesic; Otic Agent, Cerumenolytic

Use Temporary relief of pain and reduction of inflammation associated with acute congestive and serous otitis media, swimmer's ear, otitis externa; facilitates ear wax removal

Contraindications Hypersensitivity to antipyrine, benzocaine or any component; perforated tympanic membrane

Warnings Use of otic anesthetics may mask symptoms of a fulminating middle ear infection (acute otitis media); not intended for prolonged use

Adverse Reactions

Local: Burning, stinging, tenderness, edema

Miscellaneous: Hypersensitivity reactions

Usual Dosage Otic: Fill ear canal; moisten cotton pledget, place in external ear, repeat every 1-2 hours until pain and congestion is relieved; for ear wax removal instill drops 3-4 times/day for 2-3 days

Dosage Forms Solution, otic: Antipyrine 5.4% and benzocaine 1.4% (10 mL, 15 mL)

Antispas® *see* Dicyclomine Hydrochloride *on page 187*

Antithymocyte Globulin (equine) *see* Lymphocyte Immune Globulin *on page 350*

Anti-Tuss® [OTC] *see* Guaifenesin *on page 278*

Antivenin (Crotalidae) Polyvalent (kroe tal' ih day)

Synonyms Crotaline Antivenin, Polyvalent; North and South American Antisnake-bite Serum; Snake (Pit Vipers) Antivenin

Therapeutic Category Antivenin

Use For neutralization of the venoms of North and South American Crotalids: rattlesnake, copperhead, cottonmouth, tropical moccasins, Fer-de-lance, bushmaster

Pregnancy Risk Factor C

Contraindications Not effective against the venoms of coral snakes

Warnings Desensitization may need to be performed on patients with positive skin test reaction or history of sensitivity to equine serum

Precautions Patients with a negative skin test may still react when antivenin is administered; skin test should not be performed unless antivenin is to be used

Adverse Reactions

Cardiovascular: Shock, edema of the face

Central nervous system: Apprehension, peripheral neuritis

Dermatologic: Urticaria

Musculoskeletal: Muscle weakness

Respiratory: Dyspnea

Miscellaneous: Anaphylaxis, serum sickness

Stability Avoid storage temperatures >37°C; reconstituted solutions should be used within 48 hours

Usual Dosage Initial intradermal sensitivity test. The entire initial dose of antivenin should be administered as soon as possible to be most effective (within 4 hours after the bite).

Children and Adults: I.V.:

Minimal envenomation: 20-40 mL

Moderate envenomation: 50-90 mL

Severe envenomation: 100-150 mL

Additional doses of antivenin are based on clinical response to the initial dose. If swelling continues to progress, symptoms increase in severity, hypotension occurs, or decrease in hematocrit appears, an additional 10-50 mL should be administered.

Administration Antivenin may be given I.M. for minimal envenomation. I.V. administration of antivenin is preferred for moderate to severe envenomation or in the presence of shock; for I.V. infusion, prepare a 1:1 to 1:10 dilution of reconstituted antivenin in normal saline or D_5W; infuse the initial 5-10 mL dilution over 3-5 minutes while carefully observing the patient for signs and symptoms of sensitivity reactions. If no reaction occurs, continue infusion at a safe I.V. fluid delivery rate.

Monitoring Parameters Vital signs, hematocrit

Patient Information When reactions occur, immediate sensitivity reactions usually occur within 30 minutes after administration; serum-sickness reaction may occur 5-24 days after a dose

Nursing Implications **Do not inject into a finger or toe**; epinephrine should be available

Additional Information Intradermal skin test: 0.02-0.03 mL of a 1:10 dilution of antivenin in normal saline. If the patient has a history of equine serum sensitivity, administer a 1:100 or greater dilution skin test.

Dosage Forms Injection: Lyophilized serum, diluent (10 mL); one vacuum vial to yield 10 mL of serum

Antivert® *see* Meclizine Hydrochloride *on page 358*

Antrizine® *see* Meclizine Hydrochloride *on page 358*

Anusol® [OTC] *see* Hemorrhoidal Preparations *on page 282*

Anxanil® *see* Hydroxyzine *on page 298*

Apacet® [OTC] *see* Acetaminophen *on page 16*

APAP *see* Acetaminophen *on page 16*

A.P.L.® *see* Chorionic Gonadotropin *on page 134*

APPG *see* Penicillin G Procaine *on page 441*

Apresoline® *see* Hydralazine Hydrochloride *on page 290*

Aprodine® [OTC] *see* Triprolidine and Pseudoephedrine *on page 586*

Aquachloral® Supprettes® *see* Chloral Hydrate *on page 122*

AquaMEPHYTON® *see* Phytonadione *on page 458*

Aquaphyllin® *see* Theophylline *on page 554*

Aquasol A® [OTC] *see* Vitamin A *on page 603*

Aquasol E® [OTC] *see* Vitamin E *on page 605*

AquaTar® [OTC] *see* Coal Tar *on page 147*

Aqueous Procaine Penicillin G *see* Penicillin G Procaine *on page 441*

Aqueous Testosterone *see* Testosterone *on page 550*

Ara-A *see* Vidarabine *on page 599*

Arabin of Uranosyladenine *see* Vidarabine *on page 599*

Arabinosylcytosine *see* Cytarabine Hydrochloride *on page 166*

Ara-C *see* Cytarabine Hydrochloride *on page 166*

Aralen® Phosphate *see* Chloroquine Phosphate *on page 126*

Aredia™ *see* Pamidronate Disodium *on page 430*

Arfonad® *see* Trimethaphan Camsylate *on page 584*

Arginine Hydrochloride (ar' ji neen)

Brand Names R-Gene®

Therapeutic Category Diagnostic Agent, Pituitary Function; Metabolic Alkalosis Agent

(Continued)

Arginine Hydrochloride *(Continued)*

Use Pituitary function test (growth hormone); management of severe, uncompensated, metabolic alkalosis (pH ≥7.55) **after** optimizing therapy with sodium and potassium supplements

Contraindications Known hypersensitivity to arginine; renal or hepatic failure

Precautions Arginine hydrochloride is metabolized to nitrogen containing products for excretion; precaution should be taken and the temporary effect of a high nitrogen load on the kidneys should be evaluated

Adverse Reactions

Cardiovascular: Flushing (after rapid I.V. administration)
Central nervous system: Headache (after rapid I.V. administration)
Endocrine & metabolic: Hyperglycemia, hyperkalemia
Gastrointestinal: Nausea, vomiting, abdominal pain, bloating
Local: Venous irritation
Miscellaneous: Increased serum gastrin concentration

Drug Interactions Estrogen-progesterone combinations, spironolactone (potentially fatal hyperkalemia has been reported in patients with hepatic disease)

Mechanism of Action Stimulates pituitary release of growth hormone and prolactin and pancreatic release of glucagon and insulin; patients with impaired pituitary function have lower or no increase in plasma concentrations of growth hormone after administration of arginine. Arginine hydrochloride has been used for severe metabolic alkalosis due to its high chloride content.

Pharmacokinetics

Absorption: Oral: Well absorbed
Peak levels: Within 2 hours

Usual Dosage I.V.:

Growth hormone reserve test:
- Children: 500 mg/kg over 30 minutes
- Adults: 300 mL over 30 minutes

Metabolic alkalosis: Arginine dose (g) = weight (kg) x 0.1 [HCO_3^- - 24] where HCO_3^- = the patient's serum bicarbonate concentration mEq/L; give $\frac{1}{2}$ to $\frac{2}{3}$ of calculated dose and re-evaluate

Arginine hydrochloride is a fourth-line treatment for uncompensated metabolic alkalosis after sodium chloride, potassium chloride, and ammonium chloride supplementation has been optimized

To correct hypochloremia: Arginine dose (mL) = 0.4 x weight (kg) x [103-Cl^-] where Cl^- = the patient's serum chloride concentration mEq/L; give $\frac{1}{2}$ to $\frac{2}{3}$ of calculated dose and re-evaluate

Note: Arginine hydrochloride should never be used as an alternative to chloride supplementation but used in the patient who is unresponsive to sodium chloride or potassium chloride supplementation.

Administration May be infused without further dilution; maximum rate of I.V. infusion: 1 g/kg/hour (maximum: 60 g/hour)

Monitoring Parameters Acid-base status (arterial or capillary blood gases), serum electrolytes, BUN, glucose, plasma growth hormone concentrations (when evaluating growth hormone reserve)

Nursing Implications I.V. infiltration of arginine may cause necrosis and phlebitis

Dosage Forms Injection: 10% [0.475 mEq chloride/mL] (500 mL)

References

Bushinsky DA and Gennari FJ, "Life-Threatening Hyperkalemia Induced by Arginine," *Ann Intern Med*, 1978, 89(5 Pt 1):632-4.

8-Arginine Vasopressin *see* Vasopressin *on page 595*

Aristocort® Forte *see* Triamcinolone *on page 579*

Aristocort® Intralesional Suspension *see* Triamcinolone *on page 579*

Aristocort® Tablet *see* Triamcinolone *on page 579*

Aristospan® *see* Triamcinolone *on page 579*

Arm-a-Med® Isoetharine *see* Isoetharine *on page 321*

Arm-a-Med® Isoproterenol *see* Isoproterenol *on page 324*

Arm-a-Med® Metaproterenol *see* Metaproterenol Sulfate *on page 367*

Arrestin® *see* Trimethobenzamide Hydrochloride *on page 585*

Artane® *see* Trihexyphenidyl Hydrochloride *on page 583*

ASA *see* Aspirin *on page 61*

A.S.A. [OTC] *see* Aspirin *on page 61*

Ascorbic Acid (a skor' bik)

Brand Names Ascorbicap® [OTC]; C-Crystals® [OTC]; Cecon® [OTC]; Cenolate®; Cetane® [OTC]; Cevalin® [OTC]; Ce-Vi-Sol® [OTC]; Dull-C® [OTC]; Flavorcee® [OTC]; Vita-C® [OTC]

Synonyms Vitamin C

Therapeutic Category Urinary Acidifying Agent; Vitamin, Water Soluble

Use Prevention and treatment of scurvy; urinary acidification; dietary supplementation; prevention and decreasing the severity of colds

Pregnancy Risk Factor A (C if used in doses above RDA recommendation)

Contraindications Large doses during pregnancy

Adverse Reactions

Cardiovascular: Flushing

Central nervous system: Faintness, dizziness, headache, fatigue

Gastrointestinal: Nausea, vomiting, heartburn, diarrhea

Renal & genitourinary: Hyperoxaluria

Drug Interactions Aspirin, iron

Stability Injectable form should be stored under refrigeration (2°C to 8°C); protect oral dosage forms from light; ascorbic acid solution is rapidly oxidized

Mechanism of Action Necessary for collagen formation and tissue repair in the body; involved in some oxidation-reduction reactions as well as many other metabolic reactions

Pharmacokinetics

Absorption: Oral: Readily absorbed; absorption is an active process and is thought to be dose-dependent

Distribution: Widely distributed

Metabolism: Metabolized in the liver by oxidation and sulfation

Elimination: Excreted in urine; there is an individual specific renal threshold for ascorbic acid; when blood levels are high, ascorbic acid is excreted in urine, whereas when the levels are subthreshold very little if any ascorbic acid is excreted into urine

Usual Dosage Oral, I.M., I.V., S.C.:

Recommended daily allowance (RDA):

- $<$6 months: 30 mg
- 6 months to 1 year: 35 mg
- 1-3 years: 40 mg
- 4-10 years: 45 mg
- 11-14 years: 50 mg
- $>$14 years to Adults: 60 mg

Children:

- Scurvy: 100-300 mg/day in divided doses
- Urinary acidification: 500 mg every 6-8 hours
- Dietary supplement (variable): 35-100 mg/day

Adults:

- Scurvy: 100-250 mg 1-2 times/day
- Urinary acidification: 4-12 g/day in 3-4 divided doses
- Dietary supplement (variable): 50-200 mg/day
- Prevention and treatment of cold: 1-3 g/day

Test Interactions False-positive urinary glucose with cupric sulfate reagent, false-negative urinary glucose with glucose oxidase method

Additional Information Sodium content of 1 g: ~5 mEq

Dosage Forms

Capsule, timed release: 500 mg

Crystals: 4 g per teaspoonful (100 g, 500 g); 5 g per teaspoonful (180 g)

Injection: 250 mg/mL (2 mL, 30 mL); 500 mg/mL (2 mL, 50 mL)

(Continued)

Ascorbic Acid *(Continued)*

Liquid: 35 mg/0.6 mL (50 mL); 100 mg/mL (50 mL)
Lozenges: 60 mg
Powder: 4 g/teaspoonful (1000 g)
Syrup: 500 mg/5 mL (5 mL, 10 mL, 120 mL, 480 mL)
Tablet: 25 mg, 50 mg, 100 mg, 250 mg, 500 mg, 1000 mg
Tablet:
Chewable: 100 mg, 250 mg, 500 mg
Timed release: 500 mg, 1000 mg, 1500 mg

Ascorbicap® [OTC] *see* Ascorbic Acid *on previous page*

Ascriptin® [OTC] *see* Aspirin *on next page*

Asendin® *see* Amoxapine *on page 43*

Asmalix® *see* Theophylline *on page 554*

ASN-ase *see* Asparaginase *on this page*

Asparaginase (a spare' a gi nase)

Related Information
Emetogenic Potential of Single Chemotherapeutic Agents *on page 655*

Brand Names Elspar®

Synonyms A-ase; ASN-ase; Colaspase

Therapeutic Category Antineoplastic Agent

Use Treatment of acute lymphocytic leukemia, lymphoma

Pregnancy Risk Factor C

Contraindications Pancreatitis; hypersensitivity to *E. coli*, asparaginase, or any component (if a reaction to Elspar® occurs, obtain investigational Erwinia preparation from NCI and use with caution)

Warnings The US Food and Drug Administration (FDA) currently recommends that procedures for proper handling and disposal of antineoplastic agents be considered. Be prepared to treat anaphylaxis at each administration

Precautions Discontinue asparaginase at the first sign of renal failure or pancreatitis

Adverse Reactions
Cardiovascular: Hypotension
Central nervous system: Drowsiness, seizures, fever, chills, malaise, coma
Dermatologic: Rash, pruritus, urticaria
Endocrine & metabolic: Hyperglycemia, transient diabetes mellitus
Gastrointestinal: Vomiting, pancreatitis
Hematologic: Leukopenia; prolonged thrombin, prothrombin, and partial prothrombin times
Hepatic: Hepatotoxicity
Renal & genitourinary: Azotemia
Respiratory: Coughing, laryngeal spasm
Miscellaneous: Anaphylaxis

Drug Interactions Methotrexate

Stability Refrigerate; reconstituted solutions are stable for 8 hours when refrigerated; discard immediately if solution becomes cloudy; use of a 0.2 micron filter may result in some loss of potency

Mechanism of Action Inhibits protein synthesis by deaminating asparagine and depriving tumor cells of this essential amino acid

Pharmacokinetics
Absorption: Not absorbed from the GI tract, therefore, requires parenteral administration
Half-life: 8-30 hours
Elimination: Clearance is unaffected by age, renal function, or hepatic function

Usual Dosage Refer to individual protocols; perform intradermal sensitivity testing before the initial dose

Children and Adults:
I.M. (preferred route): 6000 units/m^2 3 times/week for 3 weeks for combination therapy
I.V.: 1000 units/kg/day for 10 days for combination therapy or 200 units/kg/day for 28 days if combination therapy is inappropriate

Administration I.V. must be infused over a minimum of 30 minutes

Monitoring Parameters Vital signs during administration, CBC, urinalysis, amylase, liver enzymes, prothrombin time, renal function tests, urine glucose, blood glucose

Test Interactions ↓ thyroxine and thyroxine-binding globulin

Nursing Implications Use two injection sites for I.M. doses >2 mL; appropriate agents for maintenance of an adequate airway and treatment of a hypersensitivity reaction (antihistamine, epinephrine, oxygen, I.V. corticosteroids) should be readily available

Dosage Forms Injection: 10,000 unit vial

References

Nesbit M, Chard R, Evans A, et al, "Evaluation of Intramuscular Versus Intravenous Administration of L-Asparaginase in Childhood Leukemia," *Am J Ped Hematology/Oncology*, 1979, 1:9-13.

Aspergum® [OTC] *see* Aspirin *on this page*

Aspirin (as' pir in)

Related Information

Overdose and Toxicology Information *on page 696-700*

Brand Names Anacin® [OTC]; A.S.A. [OTC]; Ascriptin® [OTC]; Aspergum® [OTC]; Bayer® Aspirin [OTC]; Bufferin® [OTC]; Easprin®; Ecotrin® [OTC]; Empirin® [OTC]; Measurin® [OTC]; Synalgos® [OTC]; ZORprin®

Synonyms Acetylsalicylic Acid; ASA

Therapeutic Category Analgesic, Non-Narcotic; Anti-inflammatory Agent; Antiplatelet Agent; Antipyretic; Nonsteroidal Anti-Inflammatory Agent (NSAID), Oral; Salicylate

Use Treatment of mild to moderate pain, inflammation and fever; may be used as a prophylaxis of myocardial infarction and transient ischemic attacks (TIA)

Pregnancy Risk Factor C (D if full-dose aspirin in 3rd trimester)

Contraindications Bleeding disorders, hypersensitivity to salicylates or other nonsteroidal anti-inflammatory drugs (NSAIDs)

Warnings Do not use aspirin in children <16 years of age for chickenpox or flu symptoms due to the association with Reye's syndrome

Precautions Use with caution in patients with impaired renal function, erosive gastritis, peptic ulcer, gout

Adverse Reactions

Dermatologic: Rash, urticaria

Gastrointestinal: Nausea, vomiting, GI distress, bleeding, ulcers

Hematologic: Inhibition of platelet aggregation

Hepatic: Hepatotoxicity

Respiratory: Bronchospasm

Drug Interactions Aspirin may ↑ methotrexate serum levels and may displace valproic acid from binding sites which can result in toxicity; warfarin and aspirin → ↑ bleeding; NSAIDs and aspirin → ↑ GI adverse effects, possible ↓ serum concentration of NSAIDs; aspirin may antagonize effects of probenecid

Stability Keep suppositories in refrigerator, do not freeze; hydrolysis of aspirin occurs upon exposure to water or moist air, resulting in salicylate and acetate, which possess a vinegar-like odor; do not use if a strong odor is present

Mechanism of Action Inhibits prostaglandin synthesis, acts on the hypothalamus heat-regulating center to reduce fever, blocks prostaglandin synthetase action which prevents formation of the platelet-aggregating substance thromboxane A_2

Pharmacokinetics

Absorption: Absorbed from the stomach and small intestine

Distribution: Readily distributes into most body fluids and tissues; hydrolyzed to salicylate (active) by esterases in the GI mucosa, red blood cells, synovial fluid and blood

Metabolism: Primarily by hepatic microsomal enzymes

Half-life: 15-20 minutes; metabolic pathways are saturable such that salicylates half-life is dose-dependent ranging from 3 hours at lower doses (300-600 mg), 5-6 hours (after 1 g) and 10 hours with higher doses

(Continued)

Aspirin *(Continued)*

Peak plasma levels: Appear in about 1-2 hours

Usual Dosage

Children:

Analgesic and antipyretic: Oral, rectal: 10-15 mg/kg/dose every 4-6 hours

Anti-inflammatory: Oral: Initial: 60-90 mg/kg/day in divided doses; usual maintenance: 80-100 mg/kg/day divided every 6-8 hours; monitor serum concentrations

Kawasaki disease: Oral: 100 mg/kg/day divided every 6 hours; after fever resolves: 8-10 mg/kg/day once daily; monitor serum concentrations

Adults:

Analgesic and antipyretic: Oral, rectal: 325-1000 mg every 4-6 hours up to 4 g/day

Anti-inflammatory: Oral: Initial: 2.4-3.6 g/day in divided doses; usual maintenance: 3.6-5.4 g/day; monitor serum concentrations

TIA: Oral: 1.3 g/day in 2-4 divided doses

Myocardial infarction prophylaxis: 160-325 mg/day

Monitoring Parameters Serum salicylate concentration with chronic use

Reference Range

Therapeutic levels: Anti-inflammatory effect: 150-300 μg/mL; analgesic and antipyretic effect: 30-50 μg/mL

Timing of serum samples: Peak levels usually occur 2 hours after normal doses but may occur 6-24 hours after acute toxic ingestion.

Salicylate serum concentrations correlate with the pharmacological actions and adverse effects observed. See table.

Serum Salicylate: Clinical Correlations

Serum Salicylate Concentration (μg/mL)	Desired Effects	Adverse Effects/ Intoxication
~100	Antiplatelet Antipyresis Analgesia	GI intolerance and bleeding, hypersensitivity, hemostatic defects
150–300	Anti–inflammatory	Mild salicylism
250–400	Treatment of rheumatic fever	Nausea/vomiting, hyperventilation, salicylism, flushing, sweating, thirst, headache, diarrhea and tachycardia
>400–500		Respiratory alkalosis, hemorrhage, excitement, confusion, asterixis, pulmonary edema, convulsions, tetany, metabolic acidosis, fever, coma, cardiovascular collapse, renal and respiratory failure

Test Interactions False-negative results for glucose oxidase urinary glucose tests (Clinistix®); false-positives using the cupric sulfate method (Clinitest®); also, interferes with Gerhardt test, VMA determination; 5-HIAA, xylose tolerance test and T_3 and T_4

Nursing Implications Administer with water, food or milk to ↓ GI effects

Dosage Forms

Capsule: Aspirin 356.4 mg and caffeine 30 mg

Suppository, rectal: 60 mg, 120 mg, 125 mg, 130 mg, 195 mg, 200 mg, 300 mg, 325 mg, 600 mg, 650 mg, 1.2 g

Tablet: 65 mg, 75 mg, 81 mg, 325 mg, 500 mg

Tablet: Aspirin 400 mg and caffeine 32 mg

Tablet:

Buffered: Aspirin 325 mg and magnesium-aluminum hydroxide 150 mg; aspirin 325 mg, magnesium hydroxide 75 mg, aluminum hydroxide 75 mg, buffered with calcium carbonate; aspirin 325 mg and magnesium-aluminum hydroxide 75 mg

Chewable, children's: 81 mg

Controlled release: 800 mg

Enteric coated: 325 mg, 500 mg, 650 mg, 975 mg

Gum: 227.5 mg

Timed release: 650 mg

Astemizole (a stem' mi zole)

Brand Names Hismanal®

Therapeutic Category Antihistamine

Use Perennial and seasonal allergic rhinitis and other allergic symptoms including urticaria

Pregnancy Risk Factor C

Contraindications Hypersensitivity to astemizole or any component; hepatic dysfunction

Adverse Reactions

Cardiovascular: Cardiac arrhythmias

Central nervous system: Drowsiness, dizziness, nervousness, headache

Gastrointestinal: Increased appetite, dry mouth

Miscellaneous: Increased weight

Drug Interactions Erythromycin, ciprofloxacin, cimetidine, ketoconazole, and disulfiram reduce hepatic metabolism which has resulted in severe, life-threatening cardiac arrhythmias

Mechanism of Action Competitively antagonizes histamine at the H_1-receptor site; preferentially binds to peripheral H_1 rather than central H_1-receptor sites resulting in a reduced sedative potential

Pharmacokinetics

Absorption: Rapidly absorbed, absorption reduced by 60% when taken with food

Distribution: Nonsedating action reportedly due to the drug's low lipid solubility and poor penetration through the blood-brain barrier

Protein binding: 97%

Metabolism: Undergoes exclusive first-pass metabolism

Half-life, biphasic:

- Distribution: 20 hours
- Elimination: 7-11 days

Peak levels: Occur after 1 hour

Elimination: Eliminated by metabolism in the liver to active and inactive metabolites

Usual Dosage

Children:

- <6 years: 0.2 mg/kg/day once daily
- 6-12 years: 5 mg/day

Children >12 years and Adults: 10-30 mg/day; give 30 mg on first day, 20 mg on second day followed by 10 mg daily as a single dose

Patient Information Take on an empty stomach, at least 2 hours after a meal or 1 hour before a meal

Additional Information Not likely to cause drowsiness

Dosage Forms Tablet: 10 mg

References

Richards DM, Brogden RN, Heel RC, et al, "Astemizole: A Review of Its Pharmacodynamic Properties ánd Therapeutic Efficacy," *Drugs*, 1984, 28:38-61.

"Safety of Terfenadine and Astemizole," *Med Lett Drugs Ther*, 1992, 34(863):9-10.

Yaffe SJ and Aranda JV, *Pediatric Pharmacology: Therapeutic Principles in Practice,* Philadelphia PA: WB Saunders Co, 1992.

AsthmaHaler® *see* Epinephrine *on page 220*

AsthmaNefrin® [OTC] *see* Epinephrine *on page 220*

Astramorph™ PF *see* Morphine Sulfate *on page 394*

Atabrine® Hydrochloride *see* Quinacrine Hydrochloride *on page 504*

Atarax® *see* Hydroxyzine *on page 298*

Atenolol (a ten' oh lole)

Related Information

Overdose and Toxicology Information *on page 696-700*

Brand Names Tenormin®

Therapeutic Category Antianginal Agent; Antihypertensive; Beta-Adrenergic Blocker

(Continued)

Atenolol *(Continued)*

Use Treatment of hypertension, alone or in combination with other agents; also used in management of angina pectoris, and as an antiarrhythmic

Pregnancy Risk Factor C

Contraindications Pulmonary edema, cardiogenic shock, bradycardia, heart block, or uncompensated congestive heart failure

Warnings Abrupt withdrawal of the drug should be avoided; drug should be discontinued over 1-2 weeks

Precautions Modify dosage in patients with renal impairment

Adverse Reactions

Cardiovascular: Bradycardia, hypotension, second or third degree A-V block

Central nervous system: Dizziness, fatigue, lethargy, headache

Respiratory: Wheezing and dyspnea have occurred when daily dosage exceeded 100 mg/day

Drug Interactions Additive effect with other hypotensive agents

Mechanism of Action Competitively blocks response to beta-adrenergic stimulation

Pharmacokinetics

Absorption: Incompletely absorbed from GI tract

Distribution: Does **not** cross the blood-brain barrier

Protein binding: Low (3% to 15%)

Half-life, beta:

Neonates: Mean: 16 hours, up to 35 hours

Children: 4.6 hours; children >10 years of age may have longer half-life (>5 hours) compared to children 5-10 years of age (<5 hours)

Adults: 6-9 hours

Prolonged half-life with renal dysfunction

Peak serum concentrations: Oral: Within 2-4 hours

Elimination: 40% excreted as unchanged drug in the urine, 50% in the feces

Moderately dialyzable (20% to 50%)

Low lipophilicity

Usual Dosage

Oral:

Children: Initial: 1-1.2 mg/kg/dose given daily; range: 0.8-1.5 mg/kg/day; maximum: 2 mg/kg/day

Adults: 50-100 mg/dose given daily

See table for dosing interval in renal impairment.

Maximum Dose	Creatinine Clearance	Frequency of Administration
50 mg or 1 mg/kg/dose	15–35 mL/min	Daily
50 mg or 1 mg/kg/dose	<15 mL/min	Every other day

I.V.: Adults: For early treatment of myocardial infarction: 5 mg slow I.V. over 5 minutes; may repeat in 10 minutes; if both doses are tolerated, may start oral atenolol 50 mg every 12 hours for 6-9 days postmyocardial infarction

Administration Administer by slow I.V. injection at a rate not to exceed 1 mg/minute; the injection can be given undiluted or diluted with a compatible I.V. solution

Monitoring Parameters Blood pressure, heart rate, fluid intake and output, daily weight, respirations

Patient Information Abrupt withdrawal of the drug should be avoided

Additional Information May potentiate hypoglycemia in a diabetic patient; may mask signs and symptoms of hypoglycemia

Dosage Forms

Injection: 0.5 mg/mL (10 mL)

Tablet: 25 mg, 50 mg, 100 mg

References

Buck ML, Wiest D, Gillette PC, et al, "Pharmacokinetics and Pharmacodynamics of Atenolol in Children," *Clin Pharmacol Ther*, 1989, 46(6):629-33.

Case CL, Trippel DL, and Gillette PC, "New Antiarrhythmic Agents in Pediatrics," *Pediatr Clin North Am*, 1989, 36(5):1293-320.

Trippel DL and Gillette PC, "Atenolol in Children With Supraventricular Tachycardia," *Am J Cardiol*, 1989, 64(3):233-6.

Trippel DL and Gillette PC, "Atenolol in Children With Ventricular Arrhythmias," *Am Heart J*, 1990, 119(6):1312-6.

ATG *see* Lymphocyte Immune Globulin *on page 350*

Atgam® *see* Lymphocyte Immune Globulin *on page 350*

Ativan® *see* Lorazepam *on page 348*

Atracurium Besylate (a tra kyoo' ree um)

Brand Names Tracrium®

Therapeutic Category Neuromuscular Blocker Agent, Nondepolarizing

Use To ease endotracheal intubation as an adjunct to general anesthesia and to relax skeletal muscle during surgery or mechanical ventilation

Pregnancy Risk Factor C

Contraindications Hypersensitivity to atracurium besylate or any component

Warnings Maintenance of an adequate airway and respiratory support is critical; contains benzyl alcohol as a preservative; use with caution in neonates

Adverse Reactions Rarely mild histamine release, cardiovascular effects are minimal and transient

Drug Interactions Enflurane and isoflurane ↑ the potency and prolong duration of neuromuscular blockade induced by atracurium by ~35% to 50%. Halothane has only a marginal effect.

Stability Refrigerate; unstable in alkaline solutions; compatible with D_5W, D_5NS, and NS; do not dilute in LR

Mechanism of Action Blocks neural transmission at the myoneural junction by binding with cholinergic receptor sites

Pharmacodynamics

Onset of action: I.V.: Within 2 minutes

Peak effect: Within 3-5 minutes; recovery begins in 20-35 minutes when anesthesia is balanced

Pharmacokinetics

Metabolism: Some metabolites are active; undergoes rapid nonenzymatic degradation (Hofman elimination) in the blood stream; additional metabolism occurs via ester hydrolysis

Half-life: Adults: 20 minutes (biphasic decline, half-life (first phase): 2 minutes)

Usual Dosage I.V.:

Children 1 month to 2 years: 0.3-0.4 mg/kg initially followed by maintenance doses of 0.3 mg/kg and 0.4 mg/kg as needed to maintain neuromuscular blockade

Children >2 years to Adults: 0.4-0.5 mg/kg then 0.08-0.1 mg/kg 20-45 minutes after initial dose to maintain neuromuscular block

Continuous infusion: 0.4-0.8 mg/kg/hour

Administration May be given without further dilution by rapid I.V. injection; for continuous infusions, dilute to a maximum concentration of 0.5 mg/mL (more concentrated solutions when diluted with I.V. fluids have reduced stability, ie, <24 hours at room temperature)

Nursing Implications Not for I.M. injection due to tissue irritation

Dosage Forms Injection: 10 mg/mL (5 mL, 10 mL)

Atropine and Diphenoxylate *see* Diphenoxylate and Atropine *on page 196*

Atropine-Care® *see* Atropine Sulfate *on this page*

Atropine Sulfate (a' troe peen)

Related Information

Compatibility of Medications Mixed in a Syringe *on page 717*

CPR Pediatric Drug Dosages *on page 614*

Overdose and Toxicology Information *on page 696-700*

Brand Names Atropine-Care®; Atropisol®; Isopto® Atropine; I-Tropine®

Therapeutic Category Anticholinergic Agent; Anticholinergic Agent, Oph-

(Continued)

Atropine Sulfate *(Continued)*

thalmic; Antidote, Organophosphate Poisoning; Antispasmodic Agent, Gastrointestinal; Bronchodilator; Ophthalmic Agent, Mydriatic

Use Preoperative medication to inhibit salivation and secretions; treatment of sinus bradycardia; management of peptic ulcer; treat exercise-induced bronchospasm; antidote for organophosphate pesticide poisoning; used to produce mydriasis and cycloplegia for examination of the retina and optic disk and accurate measurement of refractive errors; uveitis

Pregnancy Risk Factor C

Contraindications Hypersensitivity to atropine sulfate or any component; narrow-angle glaucoma; tachycardia; thyrotoxicosis; obstructive disease of the GI tract; obstructive uropathy

Precautions Use with caution in children with spastic paralysis or brain damage

Adverse Reactions

Cardiovascular: Tachycardia, palpitations

Central nervous system: Fatigue, tremor, delirium, headache, ataxia, restlessness

Dermatologic: Dry hot skin

Gastrointestinal: Impaired GI motility

Ocular: Blurred vision

Mechanism of Action Blocks the action of acetylcholine at parasympathetic sites in smooth muscle, secretory glands, and the CNS; increases cardiac output, dries secretions, antagonizes histamine and serotonin

Usual Dosage

Children:

Preanesthetic: Oral, I.M., I.V., S.C.:

<5 kg: 0.02 mg/kg/dose 30-60 minutes preop then every 4-6 hours as needed

>5 kg: 0.01-0.02 mg/kg/dose to a maximum 0.4 mg 30-60 minutes preop; minimum dose: 0.1 mg

Bradycardia: I.V., intratracheal: 0.02 mg/kg, minimum dose 0.1 mg, maximum single dose: 0.5 mg in children and 1 mg in adolescents; may repeat in 5-minute intervals to a maximum total dose of 1 mg in children or 2 mg in adolescents. (**Note:** For intratracheal administration, the dosage must be diluted with normal saline to a total volume of 1-2 mL.) When using to treat bradycardia in neonates, reserve use for those patients unresponsive to improved oxygenation.

Bronchospasm: Inhalation: 0.03-0.05 mg/kg/dose 3-4 times/day

Ophthalmic, 0.5% solution: 1-2 drops twice daily for 1-3 days before the procedure

Adults (doses of <0.5 mg have been associated with paradoxical bradycardia):

Asystole: I.V.: 1 mg; may repeat every 3-5 minutes as needed

Preanesthetic: Oral, I.M., I.V., S.C.: 0.4-0.6 mg 30-60 minutes preop

Bradycardia: I.V.: 0.5-1 mg every 5 minutes, not to exceed a total of 2 mg or 0.04 mg/kg

Bronchospasm: Inhalation: 0.025-0.05 mg/kg/dose every 4-6 hours as needed

Ophthalmic, 1% solution: 1-2 drops before the procedure

Administration Administer undiluted by rapid I.V. injection; slow injection may result in paradoxical bradycardia

Monitoring Parameters Heart rate

Dosage Forms

Injection: 0.1 mg/mL (5 mL, 10 mL); 0.3 mg/mL (1 mL, 30 mL); 0.4 mg/mL (1 mL, 20 mL, 30 mL); 0.5 mg/mL (1 mL, 5 mL, 30 mL); 0.8 mg/mL (0.5 mL, 1 mL); 1 mg/mL (1 mL, 10 mL)

Ointment, ophthalmic: 0.5% (3.5 g); 1% (3.5 g)

Solution, ophthalmic: 0.5% (5 mL); 1% (2 mL); 2% (1 mL, 2 mL); 3% (5 mL)

Tablet: 0.4 mg

Tablet, soluble: 0.4 mg, 0.6 mg

References

Emergency Cardiac Care Committee and Subcommittees, American Heart Association, "Guidelines for Cardiopulmonary Resuscitation and Emergency Cardiac Care, III: Adult Advanced Cardiac Life Support" and "VI: Pediatric Advanced Life Support," *JAMA*, 1992, 268(16):2199-241 and 2262-75.

Atropisol® *see* Atropine Sulfate *on page 65*

Atrovent® *see* Ipratropium Bromide *on page 319*

A/T/S® *see* Erythromycin *on page 226*

Augmentin® *see* Amoxicillin and Clavulanic Acid *on page 45*

Auralgan® *see* Antipyrine and Benzocaine *on page 56*

Auranofin (au rane' oh fin)

Brand Names Ridaura®

Therapeutic Category Gold Compound

Use Management of active stage of classic or definite rheumatoid arthritis in patients who do not respond to or tolerate other agents

Pregnancy Risk Factor C

Contraindications Renal disease; known hypersensitivity to auranofin; history of blood dyscrasias; congestive heart failure; exfoliative dermatitis; necrotizing enterocolitis; bone marrow aplasia, pulmonary fibrosis

Warnings Explain the possibility of adverse reactions before initiating therapy; signs of gold toxicity include decrease in hemoglobin, leukocytes, granulocytes and platelets, proteinuria, hematuria, pruritus, stomatitis or persistent diarrhea; advise patients to report any symptoms of toxicity

Adverse Reactions

Dermatologic: Dermatitis, pruritus, alopecia

Gastrointestinal: Diarrhea, loose stools, stomatitis, abdominal cramping, metallic taste

Hematologic: Thrombocytopenia, aplastic anemia, eosinophilia

Ocular: Conjunctivitis

Renal & genitourinary: Proteinuria, hematuria, nephrotic syndrome

Mechanism of Action Unknown, acts principally via immunomodulating effects and by decreasing lysosomal enzyme release; may alter cellular mechanisms by inhibiting sulfhydryl systems

Pharmacodynamics Onset of action: Therapeutic response may not be seen for 3-4 months after start of therapy

Pharmacokinetics

Absorption: Only about 20% of gold in a dose is absorbed following oral administration

Protein binding: 60%

Half-life: 21-31 days (half-life dependent upon single or multiple dosing)

Peak blood gold concentrations: Within 2 hours

Elimination: 60% of absorbed gold is eliminated in the urine while the remainder is eliminated in the feces

Usual Dosage Oral:

Children: Initial: 0.1 mg/kg/day; usual maintenance: 0.15 mg/kg/day in 1-2 divided doses; maximum: 0.2 mg/kg/day in 1-2 divided doses

Adults: 6 mg/day in 1-2 divided doses; after 3 months may be increased to 9 mg/day in 3 divided doses; if still no response after 3 months at 9 mg/day, discontinue drug

Monitoring Parameters CBC with differential, platelet count, urinalysis, baseline renal and liver function tests

Reference Range Gold: Normal: 0-0.1 μg/mL (SI: 0-0.5 μmol/L); Therapeutic: 1-3 μg/mL (SI: 5.1-15.2 μmol/L); Urine <0.1 μg/24 hours

Test Interactions May enhance the response to a tuberculin skin test

Patient Information Minimize exposure to sunlight

Nursing Implications Therapy should be discontinued if platelet count falls below 100,000/mm^3

Additional Information Metallic taste may indicate stomatitis

Dosage Forms Capsule: 3 mg = gold 29%

Auro® Ear Drops [OTC] *see* Carbamide Peroxide *on page 103*

Aurothioglucose (aur oh thye oh gloo' kose)

Brand Names Solganal®

Therapeutic Category Gold Compound

Use Adjunctive treatment in adult and juvenile active rheumatoid arthritis

Pregnancy Risk Factor C

Contraindications Renal disease; known hypersensitivity to aurothioglu-

(Continued)

Aurothioglucose *(Continued)*

cose; history of blood dyscrasias; congestive heart failure; exfoliative dermatitis; hepatic disease; colitis

Warnings Explain the possibility of adverse reactions before initiating therapy; signs of gold toxicity include: decrease in hemoglobin, leukocytes, granulocytes and platelets; proteinuria, hematuria, pruritus, stomatitis, persistent diarrhea, rash, or metallic taste; advise patients to report any symptoms of toxicity

Adverse Reactions

Central nervous system: Neuropathies
Dermatologic: Alopecia, urticaria, mild to severe dermatitis, pruritus
Gastrointestinal: Diarrhea, stomatitis, glossitis
Hematologic: Eosinophilia, leukopenia, thrombocytopenia
Hepatic: Hepatitis
Renal & genitourinary: Hematuria, proteinuria, nephrotic syndrome
Respiratory: Interstitial pneumonitis and fibrosis
Miscellaneous: Vaginitis, metallic taste

Mechanism of Action Unknown, may decrease prostaglandin synthesis or may alter cellular mechanisms by inhibiting sulfhydryl systems; may decrease lysosomal enzyme release

Pharmacokinetics

Absorption: I.M.: Erratic and slow
Distribution: Crosses the placenta; appears in breast milk
Protein binding: 95% to 99%
Metabolism: Unknown
Half-life: 3-27 days
Peak serum levels: Within 4-6 hours
Mean steady-state plasma levels: 1-10 μg/mL
Elimination: Majority ultimately eliminated in the urine (70%) and the remainder in the feces (30%)

Usual Dosage I.M. (doses should initially be given at weekly intervals):

Children: Initial: 0.25 mg/kg/dose first week; increment at 0.25 mg/kg/dose increasing with each weekly dose; maintenance: 0.75-1 mg/kg/dose weekly not to exceed 25 mg/dose to a total of 20 doses, then every 2-4 weeks

Adults: 10 mg first week; 25 mg second and third week; then 50 mg/week until 800 mg to 1 g cumulative dose has been given – if improvement occurs without adverse reactions, give 25-50 mg every 2-3 weeks, then every 3-4 weeks

Monitoring Parameters CBC with differential, platelet count, urinalysis, baseline renal and liver function tests

Reference Range Gold: Normal: 0-0.1 μg/mL (SI: 0-0.5 μmol/L); Therapeutic: 1-3 μg/mL (SI: 5.1-15.2 μmol/L); Urine $<$0.1 μg/24 hours

Patient Information Minimize exposure to sunlight

Nursing Implications Deep I.M. injection into the upper outer quadrant of the gluteal region; vial should be thoroughly shaken before withdrawing a dose. Do not administer I.V.

Dosage Forms Suspension, sterile: 50 mg/mL = gold 50% (10 mL)

Auroto® *see* Antipyrine and Benzocaine *on page 56*

Aveeno® Cleansing Bar [OTC] *see* Sulfur and Salicylic Acid *on page 545*

Aygestin® *see* Norethindrone *on page 419*

Ayr® *see* Sodium Chloride *on page 527*

Azactam® *see* Aztreonam *on page 71*

Azathioprine (ay za thye' oh preen)

Brand Names Imuran®

Therapeutic Category Antineoplastic Agent; Immunosuppressant Agent

Use Used as an adjunct with other agents in prevention of rejection of transplants; also used in severe rheumatoid arthritis unresponsive to other agents

Pregnancy Risk Factor D

Contraindications Hypersensitivity to azathioprine or any component; pregnancy and lactation

Warnings Chronic immunosuppression increases the risk of neoplasia; mutagenic potential in both men and women; may cause irreversible bone marrow depression

Precautions Use with caution in patients with liver disease, renal impairment, and those with cadaveric kidneys; modify dosage in patients with renal impairment; reduce usual dosage 25% to 33% in patients receiving both allopurinol and azathioprine concurrently

Adverse Reactions

Central nervous system: Fever
Dermatologic: Alopecia, rash
Gastrointestinal: Nausea, vomiting, anorexia, diarrhea, aphthous stomatitis
Hematologic: Bone marrow depression
Hepatic: Hepatotoxicity
Musculoskeletal: Arthralgias
Ocular: Retinopathy
Miscellaneous: Rare hypersensitivity reactions which include myalgias, rigors, maculopapular rash, dyspnea, hypotension

Drug Interactions Allopurinol inhibits metabolism of azathioprine by blocking the conversion of mercaptopurine to inactive products → ↑ azathioprine effects

Stability Reconstituted 10 mg/mL solution is stable for 24 hours at room temperature; stable in neutral or acid solutions, but is hydrolyzed to mercaptopurine in alkaline solutions

Mechanism of Action Antagonizes purine metabolism and may inhibit synthesis of DNA, RNA, and proteins; may also interfere with cellular metabolism and inhibit mitosis

Pharmacokinetics

Distribution: Crosses the placenta
Protein binding: ~30%
Metabolism: Extensively metabolized by hepatic xanthine oxidase to 6-mercaptopurine (active)
Half-life:
Parent: 12 minutes
6-mercaptopurine: 0.7-3 hours
Elimination: Small amounts are eliminated as unchanged drug; metabolites eliminated eventually in the urine
Slightly dialyzable (5% to 20%)

Usual Dosage

Children and Adults: Transplantation: Oral, I.V.: Initial: 2-5 mg/kg/day; maintenance: 1-3 mg/kg/day

Adults: Rheumatoid arthritis: Oral: 1 mg/kg/day for 6-8 weeks; increase by 0.5 mg/kg every 4 weeks until response or up to 2.5 mg/kg/day

Administration Can be administered IVP over 5 minutes at a concentration not to exceed 10 mg/mL; or azathioprine can be further diluted with normal saline or D_5W and administered by intermittent infusion over 15-60 minutes

Monitoring Parameters CBC, platelet counts, total bilirubin, alkaline phosphatase

Patient Information Response in rheumatoid arthritis may not occur for up to 3 months; inform physician of persistent sore throat, unusual bleeding or bruising, or fatigue

Dosage Forms

Injection, as sodium: 100 mg (20 mL)
Tablet: 50 mg

Extemporaneous Preparation(s) A 50 mg/mL suspension compounded from twenty (20) 50 mg tablets, distilled water, Cologel® 5 mL, and then adding 2:1 simple syrup/cherry syrup mixture to a total volume of 20 mL, was stable for 8 weeks when stored in the refrigerator

Handbook on Extemporaneous Formulations, Bethesda MD: American Society of Hospital Pharmacists, 1987.

References

Baum D, Bernstein D, Starnes VA, et al, "Pediatric Heart Transplantation at Stanford: Results of a 15-Year Experience," *Pediatrics*, 1991, 88(2):203-14.

Leichter HE, Sheth KJ, Gerlach MJ, et al, "Outcome of Renal Transplantation in Children Aged 1-5 and 6-18 Years," *Child Nephrology & Urology*, 1992(12):1-5

Azidothymidine *see* Zidovudine *on page 608*

Azithromycin

Brand Names Zithromax™

Therapeutic Category Antibiotic, Macrolide

Use Treatment of mild to moderate upper and lower respiratory tract infections, infections of the skin and skin structure, and sexually transmitted diseases due to susceptible strains of *C. trachomatis*, *M. catarrhalis*, *H. influenzae*, *S. aureus*, *S. pneumoniae*, *Mycoplasma pneumoniae*, and *C. psittaci*

Pregnancy Risk Factor B

Contraindications Hypersensitivity to azithromycin, erythromycin, or any macrolide antibiotics

Warnings Should not be used to treat pneumonia that is considered inappropriate for outpatient oral therapy; may mask or delay symptoms of incubating gonorrhea or syphilis so appropriate culture and susceptibility tests should be performed prior to initiating azithromycin; pseudomembranous colitis has been reported with use of macrolide antibiotics

Precautions Use with caution in patients with impaired hepatic function

Adverse Reactions

Cardiovascular: Angioedema

Central nervous system: Headache, dizziness

Dermatologic: Rash

Gastrointestinal: Diarrhea (3.6%), nausea (2.6%), abdominal pain (2.5%); vomiting

Hepatic: Elevation in hepatic enzymes, cholestatic jaundice

Renal & genitourinary: Nephritis, vaginitis

Drug Interactions Aluminum- and magnesium-containing antacids ↓ azithromycin peak serum levels by 24%

Mechanism of Action Inhibits bacterial RNA-dependent protein synthesis by binding to the 50S ribosomal subunit

Pharmacokinetics

Absorption: Rapidly absorbed from the GI tract

Distribution: Extensive tissue distribution

Protein binding: 7% to 50% (concentration-dependent)

Metabolism: Metabolized in the liver

Bioavailability: 37%, food decreases bioavailability

Half-life, terminal: 68 hours

Peak serum concentration: 2.3-4 hours

Elimination: 4.5% to 12% of dose is excreted in urine; 50% of dose is excreted unchanged in bile

Usual Dosage Oral:

Children: Not currently FDA approved for use in children; dosages of 10 mg/kg on day 1 followed by 5 mg/kg/day once daily on days 2-5 have been used in clinical trials

Adolescents ≥16 years and Adults:

Respiratory tract, skin and soft tissue infections: 500 mg on day 1, 250 mg/day on days 2-5

Uncomplicated chlamydial urethritis or cervicitis: Single 1 g dose

Monitoring Parameters Monitor patients receiving azithromycin and drugs known to interact with erythromycin (ie, theophylline, digoxin, anticoagulants, triazolam) since there are still very few studies examining drug-drug interactions with azithromycin; liver function tests, WBC with differential

Patient Information Take medication at least 1 hour prior to a meal or 2 hours after a meal; do not take with food

Dosage Forms Capsule, as dihydrate: 250 mg

References

Foulds G, Shepard RM, and Johnson RB, "The Pharmacokinetics of Azithromycin in Human Serum and Tissues," *J Antimicrob Chemother*, 1990, 25(Suppl A):73-82.

Steingrimsson O, Olafsson JH, Thorarinsson H, et al, "Azithromycin in the Treatment of Sexually Transmitted Disease," *J Antimicrob Chemother*, 1990, 25(Suppl A):109-14.

Azmacort™ *see* Triamcinolone *on page 579*

Azo-Standard® *see* Phenazopyridine Hydrochloride *on page 449*

AZT *see* Zidovudine *on page 608*

Azthreonam *see* Aztreonam *on this page*

Aztreonam (az' tree oh nam)

Brand Names Azactam®

Synonyms Azthreonam

Therapeutic Category Antibiotic, Miscellaneous

Use Treatment of patients with documented multidrug resistant aerobic gram-negative infection in which beta-lactam therapy is contraindicated; used for UTI, lower respiratory tract infections, septicemia, skin/skin structure infections, intra-abdominal infections and gynecological infections caused by susceptible *Enterobacteriaceae*, *H. influenzae*, and *P. aeruginosa*

Pregnancy Risk Factor B

Contraindications Hypersensitivity to aztreonam or any component

Warnings Check for hypersensitivity to other beta-lactams (hypersensitivity reactions to aztreonam have occurred rarely in patients with a history of penicillin or cephalosporin hypersensitivity); prolonged use may result in superinfection

Precautions Requires dosage reduction in renal impairment

Adverse Reactions

Cardiovascular: Hypotension
Central nervous system: Seizures, confusion
Dermatologic: Rash
Gastrointestinal: Diarrhea, nausea, vomiting, pseudomembranous colitis
Hematologic: Eosinophilia, leukopenia, neutropenia, thrombocytopenia
Hepatic: Elevation of liver enzymes
Local: Pain at injection site, thrombophlebitis

Drug Interactions Avoid antibiotics that induce beta-lactamase production (cefoxitin, imipenem)

Stability Reconstituted solution is stable 48 hours at room temperature and 7 days when refrigerated; incompatible when mixed with nafcillin, metronidazole

Mechanism of Action Binds to penicillin-binding protein 3, inhibiting bacterial cell wall synthesis during active multiplication and causing cell wall destruction

Pharmacokinetics

Absorption: I.M.: Well absorbed
Distribution: Widely distributed into body tissues and fluids; V_d:
- Neonates: 0.26-0.36 L/kg
- Children: 0.2-0.29 L/kg
- Adults: 0.2 L/kg

Protein binding: 56%
Half-life:
- Neonates:
  - <7 days, ≤2.5 kg: 5.5-9.9 hours
  - <7 days, >2.5 kg: 2.6 hours
  - 1 week to 1 month: 2.4 hours
- Children 2 months to 12 years: 1.7 hours
- Adults: 1.3-2.2 hours (half-life prolonged in renal failure)

Peak serum concentrations: Within 60 minutes after an I.M. dose
Elimination: 60% to 70% excreted unchanged in the urine and partially excreted in feces
Moderately dialyzable (20% to 50%)

Usual Dosage I.M., I.V.:

Neonates:
- Postnatal age ≤7 days:
  - ≤2000 g: 60 mg/kg/day divided every 12 hours
  - >2000 g: 90 mg/kg/day divided every 8 hours
- Postnatal age >7 days:
  - <1200 g: 60 mg/kg/day divided every 12 hours
  - 1200-2000 g: 90 mg/kg/day divided every 8 hours
  - >2000 g: 120 mg/kg/day divided every 6 hours

(Continued)

Aztreonam *(Continued)*

Children >1 month: 90-120 mg/kg/day divided every 6-8 hours
- Cystic fibrosis: 50 mg/kg/dose every 6-8 hours (ie, up to 200 mg/kg/day); maximum: 6-8 g/day

Adults:
- Urinary tract infection: 500 mg to 1 g every 8-12 hours
- Moderately severe systemic infections: 1 g I.V. or I.M. or 2 g I.V. every 8-12 hours
- Severe systemic or life-threatening infections (especially caused by *Pseudomonas aeruginosa*): I.V.: 2 g every 6-8 hours; maximum: 8 g/day

Dosing adjustment in renal impairment:
- Cl_{cr} 10-30 mL/minute: Reduce dose 50% given at the usual interval
- Cl_{cr} <10 mL/minute: Reduce dose 75% given at the usual interval

Administration Administer by IVP over 3-5 minutes at a maximum concentration of 66 mg/mL or by intermittent infusion over 20-60 minutes at a final concentration not to exceed 20 mg/mL

Monitoring Parameters Periodic liver function test

Test Interactions Urine glucose (Clinitest®)

Dosage Forms Powder for injection: 500 mg (15 mL, 100 mL); 1 g (15 mL, 100 mL); 2 g (15 mL, 100 mL)

References

Stutman HR, Chartrand SA, Tolentino T, et al, "Aztreonam Therapy for Serious Gram-Negative Infections in Children," *Am J Dis Child*, 1986, 140(11):1147-51.

Azulfidine® *see* Sulfasalazine *on page 543*

Azulfidine® EN-tabs® *see* Sulfasalazine *on page 543*

Babee® Teething Lotion [OTC] *see* Benzocaine *on page 77*

Bacampicillin Hydrochloride (ba kam pi sill' in)

Brand Names Spectrobid®

Synonyms Carampicillin Hydrochloride

Therapeutic Category Antibiotic, Penicillin

Use Treatment of susceptible bacterial infections involving the urinary tract, skin structure, upper and lower respiratory tract; activity is identical to that of ampicillin

Pregnancy Risk Factor B

Contraindications Hypersensitivity to bacampicillin or any component or penicillins; patients with infectious mononucleosis

Precautions Use with caution in patients with severe renal impairment; modify dosage in patients with renal insufficiency

Adverse Reactions
- Dermatologic: Rash
- Gastrointestinal: Nausea, diarrhea, pseudomembranous colitis
- Hematologic: Agranulocytosis
- Hepatic: Mild elevation in AST
- Miscellaneous: Hypersensitivity reactions

Drug Interactions Disulfiram

Stability Reconstituted suspension is stable for 10 days when stored in the refrigerator

Mechanism of Action Interferes with bacterial cell wall synthesis during active multiplication causing cell wall death and resultant bactericidal activity against susceptible bacteria

Pharmacokinetics Bacampicillin is an inactive prodrug that is hydrolyzed to ampicillin; area under the serum concentration time curve is 40% higher for bacampicillin than after equivalent ampicillin doses

- Protein binding: 15% to 25%
- Bioavailability: 80% to 98%
- Half-life: 65 minutes and is prolonged in patients with impaired renal function

Usual Dosage Oral:

Children: 25-50 mg/kg/day in divided doses every 12 hours

Adults: 400-800 mg every 12 hours

Dosing interval in renal impairment:
- Cl_{cr} 10-30 mL/minute: Administer every 24 hours

Cl_{cr} <10 mL/minute: Administer every 36 hours

Monitoring Parameters Renal, hepatic,and hematologic function tests

Test Interactions False-positive urine glucose with Clinitest®

Patient Information Take oral suspension 1 hour before or 2 hours after a meal

Additional Information Each mg of bacampicillin is equivalent to 700 μg of ampicillin

Dosage Forms

Powder for oral suspension: 125 mg/5 mL equivalent to 87.5 mg of ampicillin per 5 mL (70 mL)

Tablet: 400 mg equivalent to 280 mg ampicillin

Bacid® [OTC] *see Lactobacillus acidophilus* and *Lactobacillus bulgaricus on page 333*

Baciguent® [OTC] *see* Bacitracin *on this page*

Baci-IM® *see* Bacitracin *on this page*

Bacitracin (bass i tray' sin)

Brand Names AK-Tracin®; Baciguent® [OTC]; Baci-IM®

Therapeutic Category Antibiotic, Miscellaneous

Use Treatment of susceptible gram-positive bacterial infections

Pregnancy Risk Factor C

Contraindications Hypersensitivity to bacitracin or any component; I.M. use is contraindicated in patients with renal impairment

Warnings I.M. use may cause renal failure due to tubular and glomerular necrosis; **do not** administer intravenously because severe thrombophlebitis occurs; bacitracin may be absorbed from denuded areas and irrigation sites

Precautions Prolonged use may result in overgrowth of nonsusceptible organisms

Adverse Reactions

Cardiovascular: Hypotension

Dermatologic: Rash, itching

Gastrointestinal: Anorexia, nausea, vomiting, diarrhea, rectal itching and burning

Hematologic: Blood dyscrasias

Miscellaneous: Swelling of lips and face, pain, sweating, tightness of chest

Drug Interactions Nephrotoxic drugs, neuromuscular blocking agents, anesthetics

Stability Sterile powder should be stored in the refrigerator; once reconstituted, bacitracin is stable for one week under refrigeration (2°C to 8°C)

Mechanism of Action Inhibits bacterial cell wall synthesis by preventing transfer of mucopeptides into the growing cell wall

Pharmacokinetics

Absorption: Poorly absorbed from mucous membranes and intact or denuded skin; rapidly absorbed following I.M. administration

Protein binding: Minimally bound to plasma proteins

Peak serum concentrations: I.M.: Within 1-2 hours

Elimination: Slow elimination into the urine with 10% to 40% of a dose excreted within 24 hours

Usual Dosage

I.M. (not recommended):

Infants:

≤2.5 kg: 900 units/kg/day in 2-3 divided doses

>2.5 kg: 1000 units/kg/day in 2-3 divided doses

Children: 800-1200 units/kg/day divided every 8 hours

Adults: 10,000-25,000 units/dose every 6 hours; not to exceed 100,000 units/day

Children and Adults:

Topical: Apply 1-5 times/day

Ophthalmic ointment: ½" ribbon every 3-4 hours; reduce frequency of administration as the infection is brought under control

Irrigation, solution: 50-100 units/mL in normal saline, lactated Ringer's, or sterile water for irrigation; soak sponges in solution for topical compresses 1-5 times/day or as needed during surgical procedures

Monitoring Parameters I.M.: Urinalysis, renal function tests

Patient Information Ophthalmic ointment may cause blurred vision; topical

(Continued)

Bacitracin *(Continued)*

bacitracin should not be used for longer than 1 week unless directed by a physician

Nursing Implications For I.M. administration, pH of urine should be kept above 6 by using sodium bicarbonate; bacitracin sterile powder should be dissolved in 0.9% sodium chloride injection containing 2% procaine hydrochloride; do not use diluents containing parabens

Dosage Forms

Injection: 50,000 units

Ointment:

Ophthalmic: 500 units/g (1 g, 3.5 g, 454 g)

Topical: 500 units/g (1.5 g, 3.75 g, 15 g, 30 g, 120 g, 454 g)

Bacitracin and Polymyxin B Sulfate (bass i tray' sin)

Brand Names AK-Poly-Bac®; Polysporin®

Therapeutic Category Antibiotic, Ophthalmic; Antibiotic, Topical

Use Treatment of superficial infections involving the conjunctiva and/or cornea caused by susceptible organisms; prevent infection in minor cuts, scrapes and burns

Pregnancy Risk Factor C

Contraindications Hypersensitivity to polymyxin, bacitracin or any component

Precautions Prolonged use may result in overgrowth of nonsusceptible organisms

Adverse Reactions

Local: Rash, itching, burning, swelling

Ocular: Conjunctival erythema

Miscellaneous: Anaphylactoid reactions

Pharmacokinetics Absorption from intact skin or mucous membrane is insignificant

Usual Dosage Children and Adults:

Ophthalmic: Instill every 3-4 hours depending on severity of the infection

Topical: Apply a small amount of ointment or dusting of powder to the affected area 1-3 times/day

Patient Information Do not use longer than 1 week unless directed by physician; do not use topical ointment in the eyes; ophthalmic ointment may cause blurred vision

Dosage Forms

Ointment:

Ophthalmic: Bacitracin 500 units and polymyxin B sulfate 10,000 units per g (3.5 g)

Topical: Bacitracin 500 units and polymyxin B sulfate 10,000 units per g (1/32 oz, 15 g, 30 g)

Powder, topical: Bacitracin 500 units and polymyxin B sulfate 10,000 units per g (10 g)

Spray, topical: Bacitracin 10,000 units and polymyxin B sulfate 200,000 units (90 g)

Baclofen (bak' loe fen)

Brand Names Lioresal®

Therapeutic Category Skeletal Muscle Relaxant, Central Acting

Use Treatment of reversible spasticity associated with multiple sclerosis or spinal cord lesions

Pregnancy Risk Factor C

Contraindications Hypersensitivity to baclofen or any component

Warnings Abrupt withdrawal of baclofen has been reported to precipitate hallucinations and/or seizures

Precautions Use with caution in patients with seizure disorder, impaired renal function, peptic ulcer disease

Adverse Reactions

Cardiovascular: Hypotension

Central nervous system: Drowsiness, fatigue, vertigo, dizziness, psychiatric disturbances, insomnia, slurred speech, headache, ataxia, hypotonia

Dermatologic: Rash

Gastrointestinal: Nausea, constipation

Renal & genitourinary: Urinary frequency

Mechanism of Action Inhibits the transmission of both monosynaptic and polysynaptic reflexes at the spinal cord level, possibly by hyperpolarization of primary afferent fiber terminals, with resultant relief of muscle spasticity

Pharmacodynamics Muscle relaxation effects require 3-4 days and maximal clinical effects are not seen for 5-10 days

Pharmacokinetics

Absorption: Rapidly absorbed following oral administration; absorption from the GI tract is thought to be dose dependent

Protein binding: 30%

Metabolism: Minimally in the liver

Half-life: 2.5-4 hours

Peak serum levels: Within 2-3 hours

Elimination: 85% of an oral dose excreted in the urine and feces as unchanged drug

Usual Dosage Oral:

Children:

2-7 years: Initial: 10-15 mg/24 hours divided every 8 hours; titrate dose every 3 days in increments of 5-15 mg/day to a maximum of 40 mg/day

≥8 years: Titrate dosage as above to a maximum of 60 mg/day

Adults: 5 mg 3 times/day, may increase 5 mg/dose every 3 days to a maximum of 80 mg/day

Monitoring Parameters Muscle rigidity, spasticity (decrease in number and severity of spasms)

Dosage Forms Tablet: 10 mg, 20 mg

Extemporaneous Preparation(s) Make a 10 mg/mL suspension by crushing thirty (30) 20 mg tablets; wet with glycerin, add 15 mL Cologel® and simple syrup to make a total volume of 60 mL; stable 4 days in refrigerator

Nahata MC and Hipple TF, *Pediatric Drug Formulations*, 1st ed, Harvey Whitney Books Co, 1990.

Bactocill® *see* Oxacillin Sodium *on page 425*

Bactrim™ *see* Co-trimoxazole *on page 156*

Bactrim™ DS *see* Co-trimoxazole *on page 156*

Bactroban® *see* Mupirocin *on page 397*

Baking Soda *see* Sodium Bicarbonate *on page 525*

Baldex® *see* Dexamethasone *on page 178*

BAL in Oil® *see* Dimercaprol *on page 194*

Bancap® HC *see* Hydrocodone and Acetaminophen *on page 292*

Banesin® [OTC] *see* Acetaminophen *on page 16*

Banophen® [OTC] *see* Diphenhydramine Hydrochloride *on page 195*

Barbita® *see* Phenobarbital *on page 450*

Barophen® *see* Hyoscyamine, Atropine, Scopolamine and Phenobarbital *on page 299*

Basaljel® [OTC] *see* Antacid Preparations *on page 53*

Bayer® Aspirin [OTC] *see* Aspirin *on page 61*

BCNU *see* Carmustine *on page 107*

Beclomethasone Dipropionate (be kloe meth' a sone)

Brand Names Beclovent®; Beconase®; Beconase AQ®; Vancenase®; Vancenase® AQ; Vanceril®

Therapeutic Category Anti-inflammatory Agent; Corticosteroid, Inhalant; Glucocorticoid

Use Oral inhalation is used for treatment of bronchial asthma in patients who require chronic administration of corticosteroids; nasal aerosol is used for the symptomatic treatment of seasonal or perennial rhinitis and nasal polyposis

Pregnancy Risk Factor C

Contraindications Status asthmaticus; hypersensitivity to the drug or fluorocarbons, oleic acid in the formulation

(Continued)

Beclomethasone Dipropionate *(Continued)*

Warnings Fatalities have occurred due to adrenal insufficiency in asthmatic patients during and after switching from systemic corticosteroids to aerosol steroids; during this period, aerosol steroids do not provide the systemic steroid needed to treat patients requiring stress doses (ie, patients with major stress such as trauma, surgery, or infections)

Precautions Avoid using higher than recommended dosages since suppression of hypothalamic, pituitary, or adrenal function may occur

Adverse Reactions

Central nervous system: Headache

Gastrointestinal: Dry mouth

Local: Growth of *Candida* in the mouth, throat, or nares, irritation and burning of the nasal mucosa, nasal ulceration, epistaxis, rhinorrhea, nasal stuffiness

Respiratory: Cough, sneezing

Miscellaneous: Hoarseness

Stability Do not store near heat or open flame

Mechanism of Action Controls the rate of protein synthesis, depresses the migration of polymorphonuclear leukocytes and fibroblasts, reverses capillary permeability, and stabilizes lysosomal membranes at the cellular level to prevent or control inflammation

Pharmacokinetics

Therapeutic effect: Within 1-4 weeks of use

Inhalation:

- Absorption: Readily absorbed; quickly hydrolyzed by pulmonary esterases prior to absorption
- Distribution: 10% to 25% of dose reaches respiratory tract

Oral:

- Absorption: 90%
- Distribution: Secreted into breast milk
- Protein binding: 87%
- Metabolism: Hepatic
- Half-life, terminal: 15 hours
- Elimination: Renal excretion

Usual Dosage

Aerosol inhalation:

- Oral:
  - Children 6-12 years: 1-2 inhalations 3-4 times/day, alternatively: 2-4 inhalations twice daily; not to exceed 10 inhalations/day
  - Children >12 years and Adults: 2 inhalations 3-4 times/day, not to exceed 20 inhalations/day
- Nasal:
  - Children 6-12 years: 1 spray each nostril 3 times/day
  - Children >12 years and Adults: 1 spray each nostril 2-4 times/day or 2 sprays each nostril twice daily

Aqueous inhalation, nasal: Children >6 years and Adults: 1-2 sprays each nostril twice daily

Patient Information Rinse mouth and expectorate after inhalation use to decrease chance of thrush

Nursing Implications Shake thoroughly before using; for asthmatics (to reduce chance of coughing): inhale drug slowly or use prescribed inhaled bronchodilator 5 minutes before beclomethasone

Dosage Forms

Inhalation:

- Nasal: 42 μg/inhalation (16.8 g)
- Oral: 42 μg/inhalation (16.8 g)

Spray, aqueous, nasal: Each actuation delivers 42 μg-200 metered doses (25 g)

References

Kobayashi RH, Tinkelman DG, Reese ME, et al, "Beclomethasone Dipropionate Aqueous Nasal Spray for Seasonal Allergic Rhinitis in Children," *Ann Allergy*, 1989, 62(3):205-8.

Wyatt R, Waschek J, Weinberger M, et al, "Effects of Inhaled Beclomethasone Dipropionate and Alternate-Day Prednisone on Pituitary-Adrenal Function in Children With Chronic Asthma," *N Engl J Med*, 1978, 299(25):1387-92.

Beclovent® *see* Beclomethasone Dipropionate *on page 75*

Beconase® *see* Beclomethasone Dipropionate *on page 75*

Beconase AQ® *see* Beclomethasone Dipropionate *on page 75*

Beef NPH Iletin® II *see* Insulin Preparations *on page 311*

Beef Regular Iletin® II *see* Insulin Preparations *on page 311*

Beepen-VK® *see* Penicillin V Potassium *on page 442*

Beesix® *see* Pyridoxine Hydrochloride *on page 501*

Belix® [OTC] *see* Diphenhydramine Hydrochloride *on page 195*

Bemote® *see* Dicyclomine Hydrochloride *on page 187*

Benadryl® [OTC] *see* Diphenhydramine Hydrochloride *on page 195*

Ben-Aqua® [OTC] *see* Benzoyl Peroxide *on next page*

Benemid® *see* Probenecid *on page 480*

Benoxyl® *see* Benzoyl Peroxide *on next page*

Bentyl® Hydrochloride *see* Dicyclomine Hydrochloride *on page 187*

Benylin® Cough Syrup [OTC] *see* Diphenhydramine Hydrochloride *on page 195*

Benzac W® *see* Benzoyl Peroxide *on next page*

Benzathine Benzylpenicillin *see* Penicillin G Benzathine *on page 438*

Benzathine Penicillin G *see* Penicillin G Benzathine *on page 438*

Benzazoline Hydrochloride *see* Tolazoline Hydrochloride *on page 571*

Benzene Hexachloride *see* Lindane *on page 344*

Benzhexol Hydrochloride *see* Trihexyphenidyl Hydrochloride *on page 583*

Benzocaine (ben' zoe kane)

Brand Names Americaine® [OTC]; Anbesol® Maximum Strength [OTC]; Babee® Teething Lotion [OTC]; BiCOZENE® [OTC]; Chiggertox® [OTC]; Dermoplast® [OTC]; Foille Plus® [OTC]; Hurricaine®; Orabase®-B [OTC]; Orabase®-O [OTC]; Orajel® Brace-Aid Oral Anesthetic [OTC]; Orajel® Maximum Strength [OTC]; Orajel® Mouth-Aid [OTC]; Rhulicaine® [OTC]; Rid-A-Pain® [OTC]; Solarcaine® [OTC]; Unguentine® [OTC]

Synonyms Ethyl Aminobenzoate

Therapeutic Category Local Anesthetic, Oral; Local Anesthetic, Topical

Use Temporary relief of pain associated with pruritic dermatosis, pruritus, minor burns, toothache, minor sore throat pain, canker sores, hemorrhoids, rectal fissures; anesthetic lubricant for passage of catheters and endoscopic tubes

Pregnancy Risk Factor C

Contraindications Known hypersensitivity to benzocaine, other ester-type local anesthetics, or other components in the formulation

Adverse Reactions

Hematologic: Methemoglobinemia in infants

Local: Contact dermatitis, burning, stinging, tenderness, urticaria, edema

Mechanism of Action Blocks both the initiation and conduction of nerve impulses from sensory nerves by decreasing the neuronal membrane's permeability to sodium ions, which results in inhibition of depolarization with resultant blockade of conduction

Pharmacokinetics

Absorption: Poorly absorbed after topical administration to intact skin, but well absorbed from mucous membranes and traumatized skin

Metabolism: Hydrolyzed in the plasma and to a lesser extent the liver by cholinesterase

Elimination: Excretion of the metabolites in the urine

(Continued)

Benzocaine *(Continued)*

Usual Dosage Children and Adults: Topical:

Cream, lotion, ointment: Apply a small amount on affected area as needed
Spray: To affected area as needed

Patient Information Do not eat for 1 hour after application to oral mucosa

Dosage Forms Topical:

Aerosol: 5%, 20% (60 g)
Cream: 5%, 6%
Lotion: 8%
Ointment: 5% (30 g)

Benzocaine and Antipyrine *see* Antipyrine and Benzocaine *on page 56*

Benzoyl Peroxide (ben' zoe ill)

Brand Names Ben-Aqua® [OTC]; Benoxyl®; Benzac W®; Clear By Design® [OTC]; Clearsil® [OTC]; Desquam-X®; Dry and Clear® [OTC]; Loroxide® [OTC]; Oxy-5® [OTC]; PanOxyl® [OTC]; PanOxyl®-AQ; Persa-Gel®; pHisoAc- BP® [OTC]; Vanoxide® [OTC]; Xerac™ BP [OTC]; Zeroxin®

Therapeutic Category Acne Product; Topical Skin Product

Use Adjunctive treatment of mild to moderate acne

Pregnancy Risk Factor C

Contraindications Known hypersensitivity to benzoyl peroxide, benzoic acid, or any of its components

Warnings Discontinue if burning, swelling, or undue dryness occurs

Precautions For external use only; may bleach colored fabrics; avoid contact with eyes, eyelids, lips, mucous membranes, and highly inflamed or denuded skin

Adverse Reactions Dermatologic: Irritation, contact dermatitis, dryness, erythema, peeling, stinging

Mechanism of Action Releases free-radical oxygen which oxidizes bacterial proteins in the sebaceous follicles decreasing the number of anaerobic bacteria and irritating free fatty acids

Pharmacokinetics

Absorption: ~5% absorbed through the skin
Metabolism: Major metabolite is benzoic acid
Elimination: Excreted in the urine as benzoate

Usual Dosage Children and Adults: Topical: Apply sparingly 1-3 times/day; initially apply for 15 minutes; length of exposure, strength, and frequency of application are increased as tolerated

Patient Information Shake lotion before using; cleanse skin before applying; for external use only; avoid contact with eyes and mucous membranes

Additional Information Granulation may indicate effectiveness; gels are more penetrating than creams and last longer than creams or lotions

Dosage Forms

Cleansers:
  Bar: 5% (120 g); 10% (120 g)
  Liquid: 5% (120 mL, 150 mL, 240 mL); 10% (120 mL, 150 mL)
Creams: 5% (30 g); 10% (30 g, 45 g)
Gels: 2.5% (45 g, 60 g, 90 g); 5% (45 g, 60 g, 90 g, 120 g); 10% (45 g, 60 g, 90 g, 120 g)
Lotions: 5% (30 mL, 60 mL); 5.5% (25 mL); 10% (30 mL, 60 mL)

References

Winston MH and Shalita AR, "Acne Vulgaris: Pathogenesis and Treatment," *Pediatr Clin North Am*, 1991, 38(4):889-903.

Benzquinamide Hydrochloride (benz kwin' a mide)

Brand Names Emete-Con®

Therapeutic Category Antiemetic

Use Antiemetic used to treat nausea and vomiting associated with anesthesia and surgery

Pregnancy Risk Factor Use in pregnancy is not recommended

Contraindications Hypersensitivity to benzquinamide hydrochloride or any component

Precautions I.V. administration has been associated with hypertension and transient arrhythmias. I.M. is the preferred route. Use in pregnancy is **not** recommended.

Adverse Reactions

Cardiovascular: Hypertension, hypotension, cardiac arrhythmias

Central nervous system: Drowsiness (most common), insomnia, restlessness, headache; very large doses have produced extrapyramidal symptoms

Gastrointestinal: Anorexia

Musculoskeletal: Weakness

Stability Protect from light; reconstituted parenteral solution is stable 14 days at room temperature

Mechanism of Action Mechanism is unknown, but probably acts directly on the chemoreceptor trigger zone

Pharmacodynamics

Onset of action: ~15 minutes

Duration: 3-4 hours

Pharmacokinetics

Absorption: I.M.: Rapid

Protein binding: 58%

Metabolism: Drug is mainly metabolized by the liver

Peak blood levels: Occur 30 minutes after administration

Elimination: Metabolites excreted in urine, feces, bile; <10% excreted unchanged in urine

Usual Dosage Not recommended for use in children <12 years of age as safety and efficacy have not been established

I.M.: 50 mg (0.5-1 mg/kg) may be repeated in 1 hour, then every 3-4 hours as needed

I.V.: 25 mg (0.2-0.4 mg/kg); not recommended route, see Precautions

Administration Reconstitute with 2.2 mL of sterile water (do **not** reconstitute with normal saline, ppt may develop); give either deep I.M. or by slow I.V. no faster than 25 mg/minute

Dosage Forms Injection: 50 mg

Benztropine Mesylate (benz' troe peen)

Related Information

Overdose and Toxicology Information *on page 696-700*

Brand Names Cogentin®

Therapeutic Category Anticholinergic Agent; Antiparkinson Agent

Use Adjunctive treatment of Parkinson's disease; also used in treatment of drug-induced extrapyramidal effects and acute dystonic reactions

Pregnancy Risk Factor C

Contraindications Hypersensitivity to benztropine mesylate or any component; children <3 years of age; patients with narrow-angle glaucoma

Precautions Use with caution in hot weather or during exercise

Adverse Reactions

Cardiovascular: Tachycardia

Central nervous system: Drowsiness, nervousness, hallucinations, coma, dry mouth

Gastrointestinal: Nausea, vomiting

Ocular: Blurred vision, mydriasis

Mechanism of Action Thought to partially block striatal cholinergic receptors to help balance cholinergic and dopaminergic activity

Usual Dosage

Drug-induced extrapyramidal reaction: Oral, I.M., I.V.:

- Children >3 years: 0.02-0.05 mg/kg/dose 1-2 times/day; use in children <3 years should be reserved for life-threatening emergencies
- Adults: 1-4 mg/dose 1-2 times/day

Parkinsonism: Oral: 0.5-6 mg/day in 1-2 divided doses; begin with 0.5 mg/day; increase in 0.5 mg increments at 5- to 6-day intervals to achieve the desired effect

Additional Information I.V. route should be reserved for situations when oral or I.M. are not appropriate

Dosage Forms

Injection: 1 mg/mL (2 mL)

Tablet: 0.5 mg, 1 mg, 2 mg

Benzylpenicillin Benzathine *see* Penicillin G Benzathine *on page 438*

Benzylpenicilloyl-polylysine

Brand Names Pre-Pen®

Synonyms Penicilloyl-polylysine; PPL

Therapeutic Category Diagnostic Agent, Penicillin Allergy Skin Test

Use As an adjunct in assessing the risk of administering penicillin (penicillin or benzylpenicillin) in patients with a history of clinical penicillin hypersensitivity

Pregnancy Risk Factor C

Contraindications Patients known to be extremely hypersensitive

Warnings PPL test alone does not identify those patients who react to a minor antigenic determinant and does not appear to predict reliably the occurrence of late reactions; patients may still have allergic reactions to penicillin

Adverse Reactions

Local: Pruritus, erythema, wheal, urticaria, edema

Miscellaneous: Systemic allergic reactions occur rarely

Stability Store in refrigerator; discard if left at room temperature for longer than 1 day

Mechanism of Action Elicits IgE antibodies which produce type I accelerated urticarial reactions to penicillins

Usual Dosage

Children and Adults: Scratch test: Use scratch technique with a 20-gauge needle to make 3-5 mm scratch on epidermis, apply a small drop of solution to scratch, rub in gently with applicator or toothpick. A positive reaction consists of a pale wheal surrounding the scratch site which develops within 10 minutes and ranges from 5-15 mm or more in diameter.

Intradermal test: Use intradermal test with a tuberculin syringe with a 26- to 30-gauge short bevel needle; a dose of 0.01-0.02 mL is injected intradermally. A control of 0.9% sodium chloride should be injected at least 1½" from the PPL test site. Most skin responses to the intradermal test will develop within 5-15 minutes.

Administration PPL is administered by a scratch technique or by intradermal injection. For initial testing, PPL should always be applied via the scratch technique. Do not give intradermally to patients who have positive reactions to a scratch test.

Nursing Implications Always use scratch test for initial testing

Dosage Forms Injection: 0.25 mL

Beractant (ber akt' ant)

Brand Names Survanta®

Synonyms Bovine Lung Surfactant; Natural Lung Surfactant

Therapeutic Category Lung Surfactant

Use Prevention and treatment of respiratory distress syndrome in premature infants

Prophylactic therapy in infants (body weight <1250 g) at risk for developing or with evidence of surfactant deficiency

Rescue therapy: Treatment of infants with RDS confirmed by x-ray and requiring mechanical ventilation

Warnings Rapidly affects oxygenation and lung compliance and should be restricted to a highly supervised use in a clinical setting with immediate availability of clinicians experienced with intubation and ventilatory management of premature infants. If transient episodes of bradycardia and decreased oxygen saturation occur, discontinue the dosing procedure and initiate measures to alleviate the condition.

Precautions Use of beractant in infants <600 g birth weight or >1750 g birth weight has not been evaluated

Adverse Reactions During the dosing procedure:

Cardiovascular: Transient bradycardia, vasoconstriction, hypotension, hypertension, pallor

Respiratory: Oxygen desaturation, endotracheal tube blockage, hypocarbia, hypercarbia, apnea, pulmonary air leaks, pulmonary interstitial emphysema

Miscellaneous: Increased probability of post-treatment nosocomial sepsis

Stability Refrigerate; protect from light, prior to administration warm by standing at room temperature for 20 minutes or hold in hand for 8 minutes; artificial warming methods should **not** be used; unused, unopened vials warmed to room temperature may be returned to the refrigerator within 8 hours of warming only once

Mechanism of Action Replaces deficient or ineffective endogenous lung surfactant in neonates with respiratory distress syndrome (RDS) or in neonates at risk of developing RDS. Surfactant prevents the alveoli from collapsing during expiration by lowering surface tension between air and alveolar surfaces.

Usual Dosage Intratracheal:

Prophylactic treatment: Give 4 mL/kg as soon as possible; as many as 4 doses may be administered during the first 48 hours of life, no more frequently than 6 hours apart. The need for additional doses is determined by evidence of continuing respiratory distress; if the infant is still intubated and requiring at least 30% inspired oxygen to maintain a $PaO_2 \leq 80$ torr.

Rescue treatment: Give 4 mL/kg as soon as the diagnosis of RDS is made.

Administration For intratracheal administration only. Suction infant prior to administration; inspect solution to verify complete mixing of the suspension. Administer intratracheally by instillation through a 5-French end-hole catheter inserted into the infant's endotracheal tube. Administer the dose in four 1 mL/kg aliquots. Each quarter-dose is instilled over 2-3 seconds; each quarter-dose is administered with the infant in a different position; slightly downward inclination with head turned to the right, then repeat with head turned to the left; then slightly upward inclination with head turned to the right, then repeat with head turned to the left.

Monitoring Parameters Continuous EKG and transcutaneous O_2 saturation should be monitored during administration; frequent ABG sampling is necessary to prevent postdosing hyperoxia and hypocarbia.

Nursing Implications Do not shake; if settling occurs during storage, swirl gently

Dosage Forms Suspension: 200 mg (8 mL) phospholipids

Beta-2® *see* Isoetharine *on page 321*

9-Beta-D-ribofuranosyladenine *see* Adenosine *on page 23*

Betagan® Liquifilm® *see* Levobunolol Hydrochloride *on page 337*

Betalin®S *see* Thiamine Hydrochloride *on page 559*

Betamethasone (bay ta meth' a sone)

Related Information

Topical Steroids Comparison Chart *on page 728*

Brand Names Alphatrex®; Betatrex®; Beta-Val®; Celestone®; Celestone® Soluspan®; Cel-U-Jec®; Diprolene®; Diprolene® AF; Diprosone®; Maxivate®; Selestoject®; Telador®; Uticort®; Valisone®

Synonyms Flubenisolone

Therapeutic Category Anti-inflammatory Agent; Corticosteroid, Systemic; Corticosteroid, Topical; Glucocorticoid

Use Anti-inflammatory, immunosuppressant agent, corticosteroid replacement therapy. Topical: Inflammatory dermatoses such as psoriasis, neurodermatitis, seborrheic or atopic dermatitis

Pregnancy Risk Factor C

Contraindications Systemic fungal infections; hypersensitivity to betamethasone or any component

Precautions Use with caution in patients with hypothyroidism, cirrhosis, ulcerative colitis

Adverse Reactions

Cardiovascular: Hypertension

Central nervous system: Convulsions, vertigo, confusion, headache

Dermatologic: Thin fragile skin, sterile abscess, hyperpigmentation or hypopigmentation, acne, impaired wound healing

Endocrine & metabolic: Cushingoid state, sodium retention, linear growth suppression

(Continued)

Betamethasone *(Continued)*

Gastrointestinal: Peptic ulcer
Local: Burning, itching
Musculoskeletal: Muscle weakness, osteoporosis
Ocular: Cataracts, glaucoma

Drug Interactions Barbiturates, phenytoin and rifampin will ↓ corticosteroid effects

Mechanism of Action Controls the rate of protein synthesis, depresses the migration of polymorphonuclear leukocytes and fibroblasts, reverses capillary permeability, and causes lysosomal stabilization at the cellular level to prevent or control inflammation

Pharmacokinetics Long-acting corticosteroid with minimal or no sodium retaining potential

Usual Dosage

Children:
- I.M.: 0.0175-0.125 mg base/kg/day divided every 6-12 hours **or** 0.5-7.5 mg base/m^2/day divided every 6-12 hours
- Oral: 0.0175-0.25 mg/kg/day divided every 6-8 hours **or** 0.5-7.5 mg/m^2/day divided every 6-8 hours

Adults:
- I.M.: 0.6-9 mg/day divided every 12-24 hours
- Oral: 2.4-4.8 mg/day in 2-4 doses; range: 0.6-7.2 mg/day

Topical: Apply thin film 1-3 times/day

Nursing Implications Do not give injectable suspension I.V.; do not apply to face or inguinal areas; not for use on broken skin or in areas of infection

Dosage Forms

Base (Celestone®):
- Tablet: 0.6 mg
- Syrup: 0.6 mg/5 mL

Benzoate salt (Uticort®):
- Cream: 0.025% (60 g)
- Gel: 0.025% (15 g, 60 g)
- Lotion: 0.025% (15 mL, 60 mL)

Dipropionate salt (Alphatrex®, Diprolene®, Diprosone®, Maxivate®):
- Cream: 0.05%
- Gel: 0.05%
- Lotion: 0.05%
- Ointment, topical: 0.05%

Valerate salt (Betatrex®, Beta-Val®, Valisone®):
- Cream: 0.1% (15 g, 45 g)
- Lotion: 0.1% (60 mL)
- Ointment, topical: 0.1% (15 g, 45 g)

Sodium phosphate salt (B-S-P®, Selestoject®):
- Injection: 4 mg/mL

Sodium phosphate and acetate salt (Celestone® Soluspan®):
- Injection, suspension: 6 mg/mL (3 mg of betamethasone sodium phosphate and 3 mg of betamethasone acetate per mL)

Betapen®-VK *see* Penicillin V Potassium *on page 442*

Betatrex® *see* Betamethasone *on previous page*

Beta-Val® *see* Betamethasone *on previous page*

Bethanechol Chloride (be than' e kole)

Brand Names Duvoid®; Myotonachol™; Urecholine®

Therapeutic Category Cholinergic Agent

Use Nonobstructive urinary retention and retention due to neurogenic bladder; gastroesophageal reflux

Pregnancy Risk Factor C

Contraindications Hypersensitivity to bethanechol chloride or any component; do not use in patients with mechanical obstruction of the GI or GU tract; do not use in patients with hyperthyroidism, peptic ulcer, bronchial asthma, or cardiac disease; contraindicated for I.M. or I.V. use due to severe cholinergic activity

Adverse Reactions

Cardiovascular: Hypotension, cardiac arrest, flushed skin (vasomotor response)

Gastrointestinal: Abdominal cramps, diarrhea, nausea, vomiting
Genitourinary: Urinary frequency
Respiratory: Bronchial constriction
Miscellaneous: Sweating, salivation

Drug Interactions Ganglionic blockers → critical fall in blood pressure; other cholinergic agents due to additive effects; epinephrine and other sympathomimetics, quinidine, procainamide

Mechanism of Action Stimulates cholinergic receptors in the smooth muscle of the urinary bladder and gastrointestinal tract resulting in ↑ peristalsis, ↑ GI and pancreatic secretions, bladder muscle contraction, and ↑ ureteral peristaltic waves

Pharmacodynamics
Onset of action:
Oral 30-90 minutes
S.C.: 5-15 minutes
Duration: Oral: Up to 6 hours

Pharmacokinetics
Absorption: Oral: Variable
Metabolic fate and excretion have not been determined

Usual Dosage
Children:
Oral:
Abdominal distention or urinary retention: 0.6 mg/kg/day divided 3-4 times/day
Gastroesophageal reflux: 0.1-0.2 mg/kg/dose given 30 minutes to 1 hour before each meal to a maximum of 4 times/day
S.C.: 0.12-0.2 mg/kg/day divided 3-4 times/day

Adults:
Oral: 10-50 mg 2-4 times/day
S.C.: 2.5-5 mg 3-4 times/day, up to 7.5-10 mg every 4 hours for neurogenic bladder

Dosage Forms
Injection: 5 mg/mL (1 mL)
Tablet: 5 mg, 10 mg, 25 mg, 50 mg

Biamine® *see* Thiamine Hydrochloride *on page 559*

Biaxin™ *see* Clarithromycin *on page 139*

Bicillin® L-A *see* Penicillin G Benzathine *on page 438*

Bicitra® *see* Sodium Citrate and Citric Acid *on page 528*

BiCNU® *see* Carmustine *on page 107*

BiCOZENE® [OTC] *see* Benzocaine *on page 77*

Biltricide® *see* Praziquantel *on page 474*

Bioca® [OTC] *see* Calcium Carbonate *on page 94*

Biocef® *see* Cephalexin Monohydrate *on page 120*

Biomox® *see* Amoxicillin *on page 44*

Bio-Tab® *see* Doxycycline *on page 210*

Bisacodyl (bis a koe' dill)

Brand Names Bisacodyl Uniserts®; Bisco-Lax® [OTC]; Carter's Little Pills® [OTC]; Clysodrast®; Dulcagen® [OTC]; Dulcolax® [OTC]; Fleet® Laxative [OTC]

Therapeutic Category Laxative, Stimulant

Use Treatment of constipation; colonic evacuation prior to procedures or examination

Pregnancy Risk Factor C

Contraindications Hypersensitivity to bisacodyl or any component; do not use in patients with abdominal pain, appendicitis, obstruction, nausea or vomiting; not to be used during pregnancy or lactation

Warnings Safety of bisacodyl tannex usage in children <10 years of age has not been established

Precautions Bisacodyl tannex should be used with caution in patients with ulceration of the colon

(Continued)

Bisacodyl *(Continued)*

Adverse Reactions

Endocrine & metabolic: Electrolyte and fluid imbalance (metabolic acidosis or alkalosis, hypocalcemia)

Gastrointestinal: Abdominal cramps, nausea, vomiting

Miscellaneous: Rectal burning

Mechanism of Action Stimulates peristalsis by directly irritating the smooth muscle of the intestine, possibly the colonic intramural plexus; alters water and electrolyte secretion producing net intestinal fluid accumulation and laxation

Pharmacodynamics

Onset of action:

Oral: Within 6-10 hours

Rectal: 15-60 minutes

Pharmacokinetics

Absorption: Oral, rectal: <5% absorbed systemically

Metabolism: Metabolized in the liver

Elimination: Conjugated metabolites excreted in milk, bile, and urine

Usual Dosage

Bisacodyl (Dulcolax®) tablet: Oral:

Children 3-12 years: 5-10 mg or 0.3 mg/kg/day as a single dose

Children ≥12 years and Adults: 5-15 mg/day as a single dose

Bisacodyl (Dulcolax®) suppository:

Children:

<2 years: 5 mg/day as a single dose

2-11 years: 5-10 mg/day as a single dose

Children ≥12 years and Adults: 10 mg/day as a single dose

Patient Information Do not break or chew enteric-coated tablet, swallow tablet whole; do not take within 1 hour of milk or antacids; should not be used regularly for more than 1 week

Dosage Forms

Enema: 10 mg/30 mL

Powder: 1.5 mg with tannic acid 2.5 g per packet (25s, 50s)

Suppository, rectal: 5 mg, 10 mg

Tablet, enteric coated: 5 mg

Bisacodyl Uniserts® *see* Bisacodyl *on previous page*

Bisco-Lax® [OTC] *see* Bisacodyl *on previous page*

Bistropamide *see* Tropicamide *on page 588*

Black Draught® [OTC] *see* Senna *on page 522*

Blenoxane® *see* Bleomycin Sulfate *on this page*

Bleomycin Sulfate (blee oh mye' sin)

Related Information

Emetogenic Potential of Single Chemotherapeutic Agents *on page 655*

Brand Names Blenoxane®

Synonyms BLM

Therapeutic Category Antineoplastic Agent

Use Palliative treatment of squamous cell carcinomas, testicular carcinoma and the following lymphomas: Hodgkin's, lymphosarcoma and reticulum cell sarcoma; sclerosing agent

Pregnancy Risk Factor D

Contraindications Hypersensitivity to bleomycin sulfate or any component

Warnings The US Food and Drug Administration (FDA) currently recommends that procedures for proper handling and disposal of antineoplastic agents be considered. Occurrence of pulmonary fibrosis is higher in elderly patients and in those receiving a total dose >400 units; pulmonary toxicity has occurred at a total dosage <200 units or 100 units/m^2 in younger patients; a severe idiosyncratic reaction consisting of hypotension, mental confusion, fever, chills and wheezing is possible

Precautions Use with caution in patients with renal or pulmonary impairment; dosage modification is recommended in patients with renal impairment; dosage modification may be necessary in patients with a 20% decrease from baseline in FEV, FVC, or DL_{co}; administer test dose prior to starting therapy

Adverse Reactions

Cardiovascular: Cerebrovascular accident

Central nervous system: Fever

Dermatologic: Hyperpigmentation, hyperkeratosis of hands and nails, rash, alopecia

Gastrointestinal: Stomatitis

Hematologic: Thrombocytopenia, leukopenia

Local: Phlebitis

Respiratory: Interstitial pneumonitis (10%), pulmonary fibrosis (cumulative lifetime dose should not exceed 400 units), dyspnea, tachypnea, nonproductive cough, rales

Miscellaneous: Anaphylactoid reactions

Drug Interactions Digoxin, phenytoin

Stability Refrigerate; reconstituted solution is stable for 24 hours at room temperature; incompatible with amino acid solutions, ascorbic acid, cefazolin, furosemide, diazepam, hydrocortisone, mitomycin, nafcillin, penicillin G, aminophylline

Mechanism of Action Inhibits synthesis of DNA; binds to DNA leading to single- and double-strand breaks

Pharmacokinetics

Protein binding: 1%

Half-life: Dependent upon renal function

- Children: 2.1-3.5 hours
- Adults, with normal renal function: 2-4 hours

Peak concentrations: I.M.: Within 30 minutes

Elimination: 60% to 70% of a dose excreted in the urine as active drug

Not removed by hemodialysis

Usual Dosage Refer to individual protocol

Children and Adults:

- I.M., I.V., S.C.:
  - Test dose for lymphoma patients: 1-2 units of bleomycin for the first 2 doses; monitor vital signs every 15 minutes; wait a minimum of 1 hour before administering remainder of dose
  - Treatment: 10-20 units/m^2 (0.25-0.5 units/kg) 1-2 times/week in combination regimens
- I.V. continuous infusion: 15-20 units/m^2/day for 4-5 days
- Reduce dose 50% to 75% in patients with Cl_{cr} <25 mL/minute

Adults: Intracavitary injection for pleural effusion: 15-60 units have been given

Administration Administer I.V. slowly over at least 10 minutes (no greater than 1 unit/minute) at a concentration not to exceed 3 units/mL; bleomycin for I.V. continuous infusion can be further diluted in normal saline (preferred) or D_5W

Monitoring Parameters Pulmonary function tests (total lung volume, forced vital capacity, carbon monoxide diffusion), renal function, chest x-ray; vital signs and temperature initially; CBC with differential and platelet count

Patient Information Report any coughing, shortness of breath, or wheezing to physician

Dosage Forms Powder for injection: 15 units

References

Alberts DS, Chen H-SG, Liu R, et al, "Bleomycin Pharmacokinetics in Man," *Cancer Chemother Pharmacol*, 1978, 1:177-81.

Berg SL, Grisell DL, Delaney TF, et al, "Principles of Treatment of Pediatric Solid Tumors," *Pediatr Clin North Am*, 1991, 38(2):249-67.

D'Arcy PF, "Reactions and Interactions in Handling Anticancer Drugs," *Drug Intell Clin Pharm*, 1983, 17(7-8):532-8.

Bleph®-10 *see* Sulfacetamide Sodium *on page 539*

BLM *see* Bleomycin Sulfate *on previous page*

Blocadren® *see* Timolol Maleate *on page 568*

Blood Level Sampling Time Guidelines *see page 694*

Bluboro® [OTC] *see* Aluminum Acetate *on page 33*

Bonine® [OTC] *see* Meclizine Hydrochloride *on page 358*

Boropak® *see* Aluminum Acetate *on page 33*

Bovine Lung Surfactant *see* Beractant *on page 80*

Breonesin® [OTC] *see* Guaifenesin *on page 278*

Brethaire® *see* Terbutaline Sulfate *on page 548*

Brethine® *see* Terbutaline Sulfate *on page 548*

Bretylium Tosylate (bre til' ee um)

Related Information

CPR Pediatric Drug Dosages *on page 614*

Brand Names Bretylol®

Therapeutic Category Antiarrhythmic Agent, Class III

Use Ventricular tachycardia or ventricular fibrillation; also used in the treatment of other serious ventricular arrhythmias resistant to lidocaine

Pregnancy Risk Factor C

Contraindications Digitalis intoxication induced arrhythmias

Precautions Hypotension; patients with fixed cardiac output (severe pulmonary hypertension or aortic stenosis) may experience severe hypotension due to ↓ in peripheral resistance without ability to ↑ cardiac output; reduce dose in renal failure patients

Adverse Reactions

Cardiovascular: Hypotension (incidence 50% to 75%), transient initial hypertension, increase in PVCs, bradycardia, flushing, nasal congestion

Central nervous system: Vertigo, syncope, confusion

Dermatologic: Rash

Gastrointestinal: Nausea and vomiting with rapid I.V. administration, rarely diarrhea, abdominal pain

Local: Muscle atrophy and necrosis with repeated I.M. injections at same site

Ocular: Conjunctivitis

Renal & genitourinary: Renal impairment

Miscellaneous: Hyperthermia, hiccups

Drug Interactions Other antiarrhythmic agents may potentiate or antagonize cardiac effects, toxic effects may be additive; the pressor effects of catecholamines may be enhanced by bretylium; may potentiate digitalis toxicity

Mechanism of Action Class III antiarrhythmic; after an initial release of norepinephrine at the peripheral adrenergic nerve terminals, bretylium inhibits further release by postganglionic nerve endings in response to sympathetic nerve stimulation

Pharmacodynamics

Onset of antiarrhythmic effects:

I.V.: Within 6-20 minutes

I.M.: Up to 2 hours

Maximum effect: Within 6-9 hours

Pharmacokinetics

Protein binding: 1% to 6%

Half-life, adults: 7-11 hours; increases with decreased renal function

Elimination: Excreted unchanged in the urine

Usual Dosage Note: Patients should undergo defibrillation/cardioversion before and after bretylium doses as necessary

Children:

I.M.: 2-5 mg/kg as a single dose

I.V.: 5 mg/kg, may repeat every 10-20 minutes as needed to a total of 30 mg/kg; PALS guidelines for treatment of ventricular fibrillation: initial: 5 mg/kg, then attempt electrical defibrillation; repeat with 10 mg/kg and reattempt electrical defibrillation if ventricular fibrillation persists; may repeat as needed to a total of 30 mg/kg

Maintenance dose: I.M., I.V.: 5 mg/kg every 6-8 hours

Adults:

Immediately life-threatening ventricular arrhythmias, ventricular fibrillation, unstable ventricular tachycardia:

Initial dose: I.V.: 5 mg/kg (undiluted) over 1 minute; if arrhythmias persists, give 10 mg/kg (undiluted) over 1 minute and repeat as necessary (usually at 15- to 30-minute intervals) up to a total dose of 30-35 mg/kg

Other life-threatening ventricular arrhythmias:

Initial dose: I.M., I.V.: 5-10 mg/kg, may repeat every 1-2 hours if arrhythmias persist; give I.V. dose (diluted) over 8-10 minutes

Maintenance dose: I.M.: 5-10 mg/kg every 6-8 hours; I.V. (diluted): 5-10 mg/kg every 6 hours; I.V. infusion (diluted): 1-2 mg/minute (little experience with doses >40 mg/kg/day)

Administration May give undiluted I.V. push over <30 seconds for life-threatening situations; dilute to 10 mg/mL for nonlife-threatening situations and give slow I.V. push over at least 8 minutes

Monitoring Parameters EKG, heart rate, rhythm, blood pressure

Nursing Implications I.M. route not recommended for ventricular fibrillation

Dosage Forms

Injection: 50 mg/mL (10 mL, 20 mL)

Injection, premixed in D_5W: 1 mg/mL (500 mL); 2 mg/mL (250 mL); 4 mg/mL (250 mL, 500 mL)

References

Emergency Cardiac Care Committee and Subcommittees, American Heart Association, "Guidelines for Cardiopulmonary Resuscitation and Emergency Cardiac Care, III: Adult Advanced Cardiac Life Support" and "VI: Pediatric Advanced Life Support," *JAMA*, 1992, 268(16):2199-241 and 2262-75.

Bretylol® *see* Bretylium Tosylate *on previous page*

Brevibloc® *see* Esmolol Hydrochloride *on page 229*

Brevital® Sodium *see* Methohexital Sodium *on page 373*

Bricanyl® *see* Terbutaline Sulfate *on page 548*

Bromaline® [OTC] *see* Brompheniramine and Phenylpropanolamine *on this page*

Bromanate® [OTC] *see* Brompheniramine and Phenylpropanolamine *on this page*

Bromarest® [OTC] *see* Brompheniramine Maleate *on next page*

Bromatapp® [OTC] *see* Brompheniramine and Phenylpropanolamine *on this page*

Bromphen® [OTC] *see* Brompheniramine and Phenylpropanolamine *on this page*

Brompheniramine and Phenylpropanolamine

Related Information

OTC Cold Preparations, Pediatric *on page 723-726*

Brand Names Bromaline® [OTC]; Bromanate® [OTC]; Bromatapp® [OTC]; Bromphen® [OTC]; Dimetapp® [OTC]; Myphetapp® [OTC]; Tamine® [OTC]

Synonyms Phenylpropanolamine and Brompheniramine

Therapeutic Category Antihistamine/Decongestant Combination

Use Temporary relief of nasal congestion, running nose, sneezing, and itchy, watery eyes

Pregnancy Risk Factor B

Contraindications Hypersensitivity to any of the ingredients

Warnings Swallow timed release tablets whole, do not crush or chew; may impair ability to perform hazardous activities requiring mental alertness or physical coordination

Precautions Use with caution in patients with high blood pressure, heart disease, diabetes, thyroid disease, asthma, glaucoma; antihistamines should be used cautiously in term and preterm infants due to an association with SIDS

Adverse Reactions

Cardiovascular: Palpitations

Central nervous system: Excitability, drowsiness, dizziness, headache

Dermatologic: Rash

Gastrointestinal: Anorexia, nausea, dry mouth

Hematologic: Leukopenia

Drug Interactions CNS depressants, MAOI, sympathomimetics, Rauwolfia alkaloids, TCA, ganglionic blocking agents, propranolol

(Continued)

Brompheniramine and Phenylpropanolamine *(Continued)*

Usual Dosage Oral:

Children:

- 1-6 months: 1.25 mL 3-4 times/day
- 7-24 months: 2.5 mL 3-4 times/day
- 2-4 years: 3.75 mL 3-4 times/day
- 4-12 years: 5 mL 3-4 times/day

Adults: 5-10 mL 3-4 times/day or 1 tablet twice daily

Patient Information Swallow timed-release tablets whole; do not crush or chew

Dosage Forms

Elixir: Brompheniramine maleate 2 mg and phenylpropanolamine hydrochloride 12.5 mg per 5 mL with 2.3% alcohol (120 mL)

Tablet, sustained release: Brompheniramine maleate 12 mg and phenylpropanolamine hydrochloride 75 mg

Brompheniramine Maleate (brome fen ir' a meen)

Related Information

Overdose and Toxicology Information *on page 696-700*

Brand Names Bromarest® [OTC]; Chlorphed® [OTC]; Codimal-A®; Cophene-B®; Dehist®; Diamine T.D.® [OTC]; Dimetane® [OTC]; Histaject®; Nasahist B®; ND-Stat®; Oraminic® II; Veltane®

Synonyms Parabromdylamine

Therapeutic Category Antihistamine

Use Perennial and seasonal allergic rhinitis and other allergic symptoms including urticaria

Pregnancy Risk Factor C

Contraindications Hypersensitivity to brompheniramine or any component, narrow-angle glaucoma, and bladder neck obstruction

Warnings Swallow timed release tablets whole, do not crush or chew; may impair ability to perform hazardous activities requiring mental alertness or physical coordination

Precautions Use with caution in patients with heart disease, hypertension, thyroid disease, and asthma; use with caution in term or preterm infants due to an association of antihistamine use with SIDS

Adverse Reactions

Central nervous system: Paradoxical excitability, drowsiness, dizziness

Dermatologic: Rash

Gastrointestinal: Nausea, anorexia, dry mouth

Drug Interactions CNS depressants, MAO inhibitors

Stability Solutions may crystallize if stored below 0°C, crystals will dissolve when warmed

Mechanism of Action Competes with histamine for H_1-receptor sites on effector cells in the gastrointestinal tract, blood vessels, and respiratory tract

Pharmacodynamics

Peak effect: Maximal clinical effects seen within 3-9 hours

Duration: Varies with formulation

Pharmacokinetics

Metabolism: Extensive metabolism by the liver

Half-life: 12-34 hours

Peak serum levels: Oral: Within 2-5 hours

Elimination: Excreted in the urine as inactive metabolites

Usual Dosage

Oral:

- Children:
  - <6 years: 0.125 mg/kg/dose given every 6 hours; maximum: 6-8 mg/day
  - 6-12 years: 2-4 mg every 6-8 hours; maximum: 12-16 mg/day
- Adults: 4-8 mg every 4-6 hours or 8 mg of sustained release form every 8-12 hours or 12 mg of sustained release every 12 hours; maximum: 24 mg/day

I.M., I.V., S.C.:

- Children <12 years: 0.5 mg/kg/day or 15 mg/m²/day divided every 6-8 hours
- Children >12 years and Adults: 10 mg (range: 5-20 mg) every 6-12 hours; maximum: 40 mg/day

Administration Dilute in 1-10 mL D_5W or normal saline and infuse over several minutes; the patient should be in a recumbent position during the infusion

Patient Information Avoid alcohol; take with food or milk

Nursing Implications Sustained release tablets should be swallowed whole, do not crush or chew

Dosage Forms

Elixir: 2 mg/5 mL with alcohol 3% (120 mL, 480 mL, 4000 mL)
Injection: 10 mg/mL (10 mL)
Tablet: 4 mg, 8 mg
Tablet, sustained release: 8 mg, 12 mg

Bronitin® *see* Epinephrine *on page 220*

Bronkaid® Mist [OTC] *see* Epinephrine *on page 220*

Bronkodyl® *see* Theophylline *on page 554*

Bronkometer® *see* Isoetharine *on page 321*

Bronkosol® *see* Isoetharine *on page 321*

Bufferin® [OTC] *see* Aspirin *on page 61*

Bumetanide (byoo met' a nide)

Brand Names Bumex®

Therapeutic Category Antihypertensive; Diuretic, Loop

Use Used in the management of edema secondary to congestive heart failure or hepatic or renal disease including nephrotic syndrome; may also be used alone or in combination with antihypertensives in the treatment of hypertension

Pregnancy Risk Factor C

Contraindications Hypersensitivity to bumetanide or any component; in anuria or increasing azotemia

Warnings Loop diuretics are potent diuretics; excess amounts can lead to profound diuresis with fluid and electrolyte loss; close medical supervision and dose evaluation is required

Precautions Use with caution in patients with cirrhosis

Adverse Reactions

Cardiovascular: Hypotension
Central nervous system: Dizziness, weakness, headache, encephalopathy
Endocrine & metabolic: Hyperglycemia, hypokalemia, hypochloremia
Gastrointestinal: Cramps, nausea, vomiting
Renal & genitourinary: Decreased uric acid excretion
Miscellaneous: Increased serum creatinine, alteration of liver function test results

Drug Interactions Allergy to sulfonamides may result in cross hypersensitivity to bumetanide; ↓ blood pressure, when used with other antihypertensive agents (may need to decrease dose of one or both agents); indomethacin and probenecid may decrease bumetanide's effect; ↓ lithium excretion

Stability Light sensitive, → discoloration when exposed to light

Mechanism of Action Inhibits reabsorption of sodium and chloride in the ascending loop of Henle and proximal renal tubule, interfering with the chloride binding cotransport system, thus causing increased excretion of water, sodium, chloride, magnesium, calcium, and phosphate

Pharmacodynamics

Onset of clinical effects:
- Oral, I.M.: Within 30-60 minutes
- I.V.: Within a few minutes

Duration: 6 hours

Pharmacokinetics

Protein binding: 95%
Metabolism: Partial metabolism occurs in the liver
Half-life:
- Infants <6 months: 2.5 hours (range: 1-5 hours)
- Adults: 1-1.5 hours

Elimination: Unchanged drug excreted in urine (30%)

Usual Dosage

Children: Oral, I.M., I.V.:
- <6 months: Dose not established

(Continued)

Bumetanide *(Continued)*

>6 months: Initial: 0.015 mg/kg/dose once daily or every other day; maximum dose: 0.1 mg/kg/day or 10 mg

Adults:

Oral: 0.5-2 mg/dose (10 mg/day maximum) 1-2 times/day

I.M., I.V.: 0.5-1 mg/dose (10 mg/day maximum)

Administration Give by direct I.V. injection over 1-2 minutes

Monitoring Parameters Blood pressure, serum electrolytes, renal function

Additional Information Patients with impaired hepatic function must be monitored carefully, often requiring reduced doses; larger doses may be necessary in patients with impaired renal function to obtain the same therapeutic response

Dosage Forms

Injection: 0.25 mg/mL

Tablet: 0.5 mg, 1 mg, 2 mg

Bumex® *see* Bumetanide *on previous page*

Buminate® *see* Albumin Human *on page 25*

Bupivacaine Hydrochloride (byoo piv' a kane)

Brand Names Marcaine®; Sensorcaine®

Therapeutic Category Local Anesthetic, Injectable

Use Local anesthetic (injectable) for peripheral nerve block, infiltration, sympathetic block, caudal or epidural block, retrobulbar block

Pregnancy Risk Factor C

Contraindications Hypersensitivity to bupivacaine hydrochloride or any component, para-aminobenzoic acid or parabens

Warnings Convulsions due to systemic toxicity leading to cardiac arrest have been reported, presumably following unintentional intravascular injection

Precautions Use with caution in patients with liver disease

Adverse Reactions

Cardiovascular: Cardiac arrest, hypotension, bradycardia, palpitations

Central nervous system: Seizures, restlessness, anxiety, dizziness, weakness

Gastrointestinal: Nausea, vomiting

Ocular: Blurred vision

Otic: Tinnitus

Respiratory: Apnea

Mechanism of Action Blocks both the initiation and conduction of nerve impulses by decreasing the neuronal membrane's permeability to sodium ions, which results in inhibition of depolarization with resultant blockade of conduction

Pharmacodynamics

Onset of anesthetic action: Dependent on route administered, but generally occurs within 4-10 minutes

Duration: 1.5-8.5 hours

Pharmacokinetics

Half-life (age-dependent):

Neonates: 8.1 hours

Adults: 1.5-5.5 hours

Metabolism: Metabolized in the liver

Elimination: Small amounts (~6%) excreted in the urine unchanged

Usual Dosage Dose varies with procedure, depth of anesthesia, vascularity of tissues, duration of anesthesia and condition of patient

Caudal block (with or without epinephrine):

Children: 1-3.7 mg/kg

Adults: 15-30 mL of 0.25% or 0.5%

Epidural block (other than caudal block):

Children: 1.25 mg/kg/dose

Adults: 10-20 mL of 0.25% or 0.5%

Peripheral nerve block: 5 mL dose of 0.25% or 0.5% (12.5-25 mg); maximum: 2.5 mg/kg (plain); 3 mg/kg (with epinephrine); up to a maximum of 400 mg/day

Sympathetic nerve block: 20-50 mL of 0.25% (no epinephrine) solution

Additional Information Metabisulfites (in epinephrine-containing injection)

Dosage Forms

Injection: 0.25% (10 mL, 20 mL, 30 mL, 50 mL); 0.5% (10 mL, 20 mL, 30 mL, 50 mL); 0.75% (2 mL, 10 mL, 20 mL, 30 mL)

Injection, with epinephrine (1:200,000): 0.25% (10 mL, 30 mL, 50 mL); 0.5% (1.8 mL, 3 mL, 5 mL, 10 mL, 30 mL, 50 mL); 0.75% (30 mL)

Burow's Solution *see* Aluminum Acetate *on page 33*

Busulfan (byoo sul' fan)

Related Information

Emetogenic Potential of Single Chemotherapeutic Agents *on page 655*

Brand Names Myleran®

Therapeutic Category Antineoplastic Agent

Use Chronic myelogenous leukemia and marrow-ablative conditioning regimen prior to bone marrow transplantation

Pregnancy Risk Factor D

Contraindications Hypersensitivity to busulfan or any component; failure to respond to previous courses; should not be used in pregnancy or lactation

Warnings The US Food and Drug Administration (FDA) currently recommends that procedures for proper handling and disposal of antineoplastic agents be considered

Precautions May induce severe bone marrow hypoplasia; reduce or discontinue dosage at first sign, as reflected by an abnormal decrease in any of the formed elements of the blood; use with extreme caution in patients who have recently received other myelosuppressive drugs or radiation therapy

Adverse Reactions

Central nervous system: Dizziness, seizures

Dermatologic: Hyperpigmentation, alopecia

Endocrine & metabolic: Addison-like syndrome, hyperuricemia

Gastrointestinal: Nausea, vomiting, diarrhea, mucositis

Hematologic: Myelosuppression with nadirs of 14-21 days for leukopenia and thrombocytopenia; anemia

Hepatic: Hepatic dysfunction, hepatic veno-occlusive disease

Ocular: Blurred vision

Renal & genitourinary: Hemorrhagic cystitis

Respiratory: Pulmonary fibrosis

Drug Interactions Thioguanine

Mechanism of Action Interferes with the normal function of DNA by alkylation and cross-linking the strands of DNA

Pharmacokinetics

Absorption: Oral: Well absorbed

Metabolism: Metabolized in the liver

Peak plasma levels: Oral: Within 0.5-3 hours

Elimination: 10% to 50% excreted in the urine as metabolites within 24 hours

Usual Dosage Oral (refer to individual protocols):

Children:

For remission induction of CML 0.06-0.12 mg/kg/day or 1.8-4.6 mg/m^2/day; titrate dose to maintain leukocyte count about 20,000/mm^3

BMT marrow-ablative conditioning regimen: 1 mg/kg/dose every 6 hours for 16 doses

Adults: 4-8 mg/day for remission induction of CML or 0.06 mg/kg/day; maintenance dose is controversial, range: 1-4 mg/day to 2 mg/week

Monitoring Parameters CBC with differential and platelet count, hemoglobin, liver function tests, bilirubin, alkaline phosphatase

Patient Information Report any difficulty in breathing, cough, fever, sore throat, bleeding or bruising to physician

Dosage Forms Tablet: 2 mg

References

Heard BE and Cooke RA, "Busulfan Lung," *Thorax*, 1968, 23:187-93.

Vassal G, Gouyette A, Hartmann O, et al, "Pharmacokinetics of High-Dose Busulfan in Children," *Cancer Chemother Pharmacol*, 1989, 24(6):386-90.

Byclomine® *see* Dicyclomine Hydrochloride *on page 187*

Cafergot® *see* Ergotamine *on page 225*

Caffeine, Citrated

Related Information

Overdose and Toxicology Information *on page 696-700*

Therapeutic Category Central Nervous System Stimulant, Nonamphetamine; Respiratory Stimulant

Use Central nervous system stimulant; used in the treatment of idiopathic apnea of prematurity

Pregnancy Risk Factor B

Contraindications Hypersensitivity to caffeine or any component

Warnings Parenteral caffeine is only available in the United States as a sodium benzoate salt. Due to reports of sodium benzoate inducing kernicterus by displacement of bilirubin and causing the gasping syndrome in newborns, its use should be avoided in neonates.

Precautions Use with caution in patients with a history of peptic ulcer; avoid in patients with symptomatic cardiac arrhythmias

Adverse Reactions

Cardiovascular: Cardiac arrhythmias, tachycardia, extrasystoles

Central nervous system: Insomnia, restlessness, agitation, irritability, hyperactivity, muscle tremors or twitches, jitteriness, headache

Gastrointestinal: Nausea, vomiting, gastric irritation

Drug Interactions Enhances the positive cardiac inotropic and chronotropic effects of beta-adrenergic agonists

Mechanism of Action Increases levels of 3-5-AMP by inhibiting phosphodiesterase; CNS stimulant which increases medullary respiratory center sensitivity to carbon dioxide, stimulates central inspiratory drive, and improves skeletal muscle contraction (diaphragmatic contractility); prevention of apnea may occur by competitive inhibition of adenosine

Pharmacokinetics

Distribution: V_d:
- Neonates: 0.4-1.3 L/kg
- Adults: 0.6 L/kg

Protein binding: 17%

Half-life:
- Neonates: 100 hours (range: 40-230 hours)
- Adults: 6 hours

Peak concentrations: Oral: Within 60-90 minutes

Elimination:
- Neonates <1 month: 86% excreted unchanged in urine
- Infants >1 month and Adults: Extensively liver metabolized to a series of partially demethylated xanthines and methyluric acids

Clearance:
- Neonates: 8.9 mL/kg/hour (range: 2.5-1.7)
- Adults: 94 mL/kg/hour

Usual Dosage Apnea of prematurity: Oral:

Loading dose: 10-20 mg/kg as caffeine citrate (5-10 mg/kg as caffeine base). If theophylline has been administered to the patient within the previous 3 days, a full or modified loading dose (50% to 75% of a loading dose) may be given.

Maintenance dose: 5-10 mg/kg/day as caffeine citrate (2.5-5 mg/kg/day as caffeine base) once daily starting 24 hours after the loading dose. Maintenance dose is adjusted based on patient's response, (efficacy and adverse effects), and serum caffeine concentrations.

Monitoring Parameters Heart rate, number, and severity of apnea spells

Reference Range Therapeutic concentration: 8-20μg/mL; Potentially toxic: >20 μg/mL; Toxic concentration: >50 μg/mL

Test Interactions ↑ uric acid (S), slight increase in urine levels of VMA, catecholamines

Dosage Forms Tablet: 65 mg

Extemporaneous Preparation(s) An oral solution of 10 mg/mL caffeine citrate is stable for 3 months refrigerated

Handbook on Extemporaneous Formulations, Bethesda MD: American Society of Hospital Pharmacists, 1987.

References

Kriter KE and Blanchard J, "Management of Apnea in Infants," *Clin Pharm*, 1989, 8(8):577-87.

Calamine Lotion (kal' a meen)

Therapeutic Category Topical Skin Product

Use Employed primarily as an astringent, protectant, and soothing agent for conditions such as poison ivy, poison oak, poison sumac, sunburn, insect bites, or minor skin irritations

Precautions For external use only

Adverse Reactions

Dermatologic: Rash

Local: Irritation

Usual Dosage Apply 1-4 times/day as needed; reapply after bathing

Patient Information Shake well before using; avoid contact with the eyes; do not use on open wounds or burns

Additional Information Active ingredients: Calamine, zinc oxide

Dosage Forms Lotion, topical: 120 mL

Calan® *see* Verapamil Hydrochloride *on page 597*

Calciferol™ *see* Ergocalciferol *on page 224*

Calcijex™ *see* Calcitriol *on this page*

Calcilac® [OTC] *see* Calcium Carbonate *on next page*

Calcimar® *see* Calcitonin, Salmon *on this page*

Calciparine® *see* Heparin *on page 282*

Calcitonin, Salmon (kal si toe' nin)

Brand Names Calcimar®; Miacalcin®

Therapeutic Category Antidote, Hypercalcemia

Use Treatment of Paget's disease of bone and as adjunctive therapy for hypercalcemia; also used in postmenopausal osteoporosis

Pregnancy Risk Factor B

Contraindications Hypersensitivity to salmon protein or gelatin diluent

Precautions A skin test should be performed prior to initiating therapy; the skin test is 0.1 mL of 10 unit/mL normal saline dilution of calcitonin (must be prepared) injected intradermally; observe injection site for 15 minutes for wheal or significant erythema

Adverse Reactions

Cardiovascular: Flushing of the face, swelling, nasal congestion

Central nervous system: Weakness, dizziness, headache, tingling of palms and soles, chills

Dermatologic: Rash

Gastrointestinal: Nausea, vomiting, diarrhea, anorexia

Renal & genitourinary: Diuresis

Respiratory: Shortness of breath

Mechanism of Action Structurally similar to human calcitonin; it directly inhibits osteoclastic bone resorption; promotes the renal excretion of calcium, phosphate, sodium, magnesium and potassium by decreasing tubular reabsorption; increases the jejunal secretion of water, sodium, potassium, and chloride

Usual Dosage Dosage for children not established

Adults: I.M., S.C.:

- Paget's disease: 100 units/day to start, 50 units/day or 50-100 units every 1-3 days maintenance dose
- Hypercalcemia: Initial: 4 units/kg every 12 hours; may increase up to 8 units/kg every 12 hours to a maximum of every 6 hours
- Osteogenesis imperfecta: 2 units/kg 3 times/week

Monitoring Parameters Serum electrolytes and calcium

Dosage Forms Injection: 100 units/mL (1 mL); 200 units/mL (2 mL)

Calcitriol (kal si trye' ole)

Brand Names Calcijex™; Rocaltrol®

Synonyms 1,25 dihydroxycholecalciferol

Therapeutic Category Vitamin, Fat Soluble

(Continued)

Calcitriol *(Continued)*

Use Management of hypocalcemia in patients on chronic renal dialysis; reduce elevated parathyroid hormone levels

Pregnancy Risk Factor A (D if used in doses above the recommended daily allowance)

Contraindications Hypercalcemia; vitamin D toxicity; abnormal sensitivity to the effects of vitamin D

Adverse Reactions

Cardiovascular: Increased blood pressure, cardiac arrhythmias
Central nervous system: Weakness, somnolence, headache, hyperthermia
Dermatologic: Pruritus
Endocrine & metabolic: Hypercholesterolemia, hypercalcemia
Gastrointestinal: Nausea, vomiting, constipation, anorexia, weight loss, dry mouth, pancreatitis
Hepatic: Increased liver enzymes
Musculoskeletal: Myalgia, bone pain
Ocular: Calcific conjunctivitis, photophobia
Renal & genitourinary: Polyuria, polydipsia, nocturia, uremia, albuminuria,
Miscellaneous: Metallic taste, rhinorrhea

Drug Interactions Thiazide diuretics, cholestyramine, colestipol, corticosteroids

Stability Protect from light and heat

Mechanism of Action Promotes absorption of calcium in the intestines and retention via the kidneys thereby increasing calcium levels in the serum; decreases excessive serum phosphatase levels, parathyroid hormone levels, and decreases bone resorption

Usual Dosage Individualize dosage to maintain calcium levels of 9-10 mg/dL

Renal failure:
- Children:
  - Oral: 0.25-2 μg/day have been used (with hemodialysis); 0.014-0.041 μg/kg/day (not receiving hemodialysis)
  - I.V.: 0.01-0.05 μg/kg 3 times/week if undergoing hemodialysis
- Adults:
  - Oral: 0.25 μg/day or every other day (may require 0.5-1 μg/day)
  - I.V.: 0.5 μg/day 3 times/week (may require from 0.5-3 μg/day given 3 times/week) if undergoing hemodialysis

Hypoparathyroidism/pseudohypoparathyroidism: Oral:
- Children:
  - <1 year: 0.04-0.08 μg/kg/day
  - 1-5 years: 0.25-0.75 μg/day
- Children >6 years and Adults: 0.5-2 μg/day

Vitamin D-dependent rickets: Children and Adults: Oral: 1 μg/day

Vitamin D-resistant rickets (familial hypophosphatemia): Children and Adults: Oral: Initial: 0.015-0.02 μg/kg/day; maintenance: 0.03-0.06 μg/kg/day; maximum: 2 μg/day

Hypocalcemia in premature infants: Oral: 1 μg/day for 5 days

Hypocalcemic tetany in premature infants: I.V.: 0.05 μg/kg/day for 5-12 days

Administration May be administered as a bolus dose I.V. through the catheter at the end of hemodialysis

Monitoring Parameters Serum calcium levels at least twice weekly at the onset of therapy and after each dosage adjustment; weekly for 12 weeks, then monthly after stabilization of dosage

Additional Information Calcitriol injection will degrade with prolonged exposure to light

Dosage Forms

Capsule: 0.25 μg, 0.5 μg
Injection: 1 μg/mL (1 mL); 2 μg/mL (1 mL)

Calcium Carbonate

Brand Names Alka-Mints® [OTC]; Amitone® [OTC]; Bioca® [OTC]; Calcilac® [OTC]; Cal-Guard Softgels® [OTC]; CalSup® [OTC]; Caltrate® [OTC]; Chooz® [OTC]; Dicarbosil® [OTC]; Glycate® [OTC]; Rolaids® Calcium Rich [OTC]; Suplical® [OTC]; Titralac® [OTC]; Tums® [OTC]

Therapeutic Category Antacid; Antidote, Hyperphosphatemia; Calcium Salt; Electrolyte Supplement, Oral

Use Treatment and prevention of calcium depletion; relief of acid indigestion, heartburn

Pregnancy Risk Factor C

Contraindications Hypercalcemia, renal calculi, ventricular fibrillation

Precautions Use cautiously in patients with sarcoidosis, renal or cardiac disease

Adverse Reactions

Central nervous system: Headache, mental confusion, dizziness

Endocrine & metabolic: Hypercalcemia, milk-alkali syndrome, hypophosphatemia, hypercalciuria, hypomagnesemia

Gastrointestinal: Constipation, nausea, vomiting, dry mouth

Drug Interactions Digoxin, tetracycline, may antagonize the effects of verapamil

Mechanism of Action Moderates nerve and muscle performance via action potential excitation threshold regulation

Usual Dosage Dosage is in terms of elemental calcium

Recommended daily allowance (RDA):

- <6 months: 400 mg/day
- 6-12 months: 600 mg/day
- 1-10 years: 800 mg/day
- 10-25 years: 1200 mg/day
- Adults >25 years: 800 mg/day

Hypocalcemia (dose depends on clinical condition and serum calcium level). Dose expressed in mg of elemental calcium carbonate:

- Neonates: 50-150 mg/kg/day in 4-6 divided doses; not to exceed 1 g/day
- Children: 45-65 mg/kg/day in 4 divided doses
- Adults: 1-2 g or more per day

Monitoring Parameters Serum calcium and phosphate

Additional Information 20 mEq calcium/g calcium carbonate; 400 mg calcium/g calcium carbonate

Dosage Forms Note: Elemental calcium shown in parenthesis

Capsule: 1250 mg (500 mg)

Powder: 6500 mg/packet (2400 mg/packet)

Suspension: 1250 mg/5 mL (500 mg/5 mL)

Tablet: 650 mg (260 mg); 667 mg (267 mg); 1250 mg (500 mg); 1500 mg (600 mg)

Tablet, chewable: 750 mg (300 mg); 1250 mg (500 mg)

Calcium Chloride

Related Information

CPR Pediatric Drug Dosages *on page 614*

Extravasation Treatment *on page 640*

Brand Names Cal Plus®

Therapeutic Category Calcium Salt; Electrolyte Supplement, Parenteral

Use Emergency treatment of hypocalcemic tetany; treatment of hypermagnesemia; cardiac disturbances of hyperkalemia, hypocalcemia or calcium channel blocking agent toxicity

Pregnancy Risk Factor C

Contraindications Hypercalcemia, renal calculi, ventricular fibrillation

Precautions Avoid too rapid I.V. administration; avoid extravasation; use with caution in digitalized patients, in patients with respiratory failure or acidosis, sarcoidosis, renal or cardiac disease

Adverse Reactions

Cardiovascular: Vasodilation, hypotension, bradycardia, cardiac arrhythmias, ventricular fibrillation, syncope

Central nervous system: Lethargy, coma

Dermatologic: Erythema

Endocrine & metabolic: Elevated serum amylase, hypomagnesemia, hypercalcemia, hypercalciuria

Local: Tissue necrosis

Musculoskeletal: Muscle weakness

Drug Interactions Administer cautiously to a digitalized patient, may precipitate arrhythmias; calcium may antagonize the effects of verapamil

Stability Incompatible with bicarbonates, phosphates, and sulfates

Mechanism of Action Moderates nerve and muscle performance via action potential excitation threshold regulation

(Continued)

Calcium Chloride *(Continued)*

Usual Dosage I.V. (dose expressed in mg of calcium chloride):

Cardiac arrest in the presence of hyperkalemia or hypocalcemia, magnesium toxicity, or calcium antagonist toxicity:

Infants and Children: 20 mg/kg; may repeat in 10 minutes if necessary

Adults: 2-4 mg/kg; may repeat in 10 minutes if necessary

Hypocalcemia:

Infants and Children: 10-20 mg/kg/dose, repeat every 4-6 hours if needed

Adults: 500 mg to 1 g/dose every 6 hours

Hypocalcemia secondary to citrated blood transfusion: Give 0.45 mEq **elemental** calcium for each 100 mL citrated blood infused

Tetany:

Infants and Children: 10 mg/kg over 5-10 minutes. May repeat after 6 hours or follow with an infusion with a maximum dose of 200 mg/kg/day

Adults: 1 g over 10-30 minutes; may repeat after 6 hours

Administration Rapid I.V. injection at a maximum rate of 50 mg/minute; for I.V. infusion, dilute to a maximum concentration of 20 mg/mL and infuse over 1 hour or no greater than 45-90 mg/kg/hour (0.6-1.2 mEq/kg/hour)

Monitoring Parameters Serum calcium (ionized calcium preferred if available, see Additional Information), phosphate, magnesium, heart rate, EKG

Nursing Implications Do not inject calcium chloride I.M. or administer subcutaneously since severe necrosis and sloughing may occur. Extravasation of calcium chloride can also result in severe necrosis and sloughing. Do not use scalp vein or small hand or foot veins for I.V. administration

Additional Information Due to a poor correlation between the serum ionized calcium (free) and total serum calcium, particularly in states of low albumin or acid/base imbalances, direct measurement of ionized calcium is recommended. In low albumin states, the corrected **total** serum calcium may be estimated by this equation (assuming a normal albumin of 4 g/dL); corrected total calcium = total serum calcium + 0.8 (4- measured serum albumin)

Dosage Forms Injection: 100 mg/mL (10 mL) (1.4 mEq calcium/mL)

Calcium Disodium Edathamil *see* Edetate Calcium Disodium *on page 215*

Calcium Disodium Edetate *see* Edetate Calcium Disodium *on page 215*

Calcium Disodium Versenate® *see* Edetate Calcium Disodium *on page 215*

Calcium Edetate *see* Edetate Calcium Disodium *on page 215*

Calcium EDTA *see* Edetate Calcium Disodium *on page 215*

Calcium Glubionate (gloo bye' oh nate)

Brand Names Neo-Calglucon® [OTC]

Therapeutic Category Calcium Salt

Use Treatment and prevention of calcium depletion

Pregnancy Risk Factor C

Contraindications Hypercalcemia, renal calculi, ventricular fibrillation

Precautions Use cautiously in patients with sarcoidosis, renal or cardiac disease

Adverse Reactions

Central nervous system: Dizziness, headache, mental confusion

Endocrine & metabolic: Hypercalcemia, hypercalciuria, milk-alkali syndrome, hypomagnesemia, hypophosphatemia

Gastrointestinal: GI irritation, diarrhea, constipation, dry mouth

Drug Interactions Digoxin, tetracycline, may antagonize effects of verapamil

Mechanism of Action Moderates nerve and muscle performance via action potential excitation threshold regulation

Usual Dosage Dose expressed in mg of calcium glubionate

Neonatal hypocalcemia: 1200 mg/kg/day in 4-6 divided doses

Maintenance: Infants and Children: 600-2000 mg/kg/day in 4 divided doses up to a maximum of 9 g/day

Elemental Calcium Content of Calcium Salts

Calcium Salt	% Calcium	mEq Calcium/g
Calcium carbonate	40	20
Calcium chloride	27.3	13.6
Calcium glubionate	6.5	3.3
Calcium gluceptate	8.2	4.1
Calcium gluconate	9.3	4.6
Calcium lactate	13	12

Adults: 6-18 g/day in divided doses. See table.

Monitoring Parameters Serum calcium, magnesium, phosphate

Dosage Forms Syrup: 1.8 g/5 mL (480 mL) (115 mg calcium/mL)

Calcium Gluceptate (gloo sep' tate)

Therapeutic Category Calcium Salt

Use Emergency treatment of hypocalcemia; treatment of hypermagnesemia; cardiac disturbances of hyperkalemia; hypocalcemia, or calcium channel blocker toxicity

Pregnancy Risk Factor C

Contraindications Ventricular fibrillation, renal calculi, hypercalcemia

Precautions Avoid too rapid I.V. administration; avoid extravasation; use with caution in digitalized patients, in patients with respiratory failure or acidosis, sarcoidosis, renal or cardiac disease

Adverse Reactions

Cardiovascular: Vasodilation, hypotension, bradycardia, cardiac arrhythmias, ventricular fibrillation, syncope

Central nervous system: Lethargy, coma, mental confusion

Dermatologic: Erythema

Endocrine & metabolic: Elevated serum amylase, hypomagnesemia, hypercalcemia, hypercalciuria

Local: Tissue necrosis

Musculoskeletal: Muscle weakness

Drug Interactions Administer cautiously to a digitalized patient, may precipitate arrhythmias; calcium may antagonize the effects of verapamil

Stability Admixture incompatibilities: Carbonates, phosphates, sulfates

Mechanism of Action Moderates nerve and muscle performance via action potential excitation threshold regulation

Usual Dosage I.V. (dose expressed in mg of calcium gluceptate):

Cardiac resuscitation in the presence of hypocalcemia, hyperkalemia, magnesium toxicity, or calcium channel blocker toxicity:

Children: 110 mg/kg/dose

Adults: 1.1-1.54 g (5-7 mL)

Hypocalcemia:

Children: 200-500 mg/kg/day divided every 6 hours

Adults: 500 mg to 1.1 g/dose as needed

After citrated blood administration: Children and Adults: 0.4 mEq/100 mL blood infused

Administration Rapid I.V. injection at a maximum rate of 50 mg/minute; for I.V. infusion, dilute to a maximum concentration of 55 mg/mL and infuse over 1 hour or no greater than 150-300 mg/kg/hour (0.6-1.2 mEq calcium/kg/hour)

Monitoring Parameters Serum calcium (ionized calcium preferred if available, see Additional Information), magnesium, phosphate, heart rate, EKG

Additional Information Due to a poor correlation between the serum ionized calcium (free) and total serum calcium, particularly in states of low albumin or acid/base imbalances, direct measurement of ionized calcium is recommended. In low albumin states, the corrected **total** serum calcium may be estimated by this equation (assuming a normal albumin of 4 g/dL); corrected total calcium = total serum calcium + 0.8 (4- measured serum albumin)

Dosage Forms Injection: 220 mg/mL = 0.9 mEq/mL (5 mL)

Calcium Gluconate (gloo' koe nate)

Related Information

Extravasation Treatment *on page 640*

Therapeutic Category Calcium Salt; Electrolyte Supplement, Oral; Electrolyte Supplement, Parenteral

Use Treatment and prevention of hypocalcemia, hypermagnesemia, cardiac disturbances of hyperkalemia, hypocalcemia, or calcium channel blocker toxicity

Pregnancy Risk Factor C

Contraindications Hypercalcemia, renal calculi, ventricular fibrillation

Precautions Avoid too rapid I.V. administration and extravasation; use with caution in digitalized patients, in patients with respiratory failure or acidosis, sarcoidosis, renal or cardiac disease

Adverse Reactions

Cardiovascular: Vasodilation, hypotension, bradycardia, cardiac arrhythmias, ventricular fibrillation, syncope

Central nervous system: Lethargy, coma, mental confusion

Dermatologic: Erythema

Endocrine & metabolic: Elevated serum amylase, hypomagnesemia, hypercalcemia, hypercalciuria

Local: Tissue necrosis

Musculoskeletal: Muscle weakness

Drug Interactions Administer cautiously to a digitalized patient, may precipitate arrhythmias; calcium may antagonize the effects of verapamil

Stability Incompatible with bicarbonates, phosphates, and sulfates

Mechanism of Action Moderates nerve and muscle performance via action potential excitation threshold regulation

Usual Dosage I.V.:

Hypocalcemia:

- Neonates: 200-800 mg/kg/day as a continuous infusion or in 4 divided doses
- Infants and Children: 200-500 mg/kg/day as a continuous infusion or in 4 divided doses
- Adults: 2-15 g/24 hours as a continuous infusion or in divided doses

Hypocalcemia secondary to citrated blood infusion: Give 0.45 mEq **elemental** calcium for each 100 mL citrated blood infused

Calcium antagonist toxicity, magnesium intoxication; cardiac arrest in the presence of hyperkalemia or hypocalcemia:

- Infants/children: 100 mg/kg/dose (maximum: 3 g/dose)
- Adults: 500-800 mg; maximum: 3 g

Tetany:

- Neonates: 100-200 mg/kg/dose, may follow with 500 mg/kg/day in 3-4 divided doses or as an infusion
- Infants and Children: 100-200 mg/kg/dose over 5-10 minutes; may repeat after 6 hours or follow with an infusion of 500 mg/kg/day
- Adults: 1-3 g may be administered until therapeutic response occurs

Administration Rapid I.V. injection at a maximum rate of 50 mg/minute; for I.V. infusion, dilute to a maximum concentration of 50 mg/mL and infuse over 1 hour or no greater than 120-240 mg/kg/hour (0.6-1.2 mEq calcium/kg/hour)

Monitoring Parameters Serum calcium (ionized calcium preferred if available, see Additional Information), magnesium, phosphate, heart rate, EKG

Nursing Implications Do not administer I.M. or S.C.

Additional Information One (1) g calcium gluconate = 90 mg elemental calcium = 4.8 mEq calcium; due to a poor correlation between the serum ionized calcium (free) and total serum calcium, particularly in states of low albumin or acid/base imbalances, direct measurement of ionized calcium is recommended. If ionized calcium is unavailable, in low albumin states, the corrected **total** serum calcium may be estimated by this equation (assuming a normal albumin of 4 g/dL); corrected total calcium = total serum calcium + 0.8 (4- measured serum albumin)

Dosage Forms Injection: 10% = 100 mg/mL = 0.45 mEq calcium/mL (10 mL)

Calcium Lactate (lak' tate)

Therapeutic Category Calcium Salt

Use Treatment and prevention of calcium depletion

Pregnancy Risk Factor C

Contraindications Hypercalcemia, renal calculi, ventricular fibrillation

Precautions Use cautiously in patients with sarcoidosis, renal insufficiency, cardiac disease, or digitalized patients

Adverse Reactions

Central nervous system: Headache, mental confusion, dizziness

Endocrine & metabolic: Hypercalcemia, milk-alkali syndrome, hypophosphatemia, hypercalciuria, hypomagnesemia

Gastrointestinal: Constipation, nausea, dry mouth, vomiting

Drug Interactions Digoxin, tetracycline, may antagonize the effects of verapamil

Mechanism of Action Moderates nerve and muscle performance via action potential excitation threshold regulation

Usual Dosage Oral:

Infants: 400-500 mg/kg/day divided every 4-6 hours

Children: 500 mg/kg/day divided every 6-8 hours; maximum daily dose: 9 g

Adults: 1.5-3 g divided every 8 hours

Monitoring Parameters Serum calcium, magnesium, phosphate

Additional Information 1 g = 130 mg elemental calcium

Dosage Forms Tablet: 325 mg, 650 mg

Calcium Leucovorin *see* Leucovorin Calcium *on page 335*

Calcium Undecylenate *see* Undecylenic Acid and Derivatives *on page 590*

CaldeCORT® *see* Hydrocortisone *on page 293*

Caldesene® [OTC] *see* Undecylenic Acid and Derivatives *on page 590*

Cal-Guard Softgels® [OTC] *see* Calcium Carbonate *on page 94*

Calm-X® [OTC] *see* Dimenhydrinate *on page 193*

Cal Plus® *see* Calcium Chloride *on page 95*

CalSup® [OTC] *see* Calcium Carbonate *on page 94*

Caltrate® [OTC] *see* Calcium Carbonate *on page 94*

Camphorated Tincture of Opium *see* Paregoric *on page 435*

Cank-aid® [OTC] *see* Carbamide Peroxide *on page 103*

Capital® and Codeine *see* Acetaminophen and Codeine Phosphate *on page 17*

Capoten® *see* Captopril *on next page*

Capsaicin (kap say' sin)

Brand Names Zostrix® [OTC]; Zostrix-HP® [OTC]

Therapeutic Category Topical Skin Product

Use Capsaicin is FDA approved for the topical treatment of pain associated with postherpetic neuralgia, rheumatoid arthritis, osteoarthritis, diabetic neuropathy, and postsurgical pain.

Unlabeled uses: Treatment of pain associated with psoriasis, chronic neuralgias unresponsive to other forms of therapy, and intractable pruritus

Contraindications Hypersensitivity to capsaicin or any component

Warnings Avoid contact with eyes, mucous membrane, or with damaged or irritated skin

Precautions Since warm water or excessive sweating may intensify the localized burning sensation after capsaicin application, the affected area should not be tightly bandaged or exposed to direct sunlight or a heat lamp

Adverse Reactions

Local: Itching, burning, or stinging sensation, erythema

Respiratory: Cough

Mechanism of Action Induces release of substance P, the principal chemomediator of pain impulses from the periphery to the CNS, from peripheral sensory neurons. After repeated application, capsaicin depletes the neuron of substance P and prevents reaccumulation.

Pharmacodynamics

Onset of action: Pain relief is usually seen within 14-28 days of regular topical application; maximal response may require 4-6 weeks of continuous therapy

(Continued)

Capsaicin *(Continued)*

Duration: Several hours

Usual Dosage Children ≥2 years and Adults: Topical: Apply to affected area at least 3-4 times/day; application frequency less than 3-4 times/day prevents the total depletion, inhibition of synthesis, and transport of substance P resulting in decreased clinical efficacy and increased local discomfort

Patient Information For external use only. Avoid washing treated areas for 30 minutes after application; should not be applied to wounds or damaged skin; avoid eye and mucous membrane exposure

Nursing Implications Wash hands with soap and water after applying to avoid spreading cream to eyes or other sensitive areas of the body

Additional Information In patients with severe and persistent local discomfort, pretreatment with topical lidocaine 5% ointment or concurrent oral analgesics for the first 2 weeks of therapy have been effective in alleviating the initial burning sensation and enabling continuation of topical capsaicin

Dosage Forms Cream: 0.025% (45 g, 90 g); 0.075% (30 g, 60 g)

References

Bernstein JE, Korman NJ, Bickers DR, et al, "Topical Capsaicin Treatment of Chronic Postherpetic Neuralgia," *J Am Acad Dermatol*, 1989, 21(2 Pt 1):265-70.

Captopril (kap' toe pril)

Brand Names Capoten®

Therapeutic Category Angiotensin Converting Enzyme (ACE) Inhibitors; Antihypertensive

Use Management of hypertension and treatment of congestive heart failure

Pregnancy Risk Factor D

Contraindications Hypersensitivity to captopril or any component

Warnings ACE inhibitor can cause injury and death to the developing fetus when used during the second and third trimester of pregnancy

Precautions Use with caution and modify dosage in patients with renal impairment; use with caution in patients with collagen vascular disease

Adverse Reactions

Cardiovascular: Hypotension, tachycardia
Dermatologic: Rash
Endocrine & metabolic: Hyperkalemia
Hematologic: Neutropenia, agranulocytosis,
Respiratory: Transient cough
Renal & genitourinary: Increased BUN and serum creatinine, proteinuria
Miscellaneous: Loss of taste perception, angioedema

Drug Interactions Captopril + potassium sparing diuretics → additive hyperkalemic effect; captopril + indomethacin or nonsteroidal anti-inflammatory agents → reduced antihypertensive response to captopril

Stability Unstable in aqueous solutions

Mechanism of Action Competitive inhibitor of angiotensin converting enzyme (ACE); prevents conversion of angiotensin I to angiotensin II, a potent vasoconstrictor; results in lower levels of angiotensin II which causes an increase in plasma renin activity and a reduction in aldosterone secretion

Pharmacodynamics

Onset of action: Decrease in blood pressure within 15 minutes; maximum effect: 60-90 minutes; may require several weeks of therapy before full hypotensive effect is seen

Duration: Dose related

Pharmacokinetics

Absorption: 60% to 75%
Distribution: 7 L/kg
Protein binding: 25% to 30%
Metabolism: 50% metabolized
Half-life:
- Infants with congestive heart failure: 3.3 hours with range: 1.2-12.4 hours
- Children: 1.5 hours with range: 0.98-2.3 hours
- Normal adults (dependent upon renal and cardiac function): 1.9 hours
- Adults with congestive heart failure: 2.06 hours
- Anuria: 20-40 hours

Peak serum levels: Within 1-2 hours

Elimination: 95% excreted in the urine in 24 hours

Usual Dosage Note: Dosage must be titrated according to patient's response; use lowest effective dose. Oral:

Neonates: Initial: 0.05-0.1 mg/kg/dose every 8-24 hours; titrate dose up to 0.5 mg/kg/dose given every 6-24 hours

Infants: Initial: 0.15-0.3 mg/kg/dose; titrate dose upward to maximum of 6 mg/kg/day in 1-4 divided doses; usual required dose: 2.5-6 mg/kg/day

Children: Initial: 0.5 mg/kg/dose; titrate upward to maximum of 6 mg/kg/day in 2-4 divided doses

Older children: Initial: 6.25-12.5 mg/dose every 12-24 hours; titrate upward to maximum of 6 mg/kg/day

Adolescents and Adults: Initial: 12.5-25 mg/dose given every 8-12 hours; increase by 25 mg/dose to maximum of 450 mg/day

Dosing adjustment in renal impairment: Reduce dose and give every 8-12 hours

Monitoring Parameters BUN, serum creatinine, renal function, urine dipstick for protein, complete leukocyte count, blood pressure, serum potassium

Nursing Implications Give at least 1 hour before meals

Additional Information Severe hypotension may occur in patients who are sodium and/or volume depleted

Dosage Forms Tablet: 12.5 mg, 25 mg, 50 mg, 100 mg

Extemporaneous Preparation(s) Stability in aqueous solution is temperature dependent and related to geographical source and chemical (metal) content of tap water used. A 1 mg/mL solution (made by crushing a 25 mg tablet and adding it to 25 mL of tap water from Edmonton, Alberta, Canada) has been found to be stable for 27 days at 5°C, 11.8 days at 25°C, 3.6 days at 50°C, and 2.1 days at 75°C. However, captopril 1 mg/mL in tap water from Rochester, New York was extremely unstable. Captopril 1 mg/mL in sterile water for irrigation was stable for at least 3 days when kept refrigerated. Other factors not yet identified may influence captopril oxidation in aqueous solution. Powder papers can be made; powder papers are stable for 12 weeks when stored at room temperature.

Anaizi NH and Swenson C, "Instability of Aqueous Captopril Solutions," *Am J Hosp Pharm*, 1993, 50:486-8.

Pereira CM and Tam YK, "Stability of Captopril in Tap Water," *Am J Hosp Pharm*, 1992, 49(3):612-5.

Taketomo CK, Chu SA, Cheng MH, et al, "Stability of Captopril in Powder Papers Under Three Storage Conditions," *Am J Hosp Pharm*, 1990, 47(8):1799-801.

References

Friedman WF and George BL, "New Concepts and Drugs in the Treatment of Congestive Heart Failure," *Pediatr Clin North Am*, 1984, 31(6):1197-227.

Levy M, Koren G, Klein J, et al, "Captopril Pharmacokinetics, Blood Pressure Response and Plasma Renin Activity in Normotensive Children With Renal Scarring," *Dev Pharmacol Ther*, 1991, 16(4):185-93.

Mirkin BL and Newman TJ, "Efficacy and Safety of Captopril in the Treatment of Severe Childhood Hypertension: Report of the International Collaborative Study Group," *Pediatrics*, 1985, 75(6):1091-100.

Pereira CM, Tam YK, Collins-Nakai RL, "The Pharmacokinetics of Captopril in Infants With Congestive Heart Failure," *Ther Drug Monit*, 1991, 13(3):209-14.

Carafate® *see* Sucralfate *on page 538*

Carampicillin Hydrochloride *see* Bacampicillin Hydrochloride *on page 72*

Carbamazepine (kar ba maz' e peen)

Related Information

Blood Level Sampling Time Guidelines *on page 694-695*

Overdose and Toxicology Information *on page 696-700*

Brand Names Epitol®; Tegretol®

Therapeutic Category Anticonvulsant

(Continued)

Carbamazepine *(Continued)*

Use Prophylaxis of generalized tonic-clonic, partial (especially complex partial), and mixed partial or generalized seizure disorder; may be used to relieve pain in trigeminal neuralgia or diabetic neuropathy; has been used to treat bipolar disorders

Pregnancy Risk Factor C

Contraindications Hypersensitivity to carbamazepine or any component; may have cross sensitivity with tricyclic antidepressants; should not be used in any patient with bone marrow depression

Warnings Potentially fatal blood cell abnormalities have been reported following treatment; early detection of hematologic change is important; advise patients of early signs and symptoms which are: fever, sore throat, mouth ulcers, infections, easy bruising, petechial or purpuric hemorrhage

Precautions MAO inhibitors should be discontinued for a minimum of 14 days before carbamazepine is begun; administer with caution to patients with history of cardiac damage, hepatic disease, or renal failure

Adverse Reactions

Cardiovascular: Edema, congestive heart failure, syncope

Central nervous system: Sedation, dizziness, fatigue, slurred speech, ataxia

Dermatologic: Rash

Endocrine & metabolic: Hyponatremia

Gastrointestinal: Nausea

Hematologic: Neutropenia (can be transient), aplastic anemia, agranulocytosis

Hepatic: Hepatitis

Ocular: Nystagmus, diplopia

Renal & genitourinary: Urinary retention

Drug Interactions Erythromycin, isoniazid, propoxyphene, verapamil, diltiazem, and cimetidine may inhibit hepatic metabolism of carbamazepine with resultant ↑ of carbamazepine serum concentrations and toxicity; carbamazepine may induce the metabolism of warfarin, doxycycline, oral contraceptives, phenytoin, theophylline, benzodiazepines, ethosuximide, valproic acid, corticosteroids and thyroid hormones

Mechanism of Action May depress activity in the nucleus ventralis of the thalamus or decrease synaptic transmission or decrease summation of temporal stimulation leading to neural discharge, by limiting influx of sodium ions across cell membrane; other unknown mechanisms; stimulates the release of ADH and potentiates its action in promoting reabsorption of water; chemically related to tricyclic antidepressants; in addition to anticonvulsant effects, carbamazepine has anticholinergic, antineuralgic, antidiuretic, muscle relaxant and antiarrhythmic properties

Pharmacokinetics

Absorption: Slowly absorbed from the GI tract

Distribution: V_d:
- Neonates: 1.5 L/kg
- Children: 1.9 L/kg
- Adults: 0.59-2 L/kg

Protein binding: 75% to 90%; protein binding may be decreased in newborns

Induces liver enzymes to increase metabolism and shorten half-life over time

Metabolism: Metabolized in liver to active epoxide metabolite

Bioavailability, oral: 85%

Half-life:
- Initial: 18-55 hours
- Multiple dosing:
  - Children: 8-14 hours
  - Adults: 12-17 hours

Peak levels: Unpredictable, within 4-8 hours

Elimination: 1% to 3% excreted unchanged in urine

Usual Dosage Dosage must be adjusted according to patient's response and serum concentrations. Oral:

Children:
- <6 years: Initial: 5 mg/kg/day; dosage may be increased every 5-7 days to 10 mg/kg/day; then up to 20 mg/kg/day if necessary; administer in 2-4 divided doses/day

6-12 years: Initial: 100 mg twice daily or 10 mg/kg/day in 2 divided doses; increase by 100 mg/day at weekly intervals until therapeutic levels achieved; usual maintenance: 15-30 mg/kg/day in 2-4 divided doses/day

Children >12 years and Adults: 200 mg twice daily to start, increase by 200 mg/day at weekly intervals until therapeutic levels achieved; usual dose: 800-1200 mg/day in 3-4 divided doses; some patients have required up to 1.6-2.4 g/day

Dosing adjustment in renal impairment: Cl_{cr} <10 mL/minute: Administer 75% of recommended dose; monitor serum levels

Monitoring Parameters CBC with platelet count, liver function tests, serum drug concentration; observe patient for excessive sedation especially when instituting or increasing therapy

Reference Range Therapeutic: 4-12 μg/mL (SI: 17-51 μmol/L). Patients who require higher levels (8-12 μg/mL (SI: 34-51 μmol/L)) should be carefully monitored. Side effects (especially CNS) occur commonly at higher levels. If other anticonvulsants are given therapeutic range is 4-8 μg/mL (SI: 17-34 μmol/L).

Nursing Implications Shake suspension well before use

Additional Information Suspension dosage should be given on a 3-4 times/day schedule vs tablet which can be given 2-4 times/day; carbamazepine is not effective in absence, myoclonic or akinetic seizures; exacerbation of certain seizure types have been seen after initiation of carbamazepine therapy in children with mixed seizure disorders

Investigationally, loading doses of the suspension (10 mg/kg for children <12 years of age and 8 mg/kg for children >12 years) were given (via NG or ND tubes followed by 5-10 mL of water to flush through tube) to PICU patients with frequent seizures/status; 5 of 6 patients attained mean Cp of 4.3 μg/mL and 7.3 μg/mL at 1 and 2 hours postload; concurrent enteral feeding or ileus may delay absorption

Dosage Forms

Suspension, oral (citrus-vanilla flavor): 100 mg/5 mL (450 mL)

Tablet: 200 mg

Tablet, chewable: 100 mg

References

Gilman JT, "Carbamazepine Dosing for Pediatric Seizure Disorders: The Highs and Lows," *DICP*, 1991, 25(10):1109-12.

Miles MV, Lawless ST, Tennison MB, et al, "Rapid Loading of Critically Ill Patients With Carbamazepine Suspension," *Pediatrics*, 1990, 86(2):263-6.

Carbamide Peroxide (kar' ba mide)

Brand Names Auro® Ear Drops [OTC]; Cank-aid® [OTC]; Debrox® [OTC]; Gly-Oxide® [OTC]; Murine® Ear Drops [OTC]; Orajel® Brace-Aid Rinse [OTC]; Proxigel® [OTC]

Synonyms Urea Peroxide

Therapeutic Category Otic Agent, Cerumenolytic

Use Relief of minor inflammation of gums, oral mucosal surfaces and lips including canker sores and dental irritation; emulsify and disperse ear wax; adjunct in oral hygiene

Pregnancy Risk Factor C

Contraindications Otic preparation should not be used in patients with a perforated tympanic membrane or following otic surgery; ear drainage, ear pain, or rash in the ear; dizziness; oral preparation should not be used for self medication in children <3 years of age

Warnings With prolonged use of oral carbamide peroxide, there is a potential for overgrowth of opportunistic organisms; damage to periodontal tissues; delayed wound healing

Adverse Reactions

Central nervous system: Dizziness

Dermatologic: Rash

Local: Irritation, tenderness, pain, redness

Stability Protect from heat and direct light

Mechanism of Action Carbamide peroxide releases hydrogen peroxide which serves as a source of nascent oxygen upon contact with catalase; deodorant action is probably due to inhibition of odor-causing bacteria; softens impacted cerumen due to its foaming action

(Continued)

Carbamide Peroxide *(Continued)*

Pharmacodynamics Onset of effect: Slight disintegration of hard ear wax in 24 hours

Usual Dosage Children and Adults:

Oral:

Solution: Apply several drops undiluted to affected area of the mouth 4 times/day and at bedtime for up to 7 days, expectorate after 2-3 minutes; as an adjunct to oral hygiene after brushing, swish 10 drops for 2-3 minutes, then expectorate

Gel: Massage on affected area 4 times/day

Otic: Solution: Instill 5-10 drops twice daily for up to 4 days in children ≥12 years or adults; keep drops in ear for several minutes by keeping head tilted or placing cotton in ear. In children <12 years, individualize the dose according to patient size; 3 drops (range: 1-5 drops) twice daily for up to 4 days

Patient Information Contact physician if dizziness or otic redness, rash, irritation, tenderness, pain, drainage or discharge develop; do not use in the eye

Nursing Implications Drops foam on contact with ear wax

Additional Information Otic preparation should not be used for >4 days; oral preparation should not be used for >7 days

Dosage Forms

Gel, oral: 11% (36 g)

Solution:

Oral: 10% in glycerin (15 mL, 22.5 mL, 30 mL, 60 mL)

Otic: 6.5% in glycerin (15 mL)

Carbenicillin Indanyl Sodium (kar ben i sill' in)

Brand Names Geocillin®

Synonyms Carindacillin

Therapeutic Category Antibiotic, Penicillin

Use Treatment of urinary tract infections, asymptomatic bacteriuria, or prostatitis caused by susceptible strains of *Pseudomonas aeruginosa*, indole-positive *Proteus*, and *Enterobacter*

Pregnancy Risk Factor B

Contraindications Hypersensitivity to carbenicillin or any component, penicillins or cephalosporins

Warnings Oral carbenicillin should be limited to treatment of urinary tract infections

Precautions Do not use in patients with severe renal impairment (Cl_{cr} <10 mL/minute)

Adverse Reactions

Dermatologic: Rash, urticaria, pruritus

Gastrointestinal: Nausea, vomiting, diarrhea, abdominal cramps

Hematologic: Eosinophilia, hemolytic anemia, neutropenia, thrombocytopenia

Hepatic: Elevation in liver enzymes, hepatotoxicity

Miscellaneous: Furry tongue

Drug Interactions Probenecid, lithium

Mechanism of Action Interferes with bacterial cell wall synthesis during active multiplication

Pharmacokinetics

Absorption: Oral: 30% to 40%; in patients with normal renal function, serum concentrations of carbenicillin following oral absorption are inadequate for the treatment of systemic infections

Protein binding: 50%

Half-life:

Neonates:

<7 days, ≤2.5 kg: 4 hours

<7 days, >2.5 kg: 2.7 hours

Children: 0.8-1.8 hours

Adults: 60-90 minutes and is prolonged to 10-20 hours with renal insufficiency

Peak levels: Within 30-120 minutes

Elimination: Carbenicillin and its metabolites are excreted in the urine; ~80% to 99% of the dose is excreted unchanged in the urine

Moderately dialyzable (20% to 50%)

Usual Dosage Oral:

Children: 30-50 mg/kg/day divided every 6 hours; maximum dose: 2-3 g/day

Adults: 1-2 tablets every 6 hours

Monitoring Parameters Renal, hepatic, and hematologic function tests

Test Interactions False-positive urine or serum proteins; false-positive urine glucose (Clinitest®)

Patient Information Tablets have a bitter taste

Additional Information Sodium content of 382 mg tablet: 23 mg

Dosage Forms Tablet, film coated: 382 mg

Carbinoxamine and Pseudoephedrine

(kar bi nox' a meen)

Brand Names Rondec® Drops; Rondec® Filmtab®; Rondec® Syrup; Rondec-TR®

Therapeutic Category Antihistamine/Decongestant Combination

Use Temporary relief of nasal congestion, running nose, sneezing, itching of nose or throat, and itchy, watery eyes due to the common cold, hay fever, or other respiratory allergies

Pregnancy Risk Factor C

Contraindications Hypersensitivity to carbinoxamine or pseudoephedrine or any component; severe hypertension or coronary artery disease, MAO inhibitor therapy, GI or GU obstruction, narrow-angle glaucoma; avoid use in premature or term infants due to a possible association with SIDS

Warnings May impair ability to perform hazardous activities requiring mental alertness or physical coordination

Precautions Use with caution in patients with mild to moderate hypertension, heart disease, diabetes, asthma, thyroid disease, or prostatic hypertrophy

Adverse Reactions

Cardiovascular: Hypertension, tachycardia, arrhythmias

Central nervous system: Sedation, CNS stimulation, headache, seizures, weakness

Gastrointestinal: Nausea, vomiting, dry mouth, anorexia, diarrhea, heart burn

Genitourinary: Polyuria, dysuria

Ocular: Diplopia

Drug Interactions MAO inhibitors, alpha- and beta-adrenergic blocking agents, other sympathomimetics, sedatives, alcohol, barbiturates, and other CNS depressants

Mechanism of Action Carbinoxamine competes with histamine for H_1-receptor sites on effector cells in the gastrointestinal tract, blood vessels, and respiratory tract

Usual Dosage Oral:

Children (may dose according to pseudoephedrine component): 4 mg/kg/day **or**

Drops:

1-3 months: ¼ dropperful (0.25 mL) 4 times/day

3-6 months: ½ dropperful (0.5 mL) 4 times/day

6-9 months: ¾ dropperful (0.75 mL) 4 times/day

9-18 months: 1 dropperful (1 mL) 4 times/day

Syrup or tablet:

18 months to 6 years: 2.5 mL 4 times/day

6-12 years: 5 mL or 1 tablet 4 times/day

Extended release tablet:

Children >12 years and Adults: 1 tablet 2 times/day

Patient Information May cause drowsiness, impaired coordination, or judgment; may cause blurred vision; may also cause CNS excitation and difficulty sleeping

Nursing Implications Raise bed rails; institute safety measures; assist with ambulation

Additional Information Do not crush or chew extended release tablets

Dosage Forms

Drops: Carbinoxamine maleate 2 mg and pseudoephedrine hydrochloride 25 mg per mL (30 mL with dropper)

(Continued)

Carbinoxamine and Pseudoephedrine *(Continued)*

Syrup: Carbinoxamine maleate 4 mg and pseudoephedrine hydrochloride 60 mg per 5 mL

Tablet:

Film-coated: Carbinoxamine maleate 4 mg and pseudoephedrine hydrochloride 60 mg

Sustained release: Carbinoxamine maleate 8 mg and pseudoephedrine hydrochloride 120 mg

Carboplatin (kar' boe pla tin)

Brand Names Paraplatin®

Synonyms CBDCA

Therapeutic Category Antineoplastic Agent

Use Palliative treatment of ovarian carcinoma; also used in the treatment of small cell lung cancer, squamous cell carcinoma of the esophagus; solid tumors of the bladder, cervix and testes; pediatric brain tumor, neuroblastoma

Pregnancy Risk Factor D

Contraindications Hypersensitivity to carboplatin, cisplatin, or other platinum-containing compounds, or mannitol; severe bone marrow depression or excessive bleeding

Warnings The US Food and Drug Administration (FDA) currently recommends that procedures for proper handling and disposal of antineoplastic agents be considered

Precautions Bone marrow depression, which may be severe, and vomiting are dose related; high doses have also resulted in severe abnormalities of liver function; reduce dosage in patients with bone marrow suppression and impaired renal function (creatinine clearance values <60 mL/minute)

Adverse Reactions

Central nervous system: Peripheral neuropathy, pain, asthenia

Dermatologic: Urticaria, rash, alopecia

Endocrine & metabolic: Electrolyte abnormalities such as hypocalcemia and hypomagnesemia

Gastrointestinal: Nausea, vomiting

Hematologic: Neutropenia, leukopenia, thrombocytopenia (platelet count reaches a nadir between 14-21 days), anemia

Hepatic: Abnormal liver function tests

Otic: Ototoxicity in 1% of patients

Renal & genitourinary: Nephrotoxicity

Drug Interactions Nephrotoxic drugs (increased renal toxicity)

Stability Store unopened vials at room temperature; protect from light; after reconstitution, solutions are stable for 8 hours; solutions diluted in D_5W for infusion are stable for 24 hours; aluminum reacts with carboplatin resulting in a precipitate

Mechanism of Action Possible cross-linking and interference with the function of DNA

Pharmacokinetics

Distribution: V_d: 16 L/kg

Protein binding: 0%; however, platinum is 30% protein bound

Half-life: Patients with Cl_{cr} >60 mL/minute: 2.5-5.9 hours

Elimination: ~60% to 80% is excreted renally

Usual Dosage I.V. (refer to individual protocols):

Children:

Solid tumor: 560 mg/m^2 once every 4 weeks

Brain tumor: 175 mg/m^2 once weekly for 4 weeks with a 2-week recovery period between courses; dose is then adjusted on platelet count and neutrophil count values

Adults: Single agent: 360 mg/m^2 once every 4 weeks; dose is then adjusted on platelet count and neutrophil count values

Administration Administer by I.V. intermittent infusion over 15 minutes to 1 hour, or by continuous infusion (continuous infusion regimens may be less toxic than the bolus route); reconstituted carboplatin 10 mg/mL should be further diluted to a final concentration of 0.5-2 mg/mL with D_5W or NS for administration

Monitoring Parameters CBC with differential and platelet count, serum electrolytes, urinalysis, creatinine clearance, liver function tests

Nursing Implications Needle or intravenous administration sets containing aluminum parts should not be used in the administration or preparation of carboplatin (aluminum can interact with carboplatin resulting in precipitate formation and loss of potency)

Dosage Forms Powder for injection, lyophilized: 50 mg, 150 mg, 450 mg

References

Lovett D, Kelsen D, Eisenberger M, et al, "A Phase II Trial of Carboplatin and Vinblastine in the Treatment of Advanced Squamous Cell Carcinoma of the Esophagus," *Cancer*, 1991, 67(2):354-6.

Oguri S, Sakakibara T, Mase H, et al, "Clinical Pharmacokinetics of Carboplatin," *J Clin Pharmacol*, 1988, 28(3):208-15.

Reece PA, Stafford I, Abbott RI, et al, "Two- Versus 24-Hour Infusion of Cisplatin: Pharmacokinetic Considerations," *J Clin Oncol*, 1989, 7(2):270-5.

Zeltzer PM, Epport K, Nelson MD Jr, et al, "Prolonged Response to Carboplatin in an Infant With Brain Stem Glioma," *Cancer*, 1991, 67(1):43-7.

Cardioquin® *see* Quinidine *on page 505*

Carindacillin *see* Carbenicillin Indanyl Sodium *on page 104*

Carmustine (kar mus' teen)

Related Information

Emetogenic Potential of Single Chemotherapeutic Agents *on page 655*

Brand Names BiCNU®

Synonyms BCNU

Therapeutic Category Antineoplastic Agent

Use Palliative treatment of brain tumors, multiple myeloma, Hodgkin's disease and non-Hodgkin's lymphomas, melanoma, and lung cancer

Pregnancy Risk Factor D

Contraindications Hypersensitivity to carmustine or any component

Warnings The US Food and Drug Administration (FDA) currently recommends that procedures for proper handling and disposal of antineoplastic agents be considered. Bone marrow depression, notably thrombocytopenia and leukopenia, may lead to bleeding and overwhelming infection in an already compromised patient; myelosuppressive effects will last for at least 6 weeks after a dose, do not give courses more frequently than every 6 weeks because the toxicity is cumulative; pulmonary toxicity is more common in patients receiving a cumulative dose >1400 mg/m^2

Precautions Administer with caution to patients with depressed platelet, leukocyte or erythrocyte counts; dosage reduction is recommended in patients with compromised bone marrow function (decreased leukocyte and platelet counts)

Adverse Reactions

Cardiovascular: Flushing
Dermatologic: Dermatitis
Gastrointestinal: Nausea, vomiting
Hematologic: Myelosuppression with nadir at 28 days
Hepatic: Hepatotoxicity
Local: Pain and thrombophlebitis at injection site
Renal & genitourinary: Renal failure
Respiratory: Pulmonary fibrosis

Drug Interactions Cimetidine (potentiates myelosuppressive effects)

Stability Store in refrigerator, protect from light and heat; stable for 8 hours at room temperature, 24 hours when refrigerated, or 48 hours when refrigerated after further dilution in D_5W or NS in a glass bottle to a concentration of 0.2 mg/mL; incompatible with sodium bicarbonate

Mechanism of Action Interferes with the normal function of DNA by alkylation and cross-linking the strands of DNA, and by possible protein modification

Pharmacokinetics

Distribution: Readily crosses the blood-brain barrier since it is highly lipid soluble, distributes into breast milk
Protein binding: 75%
Metabolism: Rapidly metabolized
Half-life, terminal: 20-70 minutes (active metabolites may persist for days)
Elimination: ~60% to 70% excreted in the urine and 6% to 10% excreted as CO_2 by the lungs

(Continued)

Carmustine *(Continued)*

Usual Dosage I.V. infusion (refer to individual protocols):

Children: 200-250 mg/m^2 every 4-6 weeks as a single dose

Adults: 150-200 mg/m^2 every 6 weeks as a single dose or divided into 75-100 mg/m^2/dose on 2 successive days; next dose is to be determined based on hematologic response to the previous dose

Administration Further dilute the 3.3 mg of carmustine per mL solution with normal saline or D_5W and administer by I.V. infusion over 1-2 hours to prevent vein irritation

Monitoring Parameters CBC with differential and platelet count; pulmonary function, liver function, and renal function tests

Nursing Implications Must administer in glass containers; do not mix with solutions containing sodium bicarbonate; accidental skin contact may cause transient burning and brown discoloration of the skin

Additional Information Myelosuppressive effects:

WBC: Moderate (nadir: 5-6 weeks)

Platelets: Severe (nadir: 4-5 weeks)

Dosage Forms Powder for injection: 100 mg/vial packaged with 3 mL of absolute alcohol for use as a diluent

References

Aronin PA, Mahaley MS, Rudnick SA, et al, "Prediction of BCNU Pulmonary Toxicity in Patients With Malignant Gliomas," *N Engl J Med*, 1980, 303(4):183-8.

Colvin M, Hartner J and Summerfield M, "Stability of Carmustine in the Presence of Sodium Bicarbonate," *Am J Hosp Pharm*, 1980, 37(5):677-8.

Carnitor® *see* Levocarnitine *on page 338*

Carter's Little Pills® [OTC] *see* Bisacodyl *on page 83*

Casanthranol and Docusate *see* Docusate and Casanthranol *on page 203*

Cascara Sagrada (kas kar' a)

Therapeutic Category Laxative, Stimulant

Use Temporary relief of constipation; sometimes used with milk of magnesia ("black and white" mixture)

Pregnancy Risk Factor C

Contraindications Nausea, vomiting, abdominal pain, fecal impaction, intestinal obstruction, GI bleeding, appendicitis, congestive heart failure

Warnings Long-term use may result in laxative dependence

Adverse Reactions

Cardiovascular: Faintness

Endocrine & metabolic: Electrolyte and fluid imbalance

Gastrointestinal: Abdominal cramps, nausea, diarrhea

Renal & genitourinary: Discolors urine reddish pink or brown

Stability Protect from light and heat

Mechanism of Action Direct chemical irritation of the intestinal mucosa resulting in an increased rate of colonic motility and change in fluid and electrolyte secretion

Pharmacodynamics Onset of action: 6-10 hours

Pharmacokinetics

Absorption: Oral: Small amount absorbed from small intestine

Metabolism: Metabolized in the liver

Usual Dosage Oral (aromatic fluid extract):

Infants: 1.25 mL/day (range 0.5-1.5 mL) as needed

Children 2-11 years: 2.5 mL/day (range 1-3 mL) as needed

Children ≥12 years and Adults: 5 mL/day (range 2-6 mL) as needed at bedtime

Patient Information Should not be used regularly for more than 1 week

Additional Information Cascara sagrada fluid extract is 5 times more potent than cascara sagrada aromatic fluid extract

Dosage Forms

Liquid, aromatic fluid extract: 5 mL, 120 mL

Tablet: 325 mg

Castor Oil (kas' tor)

Brand Names Alphamul® [OTC]; Emulsoil® [OTC]; Neoloid® [OTC]; Purge® [OTC]

Synonyms Oleum Ricini

Therapeutic Category Laxative, Stimulant

Use Preparation for rectal or bowel examination or surgery; rarely used to relieve constipation

Pregnancy Risk Factor X

Contraindications Known hypersensitivity to castor oil; nausea, vomiting, abdominal pain, fecal impaction, GI bleeding, appendicitis, congestive heart failure, menstruation, dehydration

Warnings Long-term use may result in laxative dependence

Adverse Reactions

Central nervous system: Dizziness

Endocrine & metabolic: Electrolyte disturbance

Gastrointestinal: Abdominal cramps, nausea, diarrhea

Stability Protect from heat (castor oil emulsion should be protected from freezing)

Mechanism of Action Acts primarily in the small intestine; hydrolyzed to ricinoleic acid which reduces net absorption of fluid and electrolytes and stimulates peristalsis

Pharmacodynamics Onset of action: Oral: Within 2-6 hours

Usual Dosage Oral:

Castor oil:
- Infants <2 years: 1-5 mL or 15 mL/m^2/dose as a single dose
- Children 2-11 years: 5-15 mL as a single dose
- Children ≥12 years and Adults: 15-60 mL as a single dose

Emulsified castor oil:
- Infants: 2.5-7.5 mL/dose
- Children:
  - <2 years: 5-15 mL/dose
  - 2-11 years: 7.5-30 mL/dose
- Children ≥12 years and Adults: 30-60 mL/dose

Monitoring Parameters I & O, serum electrolytes, stool frequency

Nursing Implications Do not administer at bedtime because of rapid onset of action; chill or give with juice or carbonated beverage to improve palatability

Dosage Forms

Emulsion, oral: 36.4%, 60%, 67%, 95%

Liquid: 95%, 100%

Catapres® *see* Clonidine *on page 143*

Catapres-TTS® *see* Clonidine *on page 143*

CBDCA *see* Carboplatin *on page 106*

CCNU *see* Lomustine *on page 347*

C-Crystals® [OTC] *see* Ascorbic Acid *on page 59*

CDDP *see* Cisplatin *on page 137*

Ceclor® *see* Cefaclor *on this page*

Cecon® [OTC] *see* Ascorbic Acid *on page 59*

CeeNU® *see* Lomustine *on page 347*

Cefaclor (sef' a klor)

Brand Names Ceclor®

Therapeutic Category Antibiotic, Cephalosporin (Second Generation)

Use Infections caused by susceptible organisms including *Staph aureus* and *H. influenzae*; treatment of infections involving the respiratory tract, otitis media, sinusitis, skin and skin structure, bone and joint, and urinary tract

Pregnancy Risk Factor B

Contraindications Hypersensitivity to cefaclor or any component, cephalosporins, or penicillins

Warnings Prolonged use may result in superinfection

Precautions Use with caution in patients with impaired renal function or a history of colitis; modify dosage in patients with severe renal impairment

(Continued)

Cefaclor *(Continued)*

Adverse Reactions

Dermatologic: Rash, urticaria, pruritus
Gastrointestinal: Nausea, vomiting, diarrhea
Hematologic: Positive Coombs' test, eosinophilia
Miscellaneous: Serum sickness-like reaction (rash, arthralgia) which has been noted after repeated courses

Drug Interactions Probenecid

Stability Refrigerate suspension after reconstitution; discard after 14 days

Mechanism of Action Interferes with bacterial cell wall synthesis during active multiplication, causing cell wall death and resultant bactericidal activity against susceptible bacteria

Pharmacokinetics

Absorption: Oral: Well absorbed; acid stable
Distribution: Crosses the placenta; appears in breast milk
Protein binding: 25%
Half-life: 30-60 minutes (prolonged with renal impairment)
Peak serum levels:
Suspension: 45 minutes
Capsule: 60 minutes
Elimination: Most of dose (80%) is excreted unchanged in the urine
Moderately dialyzable (20% to 50%)

Usual Dosage Oral:

Children >1 month: 20-40 mg/kg/day divided every 8-12 hours; maximum dose: 2 g/day (twice daily option is for treatment of otitis media or pharyngitis)

Adults: 250-500 mg every 8 hours or daily dose can be given in 2 divided doses

Monitoring Parameters With prolonged therapy, monitor CBC and stool frequency periodically

Test Interactions Positive Coombs' [direct], false-positive urine glucose (Clinitest®), false ↑ serum or urine creatinine

Dosage Forms

Capsule: 250 mg, 500 mg
Powder for oral suspension (strawberry flavor): 125 mg/5 mL (75 mL, 150 mL); 187 mg/5 mL (50 mL, 100 mL); 250 mg/5 mL (75 mL, 150 mL); 375 mg/5 mL (50 mL, 100 mL)

References

Levine LR, "Quantitative Comparison of Adverse Reactions to Cefaclor vs Amoxicillin in a Surveillance Study," *Ped Inf Dis*, 1985, 4(4):358-61.

Cefanex® *see* Cephalexin Monohydrate *on page 120*

Cefazolin Sodium (sef a' zoe lin)

Related Information

Medications Compatible With PN Solutions *on page 649-650*

Brand Names Ancef®; Kefzol®; Zolicef®

Therapeutic Category Antibiotic, Cephalosporin (First Generation)

Use A first generation cephalosporin useful in the treatment of gram-positive bacilli and cocci (except enterococcus); some gram-negative bacilli including *E. coli*, *Proteus*, and *Klebsiella* may be susceptible

Pregnancy Risk Factor B

Contraindications Hypersensitivity to cefazolin sodium or any component, cephalosporins, or penicillins

Precautions Modify dosage in patients with renal impairment

Adverse Reactions

Central nervous system: Fever, CNS irritation, seizures
Dermatologic: Rash, urticaria
Hematologic: Positive Coombs' test, leukopenia, thrombocytopenia
Hepatic: Transient elevation of liver enzymes
Local: Thrombophlebitis

Drug Interactions Probenecid, nephrotoxic agents

Stability Reconstituted solution is stable for 24 hours at room temperature or 96 hours when refrigerated; thawed solutions of the commercially available frozen cefazolin injections are stable for 48 hours at room temperature or 10 days when refrigerated

Mechanism of Action Interferes with bacterial cell wall synthesis during active multiplication, causing cell wall death and resultant bactericidal activity against susceptible bacteria

Pharmacokinetics

Distribution: Crosses the placenta; small amounts appear in breast milk; CSF penetration is poor; penetrates bone and synovial fluid well; distributes into bile

Protein binding: 74% to 86%

Metabolism: Hepatic metabolism is minimal

Half-life: 90-150 minutes (prolonged with renal impairment)

Peak serum levels:

- I.M.: Within 0.5-2 hours
- I.V.: Within 5 minutes

Elimination: 80% to 100% is excreted unchanged in urine

Moderately dialyzable (20% to 50%)

Usual Dosage I.M., I.V.:

Neonates:

- Postnatal age ≤7 days: 40 mg/kg/day divided every 12 hours
- Postnatal age >7 days:
  - ≤2000 g: 40 mg/kg/day divided every 12 hours
  - >2000 g: 60 mg/kg/day divided every 8 hours

Infants and Children: 50-100 mg/kg/day divided every 8 hours; maximum dose: 6 g/day

Adults: 0.5-2 g every 6-8 hours; maximum dose: 12 g/day

- Dosing interval in renal impairment:
  - Cl_{cr} 10-30 mL/minute: Administer every 12 hours
  - Cl_{cr} <10 mL/minute: Administer every 24 hours

Administration Cefazolin can be administered IVP over 3-5 minutes at a maximum concentration of 100 mg/mL or I.V. intermittent infusion over 10-60 minutes at a final concentration for I.V. administration of 20 mg/mL. In fluid-restricted patients, a concentration of 138 mg/mL can be administered IVP.

Monitoring Parameters Renal function periodically when used in combination with other nephrotoxic drugs, hepatic function tests, and CBC

Test Interactions False-positive urine glucose using Clinitest®, positive Coombs' [direct], false ↑ serum or urine creatinine

Additional Information Sodium content of 1 g: 2 mEq

Dosage Forms

Infusion, premixed, in D_5W (frozen): 500 mg (50 mL); 1 g (50 mL)

Injection: 500 mg, 1 g

Powder for injection: 250 mg, 500 mg, 1 g, 5 g, 10 g, 20 g

References

Pickering LK, O'Connor DM, Anderson D, et al, "Clinical and Pharmacologic Evaluation of Cefazolin in Children," *J Infect Dis* 1973, (Suppl):S407-14.

Cefixime (sef ix' eem)

Brand Names Suprax®

Therapeutic Category Antibiotic, Cephalosporin (Third Generation)

Use Treatment of urinary tract infections, otitis media, respiratory infections due to susceptible organisms including *S. pneumoniae* and *Pyogenes*, *H. influenzae* and many *Enterobacteriaceae*; documented poor compliance with other oral antimicrobials; outpatient therapy of serious soft tissue or skeletal infections due to susceptible organisms; single-dose oral treatment of uncomplicated cervical/urethral gonorrhea due to *N. gonorrhoeae*

Pregnancy Risk Factor B

Contraindications Hypersensitivity to cefixime or cephalosporins

Warnings Prolonged use may result in superinfection

Precautions Use with caution in patients hypersensitive to penicillin, patients with impaired renal function, and patients with a history of colitis; modify dosage in patients with renal impairment

Adverse Reactions

Central nervous system: Headache, fever

Dermatologic: Skin rash

Gastrointestinal: Nausea, diarrhea (up to 15% of children), abdominal pain, pseudomembranous colitis

(Continued)

Cefixime *(Continued)*

Hepatic: Transient elevation of liver enzymes
Renal & genitourinary: Transient elevation of BUN or creatinine

Drug Interactions Probenecid

Stability After reconstitution, suspension may be stored for 14 days at room temperature

Mechanism of Action Interferes with bacterial cell wall synthesis during active multiplication, causing cell wall death and resultant bactericidal activity against susceptible bacteria

Pharmacokinetics

Absorption: Oral: 40% to 50%
Protein binding: 65%
Half-life:
  Normal renal function: 3-4 hours
  Renal failure: Up to 11.5 hours
Peak serum levels: Within 2-6 hours; peak serum concentrations are 15% to 50% higher for the oral suspension versus tablets
Elimination: 50% of the absorbed dose is excreted as active drug in the urine and 10% in bile
10% removed by hemodialysis

Usual Dosage Oral:

Children: 8 mg/kg/day divided every 12-24 hours; maximum dose: 400 mg/day

Adolescents and Adults: 400 mg/day divided every 12-24 hours
  Uncomplicated cervical/urethral gonorrhea due to *N. gonorrhoeae*: 400 mg as a single dose

Dosing adjustment in renal impairment:
  Cl_{cr} 21-60 mL/minute: Administer 75% of the standard dose
  Cl_{cr} <20 mL/minute: Administer 50% of the standard dose

Monitoring Parameters With prolonged therapy, monitor renal and hepatic function periodically

Test Interactions False-positive reaction for urine glucose using Clinitest®

Additional Information Otitis media should be treated with the suspension since it results in higher peak blood levels than the tablet

Dosage Forms

Powder for oral suspension (strawberry flavor): 100 mg/5 mL (50 mL, 100 mL)
Tablet, film coated: 200 mg, 400 mg

References

Johnson CE, Carlin SA, Super DM, et al, "Cefixime Compared With Amoxicillin for Treatment of Acute Otitis Media," *J Pediatr*, 1991, 119(1):117-22.

Cefotaxime Sodium (sef oh taks' eem)

Related Information

Medications Compatible With PN Solutions *on page 649-650*

Brand Names Claforan®

Therapeutic Category Antibiotic, Cephalosporin (Third Generation)

Use Treatment of a documented or suspected meningitis due to susceptible organisms such as *H. influenzae* and *N. meningitidis*; nonpseudomonal gram-negative rod infection in a patient at risk of developing aminoglycoside-induced nephrotoxicity and/or ototoxicity; infection due to an organism whose susceptibilities clearly favor cefotaxime over cefuroxime or an aminoglycoside

Pregnancy Risk Factor B

Contraindications Hypersensitivity to cefotaxime or any component, cephalosporins, or penicillins

Warnings Prolonged use may result in superinfection

Precautions Use with caution in patients with impaired renal function or history of colitis; modify dosage in patients with Cl_{cr} <20 mL/minute

Adverse Reactions

Central nervous system: Fever, headache
Dermatologic: Rash, pruritus
Gastrointestinal: Antibiotic-associated pseudomembranous colitis, diarrhea, nausea, vomiting
Hematologic: Positive direct Coombs' test, transient neutropenia, thrombocytopenia

Hepatic: Transient elevation of liver enzymes
Local: Phlebitis
Renal & genitourinary: Transient elevation of BUN/creatinine

Drug Interactions Probenecid

Stability Reconstituted solution is stable for 24 hours at room temperature and 10 days when refrigerated

Mechanism of Action Interferes with bacterial cell wall synthesis during active multiplication by binding to penicillin binding proteins, causing cell wall death and resultant bactericidal activity against susceptible bacteria

Pharmacokinetics

Distribution: Crosses the placenta; appears in breast milk
Protein binding: 31% to 50%
Metabolism: Partially metabolized in the liver to active metabolite, desacetylcefotaxime
Half-life:
- Desacetylcefotaxime: Adults: 1.5-1.9 hours (prolonged with renal impairment)
- Cefotaxime:
  - Neonates, premature: <1 week: 5-6 hours
  - Neonates, full term: <1 week: 2-3.4 hours; 1-4 weeks: 2 hours
  - Children: 1.5 hours
  - Adults: 1-1.5 hours (prolonged with renal and/or hepatic impairment)

Peak serum levels:
- I.M.: Within 30 minutes
- I.V.: Within ~5 minutes

Moderately dialyzable (20% to 50%)

Usual Dosage I.M., I.V.:

Neonates:
- Postnatal age ≤7 days: 100 mg/kg/day divided every 12 hours
- Postnatal age >7 days:
  - <1200 g: 100 mg/kg/day divided every 12 hours
  - ≥1200 g: 150 mg/kg/day divided every 8 hours

Infants and Children 1 month to 12 years:
- <50 kg: 100-200 mg/kg/day divided every 6-8 hours
- Meningitis: 200 mg/kg/day divided every 6 hours
- ≥50 kg: Moderate to severe infection: 1-2 g every 6-8 hours; life-threatening infection: 2 g/dose every 4 hours; maximum dose: 12 g/day

Children >12 years and Adults: 1-2 g every 6-8 hours (up to 12 g/day)

Dosing adjustment in renal impairment: Cl_{cr} <20 mL/minute: Reduce dose 50%

Administration Cefotaxime can be administered IVP over 3-5 minutes at a maximum concentration of 100 mg/mL or I.V. intermittent infusion over 15-30 minutes at a final concentration for I.V. administration of 20-60 mg/mL; in fluid-restricted patients, a concentration of 150 mg/mL can be administered IVP

Monitoring Parameters With prolonged therapy, monitor renal, hepatic, and hematologic function periodically

Test Interactions Positive Coombs' [direct]

Additional Information Sodium content of 1 g: 2.2 mEq

Dosage Forms

Infusion, premixed, in D_5W (frozen): 1 g (50 mL); 2 g (50 mL)
Powder for injection: 1 g, 2 g, 10 g

References

Spritzer R, Kamp HJ, Dzoljic G, et al, "Five Years of Cefotaxime Use in a Neonatal Intensive Care Unit," *Pediatr Infect Dis J*, 1990, 9(2):92-6.

Cefoxitin Sodium (se fox' i tin)

Related Information

Medications Compatible With PN Solutions *on page 649-650*

Brand Names Mefoxin®

Therapeutic Category Antibiotic, Cephalosporin (Second Generation)

Use A second generation cephalosporin less active against staphylococci and streptococci than first generation cephalosporins, but active against anaerobes including *Bacteroides fragilis*; active against gram-negative enteric bacilli including *E. coli*, *Klebsiella*, and *Proteus*; active against many strains of *N. gonorrhoeae*

(Continued)

Cefoxitin Sodium *(Continued)*

Pregnancy Risk Factor B

Contraindications Hypersensitivity to cefoxitin or any component, cephalosporins, or penicillins

Warnings Prolonged use may result in superinfection; high doses in children have been associated with an increased incidence of eosinophilia and elevation of serum AST; safety and efficacy in infants <3 months have not been established

Precautions Use with caution and modify dosage in patients with renal impairment; use with caution in patients with history of colitis

Adverse Reactions

Central nervous system: Fever, headache

Dermatologic: Rash, pruritus

Gastrointestinal: Pseudomembranous colitis, diarrhea, nausea, vomiting

Hematologic: Positive direct Coombs' test, transient leukopenia, thrombocytopenia, neutropenia, anemia, eosinophilia

Hepatic: Transient elevation of liver enzymes, AST, ALT, and alkaline phosphatase

Local: Thrombophlebitis

Renal & genitourinary: Transient elevation of BUN/creatinine

Drug Interactions Probenecid (increases serum concentration of cefoxitin)

Stability Reconstituted solution is stable for 24 hours at room temperature and for one week under refrigeration; thawed solutions of the commercially available frozen cefoxitin injections are stable for 24 hours at room temperature or 5 days when refrigerated

Mechanism of Action Bactericidal antibiotic with a mechanism similar to that of penicillins; inhibits mucopeptide synthesis in the bacterial cell wall

Pharmacokinetics

Distribution: Poorly penetrates into CSF even with inflamed meninges; crosses the placenta; small amounts appear in breast milk

Protein binding: 65% to 79%

Peak serum levels:

- I.M.: Within 20-30 minutes
- I.V.: Within 5 minutes

Half-life: 45-60 minutes, increases significantly with renal insufficiency

Elimination: Rapidly excreted as unchanged drug (85%) in the urine

Moderately dialyzable (20% to 50%)

Usual Dosage I.M., I.V.:

Infants ≥3 months and Children:

- Mild-moderate infection: 80-100 mg/kg/day divided every 6-8 hours
- Severe infection: 100-160 mg/kg/day divided every 4-6 hours
- Maximum dose: 12 g/day

Adults: 1-2 g every 6-8 hours (I.M. injection is painful)

Dosing interval in renal impairment:

- Cl_{cr} 30-50 mL/minute: Administer every 8-12 hours
- Cl_{cr} 10-30 mL/minute: Administer every 12-24 hours
- Cl_{cr} <10 mL/minute: Administer every 24-48 hours

Administration Cefoxitin can be administered IVP over 3-5 minutes at a maximum concentration of 100 mg/mL or I.V. intermittent infusion over 10-60 minutes at a final concentration for I.V. administration not to exceed 40 mg/mL

Monitoring Parameters Renal function periodically when used in combination with other nephrotoxic drugs; liver function and hematologic function tests

Test Interactions Positive Coombs' [direct]; false-positive urine glucose (Clinitest®), false ↑ in serum or urine creatinine

Additional Information Sodium content of 1 g: 2.3 mEq

Dosage Forms

Infusion, premixed, in D_5W (frozen): 1 g (50 mL); 2 g (50 mL)

Powder for injection: 1 g, 2 g, 10 g

References

Feldman WE, Moffitt S, and Sprow N, "Clinical and Pharmacokinetic Evaluation of Parenteral Cefoxitin in Infants and Children," *Antimicrob Agents Chemother*, 1980, 17(4):669-74.

Cefpodoxime Proxetil (sef pode ox' eem)

Brand Names Vantin®

Therapeutic Category Antibiotic, Cephalosporin (Second Generation)

Use Treatment of susceptible acute, community-acquired pneumonia caused by *S. pneumoniae* or non-beta-lactamase producing *H. influenzae*; acute uncomplicated gonorrhea caused by *N. gonorrhoeae*; uncomplicated skin and skin structure infections caused by *S. aureus* or *S. pyogenes*; acute otitis media caused by *S. pneumoniae*, *H. influenzae*, or *M. catarrhalis*; pharyngitis or tonsilitis; and uncomplicated urinary tract infections caused by *E coli*, *Klebsiella*, and *Proteus*

Pregnancy Risk Factor B

Contraindications Hypersensitivity to cefpodoxime or cephalosporins

Warnings Prolonged use may result in superinfection

Precautions Use with caution in patients with impaired renal function and patients with a history of colitis; modify dosage in patients with renal impairment

Adverse Reactions

Central nervous system: Headache

Dermatologic: Rash

Gastrointestinal: Nausea (3.8%), vomiting, abdominal pain, diarrhea (7.1%), pseudomembranous colitis

Hematologic: Eosinophilia, leukocytosis, thrombocytosis; decrease in hemoglobin, hematocrit; leukopenia, prolonged PT and PTT

Hepatic: Transient elevation in AST, ALT, bilirubin

Renal & genitourinary: Increase in BUN and creatinine

Miscellaneous: Vaginal fungal infections (3.3%)

Drug Interactions Antacids and H_2-receptor antagonists (reduce absorption and serum concentration of cefpodoxime); probenecid (inhibits renal excretion of cefpodoxime)

Stability After reconstitution, suspension may be stored in refrigerator for 14 days

Pharmacokinetics

Absorption: Absorption is enhanced in the presence of food or low gastric pH

Distribution: Good tissue penetration, including lung and tonsils; penetrates into pleural fluid

Protein binding: 18% to 23%

Metabolism: Following oral administration, cefpodoxime proxetil is de-esterified in the GI tract to the active metabolite, cefpodoxime

Bioavailability: Oral: 50%

Half-life: 2.2 hours (prolonged with renal impairment)

Peak levels: Within 2-3 hours

Elimination: Primarily eliminated by the kidney with 80% of dose excreted unchanged in urine in 24 hours

Usual Dosage Oral:

Children >6 months to 12 years: 10 mg/kg/day divided every 12 hours

Children ≥13 years and Adults: 100-400 mg/dose every 12 hours

Uncomplicated gonorrhea: 200 mg as a single dose

Dosing adjustment in renal impairment: Cl_{cr} <30 mL/minute: Administer every 24 hours

Monitoring Parameters Observe patient for diarrhea; with prolonged therapy, monitor renal function periodically

Test Interactions Positive direct Coombs' test

Patient Information Take with food

Additional Information Dose adjustment is not necessary in patients with cirrhosis

Dosage Forms

Granules for oral suspension (lemon creme flavor): 50 mg/5 mL (100 mL); 100 mg/5 mL (100 mL)

Tablet, film coated: 100 mg, 200 mg

References

Borin MT, "A Review of the Pharmacokinetics of Cefpodoxime Proxetil", *Drugs*, 1991, 42(Suppl 3):13-21.

Fujii R, "Clinical Trials of Cefpodoxime Proxetil Suspension in Pediatrics," *Drugs*, 1991, 42(Suppl 3):57-60.

(Continued)

Cefpodoxime Proxetil *(Continued)*

Mendelman PM, Del-Beccaro MA, McLinn SE, et al, "Cefpodoxime Proxetil Compared With Amoxicillin-Clavulante for the Treatment of Otitis Media," *J Pediatr*, 1992, 121(3):459-65.

Ceftazidime (sef' tay zi deem)

Related Information

Medications Compatible With PN Solutions *on page 649-650*

Brand Names Ceptaz™; Fortaz®; Pentacef®; Tazicef®; Tazidime®

Therapeutic Category Antibiotic, Cephalosporin (Third Generation)

Use Treatment of documented susceptible *Pseudomonas aeruginosa* infection; pseudomonal infection in patient at risk of developing aminoglycoside-induced nephrotoxicity and/or ototoxicity; empiric therapy of a febrile, granulocytopenic patient

Pregnancy Risk Factor B

Contraindications Hypersensitivity to ceftazidime or any component, cephalosporins, or penicillins

Warnings Prolonged use may result in superinfection

Precautions Use with caution and modify dosage in patients with impaired renal function; use with caution in patients with history of colitis

Adverse Reactions

Central nervous system: Fever, headache

Dermatologic: Rash, pruritus

Gastrointestinal: Pseudomembranous colitis, diarrhea, nausea, vomiting

Hematologic: Positive direct Coombs' test, transient leukopenia, thrombocytopenia, eosinophilia, thrombocytosis, hemolytic anemia

Hepatic: Transient elevation of liver enzymes

Local: Phlebitis

Renal & genitourinary: Transient elevation of BUN/creatinine

Miscellaneous: Candidiasis

Stability Reconstituted solution is stable for 24 hours at room temperature and 10 days when refrigerated; incompatible with sodium bicarbonate; potentially incompatible with aminoglycosides

Mechanism of Action Bactericidal antibiotic with a mechanism similar to that of penicillins; inhibits mucopeptide synthesis in the bacterial cell wall

Pharmacokinetics

Distribution: Widely distributed throughout the body including bone, bile, skin, CSF (diffuses into CSF at higher concentrations when the meninges are inflamed), endometrium, heart, pleural and lymphatic fluids

Protein binding: 17%

Peak serum levels: I.M.: Within 60 minutes

Half-life:

- Neonates $<$23 days: 2.2-4.7 hours
- Adults: 1-2 hours (prolonged with renal impairment)

Elimination: Eliminated by glomerular filtration with 80% to 90% of the dose excreted as unchanged drug in urine within 24 hours

Dialyzable (50% to 100%)

Usual Dosage I.M., I.V.:

Neonates:

- Postnatal age $\leq$7 days: 100 mg/kg/day divided every 12 hours
- Postnatal age $>$7 days:
  - $<$1200 g: 100 mg/kg/day divided every 12 hours
  - $\geq$1200 g: 150 mg/kg/dose divided every 8 hours

Infants and Children 1 month to 12 years: 100-150 mg/kg/day divided every 8 hours

- Meningitis: 225 mg/kg/day divided every 8 hours; maximum dose: 6 g/day

Adults: 1-2 g every 8-12 hours

- Urinary tract infections: 250-500 mg every 12 hours

Dosing interval in renal impairment:

- Cl_{cr} of 30-50 mL/minute: Administer every 12 hours
- Cl_{cr} of 10-30 mL/minute: Administer every 24 hours
- Cl_{cr} $<$10 mL/minute: Administer every 24-48 hours

Administration Any carbon dioxide bubbles that may be present in the withdrawn solution should be expelled prior to injection; ceftazidime can be administered IVP over 3-5 minutes at a maximum concentration of 100 mg/mL or I.V. intermittent infusion over 15-30 minutes at a final concentration of ≤40 mg/mL

Monitoring Parameters Renal function periodically when used in combination with aminoglycosides; with prolonged therapy also monitor hepatic and hematologic function periodically

Test Interactions Positive Coombs' [direct], false-positive urine glucose (Clinitest®)

Additional Information Sodium content of 1 g: 2.3 mEq

Dosage Forms

Infusion, premixed (frozen): 1 g (50 mL); 2 g (50 mL)

Powder for injection: 500 mg, 1 g, 2 g, 6 g, 10 g

Ceftin® *see* Cefuroxime *on next page*

Ceftriaxone Sodium (sef try ax' one)

Related Information

Medications Compatible With PN Solutions *on page 649-650*

Brand Names Rocephin®

Therapeutic Category Antibiotic, Cephalosporin (Third Generation)

Use Treatment of lower respiratory tract infections, skin and skin structure infections, bone and joint infections, intra-abdominal and urinary tract infections, sepsis and meningitis due to susceptible organisms; documented or suspected infection due to susceptible organisms in home care patients and patients without I.V. line access; treatment of documented or suspected gonococcal infection or chancroid; emergency room management of patients at high risk for bacteremia, periorbital or buccal cellulitis, salmonellosis or shigellosis and pneumonia of unestablished etiology (<5 years of age)

Pregnancy Risk Factor B

Contraindications Hypersensitivity to ceftriaxone sodium or any component, cephalosporins, or penicillins; do not use in hyperbilirubinemic neonates, particularly those who are premature since ceftriaxone is reported to displace bilirubin from albumin binding sites increasing the risk for kernicterus

Warnings Prolonged use may result in superinfection with yeasts, enterococci, *B. fragilis*, or *P. aeruginosa*

Precautions Use with caution in patients with gall bladder, biliary tract, liver, or pancreatic disease, or history of colitis

Adverse Reactions

Dermatologic: Rash

Gastrointestinal: Diarrhea, nausea, vomiting, sludging in the gallbladder, cholelithiasis, pseudomembranous colitis

Hematologic: Eosinophilia, leukopenia, anemia, thrombocytopenia, thrombocytosis, bleeding

Hepatic: Transient elevation in liver enzymes, jaundice

Renal & genitourinary: Increase in serum creatinine and BUN

Drug Interactions High-dose probenecid (decreased elimination half-life of ceftriaxone); aminoglycosides

Stability Reconstituted solution (100 mg/mL) is stable for 3 days at room temperature and 10 days when refrigerated; reconstituted solution (250 mg/mL) is stable for 24 hours at room temperature and 3 days when refrigerated

Mechanism of Action Bactericidal antibiotic with a mechanism similar to that of penicillins; inhibits mucopeptide synthesis in the bacterial cell wall

Pharmacokinetics

Distribution: Widely distributed throughout the body including gall bladder, lungs, bone, bile, CSF (diffuses into the CSF at higher concentrations when the meninges are inflamed)

Protein binding: 85% to 95%

Half-life:

- Neonates:
  - 1-4 days: 16 hours
  - 9-30 days: 9 hours
- Adults: 5-9 hours (with normal renal and hepatic function)

Peak serum levels:

- I.M.: Within 1-2 hours

(Continued)

Ceftriaxone Sodium *(Continued)*

I.V.: Within minutes

Elimination: Excreted unchanged in the urine (33% to 65%) by glomerular filtration and in feces via bile

Not dialyzable (0% to 5%)

Usual Dosage I.M., I.V.:

Neonates:

Postnatal age ≤7 days: 50 mg/kg/day given every 24 hours

Postnatal age >7 days:

≤2000 g: 50 mg/kg/day given every 24 hours

>2000 g: 75 mg/kg/day given every 24 hours

Gonococcal prophylaxis: 50 mg/kg as a single dose (dose not to exceed 125 mg)

Gonococcal infection: 50 mg/kg/day (maximum dose: 125 mg) given every 24 hours for 7 days

Infants and Children: 50-75 mg/kg/day divided every 12-24 hours

Meningitis: 100 mg/kg/day divided every 12 hours; loading dose of 75 mg/kg may be administered at the start of therapy

Chancroid, uncomplicated gonorrhea: I.M.:

<45 kg: 125 mg as a single dose

≥45 kg: 250 mg as a single dose

Adults: 1-2 g every 12-24 hours depending on the type and severity of the infection; maximum dose: 4 g/day

Dosing interval in renal impairment: No change necessary

Administration Ceftriaxone can be administered by I.V. intermittent infusion over 10-30 minutes; final concentration for I.V. administration should not exceed 40 mg/mL; for I.M. injection, ceftriaxone can be diluted with sterile water or 1% lidocaine to a final concentration of 250 mg/mL

Monitoring Parameters CBC with differential, PT, renal and hepatic function tests periodically

Test Interactions False-positive urine glucose with Clinitest®

Additional Information Sodium content of 1 g: 3.6 mEq

Dosage Forms

Infusion, premixed (frozen): 1 g in $D_{3.8}W$ (50 mL); 2 g in $D_{2.4}W$ (50 mL)

Powder for injection: 250 mg, 500 mg, 1 g, 2 g, 10 g

References

"1989 Sexually Transmitted Diseases Treatment Guidelines," *MMWR Morb Mortal Wkly Rep*, 1989, 38(Suppl 8):1-43.

Richards DM, Heel RC, Brogden RN, et al, "Ceftriaxone: A Review of Its Antibacterial Activity, Pharmacological Properties and Therapeutic Use," *Drugs*, 1984, 27(6):469-527.

Cefuroxime (se fyoor ox' eem)

Related Information

Medications Compatible With PN Solutions *on page 649-650*

Brand Names Ceftin®; Kefurox®; Zinacef®

Therapeutic Category Antibiotic, Cephalosporin (Second Generation)

Use A second generation cephalosporin useful in infections caused by susceptible staphylococci, group B streptococci, pneumococci, *H. influenzae* (type A and B), *E. coli*, *Enterobacter*, and *Klebsiella*; treatment of susceptible infections of the lower respiratory tract, otitis media, urinary tract, skin and soft tissue, bone and joint, sepsis and gonorrhea

Pregnancy Risk Factor B

Contraindications Hypersensitivity to cefuroxime or any component, cephalosporins, or penicillins

Warnings Prolonged use may result in superinfection; safety and efficacy in infants <3 months of age have not been established

Precautions Use with caution and modify dosage in patients with renal impairment; use with caution in patients with history of colitis

Adverse Reactions

Central nervous system: Fever, headache, dizziness, vertigo

Dermatologic: Rash

Gastrointestinal: Nausea, vomiting, diarrhea, stomach cramps, GI bleeding, colitis, stomatitis

Hematologic: Positive direct Coombs' test, transient neutropenia and leukopenia, decreased hemoglobin and hematocrit
Hepatic: Transient increase in liver enzymes
Local: Pain at injection site, thrombophlebitis
Renal & genitourinary: Increase in creatinine and/or BUN
Miscellaneous: Vaginitis

Drug Interactions Probenecid (increases serum cefuroxime concentration)

Stability Potentially incompatible with aminoglycosides

Mechanism of Action Interferes with bacterial cell wall synthesis during active multiplication, causing cell wall death and resultant bactericidal activity against susceptible bacteria

Pharmacokinetics

Absorption: Increased when given with or shortly after food or infant formula
Protein binding: 33% to 50%
Bioavailability: Oral cefuroxime axetil: 37% to 52%
Half-life:
- Neonates:
  - ≤3 days: 5.1-5.8 hours
  - 6-14 days: 2-4.2 hours
  - 3-4 weeks: 1-1.5 hours
- Adults: 1-2 hours (prolonged in renal impairment)

Peak plasma levels:
- I.M.: Within 15-60 minutes
- I.V. injection: 2-3 minutes

Elimination: Primarily excreted 66% to 100% as unchanged drug in the urine by both glomerular filtration and tubular secretion
Can be removed by dialysis

Usual Dosage

I.M., I.V.:
- Children: 75-150 mg/kg/day divided every 8 hours; maximum dose: 6 g/day
- Meningitis: Not recommended (doses of 200-240 mg/kg/day divided every 6-8 hours have been used)
- Adults: 750 mg to 1.5 g/dose every 8 hours

Dosing interval in renal impairment:
- Cl_{cr} 10-20 mL/minute: Administer every 12 hours
- Cl_{cr} <10 mL/minute: Administer every 24 hours

Oral:
- Children: 30-40 mg/kg/day divided every 12 hours
- Adults: 250-500 mg twice daily

Administration Cefuroxime sodium can be administered IVP over 3-5 minutes at a maximum concentration of 100 mg/mL, or I.V. intermittent infusion over 15-30 minutes at a final concentration for administration of ≤30 mg/mL; in fluid restricted patients, a concentration of 137 mg/mL can be administered

Monitoring Parameters With prolonged therapy, monitor renal, hepatic, and hematologic function periodically

Test Interactions Positive Coombs' [direct]; false-positive urine glucose with Clinitest®

Patient Information Oral cefuroxime may be taken with food

Nursing Implications Avoid crushing the tablet due to its bitter taste

Additional Information Sodium content of 1 g: 2.4 mEq

Dosage Forms

Infusion, premixed (frozen): 750 mg in $D_{2.8}W$ (50 mL); 1.5 g in water (50 mL)
Injection, as sodium: 750 mg, 1.5 g, 7.5 g
Tablet, as axetil (Ceftin®): 125 mg, 250 mg, 500 mg

References

Nelson JD, "Cefuroxime: A Cephalosporin With Unique Applicability to Pediatric Practice," *Pediatr Infect Dis*, 1983, 2(5):394-6.

Thoene DE and Johnson CE, "Pharmacotherapy of Otitis Media," *Pharmacotherapy*, 1991, 11(3):212-21.

Celestone® *see* Betamethasone *on page 81*

Celestone® Soluspan® *see* Betamethasone *on page 81*

Celontin® *see* Methsuximide *on page 376*

Cel-U-Jec® *see* Betamethasone *on page 81*

Cenafed® [OTC] *see* Pseudoephedrine *on page 497*

Cenafed® Plus [OTC] *see* Triprolidine and Pseudoephedrine *on page 586*

Cena-K® *see* Potassium Chloride *on page 469*

Cenocort® *see* Triamcinolone *on page 579*

Cenocort® Forte *see* Triamcinolone *on page 579*

Cenolate® *see* Ascorbic Acid *on page 59*

Cephalexin Monohydrate (sef a lex' in)

Brand Names Biocef®; Cefanex®; Keflex®; Keftab®; Zartan®

Therapeutic Category Antibiotic, Cephalosporin (First Generation)

Use Treatment of susceptible bacterial infections, including those caused by group A beta-hemolytic *Streptococcus*, *Staphylococcus*, *Klebsiella pneumoniae*, *E. coli*, and *Proteus mirabilis*; used to treat susceptible infections of the respiratory tract, skin and skin structure, bone, genitourinary tract, and otitis media

Pregnancy Risk Factor B

Contraindications Hypersensitivity to cephalexin or any component, cephalosporins, or penicillins

Warnings Prolonged use may result in gastrointestinal or genitourinary superinfection

Precautions Use with caution and modify dosage in patients with renal impairment; use with caution in patients with history of colitis

Adverse Reactions

Central nervous system: Dizziness, headache, fatigue, fever

Dermatologic: Rash

Gastrointestinal: Nausea, vomiting, pseudomembranous colitis, diarrhea, cramps

Hematologic: Transient neutropenia, anemia, positive Coombs' test, eosinophilia

Hepatic: Transient elevation in liver enzymes

Drug Interactions Probenecid

Stability Refrigerate suspension after reconstitution; discard after 14 days

Mechanism of Action Bactericidal antibiotic with a mechanism similar to that of penicillins; inhibits mucopeptide synthesis in the bacterial cell wall

Pharmacokinetics

Absorption: Delayed in young children and may be decreased up to 50% in neonates

Distribution: Appears in breast milk

Protein binding: 6% to 15%

Half-life:

- Neonates: 5 hours
- Children 3-12 months: 2.5 hours
- Adults: 0.5-1.2 hours (prolonged with renal impairment)

Peak serum levels: Oral: Within 60 minutes

Elimination: 80% to 100% of a dose excreted as unchanged drug in the urine within 8 hours

Moderately dialyzable (20% to 50%)

Usual Dosage Oral:

Children: 25-100 mg/kg/day divided every 6 hours; maximum dose: 4 g/day

Adults: 250-500 mg every 6 hours

Dosing interval in renal impairment:

- Cl_{cr} 10-40 mL/minute: Administer every 8-12 hours
- Cl_{cr} <10 mL/minute: Administer every 12-24 hours

Monitoring Parameters With prolonged therapy, monitor renal, hepatic, and hematologic function periodically

Test Interactions False-positive urine glucose with Clinitest®; positive Coombs' test [direct]; false ↑ serum or urine creatinine

Nursing Implications Give on an empty stomach (ie, 1 hour prior to, or 2 hours after meals)

Dosage Forms

Capsule: 250 mg, 500 mg

Pediatric oral suspension: 100 mg/mL [5 mg/drop] (10 mL)
Powder for oral suspension: 125 mg/5 mL (5 mL unit dose, 60 mL, 100 mL, 200 mL); 250 mg/5 mL (5 mL unit dose, 100 mL, 200 mL)
Tablet: 250 mg, 500 mg, 1 g
Tablet, as hydrochloride: 250 mg, 500 mg

Cephulac® *see* Lactulose *on page 334*

Ceptaz™ *see* Ceftazidime *on page 116*

Ceredase® *see* Alglucerase *on page 29*

Cerespan® *see* Papaverine Hydrochloride *on page 433*

Cerubidine® *see* Daunorubicin Hydrochloride *on page 172*

Cerumenex® *see* Triethanolamine Polypeptide Oleate-Condensate *on page 582*

C.E.S. *see* Estrogens, Conjugated *on page 232*

Cetacort® *see* Hydrocortisone *on page 293*

Cetamide® *see* Sulfacetamide Sodium *on page 539*

Cetane® [OTC] *see* Ascorbic Acid *on page 59*

Cevalin® [OTC] *see* Ascorbic Acid *on page 59*

Ce-Vi-Sol® [OTC] *see* Ascorbic Acid *on page 59*

CG *see* Chorionic Gonadotropin *on page 134*

Charcoaid® [OTC] *see* Charcoal *on this page*

Charcoal

Brand Names Actidose-Aqua® [OTC]; Actidose® With Sorbitol [OTC]; Charcoaid® [OTC]; Charcocaps® [OTC]; Liqui-Char® [OTC]; SuperChar® [OTC]

Synonyms Activated Carbon; Activated Charcoal; Adsorbent Charcoal; Liquid Antidote; Medicinal Carbon; Medicinal Charcoal

Therapeutic Category Antidiarrheal; Antidote, Adsorbent; Antiflatulent

Use Emergency treatment in poisoning by drugs and chemicals; repetitive doses for gastric dialysis in uremia to adsorb various waste products

Pregnancy Risk Factor C

Contraindications Not effective for cyanide, mineral acids, caustic alkalis, organic solvents, iron, ethanol, methanol or lithium poisonings; do not use charcoal with sorbitol in patients with fructose intolerance; charcoal with sorbitol is not recommended in children <1 year

Warnings If charcoal in sorbitol is administered, doses should be limited to prevent excessive fluid and electrolyte losses

Precautions When using ipecac with charcoal, induce vomiting with ipecac before administering activated charcoal since charcoal adsorbs ipecac syrup; charcoal may cause vomiting which is hazardous in petroleum distillate and caustic ingestions

Adverse Reactions Gastrointestinal: Emesis, constipation, diarrhea with sorbitol, stools will turn black

Drug Interactions Do not mix with milk, ice cream, sherbet

Mechanism of Action Adsorbs toxic substances or irritants, thus inhibiting GI absorption; adsorbs intestinal gas; the addition of sorbitol results in hyperosmotic laxative action causing catharsis

Pharmacokinetics

Absorption: Not absorbed from the GI tract
Metabolism: Not metabolized
Elimination: Excreted as charcoal in the feces

Usual Dosage Oral:

Acute poisoning:

Single dose: Charcoal with sorbitol (**Note:** The use of repeated oral charcoal with sorbitol doses is not recommended):

Children 1-12 years: 1-2 g/kg or 15-30 g or approximately 5-10 times the weight of the ingested poison; 1 g absorbs 100-1000 mg of poison; in young children sorbitol should be repeated **no more** than 1-2 times/day

Adults: 30-100 g

(Continued)

Charcoal *(Continued)*

Single dose: Charcoal in water:
- Infants <1 year: 1 g/kg
- Children 1-12 years: 1-2 g/kg or 15-30 g
- Adults: 30-100 g or 1-2 g/kg

Multiple dose: Charcoal in water (doses are repeated until clinical observations and serum drug concentrations have returned to a subtherapeutic range):
- Infants <1 year: 1 g/kg every 4-6 hours
- Children 1-12 years: 1-2 g/kg or 15-30 g every 2-6 hours
- Adults: 25-50 g or 1-2 g/kg every 2-6 hours

Gastric dialysis: Adults: 20-50 g every 6 hours for 1-2 days

Patient Information Charcoal causes the stools to turn black

Additional Information 5-6 tablespoonfuls is approximately equal to 30 g of activated charcoal; minimum dilution of 240 mL water per 20-30 g activated charcoal should be mixed as an aqueous slurry

Dosage Forms

Capsule: 250 mg
Liquid, activated: 12.5 g, 15 g, 25 g, 30 g, 50 g
Powder, for suspension: 30 g, 50 g
Tablet: 325 mg

References

Farley TA, "Severe Hypernatremic Dehydration After Use of an Activated Charcoal-Sorbitol Suspension," *J Pediatr*, 1986, 109(4):719-22.

Charcocaps® [OTC] *see* Charcoal *on previous page*

Chemet® *see* Succimer *on page 537*

Cheracol® *see* Guaifenesin and Codeine *on page 279*

Chiggertox® [OTC] *see* Benzocaine *on page 77*

Chlo-Amine® [OTC] *see* Chlorpheniramine Maleate *on page 128*

Chloral *see* Chloral Hydrate *on this page*

Chloral Hydrate

Related Information

Preprocedure Sedatives in Children *on page 687-689*

Brand Names Aquachloral® Supprettes®; Noctec®

Synonyms Chloral; Hydrated Chloral; Trichloroacetaldehyde Monohydrate

Therapeutic Category Hypnotic; Sedative

Use Short-term sedative and hypnotic; sedative prior to EEG evaluations

Restrictions C-IV

Pregnancy Risk Factor C

Contraindications Hypersensitivity to chloral hydrate or any component; hepatic or renal impairment; gastritis or ulcers; severe cardiac disease

Warnings Trichloroethanol (TCE), a metabolite of chloral hydrate, is a carcinogen in mice; there is no data in humans

Precautions Use with caution in neonates, drug may accumulate with repeated use, prolonged use in neonates associated with hyperbilirubinemia; use with caution in patients with porphyria. Tolerance to hypnotic effect develops, therefore, not recommended for use >2 weeks; taper dosage to avoid withdrawal with prolonged use.

Adverse Reactions

Central nervous system: Disorientation, sedation, ataxia, excitement (paradoxical), dizziness, fever, headache
Dermatologic: Rash, urticaria
Gastrointestinal: Gastric irritation, nausea, vomiting, diarrhea, flatulence
Hematologic: Leukopenia, eosinophilia
Miscellaneous: Physical and psychological dependence may occur with prolonged use

Drug Interactions May potentiate effects of warfarin, central nervous system depressants, alcohol; vasodilation reaction (flushing, tachycardia, etc) may occur with concurrent use of alcohol; concomitant use of furosemide (I.V.) may result in flushing, diaphoresis, and blood pressure changes

Stability Sensitive to light; exposure to air causes volatilization; store in light-resistant, airtight container

Mechanism of Action Central nervous system depressant effects are due to its active metabolite trichloroethanol, mechanism unknown

Pharmacodynamics

Peak effects: Within 30-60 minutes

Duration: 4-8 hours

Pharmacokinetics

Absorption: Oral, rectal: Well absorbed

Distribution: Crosses the placenta; negligible amounts appear in breast milk

Metabolism: Rapidly metabolized to trichloroethanol (active metabolite); variable amounts metabolized in liver and kidney to trichloroacetic acid (inactive)

Half-life: Trichloroethanol (active metabolite):

- Neonates: 8.5-66 hours
- Adults: 8-11 hours

Elimination: Metabolites excreted in urine; small amounts excreted in feces via bile

Dialyzable (50% to 100%)

Usual Dosage

Neonates: Oral, rectal: 25 mg/kg/dose for sedation prior to a procedure

Children:

- Sedation, anxiety: Oral, rectal: 25-50 mg/kg/day divided every 6-8 hours, maximum: 500 mg/dose
- Prior to EEG: Oral, rectal: 25-50 mg/kg/dose, 30-60 minutes prior to EEG; may repeat in 30 minutes to maximum of 100 mg/kg or 2 g total
- Hypnotic: Oral, rectal: 50 mg/kg; maximum: 2 g/dose
- Sedation, nonpainful procedure: Oral: 50-75 mg/kg/dose 30-60 minutes prior to procedure; may repeat 30 minutes after initial dose if needed, to a total maximum dose of 120 mg/kg or 2 g total

Adults: Oral, rectal:

- Sedation, anxiety: 250 mg 3 times/day
- Hypnotic: 500-1000 mg at bedtime or 30 minutes prior to procedure, not to exceed 2 g/24 hours

Test Interactions False-positive urine glucose using Clinitest® method; may interfere with fluorometric urine catecholamine and urinary 17-hydroxycorticosteroid tests

Nursing Implications May cause irritation of skin and mucous membranes; minimize unpleasant taste and gastric irritation by administering with water or other liquid

Additional Information Not an analgesic

Dosage Forms

Capsule: 250 mg, 500 mg

Suppository, rectal: 324 mg, 500 mg, 648 mg

Syrup: 250 mg/5 mL (10 mL); 500 mg/5 mL (5 mL, 10 mL, 480 mL)

References

Kauffman RE, "Chloral Hydrate - Is It a Carcinogenic Hazard?," *Pediatr Alert*, 1991, 16(6) 21-22.

Laptook AR and Rosenfeld CR, "Chloral Hydrate Toxicity in a Preterm Infant," *Pediatr Pharmacol New York*, 1984, 4(3):161-5.

Zeltzer LK, Altman A, Cohen D, et al, "American Academy of Pediatrics Report of the Subcommittee on the Management of Pain Associated With Procedures in Children With Cancer," *Pediatrics*, 1990, 86(5 Pt 2):826-31.

Chlorambucil (klor am' byoo sil)

Related Information

Emetogenic Potential of Single Chemotherapeutic Agents *on page 655*

Brand Names Leukeran®

Therapeutic Category Antineoplastic Agent

Use Management of chronic lymphocytic leukemia, Hodgkin's and non-Hodgkin's lymphoma; management of nephrotic syndrome unresponsive to conventional therapy

Pregnancy Risk Factor D

Contraindications Hypersensitivity to chlorambucil or any component, or previous resistance

Warnings The US Food and Drug Administration (FDA) currently recommends that procedures for proper handling and disposal of antineoplastic

(Continued)

Chloramubucil *(Continued)*

agents be considered. Chlorambucil can severely suppress bone marrow function; affects human fertility; carcinogenic in humans and probably mutagenic and teratogenic as well; chromosomal damage has been documented; secondary AML may be associated with chronic therapy

Precautions Use with caution in patients with seizure disorder and bone marrow suppression; reduce initial dosage if patient has received radiation therapy, myelosuppressive drugs or has a depressed baseline leukocyte or platelet count within the previous 4 weeks

Adverse Reactions

Central nervous system: Weakness, seizures
Dermatologic: Rash
Endocrine & metabolic: Hyperuricemia
Gastrointestinal: Nausea, vomiting
Hematologic: Leukopenia, thrombocytopenia, anemia
Hepatic: Hepatotoxicity
Renal & genitourinary: Oligospermia
Respiratory: Pulmonary fibrosis

Mechanism of Action Interferes with DNA replication and RNA transcription by alkylation and cross-linking the strands of DNA

Pharmacokinetics

Absorption: Oral: Well absorbed
Protein binding: ~99%
Metabolism: Metabolized in the liver to an active metabolite
Half-life: 90 minutes
Elimination: 60% excreted in the urine within 24 hours principally as metabolites
Probably not dialyzable

Usual Dosage Oral (refer to individual protocols):

Children:
- General short courses: 0.1-0.2 mg/kg/day or 4-8 mg/m^2/day for 3-6 weeks for remission induction; maintenance therapy: 0.03-0.1 mg/kg/day
- Nephrotic syndrome: 0.1-0.2 mg/kg/day every day for 5-15 weeks with low dose prednisone
- CLL:
  - Biweekly regimen: Initial: 0.4 mg/kg dose is increased by 0.1 mg/kg every 2 weeks until a response occurs and/or myelosuppression occurs
  - Monthly regimen: Initial: 0.4 mg/kg, increase dose by 0.2 mg/kg every 4 weeks until a response occurs and/or myelosuppression occurs
- Malignant lymphomas:
  - Non-Hodgkins lymphoma: 0.1 mg/kg/day
  - Hodgkins: 0.2 mg/kg/day

Adults: 0.1-0.2 mg/kg/day for 3-6 weeks, then adjust dose on basis of blood counts

Monitoring Parameters Liver function tests, CBC, leukocyte counts, platelets, serum uric acid

Patient Information Notify physician if fever, sore throat, or bleeding occurs

Additional Information Myelosuppressive effects:

WBC: Moderate
Platelets: Moderate
Onset (days): 7
Nadir (days): 14-21

Dosage Forms Tablet, sugar coated: 2 mg

References

Baluarte HJ, Hiner L, and Grushkin AB, "Chlorambucil Dosage in Frequently Relapsing Nephrotic Syndrome: A Controlled Clinical Trial," *J Pediatr*, 1978, 92(2):295-8.

Chloramphenicol (klor am fen' i kole)

Related Information

Blood Level Sampling Time Guidelines *on page 694-695*
Medications Compatible With PN Solutions *on page 649-650*

Brand Names AK-Chlor®; Chloromycetin®; Chloroptic®; Ophthochlor®

Therapeutic Category Antibiotic, Miscellaneous; Antibiotic, Ophthalmic; Antibiotic, Otic

Use Treatment of serious infections due to organisms resistant to other less toxic antibiotics or when its penetrability into the site of infection is clinically superior to other antibiotics to which the organism is sensitive; useful in infections caused by *Bacteroides*, *H. influenzae*, *Neisseria meningitidis*, *S.* pneumoniae, *Salmonella*, and *Rickettsia*

Pregnancy Risk Factor C

Contraindications Hypersensitivity to chloramphenicol or any component

Warnings Serious and fatal blood dyscrasias have occurred after both short-term and prolonged therapy; should not be used when less potentially toxic agents are effective; prolonged use may result in superinfection

Precautions Use with caution in patients with glucose-6-phosphate dehydrogenase deficiency, impaired renal or hepatic function and in neonates; monitor serum concentrations and CBC in all patients; reduce dose in patients with hepatic and renal impairment

Adverse Reactions

Cardiovascular: Cardiotoxicity (left ventricular dysfunction); gray baby syndrome

Central nervous system: Optic neuritis, peripheral neuropathy, nightmares, headache

Dermatologic: Rash

Gastrointestinal: Diarrhea, stomatitis, enterocolitis, vomiting

Hematologic: Bone marrow depression, aplastic anemia, neutropenia, thrombocytopenia, hemolysis in patients with G-6-PD deficiency

Hepatic: Hepatitis-pancytopenia syndrome

Miscellaneous: Anaphylaxis

Drug Interactions Chloramphenicol inhibits the metabolism of chlorpropamide, phenytoin, oral anticoagulants; phenobarbital and rifampin may ↓ concentration of chloramphenicol

Stability Store ophthalmic solution in the refrigerator; reconstituted parenteral solution (100 mg/mL) is stable for 30 days at room temperature

Mechanism of Action Reversibly binds to 50S ribosomal subunits of susceptible organisms preventing amino acids from being transferred to growing peptide chains thus inhibiting protein synthesis

Pharmacokinetics

Absorption: Oral: 75% to 100%; in neonates, GI absorption of chloramphenicol palmitate is slow and erratic

Distribution: Readily crosses the placenta; appears in breast milk; distributes to most tissues and body fluids; good CSF and brain penetration

Protein binding: 60%

Metabolism: Extensive metabolism in the liver (90%) to inactive metabolites, principally by glucuronidation; chloramphenicol palmitate is hydrolyzed by lipases in the GI tract to the active base; chloramphenicol sodium succinate must be hydrolyzed by esterases to active base.

Half-life:

- Neonates:
  - 1-2 days: 24 hours
  - 10-16 days: 10 hours
- Adults: 1.6-3.3 hours (prolonged with hepatic insufficiency)

Peak serum levels: Within 30 minutes to 3 hours after an oral dose

Elimination: 5% to 15% excreted as unchanged drug in the urine and 4% excreted in bile; in neonates, 6% to 80% of the dose may be excreted unchanged in the urine

Slightly dialyzable (5% to 20%)

Usual Dosage

Neonates: Initial loading dose: I.V. (I.M. administration is not recommended): 20 mg/kg (the first maintenance dose should be given 12 hours after the loading dose)

Maintenance dose: Postnatal age:

- ≤7 days: 25 mg/kg/day once every 24 hours
- >7 days, ≤2000 g: 25 mg/kg/day once every 24 hours
- >7 days, >2000 g: 50 mg/kg/day divided every 12 hours

Meningitis: I.V.: Infants and Children: Maintenance dose: 75-100 mg/kg/day divided every 6 hours

Other infections: Oral, I.V.:

Infants and Children: 50-75 mg/kg/day divided every 6 hours; maximum daily dose: 4 g/day

(Continued)

Chloramphenicol *(Continued)*

Adults: 50 mg/kg/day in divided doses every 6 hours; maximum daily dose: 4 g/day

Children and Adults:

Ophthalmic: Apply 1-2 drops or small amount of ointment every 3-6 hours; increase interval between applications after 48 hours

Topical: Gently rub into the affected area 3-4 times/day

Administration Can be administered IVP over 5 minutes at a maximum concentration of 100 mg/mL, or I.V. intermittent infusion over 15-30 minutes at a final concentration for administration of ≤20 mg/mL

Monitoring Parameters CBC with reticulocyte and platelet counts, serum iron level, iron-binding capacity, periodic liver and renal function tests, serum drug concentration

Reference Range

Meningitis: Peak: 15-25 μg/mL; Trough: 5-15 μg/mL

Other infections: Peak: 10-20 μg/mL; Trough: 5-10 μg/mL

Patient Information Take on empty stomach with a full glass of water

Nursing Implications Draw peak level 2 hours post oral dose or draw peak levels 90 minutes after the end of a 30-minute infusion; trough levels should be drawn just prior to the next dose

Additional Information Sodium content of 1 g injection: 2.25 mEq

Three (3) major toxicities associated with chloramphenicol include:

Aplastic anemia, an idiosyncratic reaction which can occur with any route of administration; usually occurs 3 weeks to 12 months after initial exposure to chloramphenicol

Bone marrow suppression is thought to be dose-related with serum concentrations >25 μg/mL and reversible once chloramphenicol is discontinued; anemia and neutropenia may occur during the first week of therapy

Gray baby syndrome is characterized by circulatory collapse, cyanosis, acidosis, abdominal distention, myocardial depression, coma, and death; reaction appears to be associated with serum levels ≥50 μg/mL; may result from drug accumulation in patients with impaired hepatic or renal function

Dosage Forms

Capsule: 250 mg, 500 mg

Cream: 1% (30 g)

Ointment, ophthalmic: 1% (3.5 g)

Powder for injection, as sodium succinate: 100 mg/mL (1 g)

Powder for ophthalmic solution: 25 mg/vial

Solution:

Ophthalmic: 0.5% (2.5 mL, 7.5 mL, 15 mL)

Otic: 0.5% (15 mL)

Suspension, oral, as palmitate (custard flavor): 150 mg/5 mL (60 mL)

References

Nahata MC and Powell DA, "Bioavailability and Clearance of Chloramphenicol After Intravenous Chloramphenicol Succinate," *Clin Pharmacol Ther*, 1981, 30(3):368-72.

Chlorate® [OTC] *see* Chlorpheniramine Maleate *on page 128*

Chloromycetin® *see* Chloramphenicol *on page 124*

Chloroptic® *see* Chloramphenicol *on page 124*

Chloroquine Phosphate (klor' oh kwin)

Brand Names Aralen® Phosphate

Therapeutic Category Amebicide; Antimalarial Agent

Use Suppression or chemoprophylaxis of malaria; treatment of uncomplicated or mild-moderate malaria; extraintestinal amebiasis; rheumatoid arthritis

Pregnancy Risk Factor C

Contraindications Retinal or visual field changes; patients with psoriasis; known hypersensitivity to chloroquine

Precautions Use with caution in patients with liver disease, G-6-PD deficiency, or in conjunction with hepatotoxic drugs

Adverse Reactions

Cardiovascular: Hypotension, EKG changes

Central nervous system: Fatigue, personality changes, headache, confusion, agitation
Dermatologic: Pruritus, hair bleaching, skin eruptions
Gastrointestinal: Anorexia, nausea, vomiting, diarrhea, stomatitis
Hematologic: Blood dyscrasias
Ocular: Retinopathy, blurred vision

Drug Interactions Intradermally administered rabies vaccine, cimetidine

Mechanism of Action Binds to and inhibits DNA and RNA polymerase; interferes with metabolism and hemoglobin utilization by parasites; inhibits prostaglandin effects

Pharmacokinetics
Absorption: Oral: Rapid
Distribution: Crosses the placenta; appears in breast milk
Protein binding: 50% to 65%
Metabolism: Partial hepatic metabolism
Half-life: 3-5 days
Peak plasma levels: Within 1-2 hours
Elimination: ~70% of a dose is excreted unchanged in the urine; acidification of the urine increases elimination of drug; small amounts of drug may be present in the urine months following discontinuation of therapy
Minimally removed by hemodialysis

Usual Dosage Oral:
Suppression:
Children: Administer 5 mg base/kg/week on the same day each week (not to exceed 300 mg base/dose); begin 1-2 weeks prior to exposure; continue for 6-8 weeks after leaving endemic area; if suppressive therapy is not begun prior to exposure, double the initial loading dose to 10 mg base/kg and give in 2 divided doses 6 hours apart, followed by the usual dosage regimen
Adults: 300 mg/week (base) on the same day each week; begin 1-2 weeks prior to exposure; continue for 6-8 weeks after leaving endemic area; if suppressive therapy is not begun prior to exposure, double the initial loading dose to 600 mg base and give in 2 divided doses 6 hours apart, followed by the usual dosage regimen

Treatment:
Children: 10 mg base/kg (maximum: 600 mg) stat, then 5 mg base/kg 6 hours later and then once daily for 2 days
Adults: 600 mg base/dose one time, then 300 mg base/dose 6 hours later, and then once daily for 2 days

Extraintestinal amebiasis (dose expressed in mg base):
Children: 10 mg/kg once daily for 2-3 weeks (up to 300 mg base/day)
Adults: 600 mg base/day for 2 days followed by 300 mg base/day for at least 2-3 weeks

Rheumatoid arthritis: Adults: 150 mg base once daily

Monitoring Parameters Periodic CBC, examination for muscular weakness and ophthalmologic examination in patients receiving prolonged therapy

Patient Information Take with meals; tablets are bitter tasting

Dosage Forms Tablet: 250 mg [150 mg base]; 500 mg [300 mg base]

Extemporaneous Preparation(s) A 15 mg chloroquine base/mL suspension (made by pulverizing two (2) Aralen® 500 mg phosphate = 300 mg base/tablet, levigating with distilled water and Cologel®, and adding it to a 2:1 simple syrup/cherry syrup mixture to make a total volume of 40 mL) is stable for 3 days when stored in the refrigerator. Chloroquine phosphate tablets have also been mixed with chocolate syrup or enclosed in gelatin capsules to mask the bitter taste.

Handbook on Extemporaneous Formulations, Bethesda MD: American Society of Hospital Pharmacists, 1987.

Chlorothiazide (klor oh thye' a zide)

Brand Names Diuril®

Therapeutic Category Antihypertensive; Diuretic, Thiazide

Use Management of mild to moderate hypertension; edema associated with congestive heart failure, pregnancy, or nephrotic syndrome

Pregnancy Risk Factor D

Contraindications Hypersensitivity to chlorothiazide or any component;

(Continued)

Chlorothiazide *(Continued)*

cross sensitivity with other thiazides or sulfonamides; do not use in anuric patients.

Warnings The injection must not be administered subcutaneously or I.M.

Precautions Use with caution in patients with severe renal disease, impaired hepatic function

Adverse Reactions

Central nervous system: Dizziness, vertigo, paresthesias

Dermatologic: Rash, photosensitivity

Endocrine & metabolic: Hypokalemia, hypochloremic alkalosis, hyperglycemia, hyperlipidemia

Gastrointestinal: Anorexia, nausea, vomiting, cramping, diarrhea, pancreatitis, constipation

Hematologic: Rarely blood dyscrasias

Hepatic: Intrahepatic cholestasis

Musculoskeletal: Muscle weakness

Renal & genitourinary: Hyperuricemia, prerenal azotemia

Drug Interactions Nonsteroidal anti-inflammatory drug (NSAID) + chlorothiazide → decreased antihypertensive effect; additive potassium losses with steroids, amphotericin B; ↓ lithium clearance

Stability Reconstituted injection is stable for 24 hours at room temperature

Mechanism of Action Inhibits sodium reabsorption in the distal tubules causing increased excretion of sodium, chloride, potassium, bicarbonate, magnesium, phosphate, calcium (transiently) and water

Pharmacodynamics

Onset of effect: Oral: Within 2 hours

Duration:

- Oral: ~6-12 hours
- I.V.: 2 hours

Pharmacokinetics

Absorption: Oral: Poor

Half-life: Adults: 45-120 minutes

Peak serum concentrations: Within 4 hours

Elimination: Excreted unchanged in urine

Usual Dosage

Infants <6 months:

- Oral: 20-40 mg/kg/day in 2 divided doses
- I.V.: 2-8 mg/kg/day in 2 divided doses

Infants >6 months and Children:

- Oral: 20 mg/kg/day in 2 divided doses
- I.V.: 4 mg/kg/day

Adults:

- Oral: 500-2 g/day divided in 1-2 doses
- I.V.: 100-500 mg/day

Administration Dilute 500 mg vial with 18 mL sterile water; administer by direct I.V. infusion over 3-5 minutes or infusion over 30 minutes in dextrose or normal saline

Monitoring Parameters Serum electrolytes (sodium, potassium, chloride, and bicarbonate)

Nursing Implications Avoid extravasation of parenteral solution since it is extremely irritating to tissues

Dosage Forms

Powder for injection: 500 mg (20 mL)

Suspension, oral: 250 mg/5 mL (237 mL)

Tablet: 250 mg, 500 mg

Chlorphed® [OTC] *see* Brompheniramine Maleate *on page 88*

Chlorphed®-LA Nasal Solution [OTC] *see* Oxymetazoline Hydrochloride *on page 429*

Chlorpheniramine Maleate (klor fen ir' a meen)

Related Information

Overdose and Toxicology Information *on page 696-700*

Brand Names Aller-Chlor® [OTC]; Chlo-Amine® [OTC]; Chlorate® [OTC]; Chlor-Pro® [OTC]; Chlor-Trimeton® [OTC]; Phenetron®; Telachlor®; Teldrin® [OTC]

Therapeutic Category Antihistamine

Use Perennial and seasonal allergic rhinitis and other allergic symptoms including urticaria

Pregnancy Risk Factor B

Contraindications Hypersensitivity to chlorpheniramine maleate or any component; narrow-angle glaucoma, bladder neck obstruction, symptomatic prostatic hypertrophy, during acute asthmatic attacks, stenosing peptic ulcer, pyloroduodenal obstruction. Avoid use in premature and term newborns due to possible association with SIDS.

Warnings Swallow whole, do not crush or chew sustained release tablets

Adverse Reactions

Central nervous system: Drowsiness, vertigo, weakness, headache, excitability (children may be at increased risk for developing central nervous system stimulation)

Dermatologic: Dermatitis

Gastrointestinal: Nausea, dry mouth

Ocular: Diplopia, blurred vision

Renal & genitourinary: Polyuria, urinary retention

Stability Protect from light

Mechanism of Action Competes with histamine for H_1-receptor sites on effector cells in the gastrointestinal tract, blood vessels, and respiratory tract

Usual Dosage Oral, I.M., I.V., S.C.:

Children: 0.35 mg/kg/day in divided doses every 4-6 hours

2-6 years: 1 mg every 4-6 hours

6-12 years: 2 mg every 4-6 hours, not to exceed 12 mg/day or extended release 8 mg every 12 hours

Adults: 4 mg every 4-6 hours, not to exceed 24 mg/day or sustained release 8-12 mg every 12 hours

Administration Dilute in NS or dextrose; infuse I.V. slowly; the 100 mg/mL injection **is not for I.V. use**

Dosage Forms

Capsule: 12 mg

Capsule, timed release: 6 mg, 8 mg, 12 mg

Injection: 10 mg/mL (1 mL, 30 mL); 100 mg/mL (2 mL)

Syrup: 1 mg/5 mL, 2 mg/5 mL

Tablet: 4 mg

Tablet:

Chewable: 2 mg

Timed release: 8 mg, 12 mg

Chlor-Pro® [OTC] *see* Chlorpheniramine Maleate *on previous page*

Chlorpromazine Hydrochloride (klor proe' ma zeen)

Related Information

Compatibility of Medications Mixed in a Syringe *on page 717*

Overdose and Toxicology Information *on page 696-700*

Brand Names Ormazine®; Thorazine®

Therapeutic Category Antiemetic; Antipsychotic Agent; Phenothiazine Derivative

Use Treatment of nausea and vomiting; psychoses; Tourette's syndrome; mania; intractable hiccups (adults); behavioral problems (children)

Pregnancy Risk Factor C

Contraindications Hypersensitivity to chlorpromazine hydrochloride or any component; cross sensitivity with other phenothiazines may exist; avoid use in patients with narrow-angle glaucoma, bone marrow depression, severe liver or cardiac disease

Warnings Significant hypotension may occur, especially when the drug is administered parenterally; extended release capsules and injection contain benzyl alcohol; injection also contains sulfites which may cause allergic reaction

Precautions Use with caution in patients with cardiovascular disease, seizures, significant disorders or children with acute illnesses

Adverse Reactions

Cardiovascular: Hypotension (especially with I.V. use); orthostatic hypotension; tachycardia, arrhythmias

Central nervous system: Sedation, drowsiness, restlessness, anxiety, extrapyramidal reactions, pseudoparkinsonian signs and symptoms, tardive

(Continued)

Chlorpromazine Hydrochloride *(Continued)*

dyskinesia, neuroleptic malignant syndrome, seizures, altered central temperature regulation

Dermatologic: Hyperpigmentation, pruritus, rash, photosensitivity

Endocrine & metabolic: Amenorrhea, galactorrhea, gynecomastia, impotence, weight gain

Gastrointestinal: Dry mouth, constipation, GI upset

Hematologic: Agranulocytosis, leukopenia (usually in patients with large doses for prolonged periods), thrombocytopenia, hemolytic anemia, eosinophilia

Hepatic: Cholestatic jaundice (rare)

Ocular: Retinal pigmentation, blurred vision

Renal & genitourinary: Urinary retention

Miscellaneous: Anaphylactoid reactions

Drug Interactions Additive effects with other CNS depressing agents; epinephrine may cause hypotension in patients receiving chlorpromazine due to phenothiazine-induced alpha-adrenergic blockade and unopposed epinephrine B_2 action; chlorpromazine may ↑ valproic acid serum concentrations

Stability Protect oral dosage forms from light; discard solution if markedly discolored

Mechanism of Action Blocks postsynaptic mesolimbic dopaminergic receptors in the brain; exhibits a strong alpha-adrenergic blocking effect and depresses the release of hypothalamic and hypophyseal hormones

Usual Dosage

Children >6 months:

- Psychosis:
  - Oral: 0.5-1 mg/kg/dose every 4-6 hours; older children may require 200 mg/day or higher
  - I.M., I.V.: 0.5-1 mg/kg/dose every 6-8 hours; maximum I.M./I.V. dose for <5 years (22.7 kg) = 40 mg/day; maximum I.M./I.V. for 5-12 years (22.7-45.5 kg) = 75 mg/day
- Nausea and vomiting:
  - Oral: 0.5-1 mg/kg/dose every 4-6 hours as needed
  - Rectal: 1 mg/kg/dose every 6-8 hours as needed
  - I.M., I.V.: 0.5-1 mg/kg/dose every 6-8 hours; maximum dose: Same as psychosis

Adults:

- Psychosis:
  - Oral: Range: 30-800 mg/day in 1-4 divided doses, initiate at lower doses and titrate as needed; usual dose is 200 mg/day; some patients may require 1-2 g/day
  - I.M., I.V.: 25 mg initially, may repeat (25-50 mg) in 1-4 hours, gradually increase to a maximum of 400 mg/dose every 4-6 hours until patient controlled; usual dose 300-800 mg/day
- Nausea and vomiting:
  - Oral: 10-25 mg every 4-6 hours
  - Rectal: 50-100 mg every 6-8 hours
  - I.M., I.V.: 25-50 mg every 4-6 hours

Administration Do not administer S.C. (tissue damage and irritation); for direct I.V. injection, must dilute with 0.9% sodium chloride, maximum concentration 1 mg/mL, administer slow I.V. at a rate not to exceed 1 mg/minute in adults and 0.5 mg/minute in children

Monitoring Parameters Periodic eye exam with prolonged therapy; blood pressure with parenteral administration

Test Interactions False-positives for phenylketonuria, amylase, uroporphyrins, urobilinogen; possible false-negative pregnancy urinary test

Nursing Implications Dilute oral concentrate solution in juice before administration; avoid contact of oral solution or injection with skin (contact dermatitis)

Additional Information Use decreased doses in elderly or debilitated patients; dystonic reactions may be more common in patients with hypocalcemia; extrapyramidal reactions may be more common in pediatric patients, especially those with dehydration or acute illnesses (viral or CNS infections); avoid rectal administration in immunocompromised patients

Dosage Forms

Capsule, sustained action: 30 mg, 75 mg, 150 mg, 200 mg, 300 mg

Concentrate, oral: 30 mg/mL (120 mL); 100 mg/mL (60 mL, 240 mL)

Injection: 25 mg/mL (1 mL, 2 mL, 10 mL)
Suppository, rectal, as base: 25 mg, 100 mg
Syrup: 10 mg/5 mL (120 mL)
Tablet: 10 mg, 25 mg, 50 mg, 100 mg, 200 mg

Chlorpropamide (klor proe' pa mide)

Brand Names Diabinese®

Therapeutic Category Antidiabetic Agent; Hypoglycemic Agent, Oral; Sulfonylurea Agent

Use To control blood sugar in adult onset, noninsulin-dependent diabétes (type II)

Pregnancy Risk Factor D

Contraindications Cross sensitivity may exist with other hypoglycemics or sulfonamides; do not use with type I diabetes, or with severe renal, hepatic, thyroid, or other endocrine disease

Precautions Patients should be properly instructed in the early detection and treatment of hypoglycemia

Adverse Reactions

Cardiovascular: Edema
Central nervous system: Headache
Dermatologic: Rash, photosensitivity
Endocrine & metabolic: Hypoglycemia, hyponatremia
Gastrointestinal: Anorexia, nausea, vomiting, diarrhea, abdominal cramps, constipation
Hematologic: Blood dyscrasias
Hepatic: Cholestatic jaundice
Renal & genitourinary: SIADH

Drug Interactions Oral anticoagulants, hydantoins, salicylates, NSAIDs, sulfonamides, alcohol, thiazide diuretics, miconazole, barbiturates, probenecid, MAO inhibitors, desmopressin

Mechanism of Action Stimulates insulin release from the pancreatic beta cells; reduces basal hepatic glucose production; insulin sensitivity is increased at peripheral target sites

Pharmacodynamics

Peak effects: Following oral administration peak hypoglycemic effects occur within 3-6 hours
Duration: 24 hours

Pharmacokinetics

Distribution: Appears in breast milk
Protein binding: 60% to 90%
Metabolism: Extensive (~80%) in the liver
Half-life: 36 hours (range: 25-60 hours) (half-life is prolonged in the elderly or with renal disease)
Peak plasma levels: Oral: Within 2-4 hours
Elimination: 10% to 30% excreted in the urine as unchanged drug

Usual Dosage The dosage of chlorpropamide is variable and should be individualized based upon the patient's response.

Adults: Oral: Initial: 250 mg once daily; initial dose in elderly patients: 100 mg once daily; subsequent dosages may be increased or decreased by 50-125 mg/day at 3- to 5-day intervals; maximum daily dose: 750 mg

Monitoring Parameters Blood or urine glucose, urine acetone

Additional Information Long half-life may complicate recovery from excess effects; patients previously maintained on insulin at <40 units/day may be directly changed to chlorpropamide; patients previously receiving larger insulin doses should have their insulin doses decreased by 50% daily for the first few days then gradually reduced further as necessary.

Intoxications with sulfonylureas can cause hypoglycemia and are best managed with glucose administration (oral for milder hypoglycemia or by injection in more severe forms)

Signs and symptoms of overdose include low blood glucose levels, tingling of lips and tongue, tachycardia, convulsions, stupor, and coma

Dosage Forms Tablet: 100 mg, 250 mg

Chlor-Trimeton® [OTC] *see* Chlorpheniramine Maleate *on page 128*

Chlorzoxazone (klor zox' a zone)

Brand Names Paraflex®; Parafon Forte™ DSC; Remular-S®

Therapeutic Category Skeletal Muscle Relaxant, Central Acting

Use Symptomatic treatment of muscle spasm and pain associated with acute musculoskeletal conditions

Pregnancy Risk Factor C

Contraindications Known hypersensitivity to chlorzoxazone; impaired liver function

Precautions May impair ability to perform hazardous activities requiring mental alertness due to sedative potential

Adverse Reactions

Central nervous system: Drowsiness, dizziness, lightheadedness, headache, paresthesia

Dermatologic: Rash, urticaria

Gastrointestinal: Nausea, vomiting, diarrhea, GI bleeding

Hematologic: Anemia, granulocytopenia

Hepatic: Hepatitis

Drug Interactions May cause additive sedation when concomitantly administered with other CNS depressant medications

Mechanism of Action Acts on the spinal cord and subcortical levels by depressing polysynaptic reflexes

Pharmacodynamics

Onset of effects: Within 60 minutes

Duration: 3-4 hours

Pharmacokinetics

Absorption: Oral: Readily absorbed

Metabolism: Extensive in the liver by glucuronidation

Elimination: Excreted in the urine as conjugates

Usual Dosage Oral:

Children: 20 mg/kg/day or 600 mg/m^2/day in 3-4 divided doses

Adults: 250-500 mg 3-4 times/day up to 750 mg 3-4 times/day

Monitoring Parameters Periodic liver function tests

Patient Information May color urine orange or purple-red

Dosage Forms Tablet: 250 mg, 500 mg

Cholac® *see* Lactulose *on page 334*

Cholestyramine Resin (koe less' tir a meen)

Brand Names Cholybar®; Questran®; Questran® Light

Therapeutic Category Antilipemic Agent

Use Adjunct in the management of primary hypercholesterolemia; pruritus associated with elevated levels of bile acids; diarrhea associated with excess fecal bile acids; pseudomembraneous colitis

Pregnancy Risk Factor C

Contraindications Hypersensitivity to cholestyramine or any component; avoid using in complete biliary obstruction or biliary atresia

Precautions Use with caution in patients with constipation

Adverse Reactions

Dermatologic: Rash, irritation of perianal area, skin, or tongue

Endocrine & metabolic: Hyperchloremic acidosis

Gastrointestinal: Constipation, nausea, vomiting, abdominal distention and pain, malabsorption of fat-soluble vitamins

Renal & genitourinary: Increased urinary calcium excretion

Drug Interactions May decrease oral absorption of digitalis glycosides, warfarin, thyroid hormones, thiazide diuretics, propranolol, phenobarbital, and other drugs by binding to the drug in the intestine

Mechanism of Action Forms a nonabsorbable complex with bile acids in the intestine, releasing chloride ions in the process; inhibits enterohepatic reuptake of intestinal bile salts and thereby increases the fecal loss of bile salt-bound low density lipoprotein cholesterol

Usual Dosage Oral (dosages are expressed in terms of anhydrous resin):

Children: 240 mg/kg/day in 3 divided doses; need to titrate dose depending on indication

Adults: 3-4 g 3-4 times/day to a maximum of 16-32 g/day in 2-4 divided doses

Administration Do not administer the powder in its dry form; just prior to administration, mix with fluid or with applesauce; to minimize binding of concomitant medications, administer other drugs at least 1 hour before or at least 4-6 hours after cholestyramine

Additional Information Overdose may result in GI obstruction; Questran® Light contains aspartame

Dosage Forms

Bars, chewable: 4 g

Powder, for oral suspension: 4 g of resin per 9 g of powder; 4 g of resin per 5 g of powder

Choline Magnesium Trisalicylate (koe' leen)

Related Information

Overdose and Toxicology Information *on page 696-700*

Brand Names Trilisate®

Therapeutic Category Analgesic, Non-Narcotic; Anti-inflammatory Agent; Nonsteroidal Anti-Inflammatory Agent (NSAID), Oral; Salicylate

Use Management of osteoarthritis, rheumatoid arthritis, and other arthritides

Pregnancy Risk Factor C

Contraindications Hypersensitivity to salicylates or any component or other nonacetylated salicylates

Warnings Avoid use in patients with suspected varicella or influenza (salicylates have been associated with Reye's syndrome in children $<$16 years of age when used to treat symptoms of chickenpox or the flu)

Precautions Use with caution in patients with impaired renal function, erosive gastritis or peptic ulcer

Adverse Reactions

Hepatic: Hepatotoxicity

Otic: Tinnitus

Respiratory: Pulmonary edema

Drug Interactions Antacids + Trilisate® → decreased salicylate concentration; warfarin + Trilisate® → possible increased hypoprothrombinemic effect

Mechanism of Action Inhibits prostaglandin synthesis; acts on the hypothalamus heat-regulating center to reduce fever; blocks the generation of pain impulses

Pharmacokinetics

Absorption: Absorbed from stomach and small intestine

Distribution: Readily distributes into most body fluids and tissues; crosses the placenta; appears in breast milk

Half-life: Dose-dependent, ranging from 2-3 hours at low doses to 30 hours at high doses

Peak plasma levels: Within ~2 hours

Usual Dosage Oral (based on **total salicylate content**):

Children: 30-60 mg/kg/day given in 3-4 divided doses

Adults: 500 mg to 1.5 g 1-3 times/day

Monitoring Parameters Serum salicylate levels; serum magnesium with high doses or in patients with decreased renal function

Reference Range Salicylate blood levels for anti-inflammatory effect: 150-300 μg/mL; analgesia and antipyretic effect: 30-50 μg/mL

Test Interactions False-negative results for Clinistix® urine test; false positive results with Clinitest®

Nursing Implications Liquid may be mixed with fruit juice just before drinking

Dosage Forms See table.

Choline Magnesium Trisalicylate

Brand Name	Dosage Form	Total Salicylate	Choline Salicylate	Magnesium Salicylate
Trilisate®	Liquid	500 mg/5 mL	293 mg/5 mL	362 mg/5 mL
Trilisate 500®	Tablet	500 mg	293 mg	362 mg
Trilisate 750®	Tablet	750 mg	440 mg	544 mg
Trilisate 1000®	Tablet	1000 mg	587 mg	725 mg

(Continued)

Choline Magnesium Trisalicylate *(Continued)*

References

Berde C, Ablin A, Glazer J, et al, "American Academy of Pediatrics Report of the Subcommittee on Disease-Related Pain in Childhood Cancer," *Pediatrics*, 1990, 86(5 Pt 2):818-25.

Cholybar® *see* Cholestyramine Resin *on page 132*

Chooz® [OTC] *see* Calcium Carbonate *on page 94*

Chorex® *see* Chorionic Gonadotropin *on this page*

Chorionic Gonadotropin (go nad' oh troe pin)

Brand Names A.P.L.®; Chorex®; Choron®; Corgonject®; Follutein®; Glukor®; Gonic®; Pregnyl®; Profasi® HP

Synonyms CG; hCG

Therapeutic Category Ovulation Stimulator

Use Treatment of hypogonadotropic hypogonadism and prepubertal cryptorchidism; induce ovulation

Pregnancy Risk Factor X

Contraindications Hypersensitivity to chorionic gonadotropin or any component; precocious puberty, prostatic carcinoma or similar neoplasms

Warnings hCG is **not** effective in the treatment of obesity

Precautions Use with caution in patients with asthma, seizure disorders, migraine, cardiac or renal disease

Adverse Reactions

Cardiovascular: Edema

Central nervous system: Irritability, restlessness, depression, fatigue, headache, aggressive behavior

Endocrine & metabolic: Gynecomastia, precocious puberty

Local: Pain at the injection site

Musculoskeletal: Premature closure of epiphyses

Stability Following reconstitution with provided diluent, stable for 30-90 days (depending upon preparation) when stored at 2°C to 15°C

Mechanism of Action Stimulates production of gonadal steroid hormones by causing production of androgen by the testis; as a substitute for luteinizing hormone (LH) to stimulate ovulation

Usual Dosage Children: I.M.:

Prepubertal cryptorchidism: 1000-2000 units/m^2/dose 3 times/week for 3 weeks or 4000 units 3 times/week for 3 weeks

Hypogonadotropic hypogonadism: 500-1000 USP units 3 times/week for 3 weeks, followed by the same dose twice weekly for 3 weeks

Induction of ovulation: 5000-10,000 units the day following the last dose of menotropins

Reference Range Depends on application and methodology; less than 3 mIU/mL (SI: 3 units/L) usually normal (nonpregnant)

Dosage Forms Powder for injection: 200 units/mL (25 mL); 500 units/mL (10 mL); 1000 units/mL (10 mL); 2000 units/mL (10 mL)

Choron® *see* Chorionic Gonadotropin *on this page*

Chroma-Pak® *see* Trace Metals *on page 574*

Chromium *see* Trace Metals *on page 574*

Chronulac® *see* Lactulose *on page 334*

Cibalith-S® *see* Lithium *on page 345*

Ciloxan™ *see* Ciprofloxacin Hydrochloride *on page 136*

Cimetidine (sye met' i deen)

Related Information

Medications Compatible With PN Solutions *on page 649-650*

Brand Names Tagamet®

Therapeutic Category Histamine-2 Antagonist

Use Short-term treatment of active duodenal ulcers and benign gastric ulcers; long-term prophylaxis of duodenal ulcer; gastric hypersecretory states; gastroesophageal reflux

Pregnancy Risk Factor B

Contraindications Hypersensitivity to cimetidine or any component

Warnings Rapid I.V. administration may cause hypotension or cardiac arrhythmias

Precautions Modify dosage in patients with renal and/or hepatic impairment

Adverse Reactions

Cardiovascular: Bradycardia, hypotension

Central nervous system: Dizziness, mental confusion, agitation, headache

Dermatologic: Rash

Endocrine & metabolic: Gynecomastia

Gastrointestinal: Mild diarrhea

Hematologic: Neutropenia

Hepatic: Elevated AST and ALT

Musculoskeletal: Myalgia

Renal & genitourinary: Elevated creatinine

Drug Interactions Decreased elimination of lidocaine, theophylline, phenytoin, metronidazole, triamterene, procainamide, quinidine and propranolol; inhibition of warfarin metabolism, tricyclic antidepressant metabolism, diazepam elimination and cyclosporine elimination; antacids may reduce the absorption of cimetidine

Stability Do not refrigerate the injection since precipitation may occur

Mechanism of Action Competitive inhibition of histamine at H_2 receptors of the gastric parietal cells resulting in reduced gastric acid secretion

Pharmacokinetics

Distribution: Crosses the placenta; appears in breast milk

Protein binding: 20%

Bioavailability: 60% to 70%

Half-life:

- Neonates: 3.6 hours
- Children: 1.4 hours
- Adults with normal renal function: 2 hours

Peak serum levels: Oral: Within 1-2 hours

Elimination: Excreted principally as unchanged drug by the kidney; some excretion in the bile and feces

Usual Dosage

Neonates: Oral, I.M., I.V.: 5-10 mg/kg/day in divided doses every 8-12 hours

Infants: Oral, I.M., I.V.: 10-20 mg/kg/day divided every 6-12 hours

Children: Oral, I.M., I.V.: 20-40 mg/kg/day in divided doses every 6 hours

Adults:

- Short-term treatment of active ulcers:
  - Oral: 300 mg 4 times/day or 800 mg at bedtime or 400 mg twice daily for up to 8 weeks
  - I.M., I.V.: 300 mg every 6 hours; I.V. dosage should be adjusted to maintain an intragastric pH of ≥ 5
- Duodenal ulcer prophylaxis: Oral: 400-800 mg at bedtime
- Gastric hypersecretory conditions: Oral, I.M., I.V.: 300-600 mg every 6 hours; dosage not to exceed 2.4 g/day

Dosing interval in renal impairment using 5-10 mg/kg/dose: Children and Adults (titrate dose to gastric pH and Cl_{cr}):

- Cl_{cr} >40 mL/minute: Administer every 6 hours
- Cl_{cr} 20-40 mL/minute: Administer every 8 hours
- Cl_{cr} 0-20 mL/minute: Administer every 12 hours

Administration Can be administered as a slow I.V. push over a minimum of 15 minutes at a concentration not to exceed 15 mg/mL; or preferably as an I.V. intermittent or I.V. continuous infusion. Intermittent infusions are administered over 15-30 minutes at a final concentration not to exceed 6 mg/mL; for patients with an active bleed, preferred method of administration is continuous infusion

Monitoring Parameters Blood pressure and heart rate with I.V. push administration; CBC; gastric pH

Dosage Forms

Infusion, as hydrochloride, in NS: 300 mg (50 mL)

Injection, as hydrochloride: 150 mg/mL (2 mL)

Liquid, oral, as hydrochloride (mint-peach flavor): 300 mg/5 mL (5 mL, 240 mL)

(Continued)

Cimetidine *(Continued)*

Tablet: 200 mg, 300 mg, 400 mg, 800 mg

References

Lambert J, Mobassaleh M, and Grand RJ, "Efficacy of Cimetidine for Gastric Acid Suppression in Pediatric Patients," *J Pediatr*, 1992, 120(3):474-8.
Lloyd CW, Martin WJ, Taylor BD, et al, "Pharmacokinetics and Pharmacodynamics of Cimetidine and Metabolites in Critically Ill Children," *J Pediatr*, 1985, 107(2):295-300.
Lloyd CW, Martin WJ, and Taylor BD, "The Pharmacokinetics of Cimetidine and Metabolites in a Neonate," *Drug Intell Clin Pharm*, 1985, 19(3):203-5.
Somogyi A and Gugler R, "Clinical Pharmacokinetics of Cimetidine," *Clin Pharmacokinet*, 1983, 8(6):463-95.

Cipro™ *see* Ciprofloxacin Hydrochloride *on this page*

Ciprofloxacin Hydrochloride (sip roe flox' a sin)

Brand Names Ciloxan™; Cipro™

Therapeutic Category Antibiotic, Ophthalmic; Antibiotic, Quinolone

Use Treatment of documented or suspected pseudomonal infection; documented multi-drug resistant gram-negative organisms; documented infectious diarrhea due to *Campylobacter jejuni*, *Shigella*, or *Salmonella*; osteomyelitis caused by susceptible organisms in which parenteral therapy is not feasible; ocular infections caused by susceptible bacterial organisms in patients with corneal ulcers or conjunctivitis

Pregnancy Risk Factor C

Contraindications Hypersensitivity to ciprofloxacin, any component or other quinolones

Warnings Not recommended in children <18 years of age; ciprofloxacin has caused arthropathy with erosions of the cartilage in weight bearing joints of immature animals; green discoloration of teeth in newborns has been reported; prolonged use may result in superinfection

Precautions Use with caution in patients with seizure disorders or renal impairment; modify dosage in patients with renal impairment

Adverse Reactions

Central nervous system: Tremor, restlessness, dizziness, confusion, seizures, headache
Dermatologic: Rash
Gastrointestinal: Pseudomembraneous colitis, nausea, diarrhea, vomiting, GI bleeding
Hematologic: Anemia, eosinophilia, neutropenia
Hepatic: Increased liver enzymes
Local: Phlebitis (I.V.)
Musculoskeletal: Arthralgia, joint and back pain
Renal & genitourinary: Acute renal failure, increased serum creatinine and BUN

Drug Interactions Magnesium, aluminum or calcium-containing antacids and sucralfate ↓ ciprofloxacin absorption; probenecid ↓ renal clearance of ciprofloxacin and can ↑ ciprofloxacin concentrations; ciprofloxacin ↓ theophylline, warfarin, and cyclosporine clearance

Mechanism of Action Inhibits DNA-gyrase in susceptible organisms; inhibits relaxation of supercoiled DNA and promotes breakage of double-stranded DNA

Pharmacokinetics

Distribution: Crosses the placenta; appears in breast milk
Protein bound: 16% to 43%
Metabolism: Partially metabolized in the liver to active metabolites
Bioavailability: Oral: 50% to 85%
Half-life, patients with normal renal function: 3-5 hours
Peak serum levels: Oral: Within 0.5-2 hours
Elimination: 30% to 50% of a dose excreted as unchanged drug in the urine; 20% to 40% of a dose is excreted in feces primarily from biliary excretion
Only small amounts of ciprofloxacin are removed by dialysis (<10%)

Usual Dosage

Children:
- Oral: 20-30 mg/kg/day in 2 divided doses; maximum dose: 1.5 g/day
- I.V.: Doses ranging from 3.2 to 12.5 mg/kg/day divided every 12 hours have been used on a compassionate basis in patients with cystic fibrosis

Adults:

Oral: 250-750 mg every 12 hours, depending on severity of infection and susceptibility

Ophthalmic:

Corneal ulcers: 2 drops every 15 minutes for the first 6 hours, then 2 drops every 30 minutes for the remainder of the first day; instill 2 drops every hour on day 2; 2 drops every 4 hours on day 3 through 14

Bacterial conjunctivitis: 1-2 drops every 2 hours while awake for 2 days, then 1-2 drops every 4 hours while awake for the next 5 days

I.V.: 200-400 mg every 12 hours depending on severity of infection

Dosing interval in renal impairment: Cl_{cr} <30 mL/minutes: Administer every 18-24 hours

Administration Administer by slow I.V. infusion over 60 minutes to reduce the risk of venous irritation (burning, pain, erythema, and swelling); final concentration for administration should not exceed 2 mg/mL

Monitoring Parameters Patients receiving concurrent ciprofloxacin and theophylline should have serum levels of theophylline monitored; periodic renal, hepatic, and hematologic function tests

Reference Range Avoid peak serum concentrations >5 μg/mL

Patient Information Take with food to minimize GI upset; avoid antacid use; drink plenty of fluids to maintain proper hydration and urine output; may cause dizziness or lightheadedness; use caution when driving or performing tasks which require alertness

Nursing Implications Do not administer antacids with or within 4 hours of a ciprofloxacin dose

Dosage Forms

Infusion, in D_5W: 400 mg (200 mL)

Infusion, in NS or D_5W: 200 mg (100 mL)

Injection: 200 mg (20 mL); 400 mg (40 mL)

Solution, ophthalmic: 3.5 mg/mL (2.5 mL, 5 mL)

Tablet: 250 mg, 500 mg, 750 mg

References

Campoli-Richards DM, Monk JP, Price A, et al, "Ciprofloxacin: A Review of Its Antibacterial Activity, Pharmacokinetic Properties and Therapeutic Use," *Drugs*, 1988, 35(4):373-447.

Cisplatin (sis' pla tin)

Related Information

Emetogenic Potential of Single Chemotherapeutic Agents *on page 655*

Brand Names Platinol®; Platinol®-AQ

Synonyms CDDP

Therapeutic Category Antineoplastic Agent

Use Management of metastatic testicular or ovarian carcinoma, advanced bladder cancer, osteosarcoma, Hodgkin's and non-Hodgkin's lymphoma, head or neck cancer, cervical cancer, lung cancer, brain tumors, neuroblastoma; used alone or with other agents

Pregnancy Risk Factor D

Contraindications Hypersensitivity to cisplatin, platinum-containing agents, or any component; pre-existing renal impairment, hearing impairment, and myelosuppression

Warnings The US Food and Drug Administration (FDA) currently recommends that procedures for proper handling and disposal of antineoplastic agents be considered. Cumulative renal toxicity may be severe; dose-related toxicities include myelosuppression, nausea and vomiting; ototoxicity, especially pronounced in children, is manifested by tinnitus or loss of high frequency hearing and occasionally, deafness

Precautions All patients should receive adequate hydration prior to and for 24 hours after cisplatin administration, with or without mannitol and/or furosemide, to ensure good urine output and decrease the chance of nephrotoxicity; reduce dosage in renal impairment

Adverse Reactions

Cardiovascular: Bradycardia, arrhythmias

(Continued)

Cisplatin *(Continued)*

Central nervous system: Peripheral neuropathy, seizures
Dermatologic: Mild alopecia
Endocrine & metabolic: Hypomagnesemia, hypocalcemia, hypokalemia, hypophosphatemia, hyperuricemia
Gastrointestinal: Nausea, vomiting
Hematologic: Myelosuppression
Hepatic: Elevation of liver enzymes
Local: Phlebitis
Ocular: Papilledema, optic neuritis
Otic: Ototoxicity (especially pronounced in children)
Renal & genitourinary: Nephrotoxicity
Miscellaneous: Anaphylactoid reactions

Drug Interactions Aminoglycosides, amphotericin B, loop diuretics

Stability Reconstituted powder for injection is stable for 20 hours at room temperature; do not refrigerate reconstituted solution since precipitation may occur; protect from light; incompatible with sodium bicarbonate; do not infuse in solutions containing <0.2% sodium chloride

Mechanism of Action Inhibits DNA synthesis by the formation of DNA cross-links; denatures the double helix

Pharmacokinetics
Distribution: I.V.: Rapid tissue distribution
Protein binding: >90%
Metabolism: Undergoes nonenzymatic metabolism
Half-life,terminal: Free drug: 1.3 hours; total platinum: 44 hours
Elimination: 25% to 40% of a dose excreted in the urine within 5 days
Minimally removed by hemodialysis

Usual Dosage Children and Adults: I.V. (refer to individual protocols):
Intermittent dosing schedule: 37-75 mg/m^2 once every 2-3 weeks or 50-200 mg/m^2 over 4-6 hours, once every 21-28 days

Daily dosing schedule: 15-20 mg/m^2/day for 5 days every 3-4 weeks

Dosing adjustment in renal impairment:
Cl_{cr} 10-50 mL/minute: Administer 75% of dose
Cl_{cr} <10 mL/minute: Administer 50% of dose

Administration I.V.: Rate of administration has varied from a 15- to 20-minute infusion, 1 mg/minute infusion, 6- to 8-hour infusion, 24-hour infusion, or per protocol

Monitoring Parameters Renal function tests (serum creatinine, BUN, Cl_{cr}), electrolytes (particularly magnesium, calcium, potassium), hearing test, neurologic exam (with high dose), liver function tests periodically, CBC with differential and platelet count, urine output, urinalysis

Nursing Implications Needles, syringes, catheters, or I.V. administration sets that contain aluminum parts should not be used for administration of drug; I.V. prehydration required to reduce toxicity of drug

Additional Information Myelosuppressive effects:
WBC: Mild
Platelets: Mild
Onset (days): 10
Nadir (days): 18-23
Recovery (days): 21-40

Dosage Forms
Injection: 1 mg/mL (50 mL, 100 mL)
Powder for injection: 10 mg, 50 mg

References

Costello MA, Dominick C, and Clerico A, "A Pilot Study of 5-Day Continuous Infusion of High-Dose Cisplatin and Pulsed Etoposide in Childhood Solid Tumors," *Amer J Pediatr Hematol/Oncol*, 1988, 10:103-8.

Reece PA, Stafford I, Abbott RL, et al, "Two-Versus 24-Hour Infusion of Cisplatin: Pharmacokinetic Considerations," *J Clin Oncol*, 1989, 7(2):270-5.

13-*cis*-Retinoic Acid *see* Isotretinoin *on page 325*

Citrate/Citric Acid *see* Sodium Citrate and Citric Acid *on page 528*

Citrate of Magnesia *see* Magnesium Citrate *on page 352*

Citro-Nesia™ [OTC] *see* Magnesium Citrate *on page 352*

Citrovorum Factor *see* Leucovorin Calcium *on page 335*

Cla *see* Clarithromycin *on this page*

Claforan® *see* Cefotaxime Sodium *on page 112*

Clarithromycin (kla rith' roe mye sin)

Brand Names Biaxin™

Synonyms Cla

Therapeutic Category Antibiotic, Macrolide

Use Treatment of upper and lower respiratory tract infections, and infections of the skin and skin structure due to susceptible strains of *S. aureus*, *S. pyogenes*, *S. pneumoniae*, *H. influenzae*, *M. catarrhalis*, *Mycoplasma pneumoniae*, *C. trachomatis*, *Legionella* spp., and *M. avium*

Pregnancy Risk Factor C

Contraindications Hypersensitivity to clarithromycin, erythromycin, or any macrolide antibiotic

Warnings Pseudomembranous colitis has been reported with use of clarithromycin

Precautions Use with caution in patients with hepatic or renal impairment; reduce dosage or prolong dosing interval in patients with severe renal impairment with or without coexisting hepatic impairment

Adverse Reactions The incidence of adverse GI effects (diarrhea, nausea, vomiting, dyspepsia, abdominal pain) is lower (13%) compared to erythromycin treated patients (32%)

Other adverse effects reported:
Central nervous system: Headache
Dermatologic: Pruritus
Gastrointestinal: Abnormal taste, stomatitis
Hematologic: Increased prothrombin time
Hepatic: Increased liver enzymes, hyperbilirubinemia

Drug Interactions Clarithromycin has been shown to increase serum **theophylline** levels by as much as 20%. **Carbamazepine** levels have been shown to increase after a single dose of clarithromycin.

Mechanism of Action Inhibits bacterial RNA-dependent protein synthesis by binding to the 50S ribosomal subunit

Pharmacokinetics

Absorption: Rapidly absorbed from the GI tract; food delays onset of absorption and formation of active metabolite but does not affect the extent of absorption

Distribution: Widely distributed throughout the body with tissue concentrations higher than serum concentrations

Protein binding: 65% to 70%

Metabolism: Extensively metabolized in the liver to active and inactive metabolites

Bioavailability: 50%

Half-life: Dose-dependent, prolonged with renal dysfunction
- Clarithromycin:
  - 250 mg dose: 3-4 hours
  - 500 mg dose: 5-7 hours
- 14-hydroxy metabolite:
  - 250 mg dose: 5-6 hours
  - 500 mg dose: 7 hours

Time to peak serum concentration: 2-4 hours

Elimination: After a 250 mg dose, 20% is excreted unchanged in the urine, 10% to 15% is excreted as active metabolite 14-OH clarithromycin, and 4% is excreted in the feces

Usual Dosage Not currently FDA approved for use in children <12 years of age; dosages of 15 mg/kg/day divided every 12 hours have been used in clinical trials

Adults: Oral: 250 mg every 12 hours for 7-14 days for all indications except sinusitis and chronic bronchitis due to *H. influenzae*; for these indications, 500 mg every 12 hours for 7-14 days

Dosing adjustment in renal impairment: Cl_{cr} <30 mL/minute: Decrease dose by 50% to 250 mg once or twice daily

(Continued)

Clarithromycin *(Continued)*

Monitoring Parameters Monitor patients receiving clarithromycin and drugs known to interact with erythromycin (ie, theophylline, digoxin, anticoagulants, triazolam) since there are still very few studies examining drug-drug interactions with clarithromycin; liver function tests

Patient Information May be taken with or without meals

Nursing Implications Clarithromycin may be given with or without meals; flavored Maalox® can be used to mask taste; do not use "cold" flavoring vehicles (ice cream, yogurt) to administer clarithromycin, since they worsen the taste; cherry syrup decreases stability of clarithromycin

Dosage Forms Tablet, film coated: 250 mg, 500 mg

References

Chonmaitree T, Owen MJ, Patel JA, et al, "Effect of Viral Respiratory Tract Infection on Outcome of Acute Otitis Media," *J Pediatr*, 1992, 120(6):856-62.

Neu HC, "The Development of Macrolides: Clarithromycin in Perspective," *J Antimicrob Chemother*, 1991, 27(Suppl A):1-9.

Clear By Design® [OTC] *see* Benzoyl Peroxide *on page 78*

Clear Eyes® [OTC] *see* Naphazoline Hydrochloride *on page 403*

Clearsil® [OTC] *see* Benzoyl Peroxide *on page 78*

Cleocin HCl® *see* Clindamycin *on this page*

Cleocin Pediatric® *see* Clindamycin *on this page*

Cleocin Phosphate® *see* Clindamycin *on this page*

Cleocin T® *see* Clindamycin *on this page*

Clindamycin (klin da mye' sin)

Related Information

Medications Compatible With PN Solutions *on page 649-650*

Brand Names Cleocin HCl®; Cleocin Pediatric®; Cleocin Phosphate®; Cleocin T®

Therapeutic Category Acne Product; Antibiotic, Anaerobic

Use Useful agent against aerobic and anaerobic streptococci (except enterococci), most staphylococci, *Bacteroides* sp. and *Actinomyces* for treatment of respiratory tract infections, skin and soft tissue infections, sepsis, intra-abdominal infections, and infections of the female pelvis and genital tract; used topically in treatment of severe acne

Pregnancy Risk Factor B

Contraindications Hypersensitivity to clindamycin or any component; previous pseudomembranous colitis, hepatic impairment

Warnings Can cause severe and possibly fatal colitis characterized by severe persistent diarrhea, severe abdominal cramps and possibly, the passage of blood and mucus; discontinue drug if significant diarrhea occurs

Precautions Use with caution and modify dosage in patients with severe renal and/or hepatic impairment

Adverse Reactions

Cardiovascular: Hypotension

Dermatologic: Urticaria, rash, Stevens-Johnson syndrome

Gastrointestinal: Diarrhea, nausea, vomiting, pseudomembranous colitis, esophagitis

Hematologic: Eosinophilia, granulocytopenia, thrombocytopenia

Hepatic: Elevation of liver enzymes

Local: Sterile abscess at I.M. injection site, thrombophlebitis

Renal & genitourinary: Rare renal dysfunction

Drug Interactions Tubocurarine, pancuronium → ↑ neuromuscular blockade

Stability Do **not** refrigerate the reconstituted oral solution because it will thicken; oral solution stable for two weeks at room temperature following reconstitution; I.V. clindamycin is incompatible with aminophylline, tobramycin

Mechanism of Action Reversibly binds to 50S ribosomal subunits preventing peptide bond formation thus inhibiting bacterial protein synthesis; bacteriostatic or bactericidal depending on drug concentration, infection site, and organism

Pharmacokinetics

Absorption: Topical: ~10% absorbed systemically; food decreases oral absorption

Distribution: No significant levels are seen in CSF, even with inflamed meninges; crosses the placenta; distributes into breast milk

Protein binding: 94%

Bioavailability: Oral: ~90%

Half-life: 1.6-5.3 hours, average: 2-3 hours; half-life shorter in children than adults

- Neonates:
  - Premature: 8.7 hours
  - Full term: 3.6 hours

Peak serum levels:

- Oral: Within 60 minutes
- I.M.: Within 1-3 hours

Elimination: Most of the drug is eliminated by hepatic metabolism; 10% of an oral dose is excreted in urine and 3.6% is excreted in feces as active drug and metabolites

Not dialyzable (0% to 5%)

Usual Dosage

Neonates: I.V., I.M.:

- ≤7 days:
  - ≤2000 g: 10 mg/kg/day divided every 12 hours
  - >2000 g: 15 mg/kg/day divided every 8 hours
- >7 days:
  - <1200 g: 10 mg/kg/day divided every 12 hours
  - 1200-2000 g: 15 mg/kg/day divided every 8 hours
  - >2000 g: 20 mg/kg/day divided every 6-8 hours

Infants and Children:

- Oral: 10-30 mg/kg/day divided every 6 hours
- I.V., I.M.: 25-40 mg/kg/day divided every 6-8 hours

Children and Adults: Topical: Apply twice daily

Adults:

- Oral: 150-450 mg/dose every 6-8 hours; maximum dose: 1.8 g/day
- I.V., I.M.: 1.2-1.8 g/day in 2-4 divided doses; maximum dose: 4.8 g/day

Dosing interval in renal impairment: No change necessary

Administration Administer by I.V. intermittent infusion over at least 10-60 minutes, at a rate **not** to exceed 30 mg/minute; final concentration for administration should not exceed 12 mg/mL

Monitoring Parameters Observe for changes in bowel frequency; during prolonged therapy monitor CBC, liver and renal function tests periodically

Patient Information Adults: Take capsule with a full glass of water to avoid esophageal irritation; report any severe diarrhea immediately

Dosage Forms

- Capsule, as hydrochloride: 75 mg, 150 mg, 300 mg
- Gel, topical, as phosphate: 1% (7.5 g, 30 g)
- Granules for oral solution, as palmitate: 75 mg/5 mL (100 mL)
- Infusion, as phosphate: 300 mg in D_5W (50 mL); 600 mg in D_5W (50 mL)
- Injection, as phosphate: 150 mg/mL (2 mL, 4 mL, 6 mL, 60 mL)
- Solution, topical, as phosphate: 1% (30 mL, 60 mL, 480 mL)

Clinoril® *see* Sulindac *on page 546*

Clioquinol *see* Iodochlorhydroxyquin *on page 318*

Clofazimine (kloe fa' zi meen)

Brand Names Lamprene®

Therapeutic Category Antibiotic, Miscellaneous; Leprostatic Agent

Use Treatment of dapsone-resistant lepromatous leprosy (*Mycobacterium leprae*) and initial treatment of multibacillary dapsone-sensitive leprosy; erythema nodosum leprosum; *Mycobacterium avium*-intracellulare (MAI) infections

Pregnancy Risk Factor C

Precautions Well tolerated when administered in dosages ≤100 mg/day; dosages >100 mg/day should be used for as short a duration as possible; use with caution in patients with GI problems; patients with abdominal pain,

(Continued)

Clofazimine *(Continued)*

colic, nausea, vomiting, or diarrhea during clofazimine therapy may require a dosage adjustment or discontinuation of therapy

Adverse Reactions

Central nervous system: Dizziness, drowsiness

Dermatologic: Pink to brownish black discoloration of the skin and conjunctiva, dry skin, rash, pruritus

Endocrine & metabolic: Increased blood glucose

Gastrointestinal: Constipation, abdominal pain, diarrhea, nausea, vomiting, bowel obstruction, GI bleeding

Ocular: Irritation of the eyes

Drug Interactions Isoniazid

Mechanism of Action Binds preferentially to mycobacterial DNA at the guanine base to inhibit mycobacterial growth; also has some anti-inflammatory activity through an unknown mechanism

Pharmacokinetics

Absorption: Oral: 45% to 70% slowly absorbed; presence of food increases the extent of absorption

Distribution: Clofazimine remains in tissues for prolonged periods and distributes into fatty tissues of the reticuloendothelial system

Metabolism: Metabolized in the liver to three metabolites

Half-life:

- Terminal: 8 days
- Tissue: 70 days

Elimination: Excreted principally in feces; only negligible amounts excreted unchanged in the urine; small amounts excreted in sputum, saliva, and sweat

Usual Dosage Oral:

Children: Leprosy: 1 mg/kg/day every 24 hours in combination with dapsone and rifampin

Adults:

- Dapsone-resistant leprosy: 50-100 mg once daily in combination with one or more antileprosy drugs for 2 years; then alone 50-100 mg/day
- Dapsone-sensitive multibacillary leprosy: 50-100 mg once daily in combination with two or more antileprosy drugs for at least 2 years and continue until negative skin smears are obtained, then institute single drug therapy with appropriate agent
- Erythema nodosum leprosum: 100-200 mg/day for up to 3 months or longer then taper dose to 100 mg/day when possible
- MAI: Combination therapy using clofazimine 100 mg 1 or 3 times/day in combination with other antimycobacterial agents

Monitoring Parameters GI complaints

Patient Information Drug may cause a pink to brownish-black discoloration of the skin, conjunctiva, tears, sweat, urine, feces, and nasal secretions; skin discoloration reversal may take several months after discontinuation of clofazimine

Nursing Implications Administer with meals

Dosage Forms Capsule: 50 mg, 100 mg

References

Chesney PJ, "New Concepts for Antimicrobial Use in Opportunistic Infections," *Semin Pediatr Infect Dis*, 1991, 2(1):67-73.

Garrelts JC, "Clofazimine: A Review of Its Use in Leprosy and *Mycobacterium Avium* Complex Infection," *DICP*, 1991, 25(5):525-31.

Clonazepam (kloe na' ze pam)

Related Information

Overdose and Toxicology Information *on page 696-700*

Brand Names Klonopin™

Therapeutic Category Anticonvulsant; Benzodiazepine

Use Prophylaxis of absence (petit mal), petit mal variant (Lennox-Gastaut), akinetic, and myoclonic seizures

Restrictions C-IV

Pregnancy Risk Factor C

Contraindications Hypersensitivity to clonazepam, any component, or other benzodiazepines; severe liver disease, acute narrow-angle glaucoma

Precautions Use with caution in patients with chronic respiratory disease or impaired renal function; abrupt discontinuance may precipitate withdrawal symptoms, status epilepticus or seizures

Adverse Reactions

Cardiovascular: Hypotension

Central nervous system: Drowsiness, changes in behavior or personality, tremor, vertigo, confusion, memory impairment, decreased concentration, headache, ataxia

Dermatologic: Rash

Gastrointestinal: Nausea, dry mouth, vomiting, diarrhea, constipation, anorexia

Hematologic: Thrombocytopenia, anemia, leukopenia, eosinophilia

Musculoskeletal: Choreiform movements, hypotonia

Ocular: Nystagmus, blurred vision

Respiratory: Hypersalivation and bronchial hypersecretion, respiratory depression

Miscellaneous: Physical and psychological dependence

Drug Interactions CNS depressants → ↑ sedation; phenytoin, barbiturates → ↑ clonazepam clearance

Mechanism of Action Suppresses the spike and wave discharge in absence seizures by depressing nerve transmission in the motor cortex

Pharmacodynamics

Onset of effect: 20-60 minutes

Duration:

Infants and young children: Up to 6-8 hours

Adults: Up to 12 hours

Pharmacokinetics

Absorption: Oral: Well absorbed

Distribution: V_d: Adults: 1.5-4.4 L/kg

Protein binding: 85%

Metabolism: Extensively metabolized; glucuronide and sulfate conjugation

Half-life:

Children: 22-33 hours

Adults: 19-50 hours

Elimination: Metabolites excreted as glucuronide or sulfate conjugates; less than 2% excreted unchanged in urine

Usual Dosage Oral:

Children <10 years or 30 kg: Initial daily dose: 0.01-0.03 mg/kg/day (maximum: 0.05 mg/kg/day) given in 2-3 divided doses; increase by no more than 0.5 mg every third day until seizures are controlled or adverse effects seen; usual maintenance dose: 0.1-0.2 mg/kg/day divided 3 times/day; not to exceed 0.2 mg/kg/day

Adults: Initial daily dose not to exceed 1.5 mg given in 3 divided doses; may increase by 0.5-1 mg every third day until seizures are controlled or adverse effects seen; usual maintenance dose: 0.05-0.2 mg/kg; do not exceed 20 mg/day

Reference Range Relationship between serum concentration and seizure control is not well established

Proposed therapeutic levels: 20-80 ng/mL; potentially toxic concentration: >80 ng/mL

Additional Information Ethosuximide or valproic acid may be preferred for treatment of absence (petit mal) seizures; clonazepam induced behavioral disturbances may be more frequent in mentally handicapped patients

Dosage Forms Tablet: 0.5 mg, 1 mg, 2 mg

Clonidine (kloe' ni deen)

Brand Names Catapres®; Catapres-TTS®

Therapeutic Category Alpha-Adrenergic Agonist; Antihypertensive

Use Management of hypertension; aid in the diagnosis of pheochromocytoma and growth hormone deficiency; has orphan drug status for epidural use for pain control; heroin withdrawal (adults); smoking cessation therapy (adults)

Pregnancy Risk Factor C

Contraindications Hypersensitivity to clonidine hydrochloride or any component

Warnings Do not abruptly discontinue as rapid increase in blood pressure, and symptoms of sympathetic overactivity (such as ↑ heart rate, tremor, ag-

(Continued)

Clonidine *(Continued)*

itation, anxiety, insomnia, sweating, palpitations) may occur; if need to discontinue, taper dose gradually over more than 1 week

Precautions Dosage modification may be required in patients with renal impairment; use with caution in cerebrovascular disease, coronary insufficiency, renal impairment, sinus node dysfunction

Adverse Reactions

Cardiovascular: Raynaud's phenomenon, hypotension, bradycardia, palpitations, tachycardia, congestive heart failure

Central nervous system: Drowsiness, headache, dizziness, fatigue, insomnia, anxiety

Dermatologic: Rash, local skin reactions with patch

Endocrine & metabolic: Sodium and water retention

Gastrointestinal: Constipation, anorexia, dry mouth

Miscellaneous: Parotid pain

Drug Interactions Tricyclic antidepressants antagonize hypotensive effects of clonidine; beta blockers may potentiate bradycardia in patients receiving clonidine and may increase the rebound hypertension seen with clonidine withdrawal; discontinue beta blocker several days before clonidine is tapered off

Mechanism of Action Stimulates $alpha_2$-adrenoreceptors in the brain stem, thus activating an inhibitory neuron, resulting in reduced sympathetic outflow, producing a decrease in vasomotor tone and heart rate

Pharmacodynamics Oral:

Onset of effects: 30-60 minutes

Peak effects: Within 2-4 hours

Duration: 6-10 hours

Pharmacokinetics

Distribution: V_d: Adults: 2.1 L/kg

Metabolism: Hepatically metabolized to inactive metabolites

Bioavailability, oral: 75% to 95%

Half-life:

- Neonates: 44-72 hours
- Adults:
  - Normal renal function: 6-20 hours
  - Renal impairment: 18-41 hours

Elimination: 65% excreted in urine (32% unchanged) and 22% excreted in feces via enterohepatic recirculation

Usual Dosage

Children: Oral: Initial: 5-10 μg/kg/day in divided doses every 8-12 hours; increase gradually to 5-25 μg/kg/day in divided doses every 6 hours; maximum: 0.9 mg/day

Clonidine tolerance test (test of growth hormone release from the pituitary): Oral: 0.15 mg/m^2 or 4 μg/kg as a single dose

Adults:

Oral: Initial dose: 0.1 mg twice daily, usual maintenance dose: 0.2-1.2 mg/day in 2-4 divided doses; maximum recommended dose: 2.4 mg/day

Transdermal: Applied once weekly as transdermal delivery system; initial therapy with 0.1 mg/24 hours applied once every 7 days; adjust dosage based on response; hypotensive action may not begin until 2-3 days after initial application

Monitoring Parameters Blood pressure, heart rate

Nursing Implications Counsel patient/parent about compliance and danger of withdrawal reaction if doses are missed or drug is discontinued

Dosage Forms

Patch, transdermal: 1, 2, and 3 (0.1, 0.2, 0.3 mg/day to 7-day duration)

Tablet, as hydrochloride: 0.1 mg, 0.2 mg, 0.3 mg

References

Rocchini AP, "Childhood Hypertension: Etiology, Diagnosis, and Treatment," *Pediatr Clin North Am*, 1984, 31(6):1259-73.

Clopra® *see* Metoclopramide Hydrochloride *on page 381*

Clorazepate Dipotassium (klor az' e pate)

Related Information

Overdose and Toxicology Information *on page 696-700*

Brand Names Gen-XENE®; Tranxene®

Therapeutic Category Benzodiazepine

Use Treatment of generalized anxiety and panic disorders; management of alcohol withdrawal; adjunct anticonvulsant in management of partial seizures

Restrictions C-IV

Pregnancy Risk Factor D

Contraindications Hypersensitivity to clorazepate dipotassium or any component; cross sensitivity with other benzodiazepines may exist; avoid using in patients with pre-existing CNS depression, severe uncontrolled pain, or narrow-angle glaucoma

Warnings Abrupt discontinuation may cause withdrawal symptoms or seizures

Precautions Use with caution in patients with hepatic or renal disease

Adverse Reactions

Cardiovascular: Hypotension

Central nervous system: Drowsiness, dizziness, confusion, amnesia, headache, depression, ataxia

Dermatologic: Rash

Gastrointestinal: Nausea, dry mouth

Ocular: Blurred vision

Miscellaneous: Physical and psychological dependence with long-term use; long-term use may also be associated with renal or hepatic injury and reduced hematocrit

Drug Interactions Cimetidine may decrease hepatic clearance

Stability Unstable in water

Mechanism of Action Facilitates gamma aminobutyric acid (GABA)-mediated transmission inhibitory neurotransmitter action, depresses subcortical levels of CNS

Pharmacokinetics

Absorption: Rapidly decarboxylated to desmethyldiazepam (active) in acidic stomach prior to absorption

Distribution: Crosses the placenta

Metabolism: Metabolized in the liver to oxazepam (active)

Half-life, adults:

Desmethyldiazepam :48-96 hours

Oxazepam: 6-8 hours

Peak serum levels: Oral: Within 1 hour

Elimination: Excreted primarily in the urine

Usual Dosage Oral:

Children 9-12 years: Anticonvulsant: Initial: 3.75-7.5 mg/dose twice daily; increase dose by 3.75 mg at weekly intervals, not to exceed 60 mg/day in 2-3 divided doses

Children >12 years and Adults: Anticonvulsant: Initial: Up to 7.5 mg/dose 2-3 times/day; increase dose by 7.5 mg at weekly intervals; usual dose: 0.5-1 mg/kg/day; not to exceed 90 mg/day (up to 3 mg/kg/day has been used)

Adults:

Anxiety: 7.5-15 mg 2-4 times/day, or given as single dose of 15-22.5 mg at bedtime

Alcohol withdrawal: Initial: 30 mg, then 15 mg 2-4 times/day on first day; maximum daily dose: 90 mg; gradually decrease dose over subsequent days

Reference Range Therapeutic: 0.12-1 μg/mL (SI: 0.36-3.01 μmol/L)

Dosage Forms

Capsule: 3.75 mg, 7.5 mg, 15 mg

Tablet: 3.75 mg, 7.5 mg, 15 mg

Tablet, single dose: 11.25 mg, 22.5 mg

Clotrimazole (kloe trim' a zole)

Brand Names Gyne-Lotrimin® [OTC]; Lotrimin®; Lotrimin AF® [OTC]; Mycelex®; Mycelex®-G

Therapeutic Category Antifungal Agent, Oral Nonabsorbed; Antifungal Agent, Topical; Antifungal Agent, Vaginal

Use Treatment of susceptible fungal infections, including oropharyngeal candidiasis, dermatophytoses, superficial mycoses, cutaneous candidiasis,

(Continued)

Clotrimazole *(Continued)*

as well as vulvovaginal candidiasis; limited data suggests that the use of clotrimazole troches may be effective for prophylaxis against oropharyngeal candidiasis in neutropenic patients

Pregnancy Risk Factor B

Contraindications Hypersensitivity to clotrimazole or any component

Warnings Clotrimazole troches should not be used for treatment of systemic fungal infection

Precautions Safety and effectiveness of clotrimazole lozenges (troches) in children <3 years of age have not been established

Adverse Reactions

Gastrointestinal: Nausea and vomiting may occur in patients on clotrimazole troches

Hepatic: Abnormal liver function tests

Local: Mild burning, irritation, stinging of skin or vaginal area

Mechanism of Action Binds to phospholipids in the fungal cell membrane altering cell wall permeability resulting in loss of essential intracellular elements

Pharmacokinetics

Absorption: Negligible through intact skin when administered topically

Distribution: Following oral/topical administration, clotrimazole is present in saliva for up to 3 hours following 30 minutes of dissolution time in the mouth

Usual Dosage

Children >3 years and Adults:

Oral: 10 mg troche dissolved slowly 5 times/day

Topical: Apply twice daily

Children >12 years and Adults: Vaginal: 100 mg/day at bedtime for 7 days or 200 mg/day at bedtime for 3 days or 500 mg single dose; or 5 g (= 1 applicatorful) of 1% vaginal cream daily at bedtime for 7-14 days

Monitoring Parameters Periodic liver function tests during oral therapy with clotrimazole lozenges

Patient Information Lozenge (troche) must be dissolved slowly in the mouth

Dosage Forms

Cream:

Topical: 1% (15 g, 30 g, 45 g, 90 g)

Vaginal: 1% (45 g, 90 g)

Lotion: 1% (30 mL)

Solution, topical: 1% (10 mL, 30 mL)

Tablet, vaginal: 100 mg (7's); 500 mg (1's)

Troche: 10 mg

Twin pack: Tablet 500 mg (1's) and vaginal cream 1% (7 g)

Cloxacillin Sodium (klox a sill' in)

Brand Names Cloxapen®; Tegopen®

Therapeutic Category Antibiotic, Penicillin

Use Treatment of susceptible bacterial infections, notably penicillinase-producing staphylococci and streptococci causing respiratory tract, skin and skin structure, bone and joint infections

Pregnancy Risk Factor B

Contraindications Hypersensitivity to cloxacillin or any component, or penicillins

Adverse Reactions

Central nervous system: Fever

Dermatologic: Rash

Gastrointestinal: Nausea, vomiting, diarrhea

Hematologic: Eosinophilia, leukopenia, neutropenia, thrombocytopenia, agranulocytosis

Hepatic: Hepatotoxicity

Renal & genitourinary: Hematuria

Miscellaneous: Serum sickness-like reactions

Drug Interactions Probenecid

Stability Refrigerate oral solution after reconstitution; discard after 14 days; stable for 3 days at room temperature

Mechanism of Action Interferes with bacterial cell wall synthesis during active multiplication, causing cell wall death and resultant bactericidal activity against susceptible bacteria

Pharmacokinetics

Absorption: Oral: ~50%

Distribution: Crosses the placenta; appears in breast milk

Protein binding: 90% to 98%

Metabolism: Metabolized significantly in the liver to active and inactive metabolites

Half-life: 30-90 minutes (prolonged with renal impairment and in neonates)

Peak serum levels: Oral: Within 0.5-2 hours

Elimination: Excreted in the urine and through the bile

Not dialyzable (0% to 5%)

Usual Dosage Oral:

Children >1 month: 50-100 mg/kg/day in divided doses every 6 hours; up to a maximum of 4 g/day

Adults: 250-500 mg every 6 hours

Monitoring Parameters CBC with differential, urinalysis, BUN, serum creatinine, and liver enzymes

Test Interactions False-positive urine and serum proteins

Nursing Implications Administer 1 hour before or 2 hours after meals

Additional Information

Sodium content of 250 mg capsule: 0.6 mEq

Sodium content of 125 mg solution, oral: 0.48 mEq

Dosage Forms

Capsule: 250 mg, 500 mg

Powder for oral suspension: 125 mg/5 mL (100 mL, 200 mL)

Cloxapen® *see* Cloxacillin Sodium *on previous page*

Clysodrast® *see* Bisacodyl *on page 83*

Coal Tar

Brand Names AquaTar® [OTC]; Denorex® [OTC]; DHS® Tar [OTC]; Duplex® T [OTC]; Estar® [OTC]; Fototar® [OTC]; Neutrogena® T/Derm; Pentrax® [OTC]; Polytar® [OTC]; psoriGel® [OTC]; T/Gel® [OTC]; Zetar® [OTC]

Synonyms LCD

Therapeutic Category Antipsoriatic Agent, Topical; Antiseborrheic Agent, Topical

Use Used topically for controlling dandruff, seborrheic dermatitis, or psoriasis

Contraindications Known hypersensitivity to coal tar or any ingredient in the formulation

Warnings Due to a potential carcinogenic risk, do not use around the rectum or in the genital area or groin

Precautions Do not apply to acutely inflamed skin; avoid exposure to sunlight for at least 24 hours

Adverse Reactions Dermatologic: Dermatitis, folliculitis, photosensitization

Drug Interactions Tetracyclines, phenothiazines, tretinoin, and sulfonamides also have phototoxic potential

Mechanism of Action Reduces the number and size of epidermal cells produced

Usual Dosage Topical: Children and Adults:

Bath: Add appropriate amount to bath water, for adults usually 60-90 mL of a 5% to 20% solution or 15-25 mL of 30% lotion; soak 5-20 minutes, then pat dry; use once daily to one every 3 days

Shampoo: Rub shampoo onto wet hair and scalp, rinse thoroughly; repeat; leave on 5 minutes; rinse thoroughly; apply twice weekly for the first 2 weeks then once weekly or more often if needed

Skin: Apply to the affected area 1-4 times/day; decrease frequency to 2-3 times/week once condition has been controlled

Atopic dermatitis: Children: 2% to 5% coal tar cream can be applied once daily or every other day to reduce inflammation

Scalp psoriasis: Tar oil bath or coal tar solution may be painted sparingly to the lesions 3-12 hours before each shampoo

Psoriasis of the body, arms, legs: Apply at bedtime; if thick scales are present, use product with salicylic acid and apply several times during the day

(Continued)

Coal Tar *(Continued)*

Patient Information Avoid contact with eyes, genital, or rectal area; coal tar preparations frequently stain the skin and hair; avoid exposure to direct sunlight

Dosage Forms

Cream: 1% to 5%
Gel: Coal tar 5%
Lotion: 2.5% to 30%
Lotion: Coal tar 2% to 5%
Shampoo: Coal tar extract 2% with salicylic acid 2% (60 mL)
Shampoo, topical: Coal tar: 0.5% to 5%
Solution:
  Coal tar: 2.5%, 5%, 20%
  Coal tar extract: 5%
Suspension, coal tar: 30% to 33.3%

References

Hanifin JM, "Atopic Dermatitis in Infants and Children," *Pediatr Clin North Am*, 1991, 38(4):763-89.

Cocaine Hydrochloride (koe' kane)

Therapeutic Category Local Anesthetic, Topical

Use Topical anesthesia for mucous membranes

Restrictions C-II

Pregnancy Risk Factor C (X if nonmedical use)

Contraindications Systemic use, hypersensitivity to cocaine or any component

Precautions Use with caution in patients with hypertension, severe cardiovascular disease, thyrotoxicosis, and in infants; use with caution in patients with severely traumatized mucosa and sepsis in the region of intended application.

Adverse Reactions

Cardiovascular: Hypertension, tachycardia
Central nervous system: Restlessness, nervousness, euphoria, excitement, hallucinations, tremors, seizures
Gastrointestinal: Vomiting
Respiratory: Tachypnea

Drug Interactions MAO inhibitors

Stability Store in well closed, light-resistant containers

Mechanism of Action Blocks both the initiation and conduction of nerve impulses by decreasing the neuronal membrane's permeability to sodium ions. This results in inhibition of depolarization with resultant blockade of conduction; interferes with the uptake of norepinephrine by adrenergic nerve terminals producing vasoconstriction.

Pharmacodynamics Following topical administration to mucosa:

Onset of action: Within 1 minute
Peak action: Within 5 minutes
Duration: ≥30 minutes, depending upon route and dosage administered

Pharmacokinetics

Absorption: Well absorbed through mucous membranes; absorption is limited by drug induced vasoconstriction and enhanced by inflammation
Distribution: Appears in breast milk
Metabolism: Metabolized in the liver
Half-life: 75 minutes
Elimination: Excreted primarily in the urine as metabolites and unchanged drug (<10%)

Usual Dosage Topical: Use lowest effective dose; do not exceed 1 mg/kg; patient tolerance, anesthetic technique, vascularity of tissue, and area to be anesthetized will determine dose needed. Solutions >4% are not recommended due to increased risk of systemic toxicities

Monitoring Parameters Heart rate, blood pressure, respiratory rate

Nursing Implications Use only on mucous membranes of the oral, laryngeal, and nasal cavities; do not use on extensive areas of broken skin

Additional Information Cocaine intoxication of infants who are receiving breast milk from their mothers abusing cocaine has been reported

Dosage Forms

Powder: 5 g, 25 g
Solution, topical: 4% (2 mL); 10% (4 mL, 15 mL)

Tablet, soluble, for topical solution: 135 mg

References

Chasnoff IJ, Lewis DE, and Squires L, "Cocaine Intoxication in Breast-Fed Infants," *Pediatrics*, 1987, 80(6):836-8.

CodAphen® *see* Acetaminophen and Codeine Phosphate *on page 17*

Codeine (koe' deen)

Related Information

Compatibility of Medications Mixed in a Syringe *on page 717*
Narcotic Analgesics Comparison Chart *on page 721-722*
Overdose and Toxicology Information *on page 696-700*

Synonyms Methylmorphine

Therapeutic Category Analgesic, Narcotic; Antitussive

Use Treatment of mild to moderate pain; antitussive in lower doses

Restrictions C-II

Pregnancy Risk Factor C (D if used for prolonged periods or in high doses at term)

Contraindications Hypersensitivity to codeine or any component

Warnings Some preparations contain sulfites which may cause allergic reactions

Precautions Use with caution in patients with hypersensitivity reactions to other phenanthrene derivative opioid agonists (morphine, hydrocodone, hydromorphone, levorphanol, oxycodone, oxymorphone); respiratory diseases including: asthma, emphysema, COPD or severe liver or renal insufficiency

Adverse Reactions

Cardiovascular: Palpitations, hypotension, bradycardia, peripheral vasodilation
Central nervous system: CNS depression, increased intracranial pressure, dizziness, drowsiness, sedation
Dermatologic: Pruritus
Endocrine & metabolic: Antidiuretic hormone release
Gastrointestinal: Nausea, vomiting, constipation
Hepatic: Biliary tract spasm
Ocular: Miosis
Renal & genitourinary: Urinary tract spasm
Respiratory: Respiratory depression
Sensitivity reactions: Histamine release
Miscellaneous: Physical and psychological dependence

Drug Interactions CNS depressants, phenothiazines, tricyclic antidepressants may potentiate the adverse effects of codeine

Mechanism of Action Binds to opiate receptors in the CNS, causing inhibition of ascending pain pathways, altering the perception of and response to pain; causes cough supression by direct central action in the medulla; produces generalized CNS depression

Pharmacodynamics

Onset:
- Oral: 30-60 minutes
- I.M.: 10-30 minutes

Peak action:
- Oral: 60-90 minutes
- I.M.: 0.5-1 hour

Duration: 4-6 hours

Pharmacokinetics

Absorption: Oral: Adequate
Distribution: Crosses the placenta; appears in breast milk
Protein binding: 7%
Metabolism: Hepatic metabolism to morphine (active)
Half-life: 2.5-3.5 hours
Elimination: 3% to 16% excreted in the urine as unchanged drug, norcodeine, and free and conjugated morphine

Usual Dosage Doses should be titrated to appropriate analgesic effect; when changing routes of administration, note that oral dose is $\frac{2}{3}$ as effective as parenteral dose

(Continued)

Codeine *(Continued)*

Analgesic: Oral, I.M., S.C.:

Children: 0.5-1 mg/kg/dose every 4-6 hours as needed; maximum: 60 mg/dose

Adults: Usual: 30 mg/dose; range: 15-60 mg every 4-6 hours as needed

Antitussive: Oral (for nonproductive cough):

Children: 1-1.5 mg/kg/day in divided doses every 4-6 hours as needed: Alternatively dose according to age:

2-6 years: 2.5-5 mg every 4-6 hours as needed; maximum: 30 mg/day

6-12 years: 5-10 mg every 4-6 hours as needed; maximum: 60 mg/day

Adults: 10-20 mg/dose every 4-6 hours as needed; maximum: 120 mg/day

Dosing adjustment in renal impairment:

Cl_{cr} 10-50 mL/minute: Administer 75% of dose

Cl_{cr} <10 mL/minute: Administer 50% of dose

Administration Not intended for I.V. use due to large histamine release and cardiovascular effects

Monitoring Parameters Respiratory rate, heart rate, blood pressure, pain relief

Additional Information Not recommended for use for cough control in patients with a productive cough; not recommended as an antitussive for children <2 years of age; equianalgesic doses: 120 mg codeine phosphate I.M. approximately equals morphine 10 mg I.M.

Dosage Forms

Injection, as phosphate: 30 mg (1 mL, 2 mL); 60 mg (1 mL, 2 mL)

Solution, oral: 15 mg/5 mL

Tablet, as sulfate: 15 mg, 30 mg, 60 mg

Tablet, as phosphate, soluble: 30 mg, 60 mg

Tablet, as sulfate, soluble: 15 mg, 30 mg, 60 mg

Codeine and Guaifenesin *see* Guaifenesin and Codeine *on page 279*

Codeine Phosphate and Acetaminophen *see* Acetaminophen and Codeine Phosphate *on page 17*

Codimal-A® *see* Brompheniramine Maleate *on page 88*

Cogentin® *see* Benztropine Mesylate *on page 79*

Colace® [OTC] *see* Docusate *on page 202*

Colaspase *see* Asparaginase *on page 60*

Colchicine (kol' chi seen)

Therapeutic Category Anti-inflammatory Agent; Uric Acid Lowering Agent

Use Treat acute gouty arthritis attacks and to prevent recurrences of such attacks; management of familial Mediterranean fever

Pregnancy Risk Factor C

Contraindications Hypersensitivity to colchicine or any component; severe renal, GI disease, or cardiac disorders

Precautions Modify dosage in patients with renal impairment

Adverse Reactions

Central nervous system: Peripheral neuritis

Dermatologic: Rash, alopecia

Gastrointestinal: Nausea, vomiting, diarrhea, abdominal pain

Hematologic: Agranulocytosis, aplastic anemia

Hepatic: Elevation in liver enzymes

Musculoskeletal: Myopathy

Renal & genitourinary: Azoospermia, hematuria, renal damage

Drug Interactions Vitamin B_{12} (decreased absorption)

Stability I.V. colchicine is incompatible with dextrose or I.V. solutions with preservatives

Mechanism of Action Decreases leukocyte motility, decreases phagocytosis in joints, and lactic acid production, thereby reducing the deposition of urate crystals that perpetuates the inflammatory response

Pharmacokinetics

Protein binding: 10% to 31%

Metabolism: Partially deacetylated in the liver
Half-life: 12-30 minutes
Peak serum level: Oral: Within 30-120 minutes then declines for 2 hours before increasing again due to enterohepatic recycling
Elimination: Primarily excreted in the feces via bile
Not dialyzable (0% to 5%)

Usual Dosage

Prophylaxis of familial Mediterranean fever: Oral:
- Children:
  - ≤5 years: 0.5 mg/day
  - >5 years: 1-1.5 mg/day in 2-3 divided doses
- Adults: 1-2 mg/day in 2-3 divided doses

Adults:
- Oral: Acute attacks: Initial: 0.5-1.2 mg, then 0.5-0.6 mg every 1-2 hours or 1-1.2 mg every 2 hours until relief or GI side effects occur to a maximum total dose of 8 mg
- I.V.: Initial: 1-3 mg, then 0.5 mg every 6 hours until response, not to exceed 4 mg/day; if pain recurs, it may be necessary to administer a daily dose of 1 to 2 mg for several days, however, do not give more colchicine by any route for at least 7 days after a full course of I.V. therapy (4 mg), transfer to oral colchicine in a dose similar to that being given I.V.
- Prophylaxis of recurrent attacks: Oral: 0.5-0.6 mg every day or every other day

Dosing adjustment in renal impairment: Cl_{cr} <10 mL/minute: Decrease dose by 50%

Administration Administer I.V. over 2-5 minutes into tubing of free-flowing I.V. with compatible fluid

Monitoring Parameters CBC and renal function test

Test Interactions May cause false-positive results in urine tests for erythrocytes or hemoglobin

Patient Information Avoid alcohol; if taking for acute gouty attacks, discontinue if pain is relieved or if nausea, vomiting or diarrhea occur

Nursing Implications Severe local irritation can occur following S.C. or I.M. administration

Dosage Forms

Injection: 0.5 mg/mL (2 mL)
Tablet: 0.5 mg, 0.6 mg

References

Levy M, Spino M, and Read SE, "Colchicine: A State-of-the-Art Review," *Pharmacotherapy*, 1991, 11(3):196-211.

Majeed HA, Carroll JE, Khuffash FA, et al, "Long-term Colchicine Prophylaxis in Children With Familial Mediterranean Fever (Recurrent Hereditary Polyserositis)," *J Pediatr*, 1990, 116(6):997-9.

Colfosceril Palmitate (kole fos' er il)

Brand Names Exosurf® Neonatal

Synonyms Dipalmitoylphosphatidylcholine; DPPC; Synthetic Lung Surfactant

Therapeutic Category Lung Surfactant

Use Neonatal respiratory distress syndrome:
- Prophylactic therapy: Body weight <1350 g in infants at risk for developing RDS; body weight >1350 g in infants with evidence of pulmonary immaturity
- Rescue therapy: Treatment of infants with RDS based on respiratory distress not attributable to any other causes and chest radiographic findings consistent with RDS

Warnings This drug may rapidly affect oxygenation and lung compliance. If chest expansion improves substantially the ventilator PIP setting should be reduced immediately. Hyperoxia and hypocarbia (hypocarbia can decrease blood flow to the brain) may occur requiring appropriate ventilator adjustments.

Adverse Reactions Respiratory: Pulmonary hemorrhage, apnea, mucous plugging, decrease in transcutaneous O_2 of >20%

Stability Reconstituted suspension is stable 12 hours after reconstitution; **do not refrigerate**

(Continued)

Colfosceril Palmitate *(Continued)*

Mechanism of Action Replaces deficient or ineffective endogenous lung surfactant in neonates with respiratory distress syndrome (RDS) or in neonates at risk of developing RDS; reduces surface tension and stabilizes the alveoli from collapsing

Pharmacokinetics Absorption: Following intratracheal administration it is absorbed from the alveolus; catabolized and reutilized for further synthesis and secretion in lung tissue

Usual Dosage Intratracheal:

Prophylactic treatment: Give 5 mL/kg as soon as possible; the second and third doses should be administered at 12 and 24 hours later to those infants remaining on ventilators

Rescue treatment: Give 5 mL/kg as soon as the diagnosis of RDS is made. The second 5 mL/kg dose should be administered 12 hours later.

Administration For intratracheal administration only. Suction infant prior to administration; inspect solution to verify complete mixing of the suspension. Administer via sideport on the special ETT adapter without interrupting mechanical ventilation. Administer the dose in two 2.5 mL/kg aliquots. Each half-dose is instilled slowly over 1-2 minutes in small bursts with each inspiration. After the first 2.5 mL/kg dose turn the infants head and torso 45° right for 30 seconds, then return to the midline position and administer the second dose as above. Following the second dose, turn the infant's head and torso 45° to the left for 30 seconds and return the infant to the midline position.

Monitoring Parameters Continuous EKG and transcutaneous O_2 saturation should be monitored during administration; frequent ABG sampling is necessary to prevent postdosing hyperoxia and hypocarbia.

Nursing Implications Use only the preservative free sterile water for injection to reconstitute the drug (provided with the drug)

Dosage Forms Suspension, intratracheal: 108 mg (10 mL)

Colonic Lavage Solution *see* Polyethylene Glycol-Electrolyte Solution *on page 466*

Colovage® *see* Polyethylene Glycol-Electrolyte Solution *on page 466*

CoLyte® *see* Polyethylene Glycol-Electrolyte Solution *on page 466*

Comfort® [OTC] *see* Naphazoline Hydrochloride *on page 403*

Compatibility of Medications Mixed in a Syringe *see page 717*

Compazine® *see* Prochlorperazine *on page 484*

Compound F *see* Hydrocortisone *on page 293*

Compound S *see* Zidovudine *on page 608*

Concentraid® *see* Desmopressin Acetate *on page 177*

Constant-T® *see* Theophylline *on page 554*

Constilac® *see* Lactulose *on page 334*

Constulose® *see* Lactulose *on page 334*

Contuss® *see* Guaifenesin, Phenylpropanolamine, and Phenylephrine *on page 280*

Cophene-B® *see* Brompheniramine Maleate *on page 88*

Copper *see* Trace Metals *on page 574*

Cordarone® *see* Amiodarone Hydrochloride *on page 39*

Corgard® *see* Nadolol *on page 399*

Corgonject® *see* Chorionic Gonadotropin *on page 134*

Cortaid® [OTC] *see* Hydrocortisone *on page 293*

Cortatrigen® *see* Neomycin, (Bacitracin) Polymyxin B and Hydrocortisone *on page 406*

Cort-Dome® *see* Hydrocortisone *on page 293*

Cortef® *see* Hydrocortisone *on page 293*

Corticotropin (kor ti koe troe' pin)

Brand Names Acthar®; H.P. Acthar® Gel

Synonyms ACTH; Adrenocorticotropic Hormone; Corticotropin, Repository

Therapeutic Category Adrenal Corticosteroid; Diagnostic Agent, Adrenocortical Insufficiency

Use Infantile spasms; diagnostic aid in adrenocortical insufficiency; acute exacerbations of multiple sclerosis; severe muscle weakness in myasthenia gravis

Pregnancy Risk Factor C

Contraindications Scleroderma, osteoporosis, systemic fungal infections, ocular herpes simplex, peptic ulcer, hypertension, congestive heart failure, hypersensitivity to corticotropins, porcine proteins, or any component

Warnings May mask signs of infection; do not administer live vaccines; long-term therapy in children may retard bone growth; acute adrenal insufficiency may occur with abrupt withdrawal after chronic use or with stress

Precautions Use with caution in patients with hypothyroidism, cirrhosis, thromboembolic disorders, seizure disorders or renal insufficiency

Adverse Reactions

Central nervous system: Seizures, mood swings, headache, pseudotumor cerebri

Dermatologic: Skin atrophy, bruising, hyperpigmentation, acne, hirsutism

Endocrine & metabolic: Amenorrhea, sodium and water retention, Cushing's syndrome, hyperglycemia, bone growth suppression

Gastrointestinal: Abdominal distention, ulcerative esophagitis, pancreatitis

Musculoskeletal: Muscle wasting

Miscellaneous: Hypersensitivity reactions, including anaphylaxis

Drug Interactions NSAIDs, loop diuretics, thiazide diuretics, amphotericin B

Stability Store repository injection in the refrigerator; warm gel before administration

Mechanism of Action Stimulates the adrenal cortex to secrete adrenal steroids (including hydrocortisone, cortisone), androgenic substances, and a small amount of aldosterone

Pharmacodynamics

Peak effect on cortisol levels:

- I.M., I.V. (aqueous): Within 1 hour
- I.M., S.C. (gel): 3-12 hours
- I.M. (zinc): 7-24 hours

Duration:

- Aqueous: 2-4 hours
- Repository: 10-25 hours, up to 3 days

Pharmacokinetics

Absorption: I.M. (repository): Over 8-16 hours

Half-life: 15 minutes

Elimination: Excreted in urine

Usual Dosage

Children:

Anti-inflammatory/immunosuppressant:

- I.M., I.V., S.C. (aqueous): 1.6 units/kg/day or 50 units/m^2/day divided every 6-8 hours
- I.M. (gel): 0.8 units/kg/day or 25 units/m^2/day divided every 12-24 hours

Infantile spasms: Various regimens have been used. Some neurologists recommend low-dose ACTH (5-40 units/day) for short periods (1-6 weeks), while others recommend larger doses of ACTH (40-160 units/day) for long periods of treatment (3-12 months). Well designed comparative dosing studies are needed. Example of low dose regimen:

Initial: I.M. (gel): 20 units/day for 2 weeks, if patient responds, taper and discontinue; if patient does not respond, increase dose to 30 units/day for 4 weeks then taper and discontinue

I.M. usual dose (gel): 20-40 units/day or 5-8 units/kg/day in 1-2 divided doses; range: 5-160 units/day

Adults:

Acute exacerbation of multiple sclerosis: I.M.: 80-120 units/day in divided doses for 2-3 weeks

(Continued)

Corticotropin *(Continued)*

Diagnostic purposes:
I.M.: 25 units
I.V.: 10-25 units in 500 mL (NS or D_5W) over 8 hours
Anti-inflammatory/immunosuppressant: I.M., S.C.:
Aqueous: 20 units 4 times/day
Gel: 40-80 units every 24-72 hours

Nursing Implications Do not give zinc hydroxide suspension S.C. or I.V.; do not abruptly discontinue the medication

Additional Information The repository injection with zinc contains benzyl alcohol; cosyntropin is preferred over corticotropin for diagnostic test of adrenocortical insufficiency (cosyntropin is less allergenic and test is shorter in duration); oral prednisone (2 mg/kg/day) was as effective as I.M. ACTH gel (20 units/day) in controlling infantile spasms.

Dosage Forms
Injection: 25 units, 40 units
Injection, repository: 40 units/mL (1 mL, 5 mL); 80 units/mL (1 mL, 5 mL)
Injection, repository, as zinc hydroxide: 40 units

References

Hrachovy RA and Frost JD Jr, "Infantile Spasms," *Pediatr Clin North Am*, 1989, 36(2):311-29.
Hrachovy RA, Frost JD Jr, Kellaway P, et al, "Double-Blind Study of ACTH vs Prednisone Therapy in Infantile Spasms, *J Pediatr*, 1983, 103(4):641-5.

Corticotropin, Repository *see* Corticotropin *on previous page*

Cortifoam® *see* Hydrocortisone *on page 293*

Cortisol *see* Hydrocortisone *on page 293*

Cortisone Acetate (kor' ti sone)

Related Information
Systemic Corticosteroids Comparison Chart *on page 727*

Brand Names Cortone® Acetate

Therapeutic Category Adrenal Corticosteroid; Anti-inflammatory Agent; Corticosteroid, Systemic; Glucocorticoid

Use Management of adrenocortical insufficiency

Pregnancy Risk Factor D

Contraindications Serious infections, except septic shock or tuberculous meningitis; known hypersensitivity to corticosteroids; systemic fungal or viral infections

Warnings May retard bone growth; acute adrenal insufficiency may occur with abrupt withdrawal after long term therapy or with stress

Precautions Use with caution in patients with hypothyroidism, cirrhosis, hypertension, congestive heart failure, ulcerative colitis, thromboembolic disorders, osteoporosis, peptic ulcer, diabetes mellitus, seizure disorders

Adverse Reactions
Cardiovascular: Edema, hypertension
Central nervous system: Vertigo, seizures, headache, psychoses, pseudotumor cerebri
Dermatologic: Acne, skin atrophy
Endocrine & metabolic: Cushing's syndrome, pituitary-adrenal axis suppression, growth suppression, glucose intolerance, hypokalemia, alkalosis
Gastrointestinal: Peptic ulcer, nausea, vomiting
Musculoskeletal: Muscle weakness, osteoporosis, fractures
Ocular: Cataracts, glaucoma

Drug Interactions Barbiturates, phenytoin, rifampin, salicylates, live virus vaccines, estrogens, NSAID, diuretics (potassium depleting), anticholinesterase agents, warfarin

Mechanism of Action Decreases inflammation by suppression of migration of polymorphonuclear leukocytes and reversal of increased capillary permeability

Pharmacodynamics
Peak effect:
Oral: Within 2 hours
I.M.: Within 20-48 hours

Duration: 30-36 hours

Pharmacokinetics

Absorption: I.M.: Slow rate of absorption, over 24-48 hours

Distribution: Crosses the placenta; appears in breast milk; distributes to muscles, liver, skin, intestines, and kidneys

Metabolism: Metabolized in the liver to inactive metabolites

Half-life: 30 minutes

Elimination: Excreted in bile and urine

Usual Dosage Depends upon the condition being treated and the response of the patient. Supplemental doses may be warranted during times of stress in the course of withdrawing therapy.

Children:

Anti-inflammatory or immunosuppressive:

Oral: 2.5-10 mg/kg/day or 20-300 mg/m^2/day in divided doses every 6-8 hours

I.M.: 1-5 mg/kg/day or 14-375 mg/m^2/day in divided doses every 12-24 hours

Physiologic replacement:

Oral: 0.5-0.75 mg/kg/day or 20-25 mg/m^2/day in divided doses every 8 hours

I.M.: 0.25-0.35 mg/kg/day or 12.5 mg/m^2/day once daily

Stress coverage for surgery: I.M.: 1 and 2 days before preanesthesia, and 1-3 days after surgery: 50-62.5 mg/m^2/day; 4 days after surgery: 31-50 mg/m^2/day; 5 days after surgery, resume presurgical corticosteroid dose

Adults: Oral, I.M.: 20-300 mg/day divided every 12-24 hours

Administration Administer I.M. daily dose before 9 AM to minimize adrenocortical suppression

Patient Information Take with meals, food, or milk

Nursing Implications I.M. use only, not to be given I.V.; shake vial before withdrawing dose

Additional Information Insoluble in water

Dosage Forms

Injection: 50 mg/mL (10 mL)

Tablet: 5 mg, 10 mg, 25 mg

Cortisporin® Cream *see* Neomycin, (Bacitracin) Polymyxin B and Hydrocortisone *on page 406*

Cortisporin® Ophthalmic Suspension *see* Neomycin, (Bacitracin) Polymyxin B and Hydrocortisone *on page 406*

Cortisporin® Otic *see* Neomycin, (Bacitracin) Polymyxin B and Hydrocortisone *on page 406*

Cortone® Acetate *see* Cortisone Acetate *on previous page*

Cortrosyn® *see* Cosyntropin *on this page*

Cosmegen® *see* Dactinomycin *on page 169*

Cosyntropin (koe sin troe' pin)

Brand Names Cortrosyn®

Synonyms Synacthen; Tetracosactide

Therapeutic Category Adrenal Corticosteroid; Diagnostic Agent, Adrenocortical Insufficiency

Use Diagnostic test to differentiate primary adrenal from secondary (pituitary) adrenocortical insufficiency

Pregnancy Risk Factor C

Contraindications Known hypersensitivity to cosyntropin

Precautions Use with caution in patients with pre-existing allergic disease or a history of allergic reactions to corticotropin

Adverse Reactions

Endocrine & metabolic: Decreased carbohydrate tolerance; increased requirements for insulin or oral hypoglycemic agents in diabetics; activation of latent diabetes mellitus

Miscellaneous: Hypersensitivity reactions, including anaphylaxis

Drug Interactions Cortisone, hydrocortisone, estrogens, spironolactone

(Continued)

Cosyntropin *(Continued)*

Stability Reconstituted solution is stable for 24 hours at room temperature and 21 days when refrigerated; for I.V. infusion in NS or D_5W solution is stable for 12 hours at room temperature

Mechanism of Action Stimulates the adrenal cortex to secrete adrenal steroids (including hydrocortisone, cortisone), androgenic substances, and a small amount of aldosterone

Pharmacodynamics I.M., I.V.:

Onset of action: Plasma cortisol levels rise in healthy individuals in 5 minutes

Peak levels: Within 45-60 minutes

Pharmacokinetics

Distribution: Does not cross placenta

Metabolism: Unknown

Usual Dosage

Adrenocortical insufficiency: I.M., I.V.:
- Neonates: 0.015 mg/kg/dose
- Children <2 years: 0.125 mg
- Children >2 years and Adults: 0.25 mg

When greater cortisol stimulation is needed, an I.V. infusion may be used:
- Children >2 years and Adults: 0.25 mg administered over 4-8 hours (usually 6 hours)

Congenital adrenal hyperplasia evaluation: 1 mg/m^2/dose up to a maximum of 1 mg

Administration Give I.V. doses over 2 minutes

Reference Range Normal baseline cortisol >5 μg/dL (SI: 138 nmol/L); increase in serum cortisol 30 minutes after cosyntropin injection of >7 μg/dL (SI: 193 nmol/L) or peak response 30 minutes after cosyntropin injection of >18 μg/dL (SI: 497 nmol/L).

Nursing Implications Patient should not receive corticosteroids or spironolactone the day prior and the day of the test

Additional Information Each 0.25 mg of cosyntropin is equivalent to 25 units of corticotropin

Dosage Forms Powder for injection: 0.25 mg

Cotazym® *see* Pancrelipase *on page 431*

Cotazym-S® *see* Pancrelipase *on page 431*

Cotrim® *see* Co-trimoxazole *on this page*

Cotrim® DS *see* Co-trimoxazole *on this page*

Co-trimoxazole

Brand Names Bactrim™; Bactrim™ DS; Cotrim®; Cotrim® DS; Septra®; Septra® DS; Sulfamethoprim®; Sulfatrim®; Sulfatrim® DS; Uroplus® DS; Uroplus® SS

Synonyms SMX-TMP; Sulfamethoxazole and Trimethoprim; TMP-SMX; Trimethoprim and Sulfamethoxazole

Therapeutic Category Antibiotic, Sulfonamide Derivative

Use Oral treatment of urinary tract infections, acute otitis media in children, acute exacerbations of chronic bronchitis in adults; prophylaxis of *Pneumocystis carinii* pneumonitis (PCP); I.V. treatment of documented PCP, empiric treatment of highly suspected PCP in immune compromised patients; treatment of documented or suspected shigellosis, typhoid fever, *Nocardia asteroides* infection in patients who are NPO; and xanthomonas maltophilia infection

Pregnancy Risk Factor C

Contraindications Hypersensitivity to any sulfa drug or any component; porphyria; megaloblastic anemia due to folate deficiency; infants <2 months of age

Warnings Fatalities associated with sulfonamides, although rare, have occurred due to severe reactions including Stevens-Johnson syndrome, toxic epidermal necrolysis, hepatic necrosis, agranulocytosis, aplastic anemia and other blood dyscrasias; discontinue use at first sign of rash or any sign of adverse reaction

Precautions Use with caution in patients with G-6-PD deficiency, impaired renal or hepatic function; adjust dosage in patients with renal impairment

Adverse Reactions

Central nervous system: Confusion, depression, hallucinations, seizures, fever, ataxia

Dermatologic: Rash (more common in patients taking large dosages or in patients with AIDS), erythema multiforme, epidermal necrolysis, Stevens-Johnson syndrome

Gastrointestinal: Nausea, vomiting, glossitis, stomatitis, diarrhea, pseudomembranous colitis, pancreatitis, splenomegaly

Hematologic: Thrombocytopenia, megaloblastic anemia, granulocytopenia, aplastic anemia, hemolysis (with G-6-PD deficiency)

Hepatic: Hepatitis, kernicterus in neonates

Local: Local irritation, pain, phlebitis

Renal & genitourinary: interstitial nephritis

Miscellaneous: Serum sickness

Drug Interactions Warfarin, phenytoin (↓ clearance); methotrexate (displaced from protein binding sites)

Stability Do not refrigerate concentrate for injection; for I.V. administration, a 1:25 dilution is stable for 6 hours, 1:20 dilution is stable for 4 hours, 1:15 or 1:10 dilution is stable for 2 hours at room temperature

Mechanism of Action Sulfamethoxazole interferes with bacterial folic acid synthesis and growth via inhibition of dihydrofolic acid formation from para-aminobenzoic acid; trimethoprim inhibits dihydrofolic acid reduction to tetrahydrofolate resulting in sequential inhibition of enzymes of the folic acid pathway

Pharmacokinetics

Absorption: Oral: Almost completely absorbed (90% to 100%)

Distribution: Crosses the placenta; distributes into breast milk and joint fluid

Protein binding:

- TMP: 45%
- SMX: 68%

Metabolism:

- TMP: Metabolized to oxide and hydroxylated metabolites
- SMX: N-acetylated and glucuronidated

Half-life:

- SMX: 9 hours, prolonged in renal failure
- TMP: 6-17 hours, prolonged in renal failure

Peak serum levels: Oral: Within 1-4 hours

Elimination: Both are excreted in the urine as metabolites and unchanged drug

Usual Dosage Oral, I.V. (dosage recommendations are based on the trimethoprim component):

Children >2 months:

- Mild-moderate infections: 6-10 mg TMP/kg/day in divided doses every 12 hours
- Serious infection/*Pneumocystis*: 15-20 mg TMP/kg/day in divided doses every 6 hours
- Urinary tract infection prophylaxis: 2 mg TMP/kg/dose daily
- Prophylaxis of *Pneumocystis*: 5-10 mg TMP/kg/day or 150 mg TMP/m^2/day in divided doses every 12 hours 3 days/week; dose should not exceed 320 mg trimethoprim and 1600 mg sulfamethoxazole/day

Adults: Urinary tract infection/chronic bronchitis: 1 double strength tablet every 12 hours for 10-14 days

Dosing adjustment in renal impairment (frequency may need to be adjusted): Cl_{cr} 15-30 mL/minute: Reduce dose by 50%

Administration Infuse I.V. co-trimoxazole over 60-90 minutes; must be further diluted 1:25 (5 mL drug to 125 mL diluent, ie, D_5W); in patients who require fluid restriction, a 1:15 dilution (5 mL drug to 75 mL diluent, ie, D_5W) or a 1:10 dilution (5 mL drug to 50 mL diluent, ie, D_5W) can be administered

Monitoring Parameters CBC, renal function test, liver function test, urinalysis

Patient Information Maintain adequate fluid intake

Additional Information Injection vehicle contains benzyl alcohol and sodium metabisulfite; folinic acid should be given if bone marrow depression occurs

Dosage Forms

Injection: Sulfamethoxazole 80 mg and trimethoprim 16 mg per mL (5 mL, 10 mL, 20 mL, 30 mL, 50 mL)

(Continued)

Co-trimoxazole *(Continued)*

Suspension, oral: Sulfamethoxazole 200 mg and trimethoprim 40 mg per 5 mL (20 mL, 100 mL, 150 mL, 200 mL, 480 mL)
Tablet: Sulfamethoxazole 400 mg and trimethoprim 80 mg
Tablet, double strength: Sulfamethoxazole 800 mg and trimethoprim 160 mg

References

Hughes WT, "*Pneumocystis carinii* Pneumonia: New Approaches to Diagnosis, Treatment, and Prevention," *Pediatr Infect Dis J*, 1991, 10(5):391-9.

Coumadin® *see* Warfarin Sodium *on page 607*

CPM *see* Cyclophosphamide *on page 162*

CPR Pediatric Drug Dosages *see page 614*

Creon® *see* Pancreatin *on page 430*

Cromoglycic Acid *see* Cromolyn Sodium *on this page*

Cromolyn Sodium (kroe' moe lin)

Brand Names Gastrocrom®; Intal®; Nasalcrom®; Opticrom®
Synonyms Cromoglycic Acid; Disodium Cromoglycate; DSCG
Therapeutic Category Inhalation, Miscellaneous
Use An adjunct in the prophylaxis of allergic disorders, including rhinitis, conjunctivitis, and asthma; inhalation product may be used for prevention of exercise-induced bronchospasm; systemic: mastocytosis, food allergy, and treatment of inflammatory bowel disease
Pregnancy Risk Factor B
Contraindications Hypersensitivity to cromolyn or any component; acute asthma attacks
Warnings Aerosol inhalant should not be used in patients with cardiac arrhythmias
Precautions Use with caution in patients with renal and hepatic impairment
Adverse Reactions
Central nervous system: Dizziness, headache
Dermatologic: Rash, urticaria
Gastrointestinal: Nausea, vomiting, diarrhea
Local: Nasal burning, hoarseness
Musculoskeletal: Joint pain
Ocular: Ocular stinging, lacrimation
Respiratory: Coughing, wheezing, throat irritation, eosinophilic pneumonia, pulmonary infiltrates
Stability Protect from direct light and heat; nebulization solution is compatible with beta-agonists, anticholinergic solutions, acetylcysteine and normal saline; incompatible with alkaline solutions, calcium and magnesium salts
Mechanism of Action Prevents the mast cell release of histamine, leukotrienes and slow-reacting substance of anaphylaxis by inhibiting degranulation after contact with antigens
Pharmacodynamics Not effective for immediate relief of symptoms in acute asthmatic attacks; must be used at regular intervals for 2-4 weeks to be effective
Pharmacokinetics
Absorption:
Oral: 0.5% to 2%
Inhalation: ~8% of dose reaches the lungs upon inhalation of the powder and is well absorbed
Half-life: 80-90 minutes
Peak serum levels: Within 15 minutes after inhalation
Elimination: Equally excreted unchanged in the urine and the feces (via bile); small amounts after inhalation are exhaled
Usual Dosage
Children:
Inhalation (taper frequency to the lowest effective dose):
Nebulization solution: >2 years: 20 mg 4 times/day
Metered spray: >5 years: 2 inhalations 4 times/day or Spinhaler® 20 mg 4 times/day
For prevention of exercise-induced bronchospasm:
Metered spray: Single dose of 2 inhalations
Nasal: >6 years: 1 spray in each nostril 3-4 times/day

Ophthalmic: >4 years: 1-2 drops 4-6 times/day

Adults:

Inhalation (Spinhaler®): 20 mg 4 times/day
Metered spray: 2 inhalations 4 times/day
Nasal: 1 spray in each nostril 3-4 times/day
Ophthalmic: 1-2 drops 4-6 times/day

Systemic mastocytosis: Oral:

Infants and Children <2 years: 20 mg/kg/day in 4 divided doses; may increase in patients 6 months to 2 years of age if benefits not seen after 2-3 weeks; do not exceed 30 mg/kg/day
Children 2-12 years: 100 mg 4 times/day; not to exceed 40 mg/kg/day
Adults: 200 mg 4 times/day

Food allergy and inflammatory bowel disease: Oral:

Children: 100 mg 4 times/day 15-20 minutes before meals, not to exceed 40 mg/kg/day
Adults: 200 mg 4 times/day 15-20 minutes before meal, up to 400 mg 4 times/day

Administration For oral use, cromolyn powder is dissolved in water and taken at least 30 minutes before meals; do not mix with food, fruit juice, or milk

Monitoring Parameters Periodic pulmonary function tests

Additional Information Reserve systemic use in children <2 years of age for severe disease; avoid systemic use in premature infants

Dosage Forms

Capsule, oral: 100 mg
Inhalation, oral: 800 μg/spray (8.1 g)
Solution, for nebulization: 10 mg/mL (2 mL)
Solution:
Nasal: 40 mg/mL (13 mL)
Ophthalmic: 40 mg/mL (10 mL)

Crotaline Antivenin, Polyvalent *see* Antivenin (Crotalidae) Polyvalent *on page 56*

Crotamiton (kroe tam' i tonn)

Brand Names Eurax®

Therapeutic Category Scabicidal Agent

Use Treatment of scabies (*Sarcoptes scabiei*) in infants and children

Pregnancy Risk Factor C

Contraindications Hypersensitivity to crotamiton or other components; patients who manifest a primary irritation response to topical medications

Precautions Avoid contact with face, eyes, mucous membranes, and urethral meatus; do not apply to acutely inflamed or raw skin

Adverse Reactions

Dermatologic: Pruritus, contact dermatitis
Local: Irritation

Usual Dosage Scabicide: Topical: Children and Adults: Wash thoroughly and scrub away loose scales, then towel dry; apply a thin layer and massage drug onto skin of the entire body from the neck to the toes (with special attention to skin folds, creases, and interdigital spaces). Follow by a repeat application in 24 hours. Take a cleansing bath 48 hours after the final application. Treatment may be repeated after 7-10 days if mites appear.

Patient Information For topical use only; all contaminated clothing and bed linen should be washed to avoid reinfestation

Nursing Implications Lotion: Shake well before using

Additional Information Treatment may be repeated after 7-10 days if live mites are still present

Dosage Forms

Cream: 10% (60 g)
Lotion: 10% (60 mL, 480 mL)

References

Eichenfield LF, Honig PJ, "Blistering Disorders in Childhood," *Pediatr Clin North Am*, 1991, 38(4):959-76.

Hogan DJ, Schachner L, Tanglertsampan C, "Diagnosis and Treatment of Childhood Scabies and Pediculosis," *Pediatr Clin North Am*, 1991, 38(4):941-57.

Cruex® [OTC] *see* Undecylenic Acid and Derivatives *on page 590*

Crystalline Penicillin *see* Penicillin G Potassium or Sodium Salts *on page 440*

Crystal Violet *see* Gentian Violet *on page 270*

Crysticillin® A.S. *see* Penicillin G Procaine *on page 441*

CSA *see* Cyclosporine *on page 164*

C-Solve-2® *see* Erythromycin *on page 226*

CTX *see* Cyclophosphamide *on page 162*

Cuprimine® *see* Penicillamine *on page 437*

Curretab® *see* Medroxyprogesterone Acetate *on page 359*

Cyanocobalamin (sye an oh koe bal' a min)

Brand Names Redisol®; Rubramin-PC®

Synonyms Vitamin B_{12}

Therapeutic Category Vitamin, Water Soluble

Use Pernicious anemia; vitamin B_{12} deficiency; increased B_{12} requirements due to pregnancy, thyrotoxicosis, hemorrhage, malignancy, liver or kidney disease

Pregnancy Risk Factor A (C if dose exceeds RDA recommendation)

Contraindications Hypersensitivity to cyanocobalamin or any component, cobalt; patients with hereditary optic nerve atrophy

Precautions Serum potassium concentrations should be monitored early as severe hypokalemia has occurred after the conversion of megaloblastic anemia to normal erythropoiesis

Adverse Reactions

Cardiovascular: Peripheral vascular thrombosis
Dermatologic: Itching, urticaria
Endocrine & metabolic: Hypokalemia
Gastrointestinal: Diarrhea
Miscellaneous: Allergic reactions

Drug Interactions Neomycin, colchicine, chloramphenicol, anticonvulsants

Stability Protect from light

Mechanism of Action Coenzyme for various metabolic functions, including fat and carbohydrate metabolism and protein synthesis, used in cell replication and hematopoiesis

Pharmacokinetics

Absorption: Oral: Drug is absorbed from the terminal ileum in the presence of calcium; for absorption to occur, gastric "intrinsic factor" must be present to transfer the compound across the intestinal mucosa

Distribution: Bound to transcobalamin II; principally stored in the liver, also stored in the kidneys and adrenals

Metabolism: Converted in the tissues to active coenzymes methylcobalamin and deoxyadenosylcobalamin

Usual Dosage I.M. or deep S.C. (oral is not generally recommended due to poor absorption and I.V. is not recommended due to more rapid elimination)

Recommended daily allowance (RDA):
Children: 0.3-2 μg
Adults: 2 μg

Pernicious anemia, congenital (if evidence of neurologic involvement): 1000 μg/day for at least 2 weeks; maintenance: 50 μg/month

Children: 30-50 μg/day for 2 or more weeks (to a total dose of 1000-5000 μg), then follow with 100 μg monthly as maintenance dosage

Adults: 100 μg/day for 6-7 days; if improvement, give same dose on alternate days for 7 doses; then every 3-4 days for 2-3 weeks; once hematologic values have returned to normal, maintenance dosage: 100 μg/month **Note:** Use only parenteral therapy as oral therapy is not dependable

Vitamin B_{12} deficiency:

Children: 100 μg/day for 10-15 days (total dose of 1-1.5 mg), then once or twice weekly for several months; may taper to 60 μg every month

Adults: Initial: 30 μg/day for 5-10 days; maintenance: 100-200 μg/month

Monitoring Parameters Serum potassium, erythrocyte and reticulocyte count, hemoglobin, hematocrit

Dosage Forms

Injection: 30 μg/mL (30 mL); 100 μg/mL (1 mL, 10 mL, 30 mL); 1000 μg/mL (1 mL, 10 mL, 30 mL)

Tablet: 25 μg, 50 μg, 100 μg, 250 μg, 500 μg, 1000 μg

Cyclobenzaprine Hydrochloride (sye kloe ben' za preen)

Brand Names Flexeril®

Therapeutic Category Skeletal Muscle Relaxant, Central Acting

Use Treatment of muscle spasm associated with acute painful musculoskeletal conditions; supportive therapy in tetanus

Pregnancy Risk Factor B

Contraindications Hypersensitivity to cyclobenzaprine or any component; hyperthyroidism, congestive heart failure, arrhythmias, heart block

Precautions Use with caution in patients with urinary retention, angle-closure glaucoma

Adverse Reactions

Cardiovascular: Tachycardia, hypotension, arrhythmias

Central nervous system: Drowsiness, headache, dizziness, fatigue, asthenia, nervousness, confusion

Dermatologic: Rash

Gastrointestinal: Dyspepsia, nausea, constipation, dry mouth, vomiting, diarrhea

Ocular: Blurred vision

Miscellaneous: Unpleasant taste

Drug Interactions MAO inhibitors

Mechanism of Action Centrally acting skeletal muscle relaxant pharmacologically related to tricyclic antidepressants; reduces tonic somatic motor activity influencing both alpha and gamma motor neurons

Pharmacodynamics

Onset of action: Within 1 hour

Duration: 12-24 hours

Pharmacokinetics

Absorption: Oral: Completely absorbed

Metabolism: Hepatic

Peak serum levels: Within 3-8 hours

Elimination: Excreted primarily renally as inactive metabolites and in the feces (via bile) as unchanged drug; may undergo enterohepatic recycling

Usual Dosage Oral:

Children: Dosage has not been established

Adults: 20-40 mg/day in 2-4 divided doses; maximum dose: 60 mg/day

Dosage Forms Tablet: 10 mg

Cyclogyl® *see* Cyclopentolate Hydrochloride *on this page*

Cyclopentolate Hydrochloride (sye kloe pen' toe late)

Brand Names AK-Pentolate®; Cyclogyl®; I-Pentolate®

Therapeutic Category Anticholinergic Agent, Ophthalmic; Ophthalmic Agent, Mydriatic

Use Diagnostic procedures requiring mydriasis and cycloplegia

Pregnancy Risk Factor C

Contraindications Narrow-angle glaucoma; known hypersensitivity to cyclopentolate

Warnings Avoid using concentrations of 1% or greater in children <1 year of age due to stimulation of severe hypertension

Adverse Reactions Central nervous system and cardiovascular reactions most commonly seen in children after receiving 2% solution:

Cardiovascular: Tachycardia

Central nervous system: Psychotic and behavioral disturbances manifested by ataxia, restlessness, hallucinations, psychosis, hyperactivity, seizures, incoherent speech

Local: Burning sensation

Ocular: Increase in intraocular pressure, loss of visual accommodation

Miscellaneous: Allergic reactions

Mechanism of Action Prevents the muscle of the ciliary body and the

(Continued)

Cyclopentolate Hydrochloride *(Continued)*

sphincter muscle of the iris from responding to cholinergic stimulation, causing mydriasis and cycloplegia

Pharmacodynamics

Peak effects:

Cycloplegia: 15-60 minutes

Mydriasis: Within 15-60 minutes, with recovery taking up to 24 hours

Usual Dosage

Infants: 1 drop of 0.5% into each eye 5-10 minutes before examination

Children: 1 drop of 0.5% or 1% in eye followed by 1 drop of 0.5% or 1% in 5 minutes, if necessary, approximately 40-50 minutes before procedure

Adults: 1 drop of 1% followed by another drop in 5 minutes; approximately 40-50 minutes prior to the procedure, may use 2% solution in heavily pigmented iris

Administration To avoid excessive systemic absorption, finger pressure should be applied on the lacrimal sac during and for 1-2 minutes following application

Additional Information Pilocarpine ophthalmic drops applied after the examination may reduce recovery time to 3-6 hours

Dosage Forms Solution, ophthalmic: 0.5% (2 mL, 5 mL, 15 mL); 1% (2 mL, 5 mL, 15 mL); 2% (2 mL, 5 mL, 15 mL)

Cyclophosphamide (sye kloe foss' fa mide)

Related Information

Emetogenic Potential of Single Chemotherapeutic Agents *on page 655*

Medications Compatible With PN Solutions *on page 649-650*

Brand Names Cytoxan®; Neosar®

Synonyms CPM; CTX; CYT

Therapeutic Category Antineoplastic Agent

Use Management of Hodgkin's disease, malignant lymphomas, multiple myeloma, leukemias, sarcomas, mycosis fungoides, neuroblastoma, ovarian carcinoma, breast carcinoma, a variety of other tumors; nephrotic syndrome, lupus erythematosus, severe rheumatoid arthritis, and rheumatoid vasculitis

Pregnancy Risk Factor D

Contraindications Hypersensitivity to cyclophosphamide or any component

Warnings The US Food and Drug Administration (FDA) currently recommends that procedures for proper handling and disposal of antineoplastic agents be considered

Precautions Use with caution in patients with bone marrow depression and impaired renal or hepatic function; modify dosage in patients with renal impairment or compromised bone marrow function. Patients with compromised bone marrow function may require a 33% to 50% reduction in initial dose

Adverse Reactions

Cardiovascular: Cardiotoxicity with high dose therapy

Dermatologic: Alopecia

Endocrine & metabolic: Hypokalemia, amenorrhea, SIADH, hyperuricemia

Gastrointestinal: Nausea, vomiting, taste distortion

Hematologic: Leukopenia nadir at 8-15 days, hemolytic anemia, myelosuppression, positive Coombs' test

Renal & genitourinary: Hemorrhagic cystitis, oligospermia

Respiratory: Interstitial pulmonary fibrosis

Miscellaneous: Nasal stuffiness

Drug Interactions Barbiturates, allopurinol, chloramphenicol, imipramine, phenothiazines; succinylcholine (prolonged neuromuscular blocking activity)

Stability Reconstituted I.V. solution is stable for 24 hours at room temperature

Mechanism of Action Interferes with the normal function of DNA by alkylation and cross-linking the strands of DNA, and by possible protein modification

Pharmacokinetics

Absorption: Completely absorbed from the GI tract

Distribution: Crosses the placenta; appears in breast milk; distributes throughout the body including the brain and CSF

Protein binding: 20%; metabolite: 50%

Metabolism: Metabolized in the liver to active metabolite

Half-life: 4-6.5 hours

Peak serum levels: Oral: Within 1 hour

Elimination: Excreted in the urine as unchanged drug (<30%) and as metabolites (85% to 90%)

Moderately dialyzable (20% to 50%)

Usual Dosage Refer to individual protocols

Children with no hematologic problems:

Induction:

Oral: 2-8 mg/kg/day (100-300 mg/m^2/day)

I.V.: 10-20 mg/kg/day divided once daily

Maintenance: Oral: 2-5 mg/kg (50-150 mg/m^2) twice weekly

Pediatric solid tumors: I.V.: 250-1800 mg/m^2 once daily for 1-4 days every 21-28 days

Adults with no hematologic problems:

Induction:

Oral: 1-5 mg/kg/day

I.V.: 40-50 mg/kg (1.5-1.8 g/m^2) in divided doses over 2-5 days

Maintenance:

Oral: 1-5 mg/kg/day

I.V.: 10-15 mg/kg (350-550 mg/m^2) every 7-10 days or 3-5 mg/kg (110-185 mg/m^2) twice weekly

Dosing adjustment in renal impairment:

Cl_{cr} 25-50 mL/minute: Decrease dose by 50%

Cl_{cr} <25 mL/minute: Avoid use

Children and Adults:

SLE: I.V.: 500-750 mg/m^2 every month; maximum: 1 g/m^2

JRA/vasculitis: I.V.: 10 mg/kg every 2 weeks

BMT conditioning regimen: I.V.: 50 mg/kg/day once daily for 3-4 days

Nephrotic syndrome: Oral: 2-3 mg/kg/day every day for up to 12 weeks when corticosteroids are unsuccessful

Administration Can be administered IVP, I.V. intermittent, or continuous infusion at a final concentration for administration of 20-25 mg/mL

Monitoring Parameters CBC with differential and platelet count, ESR, BUN, urinalysis, serum electrolytes, serum creatinine

Patient Information Maintain high fluid intake and urine output

Nursing Implications Encourage adequate hydration and frequent voiding to help prevent hemorrhagic cystitis

Additional Information May be used in combination with a prophylactic agent for hemorrhagic cystitis, such as mesna

Myelosuppressive effects:

WBC: Moderate

Platelets: Moderate

Onset (days): 7

Nadir (days): 8-14

Recovery (days): 21

Dosage Forms

Powder for injection: 100 mg, 200 mg, 500 mg, 1 g, 2 g

Tablet: 25 mg, 50 mg

References

Bostrom BC, Weisdorf DJ, Kim TH, et al, "Bone Marrow Transplantation for Advanced Acute Leukemia: A Pilot Study of High-Energy Total Body Irradiation, Cyclophosphamide and Continuous Infusion Etoposide," *Bone Marrow Transplant*, 1990, 5(2):83-9.

McCune WJ, Golbus J, Zeldes W, et al, "Clinical and Immunologic Effects of Monthly Administration of Intravenous Cyclophosphamide in Severe Systemic Lupus Erythematosus," *N Engl J Med*, 1988, 318(22):1423-31.

Cycloserine (sye kloe ser' een)

Brand Names Seromycin® Pulvules®

Therapeutic Category Antibiotic, Miscellaneous; Antitubercular Agent

Use Adjunctive treatment in pulmonary or extrapulmonary tuberculosis; treatment of acute urinary tract infections caused by *E. coli* or *Enterobacter* sp when less toxic conventional therapy has failed or is contraindicated

Pregnancy Risk Factor C

Contraindications Known hypersensitivity to cycloserine; epilepsy, depression, severe anxiety or psychosis, severe renal insufficiency, chronic alcoholism

Precautions Dosage must be adjusted in patients with renal impairment

Adverse Reactions

Cardiovascular: Cardiac arrhythmias

Central nervous system: Drowsiness, headache, dizziness, tremor, vertigo, seizures, confusion, psychosis, paresis, coma

Dermatologic: Rash

Endocrine & metabolic: Vitamin B_{12} deficiency, folate deficiency

Hepatic: Elevated liver enzymes

Drug Interactions Cycloserine inhibits metabolism of phenytoin; alcohol may increase risk of seizures

Mechanism of Action Inhibits bacterial cell wall synthesis by competing with amino acid (D-alanine) for incorporation into the bacterial cell wall

Pharmacokinetics

Absorption: ~70% to 90% absorbed from the GI tract

Distribution: Crosses the placenta; appears in breast milk

Half-life: Patients with normal renal function: 10 hours

Peak serum levels: Within 3-4 hours

Elimination: 60% to 70% of an oral dose is excreted unchanged in urine by glomerular filtration within 72 hours, small amounts excreted in feces, remainder is metabolized

Usual Dosage Oral:

Tuberculosis:

Children: 10-20 mg/kg/day divided every 12 hours up to 1000 mg/day

Adults: Initial: 250 mg every 12 hours for 14 days, then give 500 mg to 1 g/day in 2 divided doses

Urinary tract infection: Adults: 250 mg every 12 hours for 14 days

Monitoring Parameters Periodic renal, hepatic, hematological tests, and plasma cycloserine concentrations

Reference Range Adjust dosage to maintain blood cycloserine concentrations <30 µg/mL

Patient Information May cause drowsiness

Nursing Implications Some of the neurotoxic effects may be relieved or prevented by the concomitant administration of pyridoxine

Dosage Forms Capsule: 250 mg

Cyclosporine (sye' kloe spor een)

Related Information

Blood Level Sampling Time Guidelines *on page 694-695*

Brand Names Sandimmune®

Synonyms CSA

Therapeutic Category Immunosuppressant Agent

Use Immunosuppressant used with corticosteroids to prevent graft vs host disease in patients with kidney, liver, heart, and bone marrow transplants

Pregnancy Risk Factor C

Contraindications Hypersensitivity to cyclosporine or any component

Warnings Administer with adrenal corticosteroids; infection and possible development of lymphoma may result; adjust dosage to avoid toxicity or possible organ rejection via cyclosporine blood level monitoring

Precautions Modify dosage in patients with hepatic and renal dysfunction

Adverse Reactions

Cardiovascular: Hypertension, hypotension, tachycardia, warmth, flushing

Central nervous system: Seizure, tremors, paresthesias, headache

Dermatologic: Hirsutism, gingival hyperplasia

Endocrine & metabolic: Hyperkalemia, hypomagnesemia, hyperuricemia, hyperlipidemia

Gastrointestinal: Abdominal discomfort
Hepatic: Hepatotoxicity
Musculoskeletal: Myositis
Renal & genitourinary: Nephrotoxicity
Respiratory: Respiratory distress
Miscellaneous: Lymphoproliferative disorder, increased susceptibility to infection, sensitivity to temperature extremes; anaphylaxis (may be due to polyoxyl 35 castor oil vehicle in the injectable solution)

Drug Interactions Ketoconazole, fluconazole, erythromycin, diltiazem, and methylprednisolone: ↑ plasma concentration of cyclosporine; rifampin, phenytoin, phenobarbital and TMP/SMZ ↓ plasma concentration of cyclosporine

Stability Do **not** store oral solution in the refrigerator, store oral solution only in original container and use contents within 2 months after opening; I.V. cyclosporine prepared in normal saline is stable 6 hours in PVC or 12 hours in a glass container; cyclosporine diluted in D_5W is stable 24 hours in PVC or glass containers

Mechanism of Action Inhibition of production and release of interleukin II and inhibits interleukin II-induced activation of resting T-lymphocytes

Pharmacokinetics

Absorption: Oral: Incomplete and erratic; larger oral doses of cyclosporine are needed in pediatric patients versus adults due to a shorter bowel length resulting in limited intestinal absorption
Distribution: Extensively distributed throughout the body primarily in liver, pancreas, and lungs; distributes into breast milk
Protein binding: 90% of dose binds to blood proteins
Metabolism: Metabolized by mixed function oxidase enzymes in the liver
Bioavailability in pediatric renal transplant patients: 31%; gut dysfunction, commonly seen in BMT recipients reduces oral bioavailability further
Half-life, adults: 19-40 hours
Peak plasma concentrations: Oral: Achieved in 3-4 hours
Elimination: Excreted primarily in the bile; clearance is more rapid in pediatric patients than in adults; clearance is decreased in patients with liver disease

Usual Dosage Children and Adults:

Oral: Initial: 14-18 mg/kg/dose administered 4-12 hours prior to organ transplantation; maintenance: 5-15 mg/kg/day divided every 12-24 hours postoperatively; maintenance dose is usually tapered to 3-10 mg/kg/day
I.V.: Initial: 5-6 mg/kg/dose administered 4-12 hours prior to organ transplantation; maintenance: 2-10 mg/kg/day in divided doses every 8-12 hours; patients should be switched to oral cyclosporine as soon as possible

Administration I.V. cyclosporine can be administered by I.V. intermittent infusion or continuous infusion; for intermittent infusion, administer over 2-6 hours at a final concentration not to exceed 2.5 mg/mL

Monitoring Parameters Blood/serum drug level (trough), renal and hepatic function tests, serum electrolytes, blood pressure, heart rate

Reference Range Reference ranges are method dependent and specimen dependent; use the same analytical method consistently; trough levels should be obtained immediately prior to next dose

Therapeutic: Not well defined, dependent on organ transplanted, time after transplant, organ function and CSA toxicity. Empiric therapeutic concentration ranges for trough cyclosporine concentrations:
Kidney: 100-200 ng/mL (serum, RIA)
BMT: 100-250 ng/mL (serum, RIA)
Heart: 100-200 ng/mL (serum, RIA)
Liver: 100-400 ng/mL (blood, HPLC)

Method dependent (optimum cyclosporine trough concentrations):
Serum, RIA: 150-300 ng/mL; 50-150 ng/mL (late post-transplant period)
Whole blood, RIA: 250-800 ng/mL; 150-450 ng/mL (late post-transplant period)
Whole blood, HPLC: 100-500 ng/mL

Test Interactions Cyclosporine adsorbs to silicone; specific whole blood, HPLC assay for cyclosporine may be falsely elevated if sample is drawn from the same central venous line through which dose was administered (even if flush has been administered and/or dose was given hours before)

Nursing Implications Use glass dropper or container (not plastic or styrofoam) when administering this medication orally; mix with milk, chocolate

(Continued)

Cyclosporine *(Continued)*

milk, or orange juice (preferably at room temperature) to improve palatability, stir well and drink at once; do not allow to stand before drinking; rinse with more diluent to ensure that the total dose is taken; after use, dry outside of pipette, do not rinse with water or other cleaning agents; adequate airway and other supportive measures and agents for treating anaphylaxis should be present when I.V. cyclosporine is given.

Dosage Forms

Capsule: 25 mg, 100 mg
Injection: 50 mg/mL (5 mL)
Solution, oral: 100 mg/mL (50 mL)

References

Burckart GJ, Canafax DM, Yee GC, "Cyclosporine Monitoring," *Drug Intell Clin Pharm*, 1986, 20(9):649-52.

Wandstrat TL, Schroeder TJ, and Myre SA, "Cyclosporine Pharmacokinetics in Pediatric Transplant Recipients," *Ther Drug Monit*, 1989, 11(5):493-6.

Cycrin® *see* Medroxyprogesterone Acetate *on page 359*

Cyklokapron® *see* Tranexamic Acid *on page 577*

Cylert® *see* Pemoline *on page 436*

Cyproheptadine Hydrochloride (si proe hep' ta deen)

Related Information

Overdose and Toxicology Information *on page 696-700*

Brand Names Periactin®

Therapeutic Category Antihistamine

Use Perennial and seasonal allergic rhinitis and other allergic symptoms including urticaria

Pregnancy Risk Factor B

Contraindications Hypersensitivity to cyproheptadine or any component; narrow-angle glaucoma, bladder neck obstruction, acute asthmatic attack, stenosing peptic ulcer, GI tract obstruction, those on MAO inhibitors; avoid use in premature and term newborns due to potential association with SIDS

Precautions May impair ability to perform hazardous duties requiring mental alertness or physical coordination

Adverse Reactions

Cardiovascular: Tachycardia
Central nervous system: Sedation, CNS stimulation, seizures
Gastrointestinal: Appetite stimulation, dry mouth
Hematologic: Hemolytic anemia, leukopenia, thrombocytopenia
Miscellaneous: Allergic reactions

Drug Interactions MAO inhibitors

Mechanism of Action A potent antihistamine and serotonin antagonist, competes with histamine for H_1-receptor sites on effector cells in the gastrointestinal tract, blood vessels, and respiratory tract

Pharmacokinetics

Absorption: Well absorbed
Metabolism: Extensively by conjugation

Usual Dosage Oral:

Children: 0.25 mg/kg/day in 2-3 divided doses or
- 2-6 years: 2 mg every 8-12 hours (not to exceed 12 mg/day)
- 7-14 years: 4 mg every 8-12 hours (not to exceed 16 mg/day)

Adults: 4 mg every 8 hours (not to exceed 0.5 mg/kg/day)

Test Interactions Diagnostic antigen skin tests

Dosage Forms

Syrup: 2 mg/5 mL with alcohol 5% (473 mL)
Tablet: 4 mg

CYT *see* Cyclophosphamide *on page 162*

Cytarabine Hydrochloride (sye tare' a been)

Related Information

Emetogenic Potential of Single Chemotherapeutic Agents *on page 655*

Medications Compatible With PN Solutions *on page 649-650*

Brand Names Cytosar-U®

Synonyms Arabinosylcytosine; Ara-C; Cytosine Arabinosine Hydrochloride

Therapeutic Category Antineoplastic Agent

Use Used in combination regimens for the treatment of leukemias and non-Hodgkin's lymphomas

Pregnancy Risk Factor D

Contraindications Hypersensitivity to cytarabine or any component

Warnings The US Food and Drug Administration (FDA) currently recommends that procedures for proper handling and disposal of antineoplastic agents be considered. Must monitor for drug toxicity; drug toxicity includes bone marrow depression with leukopenia, thrombocytopenia and anemia along with nausea, vomiting, diarrhea, abdominal pain, oral ulceration and hepatic dysfunction

Precautions Marked bone marrow depression necessitates dosage reduction or a reduction in the number of days of administration; with severe hepatic dysfunction, dosage may need to be reduced

Adverse Reactions

Cardiovascular: Cardiomegaly

Central nervous system: Headache, peripheral neuropathy, malaise, confusion, seizures, fever, ataxia; cerebral and cerebellar dysfunction (somnolence, personality changes, coma)

Dermatologic: Alopecia, rash

Gastrointestinal: Nausea, vomiting, oral and anal inflammation with ulceration, anorexia, diarrhea

Hematologic: Myelosuppression

Hepatic: Hepatic dysfunction

Musculoskeletal: Myalgia, bone pain

Ocular: Conjunctivitis, hemorrhagic conjunctivitis, corneal toxicity

Respiratory: Syndrome of sudden respiratory distress progressing to pulmonary edema and diffuse interstitial pneumonitis have been reported with high-dose regimens

Miscellaneous: Ara-C syndrome (fever, myalgia, bone pain, rash, conjunctivitis, malaise occurring 6-12 hours after administration)

Drug Interactions ↓ digoxin oral tablet absorption

Stability Reconstituted solutions containing 20 or up to 100 mg/mL cytarabine are stable for 48 hours at room temperature; I.T. Ara-C is compatible with methotrexate and hydrocortisone mixed in the same syringe

Mechanism of Action Incorporated into DNA; inhibits DNA synthesis; cell cycle-specific for the S phase of cell division

Pharmacokinetics

Distribution: Penetrates the CSF in limited amounts

Protein binding: 10%

Metabolism: Metabolized primarily in the liver

Half-life, terminal: 1-3 hours

Elimination: ~80% of a dose excreted in the urine as metabolites within 24 hours

Usual Dosage Children and Adults (refer to individual protocols):

Induction remission:

- I.V.: 200 mg/m^2/day for 5 days at 2-week intervals as a single agent; in combination chemotherapy, 100-200 mg/m^2/day for 5- to 10-day therapy course or every day until remission; given as an I.V. continuous drip or in 2 divided doses/day
- I.T.: 5-75 mg/m^2 every 2-7 days until CNS findings normalize

Maintenance remission:

- I.V.: 70-200 mg/m^2/day for 2-5 days at monthly intervals
- I.M., S.C.: 1-1.5 mg/kg single dose for maintenance at 1- to 4-week intervals
- I.T.: 5-75 mg/m^2 every 2-7 days until CNS findings normalize
- Ara-C:
  - <1 year: 20 mg
  - 1-2 years: 30 mg
  - 2-3 years: 50 mg
  - >3 years: 70 mg

High-dose therapies: Doses as high as 3 g/m^2 have been used for refractory leukemias or refractory non-Hodgkins lymphoma (dosages of 3 g/m^2 every 12 hours for 4-6 doses have been used)

(Continued)

Cytarabine Hydrochloride *(Continued)*

Administration Can be administered I.M., IVP, I.V. infusion, or S.C. at a concentration not to exceed 100 mg/mL; high-dose regimens are usually administered by I.V. infusion over 1-3 hours or as I.V. continuous infusion; for I.T. use, reconstitute with preservative free saline or preservative free lactated Ringer's solution.

Monitoring Parameters Liver function tests, CBC with differential and platelet count, serum creatinine, BUN, serum uric acid

Patient Information Notify physician of any fever, sore throat, bleeding, or bruising

Nursing Implications Administer corticosteroid eye drops around the clock prior to, during, and after high-dose Ara-C for prophylaxis of conjunctivitis; pyridoxine has been administered on days of high-dose Ara-C therapy for prophylaxis of CNS toxicity.

Additional Information Myelosuppressive effects:

WBC: Severe
Platelets: Severe
Onset (days): 4-7
Nadir (days): 14-18
Recovery (days): 21-28

Dosage Forms Powder for injection: 100 mg, 500 mg, 1 g, 2 g

References

Grossman L, Baker MA, Sutton DM, et al, "Central Nervous System Toxicity of High-Dose Cytosine Arabinoside," *Med Pediatr Oncol*, 1983, 11(4):246-50.

Cytosar-U® *see* Cytarabine Hydrochloride *on page 166*

Cytosine Arabinosine Hydrochloride *see* Cytarabine Hydrochloride *on page 166*

Cytovene® *see* Ganciclovir *on page 267*

Cytoxan® *see* Cyclophosphamide *on page 162*

D-3-Mercaptovaline *see* Penicillamine *on page 437*

Dacarbazine (da kar' ba zeen)

Related Information

Emetogenic Potential of Single Chemotherapeutic Agents *on page 655*

Brand Names DTIC-Dome®

Synonyms DIC; Imidazole Carboxamide

Therapeutic Category Antineoplastic Agent

Use Metastatic malignant melanoma; in combination with other agents in Hodgkin's disease; has been used for soft tissue sarcomas and neuroblastomas

Pregnancy Risk Factor C

Contraindications Hypersensitivity to dacarbazine or any component

Warnings The US Food and Drug Administration (FDA) currently recommends that procedures for proper handling and disposal of antineoplastic agents be considered. Hematopoietic depression is common; hepatic necrosis is also possible

Precautions Use with caution in patients with bone marrow depression, renal and/or hepatic impairment; dosage reduction may be necessary in patients with renal or hepatic insufficiency; avoid extravasation of the drug

Adverse Reactions

Cardiovascular: Facial flushing
Central nervous system: Malaise, paresthesias, headache, fever
Dermatologic: Alopecia, rash
Gastrointestinal: Anorexia, nausea, vomiting, metallic taste
Hematologic: Myelosuppression (nadir: 2-4 weeks)
Hepatic: Hepatotoxicity
Local: Pain and burning at infusion site, thrombophlebitis
Musculoskeletal: Myalgia
Miscellaneous: Sinus congestion, flu-like syndrome, anaphylactic reactions

Drug Interactions Phenytoin, phenobarbital

Stability Store in refrigerator, protect from light; reconstituted dacarbazine solution 10 mg/mL is stable for 72 hours when refrigerated or 8 hours at room temperature; dacarbazine is incompatible with hydrocortisone sodium succinate

Mechanism of Action Alkylating agent which forms methylcarbonium ions that attack nucleophilic groups in DNA; cross-links strands of DNA resulting in the inhibition of DNA and RNA synthesis

Pharmacokinetics

Protein binding: Minimal, 5%

Metabolism: Metabolized in the liver by microsomal enzymes; metabolites may also have an antineoplastic effect

Half-life (biphasic): Initial: 20-40 minutes; terminal: 5 hours (in patients with normal renal/hepatic function)

Elimination: ~30% to 50% of a dose is excreted in the urine by tubular secretion, 15% to 25% is excreted as unchanged drug

Usual Dosage I.V. (refer to individual protocols):

Children:

Pediatric solid tumors: 200-470 mg/m^2/day over 5 days every 21-28 days

Pediatric neuroblastoma: 800-900 mg/m^2 as a single dose every 3-4 weeks in combination therapy

Adults:

Malignant melanoma: 2-4.5 mg/kg/day for 10 days, repeat in 4 weeks or may use 250 mg/m^2/day for 5 days, repeat in 3 weeks

Hodgkin's disease: 150 mg/m^2/day for 5 days, repeat every 4 weeks or 375 mg/m^2 on day 1, repeat in 15 days of each 28-day cycle in combination with other agents

Administration Administer by slow IVP over 2-3 minutes at a concentration not to exceed 10 mg/mL or by I.V. infusion over 15-30 minutes

Monitoring Parameters CBC with differential, erythrocytes and platelet count; liver function tests

Nursing Implications Local pain, burning sensation, and irritation at the injection site may be relieved by local application of hot packs, slowing the I.V. rate, or further dilution in I.V. fluid

Dosage Forms Injection: 100 mg, 200 mg, 500 mg

References

Berg SL, Grisell DL, DeLaney TF, et al, "Principles of Treatment of Pediatric Solid Tumors," *Pediatr Clin North Am*, 1991, 38(2):249-67.

Finkelstein JZ, Albo V, Ertel I, et al, "5-(3,3-Dimethyl-l-triazeno) imidazole-4-carboxamide (NSC-45388) in the Treatment of Solid Tumors in Children," *Cancer Chemother Rep*, 1975, 59(2):351-7.

Mutz ID and Urban CE, "Dimethyl-triazeno-carboxamide (DTIC) in Combination Chemotherapy for Childhood Neuroblastoma," *Wien Klin Wochenschr*, 1978, 90(23):867-70.

Dactinomycin (dak ti noe mye' sin)

Brand Names Cosmegen®

Synonyms ACT; Actinomycin D

Therapeutic Category Antineoplastic Agent

Use Management, either alone or with other treatment modalities of Wilms' tumor, rhabdomyosarcoma, neuroblastoma, retinoblastoma, Ewing's sarcoma, trophoblastic neoplasms, testicular carcinoma, and other malignancies

Pregnancy Risk Factor C

Contraindications Hypersensitivity to dactinomycin or any component; patients with chickenpox or herpes zoster; avoid in infants <6 months of age since the incidence of adverse effects is increased in infants

Warnings The US Food and Drug Administration (FDA) currently recommends that procedures for proper handling and disposal of antineoplastic agents be considered. Dactinomycin is extremely irritating to tissues. If extravasation occurs during I.V. use, severe damage to soft tissues may occur leading to necrosis, pain, and ulceration.

Precautions Use with caution in patients with hepatobiliary dysfunction or in patients who have received radiation therapy; reduce dosage in patients receiving concurrent radiation therapy

Adverse Reactions

Dermatologic: Alopecia, erythema, hyperpigmentation of skin, desquamation

(Continued)

Dactinomycin *(Continued)*

Endocrine & metabolic: Hypocalcemia
Gastrointestinal: Anorexia, vomiting, diarrhea, stomatitis, proctitis
Hematologic: Myelosuppression (nadir: 2-3 weeks)
Hepatic: Hepatitis
Local: Soft tissue damage with extravasation
Miscellaneous: Anaphylactoid reaction

Drug Interactions Dactinomycin potentiates the effects of radiation therapy

Stability Binds to cellulose filters, therefore, avoid in-line filtration; adsorbs to glass and plastic so dactinomycin should not be given by continuous or intermittent infusion; use of a diluent containing preservatives for reconstitution may result in a precipitate

Mechanism of Action Binds to the guanine portion of DNA intercalating between guanine and cytosine base pairs inhibiting DNA and RNA synthesis

Pharmacokinetics

Distribution: Crosses the placenta
Half-life: 36 hours
Peak serum levels: I.V.: Within 2-5 minutes
Elimination: ~10% of a dose is excreted as unchanged drug in the urine while 50% appears in the bile

Usual Dosage Dosage should be based on body surface area in obese or edematous patients

Children >6 months and Adults: I.V. (refer to individual protocols): 15 μg/kg/day or 400-600 μg/m^2/day for 5 days, may repeat every 3-6 weeks; or 2.5 mg/m^2 given in divided doses over 1 week; 0.75-2 mg/m^2 as a single dose given at intervals of 1-4 weeks has been used

Administration Administer IVP over a few minutes at a concentration not to exceed 500 μg/mL through a freely flowing I.V.

Monitoring Parameters CBC with differential and platelet count, liver function tests and renal function tests

Patient Information Notify physician if fever, sore throat, bleeding, or bruising occurs

Nursing Implications For I.V. administration only; since drug is extremely irritating to tissues, **do not give I.M. or S.C.**

Dosage Forms Powder for injection, lyophilized: 0.5 mg

References

Berg SL, Grisell DL, DeLaney TF, et al, "Principles of Treatment of Pediatric Solid Tumors," *Pediatr Clin North Am*, 1991, 38(2):249-67.
Carli M, Pastore G, Perilongo G, et al, "Tumor Response and Toxicity After Single High-Dose Versus Standard Five-Day Divided Dose Dactinomycin in Childhood Rhabdomyosarcoma," *J Clin Oncol*, 1988, 6(4):654-8.

Dalalone L.A.® *see* Dexamethasone *on page 178*
Dalcaine® *see* Lidocaine Hydrochloride *on page 342*
Dalmane® *see* Flurazepam Hydrochloride *on page 260*
***d*-Alpha Tocopherol** *see* Vitamin E *on page 605*
Dantrium® *see* Dantrolene Sodium *on this page*

Dantrolene Sodium (dan' troe leen)

Brand Names Dantrium®

Therapeutic Category Antidote, Malignant Hyperthermia; Hyperthermia, Treatment; Skeletal Muscle Relaxant, Direct Acting

Use Treatment of spasticity associated with upper motor neuron disorders such as spinal cord injury, stroke, cerebral palsy, or multiple sclerosis; also used as treatment of malignant hyperthermia

Pregnancy Risk Factor C

Contraindications Active hepatic disease; should not be used where spasticity is used to maintain posture or balance

Warnings Has potential for hepatotoxicity; overt hepatitis has been most frequently observed between the third and twelfth month of therapy; hepatic injury appears to be greater in females and in patients >35 years of age

Precautions Use with caution in patients with impaired cardiac or pulmonary function

Adverse Reactions

Cardiovascular/respiratory: Pleural effusion with pericarditis

Central nervous system: Seizures, drowsiness, dizziness, lightheadedness, confusion, headache, fatigue, speech disturbances

Dermatologic: Rash

Gastrointestinal: Diarrhea, nausea, vomiting, severe constipation

Hepatic: Hepatitis

Musculoskeletal: Muscle weakness

Ocular: Visual disturbances

Renal & genitourinary: Urinary retention

Drug Interactions Verapamil (associated with ventricular fibrillation and cardiovascular collapse when used concomitantly with I.V. dantrolene; animal study, relevance in humans remains to be determined)

Stability Protect from light; use within 6 hours; incompatible with dextrose, normal saline, or bacteriostatic water for injection; precipitates when placed in glass containers for infusion

Mechanism of Action Acts directly on skeletal muscle by interfering with release of calcium ion from the sarcoplasmic reticulum; prevents or reduces the increase in myoplasmic calcium ion concentration that activates the acute catabolic processes associated with malignant hyperthermia

Pharmacokinetics

Absorption: Oral: 35%

Metabolism: Extensive

Half-life:

Children: 7.3 hours

Adults: 8.7 hours

Usual Dosage

Spasticity: Oral:

Children: Initial: 0.5 mg/kg/dose twice daily, increase frequency to 3-4 times/day at 4- to 7-day intervals, then increase dose by 0.5 mg/kg to a maximum of 3 mg/kg/dose 2-4 times/day up to 400 mg/day

Adults: 25 mg/day to start, increase frequency to 3-4 times/day, then increase dose by 25 mg every 4-7 days to a maximum of 100 mg 2-4 times/day or 400 mg/day

Hyperthermia: Children and Adults:

Oral: 4-8 mg/kg/day in 4 divided doses given 1-2 days prior to surgery for those patients at risk; to prevent recurrence, this dosage may be used for up to 3 days after crisis

I.V.: 1 mg/kg; may repeat as needed to a cumulative dose of 10 mg/kg (mean effective dose is 2.5 mg/kg), then switch to oral dosage; may also be administered over 1 hour beginning 1.25 hours before surgery for patients at risk

Administration Reconstitute by adding 60 mL sterile water (**not bacteriostatic water for injection**); give by rapid I.V. injection; for infusion, **do not** further dilute with normal saline or dextrose; place solution in plastic container for continuous infusion

Monitoring Parameters Baseline and periodic liver function tests

Patient Information Avoid unnecessary exposure to sunlight

Nursing Implications Avoid extravasation as is a tissue irritant

Dosage Forms

Capsule: 25 mg, 50 mg, 100 mg

Powder for injection: 20 mg

Extemporaneous Preparation(s) A 5 mg/mL suspension may be made by adding five (5) 100 mg capsules to a citric acid solution (150 mg citric acid powder in 10 mL water) and then adding syrup to a total volume of 100 mL; stable 2 days in refrigerator

Nahata MC and Hipple TF, *Pediatric Drug Formulations*, 1st ed, Harvey Whitney Books Co, 1990.

Dapa® [OTC] *see* Acetaminophen *on page 16*

Daraprim® *see* Pyrimethamine *on page 502*

Darvocet-N® *see* Propoxyphene and Acetaminophen *on page 492*

Darvocet-N® 100 *see* Propoxyphene and Acetaminophen *on page 492*

Darvon® *see* Propoxyphene *on page 491*

Darvon-N® *see* Propoxyphene *on page 491*

Datril® [OTC] *see* Acetaminophen *on page 16*

Daunomycin *see* Daunorubicin Hydrochloride *on this page*

Daunorubicin Hydrochloride (daw noe roo' bi sin)

Related Information

Extravasation Treatment *on page 640*

Brand Names Cerubidine®

Synonyms Daunomycin; DNR; Rubidomycin Hydrochloride

Therapeutic Category Antineoplastic Agent

Use In combination with other agents in the treatment of leukemias (ALL, ANL)

Pregnancy Risk Factor D

Contraindications Hypersensitivity to daunorubicin or any component; congestive heart failure or arrhythmias; pre-existing bone marrow suppression

Warnings The US Food and Drug Administration (FDA) currently recommends that procedures for proper handling and disposal of antineoplastic agents be considered. I.V. use only, severe local tissue necrosis will result if extravasation occurs; irreversible myocardial toxicity may occur as total dosage approaches 550 mg/m^2 in adults, 400 mg/m^2 in patients receiving chest radiation; 300 mg/m^2 in children >2 years of age or 10 mg/kg in children <2; this may occur during therapy or several months after therapy; total cumulative dose should take into account previous or concomitant treatment with cardiotoxic agents or irradiation of chest; severe myelosuppression is possible when used in therapeutic doses

Precautions Reduce dosage in patients with hepatic, biliary, or renal impairment

Adverse Reactions

Cardiovascular: Cardiotoxicity

Central nervous system: Fever, chills

Dermatologic: Alopecia, pigmentation of nail beds, urticaria

Endocrine & metabolic: Hyperuricemia

Gastrointestinal: Stomatitis, esophagitis, nausea, vomiting

Hematologic: Myelosuppression

Hepatic: Elevation in serum bilirubin, AST, and alkaline phosphatase

Local: Severe tissue necrosis with extravasation

Stability Reconstituted solution should be protected from sunlight; reconstituted solution is stable for 48 hours when refrigerated and 24 hours at room temperature; unstable in solutions with a pH >8; incompatible with heparin, sodium bicarbonate, 5-FU, and dexamethasone

Mechanism of Action Inhibition of DNA and RNA synthesis, by intercalating between DNA base pairs and by steric obstruction; is not cell cycle-specific for the S phase of cell division

Pharmacokinetics

Distribution: Widely distributed in tissues such as spleen, heart, kidneys, liver, and lungs; does not cross the blood-brain barrier; crosses the placenta

Metabolism: Metabolized to daunorubicinol (active)

Half-life, terminal: 14-18.5 hours

Daunorubicinol, active metabolite: 24-48 hours

Elimination: 40% of a dose is excreted in the bile while ~25% is excreted in the urine as metabolite and unchanged drug

Usual Dosage I.V. (refer to individual protocols):

Children:

ALL combination therapy: Remission induction: 25-45 mg/m^2 on day 1 every week for 4 cycles or 30-45 mg/m^2/day for 3 days

<2 years or <0.5 m^2: 1 mg/kg per protocol with frequency dependent on regimen employed

Adults: 30-60 mg/m^2/day for 3-5 days, repeat dose in 3-4 weeks; total cumulative dose should not exceed 400-600 mg/m^2

Single agent induction for AML: 60 mg/m^2/day for 3 days; repeat every 3-4 weeks

Combination therapy induction for AML: 45 mg/m^2/day for 3 days; Subsequent courses: Every day for 2 days

ALL combination therapy: Remission induction: 45 mg/m^2 on days 1, 2, and 3 of induction course

Dosing adjustment in hepatic or renal impairment: Reduce dose 25% in patients with serum bilirubin of 1.2-3 mg/dL; reduce dose 50% in patients with serum bilirubin and/or creatinine >3 mg/dL

Administration Administer IVP diluting the reconstituted dose in 10-15 mL normal saline and administering over 2-3 minutes into the tubing of a rapidly infusing I.V. solution of D_5W or NS; daunorubicin has also been diluted in 100 mL of D_5W or NS and infused over 30-45 minutes

Monitoring Parameters CBC with differential and platelet count, liver function test, EKG, ventricular ejection fraction, renal function test

Patient Information Transient red/orange discoloration of urine can occur for up to 48 hours after a dose; notify physician if fever, sore throat, bleeding, or bruising occurs

Nursing Implications Drug is very irritating, do not inject I.M. or S.C.; avoid extravasation; for extravasation, infiltrate area with hydrocortisone and/or sodium bicarbonate and apply cold packs for 15 minutes 4 times/day

Additional Information Myelosuppressive effects:

WBC: Severe
Platelets: Severe
Onset (days): 7
Nadir (days): 10-14
Recovery (days): 21-28

Dosage Forms Powder for injection, lyophilized: 20 mg

References

Crom WR, Glynn-Barnhart AM, Rodman JH, et al, "Pharmacokinetics of Anticancer Drugs in Children," *Clin Pharmacokinet*, 1987, 12(3):168-213.

Dazamide® *see* Acetazolamide *on page 18*

DDAVP® *see* Desmopressin Acetate *on page 177*

DDI *see* Didanosine *on page 188*

1-Deamino-8-D-Arginine Vasopressin *see* Desmopressin Acetate *on page 177*

Debrox® [OTC] *see* Carbamide Peroxide *on page 103*

Decadron® *see* Dexamethasone *on page 178*

Decadron®-LA *see* Dexamethasone *on page 178*

Decadron® Turbinaire® *see* Dexamethasone *on page 178*

Decaject-L.A.® *see* Dexamethasone *on page 178*

Decaspray® *see* Dexamethasone *on page 178*

Declomycin® *see* Demeclocycline Hydrochloride *on page 175*

Decofed® Syrup [OTC] *see* Pseudoephedrine *on page 497*

Deferoxamine Mesylate (de fer ox' a meen)

Brand Names Desferal® Mesylate

Therapeutic Category Antidote, Aluminum Toxicity; Antidote, Iron Toxicity

Use Acute iron intoxication; chronic iron overload secondary to multiple transfusions; diagnostic test for iron overload; used investigationally in the treatment of aluminum accumulation in renal failure

Pregnancy Risk Factor C

Contraindications Patients with anuria

Precautions Use with caution in patients with severe renal disease, pyelonephritis

Adverse Reactions

Cardiovascular: Flushing, hypotension, tachycardia, shock, swelling
Central nervous system: Fever
Dermatologic: Erythema, urticaria, pruritus, rash, cutaneous wheal formation
Gastrointestinal: Abdominal discomfort, diarrhea
Musculoskeletal: Leg cramps
Ocular: Blurred vision, cataracts
Otic: Hearing loss
Miscellaneous: Anaphylaxis, possible increased risk of fungal and *Y. enterocolitica* infections

(Continued)

Deferoxamine Mesylate *(Continued)*

Stability Protect from light

Mechanism of Action Complexes with trivalent ions (ferric ions) to form ferrioxamine, which is removed by the kidneys

Pharmacokinetics

Absorption: Oral: <15%

Metabolism: Metabolized in the liver to ferrioxamine

Half-life:

Deferoxamine: 6.1 hours

Ferrioxamine: 5.8 hours

Elimination: Renal excretion of the metabolite and unchanged drug

Usual Dosage

Children:

Acute iron intoxication:

I.M.: 90 mg/kg/dose every 8 hours; maximum: 6 g/day

I.V.: 15 mg/kg/hour; maximum: 6 g/day

Chronic iron overload:

I.V.: 15 mg/kg/hour; maximum: 6 g/day

S.C. infusion via a portable, controlled infusion device: 20-40 mg/kg/day over 8-12 hours

Aluminum induced bone disease: 20-40 mg/kg every hemodialysis treatment, frequency dependent on clinical status of the patient

Adults:

Acute iron intoxication:

I.M.: 1 g stat, then 0.5 g every 4 hours for two doses, additional doses of 0.5 g every 4-12 hours up to 6 g/day may be needed depending upon the clinical response

I.V.: 15 mg/kg/hour; maximum: 6 g/day

Chronic iron overload:

I.M.: 0.5-1 g/day

S.C. infusion via a portable, controlled infusion device: 1-2 g/day over 8-24 hours

Administration Add 2 mL sterile water to 500 mg vial; for I.M. or S.C. administration, no further dilution is required; for I.V. infusion, dilute in dextrose, normal saline, or lactated Ringer's; 10 mg/mL (maximum: 25 mg/mL); maximum rate of infusion: 15 mg/kg/hour

Monitoring Parameters Serum iron, total iron binding capacity; ophthalmologic exam and audiometry with chronic use

Nursing Implications May cause the urine to turn a reddish color

Additional Information Has been used investigationally as a single 40 mg/kg I.V. dose over 2 hours, to promote mobilization of aluminum from tissue stores as an aid in the diagnosis of aluminum-associated osteodystrophy

Dosage Forms Injection: 500 mg

References

Bentur Y, McGuigan M, and Koren G, "Deferoxamine (Desferrioxamine): New Toxicities for an Old Drug," *Drug Saf*, 1991, 6(1):37-46.

Freedman MH, Olivieri N, Benson L, et al, "Clinical Studies on Iron Chelation in Patients With Thalassemia Major," *Haematologica*, 1990, 75(Suppl 5):74-83.

Giardina PJ, Grady RW, Ehlers KH, et al, "Current Therapy of Cooley's Anemia: A Decade of Experience With Subcutaneous Desferrioxamine," *Ann N Y Acad Sci*, 1990, 612:275-85.

Pippard MJ, "Iron Metabolism and Iron Chelation in the Thalassemia Disorders," *Haematologica*, 1990, 75(Suppl 5):66-71.

Degest® 2 [OTC] *see* Naphazoline Hydrochloride *on page 403*

Dehist® *see* Brompheniramine Maleate *on page 88*

Delatest® *see* Testosterone *on page 550*

Delatestryl® *see* Testosterone *on page 550*

Delaxin® *see* Methocarbamol *on page 372*

Delestrogen® *see* Estradiol *on page 231*

Delta-Cortef® *see* Prednisolone *on page 476*

Deltacortisone *see* Prednisone *on page 477*

Deltadehydrocortisone *see* Prednisone *on page 477*

Deltahydrocortisone *see* Prednisolone *on page 476*

Deltasone® *see* Prednisone *on page 477*

Demeclocycline Hydrochloride (dem e kloe sye' kleen)

Brand Names Declomycin®

Synonyms Demethylchlortetracycline

Therapeutic Category Antibiotic, Tetracycline Derivative

Use Treatment of susceptible bacterial infections (acne, gonorrhea, pertussis and urinary tract infections) caused by both gram-negative and gram-positive organisms; used when penicillin is contraindicated; the treatment of chronic syndrome of inappropriate antidiuretic hormone secretion

Pregnancy Risk Factor D

Contraindications Hypersensitivity to demeclocycline, tetracyclines, or any component

Warnings Photosensitivity reactions occur frequently with this drug, avoid prolonged exposure to sunlight; do not use tanning equipment. Do not administer to children ≤8 years of age; use of tetracyclines during tooth development may cause permanent discoloration of the teeth and enamel hypoplasia; prolonged use may result in superinfection

Precautions Modify dosage in patients with impaired renal function

Adverse Reactions

Central nervous system: Paresthesia; increased intracranial pressure, bulging fontanels in infants

Dermatologic: Dermatologic effects, photosensitivity

Endocrine & metabolic: Diabetes insipidus syndrome

Gastrointestinal: Nausea, vomiting, diarrhea

Renal & genitourinary: Azotemia

Miscellaneous: Superinfections

Drug Interactions Do not administer with antacids, milk or dairy products, zinc, and iron preparations → ↓ absorption of demeclocycline

Stability Outdated tetracyclines have caused a Fanconi-like syndrome

Mechanism of Action Inhibits protein synthesis by binding with the 30S and possibly the 50S ribosomal subunit(s) of susceptible bacteria; may also cause alterations in the cytoplasmic membrane

Pharmacodynamics Onset of action for diuresis in SIADH: Several days

Pharmacokinetics

Absorption: ~50% to 80% of a dose is absorbed from the GI tract; food and dairy products reduce absorption

Protein binding: 41% to 50%

Metabolism: Small amounts metabolized in the liver to inactive metabolites; enterohepatically recycled

Half-life: 10-17 hours (prolonged with reduced renal function)

Peak serum levels: Oral: Within 3-6 hours

Elimination: Excreted as unchanged drug (42% to 50%) in the urine

Usual Dosage Oral:

Children >8 years: 8-12 mg/kg/day divided every 6-12 hours

Adults: 150 mg 4 times/day or 300 mg twice daily

Uncomplicated gonorrhea: 600 mg stat, 300 mg every 12 hours for 4 days (3 g total)

SIADH: 900-1200 mg/day or 13-15 mg/kg/day divided every 6-8 hours initially, then decrease to 600-900 mg/day

Monitoring Parameters CBC, renal and hepatic function tests

Test Interactions May interfere with tests for urinary glucose (false-negative urine glucose using Clinistix®, Tes-Tape®)

Patient Information Avoid prolonged exposure to sunlight or sunlamps; avoid taking antacids before tetracyclines

Nursing Implications Administer 1 hour before or 2 hours after food or milk; give with plenty of fluids

Dosage Forms

Capsule: 150 mg

Tablet: 150 mg, 300 mg

(Continued)

Demeclocycline Hydrochloride *(Continued)*

References

Abdi EA and Bishop S, "The Syndrome of Inappropriate Antidiuretic Hormone Secretion With Carcinoma of the Tongue," *Med Pediatr Oncol*, 1988, 16(3):210-5.

Troyer AD, "Demeclocycline, Treatment for Syndrome of Inappropriate Antidiuretic Hormone Secretion," *JAMA*, 1977, 237(25):2723-6.

Demerol® *see* Meperidine Hydrochloride *on page 362*

4-Demethoxydaunorubicin *see* Idarubicin Hydrochloride *on page 301*

Demethylchlortetracycline *see* Demeclocycline Hydrochloride *on previous page*

Denorex® [OTC] *see* Coal Tar *on page 147*

Depakene® *see* Valproic Acid and Derivatives *on page 592*

Depakote® *see* Valproic Acid and Derivatives *on page 592*

Depen® *see* Penicillamine *on page 437*

depGynogen® *see* Estradiol *on page 231*

depMedalone® *see* Methylprednisolone *on page 379*

Depo®-Estradiol *see* Estradiol *on page 231*

Depogen® *see* Estradiol *on page 231*

Depoject® *see* Methylprednisolone *on page 379*

Depo-Medrol® *see* Methylprednisolone *on page 379*

Deponit® *see* Nitroglycerin *on page 415*

Depopred® *see* Methylprednisolone *on page 379*

Depo-Provera® *see* Medroxyprogesterone Acetate *on page 359*

Depotest® *see* Testosterone *on page 550*

Depo®-Testosterone *see* Testosterone *on page 550*

Derma-Smoothe/FS® *see* Fluocinolone Acetonide *on page 254*

Dermolate® [OTC] *see* Hydrocortisone *on page 293*

Dermoplast® [OTC] *see* Benzocaine *on page 77*

Desenex® [OTC] *see* Tolnaftate *on page 573*

Desferal® Mesylate *see* Deferoxamine Mesylate *on page 173*

Desipramine Hydrochloride (dess ip' ra meen)

Related Information

Overdose and Toxicology Information *on page 696-700*

Brand Names Norpramin®; Pertofrane®

Therapeutic Category Antidepressant, Tricyclic

Use Treatment of various forms of depression, often in conjunction with psychotherapy

Pregnancy Risk Factor C

Contraindications Hypersensitivity to desipramine (cross-sensitivity with other tricyclic antidepressants may occur); patients receiving MAO inhibitors within past 14 days; narrow-angle glaucoma

Warnings Some formulations contain tartrazine which may cause allergic reaction; do not discontinue abruptly in patients receiving long term high dose therapy

Precautions Use with caution in patients with cardiovascular disease, conduction disturbances, urinary retention; seizure disorders, hyperthyroidism or those receiving thyroid replacement

Adverse Reactions Less sedation and anticholinergic adverse effects than amitriptyline or imipramine

Cardiovascular: Arrhythmias, hypotension

Central nervous system: Sedation, confusion, dizziness

Dermatologic: Photosensitivity

Endocrine & metabolic: SIADH

Gastrointestinal: Constipation, nausea, vomiting, weight gain, dry mouth

Hematologic: Blood dyscrasias

Hepatic: Hepatitis
Ocular: Blurred vision, increases intraocular pressure
Otic: Tinnitus
Renal & genitourinary: Urinary retention
Miscellaneous: Hypersensitivity reactions

Drug Interactions May ↓ effects of guanethidine and clonidine; may ↑ effects of CNS depressants, adrenergic agents, anticholinergic agents; with MAO inhibitors hyperpyrexia, tachycardia, hypertension, seizures, and death may occur; interactions similar to other tricyclics may occur

Mechanism of Action Increases the synaptic concentration of serotonin and/or norepinephrine in the central nervous system by inhibition of their reuptake by the presynaptic neuronal membrane

Pharmacodynamics Maximum antidepressant effects: After more than 2 weeks

Pharmacokinetics

Absorption: Well absorbed from the GI tract
Protein binding: 90%
Metabolism: Metabolized in the liver
Half-life, adults: 12-57 hours
Elimination: 70% excreted in the urine

Usual Dosage Oral:

Children 6-12 years: 10-30 mg/day or 1-5 mg/kg/day in divided doses; do not exceed 5 mg/kg/day

Adolescents: Initial: 25-50 mg/day; gradually ↑ to 100 mg/day in single or divided doses; maximum: 150 mg/day

Adults: Initial: 75 mg/day in divided doses; ↑ gradually to 150-200 mg/day in divided or single dose; maximum: 300 mg/day

Monitoring Parameters Blood pressure, heart rate, mental status

Reference Range Therapeutic: 150-300 ng/mL (SI: 560-1125 nmol/L); possible toxicity: >300 ng/mL (SI: 1070 nmol/L); Toxic: >1000 ng/mL (SI: >3750 nmol/L)

Dosage Forms

Capsule: 25 mg, 50 mg
Tablet: 10 mg, 25 mg, 50 mg, 75 mg, 100 mg, 150 mg

Desmopressin Acetate (des moe press' in)

Brand Names Concentraid®; DDAVP®

Synonyms 1-Deamino-8-D-Arginine Vasopressin

Therapeutic Category Antihemophilic Agent; Hemostatic Agent; Vasopressin Analog, Synthetic; Vitamin, Fat Soluble

Use Treatment of diabetes insipidus and controlling bleeding in certain types of hemophilia

Pregnancy Risk Factor B

Contraindications Hypersensitivity to desmopressin or any component; avoid using in patients with type IIB or platelet-type von Willebrand's disease

Adverse Reactions

Cardiovascular: Facial flushing, increase in blood pressure, nasal congestion
Central nervous system: Headache
Gastrointestinal: Nausea, abdominal cramps
Local: Pain at the injection site
Renal & genitourinary: Water intoxication, hyponatremia, vulval pain

Drug Interactions Lithium, chlorpropamide, fludrocortisone, clofibrate

Stability Refrigerate

Mechanism of Action Enhances reabsorption of water in the kidneys by increasing cellular permeability of the collecting ducts; possibly causes smooth muscle constriction with resultant vasoconstriction; dose-dependent increase in plasma factor VIII and plasminogen activator

Pharmacodynamics

Intranasal administration:
Onset of ADH effects: Within 1 hour
Peak effect: Within 1-5 hours
Duration: 5-21 hours

(Continued)

Desmopressin Acetate *(Continued)*

I.V. infusion:
Onset of increased factor VIII activity: Within 15-30 minutes
Peak effect: 90 minutes to 3 hours

Pharmacokinetics
Absorption: 10% to 20% of a dose absorbed following nasal administration
Metabolism: Unknown
Half-life:
Mean initial: 7.8 minutes
Terminal: 75.5 minutes (range: 0.4-4 hours)

Usual Dosage
Children:
Diabetes insipidus: 3 months to 12 years: Intranasal: Initial: 5 μg/day divided 1-2 times/day; range: 5-30 μg/day divided 1-2 times/day
Hemophilia: >3 months: I.V.: 0.3 μg/kg; may repeat dose if needed; begin 30 minutes before procedure
Nocturnal enuresis: ≥6 years: Intranasal: Initial: 20 μg at bedtime; range: 10-40 μg
Children >12 years and Adults:
Diabetes insipidus: I.V., S.C.: 2-4 μg/day in 2 divided doses or $\frac{1}{10}$ of the maintenance intranasal dose; intranasal: 5-40 μg/day 1-3 times/day
Hemophilia: I.V.: 0.3 μg/kg by slow infusion, begin 30 minutes before procedure

Administration Dilute to a maximum concentration of 0.5 μg/mL in normal saline and infuse over 15-30 minutes

Monitoring Parameters Blood pressure and pulse should be monitored during I.V. infusion
Diabetes insipidus: Fluid intake, urine volume, specific gravity, plasma and urine osmolality, serum electrolytes
Hemophilia: Factor VIII antigen levels, APTT

Patient Information Avoid overhydration

Additional Information If desmopressin I.V. is given preoperatively, administer 30 minutes prior to surgery; avoid spray use in children due to difficulty in titrating dosage

Dosage Forms
Injection: 4 μg/mL (1 mL)
Solution, nasal: 100 μg/mL (2.5 mL, 5 mL)

Desquam-X® *see* Benzoyl Peroxide *on page 78*

Desyrel® *see* Trazodone *on page 577*

Dexacidin® *see* Dexamethasone, Neomycin and Polymyxin B *on page 180*

Dexamethasone (dex a meth' a sone)

Related Information
Systemic Corticosteroids Comparison Chart *on page 727*

Brand Names Aeroseb-Dex®; AK-Dex®; Baldex®; Dalalone L.A.®; Decadron®; Decadron®-LA; Decadron® Turbinaire®; Decaject-L.A.®; Decaspray®; Dexasone- L.A.®; Dexone®; Dexone L.A.®; Hexadrol®; I-Methasone®; Maxidex®; Solurex L.A.®

Therapeutic Category Antiemetic; Anti-inflammatory Agent; Corticosteroid, Inhalant; Corticosteroid, Ophthalmic; Corticosteroid, Systemic; Corticosteroid, Topical; Glucocorticoid

Use Used systemically and locally for chronic inflammation, allergic, hematologic, neoplastic, and autoimmune diseases; may be used in management of cerebral edema, septic shock, and as a diagnostic agent

Pregnancy Risk Factor C

Contraindications Active untreated infections; viral, fungal, or tuberculous diseases of the eye

Warnings Fatalities have occurred due to adrenal insufficiency in asthmatic patients during and after transfer from systemic corticosteroids to aerosol steroids; during this period, aerosol steroids do **not** provide the systemic steroid needed to treat patients having trauma, surgery or infections; may retard bone growth

Precautions Use with caution in patients with hypothyroidism, cirrhosis, hypertension, congestive heart failure, ulcerative colitis, thromboembolic disorders

Adverse Reactions

Cardiovascular: Edema, hypertension

Central nervous system: Headache, vertigo, seizures, psychosis, pseudotumor cerebri

Dermatologic: Acne, skin atrophy

Endocrine & metabolic: Pituitary-adrenal axis suppression, growth suppression, glucose intolerance, hypokalemia, alkalosis

Gastrointestinal: Peptic ulcer, nausea, vomiting

Musculoskeletal: Muscle weakness, osteoporosis, fractures, Cushing's syndrome

Ocular: Cataracts, glaucoma

Drug Interactions Barbiturates, phenytoin, rifampin, salicylates, vaccines, toxoids

Mechanism of Action Decreases inflammation by suppression of migration of polymorphonuclear leukocytes and reversal of increased capillary permeability; suppresses normal immune response

Pharmacodynamics Duration: Metabolic effects can last for 72 hours

Pharmacokinetics

Metabolism: Metabolized in the liver

Peak serum levels:

Oral: Within 1-2 hours

I.M.: Within 8 hours

Elimination: Excreted in the urine and bile

Usual Dosage

Children:

Airway edema or extubation: Oral, I.M., I.V.: 0.5-2 mg/kg/day in divided doses every 6 hours; begin 24 hours prior to extubation and continue for 4-6 doses after extubation

Antiemetic (chemotherapy induced): I.V.: Initial: 10 mg/m^2/dose (maximum: 20 mg) then 5 mg/m^2/dose every 6 hours

Anti-inflammatory: Oral, I.M., I.V.: 0.08-0.3 mg/kg/day or 2.5-10 mg/m^2/day in divided doses every 6-12 hours

Bacterial meningitis: Infants and children >2 months: I.V.: 0.6 mg/kg/day divided every 6 hours for the first 4 days of antibiotic treatment; start dexamethasone at the time of the first dose of antibiotic

Cerebral edema: Oral, I.M., I.V.: Loading dose: 1-2 mg/kg/dose as a single dose; maintenance: 1-1.5 mg/kg/day (maximum: 16 mg/day) in divided doses every 4-6 hours

Ophthalmic: Instill 3-4 times/day

Physiologic replacement: Oral, I.M., I.V.: 0.03-0.15 mg/kg/day or 0.6-0.75 mg/m^2/day in divided doses every 6-12 hours

Adults:

ANLL protocol: I.V.: 2 mg/m^2/dose every 8 hours for 12 doses

Anti-inflammatory: Oral, I.M., I.V.: 0.75-9 mg/day in divided doses every 6-12 hours

Cerebral edema: I.V.: Initial: 10 mg then 4 mg I.M./I.V. every 6 hours

Diagnosis for Cushing's syndrome: Oral: 1 mg at 11 PM, draw blood at 8 AM

Administration Administer undiluted solution IVP over 1-4 minutes if dose is <10 mg; high dose therapy must be administered by I.V. intermittent infusion over 15-30 minutes

Monitoring Parameters Hemoglobin, occult blood loss, serum potassium and glucose

Reference Range Dexamethasone suppression test, overnight: 8 AM cortisol less than 6 μg/100 mL (dexamethasone 1 mg)

Nursing Implications Give after meals or with food or milk

Additional Information Due to long duration of effect, not suitable for every other day dosing

Dosage Forms

Aerosol:

Nasal, as sodium phosphate: 0.1 mg/spray (12.6 g)

Oral: Each actuation delivers 84 μg (12.6 g)

Topical: 0.01% (58 g); 0.04% (25 g)

Cream, as sodium phosphate: 0.1% (15 g, 30 g)

Elixir: 0.5 mg/5 mL (100 mL, 273 mL)

Gel, topical: 0.01% (30 g)

(Continued)

Dexamethasone *(Continued)*

Injection, as acetate: 8 mg/mL (1 mL, 5 mL); 16 mg/mL (1 mL, 5 mL)
Injection, as sodium phosphate: 4 mg/mL (1 mL, 5 mL, 10 mL, 25 mL, 30 mL); 10 mg/mL (1 mL, 10 mL); 20 mg/mL (5 mL)
Ointment, ophthalmic, as sodium phosphate: 0.05% (3.5 g)
Solution:
Concentrate: 0.5 mg/0.5 mL (30 mL)
Oral: 0.5 mg/5 mL (5 mL, 20 mL, 500 mL)
Suspension, ophthalmic, as sodium phosphate: 0.1% with methylcellulose 0.5% (15 mL)
Tablet: 0.25 mg, 0.5 mg, 0.75 mg, 1 mg, 1.5 mg, 2 mg, 4 mg, 6 mg

References

American Academy of Pediatrics Committee on Infectious Diseases, "Dexamethasone Therapy for Bacterial Meningitis in Infants and Children," *Pediatrics*, 1990, 86(1):130-3.
Bahal N and Nahata MC, "The Role of Corticosteroids in Infants and Children With Bacterial Meningitis," *DICP*, 1991, 25(5):542-5.

Dexamethasone, Neomycin and Polymyxin B

Brand Names AK-Trol®; Dexacidin®; Dexasporin®; Infectrol®; Maxitrol®; Ocu-Trol®
Therapeutic Category Antibiotic, Ophthalmic; Corticosteroid, Ophthalmic
Use For steroid-responsive inflammatory ocular conditions in which a corticosteroid is indicated and where bacterial infection or a risk of bacterial infection exists
Pregnancy Risk Factor C
Contraindications Hypersensitivity to dexamethasone, polymyxin, neomycin or any component; viral diseases of the cornea and conjunctiva; mycobacterial infection of the eye; fungal disease of ocular structures; dendritic keratitis; use after uncomplicated removal of a corneal foreign body
Warnings Prolonged use may result in glaucoma, defects in visual acuity, posterior subcapsular cataract formation, and secondary ocular infections
Adverse Reactions
Dermatologic: Contact dermatitis, cutaneous sensitization (sensitivity to topical neomycin has been reported to occur in 5% to 15% of patients)
Local: Pain, stinging
Ocular: Development of glaucoma, cataract, increased intraocular pressure, optic nerve damage, visual defects, blurred vision
Miscellaneous: Delayed wound healing, secondary infections
Usual Dosage Children and Adults: Ophthalmic:
Solution: 1-2 drops into affected eye(s) every 4-6 hours; in severe disease drops may be used hourly and tapered to discontinuation
Ointment: Instill a small amount (~½") in the affected eye 3-4 times/day or apply at bedtime as an adjunct with drops
Monitoring Parameters Intraocular pressure with use >10 days
Patient Information May cause temporary blurring of vision or stinging following administration
Nursing Implications Shake well before using
Dosage Forms
Ointment, ophthalmic: Dexamethasone 0.1%, neomycin sulfate 3.5 mg, and polymyxin B sulfate 10,000 units per g (3.5 g)
Suspension, ophthalmic: Dexamethasone 0.1%, neomycin sulfate 3.5 mg, and polymyxin B sulfate 10,000 units per mL (5 mL)

Dexasone- L.A.® *see* Dexamethasone *on page 178*

Dexasporin® *see* Dexamethasone, Neomycin and Polymyxin B *on this page*

Dexedrine® *see* Dextroamphetamine Sulfate *on this page*

Dexone® *see* Dexamethasone *on page 178*

Dexone L.A.® *see* Dexamethasone *on page 178*

Dextroamphetamine Sulfate (dex troe am fet' a meen)

Brand Names Dexedrine®; Ferndex®
Therapeutic Category Amphetamine; Anorexiant; Central Nervous System Stimulant, Amphetamine

Use Attention deficit disorder with hyperactivity (ADDH); narcolepsy

Restrictions C-II

Pregnancy Risk Factor C

Contraindications Hypersensitivity to dextroamphetamine or any component; advanced arteriosclerosis, hypertension, hyperthyroidism, glaucoma, MAO inhibitors

Warnings Has high potential for abuse; use in weight reduction programs only when alternative therapy has been ineffective; prolonged administration may lead to drug dependence

Precautions Use with caution in patients with psychopathic personalities

Adverse Reactions

- Cardiovascular: Hypertension, tachycardia, palpitations, cardiac arrhythmias
- Central nervous system: Insomnia, headache, nervousness, dizziness, irritability, tremor, depression
- Endocrine & metabolic: Growth suppression
- Gastrointestinal: Anorexia, nausea, vomiting, diarrhea, abdominal cramps, metallic taste, dry mouth
- Musculoskeletal: Movement disorders

Drug Interactions May ↓ effect of methyldopa; may ↑ serum concentration of tricyclic antidepressants; may precipitate hypertensive crisis in patients receiving MAO inhibitors and arrhythmias in patients receiving general anesthetics

Mechanism of Action Blocks reuptake of dopamine and norepinephrine from the synapse, thus increases the amounts of circulating dopamine and norepinephrine in cerebral cortex to reticular activating system; inhibits the action of monoamine oxidase and causes catecholamines to be released

Pharmacodynamics Onset of action: Oral: 60-90 minutes

Pharmacokinetics

- Metabolism: Metabolized in the liver
- Half-life, adults: 34 hours (pH dependent)
- Peak serum levels: Oral: Within 3 hours
- Elimination: Excreted in the urine as unchanged drug and inactive metabolites

Usual Dosage Oral:

- Narcolepsy:
  - Children 6-12 years: Initial: 5 mg/day, may increase at 5 mg increments in weekly intervals until side effects appear; maximum dose: 60 mg/day
  - Children >12 and Adults: Initial: 10 mg/day, may increase at 10 mg increments in weekly intervals until side effects appear; maximum: 60 mg/day
- Attention deficit disorder:
  - Children:
    - 3-5 years: Initial: 2.5 mg/day given every morning; increase by 2.5 mg/day in weekly intervals until optimal response is obtained, usual range is 0.1-0.5 mg/kg/dose every morning with maximum of 40 mg/day
    - ≥6 years: 5 mg once or twice daily; increase in increments of 5 mg/day at weekly intervals until optimal response is reached, usual range is 0.1-0.5 mg/kg/dose every morning (5-20 mg/day) with maximum of 40 mg/day
- Exogenous obesity: Children >12 years and Adults: 5-30 mg/day in divided doses of 5-10 mg given 30-60 minutes before meals

Nursing Implications Daily dose may be given in 1-3 divided doses/day; sustained release preparations should be used for once daily dosing; last daily dose should be given 6 hours before retiring; do not crush or allow patient to chew sustained release preparations

Additional Information 5 mg tablets and 5 mg, 10 mg, and 15 mg Dexedrine® Spansule® capsules contain tartrazine; treatment for ADDH should include "drug holiday" or periodic discontinuation in order to assess the patient's requirements and to decrease tolerance and limit suppression of linear growth and weight

Dosage Forms

- Capsule, sustained release: 5 mg, 10 mg, 15 mg
- Elixir (orange flavor): 5 mg/mL (480 mL)
- Tablet: 5 mg, 10 mg

Dextromethorphan and Guaifenesin *see* Guaifenesin and Dextromethorphan *on page 279*

Dey-Dose® Isoproterenol *see* Isoproterenol *on page 324*

Dey-Dose® Metaproterenol *see* Metaproterenol Sulfate *on page 367*

Dey-Lute® Isoetharine *see* Isoetharine *on page 321*

DHAD *see* Mitoxantrone Hydrochloride *on page 393*

DHPG Sodium *see* Ganciclovir *on page 267*

DHS® Tar [OTC] *see* Coal Tar *on page 147*

DHT™ *see* Dihydrotachysterol *on page 192*

Diaβeta® *see* Glyburide *on page 272*

Diabinese® *see* Chlorpropamide *on page 131*

Dialose® [OTC] *see* Docusate *on page 202*

Diamine T.D.® [OTC] *see* Brompheniramine Maleate *on page 88*

Diamox® *see* Acetazolamide *on page 18*

Diaqua® *see* Hydrochlorothiazide *on page 291*

Diazepam (dye az' e pam)

Related Information

Overdose and Toxicology Information *on page 696-700*

Preprocedure Sedatives in Children *on page 687-689*

Brand Names Valium®; Valrelease®; Zetran®

Therapeutic Category Antianxiety Agent; Anticonvulsant; Benzodiazepine; Sedative

Use Management of general anxiety disorders, panic disorders, and to provide preoperative sedation, light anesthesia, and amnesia; treatment of status epilepticus, alcohol withdrawal symptoms; used as a skeletal muscle relaxant

Restrictions C-IV

Pregnancy Risk Factor D

Contraindications Hypersensitivity to diazepam or any component; there may be a cross sensitivity with other benzodiazepines; do not use in a comatose patient, in those with pre-existing CNS depression, respiratory depression, narrow-angle glaucoma, or severe uncontrolled pain.

Warnings Rapid I.V. push may cause sudden respiratory depression, apnea, or hypotension

Precautions Use with caution in patients receiving other CNS depressants, patients with low albumin, hepatic dysfunction, and in the elderly and young infants; use with extreme caution in neonates; injection contains sodium benzoate and benzoic acid which may displace bilirubin from protein binding sites and at larger doses can cause the gasping syndrome; neonates have decreased metabolism of diazepam and desmethyldiazepam (active metabolite), both can accumulate with use and cause increased toxicity

Adverse Reactions

Cardiovascular: Cardiac arrest, hypotension, bradycardia, cardiovascular collapse

Central nervous system: Drowsiness, confusion, dizziness, ataxia, amnesia, slurred speech, impaired coordination, paradoxical excitement or rage (rare)

Local: Phlebitis, pain with injection

Ocular: Blurred vision, diplopia

Respiratory: Decrease in respiratory rate; apnea, laryngospasm

Miscellaneous: Physical and psychological dependence with prolonged use

Drug Interactions CNS depressants (alcohol, barbiturates, opioids) may enhance sedation and respiratory depression of diazepam; enzyme inducers may increase the hepatic metabolism of diazepam; cimetidine may decrease the metabolism of diazepam; valproic acid may displace diazepam from binding sites which may result an increase in sedative effects

Stability Do not mix I.V. product with other medications; protect I.V. product from light

Mechanism of Action Depresses all levels of the CNS, including the limbic and reticular formation, probably through the increased action of gamma-aminobutyric acid (GABA), which is a major inhibitory neurotransmitter in the brain

Pharmacodynamics Status epilepticus: I.V.:
- Onset of action: Almost immediate
- Duration: 20-30 minutes

Pharmacokinetics
- Absorption:
  - Oral: 85% to 100%
  - I.M.: Poorly absorbed
- Protein binding: 98%
- Metabolism: Metabolized in liver
- Half-life, adults: 20-50 hours, increased half-life in neonates, elderly, and those with severe hepatic disorders; active major metabolite is desmethyldiazepam which has a half-life of 50-100 hours and can be prolonged in neonates

Usual Dosage
- Children:
  - Conscious sedation for procedures: Oral: 0.2-0.3 mg/kg (maximum: 10 mg) 45-60 minutes prior to procedure
  - Sedation or muscle relaxation or anxiety:
    - Oral: 0.12-0.8 mg/kg/day in divided doses every 6-8 hours
    - I.M., I.V.: 0.04-0.3 mg/kg/dose every 2-4 hours to a maximum of 0.6 mg/kg within an 8-hour period if needed
  - Status epilepticus: I.V.:
    - Infants 30 days to 5 years: 0.05-0.3 mg/kg/dose given over 2-3 minutes, every 15-30 minutes to a maximum total dose of 5 mg; repeat in 2-4 hours as needed **or** 0.2-0.5 mg/dose every 2-5 minutes to a maximum total dose of 5 mg
    - >5 years: 0.05-0.3 mg/kg/dose given over 2-3 minutes, every 15-30 minutes to a maximum total dose of 10 mg; repeat in 2-4 hours as needed **or** 1 mg/dose every 2-5 minutes to a maximum of 10 mg;
  - Rectal: 0.5 mg/kg then 0.25 mg/kg in 10 minutes if needed
- Adolescents: Conscious sedation for procedures:
  - Oral: 10 mg
  - I.V.: 5 mg; may repeat with ½ dose if needed
- Adults:
  - Anxiety:
    - Oral: 2-10 mg 2-4 times/day
    - I.M., I.V.: 2-10 mg, may repeat in 3-4 hours if needed
  - Skeletal muscle relaxation:
    - Oral: 2-10 mg 2-4 times/day
    - I.M., I.V.: 5-10 mg, may repeat in 2-4 hours
  - Status epilepticus: I.V.: 5-10 mg every 10-20 minutes up to 30 mg in an 8-hour period; may repeat in 2-4 hours

Administration In infants and children, do not exceed 1-2 mg/minute IVP; adult maximum infusion rate: 5 mg/minute; rapid injection may cause respiratory depression or hypotension

Monitoring Parameters Heart rate, respiratory rate, blood pressure with I.V. use

Reference Range Effective therapeutic range not well established. Proposed therapeutic: Diazepam: 0.2-1.5 μg/mL (SI: 0.7-5.3 μmol/L); N-desmethyldiazepam (nordiazepam): 0.1-0.5 μg/mL (SI: 0.35-1.8 μmol/L)

Test Interactions False-negative urinary glucose determinations when using Clinistix® or Diastix®

Additional Information Diazepam does not have any analgesic effects

Dosage Forms
- Capsule, sustained release: 15 mg
- Injection: 5 mg/mL (1 mL, 2 mL, 5 mL, 10 mL)
- Solution, oral (wintergreen-spice flavor): 5 mg/5 mL (5 mL, 10 mL, 500 mL)
- Solution, oral concentrate: 5 mg/mL (30 mL)
- Tablet: 2 mg, 5 mg, 10 mg

References

Zeltzer LK, Altman A, Cohen D, et al, "Report of the Subcommittee on the Management of Pain Associated With Procedures in Children With Cancer," *Pediatrics*, 1990, 86(5 Pt 2):826-31.

Diazoxide (dye az ox' ide)

Brand Names Hyperstat® I.V.; Proglycem®

Therapeutic Category Antihypertensive; Antihypoglycemic Agent

Use I.V.: Emergency lowering of blood pressure; Oral: Hypoglycemia related to islet cell adenoma, carcinoma, hyperplasia, or adenomatosis, nesidioblastosis, leucine sensitivity, or extrapancreatic malignancy

Pregnancy Risk Factor C

Contraindications Hypersensitivity to diazoxide, thiazides, or other sulfonamide derivatives; aortic coarctation, arteriovenous shunts, dissecting aortic aneurysm

Precautions Diabetes mellitus, renal or liver disease, coronary artery disease, or cerebral vascular insufficiency

Adverse Reactions

Cardiovascular: Hypotension, tachycardia, flushing

Central nervous system: Dizziness, weakness, seizure, headache

Dermatologic: Rash, hirsutism

Endocrine & metabolic: Hyperglycemia, ketoacidosis, inhibition of labor, sodium and water retention

Gastrointestinal: Nausea, vomiting, anorexia, constipation

Hematologic: Leukopenia, thrombocytopenia

Local: Pain, burning, cellulitis/phlebitis upon extravasation

Renal & genitourinary: Hyperuricemia

Miscellaneous: Extrapyramidal symptoms and development of abnormal facies with chronic oral use

Drug Interactions Diuretics and hypotensive agents may potentiate diazoxide adverse effects; diazoxide may ↑ phenytoin metabolism or free fraction; diazoxide may ↓ warfarin protein binding

Stability Protect from light, heat, and freezing; avoid using darkened solutions

Mechanism of Action Inhibits insulin release from the pancreas; produces direct smooth muscle relaxation of the peripheral arterioles which results in decrease in blood pressure and reflex increase in heart rate and cardiac output

Pharmacodynamics

Hyperglycemic effects (oral):

- Onset of action: Within 1 hour
- Duration (normal renal function): 8 hours

Hypotensive effects (I.V.):

- Peak: Within 5 minutes
- Duration: Usually 3-12 hours

Pharmacokinetics

Protein binding: 90%

Half-life:

- Children: 9-24 hours
- Adults: 20-36 hours

Elimination: 50% excreted unchanged in urine

Usual Dosage

Hyperinsulinemic hypoglycemia: Oral: (**Note**: Use lower dose listed as initial dose)

- Newborns and Infants: 8-15 mg/kg/day in divided doses every 8-12 hours
- Children and Adults: 3-8 mg/kg/day in divided doses every 8-12 hours

Hypertension: I.V.: Children and Adults: 1-3 mg/kg (maximum: 150 mg in a single injection); repeat dose in 5-15 minutes until blood pressure adequately reduced; repeat administration every 4-24 hours; monitor blood pressure closely

Administration Do not give I.M. or S.C.; give I.V. (undiluted) by rapid I.V. injection over a period of 30 seconds or less

Monitoring Parameters Blood pressure, blood glucose

Nursing Implications Shake suspension well before using

Additional Information Patients may require a diuretic with repeated I.V. doses.

Dosage Forms

Capsule: 50 mg

Injection: 15 mg/mL (1 mL, 20 mL)

Suspension, oral (chocolate-mint flavor): 50 mg/mL (30 mL)

Dibent® *see* Dicyclomine Hydrochloride *on page 187*

Dibenzyline® *see* Phenoxybenzamine Hydrochloride *on page 451*

Dibucaine (dye' byoo kane)

Brand Names Nupercainal® [OTC]

Therapeutic Category Local Anesthetic, Topical

Use Fast, temporary relief of pain and itching due to hemorrhoids, minor burns, other minor skin conditions

Pregnancy Risk Factor C

Contraindications Known hypersensitivity to amide-type anesthetics

Warnings Products may contain sulfites; avoid use in sensitive individuals

Adverse Reactions

Cardiovascular: Edema

Dermatologic: Urticaria, cutaneous lesions, burning, tenderness, irritation, inflammation, contact dermatitis

Mechanism of Action Blocks both the initiation and conduction of nerve impulses by decreasing the neuronal membrane's permeability to sodium ions, which results in inhibition of depolarization with resultant blockade of conduction

Pharmacodynamics

Onset of action: Within 15 minutes

Duration: 2-4 hours

Pharmacokinetics Absorption: Poorly absorbed through intact skin, but well absorbed through mucous membranes and excoriated skin

Usual Dosage Children and Adults:

Topical: Apply gently to the affected areas; no more than 30 g for adults or 7.5 g for children should be used in any 24-hour period

Rectal: Hemorrhoids: Insert ointment into rectum using a rectal applicator; administer each morning, evening, and after each bowel movement

Nursing Implications Do not use near the eyes or over denuded surfaces or blistered areas

Dosage Forms

Cream: 0.5% (45 g)

Ointment, topical: 1% (30 g, 60 g)

DIC *see* Dacarbazine *on page 168*

Dicarbosil® [OTC] *see* Calcium Carbonate *on page 94*

Dichysterol *see* Dihydrotachysterol *on page 192*

Diclofenac Sodium (dye kloe' fen ak)

Brand Names Voltaren®

Therapeutic Category Analgesic, Non-Narcotic; Anti-inflammatory Agent; Nonsteroidal Anti-Inflammatory Agent (NSAID), Ophthalmic; Nonsteroidal Anti-Inflammatory Agent (NSAID), Oral

Use Acute and chronic treatment of rheumatoid arthritis, ankylosing spondylitis, and osteoarthritis; also used for juvenile rheumatoid arthritis, gout, dysmenorrhea and pain relief

Pregnancy Risk Factor B

Contraindications Known hypersensitivity to diclofenac, any component, aspirin or other nonsteroidal anti-inflammatory drugs (NSAIDs); porphyria

Precautions Use with caution in patients with congestive heart failure, hypertension, ↓ renal or hepatic function, history of GI disease, or those receiving anticoagulants

Adverse Reactions

Cardiovascular: Fluid retention

Central nervous system: Dizziness, headache

Dermatologic: Rash, pruritus

Gastrointestinal: Abdominal pain, indigestion, peptic ulcer, GI bleeding, GI perforation, constipation, diarrhea

Hematologic: Agranulocytosis, aplastic anemia (rare), inhibition of platelet aggregation

Hepatic: Elevation of ALT or AST, possible hepatitis

Otic: Tinnitus

Renal & genitourinary: Renal impairment, nephrotic-like syndrome

Drug Interactions Diclofenac may ↑ serum concentrations of digoxin, me-

(Continued)

Diclofenac Sodium *(Continued)*

thotrexate and lithium; may increase nephrotoxicity of cyclosporin; may decrease diuretic and antihypertensive effects of thiazides and furosemides; diclofenac + potassium-sparing diuretics → ↑ serum potassium; concomitant insulin or oral hypoglycemic agents → ↑ or ↓ serum glucose; aspirin may ↓ serum concentration of diclofenac (combination not recommended)

Mechanism of Action Inhibits prostaglandin synthesis by decreasing the activity of the enzyme, cyclo-oxygenase, which results in decreased formation of prostaglandin precursors

Usual Dosage Oral:

Children: 2-3 mg/kg/day divided 2-4 times/day

Adults:

Rheumatoid arthritis: 150-200 mg/day in 2-4 divided doses
Osteoarthritis: 100-150 mg/day in 2-3 divided doses
Ankylosing spondylitis: 100-125 mg/day in 4-5 divided doses

Monitoring Parameters CBC, liver enzymes; monitor urine output and BUN/serum creatinine in patients receiving diuretics

Nursing Implications Do not crush tablets

Additional Information Vomiting, drowsiness, and acute renal failure have been reported with overdoses

Dosage Forms Tablet, enteric coated: 25 mg, 50 mg, 75 mg

References

Brogden RN, Heel RC, Pakes GE, et al, "Diclofenac Sodium: A Review of Its Pharmacological Properties and Therapeutic Use in Rheumatic Diseases and Pain of Varying Origin," *Drugs*, 1980, 20(1):24-48.

Haapasaari J, Wuolijoki E, and Ylijoki H, "Treatment of Juvenile Rheumatoid Arthritis With Diclofenac Sodium" *Scand J Rheumatol*, 1983, 12(4):325-30.

Dicloxacillin Sodium (dye klox a sill' in)

Brand Names Dycill®; Dynapen®; Pathocil®

Therapeutic Category Antibiotic, Penicillin

Use Treatment of skin and soft tissue infections, pneumonia and follow-up therapy of osteomyelitis caused by susceptible penicillinase-producing staphylococci

Pregnancy Risk Factor B

Contraindications Known hypersensitivity to dicloxacillin, penicillin, or any components

Warnings Elimination is prolonged in neonates

Adverse Reactions

Central nervous system: Fever
Dermatologic: Rash
Gastrointestinal: Nausea, vomiting, diarrhea, *C. difficile* colitis
Hematologic: Eosinophilia, neutropenia, leukopenia, thrombocytopenia
Hepatic: Elevation in liver enzymes
Miscellaneous: Serum sickness-like reaction

Stability Reconstituted dicloxacillin suspension is stable for 7 days at room temperature or 14 days if refrigerated

Mechanism of Action Interferes with bacterial cell wall synthesis during active multiplication, causing cell wall death and resultant bactericidal activity against susceptible bacteria

Pharmacokinetics

Absorption: 35% to 76% of a dose is absorbed from the GI tract; food decreases the rate and extent of absorption

Distribution: Crosses the placenta; distributes into breast milk

Protein binding: 96%

Half-life: 0.6-0.8 hours, half-life is slightly prolonged in patients with renal impairment

Peak serum levels: Within 0.5-2 hours

Elimination: Prolonged in neonates; partially eliminated by the liver and excreted in the bile; 56% to 70% is eliminated in the urine as unchanged drug

Not dialyzable (0% to 5%)

Usual Dosage Oral:

Children <40 kg: 12.5-50 mg/kg/day divided every 6 hours; doses of 50-100 mg/kg/day in divided doses every 6 hours have been used for follow-up therapy of osteomyelitis

Children >40 kg and Adults: 125-500 mg every 6 hours

Monitoring Parameters Periodic monitoring of CBC, BUN, serum creatinine, urinalysis, and liver enzymes during prolonged therapy

Nursing Implications Administer 1 hour before or 2 hours after meals

Additional Information

Sodium content of 250 mg capsule: 0.6 mEq

Sodium content of 5 mL suspension: 2.9 mEq

Dosage Forms

Capsule: 125 mg, 250 mg, 500 mg

Powder for oral suspension: 62.5 mg/5 mL (80 mL, 100 mL, 200 mL)

Dicyclomine Hydrochloride (dye sye' kloe meen)

Related Information

Overdose and Toxicology Information *on page 696-700*

Brand Names Antispas®; Bemote®; Bentyl® Hydrochloride; Byclomine®; Dibent®; Di-Spaz®; Neoquess®

Synonyms Dicycloverine Hydrochloride

Therapeutic Category Anticholinergic Agent; Antispasmodic Agent, Gastrointestinal

Use Treatment of functional disturbances of GI motility such as irritable bowel syndrome

Pregnancy Risk Factor B

Contraindications Hypersensitivity to any anticholinergic drug; narrow-angle glaucoma, tachycardia, GI obstruction, obstruction of the urinary tract, myasthenia gravis; should not be used in infants <6 months of age

Precautions Use with caution in patients with hepatic or renal disease, ulcerative colitis, hyperthyroidism, cardiovascular disease, hypertension

Adverse Reactions

Cardiovascular: Tachycardia, palpitations

Central nervous system: Seizures, coma, nervousness, excitement, confusion, insomnia, headache

Gastrointestinal: Nausea, vomiting, constipation, dry mouth

Musculoskeletal: Muscular hypotonia

Ocular: Blurred vision

Renal & genitourinary: Urinary retention

Respiratory: Respiratory distress, asphyxia

Drug Interactions Additive adverse effects when given with medications with anticholinergic effects; may alter GI absorption of various drugs due to prolonged GI transit time; antacids

Stability Protect from light

Mechanism of Action Blocks the action of acetylcholine at parasympathetic sites in smooth muscle, secretory glands and the CNS

Pharmacodynamics

Onset of effects: 1-2 hours

Duration: Up to 4 hours

Pharmacokinetics

Absorption: Oral: Well absorbed

Half-life:

- Initial phase: 1.8 hours
- Terminal phase: 9-10 hours

Elimination: 80% eliminated in urine

Usual Dosage

Infants >6 months: Oral: 5 mg/dose 3-4 times/day

Children: Oral: 10 mg/dose 3-4 times/day

Adults:

- Oral: 160 mg/day in 4 equally divided doses; however, because of its side effects begin with 80 mg/day in 4 equally divided doses, then increase up to 160 mg/day
- I.M.: 20 mg/dose 4 times/day; oral therapy should replace I.M. therapy as soon as possible

Dosage Forms

Capsule: 10 mg, 20 mg

Injection: 10 mg/mL (2 mL, 10 mL)

Syrup: 10 mg/5 mL (118 mL, 473 mL, 946 mL)

Tablet: 20 mg

Dicycloverine Hydrochloride *see* Dicyclomine Hydrochloride *on previous page*

Didanosine (dye dan' oh seen)

Brand Names Videx®

Synonyms DDI; Dideoxyinosine

Therapeutic Category Antiviral Agent, Oral

Use Treatment of patients with advanced HIV infection who are resistant to zidovudine therapy or in those patients with zidovudine intolerance

Pregnancy Risk Factor B

Contraindications Hypersensitivity to didanosine or any component

Warnings Major clinical toxicities of didanosine include pancreatitis and peripheral neuropathy; risk factors for developing pancreatitis include a previous history of the condition, concurrent cytomegalovirus or *Mycobacterium avium* intracellulare infection, and concomitant use of pentamidine or co-trimoxazole. May cause retinal depigmentation in children receiving doses >300 mg/m²/day

Precautions Use with caution in patients with phenylketonuria, patients on sodium-restricted diets, and patients with renal or hepatic impairment; adjust dosage in patients with renal impairment or peripheral neuropathy; discontinue didanosine if clinical signs of pancreatitis occur; only after pancreatitis has been ruled out should dosing be resumed

Adverse Reactions

- Central nervous system: Headache (32% to 36%), peripheral neuropathy (34%), asthenia, insomnia, malaise, CNS depression, fever
- Dermatologic: Rash, pruritus, alopecia
- Endocrine & metabolic: Hypokalemia, hyperuricemia
- Gastrointestinal: Diarrhea (18%), nausea, vomiting, anorexia, stomatitis, pancreatitis (9%), abdominal pain
- Hepatic: Elevated liver enzymes, hepatic failure
- Ocular: Retinal depigmentation
- Respiratory: Cough, dyspnea

Drug Interactions Decreases absorption of ketoconazole, ciprofloxacin, tetracyclines

Stability Undergoes rapid degradation when exposed to an acidic environment; tablets dispersed in water are stable for 1 hour at room temperature; reconstituted buffered solution is stable for 4 hours at room temperature; reconstituted unbuffered solution is stable for 30 days if refrigerated; unbuffered powder for oral solution must be reconstituted and mixed with an equal volume of antacid at time of preparation

Mechanism of Action Converted within the cell to an active metabolite, dideoxyadenosine triphosphate which serves as a substrate and inhibitor of viral RNA-directed DNA polymerase resulting in suppression of retrovirus replication

Pharmacokinetics

- Distribution: Distributes into CSF
  - V_d:
    - Children: 35.6 L/m²
    - Adults: 18.4-60.7 L/m²
- Protein binding: <5%
- Bioavailability: Children and Adolescents: 21% (ranges from 2% to 89%); variable and affected by the presence of food in the GI tract, gastric pH, and the dosage form administered
- Half-life:
  - Children and Adolescents: 0.8 hours
  - Adults: 1.3-1.6 hours
- Elimination: 50% of dose is eliminated renally

Usual Dosage Oral:

- Children: Dosing is based on body surface area (m²):
  - <1 year or ≤0.4 m²: 100-300 mg/m²/day divided every 12 hours (single tablet/dose twice daily)
  - ≥1 year: 100-300 mg/m²/day divided every 12 hours using 2 tablets/dose
- Children ≥35 kg and Adults: Dosing is based on patient weight with an initial recommended dose of 5-10 mg/kg/day divided every 12 hours:
  - 35-49 kg: 125 mg every 12 hours using 2 tablets/dose
    - Buffered oral solution: 167 mg every 12 hours

50-74 kg: 200 mg every 12 hours using 2 tablets/dose
Buffered oral solution: 250 mg every 12 hours
≥75 kg: 300 mg every 12 hours using 2 tablets/dose
Buffered oral solution: 375 mg every 12 hours

Monitoring Parameters Serum potassium, uric acid, creatinine; hemoglobin, CBC with neutrophil, and platelet count, CD_4 cells; liver function tests, amylase; weight gain; perform dilated retinal exam every 6 months

Patient Information Tablets should be chewed, crushed, or dispersed in water for oral administration; do not mix with fruit juice or other acid-containing liquid; take on an empty stomach at least 1 hour before or 2 hours after meals; the buffered powder vehicle may contribute to the development of diarrhea

Additional Information

Contents of each tablet: 11.5 mEq of sodium, 15.7 mEq of magnesium, along with phenylalanine; tablets are buffered with dihydroxyaluminum sodium carbonate, magnesium hydroxide, and sodium citrate

Sodium content of each packet of buffered powder for oral solution: 60 mEq

Dosage Forms

Powder for oral solution:
Buffered (single dose packet): 100 mg, 167 mg, 250 mg, 375 mg
Pediatric: 2 g, 4 g

Tablet, buffered, chewable (mint flavor): 25 mg, 50 mg, 100 mg, 150 mg

References

Balis FM, Pizzo PA, Butler KM, et al, "Clinical Pharmacology of 2', 3'-Dideoxyinosine in Human Immunodeficiency Virus-Infected Children," *J Infect Dis*, 1992, 165(1):99-104.

Butler KM, Husson RN, Balis FM, et al, "Dideoxyinosine in Children With Symptomatic Human Immunodeficiency Virus Infection," *N Engl J Med*, 1991, 324(3):137-44.

Dideoxyinosine *see* Didanosine *on previous page*

Didronel® *see* Etidronate Disodium *on page 236*

Diflucan® *see* Fluconazole *on page 248*

Digibind® *see* Digoxin Immune Fab *on page 191*

Digoxin (di jox' in)

Related Information

Blood Level Sampling Time Guidelines *on page 694-695*
Medications Compatible With PN Solutions *on page 649-650*
Overdose and Toxicology Information *on page 696-700*

Brand Names Lanoxicaps®; Lanoxin®

Therapeutic Category Antiarrhythmic Agent, Miscellaneous; Cardiac Glycoside

Use Treatment of congestive heart failure; slows the ventricular rate in tachyarrhythmias such as atrial fibrillation, atrial flutter, supraventricular tachycardia

Pregnancy Risk Factor A

Contraindications Hypersensitivity to digoxin or any component; A-V block, idiopathic hypertrophic subaortic stenosis, or constrictive pericarditis

Warnings Use with caution in patients with hypoxia, hypothyroidism, acute myocarditis

Precautions Dosage reduction required in patients with renal impairment

Adverse Reactions

Cardiovascular: Sinus bradycardia, A-V block, S-A block, atrial or nodal ectopic beats, ventricular arrhythmias, bigeminy, trigeminy, atrial tachycardia with A-V block

Central nervous system: Drowsiness, fatigue, headache, lethargy, neuralgia, vertigo, disorientation

Endocrine & metabolic: Hyperkalemia with acute toxicity

Gastrointestinal: Vomiting, nausea, feeding intolerance, abdominal pain, diarrhea

Ocular: Blurred vision, halos, yellow or green vision, diplopia, photophobia, flashing lights

Drug Interactions Antacids, kaolin-pectin, cholestyramine, and metoclopramide may ↓ absorption of digoxin; quinidine, indomethacin, verapamil,

(Continued)

Digoxin *(Continued)*

amiodarone, erythromycin, propafenone, tetracycline, and spironolactone may ↑ digoxin serum concentration; penicillamine may ↓ digoxin's pharmacologic effects

Stability Solution compatibility: D_5W, $D_{10}W$, NS, sterile water for injection (when diluted 4-fold or greater); do not mix with other drugs

Mechanism of Action Increases the influx of calcium ions, from extracellular to intracellular cytoplasm by inhibition of sodium and potassium ion movement across the myocardial membranes; this increase in calcium ions results in a potentiation of the activity of the contractile heart muscle fibers and an increase in the force of myocardial contraction (positive inotropic effect); inhibits adenosine triphosphatase (ATPase); decreases conduction through the S-A and A-V nodes

Pharmacodynamics

Onset of effects:
- Oral: 1-2 hours
- I.V.: 5-30 minutes

Maximum effect:
- Oral: 2-8 hours
- I.V.: 1-4 hours

Duration (adults): 3-4 days

Pharmacokinetics

Distribution: V_d:
- Neonates, full term: 7.5-10 L/kg
- Children: 16 L/kg
- Adults: 7 L/kg; decreased V_d with renal disease

Bioavailability (dependent upon formulation):
- Elixir: 70% to 85%
- Tablets: 60% to 80%
- Capsules: 90% to 100%

Half-life (dependent upon age, renal and cardiac function)
- Elimination:
  - Premature: 61-170 hours
  - Neonates, full term: 35-45 hours
  - Infants: 18-25 hours
  - Children: 35 hours
  - Adults: 38-48 hours
  - Anephric adults: >4.5 days

Elimination: 50% to 70% excreted unchanged in urine

Usual Dosage See table.

Dosage Recommendations for Digoxin*

Age	Total Digitalizing Dose† (μg/kg)		Daily Maintenance Dose‡ (μg/kg)	
	P.O.	I.V. or I.M.	P.O.	I.V. or I.M.
Preterm infant	20–30	15–25	5–7.5	4–6
Full term infant	25–35	20–30	6–10	5–8
1 mo–2 y	35–60	30–50	10–15	7.5–12
2–5 y	30–40	25–35	7.5–10	6–9
5–10 y	20–35	15–30	5–10	4–8
>10 y	10–15	8–12	2.5–5	2–3
Adults	0.75–1.5 mg	0.5–1 mg	0.125–0.5 mg	0.1–0.4 mg

*Based on lean body weight and normal renal function for age. Decrease dose in patients with ↓ renal function.

†Give one-half of the total digitalizing dose (TDD) in the initial dose, then give one-quarter of the TDD in each of two subsequent doses at 8–12 hour intervals. Obtain EKG 6 hours after each dose to assess potential toxicity.

‡Divided every 12 hours in infants and children <10 years old. Given once daily to children >10 years and adults.

Administration Administer I.V. doses slowly over 5 minutes; I.M. route not usually recommended due to local irritation, pain, and tissue damage

Monitoring Parameters Heart rate and rhythm, periodic EKGs to assess both desired effects and signs of toxicity; follow closely (especially in patients receiving diuretics or amphotericin) for decreased serum potassium and magnesium, or increased calcium all of which predispose to digoxin toxicity; assess renal function; be aware of drug interactions; obtain serum drug concentrations at least 8-12 hours after a dose. (Preferably prior to next scheduled dose.)

Reference Range Therapeutic: 0.8-2 ng/mL (SI: 1.0-2.6 nmol/L); adults: <0.5 ng/mL (SI: 0.6 nmol/L) probably indicates underdigitalization unless there are special circumstances. Toxicity usually associated with levels >2 ng/mL (SI: >2.6 nmol/L). **Note**: Serum concentration must be used in conjunction with clinical symptoms and EKG, to confirm diagnosis of digoxin intoxication.

Additional Information Digoxin-like immunoreactive substance (DLIS) may cross react with digoxin immunoassay. DLIS has been found in patients with renal and liver disease, congestive heart failure, neonates, and pregnant women (third trimester)

Dosage Forms

Capsule: 50 μg, 100 μg, 200 μg
Elixir, pediatric: 50 μg/mL (60 mL)
Injection: 250 μg/mL (1 mL, 2 mL)
Injection, pediatric: 100 μg/mL (1 mL)
Tablet: 125 μg, 250 μg, 500 μg

References

Bendayan R and McKenzie MW, "Digoxin Pharmacokinetics and Dosage Requirements in Pediatric Patients," *Clin Pharm*, 1983, 2(3):224-35.

Park MK, "Use of Digoxin in Infants and Children With Specific Emphasis on Dosage," *J Pediatr*, 1986, 108(6):871-7.

Digoxin Immune Fab

Brand Names Digibind®

Synonyms Antidigoxin Fab Fragments

Therapeutic Category Antidote, Digoxin

Use Treatment of potentially life-threatening digoxin or digitoxin intoxication in carefully selected patients

Pregnancy Risk Factor C

Contraindications Hypersensitivity to ovine (sheep) proteins; renal or cardiac failure

Warnings Hypokalemia may develop rapidly once therapy is begun; monitor serum potassium levels closely

Adverse Reactions

Cardiovascular: Worsening of low cardiac output or congestive heart failure, rapid ventricular response in patients with atrial fibrillation as digoxin is withdrawn
Dermatologic: Urticarial rash
Endocrine & metabolic: Hypokalemia
Miscellaneous: Facial swelling and redness

Stability Reconstituted solutions are stable 4 hours at 2°C to 8°C

Mechanism of Action Binds with molecules of free (unbound) digoxin or digitoxin and then is removed from the body by renal excretion

Pharmacodynamics Onset of action: Improvement in signs and symptoms occurs within 2-30 minutes following I.V. infusion

Pharmacokinetics

Half-life: 15-20 hours, prolonged in patients with renal impairment
Elimination: Eliminated renally with levels declining to undetectable amounts within 5-7 days

Usual Dosage To determine the dose of digoxin immune Fab, first determine the total body load of digoxin (TBL) as follows (using either an approximation of the amount ingested or a postdistribution serum digoxin concentration (C)):

TBL of digoxin (in mg) = C (in ng/mL) x 5.6 x body weight (in kg)/1000
or
TBL = mg of digoxin ingested (as tablets or elixir) x 0.8

Dose of digoxin immune Fab (in mg) I.V. = TBL x 66.7
See tables on following page.

(Continued)

Digoxin Immune Fab *(Continued)*

Infants and Children Dose Estimates of Digibind® (in mg) From Serum Digoxin Concentration

Patient Weight (kg)	Serum Digoxin Concentration (ng/mL)						
	1	2	4	8	12	16	20
1	0.5 mg*	1 mg*	1.5 mg*	3 mg	5 mg	6 mg	8 mg
3	1 mg*	2 mg*	5 mg	9 mg	13 mg	18 mg	22 mg
5	2 mg*	4 mg	8 mg	15 mg	22 mg	30 mg	40 mg
10	4 mg	8 mg	15 mg	30 mg	40 mg	60 mg	80 mg
20	8 mg	15 mg	30 mg	60 mg	80 mg	120 mg	160 mg

*Dilution of reconstituted vial to 1 mg/mL may be desirable.

Adult Dose Estimate of Digibind® (in # of Vials) From Serum Digoxin Concentration

Patient Weight (kg)	Serum Digoxin Concentration (ng/mL)						
	1	2	4	8	12	16	20
40	0.5 v*	1 v	2 v	3 v	5 v	6 v	8 v
60	0.5 v	1 v	2 v	5 v	7 v	9 v	11 v
70	1 v	2 v	3 v	5 v	8 v	11 v	13 v
80	1 v	2 v	3 v	6 v	9 v	12 v	15 v
100	1 v	2 v	4 v	8 v	11 v	15 v	19 v

* v = vials.

Administration Digoxin immune fab is reconstituted by adding 4 mL sterile water, resulting in 10 mg/mL for I.V. infusion, the reconstituted solution may be further diluted with NS to a convenient volume (eg, 1 mg/mL); infuse over 15-30 minutes; to remove protein aggregates, 0.22 micron in-line filter is needed

Monitoring Parameters Serum potassium; serum digoxin level prior to therapy; continuous EKG monitoring

Additional Information Serum digoxin levels drawn prior to therapy may be difficult to evaluate if 6-8 hours have not elapsed after the last dose of digoxin (time to equilibration between serum and tissue); digoxin immune Fab fragments may interfere with digoxin measurements depending upon the assay used. For individuals at increased risk of sensitivity (see Contraindications) an intradermal or scratch technique skin test using a 1:100 dilution of reconstituted digoxin immune Fab diluted in normal saline has been used. Skin test volume is 0.1 mL of 1:100 dilution; evaluate after 20 minutes.

Dosage Forms Injection, lyophilized: 40 mg

References

Hickey AR, Wenger TL, Carpenter VP, et al, "Digoxin Immune Fab Therapy in the Management of Digitalis Intoxication: Safety and Efficacy Results of an Observational Surveillance Study," *J Am Coll Cardiol*, 1991, 17(3):590-8.

Dihydrotachysterol (dye hye droe tak iss' ter ole)

Brand Names DHT™; Hytakerol®

Synonyms Dichysterol

Therapeutic Category Vitamin, Fat Soluble

Use Treatment of hypocalcemia associated with hypoparathyroidism; prophylaxis of hypocalcemic tetany following thyroid surgery; suppress hyperparathyroidism and treat renal osteodystrophy in patients with chronic renal failure

Pregnancy Risk Factor A (D if used in doses above the recommended daily allowance)

Contraindications Hypercalcemia, known hypersensitivity to dihydrotachysterol

Warnings Use cautiously in patients with renal stones, renal failure, and heart disease

Adverse Reactions Related to accompanying hypercalcemia

Central nervous system: Convulsions
Endocrine & metabolic: Hypercalcemia
Gastrointestinal: Nausea, vomiting, anorexia, weight loss
Hematologic: Anemia
Musculoskeletal: Metastatic calcification, weakness
Renal & genitourinary: Renal damage, polyuria, polydipsia

Drug Interactions Cholestyramine, clofibrate, thiazides, phenobarbital, phenytoin, cardiac glycosides

Mechanism of Action Stimulates calcium and phosphate absorption from the small intestine, promotes secretion of calcium from bone to blood

Pharmacodynamics

Maximum hypercalcemic effects: Within 2 weeks
Duration: As long as 9 weeks

Pharmacokinetics Absorption: Well absorbed from the GI tract

Usual Dosage Oral:

Hypoparathyroidism:
- Neonates: 0.05-0.1 mg/day
- Infants and young Children: Initial: 1-5 mg/day for 4 days, then 0.5-1.5 mg/day
- Older Children and Adults: Initial: 0.75-2.5 mg/day for 4 days, then 0.2-1 mg/day; maximum: 1.5 mg/day

Nutritional rickets: 0.5 mg as a single dose or 13-50 μg/day until healing occurs

Renal osteodystrophy:
- Children and Adolescents: 0.1-0.5 mg/day
- Adults: 0.1-0.6 mg/day

Monitoring Parameters Serum calcium and phosphate

Dosage Forms

Capsule: 0.125 mg
Solution:
- Concentrate: 0.2 mg/mL (30 mL)
- Oral: 0.2 mg/5 mL (500 mL)
- Oral, in oil: 0.25 mg/mL (15 mL)

Tablet: 0.125 mg, 0.2 mg, 0.4 mg

1,25 dihydroxycholecalciferol *see* Calcitriol *on page 93*

Diiodohydroxyquin *see* Iodoquinol *on page 318*

Dilantin® *see* Phenytoin *on page 455*

Dilaudid® *see* Hydromorphone Hydrochloride *on page 295*

Dilaudid® Cough Syrup *see* Hydromorphone Hydrochloride *on page 295*

Dilocaine® *see* Lidocaine Hydrochloride *on page 342*

Dimenhydrinate (dye men hye' dri nate)

Related Information

Overdose and Toxicology Information *on page 696-700*

Brand Names Calm-X® [OTC]; Dimetabs®; Dinate®; Dramamine® [OTC]; Hydrate®; Marmine® [OTC]; Nico-Vert®; TripTone® Caplets® [OTC]; Vertab® [OTC]; Wehamine®

Therapeutic Category Antiemetic; Antihistamine

Use Treatment and prevention of nausea, vertigo, and vomiting associated with motion sickness

Pregnancy Risk Factor B

Contraindications Hypersensitivity to dimenhydrinate or any component

Precautions Sedation may impair ability to perform hazardous tasks requiring mental alertness; use with caution in patients with a history of seizure disorder; chewable tablets contain the dye tartrazine which may cause allergic reactions in sensitive individuals (particularly if sensitive to aspirin)

Adverse Reactions

Cardiovascular: Hypotension
Central nervous system: Drowsiness, headache, paradoxical CNS stimulation, dizziness

(Continued)

Dimenhydrinate *(Continued)*

Gastrointestinal: Anorexia, dry mouth and mucous membranes
Local: Pain at the injection site
Ocular: Blurred vision
Otic: Tinnitus
Renal & genitourinary: Urinary frequency

Drug Interactions Enhances sedative effects of other CNS depressants, may potentiate anticholinergic effects; may mask early signs and symptoms of ototoxicity in patients on aminoglycosides, Lasix®, etc

Mechanism of Action Competes with histamine for H_1-receptor sites on effector cells in the gastrointestinal tract, blood vessels, and respiratory tract; diminish vestibular stimulation and depress labyrinthine function function through its central anticholinergic activity

Pharmacodynamics
Onset of action:
Oral: Within 15-30 minutes
I.M.: 20-30 minutes
I.V.: Immediate
Duration: ~3-6 hours

Pharmacokinetics
Absorption: Well absorbed from the GI tract
Distribution: Small amounts appear in breast milk
Metabolism: Extensively metabolized in the liver

Usual Dosage Oral, I.M., I.V.:
Children:
2-5 years: 12.5-25 mg every 6-8 hours, maximum: 75 mg/day
6-12 years: 25-50 mg every 6-8 hours, maximum: 75 mg/day
or
Alternately: 5 mg/kg/day in 4 divided doses, not to exceed 300 mg/day

Adults: 50-100 mg every 4-6 hours, not to exceed 400 mg/day

Administration Dilute to a maximum concentration of 5 mg/mL in normal saline and infuse over 2 minutes

Dosage Forms
Capsule: 50 mg
Injection: 50 mg/mL (1 mL, 5 mL, 10 mL)
Liquid: 12.5 mg/4 mL
Tablet: 50 mg
Tablet, chewable: 50 mg

Dimercaprol (dye mer kap' role)

Brand Names BAL in Oil®

Therapeutic Category Antidote, Arsenic Toxicity; Antidote, Gold Toxicity; Antidote, Lead Toxicity; Antidote, Mercury Toxicity

Use Antidote to gold, arsenic, and mercury poisoning; adjunct to edetate calcium disodium in lead poisoning

Pregnancy Risk Factor C

Contraindications Hepatic insufficiency; do not use in iron, cadmium, or selenium poisoning

Precautions Use with caution in patients with renal impairment or hypertension; produces hemolysis in persons with G-6-PD deficiency

Adverse Reactions
Cardiovascular: Hypertension, tachycardia
Central nervous system: Nervousness, fever, headache
Gastrointestinal: Vomiting, nausea
Hematologic: Transient neutropenia
Local: Pain at the injection site
Ocular: Blepharospasm
Renal & genitourinary: Nephrotoxicity
Miscellaneous: Salivation, burning sensation of the lips, mouth, throat, eyes

Mechanism of Action Sulfhydryl group combines with ions of various heavy metals to form relatively stable, nontoxic, soluble chelates which are excreted in the urine

Pharmacokinetics
Distribution: Distributes to all tissues including the brain
Metabolism: Rapidly metabolized to inactive products
Peak levels: Obtained in 30-60 minutes
Elimination: Excreted in the urine and feces via bile

Usual Dosage Children and Adults: I.M.:

Mild arsenic and gold poisoning: 2.5 mg/kg/dose every 6 hours for two days, then every 12 hours on the third day, and once daily thereafter for 10 days

Severe arsenic and gold poisoning: 3 mg/kg/dose every 4 hours for two days then every 6 hours on the third day, then every 12 hours thereafter for 10 days

Mercury poisoning: 5 mg/kg initially followed by 2.5 mg/kg/dose 1-2 times/day for 10 days

Lead poisoning (use with edetate calcium disodium):
- Mild: 3 mg/kg/dose every 4 hours for 5-7 days
- Severe: 4 mg/kg/dose every 4 hours in combination with edetate calcium disodium

Monitoring Parameters Specific heavy metal levels, urine pH

Nursing Implications Urine should be kept alkaline; give undiluted, deep I.M.

Dosage Forms Injection: 100 mg/mL (3 mL)

Dimetabs® *see* Dimenhydrinate *on page 193*

Dimetane® [OTC] *see* Brompheniramine Maleate *on page 88*

Dimetapp® [OTC] *see* Brompheniramine and Phenylpropanolamine *on page 87*

Dimethoxyphenyl Penicillin Sodium *see* Methicillin Sodium *on page 370*

β,β-Dimethylcysteine *see* Penicillamine *on page 437*

Dinate® *see* Dimenhydrinate *on page 193*

Diocto® [OTC] *see* Docusate *on page 202*

Diocto-C® [OTC] *see* Docusate and Casanthranol *on page 203*

Dioctyl Calcium Sulfosuccinate *see* Docusate *on page 202*

Dioctyl Potassium Sulfosuccinate *see* Docusate *on page 202*

Dioctyl Sodium Sulfosuccinate *see* Docusate *on page 202*

Dioeze® [OTC] *see* Docusate *on page 202*

Dioval® *see* Estradiol *on page 231*

Dipalmitoylphosphatidylcholine *see* Colfosceril Palmitate *on page 151*

Diphen® Cough [OTC] *see* Diphenhydramine Hydrochloride *on this page*

Diphenhydramine Hydrochloride (dye fen hye' dra meen)

Related Information

Compatibility of Medications Mixed in a Syringe *on page 717*
OTC Cold Preparations, Pediatric *on page 723-726*
Overdose and Toxicology Information *on page 696-700*

Brand Names AllerMax® [OTC]; Banophen® [OTC]; Belix® [OTC]; Benadryl® [OTC]; Benylin® Cough Syrup [OTC]; Diphen® Cough [OTC]; Dormin® [OTC]; Genahist®; Nidryl® [OTC]; Nordryl®; Nytol® [OTC]; Sleep-eze 3® [OTC]; Sleepinal® [OTC]; Sominex® [OTC]; Tusstat®; Twilite® [OTC]

Therapeutic Category Antidote, Hypersensitivity Reactions; Antihistamine; Sedative

Use Symptomatic relief of allergic symptoms caused by histamine release which include nasal allergies and allergic dermatosis; mild nighttime sedation, prevention of motion sickness, as an antitussive; treatment of phenothiazine-induced dystonic reactions

Pregnancy Risk Factor C

Contraindications Hypersensitivity to diphenhydramine or any component; should not be used in acute attacks of asthma

Precautions Use with caution in patients with angle-closure glaucoma, peptic ulcer, urinary tract obstruction, hyperthyroidism; antihistamines should be used cautiously in preterm and term infants due to a possible association with SIDS

(Continued)

Diphenhydramine Hydrochloride *(Continued)*

Adverse Reactions

Cardiovascular: Hypotension, palpitations

Central nervous system: Sedation, dizziness, paradoxical excitement, fatigue, insomnia, tremor

Gastrointestinal: Nausea, vomiting, dry mouth and mucous membranes

Ocular: Blurred vision

Renal & genitourinary: Urinary retention

Drug Interactions Additive sedation when given with drugs which depress the central nervous system

Mechanism of Action Competes with histamine for H_1-receptor sites on effector cells in the gastrointestinal tract, blood vessels, and respiratory tract

Pharmacodynamics

Maximum sedative effect: 1-3 hours after administration

Duration of action: 4-7 hours

Pharmacokinetics

Absorption: Oral: Well absorbed but 40% to 60% of an oral dose reaches the systemic circulation due to first-pass metabolism

Protein-binding: 78%

Metabolism: Extensively metabolized in the liver

Half-life: 2-8 hours

Peak serum levels: Occur in 2-4 hours

Usual Dosage Oral, I.M., I.V.:

Children: 5 mg/kg/day or 150 mg/m^2/day in divided doses every 6-8 hours, not to exceed 300 mg/day

Adults: 10-50 mg in a single dose every 4 hours, not to exceed 400 mg/day

Topical creams, lotions containing 1% to 2% diphenhydramine may be applied 3-4 times/day

Administration Dilute to a maximum concentration of 25 mg/mL and infuse over 10-15 minutes (maximum rate of infusion: 25 mg/minute)

Test Interactions May suppress the wheal and flare reactions to skin test antigens

Dosage Forms

Capsule: 25 mg, 50 mg

Cream: 1%, 2%

Elixir: 12.5 mg/5 mL

Injection: 10 mg/mL; 50 mg/mL

Lotion: 1% (75 mL)

Solution, topical spray: 1% (60 mL)

Syrup: 12.5 mg/5 mL

Tablet: 25 mg, 50 mg

Diphenoxylate and Atropine (dye fen ox' i late)

Brand Names Lofene®; Logen®; Lomanate®; Lomodix®; Lomotil®; Lonox®; Low-Quel®

Synonyms Atropine and Diphenoxylate

Therapeutic Category Antidiarrheal

Use Treatment of diarrhea

Restrictions C-V

Pregnancy Risk Factor C

Contraindications Hypersensitivity to diphenoxylate, atropine or any component; severe liver disease, jaundice, dehydrated patient, and narrow-angle glaucoma; do not use in children <2 years of age

Warnings Reduction of intestinal motility may be deleterious in diarrhea resulting from *Shigella*, *Salmonella*, toxigenic strains of *E. coli* and from pseudomembranous enterocolitis associated with broad spectrum antibiotics; children (especially those with Down's syndrome) may develop signs of atropinism (dry skin and mucous membranes, thirst, hyperthermia, tachycardia, urinary retention, flushing) even at the recommended dosages

Precautions Use with extreme caution in patients with dehydration, cirrhosis, hepatorenal disease, renal dysfunction, and acute ulcerative colitis

Adverse Reactions

Cardiovascular: Tachycardia

Central nervous system: Sedation, dizziness, euphoria, weakness, headache, hyperthermia

Dermatologic: Pruritus, urticaria
Gastrointestinal: Nausea, vomiting, abdominal discomfort, paralytic ileus, pancreatitis, dry mouth
Ocular: Blurred vision
Renal & genitourinary: Urinary retention
Respiratory: Respiratory depression (young children may be at greater risk)
Miscellaneous: Physical and psychological dependence with prolonged use

Drug Interactions MAO inhibitors, CNS depressants, alcohol

Mechanism of Action Diphenoxylate inhibits excessive GI motility and GI propulsion; commercial preparations contain a subtherapeutic amount of atropine to discourage abuse

Pharmacodynamics
Onset of action: Within 45-60 minutes
Peak effect: Within 2 hours
Duration: 3-4 hours
Tolerance to antidiarrheal effects may occur with prolonged use

Pharmacokinetics
Absorption: Oral: Well absorbed
Metabolism: Extensively metabolized in the liver to diphenoxylic acid (active)
Half-life:
Diphenoxylate: 2.5 hours
Diphenoxylic acid: 12-24 hours
Peak plasma concentrations: Occur at 2 hours
Elimination: Excreted primarily in the feces (via bile) and ~14% is excreted in the urine; <1% excreted unchanged in urine

Usual Dosage Oral (as diphenoxylate):
Children: Liquid: 0.3-0.4 mg/kg/day in 2-4 divided doses **or**
<2 years: Not recommended
2-5 years: 2 mg 3 times/day
5-8 years: 2 mg 4 times/day
8-12 years: 2 mg 5 times/day
Note: Do not exceed recommended doses; reduce dose as soon as symptoms are initially controlled; maintenance doses may be as low as 25% of initial dose; if no improvement within 48 hours of therapy, diphenoxylate is not likely to be effective.

Adults: 15-20 mg/day in 3-4 divided doses; maintenance: 5-15 mg/day in 2-3 divided doses

Monitoring Parameters Bowel frequency, signs and symptoms of atropinism

Dosage Forms
Solution, oral: Diphenoxylate hydrochloride 2.5 mg and atropine sulfate 0.025 mg per 5 mL (60 mL)
Tablet: Diphenoxylate hydrochloride 2.5 mg and atropine sulfate 0.025 mg

Diphenylan Sodium® *see* Phenytoin *on page 455*

Diphenylhydantoin *see* Phenytoin *on page 455*

Diphtheria and Tetanus Toxoids *see* Immunization Guidelines *on page 660-667*

Diphtheria, Tetanus Toxoids and Accellular Pertussis Vaccine *see* Immunization Guidelines *on page 660-667*

Diphtheria, Tetanus Toxoids and Whole-cell Pertussis Vaccine *see* Immunization Guidelines *on page 660-667*

Dipivalyl Epinephrine *see* Dipivefrin Hydrochloride *on this page*

Dipivefrin Hydrochloride (dye pi' ve frin)

Brand Names Propine®

Synonyms Dipivalyl Epinephrine; DPE

Therapeutic Category Adrenergic Agonist Agent, Ophthalmic; Ophthalmic Agent, Vasoconstrictor

Use Reduce elevated intraocular pressure in chronic open-angle glaucoma; also used to treat ocular hypertension

Pregnancy Risk Factor B

Contraindications Hypersensitivity to dipivefrin, ingredients in the formula-

(Continued)

Dipivefrin Hydrochloride *(Continued)*

tion, or epinephrine; contraindicated in patients with angle-closure glaucoma

Precautions Use with caution in patients with vascular hypertension or cardiac disorders and in aphakic patients

Adverse Reactions

Central nervous system: Headache

Local: Burning, stinging

Ocular: Ocular congestion, photophobia, mydriasis, blurred vision, ocular pain, bulbar conjunctival follicles, blepharoconjunctivitis, cystoid macular edema

Drug Interactions Effects of lowering IOP may be additive when used with topical miotics, timolol, betaxolol, or carbonic anhydrase inhibitors

Stability Protect from light and avoid exposure to air; discolored or darkened solutions indicate loss of potency

Mechanism of Action Dipivefrin is a prodrug of epinephrine which is the active agent that stimulates alpha- and/or beta-adrenergic receptors increasing aqueous humor outflow

Pharmacodynamics

Onset of action:

Ocular pressure effects: Within 30 minutes

Mydriasis: Within 30 minutes

Duration:

Ocular pressure effects: 12 hours or longer

Mydriasis: Several hours

Pharmacokinetics Absorption: Rapidly absorbed into the aqueous humor; converted to epinephrine

Usual Dosage Children and Adults: Ophthalmic: Initial: 1 drop every 12 hours

Monitoring Parameters Intraocular pressure

Patient Information Discolored solutions should be discarded; may cause burning or stinging, blurred vision, and sensitivity to light

Additional Information Contains sodium metabisulfite

Dosage Forms Solution, ophthalmic: 0.1% (5 mL, 10 mL, 15 mL)

Diprolene® *see* Betamethasone *on page 81*

Diprolene® AF *see* Betamethasone *on page 81*

Dipropylacetic Acid *see* Valproic Acid and Derivatives *on page 592*

Diprosone® *see* Betamethasone *on page 81*

Dipyridamole (dye peer id' a mole)

Brand Names Persantine®

Therapeutic Category Antiplatelet Agent; Vasodilator, Coronary

Use Maintain patency after surgical grafting procedures including coronary artery bypass; with warfarin to decrease thrombosis in patients after artificial heart valve replacement; for chronic management of angina pectoris; with aspirin to prevent coronary artery thrombosis; in combination with aspirin or warfarin to prevent other thromboembolic disorders

Pregnancy Risk Factor C

Contraindications Hypersensitivity to dipyridamole or any component

Precautions May further decrease blood pressure in patients with hypotension due to peripheral vasodilation

Adverse Reactions

Cardiovascular: Vasodilatation, flushing, syncope

Central nervous system: Dizziness, headache (dose related), weakness

Dermatologic: Rash, pruritus

Gastrointestinal: Abdominal distress, nausea, vomiting, diarrhea

Drug Interactions Heparin

Mechanism of Action Inhibits the activity of adenosine deaminase and phosphodiesterase, which causes an accumulation of adenosine, adenine nucleotides, and cyclic AMP; these mediators then inhibit platelet aggregation and may cause vasodilation; may also stimulate release of prostacyclin or PGD_2; causes coronary vasodilation

Pharmacokinetics Oral:

Absorption: Readily absorbed from the GI tract

Distribution: V_d: Adults: 2-3 L/kg

Protein binding: 91% to 99%

Metabolism: Concentrated and metabolized in the liver

Half-life, terminal: 10-12 hours

Bioavailability: Ranges from 37% to 66%

Peak serum levels: Within 2-2.5 hours

Elimination: Excreted in feces via bile as glucuronide conjugates and unchanged drug

Usual Dosage

Children: Oral: 3-6 mg/kg/day in 3 divided doses; doses of 4-10 mg/kg/day have been used investigationally to treat proteinuria in pediatric renal disease

Adults: Oral: 75-400 mg/day in 3-4 divided doses

Dipyridamole stress test (for evaluation of myocardial perfusion): I.V.: 0.142 mg/kg/minute for a total of 4 minutes (0.57 mg/kg total); adult maximum: 60 mg. Inject thallium 201 within 5 minutes after end of injection of dipyridamole.

Platelet aggregation inhibitor: I.V. infusion: Adults: 250 mg/day at a rate of 10 mg/hour; maximum: 400 mg/day (use lower doses with aspirin)

Administration I.V.: Dilute in at least a 1:2 ratio with NS, ½NS, or D_5W; infusion of undiluted dipyridamole may cause local irritation

Monitoring Parameters Blood pressure, heart rate

Additional Information Dipyridamole may also be given 2 days prior to open heart surgery to prevent platelet activation by extracorporeal bypass pump

Dosage Forms

Injection: 10 mg/2 mL

Tablet: 25 mg, 50 mg, 75 mg

References

Rao PS, Solymar L, Mardini MK, et al, "Anticoagulant Therapy in Children With Prosthetic Valves," *Ann Thorac Surg*, 1989, 47(4):589-92.

Ueda N, Kawaguchi S, Niinomi Y, et al, "Effect of Dipyridamole Treatment on Proteinuria in Pediatric Renal Disease," *Nephron*, 1986, 44(3):174-9.

Disanthrol® [OTC] *see* Docusate and Casanthranol *on page 203*

Disodium Cromoglycate *see* Cromolyn Sodium *on page 158*

***d*-Isoephedrine Hydrochloride** *see* Pseudoephedrine *on page 497*

Disonate® [OTC] *see* Docusate *on page 202*

Disopyramide Phosphate (dye soe peer' a mide)

Brand Names Norpace®

Therapeutic Category Antiarrhythmic Agent, Class Ia

Use Suppression and prevention of unifocal and multifocal ventricular premature complexes, coupled ventricular premature complexes, and/or paroxysmal ventricular tachycardia; also effective in the conversion and prevention of recurrence of atrial fibrillation, atrial flutter, and paroxysmal atrial tachycardia

Pregnancy Risk Factor C

Contraindications Pre-existing second or third degree A-V block; cardiogenic shock or known hypersensitivity to the drug

Precautions Pre-existing urinary retention, family history or existing angle-closure glaucoma, myasthenia gravis, hypotension during initiation of therapy, congestive heart failure unless caused by an arrhythmia, widening of QRS complex during therapy or lengthening of QT interval (>25% to 50% of baseline QRS complex or QT interval), sick-sinus syndrome, WPW or bundle branch block; may ↑ ventricular rate in patients with atrial flutter who have not received digoxin; renal or hepatic impairment require decrease in dosage

Adverse Reactions

Cardiovascular: Congestive heart failure, edema, weight gain, dyspnea, chest pain, syncope and hypotension, conduction disturbances including A-V block, widening QRS complex and lengthening of QT interval

(Continued)

Disopyramide Phosphate *(Continued)*

Central nervous system: Fatigue, headache, malaise, nervousness, acute psychosis, depression, dizziness, weakness,
Dermatologic: Generalized rashes
Endocrine & metabolic: Hypoglycemia, ↑ cholesterol and triglycerides; may initiate contractions of pregnant uterus; hyperkalemia may enhance toxicities
Gastrointestinal: Dry mouth, constipation, nausea, vomiting, diarrhea, pain, gas, anorexia
Hepatic: Elevated liver enzymes; hepatic cholestasis
Ocular: Blurred vision
Renal & genitourinary: Urinary retention/hesitancy
Miscellaneous: Dry nose, eyes and throat

Drug Interactions Hepatic microsomal enzyme inducing agents (ie, phenytoin, phenobarbital, rifampin) may increase metabolism of disopyramide; erythromycin may ↑ disopyramide serum concentrations

Mechanism of Action Class IA antiarrhythmic: Decreases myocardial excitability and conduction velocity; reduces disparity in refractory between normal and infarcted myocardium; possesses anticholinergic, peripheral vasoconstrictive and negative inotropic effects

Pharmacodynamics
Onset of action: 30-210 minutes
Duration: 1.5-8.5 hours

Pharmacokinetics
Protein binding: Concentration dependent, stereoselective, and ranges from 20% to 60%
Distribution: V_d: Children: 1 L/kg
Metabolism: Metabolized in the liver to inactive metabolites
Bioavailability: 60% to 83%
Half-life:
Children: 3.15 hours
Adults: 4-10 hours, increased half-life with hepatic or renal disease
Elimination: Excreted 40% to 60% unchanged in urine and 10% to 15% in feces; clearance in children: 3.76 mL/minute/kg; clearance is greater and half life shorter in children vs adults

Usual Dosage Oral:
Children (start with lower dose listed):
<1 year: 10-30 mg/kg/24 hours in 4 divided doses
1-4 years: 10-20 mg/kg/24 hours in 4 divided doses
4-12 years: 10-15 mg/kg/24 hours in 4 divided doses
12-18 years: 6-15 mg/kg/24 hours in 4 divided doses

Adults:
<50 kg: 100 mg every 6 hours or 200 mg every 12 hours (controlled release)
>50 kg: 150 mg every 6 hours or 300 mg every 12 hours (controlled release); if no response, may increase to 200 mg every 6 hours; maximum dose required for patients with severe refractory ventricular tachycardia is 400 mg every 6 hours

Adult dosing adjustment in renal impairment: 100 mg (nonsustained release) given at the following intervals: See table.

Creatinine Clearance (mL/min)	Dosage Interval
30–40	q8h
15–30	q12h
<15	q24h

Monitoring Parameters Blood pressure, EKG, drug level; especially important to monitor EKG in patients with hepatic or renal disease, heart disease, or others with increased risk of adverse effects

Reference Range Therapeutic: Atrial arrhythmias: 2.8-3.2 μg/mL (SI: 8.3-9.4 μmol/L); Ventricular arrhythmias: 3.3-7.5 μg/mL (SI: 9.7-22 μmol/L); Toxic: >7 μg/mL (SI: >20.7 μmol/L)

Nursing Implications Do not crush, break, or chew controlled release capsules

Dosage Forms

Capsule: 100 mg, 150 mg

Capsule, sustained action: 100 mg, 150 mg

Extemporaneous Preparation(s) Extemporaneous suspension in cherry syrup (1-10 mg/mL) is stable for 4 weeks refrigerated in an amber glass bottle; shake well before use; do not use extended release capsules for this suspension

Handbook on Extemporaneous Formulations, Bethesda MD: American Society of Hospital Pharmacists, 1987, 20.

References

Chiba K, Koike K, Nakamoto M, et al, "Steady-State Pharmacokinetics and Bioavailability of Total and Unbound Disopyramide in Children With Cardiac Arrhythmias," *Ther Drug Monit*, 1992, 14(2):112-8.

Echizen H, Takahashi H, Nakamura H, et al, "Stereoselective Disposition and Metabolism of Disopyramide in Pediatric Patients," *J Pharmacol Exp Ther*, 1991, 259(3):953-60.

Di-Spaz® *see* Dicyclomine Hydrochloride *on page 187*

Dispos-a-Med® Isoproterenol *see* Isoproterenol *on page 324*

Ditropan® *see* Oxybutynin Chloride *on page 427*

Diulo® *see* Metolazone *on page 382*

Diuril® *see* Chlorothiazide *on page 127*

Divalproex Sodium *see* Valproic Acid and Derivatives *on page 592*

Dizmiss® [OTC] *see* Meclizine Hydrochloride *on page 358*

Dizymes® *see* Pancreatin *on page 430*

***dl*-Alpha Tocopherol** *see* Vitamin E *on page 605*

***D*-Mannitol** *see* Mannitol *on page 355*

4-DMDR *see* Idarubicin Hydrochloride *on page 301*

DNR *see* Daunorubicin Hydrochloride *on page 172*

Dobutamine Hydrochloride (doe byoo' ta meen)

Related Information

Emergency Pediatric Drip Calculations *on page 615*

Extravasation Treatment *on page 640*

Medications Compatible With PN Solutions *on page 649-650*

Brand Names Dobutrex®

Therapeutic Category Adrenergic Agonist Agent; Sympathomimetic

Use Short term management of patients with cardiac decompensation

Pregnancy Risk Factor C

Contraindications Hypersensitivity to sulfites (commercial preparation contains sodium bisulfite); patients with idiopathic hypertrophic subaortic stenosis

Warnings Potent drug; must be diluted prior to use. Patient's hemodynamic status should be monitored.

Precautions Hypovolemia should be corrected prior to use; infiltration causes local inflammatory changes, extravasation may cause dermal necrosis

Adverse Reactions

Cardiovascular: Ectopic heartbeats, increased heart rate, chest pain, angina, palpitations, elevation in blood pressure; in higher doses ventricular tachycardia or arrhythmias may be seen; patients with atrial fibrillation or flutter are at risk of developing a rapid ventricular response

Central nervous system: Tingling sensation, paresthesia, headache

Gastrointestinal: Nausea, vomiting

Musculoskeletal: Mild leg cramps

Respiratory: Dyspnea

Drug Interactions Beta-adrenergic blocking agents, general anesthetics

Stability Stable in various solutions for 24 hours; incompatible with alkaline solutions, do not give through same I.V. line as heparin, sodium bicarbon-

(Continued)

Dobutamine Hydrochloride *(Continued)*

ate, cefazolin, or penicillin; compatible when coadministered with dopamine, epinephrine, isoproterenol, and lidocaine; pink discoloration of dobutamine hydrochloride indicates slight oxidation, but no significant loss of potency if administered within the recommended time period

Mechanism of Action Stimulates $beta_1$-adrenergic receptors, causing increased contractility and heart rate, with little effect on $beta_2$ or alpha receptors

Pharmacodynamics

Onset of action: Following I.V. administration activity appears in 1-10 minutes

Peak effect: Within 10-20 minutes

Pharmacokinetics

Metabolism: Metabolized in tissues and the liver to inactive metabolites

Half-life: 2 minutes

Usual Dosage I.V. infusion:

Neonates: 2-15 μg/kg/minute, titrate to desired response

Children: 2.5-15 μg/kg/minute, titrate to desired response; maximum: 40 μg/kg/minute

Adults: 2.5-15 μg/kg minute; maximum: 40 μg/kg/minute, titrate to desired response

Administration Dilute in dextrose or normal saline; maximum recommended concentration: 6000 μg/mL (6 mg/mL); rate of infusion (mL/hour) = dose (μg/kg/minute) x weight (kg) x 60 minutes/hour divided by the concentration (μg/mL)

Monitoring Parameters EKG, heart rate, CVP, RAP, MAP, urine output; if pulmonary artery catheter is in place, monitor CI, PCWP, and SVR. Dobutamine lowers central venous pressure and wedge pressure but has little effect on pulmonary vascular resistance.

Nursing Implications Administer into large vein; use infusion device to control rate of flow

Dosage Forms Injection: 250 mg (20 mL)

Dobutrex® *see* Dobutamine Hydrochloride *on previous page*

Docusate (dok' yoo sate)

Brand Names Colace® [OTC]; Dialose® [OTC]; Diocto® [OTC]; Dioeze® [OTC]; Disonate® [OTC]; Doxinate® [OTC]; Kasof® [OTC]; Modane® Soft [OTC]; Pro-Sof® [OTC]; Surfak® [OTC]

Synonyms Dioctyl Calcium Sulfosuccinate; Dioctyl Potassium Sulfosuccinate; Dioctyl Sodium Sulfosuccinate; DOSS; DSS

Therapeutic Category Laxative, Surfactant; Stool Softener

Use Stool softener in patients who should avoid straining during defecation and constipation associated with hard, dry stools

Pregnancy Risk Factor C

Contraindications Concomitant use of mineral oil; intestinal obstruction, acute abdominal pain, nausea, vomiting; hypersensitivity to docusate or any component

Adverse Reactions

Gastrointestinal: Intestinal obstruction, diarrhea, abdominal cramping

Local: Throat irritation

Drug Interactions Mineral oil, phenolphthalein, aspirin

Mechanism of Action Reduces surface tension of the oil-water interface of the stool resulting in enhanced incorporation of water and fat allowing for stool softening

Pharmacodynamics Onset of action: 12-72 hours

Usual Dosage

Infants and Children <3 years: Oral: 10-40 mg/day in 1-4 divided doses

Children: Oral:

- 3-6 years: 20-60 mg/day in 1-4 divided doses
- 6-12 years: 40-150 mg/day in 1-4 divided doses

Adolescents and Adults: Oral: 50-400 mg/day in 1-4 divided doses

Older Children and Adults: Rectal: Add 50-100 mg of docusate liquid to enema fluid (saline or water); give as retention or flushing enema

Patient Information Adults: Docusate should be taken with a full glass of water

Nursing Implications Docusate liquid should be given with milk, fruit juice, or infant formula to mask the bitter taste

Additional Information Docusate sodium 5-10 mg/mL liquid instilled in the ear as a cerumenolytic produces substantial ear wax disintegration within 15 minutes and complete disintegration after 24 hours

Dosage Forms

Capsule, as calcium: 50 mg, 240 mg
Capsule, as potassium: 100 mg, 240 mg
Capsule, as sodium: 50 mg, 100 mg, 240 mg, 250 mg
Liquid, as sodium: 50 mg/5 mL (30 mL, 480 mL)
Solution, oral, as sodium: 50 mg/mL (60 mL, 4000 mL)
Syrup, as sodium: 16.7 mg/5 mL (30 mL); 20 mg/5 mL (15 mL, 30 mL, 60 mL, 240 mL, 473 mL)
Tablet, as sodium: 100 mg

References

Chen DA and Caparosa RJ, "A Nonprescription Cerumenolytic," *Am J Otology*, 1991, 12(6):475-6.

Docusate and Casanthranol

Brand Names Diocto-C® [OTC]; Disanthrol® [OTC]; Peri-Colace® [OTC]; Peri-DOS® [OTC]

Synonyms Casanthranol and Docusate; DSS With Casanthranol

Therapeutic Category Laxative, Surfactant; Stool Softener

Use Treatment of constipation generally associated with dry, hard stools and decreased intestinal motility

Pregnancy Risk Factor C

Contraindications Concomitant use of mineral oil; intestinal obstruction; acute abdominal pain; nausea, vomiting; hypersensitivity to docusate or casanthranol

Warnings Do not use when abdominal pain, nausea, or vomiting are present

Precautions Habit-forming, may result in laxative dependence and loss of normal bowel function with prolonged use

Adverse Reactions

Dermatologic: Rash
Gastrointestinal: Intestinal obstruction, diarrhea, abdominal cramping
Local: Throat irritation

Drug Interactions Mineral oil, phenolphthalein, aspirin

Pharmacodynamics Onset of action: 8-12 hours after administration but may require up to 24 hours

Usual Dosage Oral:

Children: 5-15 mL of syrup at bedtime or 1 capsule at bedtime

Adults: 1-2 capsules or 15-30 mL syrup at bedtime, may be increased to 2 capsules or 30 mL twice daily or 3 capsules at bedtime

Monitoring Parameters Bowel frequency

Dosage Forms

Capsule: Docusate potassium 100 mg and casanthranol 30 mg
Capsule: Docusate sodium 100 mg and casanthranol 30 mg
Syrup: Docusate sodium 20 mg and casanthranol 10 mg per 5 mL (240 mL, 480 mL, 4000 mL)

Doktors® Nasal Solution [OTC] *see* Phenylephrine Hydrochloride *on page 453*

Dolacet® *see* Hydrocodone and Acetaminophen *on page 292*

Dolene® *see* Propoxyphene *on page 491*

Dolophine® *see* Methadone Hydrochloride *on page 368*

Domeboro® [OTC] *see* Aluminum Acetate *on page 33*

Donnatal® *see* Hyoscyamine, Atropine, Scopolamine and Phenobarbital *on page 299*

Donnazyme® *see* Pancreatin *on page 430*

Dopamine Hydrochloride (doe' pa meen)

Related Information

Emergency Pediatric Drip Calculations *on page 615*
Extravasation Treatment *on page 640*
Medications Compatible With PN Solutions *on page 649-650*

Brand Names Intropin®

Therapeutic Category Adrenergic Agonist Agent; Sympathomimetic

Use Adjunct in the treatment of shock which persists after adequate fluid volume replacement

Pregnancy Risk Factor C

Contraindications Hypersensitivity to sulfites (commercial preparation contains sodium bisulfite); pheochromocytoma, or ventricular fibrillation

Warnings Potent drug; must be diluted prior to use. Patient's hemodynamic status should be monitored.

Precautions Blood volume depletion should be corrected, if possible, before starting dopamine therapy. Dopamine must not be used as sole therapy in hypovolemic patients. Extravasation may cause tissue necrosis (treat extravasation with phentolamine)

Adverse Reactions

Cardiovascular: Ectopic heartbeats, tachycardia, vasoconstriction, cardiac conduction abnormalities, widened QRS complex, hypertension, ventricular arrhythmias, gangrene of the extremities (with high doses for prolonged periods or even with low doses in patients with occlusive vascular disease)

Central nervous system: Anxiety, headache

Gastrointestinal: Nausea, vomiting

Musculoskeletal: Piloerection

Renal & genitourinary: Decreased urine output, azotemia

Respiratory: Dyspnea

Drug Interactions Dopamine's effects are prolonged and intensified by MAO inhibitors, alpha- and beta-adrenergic blockers, general anesthetics, phenytoin

Stability Protect from light; solutions that are darker than slightly yellow should not be used; incompatible with alkaline solutions or iron salts; compatible when coadministered with dobutamine, epinephrine, isoproterenol, and lidocaine

Mechanism of Action Stimulates both adrenergic and dopaminergic receptors, lower doses are mainly dopaminergic stimulating and produce renal and mesenteric vasodilation, higher doses stimulate both dopaminergic and $beta_1$-adrenergic receptors and produce cardiac stimulation and renal vasodilation, large doses stimulate alpha-adrenergic receptors primarily

Pharmacodynamics

Onset of action: Adults: 5 minutes

Duration: Due to its short duration of action (<10 minutes) a continuous infusion must be used

Pharmacokinetics

Metabolism: Metabolized in the plasma, kidneys, and liver 75% to inactive metabolites by monoamine oxidase and 25% to norepinephrine (active)

Half-life: 2 minutes

Clearance: Neonatal clearance varies and appears to be age related. Clearance is more prolonged with combined hepatic and renal dysfunction. Dopamine has exhibited nonlinear kinetics in children; dose changes in children may not achieve steady-state for approximately 1 hour rather than 20 minutes seen in adults.

Usual Dosage I.V. infusion:

Neonates: 1-20 μg/kg/minute continuous infusion, titrate to desired response

Children: 1-20 μg/kg/minute, maximum: 50 μg/kg/minute continuous infusion, titrate to desired response

Adults: 1 μg/kg/minute up to 50 μg/kg/minute, titrate to desired response

If dosages >20-30 μg/kg/minute are needed, a more direct acting pressor may be more beneficial (ie, epinephrine, norepinephrine)

The hemodynamic effects of dopamine are dose-dependent:

Low dosage: 1-5 μg/kg/minute, increased renal blood flow and urine output

Intermediate dosage: 5-15 μg/kg/minute, increased renal blood flow, heart rate, cardiac contractility, and cardiac output

High dosage: >15 μg/kg/minute, alpha-adrenergic effects begin to predominate, vasoconstriction, increased blood pressure

Administration Must be diluted prior to administration; maximum concentration: 6000 μ/mL (6 mg/mL); rate of infusion (mL/hour) = dose (μg/kg/minute) x weight (kg) x 60 minutes/hour divided by concentration (μg/mL)

Monitoring Parameters EKG, heart rate, CVP, RAP, MAP, urine output; if pulmonary artery catheter is in place, monitor CI, PWCP, SVR, and PVR

Nursing Implications Administer into large vein to prevent the possibility of extravasation; use infusion device to control rate of flow; administration into an umbilical arterial catheter is **not** recommended

Dosage Forms

Infusion, in D_5W: 0.8 mg/mL (250 mL, 500 mL); 1.6 mg/mL (250 mL, 500 mL); 3.2 mg/mL (250 mL, 500 mL)

Injection: 40 mg/mL (5 mL, 10 mL, 20 mL); 80 mg/mL (5 mL, 20 mL); 160 mg/mL (5 mL)

References

Banner W, Jr, Vernon DD, Dean JM, et al, "Nonlinear Dopamine Pharmacokinetics in Pediatric Patients," *J Pharmacol Exp Ther*, 1989, 249(1):131-3.

Dopar® *see* Levodopa *on page 338*

Dopram® *see* Doxapram Hydrochloride *on next page*

Dorcol® [OTC] *see* Acetaminophen *on page 16*

Dormin® [OTC] *see* Diphenhydramine Hydrochloride *on page 195*

Doryx® *see* Doxycycline *on page 210*

DOSS *see* Docusate *on page 202*

Doxacurium Chloride (dox a kyoo' rium)

Brand Names Nuromax® Injection

Therapeutic Category Neuromuscular Blocker Agent, Nondepolarizing; Skeletal Muscle Relaxant, Long Acting

Use Doxacurium is indicated for use as an adjunct to general anesthesia. It provides skeletal muscle relaxation during surgery or endotracheal intubation; increases pulmonary compliance during mechanical ventilation

Pregnancy Risk Factor C

Contraindications Patients with known hypersensitivity

Warnings Ventilation must be supported during neuromuscular blockade

Precautions Contains benzyl alcohol; avoid use in infants

Adverse Reactions The most frequent adverse reactions appear as an extension of the agent's neuromuscular blocking actions. This may vary from skeletal muscle weakness to profound and prolonged skeletal muscle paralysis resulting in respiratory insufficiency and apnea. Neuromuscular blocking agents may have a profound effect in patients with neuromuscular diseases (ie, myasthenia gravis). In these patients, a prolonged neuromuscular block and inadequate reversal of neuromuscular blockade are possible.

Musculoskeletal: Skeletal muscle weakness

Respiratory: Respiratory insufficiency and apnea

Drug Interactions Phenytoin, carbamazepine (↓ neuromuscular blockade); tetracycline, aminoglycosides, magnesium, lithium, halothane, enflurane, local anesthetics, procainamide, quinidine, isoflurane (↑ neuromuscular blockade)

Stability Stable for 24 hours at room temperature when diluted, up to 0.1 mg/mL in dextrose 5% or normal saline; compatible with sufentanil, alfentanil, and fentanyl

Mechanism of Action Doxacurium is a long-acting nondepolarizing skeletal muscle relaxant. The drug is a bis-quaternary benzylisoquinolinium diester, with a chemical structure similar to that of atracurium. Similar to other nondepolarizing neuromuscular blocking agents, doxacurium produces muscle relaxation by competing with acetylcholine for cholinergic receptor sites on the postjunctional membrane; significant presynaptic depressant activity is also observed.

Pharmacodynamics

Onset of effects: 5-11 minutes

Duration: 30 minutes (range: 12-54 minutes)

(Continued)

Doxacurium Chloride *(Continued)*

Pharmacokinetics

Protein binding: 30%

Elimination: Primarily excreted as unchanged drug via the kidneys and biliary tract

Usual Dosage I.V. (in obese patients, use ideal body weight):

Children 2-12 years: Initial: 0.03-0.05 mg/kg/dose; maintenance: 0.005-0.01 mg/kg after 30-45 minutes

Children >12 years and Adults: Initial: 0.025-0.05 mg/kg/dose; maintenance: 0.005-0.01 mg/kg/dose every 60-100 minutes

Administration May be given rapid I.V. injection undiluted

Additional Information Doxacurium is a long-acting nondepolarizing neuromuscular blocker with virtually no cardiovascular side effects. The characteristics of this agent make it especially useful in procedures requiring careful maintenance of hemodynamic stability for prolonged periods; reduce dosage in renal or hepatic impairment

Dosage Forms Injection: 1 mg/mL (5 mL)

Doxapram Hydrochloride (dox' a pram)

Brand Names Dopram®

Therapeutic Category Central Nervous System Stimulant, Nonamphetamine; Respiratory Stimulant

Use Respiratory and CNS stimulant

Pregnancy Risk Factor B

Contraindications Hypersensitivity to doxapram or any component; epilepsy, cerebral edema, head injury, asthma or restrictive pulmonary disease, pheochromocytoma, cardiovascular or coronary artery disease, hypertension, hyperthyroidism, cardiac arrhythmias

Warnings Should be used with caution in newborns as the U.S. product contains benzyl alcohol (0.9%); recommended doses of doxapram for neonates will deliver 5.4-27 mg/kg/day of benzyl alcohol; large amounts of benzyl alcohol (>100 mg/kg/day) have been associated with fatal toxicity (gasping syndrome); the use of doxapram in newborns should be reserved for neonates who are unresponsive to the treatment of apnea with therapeutic serum concentrations of theophylline or caffeine

Adverse Reactions

Cardiovascular: Hypertension (dose related), tachycardia, arrhythmias, hypotension, flushing, feeling of warmth

Central nervous system: CNS stimulation, tremor, restlessness, lightheadedness, jitters, hallucinations, irritability, seizures, headache, hyperpyrexia

Hematologic: Hemolysis

Gastrointestinal: Abdominal distension, nausea, vomiting, retching

Local: Phlebitis

Musculoskeletal: Hyperreflexia

Ocular: Lacrimation, mydriasis

Respiratory: Coughing, laryngospasm, dyspnea

Miscellaneous: Sweating

Drug Interactions Sympathomimetic drugs and MAO inhibitors may cause significant ↑ in blood pressure; general anesthetics

Stability Incompatible with aminophylline, sodium bicarbonate, thiopental sodium

Mechanism of Action Stimulates respiration through action on respiratory center in medulla or through reflex stimulation of carotid, aortic, or other peripheral chemoreceptors

Pharmacodynamics Following I.V. injection:

Onset of respiratory stimulation: Within 20-40 seconds

Peak effect: Within 1-2 minutes

Duration: 5-12 minutes

Pharmacokinetics

Metabolism: Extensively liver metabolized

Distribution: V_d: Neonates: 4-7.3 L/kg

Half-life:

Neonates, premature: 6.6-8.2 hours

Adults: Mean: 3.4 hours

Clearance: Neonates: 0.44-0.7 L/kg/hour

Usual Dosage I.V.:

Neonatal apnea (apnea of prematurity): Initial loading dose: 2.5-3 mg/kg followed by a continuous infusion of 1 mg/kg/hour titrated to the lowest rate at which apnea is controlled (maximum: 2.5 mg/kg/hour)

Adults: Respiratory depression following anesthesia:

Initial: 0.5-1 mg/kg; may repeat at 5-minute intervals; maximum total dose: 2 mg/kg

I.V. infusion: Initial: 5 mg/minute until adequate response or adverse effects seen; ↓ to 1-3 mg/minute; usual total dose: 0.5-4 mg/kg or 300 mg

Administration Dilute loading dose to a maximum concentration of 2 mg/mL and infuse over 15-30 minutes; for infusion, dilute in normal saline or dextrose to 1 mg/mL (maximum: 2 mg/mL)

Monitoring Parameters Blood pressure, heart rate, deep tendon reflexes; for apnea: number and duration of apnea episodes

Nursing Implications Irritating to tissues; avoid extravasation

Additional Information Initial studies suggest a therapeutic range of at least 1.5 mg/L; toxicity becomes frequent at serum levels >5 mg/L

Dosage Forms Injection: 20 mg/mL (20 mL)

References

Barrington KJ, Finer NN, Torok-Both G, et al, "Dose-Response Relationship of Doxapram in the Therapy for Refractory Idiopathic Apnea of Prematurity," *Pediatrics*, 1987, 80(1):22-7.

Doxepin Hydrochloride (dox' e pin)

Related Information

Overdose and Toxicology Information *on page 696-700*

Brand Names Adapin®; Sinequan®

Therapeutic Category Antianxiety Agent; Antidepressant, Tricyclic

Use Treatment of various forms of depression, usually in conjunction with psychotherapy; treatment of anxiety disorders; analgesic for certain chronic and neuropathic pain

Pregnancy Risk Factor C

Contraindications Hypersensitivity to doxepin or any component (cross-sensitivity with other tricyclic antidepressants may occur); narrow-angle glaucoma

Warnings Do not discontinue abruptly in patients receiving chronic high dose therapy

Precautions Use with caution in patients with cardiovascular disease, conduction disturbances, seizure disorders, urinary retention, hyperthyroidism or those receiving thyroid replacement; avoid use during lactation; use with caution in pregnancy

Adverse Reactions Pronounced sedation and anticholinergic adverse effects may occur

Cardiovascular: Hypotension, arrhythmias

Central nervous system: Sedation, confusion, dizziness

Dermatologic: Photosensitivity

Endocrine & metabolic: SIADH

Gastrointestinal: Constipation, nausea, vomiting, dry mouth

Hematologic: Blood dyscrasias

Hepatic: Hepatitis

Ocular: Blurred vision

Otic: Tinnitus

Renal & genitourinary: Urinary retention

Miscellaneous: Hypersensitivity reactions

Drug Interactions MAO inhibitors, guanethidine, clonidine

Stability Protect from light

Mechanism of Action Increases the synaptic concentration of serotonin and/or norepinephrine in the central nervous system by inhibition of their reuptake by the presynaptic neuronal membrane

Pharmacodynamics Maximum antidepressant effects: Usually occur after >2 weeks; anxiolytic effects may occur sooner

Pharmacokinetics

Distribution: Crosses the placenta; appears in breast milk

Protein binding: 80% to 85%

Metabolism: Hepatically metabolized to metabolites, including desmethyldoxepin (active)

(Continued)

Doxepin Hydrochloride *(Continued)*

Half-life, adults: 6-8 hours
Elimination: Renal excretion

Usual Dosage Oral:

Adolescents: Initial: 25-50 mg/day in single or divided doses; gradually increase to 100 mg/day

Adults: Initial: 30-150 mg/day at bedtime or in 2-3 divided doses; may increase up to 300 mg/day; single dose should not exceed 150 mg; select patients may respond to 25-50 mg/day

Administration Oral concentrate should be diluted in 120 mL of water, milk, juice (but not grape juice) prior to administration; do **not** mix with carbonated beverages (physically incompatible)

Monitoring Parameters Blood pressure, heart rate, mental status, weight

Reference Range Utility of serum level monitoring controversial. Therapeutic concentration: Doxepin plus desmethyldoxepin: 110-250 ng/mL (SI: 4-9 nmol/L); Toxic concentration: >300 ng/mL (SI: 11 nmol/L)

Dosage Forms

Capsule: 10 mg, 25 mg, 50 mg, 75 mg, 100 mg, 150 mg
Concentrate, oral: 10 mg/mL (120 mL)

Doxinate® [OTC] *see* Docusate *on page 202*

Doxorubicin Hydrochloride (dox oh roo' bi sin)

Related Information

Emetogenic Potential of Single Chemotherapeutic Agents *on page 655*
Extravasation Treatment *on page 640*

Brand Names Adriamycin PFS™; Adriamycin RDF™; Rubex®

Synonyms ADR; Hydroxydaunomycin Hydrochloride

Therapeutic Category Antineoplastic Agent

Use Treatment of various solid tumors including ovarian, breast, and bladder tumors; various lymphomas and leukemias (ANL, ALL), soft tissue sarcomas, neuroblastoma, osteosarcoma

Pregnancy Risk Factor D

Contraindications Hypersensitivity to doxorubicin or any component, severe congestive heart failure, cardiomyopathy, pre-existing myelosuppression; patients who have received a total dose of 550 mg/m^2 of doxorubicin or 400 mg/m^2 in patients with previous or concomitant treatment with daunorubicin, cyclophosphamide, or irradiation of the cardiac region

Warnings The US Food and Drug Administration (FDA) currently recommends that procedures for proper handling and disposal of antineoplastic agents be considered. **I.V. use only,** severe local tissue necrosis will result if extravasation occurs; irreversible myocardial toxicity may occur as total dosage approaches 550 mg/m^2; severe myelosuppression is also possible

Precautions Modify dosage in patients with impaired hepatic function

Adverse Reactions

Cardiovascular: Congestive heart failure, cardiotoxicity (transient type with abnormal EKG and arrhythmias, or a chronic, cumulative, dose-dependent type which progresses to congestive heart failure), cardiorespiratory decompensation, facial flushing
Dermatologic: Alopecia, hyperpigmentation of nail beds
Endocrine & metabolic: Hyperuricemia
Gastrointestinal: Stomatitis, esophagitis, nausea, vomiting, mucositis
Hematologic: Leukopenia (nadir: 10-14 days)
Local: Tissue necrosis upon extravasation, erythematous streaking along the vein if administered too rapidly

Drug Interactions May potentiate the toxicity of cyclophosphamide, mercaptopurine

Stability Store vials containing powder at room temperature, refrigerate vials containing liquid; reconstituted vials stable for 24 hours at room temperature and 48 hours if refrigerated. Incompatible with hydrocortisone, fluorouracil, sodium bicarbonate, aminophylline, heparin, cephalothin, dexamethasone; unstable in solutions with a pH <3 or >7

Mechanism of Action Inhibits DNA and RNA synthesis by intercalating between DNA base pairs and by steric obstruction; active throughout entire cell cycle

Pharmacokinetics

Distribution: Distributes into breast milk; does not penetrate into CSF

Protein binding: 75%

Metabolism: Metabolized in both the liver and in plasma to both active and inactive metabolites

Half-life:

Primary: 30 minutes

Secondary: 3-3.5 hours for its metabolites

Terminal: 17-30 hours for doxorubicin and its metabolites

Elimination: Undergoes triphasic elimination; 80% eventually excreted in bile and feces; <5% excreted in urine, primarily as unchanged drug

Usual Dosage Patient's ideal weight should be used to calculate body surface area: I.V. (refer to individual protocols):

Children: 35-75 mg/m^2 as a single dose, repeat every 21 days; or 20-30 mg/m^2 once weekly; or 45-90 mg/m^2 given as a continuous infusion over 24-96 hours

Adults: 60-75 mg/m^2 as a single dose, repeat every 21 days; or 20-30 mg/m^2/day for 2-3 days, repeat in 4 weeks or 20 mg/m^2 once weekly

Lower dose regimens should be given to patients with decreased bone marrow reserve, prior therapy or marrow infiltration with malignant cells

Dosing adjustment in hepatic impairment:

Bilirubin 1.2-3 mg/dL: Reduce dose 50%

Bilirubin >3 mg/dL: Reduce dose 75%

Administration Administer slow IVP at a rate no faster than over 3-5 minutes or by I.V. infusion over 1-4 hours at a concentration not to exceed 2 mg/mL

Monitoring Parameters CBC with differential, erythrocyte and platelet count; echocardiogram, liver function tests including AST, ALT, alkaline phosphatase, and bilirubin; observe I.V. injection site for infiltration and vein irritation

Patient Information Transient red/orange discoloration of urine can occur for up to 48 hours after a dose; notify physician if fever, sore throat, bleeding, or bruising occurs

Nursing Implications Local erythematous streaking along the vein and/or facial flushing may indicate too rapid a rate of administration; drug is very irritating; avoid extravasation; if extravasation occurs, apply cold packs. Local infiltration with a corticosteroid and irrigating the site with normal saline may also be helpful.

Additional Information Myelosuppressive effects:

WBC: Moderate

Platelets: Moderate

Onset (days): 7

Nadir (days): 10-14

Recovery (days): 21-28

Dosage Forms

Injection:

Aqueous, with NS: 2 mg/mL (5 mL, 10 mL, 25 mL)

Preservative free: 2 mg/mL (5 mL, 10 mL, 25 mL, 100 mL)

Powder for injection, lyophilized: 10 mg, 20 mg, 50 mg, 100 mg

Powder for injection, lyophilized, rapid dissolution formula: 10 mg, 20 mg, 50 mg, 150 mg

References

Berg SL, Grisell DL, DeLaney TF, et al, "Principles of Treatment of Pediatric Solid Tumors," *Pediatr Clin North Am*, 1991, 38(2):249-67.

Ishii E, Hara T, Ohkubo K, et al, "Treatment of Childhood Acute Lymphoblastic Leukemia With Intermediate Dose Cytosine Arabinoside and Adriamycin," *Med Pediatr Oncol*, 1986, 14(2):73-7.

Legha SS, Benjamin RS, Mackay B, et al, "Reduction of Doxorubicin Cardiotoxicity by Prolonged Continuous Intravenous Infusion," *Ann Intern Med*, 1982, 96(2):133-9.

Doxy-200® *see* Doxycycline *on next page*

Doxy-Caps® *see* Doxycycline *on next page*

Doxychel® *see* Doxycycline *on next page*

Doxycycline (dox i sye' kleen)

Brand Names Bio-Tab®; Doryx®; Doxy-200®; Doxy-Caps®; Doxychel®; Doxy-Tabs®; Dynacin®; Monodox®; Vibramycin®; Vibra-Tabs®

Synonyms Doxycycline Hyclate; Doxycycline Monohydrate

Therapeutic Category Antibiotic, Tetracycline Derivative

Use Used principally in the treatment of infections caused by susceptible *Rickettsia*, *Chlamydia*, and *Mycoplasma* along with uncommon susceptible gram-negative and gram-positive organisms

Pregnancy Risk Factor D

Contraindications Hypersensitivity to doxycycline, tetracycline or any component; children <8 years; severe hepatic dysfunction

Warnings Photosensitivity reaction may occur with this drug; avoid prolonged exposure to sunlight or tanning equipment. Do not administer to children <8 years of age; use of tetracyclines during tooth development may cause permanent discoloration of the teeth and enamel hypoplasia; prolonged use may result in superinfection

Adverse Reactions

Central nervous system: Increased intracranial pressure, bulging fontanels in infants

Dermatologic: Rash, photosensitivity

Gastrointestinal: Nausea, diarrhea, esophagitis and esophageal ulceration with the hyclate salt formulation

Hematologic: Neutropenia, eosinophilia

Hepatic: Hepatotoxicity

Local: Phlebitis

Miscellaneous: May cause discoloration of teeth in children

Drug Interactions Antacids containing aluminum, calcium or magnesium, and iron and bismuth subsalicylate may decrease doxycycline bioavailability; barbiturates, phenytoin, and carbamazepine decrease doxycycline's half-life

Stability Reconstituted oral doxycycline suspension is stable for 2 weeks at room temperature; I.V. doxycycline solutions must be protected from direct sunlight

Mechanism of Action Inhibits protein synthesis by binding with the 30S and possibly the 50S ribosomal subunit(s) of susceptible bacteria; may also cause alterations in the cytoplasmic membrane

Pharmacokinetics

Absorption: Almost completely absorbed from the GI tract; absorption can be reduced by food or milk by 20%

Distribution: Appears in breast milk

Protein binding: 90%

Metabolism: Not metabolized in the liver, instead it is partially inactivated in the GI tract by chelate formation

Half-life: 12-15 hours (usually increases to 22-24 hours with multiple dosing)

Peak serum levels: Oral: Within 1.5-4 hours

Elimination: Excreted in the urine (23%) and feces (30%)

Not dialyzable (0% to 5%)

Usual Dosage Oral, I.V.:

Children ≥8 years: 2-5 mg/kg/day in 1-2 divided doses, not to exceed 200 mg/day

Adults: 100-200 mg/day in 1-2 divided doses

Administration Administer by slow I.V. intermittent infusion over a minimum of 1-2 hours at a concentration not to exceed 1 mg/mL (can be infused over 1-4 hours); concentrations <0.1 mg/mL are not recommended

Monitoring Parameters Periodic monitoring of renal, hepatic, and hematologic function tests

Test Interactions False-negative urine glucose using Clinistix®, Tes-Tape®

Patient Information Avoid unnecessary exposure to sunlight; do not take with antacids, iron products, or dairy products; take capsules or tablets with adequate amounts of fluid

Nursing Implications Check for signs of phlebitis; I.V. doxycycline should not be given I.M. or S.C.; avoid extravasation

Dosage Forms

Capsule, as hyclate: 50 mg, 100 mg

Capsule, coated pellets, as hyclate: 100 mg

Powder for injection, as hyclate: 100 mg, 200 mg

Powder for oral suspension, as monohydrate (raspberry flavor): 25 mg/5 mL (60 mL)
Syrup, as calcium (raspberry-apple flavor): 50 mg/5 mL (30 mL, 473 mL)
Tablet, as hyclate: 50 mg, 100 mg

Doxycycline Hyclate *see* Doxycycline *on previous page*

Doxycycline Monohydrate *see* Doxycycline *on previous page*

Doxy-Tabs® *see* Doxycycline *on previous page*

DPA *see* Valproic Acid and Derivatives *on page 592*

DPE *see* Dipivefrin Hydrochloride *on page 197*

D-Penicillamine *see* Penicillamine *on page 437*

DPH *see* Phenytoin *on page 455*

DPPC *see* Colfosceril Palmitate *on page 151*

Dramamine® [OTC] *see* Dimenhydrinate *on page 193*

Drisdol® *see* Ergocalciferol *on page 224*

Dristan® Long Lasting Nasal Solution [OTC] *see* Oxymetazoline Hydrochloride *on page 429*

Drixoral® Non-Drowsy [OTC]' *see* Pseudoephedrine *on page 497*

Dronabinol (droe nab' i nol)

Brand Names Marinol®

Synonyms Tetrahydrocannabinol, THC

Therapeutic Category Antiemetic

Use Used when conventional antiemetics fail to relieve the nausea and vomiting associated with cancer chemotherapy

Restrictions C-II

Pregnancy Risk Factor B

Contraindications Use only for cancer chemotherapy-induced nausea; should not be used in patients with a history of schizophrenia or in patients with known hypersensitivity to dronabinol, marijuana, or sesame oil

Precautions Use with caution in patients with heart disease, hepatic disease, or seizure disorders; reduce dosage in patients with severe hepatic impairment; may impair ability to perform hazardous tasks requiring mental alertness or physical coordination

Adverse Reactions

Cardiovascular: Orthostatic hypotension, tachycardia
Central nervous system: Drowsiness, dizziness, vertigo, difficulty concentrating, mood change, euphoria, detachment, depression, anxiety, paranoia, hallucinations
Gastrointestinal: Dry mouth

Drug Interactions Alcohol, CNS depressants, psychotomimetic substances, sedatives, barbiturates may result in additive drowsiness

Stability Store in a cool place

Mechanism of Action Not well defined, probably inhibits the vomiting center in the medulla oblongata

Pharmacokinetics

Absorption: Oral: Erratic; 10% to 20% absorption
Protein binding: 97% to 99%
Metabolism: Extensive first-pass metabolism; metabolized in the liver to several metabolites some of which are active
Half-life:
Biphasic: Alpha: 4 hours
Terminal: 25-36 hours
Peak serum levels: Within 2-3 hours
Elimination: Biliary excretion is the major route of elimination

Usual Dosage Children and Adults: Oral: 5 mg/m^2 1-3 hours before chemotherapy, then give 5 mg/m^2/dose every 2-4 hours after chemotherapy for a total of 4-6 doses/day; dose may be increased up to a maximum of 15 mg/m^2 per dose if needed (dosage may be increased in 2.5 mg/m^2 increments)

Monitoring Parameters Heart rate, blood pressure

Patient Information Avoid activities such as driving which require motor coordination

(Continued)

Dronabinol *(Continued)*

Dosage Forms Capsule: 2.5 mg, 5 mg, 10 mg

References

Lane M, Smith FE, Sullivan RA, et al, "Dronabinol and Prochlorperazine Alone and in Combination as Antiemetic Agents for Cancer Chemotherapy," *Am J Clin Oncol*, 1990, 13(6):480-4.

Droperidol (droe per' i dole)

Related Information

Compatibility of Medications Mixed in a Syringe *on page 717*

Brand Names Inapsine®

Therapeutic Category Antiemetic

Use As a tranquilizer and antiemetic in surgical and diagnostic procedures; antiemetic for cancer chemotherapy; preoperative medication

Pregnancy Risk Factor C

Contraindications Hypersensitivity to droperidol or any component

Precautions Use with caution in patients with impaired hepatic or renal function

Adverse Reactions

Cardiovascular: Hypotension, tachycardia

Central nervous system: Dystonic reactions, akathisia, oculogyric crisis, anxiety, hyperactivity, drowsiness, dizziness, hallucinations, chills

Respiratory: Laryngospasm, bronchospasm

Drug Interactions Other CNS depressants → additive effects (CNS, respiratory depression, etc); droperidol plus fentanyl or other other analgesics → ↑ blood pressure; conduction anesthesia may ↑ hypotension; droperidol plus epinephrine → ↓ blood pressure due to alpha-adrenergic blockade effects of droperidol

Mechanism of Action Alters the action of dopamine in the CNS, at subcortical levels, to produce sedation

Pharmacodynamics

Peak effects: Parenteral: Within 30 minutes

Duration: 2-4 hours (up to 12 hours)

Pharmacokinetics

Metabolism: Metabolized in the liver

Half-life, adults: 2.3 hours

Elimination: Excreted in the urine (75%) and feces (22%)

Usual Dosage Titrate carefully to desired effect

Children 2-12 years:

- Premedication: I.M.: 0.088-0.165 mg/kg
- Adjunct to general anesthesia: I.V. induction: 0.088-0.165 mg/kg
- Nausea and vomiting: I.M., I.V.: 0.05-0.06 mg/kg/dose every 4-6 hours as needed

Adults:

- Premedication: I.M.: 2.5-10 mg 30-60 minutes preoperatively
- Adjunct to general anesthesia: I.V. induction: 0.22-0.275 mg/kg; maintenance: 1.25-2.5 mg/dose
- Alone in diagnostic procedures: I.M.: Initial: 2.5-10 mg 30-60 minutes before, then 1.25-2.5 mg if needed
- Nausea and vomiting: I.M., I.V.: 2.5-5 mg/dose every 3-4 hours as needed

Administration I.V. over 2-5 minutes

Monitoring Parameters Blood pressure, heart rate, respiratory rate

Additional Information Does not possess analgesic effects; has little or no amnesic properties

Dosage Forms Injection: 2.5 mg/mL (1 mL, 2 mL, 5 mL, 10 mL)

Droperidol and Fentanyl (droe per' i dole)

Related Information

Overdose and Toxicology Information *on page 696-700*

Brand Names Innovar®

Synonyms Fentanyl and Droperidol

Therapeutic Category Analgesic, Narcotic

Use To produce and maintain analgesia and sedation during diagnostic or surgical procedures (neuroleptanalgesia and neuroleptanesthesia); adjunct to general anesthesia

Restrictions C-II
Pregnancy Risk Factor C
Contraindications Hypersensitivity to droperidol or fentanyl, patients who have taken MAO inhibitors within 14 days
Warnings Rapid I.V. injection can cause muscle rigidity, particularly involving those muscles of respiration.
Precautions Use with caution in patients with impaired hepatic, renal, or respiratory function and those with pre-existing cardiac bradyarrhythmias
Adverse Reactions
Cardiovascular: Hypotension, hypertension, bradycardia
Central nervous system: Postoperative drowsiness, dysphoria, disorientation, restlessness, delirium, extrapyramidal symptoms
Endocrine & metabolic: Hyperglycemia
Gastrointestinal: Nausea, vomiting
Musculoskeletal: Muscular rigidity
Ocular: Miosis
Respiratory: Respiratory depression, apnea
Miscellaneous: Hypothermia, shivering
Drug Interactions CNS depressant drugs → additive effects; MAO inhibitors
Mechanism of Action See individual monographs for Droperidol and Fentanyl Citrate
Usual Dosage
Children:
Premedication: I.M.: 0.03 mL/kg 30-60 minutes prior to procedure
Adjunct to general anesthesia: I.V.: Total dose: 0.05 mL/kg as slow infusion (1 mL/1-2 minutes) until sleep occurs

Adults:
Premedication: I.M.: 0.5-2 mL 30-60 minutes prior to surgery
Adjunct to general anesthesia: I.V.: 0.09-0.11 mL/kg as slow infusion (1 mL/1-2 minutes) until sleep occurs
Monitoring Parameters Vital signs, oxygen saturation, blood pressure
Nursing Implications An opioid antagonist, resuscitative and intubation equipment, and oxygen should be available
Dosage Forms Injection: Droperidol 2.5 mg and fentanyl 50 μg per mL (2 mL, 5 mL)

Drotic® *see* Neomycin, (Bacitracin) Polymyxin B and Hydrocortisone *on page 406*

Dry and Clear® [OTC] *see* Benzoyl Peroxide *on page 78*

DSCG *see* Cromolyn Sodium *on page 158*

DSS *see* Docusate *on page 202*

DSS With Casanthranol *see* Docusate and Casanthranol *on page 203*

DTIC-Dome® *see* Dacarbazine *on page 168*

***d*-Tubocurarine Chloride** *see* Tubocurarine Chloride *on page 589*

Dulcagen® [OTC] *see* Bisacodyl *on page 83*

Dulcolax® [OTC] *see* Bisacodyl *on page 83*

Dull-C® [OTC] *see* Ascorbic Acid *on page 59*

DuoCet™ *see* Hydrocodone and Acetaminophen *on page 292*

Duo-Trach® *see* Lidocaine Hydrochloride *on page 342*

Duphalac® *see* Lactulose *on page 334*

Duplex® T [OTC] *see* Coal Tar *on page 147*

Dura-Estrin® *see* Estradiol *on page 231*

Duragesic™ *see* Fentanyl Citrate *on page 240*

Dura-Gest® *see* Guaifenesin, Phenylpropanolamine, and Phenylephrine *on page 280*

Duralone® *see* Methylprednisolone *on page 379*

Duramorph® *see* Morphine Sulfate *on page 394*

Duratears® [OTC] *see* Ocular Lubricant *on page 423*

Duratest® *see* Testosterone *on page 550*

Durathate® *see* Testosterone *on page 550*

Duration® Nasal Solution [OTC] *see* Oxymetazoline Hydrochloride *on page 429*

Duvoid® *see* Bethanechol Chloride *on page 82*

Dycill® *see* Dicloxacillin Sodium *on page 186*

Dyclone® *see* Dyclonine Hydrochloride *on this page*

Dyclonine Hydrochloride (dye' kloe neen)

Brand Names Dyclone®; Sucrets® [OTC]

Therapeutic Category Local Anesthetic, Oral

Use As a local anesthetic prior to laryngoscopy, bronchoscopy, or endotracheal intubation; used topically for temporary relief of pain associated with oral mucosa, skin, episiotomy, or anogenital lesions; the 0.5% topical solution may be used to block the gag reflex, and to relieve the pain of oral ulcers or stomatitis

Pregnancy Risk Factor C

Contraindications Contraindicated in patients allergic to chlorobutanol (preservative used in dyclonine) or dyclonine

Warnings Resuscitative equipment, oxygen and resuscitative drugs should be immediately available when dyclonine topical solution is administered to mucous membranes

Precautions Use with caution in patients with sepsis or traumatized mucosa in the area of application to avoid rapid systemic absorption; may impair swallowing and enhance the danger of aspiration; use with caution in patients with shock or heart block

Adverse Reactions

Cardiovascular: Hypotension, bradycardia, respiratory arrest, cardiac arrest

Central nervous system: Excitation, drowsiness, nervousness, dizziness, seizures

Dermatologic: Rash, urticaria

Local: Slight irritation and stinging may occur when applied, swelling

Ocular: Blurred vision

Miscellaneous: Allergic reactions

Excessive dosage and rapid absorption may result in the adverse CNS and cardiovascular effects,

Mechanism of Action Blocks impulses at peripheral nerve endings in skin and mucous membranes by altering cell membrane permeability to ionic transfer

Pharmacodynamics

Onset of local anesthesia: 2-10 minutes

Duration: 30-60 minutes

Usual Dosage Children and Adults: Topical solution:

Mouth sores: 5-10 mL of 0.5% or 1% to oral mucosa (swab or swish and then spit) 3-4 times/day as needed; maximum single dose: 200 mg (40 mL of 0.5% solution or 20 mL of 1% solution); solution may be diluted 1:1 with water

Sore throat pain: Slowly dissolve lozenge in mouth every 2 hours if necessary

Bronchoscopy: Use 2 mL of the 1% solution or 4 mL of the 0.5% solution sprayed onto the larynx and trachea every 5 minutes until the reflex has been abolished

Patient Information Food should not be ingested for 60 minutes following application in the mouth or throat area; numbness of the tongue and buccal mucosa may result in increased risk of biting trauma; may impair swallowing

Nursing Implications Administer 60 minutes prior to oral food or fluids; use the lowest dose needed to provide effective anesthesia; not for injection; do not apply nasally or to the eye

Dosage Forms

Lozenges: 1.2 mg, 3 mg

Solution, topical: 0.1%, 0.5%, 1%

References

Carnel SB, Blakeslee DB, Oswald SG, et al, "Treatment of Radiation- and Chemotherapy-Induced Stomatitis," *Otolaryngol Head Neck Surg*, 1990, 102(4):326-30.

Dynacin® *see* Doxycycline *on page 210*

Dynapen® *see* Dicloxacillin Sodium *on page 186*

Dyrenium® *see* Triamterene *on page 580*

Easprin® *see* Aspirin *on page 61*

Econazole Nitrate (e kone' a zole)

Brand Names Spectazole™

Therapeutic Category Antifungal Agent, Topical

Use Topical treatment of tinea pedis, tinea cruris, tinea corporis, tinea versicolor, and cutaneous candidiasis

Pregnancy Risk Factor C

Contraindications Known hypersensitivity to econazole or any component

Warnings Not for ophthalmic or intravaginal use

Precautions Discontinue the drug if sensitivity or chemical irritation occurs

Adverse Reactions

Dermatologic: Pruritus, erythema

Local: Burning, stinging

Mechanism of Action Alters fungal cell wall membrane permeability; may interfere with RNA and protein synthesis, and lipid metabolism

Pharmacokinetics

Absorption: Following topical administration <10% is percutaneously absorbed

Metabolism: Metabolized in the liver to >20 metabolites

Elimination: <1% of an applied dose recovered in the urine or feces

Usual Dosage Children and Adults: Topical: Apply a sufficient amount to cover affected areas. For tinea cruris, corporis, pedis, and cutaneous candidiasis: Apply twice daily; tinea versicolor: once daily

Patient Information For external use only

Additional Information Candidal infections and tinea cruris, versicolor, and corporis should be treated for 2 weeks and tinea pedis for 1 month; occasionally, longer treatment periods may be required

Dosage Forms Cream: 1% (15 g, 30 g, 85 g)

Econopred® *see* Prednisolone *on page 476*

Econopred® Plus *see* Prednisolone *on page 476*

Ecotrin® [OTC] *see* Aspirin *on page 61*

Edecrin® *see* Ethacrynic Acid *on page 233*

Edetate Calcium Disodium (ed' e tate)

Brand Names Calcium Disodium Versenate®

Synonyms Calcium Disodium Edathamil; Calcium Disodium Edetate; Calcium Edetate; Calcium EDTA

Therapeutic Category Antidote, Lead Toxicity

Use Treatment of acute and chronic lead poisoning; also used as an aid in the diagnosis of lead poisoning

Pregnancy Risk Factor C

Contraindications Severe renal disease, anuria

Warnings Do not exceed recommended daily dose; avoid rapid I.V. infusion in the management of lead encephalopathy, intracranial pressure may be increased to lethal levels

Precautions Renal tubular necrosis and fatal nephrosis may occur, especially with high doses; establish urine flow prior to administration

Adverse Reactions

Cardiovascular: Hypotension, nasal congestion, arrhythmias, EKG changes

Central nervous system: Numbness, tingling, fever, headache, chills

Dermatologic: Skin lesions

Endocrine & metabolic: Hypercalcemia

Gastrointestinal: GI upset

Hematologic: Transient marrow suppression

(Continued)

Edetate Calcium Disodium *(Continued)*

Local: Pain at injection site following I.M. injection, thrombophlebitis following I.V. infusion (when concentration >5 mg/mL)

Ocular: Lacrimation

Renal & genitourinary: Renal tubular necrosis, proteinuria, microscopic hematuria

Respiratory: Sneezing

Drug Interactions Do not use simultaneously with zinc insulin preparations, do not mix in the same syringe with dimercaprol

Stability Dilute with 0.9% sodium chloride or D_5W; physically incompatible with $D_{10}W$, Lactated Ringer's, Ringer's

Mechanism of Action Calcium is displaced by divalent and trivalent heavy metals, forming a nonionizing soluble complex that is excreted in the urine

Pharmacodynamics When administered I.V., urinary excretion of chelated lead begins in 1 hour and peak excretion of chelated lead occurs within 24-48 hours

Pharmacokinetics

Absorption: I.M., S.C.: Well absorbed

Distribution: Distributed into extracellular fluid; minimal CSF penetration

Half-life, plasma:

I.M.: 1.5 hours

I.V.: 20 minutes

Elimination: Rapidly excreted in urine as metal chelates or unchanged drug, ↓ GFR decreases elimination

Usual Dosage Children: I.M., I.V. (several regimens have been recommended):

Diagnosis of lead poisoning: Mobilization test:

Children: 500 mg/m²/dose, (maximum: 1 g) as a single dose or divided into 2 doses I.M.

Adults: 500 mg/m²/dose

Note: Urine is collected for 24 hours after first EDTA dose and analyzed for lead content; if the ratio of μg of lead in urine to mg calcium EDTA given is >1, then test is considered positive; for convenience, an 8-hour urine collection may be done after a 500 mg/m² dose; a positive test occurs if the ratio of lead excretion to mg calcium EDTA >0.5-0.6.

Treatment of lead poisoning: Children and Adults:

Symptoms of lead encephalopathy and/or blood lead level >70 μg/dL: 1.5 g/m² I.V. as either an 8-24 hour infusion or divided into 2 doses every 12 hours **or** 250 mg/m²/dose I.M. every 4 hours, treat 5 days; give in conjunction with dimercaprol

Symptomatic lead poisoning **without** encephalopathy **or** asymptomatic with blood lead level >70 μg/dL:

I.V.: 1 g/m² as an 8-24 hour infusion or divided every 12 hours **or** I.M.: 167 mg/m² every 4 hours; treat 3-5 days; treatment with dimercaprol is recommended until the blood lead level concentration <50 μg/dL

Asymptomatic **children** with blood lead level 45-69 μg/dL: 1 g/m² as an 8 to 24-hour infusion or divided into 2 doses every 12 hours

Note: Depending upon the blood lead level, additional courses may be necessary; give at least 2-4 days and preferably 2-4 weeks apart

Adults with lead nephropathy: An alternative dosing regimen reflecting the reduction in renal clearance is based upon the serum creatinine (see table):

Alternative Dosing Regimen for Adults with Renal Failure

Serum creatinine	Ca EDTA dosage
≤2 mg/dL	1 g/m²/day for 5 days
2–3	500 mg/m²/day for 5 days
3–4	500 mg/m²/dose every 48 hours for 3 doses
>4	500 mg/m²/week

Repeat these regimens monthly until lead excretion is reduced toward normal.

Administration For intermittent I.V. infusion, administer the dose I.V. over at least one hour in asymptomatic patients, 2 hours in symptomatic patients; for single daily I.V. (continuous infusion), dilute to 2-4 mg/mL in D_5W or NS and infuse over at least 8 hour, usually over 12-24 hours; for I.M. injection, 1 mL of 1% lidocaine or procaine hydrochloride may be added to each mL of EDTA calcium to minimize pain at I.M. injection site

Monitoring Parameters BUN, serum creatinine, urinalysis, fluid balance, EKG

Test Interactions If calcium EDTA is given as a continuous I.V. infusion, stop the infusion for at least 1 hour before blood is drawn for lead concentration to avoid a falsely elevated value

Additional Information If anuria, increasing proteinuria, or hematuria occurs during therapy, discontinue calcium EDTA

Dosage Forms Injection: 200 mg/mL (5 mL)

Edrophonium Chloride (ed roe foe' nee um)

Related Information

Overdose and Toxicology Information *on page 696-700*

Brand Names Enlon®; Reversol®; Tensilon®

Therapeutic Category Antidote, Neuromuscular Blocking Agent; Cholinergic Agent; Diagnostic Agent, Myasthenia Gravis

Use Diagnosis of myasthenia gravis; differentiation of cholinergic crises from myasthenia crises; reversal of nondepolarizing neuromuscular blockers; treatment of paroxysmal atrial tachycardia

Pregnancy Risk Factor C

Contraindications Hypersensitivity to edrophonium or any component (injection contains sodium sulfite and phenol), GI or GU mechanical obstruction

Precautions Use with caution in asthmatic patients and those receiving a cardiac glycoside

Adverse Reactions

Cardiovascular: Arrhythmias (especially bradycardia), hypotension
Central nervous system: Seizures
Gastrointestinal: Nausea, vomiting, diarrhea, excessive salivation
Musculoskeletal: Weakness, muscle cramps
Ocular: Diplopia, miosis
Renal & genitourinary: Urinary frequency
Respiratory: Laryngospasm, bronchospasm, respiratory paralysis
Miscellaneous: Sweating

Drug Interactions Digoxin, succinylcholine, decamethonium, nondepolarizing muscle relaxants (ie, pancuronium, vecuronium)

Mechanism of Action Inhibits destruction of acetylcholine by acetylcholinesterase. This facilitates transmission of impulses across myoneural junction and results in increased cholinergic responses such as miosis, increased tonus of intestinal and skeletal muscles, bronchial and ureteral constriction, bradycardia, and increased salivary and sweat gland secretions

Pharmacodynamics

Onset:
- I.M.: 2-10 minutes
- I.V.: 30-60 seconds

Duration:
- I.M.: 5-30 minutes
- I.V.: 5-10 minutes

Usual Dosage Usually administered I.V., however, if not possible, I.M. or S.C. may be used

Infants:
- I.M.: 0.5-1 mg
- I.V.: Initial: 0.1 mg, followed by 0.4 mg (if no response); total dose = 0.5 mg

Children:
- Diagnosis: Initial:
  - I.M.: ≤34 kg: 1 mg; >34 kg: 5 mg
  - I.V.: 0.04 mg/kg given over 1 minute followed by 0.16 mg/kg given within 45 seconds (if no response)

(Continued)

Edrophonium Chloride *(Continued)*

Titration of oral anticholinesterase therapy: 0.04 mg/kg once given 1 hour after oral intake of the drug being used in treatment; if strength improves, an increase in neostigmine or pyridostigmine dose is indicated

Adults:

Diagnosis:

I.M.: Initial: 10 mg; if cholinergic reaction occurs, give 2 mg 30 minutes later to rule out false-negative reaction

I.V.: 2 mg test dose administered over 15-30 seconds; 8 mg given 45 seconds later (if no response is seen). Test dose may be repeated after 30 minutes.

Titration of oral anticholinesterase therapy: 1-2 mg given 1 hour after oral dose of anticholinesterase; if strength improves, an increase in neostigmine or pyridostigmine dose is indicated

Differentiation of cholinergic from myasthenic crisis: I.V.: 1 mg, may repeat after one minute (**Note:** Intubation and controlled ventilation may be required if patient has cholinergic crises.)

Reversal of nondepolarizing neuromuscular blocking agents (neostigmine with atropine usually preferred): I.V.: 10 mg over 30-45 seconds, may repeat every 5-10 minutes up to 40 mg total dose

Termination of paroxysmal atrial tachycardia: I.V.: 5-10 mg

Administration Edrophonium is administered by direct I.V. injection; see Usual Dosage

Monitoring Parameters Pre- and postinjection strength (cranial musculature is most useful); heart rate, respiratory rate, blood pressure

Additional Information Overdosage can cause cholinergic crisis which may be fatal; I.V. atropine should be readily available for treatment of cholinergic reactions

Dosage Forms Injection: 10 mg/mL (1 mL, 10 mL, 15 mL)

E.E.S.® *see* Erythromycin *on page 226*

E.E.S. 400® *see* Erythromycin *on page 226*

E.E.S.® Chewable *see* Erythromycin *on page 226*

E.E.S.® Granules *see* Erythromycin *on page 226*

Effer-Syllium® [OTC] *see* Psyllium *on page 498*

Efudex® *see* Fluorouracil *on page 257*

EHDP *see* Etidronate Disodium *on page 236*

Elavil® *see* Amitriptyline Hydrochloride *on page 41*

Electrolyte Lavage Solution *see* Polyethylene Glycol-Electrolyte Solution *on page 466*

Elimite™ *see* Permethrin *on page 448*

Elixicon® *see* Theophylline *on page 554*

Elixophyllin® *see* Theophylline *on page 554*

Elixophyllin® SR *see* Theophylline *on page 554*

E-Lor® *see* Propoxyphene and Acetaminophen *on page 492*

Elspar® *see* Asparaginase *on page 60*

Emergency Pediatric Drip Calculations *see page 615*

Emete-Con® *see* Benzquinamide Hydrochloride *on page 78*

Emetogenic Potential of Single Chemotherapeutic Agents *see page 655*

Emgel® *see* Erythromycin *on page 226*

EMLA® *see* Lidocaine and Prilocaine *on page 341*

Empirin® [OTC] *see* Aspirin *on page 61*

Emulsoil® [OTC] *see* Castor Oil *on page 109*

E-Mycin® *see* Erythromycin *on page 226*

E-Mycin-E® *see* Erythromycin *on page 226*

Enalapril/Enalaprilat (e nal' a pril)

Brand Names Vasotec®

Therapeutic Category Angiotensin Converting Enzyme (ACE) Inhibitors; Antihypertensive

Use Management of mild to severe hypertension and congestive heart failure

Pregnancy Risk Factor D

Contraindications Hypersensitivity to enalapril, enalaprilat or any component

Warnings ACE inhibitor can cause injury and death to the developing fetus when used during the second and third trimesters of pregnancy

Precautions Use with caution and modify dosage in patients with renal impairment (especially renal artery stenosis), hyponatremia, hypovolemia, severe congestive heart failure or with coadministered diuretic therapy; experience in children is limited

Adverse Reactions

Cardiovascular: Hypotension, syncope
Central nervous system: Fatigue, vertigo, insomnia, dizziness, headache
Dermatologic: Rash
Endocrine & metabolic: Hypoglycemia, hyperkalemia, impotence
Gastrointestinal: Nausea, diarrhea
Hematologic: Agranulocytosis, neutropenia, anemia
Musculoskeletal: Muscle cramps
Renal & genitourinary: Deterioration in renal function
Respiratory: Cough
Miscellaneous: Loss of taste perception; angioedema

Drug Interactions Use with potassium sparing diuretics → additive hyperkalemic effect; hypotensive agent or diuretics → ↑ hypotensive effect; indomethacin may ↓ hypotensive effect

Mechanism of Action Competitive inhibitor of angiotensin converting enzyme (ACE); prevents conversion of angiotensin I to angiotensin II, a potent vasoconstrictor; results in lower levels of angiotensin II which causes an increase in plasma renin activity and a reduction in aldosterone secretion

Pharmacodynamics

Onset of action: Oral: Within 1 hour
Maximum effect: Within 4-8 hours
Duration: 12-24 hours

Pharmacokinetics

Absorption: Oral: 55% to 75% (enalapril)
Protein binding: 50% to 60%
Metabolism: Enalapril is a prodrug and undergoes biotransformation to enalaprilat in the liver
Half-life:
- Enalapril:
  - Healthy adults: 2 hours
  - CHF adults: 3.4-5.8 hours
- Enalaprilat:
  - Infants 6 weeks to 8 months: 6-10 hours
  - Adults: 35-38 hours

Peak serum levels: Oral:
- Enalapril: Within 0.5-1.5 hours
- Enalaprilat (active): Within 3-4.5 hours

Elimination: Excreted principally in the urine (60% to 80%) with some fecal excretion

Usual Dosage Use lower listed initial dose in patients with hyponatremia, hypovolemia, severe congestive heart failure, ↓ renal function, or in those receiving diuretics

Infants and Children:
- Oral: **Enalapril**: Initial: 0.1 mg/kg/day; increase as required over 2 weeks to maximum of 0.5 mg/kg/day
- I.V.: **Enalaprilat**: 5-10 μg/kg/dose administered every 8-24 hours (as determined by blood pressure readings) has been used for the treatment of neonatal hypertension; monitor patients carefully; select patients may require higher doses

Adults:
- Oral: **Enalapril**: 2.5-5 mg/day then increase as required, usually 10-40 mg/day in 1-2 divided doses

(Continued)

Enalapril/Enalaprilat *(Continued)*

I.V.: **Enalaprilat**: 0.625-1.25 mg/dose, given over 5 minutes every 6 hours

Dosing adjustment in renal impairment:

Cl_{cr} 10-50 mL/minute: Administer 75% to 100% of dose

Cl_{cr} <10 mL/minute: Administer 50% of dose

Administration I.V.: Give as I.V. infusion (undiluted solution or further diluted) over 5 minutes

Monitoring Parameters Blood pressure, renal function, WBC, serum potassium

Additional Information Severe hypotension may occur in patients who are sodium and/or volume depleted, initiate lower doses and monitor closely when starting therapy in these patients

Dosage Forms

Injection, as enalaprilat: 1.25 mg/mL (1 mL, 2 mL)

Tablet: 2.5 mg, 5 mg, 10 mg, 20 mg

References

Frenneaux M, Stewart RA, Newman CM, et al, "Enalapril for Severe Heart Failure in Infancy," *Arch Dis Child*, 1989, 64(2):219-23.

Lloyd TR, Mahoney LT, Knoedel D, et al, "Orally Administered Enalapril for Infants With Congestive Heart Failure: A Dose Finding Study," *J Pediatr*, 1989, 114(4 Pt 1):650-4.

Marcadis ML, Kraus DM, Hatzopoulos FK, et al, "Use of Enalaprilat for Neonatal Hypertension," *J Pediatr*, 1991, 119(3):505-6.

Wells TG, Bunchman TE, Kearns GL, "Treatment of Neonatal Hypertension With Enalaprilat," *J Pediatr*, 1990, 117(4):664-7.

Endep® *see* Amitriptyline Hydrochloride *on page 41*

Endocarditis Prophylaxis *see page 659*

Enlon® *see* Edrophonium Chloride *on page 217*

Enomine® *see* Guaifenesin, Phenylpropanolamine, and Phenylephrine *on page 280*

Enovil® *see* Amitriptyline Hydrochloride *on page 41*

Entex® *see* Guaifenesin, Phenylpropanolamine, and Phenylephrine *on page 280*

Entozyme® *see* Pancreatin *on page 430*

Enulose® *see* Lactulose *on page 334*

Epifrin® *see* Epinephrine *on this page*

Epinal® *see* Epinephrine *on this page*

Epinephrine (ep i nef' rin)

Related Information

CPR Pediatric Drug Dosages *on page 614*

Emergency Pediatric Drip Calculations *on page 615*

Extravasation Treatment *on page 640*

Brand Names Adrenalin®; AsthmaHaler®; AsthmaNefrin® [OTC]; Bronitin®; Bronkaid® Mist [OTC]; Epifrin®; Epinal®; EpiPen®; EpiPen® Jr; Eppy/N®; Glaucon®; Medihaler-Epi®; microNefrin®; Primatene® Mist [OTC]; Sus-Phrine®; Vaponefrin®

Synonyms Adrenaline; Epinephrine Bitartrate; Epinephrine Hydrochloride; Racemic Epinephrine

Therapeutic Category Adrenergic Agonist Agent; Antidote, Hypersensitivity Reactions; Bronchodilator; Sympathomimetic

Use Treatment of bronchospasm, anaphylactic reactions, cardiac arrest, and management of open-angle (chronic simple) glaucoma

Pregnancy Risk Factor C

Contraindications Hypersensitivity to epinephrine or any component; cardiac arrhythmias, angle closure glaucoma

Precautions Patients that are geriatric, have diabetes mellitus, cardiovascular disease (angina, tachycardia, myocardial infarction), thyroid disease, or cerebral arteriosclerosis

Adverse Reactions

Cardiovascular: Pallor, tachycardia, hypertension, increased myocardial oxygen consumption, cardiac arrhythmias, sudden death

Central nervous system: Anxiety, headache
Gastrointestinal: Nausea
Musculoskeletal: Weakness, tremor
Ocular: Precipitation of or exacerbation of narrow-angle glaucoma
Renal & genitourinary: Decreased renal and splanchnic blood flow, acute urinary retention in patients with bladder outflow obstruction

Drug Interactions Increased cardiac irritability if administered concurrently with halogenated inhalational anesthetics; beta blocking agents (ie, propranolol); alpha blocking agents (ie, phentolamine)

Stability Protect from light; incompatible with alkaline solutions (sodium bicarbonate); compatible when coadministered with dopamine and dobutamine

Mechanism of Action Stimulates alpha, beta$_1$- and beta$_2$-adrenergic receptors resulting in relaxation of smooth muscle of the bronchial tree, cardiac stimulation, and dilation of skeletal muscle vasculature; small doses can cause vasodilation via beta$_2$ vascular receptors; large doses may produce constriction of skeletal and vascular smooth muscle; decreases production of aqueous humor and increases aqueous outflow; dilates the pupil by contracting the dilator muscle

Pharmacodynamics

Onset of bronchodilation:
- S.C.: Within 5-10 minutes
- Inhalation: Within 1 minute

Peak ocular effect: Following conjunctival instillation intraocular pressures fall within 1 hour with a maximal response occurring within 4-8 hours
Duration: Ocular effects persist for 12-24 hours

Pharmacokinetics

Absorption: Orally ingested doses are rapidly metabolized in GI tract and liver; pharmacologically active concentrations are **not** achieved
Distribution: Crosses placenta but not blood-brain barrier
Elimination: Extensively metabolized in liver and other tissues by the enzymes catechol-o-methyltransferase and monoamine oxidase

Usual Dosage

Neonates: I.V., Intratracheal: 0.01-0.03 mg/kg (0.1-0.3 mL/kg of **1:10,000** solution) every 3-5 minutes as needed; dilute intratracheal doses to 1-2 mL with normal saline

Infants and Children:
- S.C.: 0.01 mg/kg (0.01 mL/kg/dose **1:1000**) not to exceed 0.5 mg **or**
- Suspension: 0.005 mL/kg/dose (1:200); not to exceed 0.15 mL every 8-12 hours
- Bradycardia:
  - I.V.: 0.01 mg/kg (0.1 mL/kg) of **1:10,000** solution (maximum: 1 mg 10 mL)
  - Intratracheal: 0.1 mg/kg (0.1 mL/kg) of **1:1000** solution; doses as high as 0.2 mg/kg may be effective
- Asystole or pulseless arrest:
  - I.V. or intraosseus: **First dose:** 0.01 mg/kg (0.1 mL/kg) of 1:10,000 solution; **Subsequent doses**: 0.1 mg/kg (0.1 mL/kg of **1:1000** solution; doses as high as 0.2 mg/kg may be effective); repeat every 3-5 minutes as needed
  - Intratracheal: 0.1 mg/kg (0.1 mL/kg) of **1:1000** solution (doses as high as 0.2 mg/kg may be effective)
- Continuous infusion rate: 1-10 μg/kg/minute; titrate dosage to desired effect
- Nebulization: 0.25-0.5 mL of 2.25% **racemic epinephrine** solution diluted in 3 mL normal saline, or L-epinephrine at an equivalent dose; racemic epinephrine 10 mg = 5 mg L-epinephrine; use lower end of dosing range for younger infants
- Ophthalmic: Instill 1-2 drops in eye(s) once or twice daily

Adults:
- Asystole: I.V.: 1 mg every 3-5 minutes; if this approach fails, alternative regimens include:
  - Intermediate: 2-5 mg every 3-5 minutes
  - Escalating: 1 mg, 3 mg, 5 mg at 3-minute intervals
  - High: 0.1 mg/kg every 3-5 minutes
- Intratracheal: 1 mg (although the optimal dose is unknown, doses of 2-2.5 times the I.V. dose may be needed)

(Continued)

Epinephrine *(Continued)*

I.M., S.C.: 0.1-0.5 mg every 10-15 minutes

Continuous infusion rate: 0.1-1 μg/kg/minute; titrate dosage to desired effect

Ophthalmic: Instill 1-2 drops in eye(s) once or twice daily; when treating open-angle glaucoma, the concentration and dosage must be adjusted to the response of the patient

Administration For continuous infusion: rate of infusion (mL/hour) = dose (μg/kg/minute) x weight (kg) x 60 minutes/hour divided by the concentration (μg/mL); maximum concentration: 64 μg/mL

Monitoring Parameters Heart rate, blood pressure, site of infusion for excessive blanching/extravasation

Nursing Implications Tissue irritant; extravasation may be treated by local small injections of a diluted phentolamine solution (mix 5 mg with 9 mL normal saline)

Dosage Forms

Aerosol, oral, as bitartrate: 0.16 mg/inhalation (10 mL, 15 mL)

Inhalation, oral, as hydrochloride: 1% (15 mL)

Injection: 0.01 mg/mL (5 mL); 0.1 mg/mL [1:10,000] (3 mL, 10 mL); 1 mg/mL [1:1000] (1 mL, 2 mL, 30 mL)

Auto-injector:

EpiPen®: Delivers 0.3 mg I.M. of epinephrine 1:1000 (2 mL)

EpiPen® Jr.: Delivers 0.15 mg I.M. of epinephrine 1:2000 (2 mL)

Suspension: 1.5 mg/0.3 mL (1:200) (0.3 mL)

Solution:

Oral nebulization, as racemic: Racemic epinephrine is equivalent to 2.25% epinephrine base (7.5 mL, 15 mL, 30 mL)

Nasal: 1 mg/mL [1:1000] (30 mL)

Ophthalmic, as borate: 0.5% (7.5 mL); 1% (7.5 mL); 2% (7.5 mL)

Ophthalmic, as hydrochloride: 0.1% (1 mL, 30 mL); 0.25% (15 mL); 0.5% (15 mL); 1% (1 mL, 10 mL, 15 mL); 2% (10 mL, 15 mL)

Topical: 0.1% (30 mL) mL, 10 mL); 0.01 mg/mL = 1:100,000 (5 mL)

Suspension: 5 mg/mL (1:200)

Solution for oral nebulization, as racemic (Vaponefrin®, microNefrin®, AsthmaNefrin®): 2.25% (7.5 mL, 15 mL, 30 mL)

Solution:

Nasal: 1 mg/mL = 1:1000 (30 mL)

Ophthalmic, as bitartrate: 1% (7.5 mL)

Ophthalmic, as borate: 0.5% (7.5 mL); 1% (7.5 mL); 2% (7.5 mL)

Ophthalmic, as hydrochloride: 0.1% (1 mL, 30 mL); 0.25% (15 mL); 0.5% (15

References

American College of Cardiology, American Heart Association Task Force, "Adult Advanced Cardiac Life Support" and "Pediatric Advanced Life Support Guidelines," *JAMA*, 1992, 268(16):2199-241 and 2262-75.

Waisman Y, Klein BL, Boenning DA, et al, "Prospective Randomized Double-Blind Study Comparing L-Epinephrine and Racemic Epinephrine Aerosols in the Treatment of Laryngotracheitis (Croup)," *Pediatrics*, 1992, 89(2):302-6.

Epinephrine Bitartrate *see* Epinephrine *on page 220*

Epinephrine Hydrochloride *see* Epinephrine *on page 220*

EpiPen® *see* Epinephrine *on page 220*

EpiPen® Jr *see* Epinephrine *on page 220*

Epitol® *see* Carbamazepine *on page 101*

EPO *see* Epoetin Alfa *on this page*

Epoetin Alfa (e poe' e tin)

Brand Names Epogen®; Procrit®

Synonyms EPO; Erythropoietin; HuEPO

Therapeutic Category Colony Stimulating Factor; Recombinant Human Erythropoietin

Use Treatment of anemia associated with chronic renal failure; anemia related to therapy with AZT-treated HIV-infected patients; anemia of prematurity

Pregnancy Risk Factor C

Contraindications Known hypersensitivity to albumin human; uncontrolled hypertension; neutropenia in newborns

Precautions Use with caution in patients with porphyria

Adverse Reactions

Cardiovascular: Hypertension, edema, chest pain

Central nervous system: Fatigue, dizziness, headache, seizure

Dermatologic: Rash

Gastrointestinal: Nausea

Musculoskeletal: Arthralgias

Miscellaneous: Hypersensitivity reactions

Mechanism of Action Induces erythropoiesis by stimulating the division and differentiation of committed erythroid progenitor cells; induces the release of reticulocytes from the bone marrow into the blood stream, where they mature to erythrocytes

Pharmacodynamics

Onset of action: Several days

Peak effect: 2-3 weeks

Pharmacokinetics

Some metabolic degradation does occur with small amounts recovered in the urine

Half-life (circulating): 4-13 hours in patients with chronic renal failure (CRF); half-life is 20% shorter in patients with normal renal function

Usual Dosage

In patients on dialysis epoetin alfa usually has been administered as an I.V. bolus 3 times/week. In patients with chronic renal failure (CRF) not on dialysis, epoetin alfa may be given either as an I.V. or S.C. injection. See table.

Epoetin Alfa: General Therapeutic Guidelines

Starting dose	50–100 units/kg 3 times/week I.V.: Dialysis patients I.V. or S.C.: nondialysis CRF patients
Reduce dose when	1. Target range is reached, or 2. Hematocrit increases >4 points in any 2–week period
Increase dose if	Hematocrit does not increase by 5 to 6 points after 8 weeks of therapy, and hematocrit is below target range
Maintenance dose	Individualize. General dosage range: 25 units/kg (3 times/week)
Target hematocrit range	30–33% (maximum: 36%)

AZT-treated HIV-infected patients: I.V., S.C.: Initial: 100 units/kg/dose 3 times/week for 8 weeks; after 8 weeks of therapy the dose can be adjusted by 50-100 units/kg increments 3 times/week to a maximum dose of 300 units/kg 3 times/week; if the hematocrit exceeds 40%, the dose should be discontinued until the hematocrit drops to 36%

Anemia of prematurity: S.C.: 25-100 units/kg/dose 3 times/week

Administration Dilute with an equal volume of normal saline and infuse over 1-3 minutes; it may be administered into the venous line at the end of the dialysis procedure

Monitoring Parameters Hematocrit, serum iron, baseline erythropoietin level, blood pressure

Additional Information Do not shake as this may denature the glycoprotein rendering the drug biologically inactive

Dosage Forms Injection, preservative free: 2000 units (1 mL); 4000 units (1 mL); 10,000 units (1 mL)

References

Blanche S, Caniglia M, Fischer A, et al, "Zidovudine Therapy in Children With Acquired Immunodeficiency Syndrome," *Am J Med*, 1988, 85(2A):203-7.

(Continued)

Epoetin Alfa *(Continued)*

Halperin DS, Wacker P, Lacourt G, et al, "Effects of Recombinant Human Erythropoietin in Infants With the Anemia of Prematurity: A Pilot Study," *J Pediatr*, 1990, 116(5):779-86.

Rhondeau SM, Christensen RD, Ross MP, et al, "Responsiveness to Recombinant Human Erythropoietin of Marrow Erythroid Progenitors From Infants With the Anemia of Prematurity," *J Pediatr*, 1988, 112(6):935-40.

Sinai-Trieman L, Salusky IB, and Fine RN, "Use of Subcutaneous Recombinant Human Erythropoietin in Children Undergoing Continuous Cycling Peritoneal Dialysis," *J Pediatr*, 1989, 114(4 Pt 1):550-4.

Epogen® *see* Epoetin Alfa *on page 222*

Eppy/N® *see* Epinephrine *on page 220*

Epsom Salts *see* Magnesium Sulfate *on page 353*

Ercaf® *see* Ergotamine *on next page*

Ergocalciferol (er goe kal sif' e role)

Brand Names Calciferol™; Drisdol®

Synonyms Activated Ergosterol; Viosterol; Vitamin D_2

Therapeutic Category Vitamin, Fat Soluble

Use Refractory rickets; hypophosphatemia; hypoparathyroidism

Pregnancy Risk Factor A

Contraindications Hypercalcemia, hypersensitivity to ergocalciferol or any component; malabsorption syndrome; evidence of vitamin D toxicity

Adverse Reactions

Cardiovascular: Hypertension, arrhythmias

Central nervous system: Drowsiness, irritability, headache

Endocrine & metabolic: Acidosis

Gastrointestinal: Nausea, vomiting, anorexia, dry mouth

Musculoskeletal: Weakness, muscle and bone pain

Renal & genitourinary: Polyuria, nephrocalcinosis

Miscellaneous: Metallic taste

Drug Interactions Cholestyramine, colestipol, thiazide diuretics, corticosteroids, cardiac glycosides

Stability Protect from light

Mechanism of Action Stimulates calcium and phosphate absorption from the small intestine, promotes secretion of calcium from bone to blood

Pharmacodynamics Peak effect occurs in ~1 month following daily doses

Pharmacokinetics Absorption: Readily absorbed from the GI tract; absorption requires intestinal levels of bile; inactive until hydroxylated in the liver and the kidney to calcifediol and then to calcitriol (most active form)

Usual Dosage Oral dosing is preferred; use I.M. only in patients with GI, liver, or biliary disease associated with malabsorption of vitamin D:

Dietary supplementation (each μg = 40 USP units):
- Premature infants: 10-20 μg/day (400-800 units), up to 750 μg/day (30,000 units)
- Infants and healthy Children: 10 μg/day (400 units)
- Adults: 10 μg/day (400 units)

Renal failure:
- Children: 100-1000 μg/day (4000-40,000 units)
- Adults: 500 μg/day (20,000 units)

Hypoparathyroidism:
- Children: 1.25-5 mg/day (50,000-200,000 units) and calcium supplements
- Adults: 625 μg to 5 mg/day (25,000-200,000 units) and calcium supplements

Vitamin D-dependent rickets:
- Children: 75-125 μg/day (3000-5000 units); maximum: 1500 μg/day
- Adults: 250 μg to 1.5 mg/day (10,000-60,000 units)

Nutritional rickets and osteomalacia:
- Children and Adults (with normal absorption): 25-125 μg/day (1000-5000 units)
- Children with malabsorption: 250-625 μg/day (10,000-25,000 units)
- Adults with malabsorption: 250-7500 μg (10,000-300,000 units)

Vitamin D-resistant rickets:

Children: Initial: 1000-2000 μg/day (400,000-800,000 units) with phosphate supplements; daily dosage is increased at 3- to 4-month intervals in 250-500 μg (10,000-20,000 units) increments

Adults: 250-1500 μg/day (10,000-60,000 units) with phosphate supplements

Monitoring Parameters Serum calcium and phosphate levels; alkaline phosphatase, BUN

Reference Range Serum calcium times phosphorus should not exceed 70 mg/dL to avoid ectopic calcification

Nursing Implications Parenteral injection for I.M. use only

Additional Information 1.25 mg ergocalciferol provides 50,000 units of vitamin D activity

Dosage Forms

Capsule: 50,000 units [1.25 mg]

Injection: 500,000 units/mL [12.5 mg/mL] (1 mL)

Solution, oral: 8000 units/mL [200 μg/mL] (60 mL)

Tablet: 50,000 units [1.25 mg]

Ergostat® *see* Ergotamine *on this page*

Ergotamine (er got' a meen)

Related Information

Overdose and Toxicology Information *on page 696-700*

Brand Names Cafergot®; Ercaf®; Ergostat®; Medihaler Ergotamine™; Wigraine®

Therapeutic Category Adrenergic Blocking Agent; Ergot Alkaloid or Derivative

Use Prevent or abort vascular headaches, such as migraine or cluster

Pregnancy Risk Factor X

Contraindications Hypersensitivity to ergotamine, caffeine or any component; peripheral vascular disease, hepatic or renal disease, hypertension, peptic ulcer disease, sepsis

Warnings Avoid during pregnancy

Adverse Reactions

Cardiovascular: Angina-like precordial pain, transient tachycardia or bradycardia, local edema, vasospasm

Dermatologic: Pruritus

Gastrointestinal: Nausea, vomiting, diarrhea

Musculoskeletal: Paresthesias of the extremities, leg cramps, myalgia, weakness

Drug Interactions Troleandomycin; erythromycin – monitor for signs of ergot toxicity

Mechanism of Action Ergot alkaloid alpha adrenergic blocker directly stimulates vascular smooth muscle to vasoconstrict peripheral and cerebral vessels; may also have antagonist effects on serotonin

Pharmacokinetics

Absorption: Oral, rectal: Erratic; absorption is enhanced by caffeine coadministration

Metabolism: Extensively metabolized in the liver

Bioavailability: Poor overall bioavailability (<5%)

Peak serum levels: Within 0.5-3 hours

Elimination: Excreted in the bile as metabolites (90%)

Usual Dosage

Older Children and Adolescents: Oral, S.L.: 1 mg at onset of attack; then 1 mg every 30 minutes as needed, up to a maximum of 3 mg per attack

Adults:

Oral (Cafergot®), S.L.: 2 mg at onset of attack; then 1-2 mg every 30 minutes as needed; maximum: 6 mg per attack; do not exceed 10 mg/week

Rectal (Cafergot® suppositories, Wigraine® suppositories, Cafergot® P-B suppositories): 2 mg at first sign of an attack; follow with second dose after 1 hour, if needed; maximum dose: 4 mg per attack; do not exceed 10 mg/week

Patient Information Any symptoms such as nausea, vomiting, numbness or tingling, and chest, muscle, or abdominal pain should be reported to the physician at the first sign of an attack; do **not** exceed recommended dosage

(Continued)

Ergotamine *(Continued)*

Additional Information In patients receiving methysergide for prophylaxis, the dose of ergotamine tartrate may have to be decreased by 50% at a minimal frequency

Dosage Forms

Aerosol, oral: 360 μg/metered spray

Suppository, rectal: Ergotamine tartrate 2 mg and caffeine 100 mg (12/box)

Tablet: Ergotamine tartrate 1 mg and caffeine 100 mg

Tablet:

- Sublingual: 2 mg
- Extended release: 0.6 mg with levorotary belladonna alkaloids 0.2 mg and phenobarbital 40 mg; 1 mg with belladonna alkaloids 0.125 mg, caffeine 100 mg, and pentobarbital 30 mg

Eryc® *see* Erythromycin *on this page*

Erycette® *see* Erythromycin *on this page*

EryDerm® *see* Erythromycin *on this page*

Erygel® *see* Erythromycin *on this page*

Erymax® *see* Erythromycin *on this page*

Ery-Tab® *see* Erythromycin *on this page*

Erythrocin® *see* Erythromycin *on this page*

Erythromycin (er ith roe mye' sin)

Related Information

Endocarditis Prophylaxis *on page 659*

Medications Compatible With PN Solutions *on page 649-650*

Brand Names AK-Mycin®; Akne-Mycin®; A/T/S®; C-Solve-2®; E.E.S.®; E.E.S. 400®; E.E.S.® Chewable; E.E.S.® Granules; Emgel®; E-Mycin®; E-Mycin-E®; Eryc®; Erycette®; EryDerm®; Erygel®; Erymax®; Ery-Tab®; Erythrocin®; E-Solve-2®; ETS-2%®; Ilosone®; Ilosone® Pulvules®; Ilotycin®; PCE®; Staticin®; T-Stat®; Wyamycin®

Synonyms Erythromycin Base; Erythromycin Estolate; Erythromycin Ethylsuccinate; Erythromycin Gluceptate; Erythromycin Lactobionate; Erythromycin Stearate

Therapeutic Category Antibiotic, Macrolide; Antibiotic, Ophthalmic

Use Treatment of pharyngitis, skin infections due to susceptible streptococci and staphylococci; other susceptible bacterial infections including mycoplasma pneumonia, *Legionella* pneumonia, diphtheria, pertussis, chancroid, *Chlamydia*, and *Campylobacter* gastroenteritis; used in conjunction with neomycin for decontaminating the bowel for surgery; dental procedure prophylaxis in penicillin allergic patients

Pregnancy Risk Factor B

Contraindications Hepatic impairment, concomitant administration with astemizole or terfenadine, known hypersensitivity to erythromycin or any components

Warnings Hepatic impairment with or without jaundice has occurred primarily in older children and adults; it may be accompanied by malaise, nausea, vomiting, abdominal colic, and fever; discontinue use if these occur; avoid using erythromycin lactobionate in neonates since formulation may contain benzyl alcohol which is associated with a fatal gasping syndrome in neonates; risk of serious cardiac arrhythmias exist in patients receiving erythromycin and astemizole or erythromycin and terfenadine

Adverse Reactions

Cardiovascular: Ventricular arrhythmias

Central nervous system: Fever, dizziness

Dermatologic: Skin rash

Gastrointestinal: Abdominal pain, cramping, nausea, vomiting, diarrhea, stomatitis

Hematologic: Eosinophilia

Hepatic: Cholestatic hepatitis, jaundice

Local: Thrombophlebitis (I.V. form)

Otic: Ototoxicity

Miscellaneous: Allergic reactions, anaphylaxis

Drug Interactions Erythromycin ↓ clearance of astemizole, terfenadine, carbamazepine, cyclosporine, and triazolam; erythromycin may ↓ theophylline clearance and ↑ theophylline's half-life by up to 60% (patients on high dose theophylline and erythromycin or who have received erythromycin for >5 days may be at higher risk); may potentiate anticoagulant effect of warfarin

Stability Erythromycin lactobionate should be reconstituted with sterile water for injection without preservatives to avoid gel formation; the reconstituted solution is stable for 2 weeks when refrigerated or 24 hours at room temperature. Erythromycin I.V. infusion solution is stable at pH 6-8.

Mechanism of Action Inhibits RNA-dependent protein synthesis at the chain elongation step; binds to the 50S ribosomal subunit resulting in blockage of transpeptidation

Pharmacokinetics

Absorption: Variable but better with salt forms like the estolate than with base form; 18% to 45% absorbed orally; ethylsuccinate may be better absorbed with food

Distribution: Crosses the placenta; distributes into body tissues, fluids, and breast milk with poor penetration into the CSF

Protein binding: 75% to 90%

Metabolism: Metabolized in the liver by demethylation

Half-life: 1.5-2 hours, prolonged with reduced renal function

Peak levels: After oral administration peak serum levels occur within 4 hours (delayed in the presence of food except when using the estolate); peak levels occur at 4 hours for the base, 3 hours for the stearate, 0.5-2.5 hours for the ethylsuccinate, 2-4 hours for the estolate

Elimination: 2% to 15% unchanged drug excreted in the urine, major excretion in the feces (via bile)

Usual Dosage

Neonates:

Oral: Postnatal age:

≤7 days: 20 mg/kg/day in divided doses every 12 hours

>7 days, <1200 g: 20 mg/kg/day in divided doses every 12 hours

>7 days, ≥1200 g: 30 mg/kg/day in divided doses every 8 hours

Ophthalmic: Prophylaxis of neonatal gonococcal or chlamydial conjunctivitis: 0.5-1 cm ribbon of ointment should be instilled into each conjunctival sac

Infants and Children:

Oral: Do not exceed 2 g/day

Base and ethylsuccinate: 30-50 mg/kg/day divided every 6-8 hours (**Note:** Due to differences in absorption, 200 mg erythromycin ethylsuccinate produces the same serum levels as 125 mg erythromycin base or estolate)

Estolate: 30-50 mg/kg/day divided every 8-12 hours

Stearate: 20-40 mg/kg/day divided every 6 hours

Endocarditis prophylaxis in penicillin allergic patients: Oral: 20 mg/kg 2 hours before procedure and 10 mg/kg 6 hours later

Pre-op bowel preparation: Oral: 20 mg/kg erythromycin base at 1, 2, and 11 PM on the day before surgery combined with mechanical cleansing of the large intestine and oral neomycin

I.V.:

Lactobionate: 20-40 mg/kg/day divided every 6 hours, not to exceed 4 g/day

Gluceptate: 20-50 mg/kg/day divided every 6 hours

Children and Adults:

Ophthalmic: Instill one or more times daily depending on the severity of the infection

Topical: Apply 2% solution over the affected area twice daily after the skin has been thoroughly washed and patted dry

Adults:

Oral:

Base: 333 mg every 8 hours

Estolate, stearate or base: 250-500 mg every 6-12 hours

Ethylsuccinate: 400-800 mg every 6-12 hours

Endocarditis prophylaxis in penicillin allergic patients: Oral: 1 g 2 hours before procedure and 500 mg 6 hours later

Pre-op bowel preparation: Oral: 1 g erythromycin base at 1, 2, and 11 PM on the day before surgery combined with mechanical cleansing of the large intestine and oral neomycin

(Continued)

Erythromycin *(Continued)*

I.V.: 15-20 mg/kg/day divided every 6 hours or given as a continuous infusion over 24 hours

Administration Administer by I.V. intermittent or continuous infusion at a concentration of 1-2.5 mg/mL; maximum concentration: 5 mg/mL; I.V. intermittent infusions can be administered over 20-60 minutes

Monitoring Parameters Liver function tests

Test Interactions False-positive urinary catecholamines

Patient Information Ethylsuccinate chewable tablets should not be swallowed whole; can take with food to decrease GI upset

Nursing Implications Do not crush enteric coated drug product

Additional Information Erythromycin has been used as a prokinetic agent to improve gastric emptying time and intestinal motility. In adults, 200 mg was infused I.V. initially followed by 250 mg orally 3 times/day 30 minutes before meals. In children, erythromycin 3 mg/kg I.V. has been infused over 60 minutes initially followed by 20 mg/kg/day orally in 3-4 divided doses before meals or before meals and at bedtime

Dosage Forms

Capsule, as estolate: 125 mg, 250 mg
Capsule, delayed release: 250 mg
Injection, gluceptate: 1 g (30 mL)
Injection, lactobionate: 500 mg, 1 g
Gel, topical: 2% (30 g)
Ointment, ophthalmic: 5 mg/g (3.5 g)
  Ointment, topical: 2% (25 g)
Solution, topical: 1.5% (60 mL); 2% (60 mL)
Suspension:
  Oral, as estolate: 125 mg/5 mL (480 mL); 250 mg/5 mL (480 mL)
  Oral, as ethylsuccinate: 200 mg/5 mL (480 mL); 400 mg/5 mL (480 mL)
  Oral drops, as estolate: 100 mg/mL (10 mL)
  Oral drops, as ethylsuccinate: 100 mg/2.5 mL (30 mL)
Swab: 2% (60s)
Tablet:
  Delayed release, as base: 250 mg, 333 mg, 500 mg
  Film coated: 250 mg, 500 mg
  Film coated, as ethylsuccinate: 400 mg
  Polymer coated particles, as base: 333 mg
  Polymer coated particles, as estolate: 500 mg
  Chewable, as estolate: 125 mg, 250 mg
  Chewable, as ethylsuccinate: 200 mg

References

Di Lorenzo C, Lachman R, and Hyman PE, "Intravenous Erythromycin for Postpyloric Intubation," *J Pediatr Gastroenterol Nutr*, 1990, 11(1):45-7.

Janssens J, Peeters TL, Vantrappen G, et al, "Improvement of Gastric Emptying in Diabetic Gastroparesis by Erythromycin," *N Engl J Med*, 1990, 322(15):1028-31.

Reid B, DiLorenzo C, Travis L, et al, "Diabetic Gastroparesis Due to Postprandial Antral Hypomotility in Childhood," *Pediatrics*, 1992, 90(1 Pt 1):43-6.

Thoene DE and Johnson CE, "Pharmacotherapy of Otitis Media," *Pharmacotherapy*, 1991, 11(3):212-21.

Erythromycin and Sulfisoxazole

Brand Names Eryzole®; Pediazole®

Synonyms Sulfisoxazole and Erythromycin

Therapeutic Category Antibiotic, Macrolide; Antibiotic, Sulfonamide Derivative

Use Treatment of susceptible bacterial infections of the upper and lower respiratory tract; otitis media in children caused by susceptible strains of *Haemophilus influenzae*; other infections in patients allergic to penicillin

Pregnancy Risk Factor C

Contraindications Hepatic dysfunction, known hypersensitivity to erythromycin or sulfonamides; infants <2 months of age (sulfas compete with bilirubin for binding sites); patients with porphyria; concomitant administration of astemizole or terfenadine

Warnings Risk of serious cardiac arrhythmias exist in patients receiving erythromycin and astemizole or erythromycin and terfenadine

Precautions Use with caution in patients with impaired renal or hepatic function, G-6-PD deficiency (hemolysis may occur)

Adverse Reactions

Central nervous system: Headache

Dermatologic: Rash, photosensitivity, Stevens-Johnson syndrome, toxic epidermal necrolysis

Gastrointestinal: Abdominal cramping, nausea, vomiting, diarrhea

Hematologic: Agranulocytosis, aplastic anemia

Hepatic: Hepatic necrosis

Renal & genitourinary: Toxic nephrosis, crystalluria

Drug Interactions Erythromycin may decrease theophylline clearance and increase theophylline's half-life by up to 60% (patients on high doses of theophylline and erythromycin or on >5 days of erythromycin may be at higher risk); erythromycin inhibits carbamazepine metabolism; erythromycin ↓ cyclosporine, triazolam, astemizole, terfenadine clearance; may potentiate anticoagulant effects of warfarin

Stability Reconstituted suspension is stable for 14 days when refrigerated

Mechanism of Action Erythromycin inhibits bacterial protein synthesis; sulfisoxazole competitively inhibits bacterial synthesis of folic acid from para-aminobenzoic acid

Pharmacokinetics

Erythromycin ethylsuccinate:

Absorption: Well absorbed from the GI tract

Distribution: Crosses the placenta; excreted in breast milk

Protein binding: 75% to 90%

Metabolism: Metabolized in the liver

Half-life: 1-1.5 hours

Elimination: Unchanged drug is excreted and concentrated in bile

Sulfisoxazole acetyl:

Absorption: Hydrolyzed in the GI tract to sulfisoxazole which is readily absorbed

Distribution: Crosses the placenta, excreted in breast milk

Protein binding: 85%

Half-life: 6 hours, prolonged in renal impairment

Elimination: 50% is excreted in the urine as unchanged drug

Usual Dosage Oral (dosage recommendation is based on the product's erythromycin content):

Children ≥2 months: 40-50 mg/kg/day in divided doses every 6-8 hours; not to exceed 2 g erythromycin or 6 g sulfisoxazole/day

Adults: 400 mg erythromycin and 1200 mg sulfisoxazole every 6 hours

Monitoring Parameters CBC and periodic liver function test

Test Interactions False-positive urinary protein

Patient Information Maintain adequate fluid intake; avoid prolonged exposure to sunlight

Dosage Forms Suspension, oral: Erythromycin ethylsuccinate 200 mg and sulfisoxazole acetyl 600 mg per 5 mL (100 mL, 150 mL, 200 mL)

Erythromycin Base *see* Erythromycin *on page 226*

Erythromycin Estolate *see* Erythromycin *on page 226*

Erythromycin Ethylsuccinate *see* Erythromycin *on page 226*

Erythromycin Gluceptate *see* Erythromycin *on page 226*

Erythromycin Lactobionate *see* Erythromycin *on page 226*

Erythromycin Stearate *see* Erythromycin *on page 226*

Erythropoietin *see* Epoetin Alfa *on page 222*

Eryzole® *see* Erythromycin and Sulfisoxazole *on previous page*

Eserine Salicylate *see* Physostigmine Salicylate *on page 457*

Esidrix® *see* Hydrochlorothiazide *on page 291*

Eskalith® *see* Lithium *on page 345*

Esmolol Hydrochloride (ess' moe lol)

Related Information

Overdose and Toxicology Information *on page 696-700*

(Continued)

Esmolol Hydrochloride *(Continued)*

Brand Names Brevibloc®

Therapeutic Category Antiarrhythmic Agent, Class II; Beta-Adrenergic Blocker

Use Supraventricular tachycardia (primarily to control ventricular rate) and hypertension (especially perioperatively)

Pregnancy Risk Factor C

Contraindications Sinus bradycardia or heart block, uncompensated congestive heart failure, cardiogenic shock, hypersensitivity to esmolol, any component, or other beta blockers

Warnings Caution should be exercised when discontinuing esmolol infusions to avoid withdrawal effects

Precautions Use with extreme caution in patients with hyper-reactive airway disease; use lowest dose possible and discontinue infusion if bronchospasm occurs; use with caution in diabetes mellitus, hypoglycemia, renal failure; avoid extravasation

Adverse Reactions

Cardiovascular: Hypotension (especially with doses >200 µg/kg/minute), bradycardia, diaphoresis

Central nervous system: Dizziness, somnolence, confusion, lethargy, Raynaud's phenomena, depression, headache

Gastrointestinal: Nausea, vomiting

Local: Phlebitis, skin necrosis after extravasation

Respiratory: Bronchoconstriction (less than propranolol, but more likely with higher doses)

Miscellaneous: Other adverse reactions similar to other beta blockers may occur

Drug Interactions Esmolol may increase serum digoxin concentrations; morphine may increase esmolol blood concentrations

Mechanism of Action Class II antiarrhythmic: Competitively blocks response to beta-adrenergic stimulation

Pharmacodynamics

Onset of action: I.V.: Beta blockade occurs within 2-10 minutes (onset of effects is quickest when loading doses are administered)

Duration: Short (10-30 minutes)

Pharmacokinetics

Protein binding: 55%

Distribution: V_d: Children: 2 L/kg

Metabolism: Metabolized in blood by esterases

Half-life:

Children: 4.5 minutes

Adults: 9 minutes

Elimination: ~69% of dose excreted in the urine as metabolites and 2% as unchanged drug

Usual Dosage Must be adjusted to individual response and tolerance

Children:

Limited information available; some centers have utilized doses of 100-500 µg/kg given over 1 minute for control of supraventricular tachycardias. One study (n=20, 2-16 years of age) used an initial dose of 600 µg/kg over 2 minutes followed by an infusion of 200 µg/kg/minute; the infusion was titrated upward by 50-100 µg/kg/minute every 5-10 minutes until a reduction of >10% in heart rate or mean blood pressure occurred. Mean dose required: 550 µg/kg/minute with a range of 300-1000 µg/kg/minute.

Loading doses of 500 µg/kg/minute over 1 minute with doses of 50-250 µg/kg/minute (mean 173) have been used in addition to nitroprusside in a small number of patients (7 patients, 7-19 years of age, median age 13 years) to treat postoperative hypertension after coarctation of aorta repair.

Adults: I.V.: Loading dose: 500 µg/kg over 1 minute; follow with a 50 µg/kg/minute infusion for 4 minutes; if response is inadequate, rebolus with another 500 µg/kg loading dose over 1 minute, and increase the maintenance infusion to 100 µg/kg/minute. Repeat this process until a therapeutic effect has been achieved or to a maximum recommended maintenance dose of 200 µg/kg/minute. Usual dosage range: 50-200 µg/kg/minute with average dose = 100 µg/kg/minute.

Administration The 250 mg/mL ampul is **not** for direct I.V. injection, but must first be diluted to a final concentration not to exceed 10 mg/mL (ie, 2.5 g in 250 mL or 5 g in 500 mL).

Monitoring Parameters Blood pressure, EKG, heart rate, respiratory rate, I.V. site

Nursing Implications Decrease infusion or discontinue if hypotension, congestive heart failure, etc occur

Dosage Forms Injection: 10 mg/mL (10 mL); 250 mg/mL (10 mL)

References

Trippel DL, Wiest DB, and Gillette PC, "Cardiovascular and Antiarrhythmic Effects of Esmolol in Children," *J Pediatr*, 1991, 119(1):142-7.

Vincent RN, Click LA, Williams HM, et al, "Esmolol As an Adjunct in the Treatment of Systemic Hypertension After Operative Repair of Coarctation of the Aorta," *Am J Cardiol*, 1990, 65(13):941-3.

Wiest DB, Trippel DL, Gillette PC, et al, "Pharmacokinetics of Esmolol in Children," *Clin Pharmacol Ther*, 1991, 49(6):618-23.

E-Solve-2® *see* Erythromycin *on page 226*

Estar® [OTC] *see* Coal Tar *on page 147*

Estivin® II [OTC] *see* Naphazoline Hydrochloride *on page 403*

Estrace® *see* Estradiol *on this page*

Estraderm® *see* Estradiol *on this page*

Estradiol (ess tra dye' ole)

Brand Names Delestrogen®; depGynogen®; Depo®-Estradiol; Depogen®; Dioval®; Dura-Estrin®; Estrace®; Estraderm®; Estro-Cyp®; Estroject-L.A.®; Estronol-LA®; Valergen®

Synonyms Estradiol Cypionate; Estradiol Valerate

Therapeutic Category Estrogen Derivative; Estrogen Derivative, Oral

Use Female hypogonadism, atrophic vaginitis, menopausal symptoms

Pregnancy Risk Factor X

Contraindications Thromboembolic disorders, active arterial thrombosis, thyroid dysfunction, blood dyscrasias

Warnings Estrogens have been reported to increase the risk of endometrial carcinoma; do not use estrogens during pregnancy

Precautions Use with caution in patients with renal or hepatic insufficiency; estrogens may cause premature closure of the epiphyses in young individuals

Adverse Reactions

Cardiovascular: Hypertension, edema, thromboembolic disorders

Central nervous system: Depression, headache

Dermatologic: Chloasma, melasma

Endocrine & metabolic: Hypercalcemia, folate deficiency, change in menstrual flow

Gastrointestinal: Nausea, vomiting

Hepatic: Cholestatic jaundice

Local: Pain at injection site; topical may cause burning or irritation

Drug Interactions Rifampin, anticoagulants, hydrocortisone

Mechanism of Action Increases the synthesis of DNA, RNA, and various proteins in target tissues; reduces the release of gonadotropin-releasing hormone from the hypothalamus; reduces FSH and LH release from the pituitary

Usual Dosage All dosage needs to be adjusted based upon the patient's response

Adolescents and Adults: Female hypogonadism:

- I.M.:
  - Cypionate: 1.5-2 mg/month
  - Valerate: 10-20 mg/month
- Oral: 1-2 mg/day in a cyclic regimen (3 weeks on drug, 1 week off)
- Transdermal: Initial: 0.05 mg patch (titrate dosage to response) applied twice weekly in a cyclic regimen

Nursing Implications Injection for I.M. use only

Dosage Forms

Cream, vaginal: 0.1 mg/g (42.5 g)

(Continued)

Estradiol *(Continued)*

Injection, as cypionate: 5 mg/mL (5 mL, 10 mL)
Injection, as valerate: 10 mg/mL (5 mL, 10 mL); 20 mg/mL (1 mL, 5 mL, 10 mL); 40 mg/mL (5 mL, 10 mL)
Tablet, micronized: 1 mg, 2 mg
Transdermal system: 0.05 mg (10 cm^2), 4 mg total estradiol; 0.1 mg (20 cm^2), 8 mg total estradiol

Estradiol Cypionate *see* Estradiol *on previous page*

Estradiol Valerate *see* Estradiol *on previous page*

Estro-Cyp® *see* Estradiol *on previous page*

Estrogenic Substances, Conjugated *see* Estrogens, Conjugated *on this page*

Estrogens, Conjugated (ess' troe jen)

Brand Names Premarin®
Synonyms C.E.S.; Estrogenic Substances, Conjugated
Therapeutic Category Estrogen Derivative; Estrogen Derivative, Oral; Estrogen Derivative, Vaginal
Use Dysfunctional uterine bleeding, hypogonadism, atrophic vaginitis
Pregnancy Risk Factor X
Contraindications Undiagnosed vaginal bleeding; hypersensitivity to estrogens or any component; thrombophlebitis, liver disease
Warnings Estrogens have been reported to increase the risk of endometrial carcinoma; do not use estrogens during pregnancy
Precautions Use with caution in patients with asthma, epilepsy, migraine, diabetes, cardiac or renal dysfunction; estrogens may cause premature closure of the epiphyses in young individuals
Adverse Reactions
Cardiovascular: Hypertension, edema, thromboembolic disorder
Central nervous system: Depression, headache
Dermatologic: Chloasma, melasma
Endocrine & metabolic: Breast tenderness, change in menstrual flow, hypercalcemia
Gastrointestinal: Nausea, vomiting
Hepatic: Cholestatic jaundice
Local: Pain at injection site
Drug Interactions Rifampin, anticoagulants, hydrocortisone
Stability Store injection in the refrigerator
Mechanism of Action Increases the synthesis of DNA, RNA, and various proteins in target tissues; reduces the release of gonadotropin-releasing hormone from the hypothalamus; reduces FSH and LH release from the pituitary
Usual Dosage Adolescents and Adults:
Hypogonadism: Oral: 2.5-7.5 mg/day for 20 days, off 10 days and repeat until menses occur

Abnormal uterine bleeding:
Stable hematocrit: Oral: 1.25 mg twice daily for 21 days; if bleeding persists after 48 hours, increase to 2.5 mg twice daily; if bleeding persists after 48 more hours, increase to 2.5 mg 4 times/day
Alternatively: Oral: 2.5-5 mg/day for 7-10 days; then decrease to 1.25 mg/day for 2 weeks
Unstable hematocrit: Oral, I.V.: 5 mg 2-4 times/day; if bleeding is profuse, 20-40 mg every 4 hours up to 24 hours may be used
Alternatively: I.V.: 25 mg every 6-12 hours until bleeding stops
Administration May also be administered intramuscularly; I.V.: Give slow I.V. to avoid flushing
Dosage Forms
Cream, vaginal: 0.625 mg/g (42.5 g)
Injection: 25 mg (5 mL)
Tablet: 0.3 mg, 0.625 mg, 0.9 mg, 1.25 mg, 2.5 mg
References

Neistein LS, "Adolescent Health Care - A Practical Guide," Baltimore-Munich: Urban & Schwarzenberg, 1984, 463-6.

Estroject-L.A.® *see* Estradiol *on page 231*

Estronol-LA® *see* Estradiol *on page 231*

Ethacrynic Acid (eth a krin' ik)

Brand Names Edecrin®

Therapeutic Category Diuretic, Loop

Use Management of edema secondary to congestive heart failure; hepatic or renal disease

Pregnancy Risk Factor D

Contraindications Hypersensitivity to ethacrynic acid or any component; hypotension, hyponatremic dehydration, metabolic alkalosis with hypokalemia, anuria, or Cl_{cr} 10 mL/minute

Warnings Loop diuretics are potent diuretics; excess amounts can lead to profound diuresis with fluid and electrolyte loss; close medical supervision and dose evaluation is required

Precautions Avoid use in patients with sever renal dysfunction, $Cl_{cr} < 10$ mL/minute

Adverse Reactions

Cardiovascular: Hypotension

Dermatologic: Rash

Endocrine & metabolic: Fluid and electrolyte imbalances (fluid depletion, hypokalemia, hyponatremia, hyperglycemia), hyperuricemia

Gastrointestinal: GI irritation, diarrhea

Hematologic: Thrombocytopenia, neutropenia, agranulocytosis

Hepatic: Abnormal liver function tests

Otic: Ototoxicity

Renal & genitourinary: Renal injury

Drug Interactions Diuretics, lithium, antidiabetic agents, hypotensive agents, probenecid, aminoglycosides, warfarin, drugs affected by or causing potassium depletion

Mechanism of Action Inhibits reabsorption of sodium and chloride in the ascending loop of Henle and distal renal tubule, interfering with the chloride binding cotransport system, thus causing increased excretion of water, sodium, chloride, magnesium, and calcium

Pharmacodynamics

Onset of action:

- Oral: Within 30 minutes
- I.V.: 5 minutes

Peak effect:

- Oral: 2 hours
- I.V.: 30 minutes

Duration:

- Oral: 6-8 hours
- I.V.: 2 hours

Pharmacokinetics

Absorption: Oral: Rapid

Protein binding: >90%

Metabolism: Metabolized in the liver to active cysteine conjugate (35% to 40%)

Elimination: Excreted in bile, 30% to 60% excreted unchanged in urine

Usual Dosage

Children:

- Oral: 1 mg/kg/dose once daily, increase at intervals of 2-3 days to a maximum of 3 mg/kg/day
- I.V.: 1 mg/kg/dose; repeat doses are not routinely recommended, however if indicated, repeat doses every 8-12 hours

Adults:

- Oral: 50-400 mg/day in 1-2 divided doses
- I.V.: 0.5-1 mg/kg/dose (maximum: 100 mg/dose); repeat doses not routinely recommended, however if indicated, repeat every 8-12 hours

Administration Dilute injection with 50 mL dextrose 5% or normal saline (1 mg/mL concentration resulting); may be injected without further dilution over a period of several minutes or infused over 20-30 minutes

Monitoring Parameters Serum electrolytes, blood pressure, renal function, hearing

(Continued)

Ethacrynic Acid *(Continued)*

Nursing Implications Tissue irritant; not to be given I.M. or S.C.

Additional Information Injection contains thimerosal

Dosage Forms

Powder for injection, as ethacrynate sodium: 50 mg (50 mL)
Tablet: 25 mg, 50 mg

Ethambutol Hydrochloride (e tham' byoo tole)

Brand Names Myambutol®

Therapeutic Category Antitubercular Agent

Use Treatment of tuberculosis and other mycobacterial diseases in conjunction with other antituberculosis agents

Pregnancy Risk Factor B

Contraindications Hypersensitivity to ethambutol or any component; optic neuritis

Warnings Use only in children whose visual acuity can accurately be determined and monitored; not recommended for use in children <13 years of age

Precautions Use with caution in patients with ocular defects or impaired renal function; dosage modification required in patients with renal impairment

Adverse Reactions

Central nervous system: Malaise, peripheral neuritis, mental confusion, fever, headache
Dermatologic: Rash, pruritus
Endocrine & metabolic: Elevated uric acid levels
Gastrointestinal: Nausea, vomiting
Hepatic: Abnormal liver function tests
Ocular: Optic neuritis, decreased visual acuity, decreased red-green color discrimination
Miscellaneous: Anaphylaxis

Mechanism of Action Suppresses mycobacteria multiplication by interfering with RNA synthesis

Pharmacokinetics

Absorption: Oral: ~80%
Distribution: Well distributed throughout the body with high concentrations in kidneys, lungs, saliva, and red blood cells
Protein binding: 20% to 30%
Metabolism: 20% metabolized by the liver to inactive metabolite
Half-life: 2.5-3.6 hours (up to 7 hours or longer with renal impairment)
Peak serum levels: Within 2-4 hours
Elimination: ~50% excreted in the urine and 20% excreted in the feces as unchanged drug
Slightly dialyzable (5% to 20%)

Usual Dosage Oral:

Children: 15 mg/kg/day once daily

Adolescents and Adults: 15-25 mg/kg/day once daily, not to exceed 2.5 g/day **or** 50 mg/kg/dose twice weekly, not to exceed 2.5 g/dose

Dosing interval in renal impairment:
Cl_{cr} 10-50 mL/minute: Administer every 24-36 hours
Cl_{cr} <10 mL/minute: Administer every 48 hours and/or reduce daily dose

Monitoring Parameters Monthly examination of visual acuity and color discrimination in patients receiving more than 15 mg/kg/day; periodic renal, hepatic, and hematologic function tests

Patient Information Report any visual changes to physician; may cause stomach upset, take with food

Dosage Forms Tablet: 100 mg, 400 mg

References

American Academy of Pediatrics, Committee on Infectious Diseases, "Chemotherapy for Tuberculosis in Infants and Children," *Pediatrics*, 1992, 89(1):161-5.

Starke JR, "Multidrug Therapy for Tuberculosis in Children," *Pediatr Infect Dis J*, 1990, 9(11):785-93.

Ethionamide (e thye on am' ide)

Brand Names Trecator®-SC

Therapeutic Category Antitubercular Agent

Use Used in conjunction with other antituberculosis agents in the treatment of tuberculosis and other mycobacterial diseases

Pregnancy Risk Factor C

Contraindications Contraindicated in patients with severe hepatic impairment or in patients who are sensitive to the drug

Precautions Use with caution in patients receiving cycloserine or isoniazid

Adverse Reactions

Cardiovascular: Postural hypotension

Central nervous system: Drowsiness, dizziness, peripheral neuritis, seizures, headache

Dermatologic: Rash

Endocrine & metabolic: Hypoglycemia, goiter, gynecomastia

Gastrointestinal: Nausea, vomiting, abdominal pain, diarrhea, anorexia, stomatitis

Hematologic: Thrombocytopenia

Hepatic: Hepatitis

Ocular: Optic neuritis

Miscellaneous: Metallic taste

Mechanism of Action Inhibits peptide synthesis

Pharmacokinetics

Distribution: Crosses the placenta; widely distributed into body tissues and fluids

Protein binding: 10%

Metabolism: Metabolized in the liver

Bioavailability: 80%

Half-life: 2-3 hours

Peak serum levels: Oral: Occur within 3 hours

Elimination: Excreted as metabolites (active and inactive) and parent drug in the urine

Usual Dosage Oral:

Children: 15-20 mg/kg/day in 2 divided doses, not to exceed 1 g/day

Adults: 500-1000 mg/day in 1-3 divided doses

Monitoring Parameters Initial and periodic serum AST and ALT

Patient Information Take with meals

Nursing Implications Neurotoxic effects may be relieved by the administration of pyridoxine

Dosage Forms Tablet: 250 mg

References

Donald PR and Seifart HI,"Cerebrospinal Fluid Concentrations of Ethionamide in Children With Tuberculous Meningitis," *J Pediatr*, 1989, 115(3):483-6.

Ethosuximide (eth oh sux' i mide)

Related Information

Blood Level Sampling Time Guidelines *on page 694-695*

Brand Names Zarontin®

Therapeutic Category Anticonvulsant

Use Management of absence (petit mal) seizures, myoclonic seizures, and akinetic epilepsy

Pregnancy Risk Factor C

Contraindications Known hypersensitivity to ethosuximide

Warnings Ethosuximide may increase tonic-clonic seizures in patients with mixed seizure disorders; ethosuximide must be used in combination with other anticonvulsants in patients with both absence and tonic-clonic seizures

Precautions Use with caution in patients with hepatic or renal disease; abrupt withdrawal of the drug may precipitate absence status; may impair mental alertness and coordination

Adverse Reactions

Central nervous system: Sedation, dizziness, lethargy, euphoria, hallucinations, insomnia, agitation, behavioral changes, headache

Dermatologic: Rashes, urticaria

Gastrointestinal: Nausea, vomiting, anorexia, abdominal pain

Hematologic: Rarely: Leukopenia, aplastic anemia, thrombocytopenia

(Continued)

Ethosuximide *(Continued)*

Miscellaneous: Hiccups; rarely SLE

Drug Interactions Phenytoin, carbamazepine, primidone, phenobarbital may increase the hepatic metabolism of ethosuximide; isoniazid may inhibit hepatic metabolism with a resultant increase in ethosuximide serum concentrations

Mechanism of Action Increases the seizure threshold and suppresses paroxysmal spike-and-wave pattern in absence seizures; depresses nerve transmission in the motor cortex

Pharmacokinetics

Distribution: V_d: Adults: 0.62-0.72 L/kg

Metabolism: ~80% is metabolized in the liver to three inactive metabolites

Half-life:

Children: 30 hours

Adults: 50-60 hours

Peak serum levels:

Capsule: Within 2-4 hours

Syrup: <2-4 hours

Elimination: Excreted slowly in the urine as metabolites (50%) and as unchanged drug (10% to 20%); small amounts excreted in the feces

Usual Dosage Oral:

Children <6 years: Initial: 15 mg/kg/day in 2 divided doses (maximum: 250 mg/dose); increase every 4-7 days; usual maintenance dose: 15-40 mg/kg/day in 2 divided doses

Children >6 years and Adults: Initial: 250 mg twice daily; increase by 250 mg/day as needed every 4-7 days up to 1.5 g/day in 2 divided doses; usual maintenance dose: 20-40 mg/kg/day in 2 divided doses

Monitoring Parameters Seizure frequency, trough serum concentrations; CBC, platelets, liver enzymes, urinalysis

Reference Range Therapeutic: 40-100 μg/mL (SI: 280-710 μmol/L); toxic: >150 μg/mL (SI: >1062 μmol/L)

Patient Information Take with food

Additional Information Considered to be drug of choice for simple absence seizures

Dosage Forms

Capsule: 250 mg

Syrup (raspberry flavor): 250 mg/5 mL (473 mL)

Ethoxynaphthamido Penicillin Sodium *see* Nafcillin Sodium *on page 400*

Ethyl Aminobenzoate *see* Benzocaine *on page 77*

Etidronate Disodium (e ti droe' nate)

Brand Names Didronel®

Synonyms EHDP; Sodium Etidronate

Therapeutic Category Antidote, Hypercalcemia; Biphosphonate

Use Symptomatic treatment of Paget's disease and heterotopic ossification due to spinal cord injury; hypercalcemia associated with malignancy

Pregnancy Risk Factor B (oral)/C (parenteral)

Contraindications Patients with serum creatinine >5 mg/dL

Precautions Dosage modification required in renal impairment

Adverse Reactions Generally dose related and most significant when taking oral doses >5 mg/kg/day

Endocrine & metabolic: Hyperphosphatemia, hypocalcemia

Gastrointestinal: Diarrhea, nausea, vomiting, occult blood in stools

Musculoskeletal: Increased risk of fractures, rachitic syndrome (found in children taking dosage >10 mg/kg/day over 1 year or longer)

Renal & genitourinary: Nephrotoxicity

Miscellaneous: Altered taste, hypersensitivity reactions

Stability When diluted in 250 mL normal saline, solutions are stable 48 hours at room temperature

Mechanism of Action Decreases bone resorption by inhibiting osteocystic osteolysis; decreases mineral release and matrix or collagen breakdown in bone

Pharmacodynamics

Onset of therapeutic effects: Within 1-3 months of therapy

Duration: Persists for 12 months without continuous therapy

Pharmacokinetics

Absorption: Dependent upon dose administered

Half-life: 8.7 hours (range: 6.9-10 hours)

Elimination: Primarily excreted as unchanged drug in the urine with unabsorbed drug eliminated in the feces

Usual Dosage

Paget's disease: Oral: 5 mg/kg/day given every day for no more than 6 months; may give 10 mg/kg/day for up to 3 months. Daily dose may be divided if adverse GI effects occur; courses of therapy should be separated by drug-free periods of at least 3 months

Heterotopic ossification with spinal cord injury: Oral: 20 mg/kg/day for 2 weeks, then 10 mg/kg/day for 10 weeks (This dosage has been used in children, however, treatment >1 year has been associated with a rachitic syndrome.)

Hypercalcemia associated with malignancy: I.V.: 7.5 mg/kg/day for 3 days; courses of therapy should be separated by at least 7 drug-free days

Administration Dilute in a minimum volume of 250 mL normal saline; infuse over at least 2 hours

Monitoring Parameters Serum calcium, phosphate, creatinine, BUN

Patient Information Maintain adequate intake of calcium and vitamin D; take medicine on an empty stomach

Dosage Forms

Injection: 50 mg/mL (6 mL)

Tablet: 200 mg, 400 mg

Etoposide (e toe poe' side)

Related Information

Emetogenic Potential of Single Chemotherapeutic Agents *on page 655*

Brand Names VePesid®

Synonyms VP-16; VP-16-213

Therapeutic Category Antineoplastic Agent

Use Treatment of testicular and lung carcinomas, malignant lymphoma, Hodgkin's disease, leukemias (ANL, ALL), neuroblastoma; etoposide has also been used in the treatment of Ewing's sarcoma, rhabdomyosarcoma, Wilms' tumor and brain tumors

Pregnancy Risk Factor D

Contraindications Hypersensitivity to etoposide or any component

Warnings The US Food and Drug Administration (FDA) currently recommends that procedures for proper handling and disposal of antineoplastic agents be considered. Severe myelosuppression with resulting infection or bleeding may occur

Precautions Dosage reduction should be considered in patients with hepatic impairment, bone marrow suppression, and renal impairment

Adverse Reactions

Cardiovascular: Hypotension, tachycardia

Central nervous system: Peripheral neuropathy, somnolence, fatigue, fever, headache, chills

Dermatologic: Alopecia

Gastrointestinal: Nausea, vomiting, diarrhea, mucositis

Hematologic: Myelosuppression, anemia (granulocyte nadir: ~7-14 days, platelet nadir: ~9-16 days)

Hepatic: Hepatotoxicity

Local: Thrombophlebitis

Respiratory: Bronchospasm

Miscellaneous: Anaphylactoid reactions

Stability Stability is concentration dependent (ie, 0.2-0.4 mg/mL = 96 or 48 hours respectively; 1 or 2 mg/mL = 2 or 1 hour respectively); at a concentration of 1 mg/mL in NS or D_5W, crystallization has occurred within 30 minutes; intact vials remain stable for 2 years at room temperature; refrigerate capsules

Mechanism of Action Inhibits mitotic activity; inhibits cells from entering prophase; inhibits DNA synthesis resulting in DNA strand breaks

Pharmacokinetics

Absorption: Oral: Large variability

(Continued)

Etoposide *(Continued)*

Distribution: CSF concentration is <5% of plasma concentration
Protein binding: 94% to 97%
Metabolism: Metabolized in the liver (with a biphasic decay)
Bioavailability: Averages 50%
Half-life, terminal:
  Children: 6-8 hours
  Adults: 4-15 hours with normal renal and hepatic function
Peak plasma concentration: Oral: Within 1-1.5 hours
Elimination: Both unchanged drug and metabolites are excreted in the urine and a small amount (2% to 16%) excreted in feces; up to 55% of an I.V. dose is excreted unchanged in urine in children

Usual Dosage Refer to individual protocols

Pediatric solid tumors: I.V.: 60-120 mg/m^2/day for 3-5 days every 3-6 weeks

Leukemia in children: I.V.: 100-200 mg/m^2/day for 5 days

Testicular cancer: I.V.: 50-100 mg/m^2/day on days 1-5 to 100 mg/m^2/day on days 1, 3 and 5 every 3-4 weeks for 3-4 courses

Small cell lung cancer:
  Oral: Twice the I.V. dose rounded to the nearest 50 mg given once daily if total dose ≤400 mg or in divided doses if >400 mg
  I.V.: 35 mg/m^2/day for 4 days or 50 mg/m^2/day for 5 days every 3-4 weeks

Dosing adjustment in patients with elevated serum bilirubin: Reduce dose by 50% for bilirubin >1.5 mg/dL; reduce dose by 75% for bilirubin >3 mg/dL

Administration Give I.V. infusion over at least 30-60 minutes to minimize the risk of hypotensive reactions at a final concentration for administration of 0.2-0.4 mg/mL in normal saline or D_5W

Monitoring Parameters CBC with differential and platelet count, hemoglobin, vital signs (blood pressure), bilirubin, and renal function tests

Patient Information Notify physician if fever, sore throat, painful/burning urination, bruising, bleeding or shortness of breath occurs

Nursing Implications I.T., I.P., and IVP administration is contraindicated; adequate airway and other supportive measures and agents for treating hypotension or anaphylactoid reactions should be present when I.V. etoposide is given; if necessary, the injection may be used for oral administration. Mix with orange juice, apple juice, or lemonade at a final concentration not to exceed 0.4 mg/mL

Dosage Forms

Capsule: 50 mg
Injection: 20 mg/mL (5 mL)

References

Berg SL, Grisell DL, DeLaney TF, et al, "Principles of Treatment of Pediatric Solid Tumors," *Pediatr Clin North Am*, 1991, 38(2):249-67.

Clark PL and Slevin ML, "The Clinical Pharmacology of Etoposide and Teniposide," *Clin Pharmacokinet*, 1987, 12(4):223-52.

Nishikawa A, Nakamura Y, Nobori U, et al, "Acute Monocytic Leukemia in Children. Response to VP-16-213 as a Single Agent," *Cancer*, 1987, 60(9):2146-9.

O'Dwyer PJ, Leyland-Jones B, Alonso MT, et al, "Etoposide (VP-16-213): Current Status of an Active Anticancer Drug," *N Engl J Med*, 1985, 312(11):692-700.

ETS-2%® *see* Erythromycin *on page 226*

Eurax® *see* Crotamiton *on page 159*

Eutectic Mixture of Lidocaine and Prilocaine *see* Lidocaine and Prilocaine *on page 341*

Evac-Q-Mag® [OTC] *see* Magnesium Citrate *on page 352*

Everone® *see* Testosterone *on page 550*

E-Vista® *see* Hydroxyzine *on page 298*

Exosurf® Neonatal *see* Colfosceril Palmitate *on page 151*

Exsel® *see* Selenium Sulfide *on page 521*

Extravasation Treatment *see page 640*

Ezide® *see* Hydrochlorothiazide *on page 291*

F_3T *see* Trifluridine *on page 583*

Factor VIII *see* Antihemophilic Factor, Human *on page 55*

Factor IX Complex (Human)

Brand Names AlphaNine®; Konÿne® 80; Mononine®; Profilnine® Heat-Treated; Proplex® SX-T; Proplex® T

Therapeutic Category Antihemophilic Agent; Blood Product Derivative

Use To control bleeding in patients with Factor IX deficiency (Hemophilia B or Christmas Disease); prevention/control of bleeding in hemophilia A patients with inhibitors to factor VIII

Pregnancy Risk Factor C

Contraindications Liver disease, intravascular coagulation or fibrinolysis

Precautions Use with caution in patients with liver dysfunction; risk of viral transmission is not totally eradicated, prepared from pooled human plasma

Adverse Reactions

Cardiovascular: Flushing, DIC, thrombosis following high dosages in hemophilia B patients

Central nervous system: Somnolence, tingling, fever, headache, chills

Dermatologic: Urticaria

Gastrointestinal: Nausea, vomiting

Respiratory: Tightness in chest and neck

Stability Administer within 3 hours after reconstitution; store unopened vials in refrigerator

Mechanism of Action Replaces deficient clotting factors including factors II; VII, IX, and X

Pharmacokinetics Cleared rapidly from the serum in two phases

Half-life:

First phase: 4-6 hours

Terminal: 22.5 hours

Usual Dosage Dose is expressed in terms of factor IX units; dose must be individualized; 1 unit/kg raises IX levels 1%

Children and Adults: I.V.:

Factor IX deficiency: Hospitalized patients: 20-50 units/kg/dose; may be higher in special cases; may be given every 24 hours or more often in special cases

Factor VIII inhibitor patients: 75-100 units/kg/dose; may be given every 6-12 hours

Administration I.V. administration only; rate of administration should not exceed 10 mL/minute; use filter needle to draw product into syringe

Monitoring Parameters Levels of factors II, IX, and X

Reference Range Patients with severe hemophilia will have levels of under 1%, often undetectable. Moderate forms of the disease have levels of 1% to 10% while some mild cases may have 11% to 49% of normal factor IX. Plasma concentration is about 4 mg/L.

Dosage Forms Injection: Single-dose vials with varied units

Factrel® *see* Gonadorelin *on page 276*

FAMP *see* Fludarabine Phosphate *on page 250*

Fansidar® *see* Sulfadoxine and Pyrimethamine *on page 541*

F-ara-AMP *see* Fludarabine Phosphate *on page 250*

Fat Emulsion

Related Information

Parenteral Nutrition (PN) *on page 642-648*

Brand Names Intralipid®; Liposyn®

Synonyms Intravenous Fat Emulsion

Therapeutic Category Caloric Agent

Use Source of calories and essential fatty acids for patients requiring parenteral nutrition of extended duration

Pregnancy Risk Factor B/C

Contraindications Pathologic hyperlipidemia, lipoid nephrosis, known hypersensitivity to fat emulsion and severe egg or legume (soybean) allergies

(Continued)

Fat Emulsion *(Continued)*

Precautions Caution in patients with severe liver damage, pulmonary disease, anemia, or blood coagulation disorder; use with caution in jaundiced or premature infants

Adverse Reactions

Cardiovascular: Cyanosis
Hepatic: Hyperlipemia, hepatomegaly
Local: Thrombophlebitis
Respiratory: Dyspnea
Miscellaneous: Sepsis

Stability May be stored at room temperature; do not use if emulsion appears to be oiling out

Mechanism of Action Essential for normal structure and function of cell membranes

Usual Dosage Fat emulsion should not exceed 60% of the total daily calories

Premature infants: Initial dose: 0.25-0.5 g/kg/day, increase by 0.25-0.5 g/kg/day to a maximum of 3-4 g/kg/day; maximum rate of infusion: 0.15 g/kg/hour (0.75 mL/kg/hour of 20% solution)

Infants and Children: Initial dose: 0.5-1 g/kg/day, increase by 0.5 g/kg/day to a maximum of 3-4 g/kg/day; maximum rate of infusion: 0.25 g/kg/hour (1.25 mL/kg/hour of 20% solution)

Adolescents and Adults: Initial dose: 1 g/kg/day, increase by 0.5-1 g/kg/day to a maximum of 2.5 g/kg/day; maximum rate of infusion: 0.25 g/kg/hour (1.25 mL/kg/hour of 20% solution); do not exceed 50 mL/hour (20%) or 100 mL/hour (10%)

Children and Adults: Fatty acid deficiency: 8% to 10% of total caloric intake; infuse once or twice weekly

Note: At the onset of therapy, the patient should be observed for any immediate allergic reactions such as dyspnea, cyanosis, and fever. Slower initial rates of infusion may be used for the first 10-15 minutes of the infusion (eg, 0.1 mL/minute of 10% or 0.05 mL/minute of 20% solution).

Monitoring Parameters Serum triglycerides, free fatty acids

Nursing Implications May be simultaneously infused with amino acid dextrose mixtures by means of Y-connector located near infusion site

Additional Information Both solutions are isotonic (10% =1.1 cal/mL; 20% = 2 cal/mL) and may be administered peripherally; avoid use of 10% fat emulsion in preterm infants; a greater accumulation of plasma lipids occurs due to the greater phospholipid load of the 10% fat emulsion

Dosage Forms Injection: 10% (100 mL, 250 mL, 500 mL); 20% (100 mL, 250 mL, 500 mL)

References

Haumont D, Richelle M, Deckelbaum RJ, et al, "Effect of Liposomal Content of Lipid Emulsions of Plasma Lipid Concentrations in Low Birth Weight Infants Receiving Parenteral Nutrition," *J Pediatr*, 1992, 121(5 Pt 1):759-63.

5-FC *see* Flucytosine *on page 249*

Feldene® *see* Piroxicam *on page 463*

Fenesin™ *see* Guaifenesin *on page 278*

Fentanyl and Droperidol *see* Droperidol and Fentanyl *on page 212*

Fentanyl Citrate (fen' ta nil)

Related Information

Compatibility of Medications Mixed in a Syringe *on page 717*
Narcotic Analgesics Comparison Chart *on page 721-722*
Overdose and Toxicology Information *on page 696-700*
Preprocedure Sedatives in Children *on page 687-689*

Brand Names Duragesic™; Sublimaze®

Therapeutic Category Analgesic, Narcotic; General Anesthetic

Use Sedation; relief of pain; preoperative medication; adjunct to general or regional anesthesia; management of chronic pain (transdermal product)

Restrictions C-II

Pregnancy Risk Factor B (D if used for prolonged periods or in high doses at term)

Contraindications Hypersensitivity to fentanyl or any component; increased intracranial pressure; severe respiratory depression; severe liver or renal insufficiency

Warnings Rapid I.V. infusion may result in skeletal muscle and chest wall rigidity → impaired ventilation → respiratory distress → apnea, bronchoconstriction, laryngospasm; inject slowly over 3-5 minutes; nondepolarizing skeletal muscle relaxant may be required

Precautions Use with caution in patients with bradycardia

Adverse Reactions

Cardiovascular: Hypotension, bradycardia

Central nervous system: CNS depression, drowsiness, dizziness, sedation

Dermatologic: Erythema, pruritus

Endocrine & metabolic: ADH release

Gastrointestinal: Nausea, vomiting, constipation

Hepatic: Biliary tract spasm

Local: Transdermal system: Edema, erythema, pruritus

Musculoskeletal: Skeletal and thoracic muscle rigidity especially following rapid I.V. administration

Ocular: Miosis

Renal & genitourinary: Urinary tract spasm

Respiratory: Respiratory depression

Miscellaneous: Physical and psychological dependence with prolonged use

Drug Interactions CNS depressants, phenothiazines, tricyclic antidepressants may potentiate fentanyl's adverse effects

Stability Protect from light

Mechanism of Action Binds with stereospecific receptors at many sites within the CNS, increases pain threshold, alters pain reception, inhibits ascending pain pathways

Pharmacodynamics

Onset of analgesia:

- I.M.: 7-15 minutes
- I.V.: Almost immediate

Duration:

- I.M.: 1-2 hours
- I.V.: 30-60 minutes; respiratory depressant effect may last longer than analgesic effect

Pharmacokinetics

Metabolism: Metabolized in the liver

Half-life: 2-4 hours

Elimination: Excreted in the urine primarily as metabolites and 10% as unchanged drug

Usual Dosage Doses should be titrated to appropriate effects; wide range of doses, dependent upon desired degree of analgesia/anesthesia

Children 1-12 years:

- Sedation for minor procedures/analgesia: I.M., I.V.: 1-2 μg/kg/dose; may repeat at 30- to 60-minute intervals. **Note:** Children 18-36 months of age may require 2-3 μg/kg/dose.
- Continuous sedation/analgesia: Initial I.V. bolus: 1-2 μg/kg then 1 μg/kg/hour; titrate upward; usual: 1-3 μg/kg/hour
- Transdermal: Not recommended

Children >12 years and Adults:

- Sedation for minor procedures/analgesia: I.V.: 0.5-1 μg/kg/dose; may repeat after 30-60 minutes; **or** 25-50 μg, repeat full dose in 5 minutes if needed, may repeat 4-5 times with 25 μg at 5-minute intervals if needed. **Note:** Higher doses are used for major procedures
- Preoperative sedation, adjunct to regional anesthesia, postoperative pain: I.M., I.V.: 50-100 μg/dose
- Adjunct to general anesthesia: I.M., I.V.: 2-50 μg/kg
- General anesthesia without additional anesthetic agents: I.V. 50-100 μg/kg with O_2 and skeletal muscle relaxant
- Transdermal: Initial: 25 μg/hour system; if currently receiving opiates, convert to fentanyl equivalent and administer equianalgesic dosage

(Continued)

Fentanyl Citrate *(Continued)*

Dosing adjustment in renal impairment:

Cl_{cr} 10-50 mL/minute: Administer 75% of dose

Cl_{cr} <10 mL/minute: Administer 50% of dose

Administration I.V.: Give by slow I.V. push over 3-5 minutes or by continuous infusion

Monitoring Parameters Respiratory rate, blood pressure, heart rate

Nursing Implications Patients with ↑ temperature may have ↑ fentanyl absorption transdermally, observe for adverse effects, dosage adjustment may be needed; pharmacologic and adverse effects can be seen after discontinuation of transdermal system, observe patients for at least 12 hours after transdermal product removed

Additional Information An opioid antagonist, resuscitative and intubation equipment, and oxygen should be available; fentanyl is 50-100 times as potent as morphine; morphine 10 mg I.M. = fentanyl 0.1-0.2 mg I.M.; fentanyl has less hypotensive effects than morphine or meperidine due to minimal or no histamine release; keep transdermal product (both used and unused) out of the reach of children; do **not** use soap, alcohol, or other solvents to remove transdermal gel if it accidentally touches skin as they may ↑ transdermal absorption, use copious amounts of water

Dosage Forms

Injection: 0.05 mg/mL (2 mL, 5 mL, 10 mL, 20 mL)

Transdermal system: 25 μg/hour (10 cm^2); 50 μg/hour (20 cm^2); 75 μg/hour (30 cm^2); 100 μg/hour (40 cm^2) all available in 5's

References

Billmire DA, Neale HW, and Gregory RO, "Use of I.V. Fentanyl in the Outpatient Treatment of Pediatric Facial Trauma," *J Trauma*, 1985, 25(11):1079-80.

Zeltzer LK, Altman A, Cohen D, et al, "Report of the Subcommittee on the Management of Pain Associated With Procedures in Children With Cancer," *Pediatrics*, 1990, 86(5 Pt 2):826-31.

Feosol® [OTC] *see* Ferrous Sulfate *on next page*

Feosol® Spansules® [OTC] *see* Ferrous Sulfate *on next page*

Fergon® [OTC] *see* Ferrous Gluconate *on this page*

Fer-In-Sol® [OTC] *see* Ferrous Sulfate *on next page*

Ferndex® *see* Dextroamphetamine Sulfate *on page 180*

Fero-Gradumet® [OTC] *see* Ferrous Sulfate *on next page*

Ferospace® [OTC] *see* Ferrous Sulfate *on next page*

Ferralet® [OTC] *see* Ferrous Gluconate *on this page*

Ferra-TD® [OTC] *see* Ferrous Sulfate *on next page*

Ferrous Gluconate (gloo' koe nate)

Related Information

Overdose and Toxicology Information *on page 696-700*

Brand Names Fergon® [OTC]; Ferralet® [OTC]; Simron® [OTC]

Therapeutic Category Iron Salt

Use Prevention and treatment of iron deficiency anemias

Pregnancy Risk Factor A

Contraindications Hemochromatosis, hemolytic anemia; known hypersensitivity to iron salts

Warnings Avoid use in premature infants until the vitamin E stores deficient at birth are replenished

Precautions Avoid using for >6 months, except in patients with conditions that require prolonged therapy; avoid in patients with peptic ulcer, enteritis, or ulcerative colitis; avoid in patients receiving frequent blood transfusions

Adverse Reactions

Gastrointestinal: GI irritation, epigastric pain, nausea, diarrhea, dark stool, constipation

Miscellaneous: Liquid preparations may temporarily stain the teeth

Drug Interactions Absorption of oral preparation of iron and tetracyclines are decreased when both of these drugs are given together; concurrent administration of antacids may decrease iron absorption; iron may decrease absorption of penicillamine when given at the same time. Response to iron therapy may be delayed in patients receiving chloramphenicol. Concurrent administration of ≥200 mg vitamin C per 30 mg elemental iron increases absorption of oral iron. Milk may decrease absorption of iron.

Mechanism of Action Replaces iron, found in hemoglobin, myoglobin, and enzymes; allows the transportation of oxygen via hemoglobin

Pharmacodynamics

Onset of action: The onset of hematologic response to either oral or parenteral iron salts is essentially the same; red blood cell form and color changes within 3-10 days

Peak effect: Peak reticulocytosis occurs in 5-10 days, and hemoglobin values increase within 2-4 weeks

Usual Dosage Oral (dose expressed in terms of elemental iron):

Children:

Severe iron deficiency anemia: 4-6 mg iron/kg/day in 3 divided doses

Mild to moderate iron deficiency anemia: 3 mg iron/kg/day in 1-2 divided doses

Prophylaxis: 1-2 mg iron/kg/day

Adults:

Iron deficiency: 60 mg iron twice daily up to 60 mg iron 4 times/day

Prophylaxis: 60 mg iron/day

Monitoring Parameters Serum iron, total iron binding capacity, reticulocyte count, hemoglobin

Test Interactions False-positive for blood in stool by the guaiac test

Patient Information May color the stool black; take between meals for maximum absorption; may take with food if GI upset occurs; do **not** take with milk or antacid

Additional Information When treating iron deficiency anemias, treat for 3-4 months after hemoglobin/hematocrit return to normal in order to replenish total body stores

Dosage Forms Amount of elemental iron in parenthesis

Capsule, soft gelatin: 86 mg (10 mg)

Elixir: 300 mg/5 mL (34 mg/5 mL)

Tablet: 300 mg (34 mg); 320 mg (37 mg); 325 mg (38 mg)

Recommended Daily Allowance of Iron (Dosage expressed as elemental iron)

Age	RDA
<5 mo	5 mg
5 mo–10 y	10 mg
11–18 y (male)	12 mg
11–50 y (female)	15 mg
>18 y (male)	10 mg
>50 y (female)	

Ferrous Sulfate

Related Information

Overdose and Toxicology Information *on page 696-700*

Brand Names Feosol® [OTC]; Feosol® Spansules® [OTC]; Fer-In-Sol® [OTC]; Fero-Gradumet® [OTC]; Ferospace® [OTC]; Ferra-TD® [OTC]; Mol-Iron® [OTC]

Synonyms $FeSO_4$; Iron Sulfate

Therapeutic Category Iron Salt

Use Prevention and treatment of iron deficiency anemias

Pregnancy Risk Factor A

Contraindications Hemochromatosis, hemolytic anemia; known hypersensitivity to iron salts

Warnings Avoid use in premature infants until the vitamin E stores, deficient at birth, are replenished

(Continued)

Ferrous Sulfate *(Continued)*

Precautions Avoid using for >6 months, except in patients with conditions that require prolonged therapy; avoid in patients with peptic ulcer, enteritis, or ulcerative colitis; avoid in patients receiving frequent blood transfusions

Adverse Reactions

Gastrointestinal: GI irritation, epigastric pain, nausea, diarrhea, dark stool, constipation

Miscellaneous: Liquid preparations may temporarily stain the teeth

Drug Interactions Absorption of oral preparation of iron and tetracyclines are decreased when both of these drugs are given together; concurrent administration of antacids may decrease iron absorption; iron may decrease absorption of penicillamine when given at the same time. Response to iron therapy may be delayed in patients receiving chloramphenicol. Concurrent administration of ≥200 mg vitamin C per 30 mg elemental iron increases absorption of oral iron. Milk may decrease absorption of iron.

Mechanism of Action Replaces iron, found in hemoglobin, myoglobin, and other enzymes; allows the transportation of oxygen via hemoglobin

Pharmacodynamics

Onset of action: Hematologic response to either oral or parenteral iron salts is essentially the same; red blood cell form and color changes within 3-10 days

Peak effect: Peak reticulocytosis occurs in 5-10 days, and hemoglobin values increase within 2-4 weeks

Usual Dosage Oral (dose expressed in terms of elemental iron):

Children:

- Severe iron deficiency anemia: 4-6 mg iron/kg/day in 3 divided doses
- Mild to moderate iron deficiency anemia: 3 mg iron/kg/day in 1-2 divided doses
- Prophylaxis: 1-2 mg iron/kg/day up to a maximum of 15 mg/day

Adults:

- Iron deficiency: 60 mg iron twice daily up to 60 mg iron 4 times/day or 50 mg iron (extended release) 1-2 times/day
- Prophylaxis: 60 mg iron/day

Monitoring Parameters Serum iron, total iron binding capacity, reticulocyte count, hemoglobin

Test Interactions False-positive for blood in stool by the guaiac test

Patient Information May color the stool black; take between meals for maximum absorption; may take with food if GI upset occurs; do **not** take with milk or antacid

Additional Information When treating iron deficiency anemias, treat for 3-4 months after hemoglobin/hematocrit return to normal in order to replenish total body stores

Dosage Forms Amount of elemental iron is listed in brackets

Capsule: 250 mg [50 mg]

Drops, oral: 75 mg/0.6 mL [15 mg/0.6 mL] (50 mL); 125 mg/mL [25 mg/mL] (50 mL)

Elixir: 220 mg/5 mL [44 mg/5 mL] (473 mL, 4000 mL)

Liquid: 300 mg/5 [60 mg/5 mL] mL

Syrup: 90 mg/5 mL [18 mg/5 mL]

Tablet: 195 mg [39 mg]; 300 mg [60 mg]; 325 mg [65 mg]

Tablet, timed release: 525 mg [105 mg]

$FeSO_4$ *see* Ferrous Sulfate *on previous page*

Feverall™ [OTC] *see* Acetaminophen *on page 16*

Fiberall® [OTC] *see* Psyllium *on page 498*

Filgrastim (fil gra' stim)

Brand Names Neupogen®

Synonyms G-CSF; Granulocyte Colony Stimulating Factor

Therapeutic Category Colony Stimulating Factor

Use To reduce the duration of neutropenia and the associated risk of infection in patients with nonmyeloid malignancies receiving myelosuppressive chemotherapeutic regimens associated with a significant incidence of severe neutropenia with fever; it has also been used in AIDS patients on zidovudine and in patients with noncancer chemotherapy-induced neutropenia

Pregnancy Risk Factor C

Contraindications Hypersensitivity to *E. coli* derived proteins or G-CSF

Warnings Leukocytosis (white blood cell counts of $\geq$100,000/mm^3) has been observed in approximately 2% of patients receiving G-CSF at doses >5 μg/kg/day

Precautions Do not administer 24 hours prior to or 24 hours following the administration of chemotherapy; use with caution in any malignancy with myeloid characteristics due to G-CSF's potential to act as a growth factor; use with caution in patients with gout, psoriasis; monitor patients with pre-existing cardiac conditions as cardiac events (myocardial infarctions, arrhythmias) have been reported in premarketing clinical studies. Be alert to the possibility of ARDS in septic patients.

Premature discontinuation of G-CSF therapy prior to the time of recovery from the expected neutrophil nadir is generally not recommended. A transient increase in neutrophil counts is typically seen 1-2 days after initiation of therapy. For a sustained therapeutic response, G-CSF should be continued until the post nadir absolute neutrophil count (ANC) reaches:
10,000/mm^3 in chemotherapy treated patients, or
>1000/mm^3 for 3 consecutive days in bone marrow transplant patients

Adverse Reactions

Cardiovascular: Transient decrease in blood pressure, vasculitis

Central nervous system: Fever

Dermatologic: Exacerbation of pre-existing skin disorders

Endocrine & metabolic: Reversible increase in uric acid, lactate dehydrogenase, alkaline phosphatase

Gastrointestinal: Splenomegaly, nausea

Hematologic: Thrombocytopenia

Musculoskeletal: Medullary bone pain (24% incidence) is generally dose related, localized to the lower back, posterior iliac crests, and sternum; osteoporosis

Renal & genitourinary: Hematuria, proteinuria

Stability Store in refrigerator; stable for 6 hours at room temperature; solutions with concentration $\geq$15 μg/mL in D_5W are stable for 24 hours; incompatible with salt solutions

Mechanism of Action Stimulates the production, maturation, and activation of neutrophils; G-CSF activates neutrophils to increase both their migration and cytotoxicity

Pharmacodynamics

Onset of action: Immediate transient leukopenia with the nadir occurring 5-15 minutes after an I.V. dose or 30-60 minutes after a S.C. dose followed by a sustained elevation in neutrophil levels within the first 24 hours reaching a plateau in 3-5 days

Duration: Upon discontinuation of G-CSF, ANC decreases by 50% within 2 days and returns to pretreatment levels within 1 week; white counts return to the normal range in 4-7 days

Pharmacokinetics

Distribution: V_d: 150 mL/kg

Bioavailability: Not bioavailable after oral administration

Half-life: 1.8-3.5 hours

Time to peak serum concentration: Within 2-6 hours following S.C. administration

Elimination: No evidence of drug accumulation over a 11- to 20-day period

Usual Dosage I.V., S.C. (refer to individual protocols):

Children and Adults: 5-10 μg/kg/day (~150-300 μg/m^2/day) once daily for up to 14 days until ANC = 10,000/mm^3; dose escalations at 5 μg/kg/day may be required in some individuals when response at 5 μg/kg/day is not adequate; dosages of 0.6-120 μg/kg/day have been used in children ranging in age from 3 months to 18 years

Administration Administer as a bolus S.C. injection, a short I.V. infusion (15-30 minutes) or a continuous infusion. If the final concentration of G-CSF in D_5W is <15 μg/mL, then add 2 mg albumin/mL of I.V. fluid; the solution is stable for 24 hours; albumin acts as a carrier molecule to prevent drug adsorption to the I.V. tubing. Albumin should be added to the D_5W prior to addition of G-CSF; do not shake solution to avoid foaming

Monitoring Parameters CBC with differential and platelet count, hematocrit, uric acid, urinalysis, liver function tests

(Continued)

Filgrastim *(Continued)*

Reference Range Blood samples for monitoring the hematologic effects of G-CSF should be drawn just before the next dose at least twice weekly

Patient Information Possible bone pain

Nursing Implications Bone pain management is usually successful with non-narcotic analgesic therapy

Dosage Forms Injection, preservative free: 300 μg/mL (1 mL, 1.6 mL), produced by recombinant DNA technology using an *E. coli* expression system

References

Bonilla MA, Gillio AP, Ruggeiro M, et al, "Effects of Recombinant Human Granulocyte Colony-Stimulating Factor on Neutropenia in Patients With Congenital Agranulocytosis," *N Engl J Med*, 1989, 320(24):1574-80.

Hollingshead LM, Goa KL, "Recombinant Granulocyte Colony-Stimulating Factor (rG-CSF). A Review of Its Pharmacological Properties and Prospective Role in Neutropenic Conditions," *Drugs*, 1991, 42(2):300-30.

Morstyn G, Campbell L, Lieschke G, et al, "Treatment of Chemotherapy-induced Neutropenia by Subcutaneously Administered Granulocyte Colony-Stimulating Factor With Optimization of Dose and Duration of Therapy," *J Clin Oncol*, 1989, 7(10):1554-62.

Taylor KM, Jagannath S, Spitzer G, et al, "Recombinant Human Granulocyte Colony-Stimulating Factor Hastens Granulocyte Recovery After High Dose Chemotherapy and Autologous Bone Marrow Transplantation in Hodgkin's Disease," *J Clin Oncol*, 1989, 7(12):1791-9.

Flagyl® *see* Metronidazole *on page 383*

Flarex® *see* Fluorometholone *on page 257*

Flatulex® [OTC] *see* Simethicone *on page 524*

Flavorcee® [OTC] *see* Ascorbic Acid *on page 59*

Flecainide Acetate (fle kay' nide)

Brand Names Tambocor®

Therapeutic Category Antiarrhythmic Agent, Class Ic

Use Prevention and suppression of documented life-threatening ventricular arrhythmias (ie, sustained ventricular tachycardia); controlling symptomatic, disabling supraventricular tachycardias in patients without structural heart disease

Pregnancy Risk Factor C

Contraindications Pre-existing second or third degree A-V block; right bundle branch block associated with left hemiblock (bifascicular block) or trifascicular block; cardiogenic shock, myocardial depression; known hypersensitivity to the drug

Warnings The manufacturer and FDA recommend that this drug be reserved for life-threatening ventricular arrhythmias unresponsive to conventional therapy. Its use for symptomatic nonsustained ventricular tachycardia, frequent premature ventricular complexes (PVCs), uniform and multiform PVCs and/or coupled PVCs is no longer recommended. Flecainide can worsen or cause arrhythmias with an associated risk of death. Proarrhythmic effects range from an increased number of PVCs to more severe ventricular tachycardias (ie, tachycardias that are more sustained or more resistant to conversion to sinus rhythm).

Precautions Worsening arrhythmias, pre-existing sinus node dysfunction, sick sinus syndrome, history of congestive heart failure or myocardial dysfunction; increases in PR interval ≥300 MS, QRS ≥180 MS, QT_c interval increases and/or new bundle branch block; patients with pacemakers, renal impairment and/or hepatic impairment

Adverse Reactions

Cardiovascular: Bradycardia, heart block, increased PR, QRS duration, worsening ventricular arrhythmias, congestive heart failure, palpitations, chest pain, edema

Central nervous system: Dizziness, fatigue, tremor, nervousness hypoesthesia, paresthesia, headache

Dermatologic: Rashes

Gastrointestinal: Nausea

Hematologic: Blood dyscrasias

Hepatic: Possible hepatic dysfunction

Ocular: Blurred vision
Respiratory: Dyspnea

Drug Interactions Digoxin → increased plasma digoxin concentrations; beta blockers → possible additive negative inotropic effects; alkalinizing agents (high dose antacids, carbonic anhydrase inhibitors or sodium bicarbonate) may decrease flecainide's clearance; amiodarone and cimetidine may increase flecainide serum concentrations

Mechanism of Action Class IC antiarrhythmic; slows conduction in cardiac tissue by altering transport of ions across cell membranes; causes slight prolongation of refractory periods; decreases the rate of rise of the action potential without affecting its duration; increases electrical stimulation threshold of ventricle, HIS-Purkinje system; possesses local anesthetic and moderate negative inotropic effects

Pharmacokinetics

Distribution: V_d: Adults: 5-13.4 L/kg
Protein binding: 40% to 50% (alpha$_1$ glycoprotein)
Metabolism: Metabolized in liver
Bioavailability: 85% to 90%
Half-life:
- Infants: 11-12 hours
- Children: 8 hours
- Adults: 7-22 hours, increased half-life with congestive heart failure or renal dysfunction

Peak serum levels: Oral: Within 1.5-3 hours
Elimination: Excreted in urine as unchanged drug and metabolites (10% to 50%)

Usual Dosage Oral:

Children: Initial: 3 mg/kg/day or 50-100 mg/m^2/day in 3 divided doses; usual: 3-6 mg/kg/day or 100-150 mg/m^2/day in 3 divided doses; up to 11 mg/kg/day or 200 mg/m^2/day for uncontrolled patients with subtherapeutic levels

Adults: Life-threatening ventricular arrhythmias: Initial: 100 mg every 12 hours, increase by 100 mg/day (given in 2 doses/day) every 4 days to maximum of 400 mg/day; for patients receiving 400 mg/day who are not controlled and have trough concentrations <0.6 μg/mL, dosage may be increased to 600 mg/day

Prevention of paroxysmal supraventricular arrhythmias in patients with disabling symptoms but no structural heart disease: Initial: 50 mg every 12 hours; maximum: 300 mg/day

Dosing adjustment in renal failure: Children and Adults: Decrease the usual dose by 25% to 50%

Monitoring Parameters EKG and serum concentrations

Reference Range Therapeutic: 0.2-1 μg/mL (SI: 0.4-2 μmol/L). **Note**: Pediatric patients may respond at the lower end of the recommended therapeutic range.

Dosage Forms Tablet: 50 mg, 100 mg, 150 mg

Extemporaneous Preparation(s) A 5 mg/mL suspension compounded from tablets and an oral flavored commercially available diluent (Roxane®) was stable for up to 45 days when stored at 5°C or 25°C in amber glass bottles

Wiest DB, Garner SS, and Pagacz LR, "Stability of Flecainide Acetate in an Extemporaneously Compounded Oral Suspension," *Am J Hosp Pharm*, 1992, 49(6):1467-70.

References

Perry JC, McQuinn RL, Smith RT, et al, "Flecainide Acetate for Resistant Arrhythmias in the Young: Efficacy and Pharmacokinetics," *J Am Coll Cardiol*, 1989, 14(1):185-91.

Priestley KA, Ladusans EJ, Rosenthal E, et al, "Experience With Flecainide for the Treatment of Cardiac Arrhythmias in Children," *Eur Heart J*, 1988, 9(12):1284-90.

Zeigler V, Gillette PC, Ross BA, et al, "Flecainide for Supraventricular and Ventricular Arrhythmias in Children and Young Adults," *Am J Cardiol*, 1988, 62(10 Pt 1):818-20.

Fleet® Babylax® [OTC] *see* Glycerin *on page 273*

Fleet® Enema [OTC] *see* Sodium Phosphate *on page 529*

Fleet® Laxative [OTC] *see* Bisacodyl *on page 83*

Fleet® Mineral Oil Enema [OTC] *see* Mineral Oil *on page 390*

Fleet® Phospho®-Soda [OTC] *see* Sodium Phosphate *on page 529*

Flexeril® *see* Cyclobenzaprine Hydrochloride *on page 161*

Florinef® Acetate *see* Fludrocortisone Acetate *on page 251*

Flubenisolone *see* Betamethasone *on page 81*

Fluconazole (floo koe' na zole)

Brand Names Diflucan®

Therapeutic Category Antifungal Agent, Systemic

Use Treatment of susceptible fungal infections including oropharyngeal and esophageal candidiasis; treatment of systemic candidal infections including urinary tract infection, peritonitis, and pneumonia; treatment of cryptococcal meningitis

Pregnancy Risk Factor C

Contraindications Known hypersensitivity to fluconazole or other azoles

Warnings Patients who develop abnormal liver function tests during fluconazole therapy should be monitored closely for the development of more severe hepatic injury; if clinical signs and symptoms consistent with liver disease develop that may be attributable to fluconazole, fluconazole should be discontinued

Precautions Dosage modification required in patients with impaired renal function

Adverse Reactions

Cardiovascular: Pallor

Central nervous system: Dizziness, headache (1.9%), seizures

Dermatologic: Skin rash (1.8%), exfoliative skin disorders

Endocrine & metabolic: Hypokalemia

Gastrointestinal: Nausea (3.7%), abdominal pain, vomiting, diarrhea (1.5%)

Hematologic: Eosinophilia

Hepatic: Elevated AST, ALT, or alkaline phosphatase

Drug Interactions Oral antidiabetic agents, hydrochlorothiazide, warfarin; fluconazole ↑ plasma cyclosporine and phenytoin concentrations; rifampin ↑ fluconazole metabolism

Stability Incompatible with ampicillin, calcium gluconate, ceftazidime, cefotaxime, cefuroxime, ceftriaxone, clindamycin, furosemide, imipenem, ticarcillin, and piperacillin

Mechanism of Action Interferes with cytochrome P-450 activity, decreasing ergosterol synthesis (principal sterol in fungal cell membrane) and inhibiting cell membrane formation

Pharmacokinetics

Absorption: Oral absorption is unaffected by the presence of food

Distribution: Distributes widely into body tissues and fluids including the CSF

Protein binding: 11% to 12%

Bioavailability: Oral: >90%

Half-life: 25-30 hours with normal renal function

Time to peak serum concentration: Oral: Within 2-4 hours

Elimination: 80% of dose is excreted unchanged in the urine

Usual Dosage The daily dose of fluconazole is the same for oral and I.V. administration

Efficacy of fluconazole has not been established in children; a small number of patients from ages 3-13 years and a few neonates and infants have been treated with fluconazole using doses of 3-6 mg/kg/day divided once daily. Doses as high as 12 mg/kg/day once daily have been used to treat candidiasis in immunocompromised children; 10-12 mg/kg/day doses once daily have been used prophylactically against fungal infections in pediatric bone marrow transplantation patients.

Adult doses of fluconazole: Oral, I.V.: See table for once daily dosing.

Prophylaxis against fungal infections in bone marrow transplantation patients: 400 mg/day

Dosing adjustment in renal impairment:

Cl_{cr} 21-50 mL/minute: Administer 50% of recommended dose

Cl_{cr} 11-20 mL/minute: Administer 25% of recommended dose

Indication	Day 1	Daily Therapy	Minimum Duration of Therapy
Oropharyngeal candidiasis	200 mg	100 mg	14 d
Esophageal candidiasis	200 mg	100 mg	21 d
Systemic candidiasis	400 mg	200 mg	28 d
Cryptococcal meningitis acute	400 mg	200 mg	10–12 wk after CSF culture becomes negative
relapse	200 mg	200 mg	

Administration Parenteral fluconazole must be administered by intravenous infusion over approximately 1-2 hours at a rate not to exceed 200 mg/hour and a final concentration for administration of 2 mg/mL

Monitoring Parameters Periodic liver function and renal function tests

Dosage Forms

Injection: 2 mg/mL (100 mL, 200 mL)

Tablet: 50 mg, 100 mg, 200 mg

References

Goodman JL, Winston DJ, Greenfield RA, et al, "A Controlled Trial of Fluconazole to Prevent Fungal Infections in Patients Undergoing Bone Marrow Transplantation," *N Engl J Med*, 1992, 326(13):845-51.

Lee JW, Seibel NL, Amantea M, et al, "Safety and Pharmacokinetics of Fluconazole in Children With Neoplastic Diseases," *J Pediatr*, 1992, 120(6):987-93.

Moncino MD and Gutman LT, "Severe Systemic Cryptococcal Disease in a Child: Review of Prognostic Indicators Predicting Treatment Failure and an Approach to Maintenance Therapy With Oral Fluconazole," *Pediatr Infect Dis J*, 1990, 9(5):363-8.

Viscoli C, Castagnola E, Fioredda F, et al, "Fluconazole in the Treatment of Candidiasis in Immunocompromised Children," *Antimicrob Agents Chemother*, 1991, 35(2):365-7.

Flucytosine (floo sye' toe seen)

Related Information

Blood Level Sampling Time Guidelines *on page 694-695*

Brand Names Ancobon®

Synonyms 5-FC; 5-Flurocytosine

Therapeutic Category Antifungal Agent, Systemic

Use Treatment of susceptible fungal infections including some strains of *Candida*, *Cryptococcus*, and *Torulopsis*

Pregnancy Risk Factor C

Contraindications Hypersensitivity to flucytosine or any component

Precautions Use with extreme caution in patients with renal impairment, bone marrow depression, patients with AIDS; dosage modification required in patients with impaired renal function

Adverse Reactions

Central nervous system: Confusion, sedation, headache, ataxia, hallucinations, vertigo

Dermatologic: Rash

Endocrine & metabolic: Temporary growth failure

Gastrointestinal: Nausea, vomiting, diarrhea, enterocolitis

Hematologic: Bone marrow depression, anemia, leukopenia, thrombocytopenia

Hepatic: Elevated liver enzymes, hepatitis

Renal & genitourinary: Elevation in serum creatinine and BUN

Miscellaneous: Anaphylaxis, growth failure

Drug Interactions Increased efficacy as well as toxicity (enterocolitis) with concurrent amphotericin administration

Mechanism of Action Penetrates fungal cells and is converted to fluorouracil which competes with uracil interfering with fungal RNA and protein synthesis

(Continued)

Flucytosine *(Continued)*

Pharmacokinetics

Absorption: Oral: 75% to 90%

Distribution: Distributes into CSF and bronchial secretions

Protein binding: 2% to 4%

Metabolism: Minimally metabolized

Half-life: 3-8 hours (prolonged as high as 200 hours in anuria)

Peak serum levels: Oral: Within 2-6 hours

Elimination: 75% to 90% excreted unchanged in the urine by glomerular filtration

Dialyzable (50% to 100%)

Usual Dosage Children and Adults: Oral: 50-150 mg/kg/day in divided doses every 6 hours; for patients with renal impairment, the dosage interval needs to be increased to every 12 hours for >50% decrease in renal function, or every 24 hours for >90% decrease in renal function

Monitoring Parameters Serum creatinine, BUN, alkaline phosphatase, AST, ALT, CBC; serum flucytosine concentrations

Reference Range Therapeutic levels: 25-100 μg/mL

Test Interactions Flucytosine causes markedly false elevations in serum creatinine values when the Ektachem® analyzer is used

Patient Information Take with food over a 15-minute period

Dosage Forms Capsule: 250 mg, 500 mg

Extemporaneous Preparation(s) Contents of two (2) 500 mg capsules can be suspended in distilled water to make 100 mL of 10 mg/mL suspension; suspension is stable for 1 week at room temperature when protected from light; pH of the solution should be kept between 5-6.5

Handbook on Extemporaneous Formulations, Bethesda MD: American Society of Hospital Pharmacists, 1987.

Fludara® *see* Fludarabine Phosphate *on this page*

Fludarabine Phosphate

Brand Names Fludara®

Synonyms FAMP; F-ara-AMP

Therapeutic Category Antineoplastic Agent

Use Treatment of B-cell chronic lymphocytic leukemia unresponsive to previous therapy with an alkylating agent containing regimen. Fludarabine has been tested in several types of pediatric cancers including acute lymphoblastic leukemia, solid tumors, refractory acute lymphocytic leukemia, and acute nonlymphocytic leukemia.

Pregnancy Risk Factor D

Contraindications Hypersensitivity to fludarabine phosphate or any component

Warnings The US Food and Drug Administration (FDA) currently recommends that procedures for proper handling and disposal of antineoplastic agents be considered. Dose levels of 77 mg/m^2/day and above for 5-7 days were associated with severe neurotoxicity. Severe bone marrow suppression has been observed at therapeutic doses. Hematologic function must be frequently monitored. Concomitant therapy with pentostatin may be associated with severe pulmonary toxicity.

Precautions Use with caution in patients with renal insufficiency; dosage adjustment may be needed in patients with impaired renal function or bone marrow depression

Adverse Reactions

Central nervous system: Neurotoxicity (primarily progressive demyelinating encephalopathy), somnolence, weakness

Dermatologic: Pruritus, rash

Endocrine & metabolic: Metabolic acidosis, tumor lysis syndrome

Gastrointestinal: Nausea, vomiting, diarrhea, stomatitis, metallic taste

Hematologic: Leukopenia, neutropenia, thrombocytopenia

Hepatic: Increased transaminase levels

Renal & genitourinary: Hematuria

Respiratory: Interstitial pneumonitis

Drug Interactions Cytarabine when administered with or prior to a fludarabine dose competes for deoxycytidine kinase decreasing the metabolism of F-ara-A to the active F-ara-ATP (inhibits the antineoplastic effect of fludarabine); however, administering fludarabine prior to cytarabine may stimulate activation of cytarabine

Stability Store vial in refrigerator; reconstituted 25 mg/mL fludarabine solution should be used within 8 hours after preparation since it contains no preservatives. When fludarabine is diluted in D_5W or 0.9% sodium chloride to a final concentration of 1 mg/mL, the solution is stable for 24 hours at room temperature.

Mechanism of Action F-ara-AMP is hydrolyzed in serum to F-ara-A which is phosphorylated intracellularly to the active metabolite F-ara-ATP. F-ara-ATP competes with deoxyadenosine triphosphate for incorporation into the A-sites of the DNA strand inhibiting DNA synthesis in the S-phase via inhibition of DNA polymerases and RNA reductase.

Pharmacokinetics

Distribution: Widely distributed with extensive tissue binding

Half-life: Terminal:

Children: 12.4-19 hours

Adults: 7-20 hours

Elimination: Fludarabine clearance appears to be inversely correlated with serum creatinine; at a dose of 25 mg/m^2/day for 5 days, 24% of the dose is excreted in urine; at higher doses, 41% to 60% of a dose is renally excreted

Usual Dosage Not currently FDA approved for use in children. I.V. (refer to individual protocols):

Children:

Acute leukemia: 10 mg/m^2 bolus over 15 minutes followed by a continuous infusion of 30.5 mg/m^2/day over 5 days; or 10.5 mg/m^2 bolus over 15 minutes followed by a continuous infusion of 30.5 mg/m^2/day over 48 hours followed by cytarabine has been used in clinical trials

Solid tumors: 9 mg/m^2 bolus followed by 27 mg/m^2/day continuous infusion over 5 days

Adults: 25 mg/m^2/day over 30 minutes for 5 days; courses are usually repeated every 28 days

Administration Fludarabine phosphate has been administered by intermittent I.V. infusion over 15-30 minutes and by continuous infusion; in clinical trials the loading dose has been diluted in 20 mL D_5W and administered over 15 minutes and the continuous infusion diluted to 240 mL in D_5W and administered at a constant rate of 10 mL/hour; in other clinical studies fludarabine has been diluted to a concentration of 0.25 to 1 mg/mL in D_5W or 0.9% sodium chloride.

Monitoring Parameters CBC with differential, platelet count, AST, ALT, creatinine, serum albumin, and uric acid

Patient Information Notify physician if fever, sore throat, bleeding, bruising, tachypnea, respiratory distress, or neurologic changes occur

Additional Information Myelosuppressive effects:

Granulocyte nadir: 13 days (3-25)

Platelet nadir: 16 days (2-32)

Recovery: 5-7 weeks

Dosage Forms Powder for injection, lyophilized: 50 mg

References

Avramis VI, Champagne J, Sato J, et al, "Pharmacology of Fludarabine Phosphate after a Phase I/II Trial by a Loading Bolus and Continuous Infusion in Pediatric Patients," *Cancer Res*, 1990, 50(22):7226-31.

Von Hoff DD, "Phase I Clinical Trials With Fludarabine Phosphate," *Semin Oncol*, 1990, 17(5 Suppl 8):33-8.

Fludrocortisone Acetate (floo droe kor' ti sone)

Related Information

Systemic Corticosteroids Comparison Chart *on page 727*

Brand Names Florinef® Acetate

Synonyms Fluohydrisone Acetate; Fluohydrocortisone Acetate; 9α-Fluorohydrocortisone Acetate

Therapeutic Category Mineralocorticoid

Use Addison's disease; partial replacement therapy for adrenal insufficiency and for treatment of salt-losing forms of congenital adrenogenital syndrome

Pregnancy Risk Factor C

Contraindications Known hypersensitivity to fludrocortisone; congestive heart failure, systemic fungal infections

(Continued)

Fludrocortisone Acetate *(Continued)*

Adverse Reactions

Cardiovascular: Hypertension, edema, congestive heart failure

Central nervous system: Convulsions, headache

Dermatologic: Acne, rash

Endocrine & metabolic: Hypokalemic alkalosis, suppression of growth, hyperglycemia, HPA suppression

Gastrointestinal: Peptic ulcer

Hematologic: Bruising

Musculoskeletal: Muscle weakness

Ocular: Cataracts

Mechanism of Action Promotes increased reabsorption of sodium and loss of potassium from distal tubules

Usual Dosage Oral:

Infants and Children: 0.05-0.1 mg/day

Adults: 0.05-0.2 mg/day

Monitoring Parameters Serum electrolytes, blood pressure, serum renin

Additional Information In patients with salt-losing forms of congenital adrenogenital syndrome, use along with cortisone or hydrocortisone; fludrocortisone 0.1 mg has sodium retention activity equal to DOCA® 1 mg

Dosage Forms Tablet: 0.1 mg

Flumazenil

Brand Names Mazicon™

Therapeutic Category Antidote, Benzodiazepine

Use Benzodiazepine antagonist, reverses sedative effects of benzodiazepines used in general anesthesia; management of benzodiazepine overdose; does **not** antagonize CNS effects of other GABA agonists (ethanol, barbiturates, or general anesthetics); does **not** reverse narcotics

Pregnancy Risk Factor C

Contraindications Hypersensitivity to flumazenil or benzodiazepines; patients given benzodiazepines for control of potentially life-threatening conditions (eg, control of intracranial pressure or status epilepticus); patients with signs of serious cyclic-antidepressant overdosage

Warnings Seizures may occur in patients physically dependent on benzodiazepines or in patients with serious cyclic antidepressant overdoses; higher than normal doses of benzodiazepines may be required to treat these seizures

Precautions Monitor patients for return of sedation and respiratory depression. Flumazenil should be used with caution in the intensive care unit because of increased risk of unrecognized benzodiazepine dependence in such settings.

Adverse Reactions

Cardiovascular: Arrhythmias

Central nervous system: Seizures (more common in patients physically dependent on benzodiazepines or with cyclic antidepressant overdoses), fatigue, dizziness, increased sweating, headache, agitation, emotional liability

Gastrointestinal: Nausea, vomiting

Local: Pain at injection site

Ocular: Blurred vision

Drug Interactions Use with caution in mixed drug overdose; toxic effects of other drugs (especially with cyclic antidepressants) may occur with reversal of benzodiazepine effects

Stability Compatible with D_5W, lactated Ringer's or normal saline for 24 hours; discard any unused solution after 24 hours

Mechanism of Action Antagonizes the effect of benzodiazepines on the GABA/benzodiazepine receptor complex. Flumazenil is benzodiazepine specific and does not antagonize other nonbenzodiazepine GABA agonists (including ethanol, barbiturates, general anesthetics); does not reverse the effects of opiates

Pharmacodynamics

Onset of benzodiazepine reversal: Within 1-3 minutes

Peak effect: 6-10 minutes

Duration: Usually <1 hour; duration is related to dose given and benzodiazepine plasma concentrations; reversal effects of flumazenil may wear off before effects of benzodiazepine

Pharmacokinetics

Distribution: Adults:

Initial V_d: 0.5 L/kg

V_{dss} 0.77-1.6 L/kg

Protein binding: ~50%

Half-life, adults:

Alpha: 7-15 minutes

Terminal: 41-79 minutes

Elimination: Clearance dependent upon hepatic blood flow, hepatically eliminated; <1% excreted unchanged in urine

Usual Dosage I.V.:

Children:

Reversal of conscious sedation or general anesthesia: Minimal information available; an initial dose of 0.01 mg/kg (maximum dose: 0.2 mg), then 0.005 mg/kg (maximum dose: 0.2 mg) given every minute to a maximum total dose of 1 mg has been used to reverse midazolam after circumcision in 40 children 3-12 years of age (mean: 7 years); mean total dose required: 0.024 mg/kg; further studies are needed

Management of benzodiazepine overdose: Minimal information available; a few cases have reported an initial dose of 0.01 or 0.02 mg/kg (maximum dose: 0.125 mg) with repeat doses of 0.01 mg/kg or follow up continuous infusions of 0.05 mg/hour (0.004 mg/kg/hour) or 0.05 mg/kg/hour (n=1) for 2-6 hours; further studies are needed

Adults:

Reversal of conscious sedation or general anesthesia: 0.2 mg over 15 seconds; may repeat 0.2 mg every 60 seconds up to a total of 1 mg, usual dose: 0.6-1 mg. In event of resedation, may repeat doses at 20-minute intervals with maximum 1 mg/dose given as 0.2 mg/minute, maximum of 3 mg in 1 hour.

Management of benzodiazepine overdose: 0.2 mg over 30 seconds; may give 0.3 mg dose after 30 seconds if desired level of consciousness is not obtained; additional doses of 0.5 mg can be given over 30 seconds at 1-minute intervals up to a cumulative dose of 3 mg, usual cumulative dose: 1-3 mg; rarely, patients with partial response at 3 mg may require additional titration up to total dose of 5 mg; if patient has not responded 5 minutes after cumulative dose of 5 mg, the major cause of sedation is likely not due to benzodiazepines. In the event of resedation, may repeat doses at 20-minute intervals with maximum of 1 mg/dose (given at 0.5 mg/minute); maximum: 3 mg in 1 hour.

Administration For I.V. use only; give via freely running I.V. infusion into larger vein to decrease chance of pain, phlebitis

Monitoring Parameters Respiratory rate, level of sedation

Patient Information Flumazenil does not consistently reverse amnesia; do not engage in activities requiring alertness for 18-24 hours after discharge; resedation may occur in patients on long acting benzodiazepines (such as diazepam)

Dosage Forms Injection: 0.1 mg/mL (5 mL, 10 mL)

References

Baktai G, Szekely E, Marialigeti T, et al, "Use of Midazolam (Dormicum) and Flumazenil (Anexate) in Pediatric Bronchology," *Curr Med Res Opin*, 1992, 12(9):552-9.

Jones RD, Lawson AD, Andrew LJ, et al, "Antagonism of the Hypnotic Effect of Midazolam in Children: A Randomized, Double Blind Study of Placebo and Flumazenil Administered After Midazolam-Induced Anaesthesia," *Br J Anaesth*, 1991, 66(6):660-6.

Richard P, Autret E, Bardol J, et al, "The Use of Flumazenil in a Neonate," *J Toxicol Clin Toxicol*, 1991, 29(1):137-40.

Roald OK and Dahl V, "Flunitrazepam Intoxication in a Child Successfully Treated With the Benzodiazepine Antagonist Flumazenil," *Crit Care Med*, 1989, 17(12):1355-6.

Flunisolide (floo niss' oh lide)

Brand Names AeroBid®; Nasalide®

Therapeutic Category Anti-inflammatory Agent; Corticosteroid, Inhalant; Corticosteroid, Topical; Glucocorticoid

Use Steroid-dependent asthma; nasal solution is used for seasonal or perennial rhinitis

(Continued)

Flunisolide *(Continued)*

Pregnancy Risk Factor C

Contraindications Known hypersensitivity to flunisolide; acute status asthmaticus; viral, tuberculosis, fungal or bacterial respiratory infections

Warnings Fatalities have occurred due to adrenal insufficiency in asthmatic patients during and after transfer from systemic corticosteroids to aerosol steroids; several months may be required for recovery of this syndrome; during this period, aerosol steroids do **not** provide the systemic steroid needed to treat patients having trauma, surgery or infections. When consumed in excessive quantities, systemic hypercorticism and adrenal suppression may occur; withdrawal and discontinuation of the corticosteroid should be done carefully.

Precautions Use with caution in patients with hypothyroidism, cirrhosis, hypertension, congestive heart failure, ulcerative colitis, thromboembolic disorders; do not stop medication abruptly if on prolonged therapy

Adverse Reactions

Central nervous system: Dizziness, headache

Endocrine & metabolic: Adrenal suppression

Local: Nasal burning, nasal congestion, nasal dryness, sore throat, bitter taste, *Candida* infections of the nose or pharynx, atrophic rhinitis

Respiratory: Sneezing

Drug Interactions Expected interactions similar to other corticosteroids

Mechanism of Action Decreases inflammation by suppression of migration of polymorphonuclear leukocytes and reversal of increased capillary permeability

Pharmacokinetics

Absorption: ~50% after nasal inhalation

Metabolism: Rapid in the liver to active metabolites

Half-life: 1.8 hours

Elimination: Excreted in the urine and feces

Usual Dosage

Children:

Oral inhalation: ≥4 years: 2 inhalations twice daily morning and evening

Nasal: 6-14 years: Initial: 1 spray each nostril 3 times/day or 2 sprays each nostril 2 times/day, not to exceed 4 sprays/day each nostril; maintenance: 1 spray each nostril once daily

Adults:

Oral inhalation: 2 inhalations twice daily up to 8 inhalations/day

Nasal: 2 sprays each nostril twice daily; maximum dose: 8 sprays/day in each nostril

Nursing Implications Shake well before giving; do not use Nasalide® orally; discard product after it has been opened for 3 months

Additional Information Does not contain fluorocarbons; contains polyethylene glycol vehicle

Dosage Forms Inhalant:

Nasal: 25 μg/metered spray 200 doses (25 mL)

Oral: 250 μg/metered spray 50 doses (7 g)

Fluocinolone Acetonide (floo oh sin' oh lone)

Related Information

Topical Steroids Comparison Chart *on page 728*

Brand Names Derma-Smoothe/FS®; Fluonid®; Flurosyn®; FS Shampoo®; Synalar®; Synemol®

Therapeutic Category Anti-inflammatory Agent; Corticosteroid, Topical; Glucocorticoid

Use Relief of susceptible inflammatory dermatosis

Pregnancy Risk Factor C

Contraindications Fungal infection, hypersensitivity to fluocinolone or any component, TB of skin, herpes (including varicella)

Warnings Infants and small children may be more susceptible to adrenal axis suppression from topical corticosteroid therapy; systemic effects may occur when used on large areas of the body, denuded areas, for prolonged periods of time, or with an occlusive dressing

Adverse Reactions

Dermatologic: Acne, hypopigmentation, allergic dermatitis, maceration of the skin, skin atrophy, folliculitis, hypertrichosis

Endocrine & metabolic: HPA suppression, Cushing's syndrome, growth retardation
Local: Burning, itching, irritation, dryness
Miscellaneous: Secondary infection

Mechanism of Action Not well defined topically; possesses anti-inflammatory, antiproliferative, and immunosuppressive properties

Usual Dosage Children and Adults: Topical: Apply thin layer 2-4 times/day

Additional Information Considered a moderate-potency steroid; do not use tight-fitting diapers or plastic pants on a child being treated in diaper area; do not overuse; a thin film of cream or ointment is effective; avoid contact with eyes; do not use for longer than directed

Dosage Forms
Cream: 0.01% (15 g, 30 g, 60 g, 425 g); 0.025% (15 g, 60 g, 425 g); 0.2% (12 g)
Ointment, topical: 0.025% (15 g, 30 g, 60 g, 425 g)
Oil: 0.01% (120 mL)
Shampoo: 0.01% (180 mL)
Solution, topical: 0.01% (20 mL, 60 mL)

Fluocinonide (floo oh sin' oh nide)

Related Information
Topical Steroids Comparison Chart *on page 728*

Brand Names Fluonex®; Lidex®; Lidex-E®

Therapeutic Category Anti-inflammatory Agent; Corticosteroid, Topical; Glucocorticoid

Use Inflammation of corticosteroid-responsive dermatoses

Pregnancy Risk Factor C

Contraindications Hypersensitivity to fluocinonide or any component; viral, fungal, or tubercular skin lesions; herpes (including varicella)

Warnings Infants and small children may be more susceptible to adrenal axis suppression from topical corticosteroid therapy; systemic effects may occur when used on large areas of the body, denuded areas, for prolonged periods of time, or with occlusive dressings

Adverse Reactions
Dermatologic: Acne, hypopigmentation, allergic dermatitis, maceration of the skin, skin atrophy; folliculitis, hypertrichosis
Endocrine & metabolic: HPA suppression, Cushing's syndrome, growth retardation
Local: Burning, itching, irritation, dryness
Miscellaneous: Secondary infection

Mechanism of Action Not well defined topically; possesses anti-inflammatory, antiproliferative, and immunosuppressive properties

Usual Dosage Children and Adults: Topical: Apply thin layer to affected area 2-4 times/day depending on the severity of the condition

Additional Information Considered to be a high potency steroid; do not use tight-fitting diapers or plastic pants on a child being treated in the diaper area; do not overuse; a thin film is effective; avoid contact with eyes; do not use for longer than directed; avoid use on face

Dosage Forms
Cream: 0.05% (15 g, 30 g, 60 g, 120 g)
Gel, topical: 0.05% (15 g, 30 g, 60 g, 120 g)
Ointment, topical: 0.05% (15 g, 30 g, 60 g, 120 g)
Solution, topical: 0.05% (20 mL, 60 mL)

Fluohydrisone Acetate *see* Fludrocortisone Acetate *on page 251*

Fluohydrocortisone Acetate *see* Fludrocortisone Acetate *on page 251*

Fluonex® *see* Fluocinonide *on this page*

Fluonid® *see* Fluocinolone Acetonide *on previous page*

Fluoride

Brand Names ACT® [OTC]; Fluorigard®; Fluoritab®; Flura®; Gel-Kam®; Gel-Tin®; Karidium®; Karigel®; Luride®; Luride®-SF F Lozi-Tabs®; Pediaflor®; Phos-Flur®; Prevident®; Thera-Flur® Gel

(Continued)

Fluoride *(Continued)*

Synonyms Acidulated Phosphate Fluoride; Sodium Fluoride; Stannous Fluoride

Therapeutic Category Mineral, Oral; Mineral, Oral Topical

Use Prevention of dental caries

Pregnancy Risk Factor C

Contraindications Hypersensitivity to fluoride or any component; when fluoride content of drinking water exceeds 0.7 ppm

Precautions Prolonged ingestion with excessive doses may result in dental fluorosis and osseous changes; dosage should be adjusted in proportion to the amount of fluoride in the drinking water; do **not** exceed recommended dosage

Adverse Reactions

Dermatologic: Rash

Gastrointestinal: GI upset, nausea, vomiting

Miscellaneous: Products containing stannous fluoride may stain the teeth

Drug Interactions Magnesium, aluminum, and calcium containing products may ↓ absorption of fluoride

Mechanism of Action Promotes remineralization of decalcified enamel; inhibits the cariogenic microbial process in dental plaque; increases tooth resistance to acid dissolution

Pharmacokinetics

Absorption: Absorbed in GI tract, lungs and skin; calcium, magnesium hydroxide, or aluminum hydroxide may delay absorption

Distribution: 50% of fluoride is deposited in teeth and bone after ingestion; crosses placenta; appears in breast milk; topical application works superficially on enamel and plaque

Elimination: Excreted in urine and feces

Usual Dosage Oral:

Recommended daily fluoride supplement: See table.

Fluoride Ion

Fluoride Content of Drinking Water	Daily Dose, Oral (mg)
<0.3 ppm	
Birth – 2 y	0.25
2–3 y	0.5
3–12 y	1
0.3–0.7 ppm	
Birth – 2 y	0
2–3 y	0.25
3–12 y	0.5

Dental rinse or gel:

Children 6-12 years: 5-10 mL rinse or apply to teeth and spit daily after brushing

Adults: 10 mL rinse or apply to teeth and spit daily after brushing

Patient Information Take with food (but not milk) to eliminate GI upset; with dental rinse or dental gel do **not** swallow, do **not** eat or drink for 30 minutes after use

Dosage Forms

Gel:

Oral, as sodium: 1.1%

Oral, as stannous: 0.4%

Oral, as acidulated phosphate: 1.1%; 1.2%, 1.23%

Paste, oral, as sodium: 33.3%

Solution:

Oral, as sodium: 1.1 mg/mL; 4.4 mg/mL; 4.97 mg/mL; 12.3 mg/mL; 13 mg/mL

Oral, as acidulated phosphate: 0.044%

Tablet, as sodium: 2.2 mg (1 mg fluoride ion)

Tablet, chewable, as sodium: 0.55 mg (0.25 mg fluoride ion); 1.1 mg (0.5 mg fluoride ion); 2.2 mg (1 mg fluoride ion)

Fluorigard® *see* Fluoride *on page 255*

Fluoritab® *see* Fluoride *on page 255*

9α-Fluorohydrocortisone Acetate *see* Fludrocortisone Acetate *on page 251*

Fluorometholone (flure oh meth' oh lone)

Brand Names Flarex®; Fluor-Op®; FML®; FML® Forte

Therapeutic Category Anti-inflammatory Agent; Corticosteroid, Ophthalmic; Glucocorticoid

Use Inflammatory conditions of the eye, including keratitis, iritis, cyclitis, and conjunctivitis

Pregnancy Risk Factor C

Contraindications Herpes simplex, fungal diseases, most viral diseases

Warnings Not recommended for children <2 years of age

Precautions Prolonged use may result in glaucoma, increased intraocular pressure, or other ocular damage; some products contain sulfites

Adverse Reactions

Local: Stinging, burning

Ocular: Increased intraocular pressure, open-angle glaucoma, defect in visual acuity and field of vision, cataracts

Mechanism of Action Decreases inflammation by suppression of migration of polymorphonuclear leukocytes and reversal of increased capillary permeability

Pharmacokinetics Absorption: Absorbed into aqueous humor with slight systemic absorption

Usual Dosage Children >2 years and Adults:

Ophthalmic drops: Instill 1-2 drops into conjunctival sac every hour during day, every 2 hours at night until favorable response is obtained, then use 1 drop every 4 hours; in mild or moderate inflammation: 1-2 drops into conjunctival sac 2-4 times/day.

Ointment: May be applied every 4 hours in severe cases or 1-3 times/day in mild to moderate cases.

Nursing Implications Do not discontinue without consulting physician; photosensitivity may occur; notify physician if improvement does not occur after 7-8 days

Dosage Forms Ophthalmic:

Ointment: 0.1% (3.5 g)

Suspension: 0.1% (5 mL, 10 mL, 15 mL); 0.25% (2 mL, 5 mL, 10 mL, 15 mL)

Fluor-Op® *see* Fluorometholone *on this page*

Fluoroplex® *see* Fluorouracil *on this page*

Fluorouracil (flure oh yoor' a sill)

Related Information

Emetogenic Potential of Single Chemotherapeutic Agents *on page 655*

Brand Names Adrucil®; Efudex®; Fluoroplex®; FUDR®

Synonyms 5-Fluorouracil; 5-FU

Therapeutic Category Antineoplastic Agent

Use Treatment of colon, breast, stomach, rectal, and pancreatic carcinomas; topically for management of multiple actinic keratoses

Pregnancy Risk Factor D

Contraindications Hypersensitivity to fluorouracil or any component; patients with poor nutritional status, bone marrow depression

Warnings The US Food and Drug Administration (FDA) currently recommends that procedures for proper handling and disposal of antineoplastic agents be considered; if intractable vomiting, diarrhea, or hemorrhage occurs, discontinue fluorouracil immediately

Precautions Use with caution in patients with renal or hepatic impairment

Adverse Reactions

Cardiovascular: Cardiac arrhythmias, heart failure, hypotension

Central nervous system: Headache, cerebellar ataxia, gait and speech abnormalities

Dermatologic: Alopecia, skin pigmentation, pruritic maculopapular rash partial loss of nails or hyperpigmentation of nail bed, photosensitivity

(Continued)

Fluorouracil *(Continued)*

Gastrointestinal: Diarrhea, nausea, vomiting, anorexia, GI hemorrhage, stomatitis
Hematologic: Myelosuppression
Hepatic: Hepatotoxicity
Ocular: Visual disturbances, nystagmus

Drug Interactions Cimetidine

Stability Store at room temperature; protect from light; slight discoloration of injection during storage does not affect potency; if precipitate forms, redissolve drug by heating to 140°F, shake well; allow to cool to body temperature before administration; incompatible with cytarabine, diazepam, doxorubicin, methotrexate

Mechanism of Action A pyrimidine antimetabolite that interferes with DNA synthesis by blocking the methylation of deoxyuricytic acid; incorporated into RNA, DNA

Pharmacokinetics

Absorption: Oral: Erratic
Distribution: Distributes into tumors, intestinal mucosa, liver, bone marrow, and CSF
Protein binding: <10%
Metabolism: Inactive metabolites are formed following metabolism in the liver
Bioavailability: 50% to 80%
Half-life:
Primary: 10-20 minutes
Terminal: 15-19 hours
Elimination: Biphasic elimination with 15% of a dose excreted as unchanged drug in the urine in 6 hours, and a large amount is excreted as CO_2 from the lung

Usual Dosage Children and Adults (refer to individual protocols):

I.V.: Initial: 12 mg/kg/day (maximum: 800 mg/day) for 4-5 days; maintenance: 6 mg/kg every other day for 4 doses
Single weekly bolus dose of 15 mg/kg or 500 mg/m^2 can be administered depending on the patient's reaction to the previous course of treatment; maintenance dose of 5-15 mg/kg/week as a single dose not to exceed 1 g/week

I.V. infusion: 15 mg/kg/day or 500 mg/m^2/day (maximum daily dose: 1 g) has been given by I.V. infusion over 4 hours for 5 days; 800-1200 mg/m^2 by continuous infusion over 24-120 hours

Oral: 20 mg/kg/day for 5 days every 5 weeks for colorectal carcinoma; 15 mg/kg/week for hepatoma

Topical: 5% cream twice daily

Administration Administer by direct I.V. push injection (50 mg/mL solution needs no further dilution) or by I.V. infusion; toxicity may be reduced by giving the drug as a constant infusion

Monitoring Parameters CBC with differential and platelet count, renal function tests, liver function tests

Patient Information Avoid unnecessary exposure to sunlight

Nursing Implications Wash hands immediately after topical application of the 5% cream; when given orally, administer in early morning on an empty stomach; the solution is very bitter so give with grape juice

Additional Information Myelosuppressive effects:

WBC: Mild
Platelets: Mild
Onset (days): 7-10
Nadir (days): 9-14
Recovery (days): 21

Dosage Forms

Cream, topical: 1% (30 g); 5% (25 g)
Injection, preservative free: 100 mg/mL (5 mL)
Powder for injection: 500 mg
Solution, topical: 1% (30 mL); 2% (10 mL); 5% (10 mL)

References

Balis FM, Holcenberg JS and Bleyer WA, "Clinical Pharmacokinetics of Commonly Used Anticancer Drugs," *Clin Pharmacokinet*, 1983, 8(3):202-32.

5-Fluorouracil *see* Fluorouracil *on page 257*

Fluoxetine Hydrochloride (floo ox' e teen)

Brand Names Prozac®

Therapeutic Category Antidepressant; Serotonin Antagonist

Use Treatment of major depression; preliminary studies report use for obsessive-compulsive disorders in children and adolescents

Pregnancy Risk Factor B

Contraindications Hypersensitivity to fluoxetine; patients receiving MAO inhibitors currently or in past 2 weeks

Precautions Due to limited experience, use with caution in patients with renal or hepatic impairment, seizure disorders, cardiac dysfunction; diabetes mellitus; use with caution in patients at high risk for suicide; discontinue MAO inhibitors at least 14 days before initiating fluoxetine; add or initiate other antidepressants with caution for up to 5 weeks after stopping fluoxetine

Adverse Reactions Predominate adverse effects are CNS and GI:

Central nervous system: Headache, nervousness, insomnia, drowsiness, anxiety, tremor, dizziness, fatigue, sedation; suicidal ideation, extrapyramidal reactions (rare)

Dermatologic: Excessive sweating, rash, pruritus

Endocrine & metabolic: Hypoglycemia, hyponatremia (elderly or volume depleted patients)

Gastrointestinal: Nausea, diarrhea, dry mouth, anorexia, dyspepsia, constipation

Ocular: Visual disturbances

Miscellaneous: Anaphylactoid reactions, allergies

Drug Interactions With MAO inhibitors: Hyperpyrexia, tremor, seizures, delirium, coma; with tryptophan → ↑ CNS and GI toxic effects; fluoxetine may inhibit metabolism and ↑ effects of tricyclic antidepressants, trazodone, and possibly diazepam; may antagonize buspirone effects and may displace highly protein bound drugs

Mechanism of Action Inhibits CNS neuron serotonin uptake; minimal or no effect on reuptake of norepinephrine or dopamine; does not significantly bind to alpha-adrenergic, histamine or cholinergic receptors; may therefore be useful in patients at risk from sedation, hypotension and anticholinergic effects of tricyclic antidepressants

Pharmacodynamics Peak effect: Maximum antidepressant effects usually occur after more than 4 weeks; due to long half-life, resolution of adverse reactions after discontinuation may be slow

Pharmacokinetics

Absorption: Oral: Well absorbed

Metabolism: Metabolized to norfluoxetine (active)

Half-life, adults: 2-3 days

Peak serum levels: Within 4-8 hours

Elimination: Excreted in the urine as fluoxetine (2.5% to 5%) and norfluoxetine (10%)

Usual Dosage Oral:

Children <18 years: Dose and safety not established; preliminary experience in children 6-17 years using initial doses of 20 mg/day has been reported

Adults: 20 mg/day in the morning; may increase after several weeks by 20 mg/day increments; maximum: 80 mg/day; doses >20 mg should be divided into morning and noon doses

Note: Lower doses of 5 mg/day have been used for initial treatment

Reference Range Therapeutic: Fluoxetine 100-800 ng/mL (SI: 289-2314 nmol/L); norfluoxetine 100-600 ng/mL (SI: 289-1735 nmol/L); Toxic: (Fluoxetine plus norfluoxetine): >2000 ng/mL (SI: 5784 nmol/L)

Dosage Forms

Capsule: 10 mg, 20 mg

Liquid (mint flavor): 20 mg/5 mL (120 mL)

References

Como PG and Kurlan R, "An Open-Label Trial of Fluoxetine for Obsessive-Compulsive Disorder in Gilles de la Tourette's Syndrome," *Neurology*, 1991, 41(6):872-4.

(Continued)

Fluoxetine Hydrochloride *(Continued)*

Riddle MA, Hardin MT, King R, et al, "Fluoxetine Treatment of Children and Adolescents With Tourette's and Obsessive-Compulsive Disorders: Preliminary Clinical Experience," *J Am Acad Child Adolesc Psychiatry*, 1990, 29(1):45-8.

Fluoxymesterone (floo ox i mes' te rone)

Brand Names Halotestin®

Therapeutic Category Androgen

Use Replacement of endogenous testicular hormone; in female used as palliative treatment of breast cancer, postpartum breast engorgement

Pregnancy Risk Factor X

Contraindications Serious cardiac disease, liver or kidney disease, hypersensitivity to fluoxymesterone or any component

Precautions May accelerate bone maturation without producing compensatory gain in linear growth; in prepubertal children perform radiographic examination of the hand and wrist every 6 months to determine the rate of bone maturation and to assess the effect of treatment on the epiphyseal centers

Adverse Reactions

Cardiovascular: Edema

Central nervous system: Anxiety, mental depression, paresthesia, headache

Dermatologic: Acne, hirsutism

Endocrine & metabolic: Gynecomastia, amenorrhea, hypercalcemia, female virilization

Gastrointestinal: Nausea

Hematologic: Polycythemia, suppression of clotting factors II, VII, IX, X

Hepatic: Cholestatic hepatitis

Renal & genitourinary: Priapism

Miscellaneous: Hypersensitivity reactions

Drug Interactions May potentiate the action of oral anticoagulants, may decrease blood glucose concentrations and insulin requirements in patients with diabetes

Mechanism of Action Synthetic androgenic anabolic steroid hormone responsible for the normal growth and development of male sex organs and maintenance of secondary sex characteristics

Usual Dosage Adults: Oral:

Males:

- Hypogonadism: 5-20 mg/day
- Delayed puberty: 2.5-20 mg/day for 4-6 months

Females:

- Breast carcinoma: 10-40 mg/day in divided doses
- Breast engorgement: 2.5 mg after delivery, 5-10 mg/day in divided doses for 4-5 days

Monitoring Parameters Periodic radiographic exams of hand and wrist; hemoglobin hematocrit (if receiving high dosages or long-term therapy)

Dosage Forms Tablet: 2 mg, 5 mg, 10 mg

Flura® *see* Fluoride *on page 255*

Flurazepam Hydrochloride (flure az' e pam)

Related Information

Overdose and Toxicology Information *on page 696-700*

Brand Names Dalmane®

Therapeutic Category Benzodiazepine; Hypnotic; Sedative

Use Short-term treatment of insomnia

Restrictions C-IV

Pregnancy Risk Factor D

Contraindications Hypersensitivity to flurazepam or any component (there may be cross-sensitivity with other benzodiazepines); pregnancy, pre-existing CNS depression, respiratory depression, narrow-angle glaucoma

Precautions Use with caution in patients receiving other CNS depressants, patients with low albumin, hepatic dysfunction and in the elderly

Adverse Reactions

Central nervous system: Drowsiness, dizziness, confusion; residual daytime sedation; paradoxical reactions, hyperactivity and excitement (rare), ataxia

Miscellaneous: Physical and psychological dependence with prolonged use

Drug Interactions Additive CNS depression with other CNS depressants, cimetidine may decrease and enzyme inducers may ↑ metabolism of flurazepam

Mechanism of Action Depresses all levels of the CNS, including the limbic and reticular formation, probably through the increased action of gamma-aminobutyric acid (GABA), which is a major inhibitory neurotransmitter in the brain

Pharmacodynamics Hypnotic effects:

Onset of action: 15-20 minutes

Peak: 3-6 hours

Duration: 7-8 hours

Pharmacokinetics

Metabolism: Metabolized in liver to N-desalkylflurazepam (active)

Half-life (metabolite), adults: 40-114 hours

Usual Dosage Oral:

Children:

<15 years: Dose not established

>15 years: 15 mg at bedtime

Adults: 15-30 mg at bedtime

Dosage Forms Capsule: 15 mg, 30 mg

Flurbiprofen Sodium (flure bi' proe fen)

Brand Names Ansaid®; Ocufen®

Therapeutic Category Analgesic, Non-Narcotic; Anti-inflammatory Agent; Nonsteroidal Anti-Inflammatory Agent (NSAID), Ophthalmic

Use

Ophthalmic: For inhibition of intraoperative trauma-induced miosis; the value of flurbiprofen for the prevention and management of postoperative ocular inflammation and postoperative cystoid macular edema remains to be determined

Systemic: Management of inflammatory disease and rheumatoid disorders; dysmenorrhea; pain

Pregnancy Risk Factor C

Contraindications Dendritic keratitis, hypersensitivity to flurbiprofen or any component; hypersensitivity to aspirin or other nonsteroidal anti-inflammatory drug

Warnings Use with caution in patients with history of herpes simplex, keratitis; patients who might be affected by inhibition of platelet aggregation; patients in whom asthma, rhinitis, or urticaria is precipitated by aspirin or other NSAIAs.

Precautions Use oral form with caution in renal or hepatic impairment, GI disease, cardiac disease, and patients receiving anticoagulants

Adverse Reactions

Cardiovascular: Edema

Central nervous system: Headache, fatigue, drowsiness, vertigo, tinnitus

Dermatologic: Pruritus, rash

Gastrointestinal: Abdominal discomfort, nausea, heartburn, constipation, vomiting, GI bleeding, ulcers, perforation

Hematologic: Thrombocytopenia, inhibits platelet aggregation; prolongs bleeding time; agranulocytosis

Hepatic: Hepatitis

Ocular: Slowing of corneal wound healing, mild ocular stinging, itching, burning, ocular irritation

Renal & genitourinary: Renal dysfunction

Drug Interactions

Ophthalmic: Carbachol and acetylcholine chloride may not be effective when used concurrently with flurbiprofen

Oral: Drug interactions similar to other NSAIDs may occur

Mechanism of Action Inhibits prostaglandin synthesis by decreasing the activity of the enzyme, cyclo-oxygenase, which results in decreased formation of prostaglandin precursors

(Continued)

Flurbiprofen Sodium *(Continued)*

Pharmacokinetics

Peak serum levels: Within 1.5-2 hours

Elimination: 95% of dose excreted in urine

Usual Dosage

Children and Adults: Ophthalmic: Instill 1 drop every 30 minutes starting 2 hours prior to surgery (total of 4 drops to each affected eye)

Adults: Oral:

Arthritis: 200-300 mg/day in 2-4 divided doses; maximum: 100 mg/dose; maximum: 300 mg/day

Dysmenorrhea: 50 mg 4 times/day

Monitoring Parameters Systemic: CBC, BUN, serum creatinine, liver enzymes, occult blood loss, periodic eye exams

Nursing Implications

Ophthalmic: Care should be taken to avoid contamination of the solution container tip

Oral: Administer with food, milk, or antacid to decrease GI effects

Dosage Forms

Solution, ophthalmic: 0.03% (2.5 mL, 5 mL, 10 mL)

Tablet: 50 mg, 100 mg

5-Flurocytosine *see* Flucytosine *on page 249*

Flurosyn® *see* Fluocinolone Acetonide *on page 254*

FML® *see* Fluorometholone *on page 257*

FML® Forte *see* Fluorometholone *on page 257*

Foille Plus® [OTC] *see* Benzocaine *on page 77*

Folacin *see* Folic Acid *on this page*

Folate *see* Folic Acid *on this page*

Folex® *see* Methotrexate *on page 374*

Folic Acid (foe' lik)

Brand Names Folvite®

Synonyms Folacin; Folate; Pteroylglutamic Acid

Therapeutic Category Vitamin, Water Soluble

Use Treatment of megaloblastic and macrocytic anemias due to folate deficiency

Pregnancy Risk Factor A (C if dose exceeds RDA recommendation)

Contraindications Pernicious, aplastic, or normocytic anemias

Warnings Large doses may mask the hematologic effects of B_{12} deficiency, thus obscuring the diagnosis of pernicious anemia while allowing the neurologic complications due to B_{12} deficiency to progress; injection contains benzyl alcohol (1.5%) as preservative; therefore, avoid use in premature infants

Adverse Reactions

Central nervous system: Irritability, difficulty sleeping, confusion

Gastrointestinal: GI upset

Miscellaneous: Hypersensitivity reactions

Drug Interactions May decrease phenytoin serum concentration; hematologic response antagonized by chloramphenicol; folic acid antagonists (ie, methotrexate, pyrimethamine, trimethoprim) prevent the formation of tetrahydrofolic acid (active metabolite), therefore, folic acid is not effective for the treatment of overdosage of these drugs

Mechanism of Action Precursor of tetrahydrofolic acid, a cofactor necessary for normal erythropoiesis

Pharmacodynamics Peak effect: Within 30-60 minutes following oral administration

Pharmacokinetics

Absorption: Absorbed in the proximal part of the small intestine

Elimination: Primarily excreted via liver metabolism

Usual Dosage Oral, I.M., I.V., S.C.:

Recommended daily allowance (RDA):

Neonates to 6 months: 25-35 μg

Children:

6 months to 3 years: 50 μg

4-6 years: 75 μg

7-10 years: 100 μg
11-14 years: 150 μg
Children >15 years and Adults: 200 μg

Folic acid deficiency:
Infants: 15 μg/kg/dose daily or 50 μg/day
Children: 1 mg/day initial dosage; maintenance dose: 1-10 years: 0.1-0.4 mg/day
Children >11 years and Adults: 1 mg/day initial dosage; maintenance dose: 0.5 mg/day

Administration Dilute with sterile water, dextrose or saline solution to 0.1 mg/mL; if I.M. route used, give deep I.M.

Monitoring Parameters Hemoglobin

Dosage Forms
Injection, as sodium folate: 5 mg/mL (10 mL); 10 mg/mL (10 mL)
Tablet: 0.1 mg, 0.4 mg, 0.8 mg, 1 mg

Folinic Acid *see* Leucovorin Calcium *on page 335*

Follutein® *see* Chorionic Gonadotropin *on page 134*

Folvite® *see* Folic Acid *on previous page*

5-Formyl Tetrahydrofolate *see* Leucovorin Calcium *on page 335*

Fortaz® *see* Ceftazidime *on page 116*

Foscarnet

Related Information
Medications Compatible With PN Solutions *on page 649-650*

Brand Names Foscavir®

Synonyms PFA; Phosphonoformate

Therapeutic Category Antiviral Agent, Parenteral

Use Alternative to ganciclovir for treatment of CMV infections and is possibly the preferred initial agent for the treatment of CMV retinitis except for those patients with decreased renal function; treatment of acyclovir-resistant HSV and herpes zoster infections

Pregnancy Risk Factor C

Contraindications Hypersensitivity to foscarnet or any component

Warnings Renal impairment occurs to some degree in the majority of patients treated with foscarnet; renal impairment may occur at any time and is usually reversible within 1 week following dose adjustment or discontinuation of therapy, however, several patients have died with renal failure within 4 weeks of stopping foscarnet; foscarnet is deposited in teeth and bone of young, growing animals; it has adversely affected tooth enamel development in rats; safety and effectiveness in children has not been studied

Precautions Use with caution in patients with renal impairment, patients with altered electrolyte levels, and patients with neurologic or cardiac abnormalities; adjust dose for patients with impaired renal function; discontinue treatment if serum creatinine ≥2.9 mg/dL; therapy can be restarted if serum creatinine ≤2 mg/dL

Adverse Reactions
Central nervous system: Peripheral neuropathy, fatigue, fever, headache, seizures, hallucinations
Endocrine & metabolic: Hypocalcemia, hypomagnesemia, hypokalemia, change in serum phosphorus
Gastrointestinal: Nausea, diarrhea, vomiting
Hematologic: Decreases in hemoglobin and hematocrit
Hepatic: Increases in liver enzymes
Local: Thrombophlebitis
Renal & genitourinary: Abnormal renal function including renal failure, proteinuria

Drug Interactions Pentamidine (additive hypocalcemia)

Stability Store at room temperature; refrigeration may result in crystallization of the drug; incompatible with dextrose 30%, I.V. solutions containing calcium, magnesium, vancomycin, TPN

Mechanism of Action Pyrophosphate analog which inhibits DNA synthesis by interfering with viral DNA polymerase

(Continued)

Foscarnet *(Continued)*

Pharmacokinetics

Distribution: Minimal penetration of the drug across the blood-brain barrier
Protein binding: 14% to 17%
Half-life, plasma: Adults with normal renal function: 3-4.5 hours
Terminal: 18-42 hours
Elimination: 80% to 90% is excreted unchanged in the urine

Usual Dosage Adolescents and Adults: I.V.:

Induction treatment: 180 mg/kg/day divided every 8 hours for 14-21 days
Maintenance therapy: 90-120 mg/kg/day as a single infusion once daily

Dosing interval in renal impairment: See tables.

Induction Treatment

Cl_{cr} (mL/min/kg)	mg/kg/8h
≥1.6	60
1.5	56.5
1.4	53
1.3	49.4
1.2	45.9
1.1	42.4
1	38.9
0.9	35.3
0.8	31.8
0.7	28.3
0.6	24.8
0.5	21.2
0.4	17.7

Maintenance Therapy

Cl_{cr} (mL/min/kg)	mg/kg/day
≥1.4	90–120
1.2–1.4	78–104
1–1.2	75–100
0.8–1	71–94
0.6–0.8	63–84
0.4–0.6	57–76

Administration 24 mg/mL solution can be administered without further dilution when using a central venous catheter for infusion; for peripheral vein administration, the solution **must** be diluted to a final concentration **not to exceed** 12 mg/mL; administer by I.V. infusion at a rate **not to exceed** 60 mg/kg/dose over 1 hour or 120 mg/kg/dose over 2 hours

Monitoring Parameters Serum creatinine, calcium, phosphorus, potassium, magnesium; hemoglobin

Reference Range Therapeutic for CMV: 150 μg/mL

Patient Information Report any numbness in the extremities, parethesias, or perioral tingling

Nursing Implications Provide adequate hydration with I.V. normal saline prior to and during treatment to minimize nephrotoxicity

Dosage Forms Injection: 24 mg/mL (250 mL, 500 mL)

References

Butler KM, DeSmet MD, Husson RN, et al, "Treatment of Aggressive Cytomegalovirus Retinitis With Ganciclovir in Combination With Foscarnet in a Child Infected With Human Immunodeficiency Virus," *J Pediatr*, 1992, 120(3):483-6.

Polis MA, "Foscarnet and Ganciclovir in the Treatment of Cytomegalovirus Retinitis," *J Acquir Immune Defic Syndr*, 1992, 5(Suppl 1):S3-10.

Foscavir® *see* Foscarnet *on previous page*

Fostex® [OTC] *see* Sulfur and Salicylic Acid *on page 545*

Fototar® [OTC] *see* Coal Tar *on page 147*

FS Shampoo® *see* Fluocinolone Acetonide *on page 254*

5-FU *see* Fluorouracil *on page 257*

FUDR® *see* Fluorouracil *on page 257*

Fulvicin® P/G *see* Griseofulvin *on page 277*

Fulvicin-U/F® *see* Griseofulvin *on page 277*

Fungizone® *see* Amphotericin B *on page 46*

Furadantin® *see* Nitrofurantoin *on page 414*

Furalan® *see* Nitrofurantoin *on page 414*

Furan® *see* Nitrofurantoin *on page 414*

Furanite® *see* Nitrofurantoin *on page 414*

Furazolidone (fur a zoe' li done)

Brand Names Furoxone®

Therapeutic Category Antibiotic, Miscellaneous; Antidiarrheal; Antiprotozoal

Use Treatment of bacterial or protozoal diarrhea and enteritis caused by susceptible organisms: *Giardia lamblia* and *Vibrio cholerae*

Pregnancy Risk Factor C

Contraindications Known hypersensitivity to furazolidone; concurrent use of alcohol; infants <1 month of age because of the possibility of producing hemolytic anemia; MAO inhibitors, tyramine-containing foods

Precautions Use caution in patients with G-6-PD deficiency

Adverse Reactions

Cardiovascular: Hypotension

Central nervous system: Dizziness, drowsiness, malaise, fever, headache

Dermatologic: Rash

Endocrine & metabolic: Hypoglycemia, disulfiram-like reaction after alcohol ingestion

Gastrointestinal: Nausea, vomiting, diarrhea

Hematologic: Agranulocytosis, hemolysis in patients with G-6-PD deficiency

Miscellaneous: Hypersensitivity reactions includes angioedema, hypotension, fever, urticaria, arthralgia, rash

Drug Interactions Alcohol (antabuse-like effect); adrenergic agents, tricyclic antidepressants, tyramine-containing foods, MAO inhibitors (↑ hypertensive effect)

Mechanism of Action Inhibits several vital enzymatic reactions causing antibacterial and antiprotozoal action

Pharmacokinetics

Absorption: Oral: Poorly absorbed

Metabolism: Inactivated in the intestine

Elimination: 5% of an oral dose is excreted in the urine as active drug and metabolites

Usual Dosage Oral:

Children >1 month: 5-8.8 mg/kg/day divided every 6 hours, not to exceed 400 mg/day

Adults: 100 mg 4 times/day

Monitoring Parameters CBC

Test Interactions False-positive results for urine glucose with Clinitest®

Patient Information May discolor urine to a brown tint; avoid drinking alcohol or eating tyramine-containing foods

Dosage Forms

Liquid: 50 mg/15 mL (60 mL, 473 mL)

Tablet: 100 mg

References

Murphy TV and Nelson JD, "Five vs Ten Days' Therapy With Furazolidone for Giardiasis," *Am J Dis Child*, 1983, 137(3):267-70.

Turner JA, "Giardiasis and Infections With Dientamoeba Fragilis," *Pediatr Clin North Am*, 1985, 32(4):865-80.

Furazosin *see* Prazosin Hydrochloride *on page 475*

Furomide® *see* Furosemide *on this page*

Furosemide (fur oh' se mide)

Related Information

Medications Compatible With PN Solutions *on page 649-650*

Brand Names Furomide®; Lasix®; Luramide®

Therapeutic Category Antihypertensive; Diuretic, Loop

Use Management of edema associated with congestive heart failure and hepatic or renal disease; used alone or in combination with antihypertensives in treatment of hypertension

(Continued)

Furosemide *(Continued)*

Pregnancy Risk Factor C

Contraindications Hypersensitivity to furosemide or any component; anuria

Warnings Loop diuretics are potent diuretics; excess amounts can lead to profound diuresis with fluid and electrolyte loss

Precautions Hepatic cirrhosis (rapid alterations in fluid/electrolytes may precipitate coma)

Adverse Reactions

Central nervous system: Dizziness, vertigo, headache

Dermatologic: Urticaria, photosensitivity

Endocrine & metabolic: Hypokalemia, hyponatremia, hypochloremia, alkalosis, dehydration, hyperuricemia

Gastrointestinal: Pancreatitis, nausea; oral solutions may cause diarrhea due to sorbitol content

Hematologic: Agranulocytosis, anemia, thrombocytopenia

Otic: Potential ototoxicity

Renal & genitourinary: Nephrocalcinosis, prerenal azotemia, interstitial nephritis, hypercalciuria

Drug Interactions Indomethacin, lithium, antidiabetic agents, salicylates (at therapeutic dosages), aminoglycosides (additive ototoxicity), drugs affected by potassium depletion (ie, digoxin)

Stability Protect from light

Mechanism of Action Inhibits reabsorption of sodium and chloride in the ascending loop of Henle and distal renal tubule, interfering with the chloride binding cotransport system, thus causing increased excretion of water, sodium, chloride, magnesium, and calcium

Pharmacodynamics

Onset of action:

- Oral: Within 30-60 minutes
- I.V.: 5 minutes
- I.M.: 30 minutes

Peak effect: Oral: Within 1-2 hours

Duration:

- Oral: 6-8 hours
- I.V. 2 hours

Pharmacokinetics

Absorption: 65% in patients with normal renal function, decreases to 45% in patients with renal failure

Protein binding: 98%

Half-life: Adults:

- Normal renal function: 30 minutes
- Renal failure: 9 hours

Elimination: 50% of an oral dose and 80% of an I.V. dose are excreted in the urine within 24 hours; the remainder is eliminated by other nonrenal pathways including liver metabolism and excretion of unchanged drug in the feces

Usual Dosage

Neonates, premature:

- Oral: Bioavailability is poor by this route. Doses of 1-4 mg/kg/dose 1-2 times/day have been used.
- I.M., I.V.: 1-2 mg/kg/dose given every 12-24 hours

Children: Oral, I.M., I.V.: 1-2 mg/kg/dose up to 6 mg/kg/day in divided doses every 6-12 hours

Adults: Oral, I.M., I.V.: 20-80 mg/day in divided doses every 6-12 hours up to 600 mg/day

Administration May be given undiluted direct I.V. at a maximum rate of 0.5 mg/kg/minute for doses $<$120 mg and 4 mg/minute for doses $>$120 mg; may also be diluted for infusion 1-2 mg/mL (maximum: 10 mg/mL) over 10-15 minutes (following maximum rate as above)

Monitoring Parameters Serum electrolytes, renal function, blood pressure, hearing (if high dosages used)

Dosage Forms

Injection: 10 mg/mL (2 mL, 4 mL, 5 mL, 6 mL, 8 mL, 10 mL, 12 mL)

Solution, oral: 10 mg/mL (60 mL, 120 mL); 40 mg/5 mL (5 mL, 10 mL, 500 mL)

Tablet: 20 mg, 40 mg, 80 mg

Furoxone® *see* Furazolidone *on page 265*

Gamimune® N *see* Immune Globulin, Intravenous *on page 307*

Gamma Benzene Hexachloride *see* Lindane *on page 344*

Gammagard® *see* Immune Globulin, Intravenous *on page 307*

Ganciclovir (gan sye' kloe vir)

Brand Names Cytovene®

Synonyms DHPG Sodium; GCV Sodium; Nordeoxyguanosine

Therapeutic Category Antiviral Agent, Parenteral

Use Treatment of cytomegalovirus retinitis in immunocompromised patients, as well as CMV GI infections and pneumonitis; prevention of CMV disease in transplant patients who have been diagnosed with latent or active CMV

Pregnancy Risk Factor C

Contraindications Absolute neutrophil count $<500/mm^3$; platelet count $<25,000/mm^3$; known hypersensitivity to ganciclovir or acyclovir

Warnings Ganciclovir may adversely affect spermatogenesis and fertility; due to its mutagenic potential, contraceptive precautions for female and male patients need to be followed during and for at least 90 days after therapy with the drug; ganciclovir is potentially carcinogenic

Precautions Dosage adjustment or interruption of ganciclovir therapy may be necessary in patients with neutropenia and/or thrombocytopenia and patients with impaired renal function; use with extreme caution in children since long-term safety has not been determined and due to ganciclovir's potential for long-term carcinogenic and adverse reproductive effects

Adverse Reactions

Cardiovascular: Edema, arrhythmias, hypertension

Central nervous system: Headaches, seizure, confusion, nervousness, dizziness, hallucinations, coma, fever, encephalopathy, malaise

Dermatologic: Rash, urticaria

Gastrointestinal: Nausea, vomiting, diarrhea

Hematologic: Neutropenia, thrombocytopenia, leukopenia, anemia, eosinophilia

Hepatic: Elevation in liver function tests

Local: Phlebitis

Ocular: Retinal detachment

Renal & genitourinary: Hematuria, ↑ BUN and serum creatinine

Miscellaneous: Dyspnea

Drug Interactions Zidovudine (pancytopenia), imipenem/cilastatin, immunosuppressive agents

Stability Reconstituted solution is stable for 12 hours at room temperature; **do not refrigerate**; reconstitute with sterile water **not** bacteriostatic water because parabens may cause precipitation

Mechanism of Action Ganciclovir is phosphorylated to a substrate which competitively inhibits the binding of deoxyguanosine triphosphate to DNA polymerase resulting in inhibition of viral DNA synthesis

Pharmacokinetics

Protein binding: 1% to 2%

Half-life: 1.7-5.8 hours (prolonged with impaired renal function)

Elimination: Majority (94% to 99%) excreted as unchanged drug in the urine 40% to 50% removed by a 4-hour hemodialysis

Usual Dosage Slow I.V. infusion:

Retinitis: Children >3 months and Adults:

Induction therapy: 10 mg/kg/day divided every 12 hours as a 1- to 2-hour infusion for 14-21 days

Maintenance therapy: 5 mg/kg/day as a single daily dose for 7 days/week or 6 mg/kg/day for 5 days/week

Other CMV infections: 10 mg/kg/day divided every 12 hours for 14-21 days or 7.5 mg/kg/day divided every 8 hours; maintenance therapy: 5 mg/kg/day as a single daily dose for 7 days/week or 6 mg/kg/day for 5 days/week

Dosing interval in renal impairment:

Cl_{cr} 50-79 mL/minute per 1.73 m^2: Administer 2.5 mg/kg every 12 hours

Cl_{cr} 25-49 mL/minute per 1.73 m^2: Administer 2.5 mg/kg every 24 hours

Cl_{cr} <25 mL/minute per 1.73 m^2: Administer 1.25 mg/kg every 24 hours

Administration Administer by slow I.V. infusion over at least 1 hour at a final concentration for administration not to exceed 10 mg/mL

(Continued)

Ganciclovir *(Continued)*

Monitoring Parameters CBC with differential and platelet count, urine output, serum creatinine, ophthalmologic exams

Nursing Implications Handle and dispose according to guidelines issued for cytotoxic drugs; to minimize the risk of phlebitis, infuse through a large vein with adequate blood flow; maintain adequate patient hydration

Dosage Forms Powder for injection, lyophilized: 500 mg

References

Fletcher C, Sawchuk R, Chinnock B, et al, "Human Pharmacokinetics of the Antiviral Drug DHPG," *Clin Pharmacol Ther*, 1986, 40(3):281-6.

Gudnason T, Belani KK, and Balfour HH Jr, "Ganciclovir Treatment of Cytomegalovirus Disease in Immunocompromised Children," *Pediatr Infect Dis J*, 1989, 8(7):436-40.

Gantanol® *see* Sulfamethoxazole *on page 542*

Gantrisin® *see* Sulfisoxazole *on page 544*

Garamycin® *see* Gentamicin *on this page*

Gastrocrom® *see* Cromolyn Sodium *on page 158*

Gas-X® [OTC] *see* Simethicone *on page 524*

Gaviscon® [OTC] *see* Antacid Preparations *on page 53*

G-CSF *see* Filgrastim *on page 244*

GCV Sodium *see* Ganciclovir *on previous page*

Gel-Kam® *see* Fluoride *on page 255*

Gel-Tin® *see* Fluoride *on page 255*

Genabid® *see* Papaverine Hydrochloride *on page 433*

Genac® [OTC] *see* Triprolidine and Pseudoephedrine *on page 586*

Genagesic® *see* Propoxyphene and Acetaminophen *on page 492*

Genahist® *see* Diphenhydramine Hydrochloride *on page 195*

Genapap® [OTC] *see* Acetaminophen *on page 16*

Genaspor® [OTC] *see* Tolnaftate *on page 573*

Genatuss® [OTC] *see* Guaifenesin *on page 278*

Gen-K® *see* Potassium Chloride *on page 469*

Genoptic® *see* Gentamicin *on this page*

Genpril® [OTC] *see* Ibuprofen *on page 300*

Gentacidin® *see* Gentamicin *on this page*

Gent-AK® *see* Gentamicin *on this page*

Gentamicin (jen ta mye' sin)

Related Information

Blood Level Sampling Time Guidelines *on page 694-695*
Endocarditis Prophylaxis *on page 659*
Medications Compatible With PN Solutions *on page 649-650*
Overdose and Toxicology Information *on page 696-700*

Brand Names Garamycin®; Genoptic®; Gentacidin®; Gent-AK®; Gentrasul®; G-myticin®; Jenamicin®

Therapeutic Category Antibiotic, Aminoglycoside; Antibiotic, Ophthalmic; Antibiotic, Topical

Use Treatment of susceptible bacterial infections, normally gram-negative organisms including *Pseudomonas*, *Proteus*, *Serratia*, and gram-positive *Staphylococcus*; treatment of bone infections, CNS infections, respiratory tract infections, skin and soft tissue infections, as well as abdominal and urinary tract infections, endocarditis, and septicemia; used topically to treat superficial infections of the skin or ophthalmic infections caused by susceptible bacteria

Pregnancy Risk Factor C

Contraindications Hypersensitivity to gentamicin or other aminoglycosides

Warnings Parenteral aminoglycosides are associated with significant nephrotoxicity or ototoxicity; the ototoxicity is directly proportional to the amount of drug given and the duration of treatment; tinnitus or vertigo are indications of vestibular injury and impending irreversible bilateral deafness; renal damage is usually reversible

Precautions Use with caution in neonates due to renal immaturity that results in a prolonged gentamicin half-life and in patients with pre-existing renal impairment, auditory or vestibular impairment, hypocalcemia, myasthenia gravis, and in conditions which depress neuromuscular transmission; modify dosage in patients with renal impairment and in neonates on ECMO

Adverse Reactions

Central nervous system: Neuromuscular blockade, vertigo, ataxia, gait instability

Dermatologic: Rash

Endocrine & metabolic: Hypomagnesemia

Hematologic: Granulocytopenia

Hepatic: Elevated AST, ALT

Local: Thrombophlebitis

Ocular: Nystagmus

Otic: Ototoxicity (peak >12-15 μg/mL and high trough levels) with tinnitus, hearing loss

Renal & genitourinary: Nephrotoxicity (high trough levels) with proteinuria, reduction in glomerular filtration rate, increased serum creatinine, decrease in urine specific gravity, casts in urine and possible electrolyte wasting

Drug Interactions Penicillins, cephalosporins, amphotericin B, indomethacin, cisplatin, furosemide, vancomycin may potentiate nephrotoxicity; neuromuscular blocking agents; loop diuretics may potentiate ototoxicity

Stability Incompatible with penicillins, cephalosporins, heparin

Mechanism of Action Interferes with bacterial protein synthesis by binding to 30S and 50S ribosomal subunits resulting in a defective bacterial cell membrane

Pharmacokinetics

Absorption: Not absorbed orally

Distribution: V_d: Increased in neonates and with edema, ascites, fluid overload; V_d is decreased in patients with dehydration; crosses the placenta
- Neonates: 0.4-0.6 L/kg
- Children: 0.3-0.35 L/kg
- Adults: 0.2-0.3 L/kg

Protein binding: <30%

Half-life:
- Infants:
  - <1 week: 3-11.5 hours
  - 1 week to 6 months: 3-3.5 hours
- Adults with normal renal function: 1.5-3 hours
- Anuria: 36-70 hours

Peak serum levels:
- I.M.: Within 30-90 minutes
- I.V.: 30 minutes after a 30-minute infusion

Elimination: Clearance is directly related to renal function; eliminated almost completely by glomerular filtration of unchanged drug with excretion into the urine

Dialyzable (50% to 100%)

Usual Dosage Dosage should be based on an estimate of ideal body weight

Neonates: I.M., I.V.:
- 0-4 weeks, <1200 g: 2.5 mg/kg/dose every 18-24 hours
- Postnatal age ≤7 days:
  - 1200-2000 g: 2.5 mg/kg/dose every 12-18 hours
  - >2000 g: 2.5 mg/kg/dose every 12 hours
- Postnatal age >7 days:
  - 1200-2000 g: 2.5 mg/kg/dose every 8-12 hours
  - >2000 g: 2.5 mg/kg/dose every 8 hours

Infants and Children <5 years: 2.5 mg/kg/dose every 8 hours*

Children ≥5 years: 1.5-2.5 mg/kg/dose every 8 hours
- Topical: Apply 3-4 times/day

(Continued)

Gentamicin *(Continued)*

Ophthalmic:

Solution: 1-2 drops every 2-4 hours, up to 2 drops every hour for severe infections

Ointment: 2-3 times/day

Intraventricular/intrathecal:

Newborns: 1 mg/day

Infants >3 months and Children: 1-2 mg/day

Adults: 4-8 mg/day

Adults:

I.M., I.V.: 3-6 mg/kg/day in divided doses every 8 hours

Topical: Apply 3-4 times/day

Ophthalmic:

Solution: 1-2 drops every 2-4 hours

Ointment: 2-3 times/day

Patients with renal dysfunction: 2.5 mg/kg** (Cl_{cr} <60 mL/minute/1.73 m^2)

* Some patients may require larger or more frequent doses (eg, every 6 hours) if serum levels document the need (ie, cystic fibrosis, patients with major burns, or febrile granulocytopenic patients)

** 2-3 serum level measurements should be obtained after the initial dose to measure the half-life in order to determine the frequency of subsequent doses

Administration Administer by I.V. slow intermittent infusion over 30 minutes; final concentration for administration should not exceed 10 mg/mL

Monitoring Parameters Urinalysis, urine output, BUN, serum creatinine, peak and trough serum gentamicin concentrations; hearing test

Reference Range Peak: 4-10 μg/mL; Trough: 0.5-2 μg/mL

Test Interactions Aminoglycoside levels measured in blood taken from Silastic® central line catheters can sometimes give falsely high readings

Patient Information Report any dizziness or sensations of ringing or fullness in ears to the physician

Nursing Implications Obtain drug levels after the third dose except in neonates and patients with rapidly changing renal function in whom levels need to be measured sooner; peak levels are drawn 30 minutes after the end of a 30-minute infusion; trough levels are drawn within 30 minutes before the next dose. Administer other antibiotics such as penicillins and cephalosporins at least 1 hour before or after gentamicin; provide optimal patient hydration and perfusion.

Dosage Forms

Cream, topical: 0.1% (15 g)

Infusion, in D_5W, as sulfate: 60 mg, 80 mg, 100 mg

Infusion, in NS, as sulfate: 40 mg, 60 mg, 80 mg, 90 mg, 100 mg, 120 mg

Injection, as sulfate: 40 mg/mL (1 mL, 1.5 mL, 2 mL)

Pediatric, as sulfate: 10 mg/mL (2 mL)

Intrathecal, preservative free, as sulfate: 2 mg/mL (2 mL)

Ointment:

Ophthalmic, as sulfate: 0.3% (3.5 g)

Topical: 0.1% (15 g)

Solution, ophthalmic: 0.3% (1 mL, 5 mL, 15 mL)

References

Reimche LD, Rooney, ME, Hindmarsh KW, et al, "An Evaluation of Gentamicin Dosing According to Renal Function in Neonates With Suspected Sepsis," *Am J Perinatol*, 1987, 4(3):262-5.

Shevchuk YM and Taylor DM, "Aminoglycoside Volume of Distribution in Pediatric Patients," *DICP*, 1990, 24(3):273-6.

Gentamicin and Prednisolone *see* Prednisolone and Gentamicin *on page 477*

Gentian Violet (jen' shun)

Synonyms Crystal Violet; Methylrosaniline Chloride

Therapeutic Category Antibacterial, Topical; Antifungal Agent, Topical

Use Treatment of cutaneous or mucocutaneous infections caused by *Candida albicans* and other superficial skin infections refractory to topical nystatin, clotrimazole, miconazole, or econazole

Pregnancy Risk Factor C

Contraindications Known hypersensitivity to gentian violet; ulcerated areas; patients with porphyria

Warnings May result in tattooing of the skin when applied to granulation tissue

Adverse Reactions

Gastrointestinal: Esophagitis

Local: Burning, irritation, vesicle formation, sensitivity reactions, ulceration of mucous membranes

Respiratory: Laryngitis, tracheitis may result from swallowing gentian violet solution; laryngeal obstruction following frequent or prolonged use

Mechanism of Action Tcpical antiseptic/germicide effective against some vegetative gram-positive bacteria, particularly *Staphylococcus* sp, and some yeast; it is much less effective against gram-negative bacteria and is ineffective against acid-fast bacteria

Usual Dosage Topical:

Infants: Apply 3-4 drops of a 0.5% solution under the tongue or on lesion after feedings

Children and Adults: Apply 0.5% to 2 % with cotton to lesion 2-3 times/day for 3 days, do not swallow

Patient Information Drug stains skin and clothing purple

Nursing Implications Do not apply to ulcerative lesions on the face

Additional Information 0.25% or 0.5% solution is less irritating than a 1% to 2% solution and is reported to be as effective

Dosage Forms Solution, topical: 1% (30 mL); 2% (30 mL)

Gentrasul® *see* Gentamicin *on page 268*

Gen-XENE® *see* Clorazepate Dipotassium *on page 144*

Geocillin® *see* Carbenicillin Indanyl Sodium *on page 104*

Geridium® *see* Phenazopyridine Hydrochloride *on page 449*

GG *see* Guaifenesin *on page 278*

GG-CEN® [OTC] *see* Guaifenesin *on page 278*

Glaucon® *see* Epinephrine *on page 220*

Glibenclamide *see* Glyburide *on next page*

Glucagon (gloo' ka gon)

Therapeutic Category Antihypoglycemic Agent

Use Hypoglycemia; diagnostic aid in the radiologic examination of GI tract when a hypotonic state is needed; used with some success as a cardiac stimulant in management of severe cases of beta-adrenergic blocking agent overdosage

Pregnancy Risk Factor B

Contraindications Hypersensitivity to glucagon or any component

Warnings Use with caution in patients with a history of insulinoma and/or pheochromocytoma

Adverse Reactions

Gastrointestinal: Nausea, vomiting

Miscellaneous: Hypersensitivity reactions

Stability After reconstitution, use immediately; may be kept at 5°C for up to 48 hours if necessary

Mechanism of Action Stimulates adenylate cyclase to produce increased cyclic AMP, which promotes hepatic glycogenolysis and gluconeogenesis, causing an increase in blood glucose levels; positive inotropic and chronotropic effects

Pharmacodynamics

Blood glucose effects:

Onset of action: Within 5-20 minutes

Duration: 60-90 minutes

GI tract effects:

Onset of action: Within 1-10 minutes

Duration: 12-30 minutes

Pharmacokinetics

Distribution: Extensively degraded in liver and kidneys

(Continued)

Glucagon *(Continued)*

Half-life, plasma: 3-10 minutes

Usual Dosage

Hypoglycemia or insulin shock therapy: I.M., I.V., S.C.:

Neonates: 0.3 mg/kg/dose; maximum: 1 mg/dose

Children: 0.025-0.1 mg/kg/dose, not to exceed 1 mg/dose, repeated in 20 minutes as needed

Adults: 0.5-1 mg, may repeat in 20 minutes as needed

Diagnostic aid: Adults: I.M., I.V.: 0.25-2 mg 10 minutes prior to procedure

Administration Dilute with manufacturer provided diluent resulting in 1 mg/mL; if doses exceeding 2 mg are used, dilute with sterile water instead of diluent; administer by direct I.V. injection

Monitoring Parameters Blood glucose, blood pressure

Additional Information 1 unit = 1 mg

Dosage Forms Injection: 1 mg [1 unit]; 10 mg [10 units]

Glucocerebrosidase *see* Alglucerase *on page 29*

Glukor® *see* Chorionic Gonadotropin *on page 134*

Glyate® [OTC] *see* Guaifenesin *on page 278*

Glyburide (glye' byoor ide)

Brand Names Diaβeta®; Glynase Prestab®; Micronase®

Synonyms Glibenclamide

Therapeutic Category Antidiabetic Agent; Hyperglycemic Agent; Sulfonylurea Agent

Use Management of noninsulin-dependent diabetes mellitus (type II)

Pregnancy Risk Factor B

Contraindications Hypersensitivity to glyburide or any component, or other sulfonamides

Precautions Use with caution in patients with hepatic impairment; avoid use in patients with Cl_{cr} <50 mL/minute

Adverse Reactions

Central nervous system: Paresthesia

Dermatologic: Pruritus, rash, photosensitivity

Endocrine & metabolic: Hypoglycemia

Gastrointestinal: Nausea, epigastric fullness, heartburn,

Hematologic: Leukopenia, thrombocytopenia, hemolytic anemia

Hepatic: Cholestatic jaundice

Musculoskeletal: Joint pain

Renal & genitourinary: Nocturia, SIADH effect

Drug Interactions Thiazides and beta blockers → ↓ effectiveness of glyburide; since this agent is highly protein bound, the toxic potential is increased when given concomitantly with other highly protein bound drugs, (ie, phenylbutazone, oral anticoagulants, hydantoins, salicylates, NSAIDs, sulfonamides) can ↑ hypoglycemic effects; alcohol → disulfiram reactions

Mechanism of Action Stimulates insulin release from the pancreatic beta cells; reduces glucose output from the liver; insulin sensitivity is increased at peripheral target sites

Pharmacodynamics

Onset of action: Insulin levels in the serum begin to increase within 15-60 minutes after a single oral dose

Duration: Up to 24 hours

Pharmacokinetics

Distribution: V_d: Adults: 0.125 L/kg; highest concentrations found in liver, kidneys, and intestines; appears to cross placenta

Protein binding: >99%

Metabolism: Appears to be completely metabolized to metabolites with ~2.5% to 15% activity

Half-life: 1.4-1.8 hours, may be prolonged with renal or hepatic insufficiency

Peak serum levels: Oral: Within 2-4 hours

Elimination: Excreted as metabolites in equal proportions via urine and feces

Clearance: 78 mL/kg/hour

Usual Dosage Adults: Oral: 1.25-5 mg to start then 1.25-20 mg maintenance dose/day divided in 1-2 doses

Prestab: Initial: 0.75-3 mg/day; increase by 1.5 mg/day in weekly intervals; maximum: 12 mg/day

Monitoring Parameters Blood sugar

Additional Information Not effective as sole therapy in type I diabetes mellitus, insulin is necessary

Dosage Forms

Tablet: 1.25 mg, 2.5 mg, 5 mg

Tablet, micronized (Glynase® prestab): 1.5 mg, 3 mg

Glycate® [OTC] *see* Calcium Carbonate *on page 94*

Glycerin (gli' ser in)

Brand Names Fleet® Babylax® [OTC]; Glyrol®; Ophthalgan®; Osmoglyn®; Sani-Supp® [OTC]

Synonyms Glycerol

Therapeutic Category Laxative, Hyperosmolar

Use Constipation; reduction of intraocular pressure; reduction of corneal edema; glycerin has been administered orally to reduce intracranial pressure

Pregnancy Risk Factor C

Contraindications Known hypersensitivity to glycerin

Precautions Use oral glycerin with caution in patients with cardiac, renal or hepatic disease and in diabetics

Adverse Reactions

Central nervous system: Dizziness, headache

Endocrine & metabolic: Hyperglycemia

Gastrointestinal: Diarrhea, nausea, tenesmus, cramping pain, rectal irritation

Local: Pain/irritation with ophthalmic solution (may need to apply a topical ophthalmic anesthetic before glycerin administration)

Miscellaneous: Thirst

Stability Protect from heat; freezing should be avoided

Mechanism of Action Osmotic dehydrating agent which increases osmotic pressure; draws fluid into colon and thus stimulates evacuation

Pharmacodynamics

Onset of action for glycerin suppository: 15-30 minutes

Onset of action in decreasing intraocular pressure: Within 10-30 minutes

Duration: 4-8 hours

Increased intracranial pressure decreases within 10-60 minutes following an oral dose

Duration: ~2-3 hours

Pharmacokinetics

Absorption:

Oral: Well absorbed

Rectal: Poorly absorbed

Metabolism: Primarily in the liver with 20% metabolized in the kidney

Half-life: 30-45 minutes

Peak effects: Following oral absorption, within 60-90 minutes

Elimination: Only a small percentage of drug is excreted unchanged in the urine

Usual Dosage

Constipation: Rectal:

Neonates: 0.5 mL/kg/dose

Children <6 years: 1 infant suppository 1-2 times/day as needed or 2-5 mL as an enema

Children >6 years and Adults: 1 adult suppository 1-2 times/day as needed or 5-15 mL as an enema

Children and Adults:

Reduction of intraocular pressure: Oral: 1-1.8 g/kg 1-1½ hours preoperatively; additional doses may be administered at 5-hour intervals

Reduction of intracranial pressure: Oral: 1.5 g/kg/day divided every 4 hours; 1 g/kg/dose every 6 hours has also been used

Reduction of corneal edema: Ophthalmic: Instill 1-2 drops in eye(s) every 3-4 hours

Monitoring Parameters Blood glucose, intraocular pressure

Patient Information Do not use if experiencing abdominal pain, nausea, or vomiting

(Continued)

Glycerin *(Continued)*

Nursing Implications Use caution during insertion of suppository to avoid intestinal perforation, especially in neonates

Dosage Forms

Solution:

Ophthalmic, sterile: Glycerin with chlorobutanol 0.55% (7.5 mL)

Oral: 50% (180 mL)

Rectal: 4 mL per applicator (6's)

Suppository: Glycerin with sodium stearate (infant and adult sizes)

References

Heinemeyer G, "Clinical Pharmacokinetic Considerations in the Treatment of Increased Intracranial Pressure," *Clin Pharmacokinet*, 1987, 13(1):1-25.

Rottenberg DA, Hurwitz BJ, and Posner JB, "The Effect of Oral Glycerol on Intraventricular Pressure in Man," *Neurology*, 1977, 27(7):600-8.

Glycerol *see* Glycerin *on previous page*

Glyceryl Guaiacolate *see* Guaifenesin *on page 278*

Glyceryl Trinitrate *see* Nitroglycerin *on page 415*

Glycopyrrolate (glye koe pye' roe late)

Related Information

Compatibility of Medications Mixed in a Syringe *on page 717*

Overdose and Toxicology Information *on page 696-700*

Brand Names Robinul®

Synonyms Glycopyrronium Bromide

Therapeutic Category Anticholinergic Agent; Antispasmodic Agent, Gastrointestinal

Use Adjunct in treatment of peptic ulcer disease; inhibit salivation and excessive secretions of the respiratory tract; reversal of neuromuscular blockade; control of upper airway secretions

Pregnancy Risk Factor B

Contraindications Narrow-angle glaucoma, acute hemorrhage, tachycardia, hypersensitivity to glycopyrrolate or any component; ulcerative colitis, obstructive uropathy

Warnings Infants, blondes, patients with Down's syndrome and children with spastic paralysis or brain damage may be hypersensitive to antimuscarinic effects.

Precautions Use with caution in patients with fever, hyperthyroidism, hepatic or renal disease, hypertension, congestive heart failure, GI infections, diarrhea, reflux esophagitis

Adverse Reactions

Cardiovascular: Tachycardia

Central nervous system: Drowsiness, nervousness, headache, insomnia

Dermatologic: Rash

Gastrointestinal: Dry mouth, constipation, nausea, vomiting

Ocular: Blurred vision

Renal & genitourinary: Urinary retention

Drug Interactions Phenothiazines, meperidine, tricyclic antidepressants, and quinidine will produce additive anticholinergic effects; wax-matrix potassium chloride (↑ severity of potassium-induced GI mucosal lesions); antacids (↓ absorption)

Stability Unstable at pH >6; compatible in the same syringe with atropine, benzquinamide, chlorpromazine, codeine, diphenhydramine, droperidol, fentanyl, hydromorphone, hydroxyzine, lidocaine, meperidine, promethazine, morphine, neostigmine, oxymorphone, procaine, prochlorperazine, promazine, pyridostigmine, scopolamine, triflupromazine, and trimethobenzamide

Mechanism of Action Blocks the action of acetylcholine at parasympathetic sites in smooth muscle, secretory glands

Pharmacodynamics

Onset of action:

Oral: Within 1 hour

I.M.: 15-30 minutes

I.V.: 1-10 minutes

Duration of effect:
- Oral: 8-12 hours
- Parenteral: 7 hours

Pharmacokinetics

Absorption: Oral: Poor and erratic; 10% absorption

Distribution: Does not adequately penetrate into CNS

Elimination: Excreted primarily unchanged via biliary elimination (70% to 90%)

Usual Dosage

Children:
- Control of secretions:
  - Oral: 40-100 μg/kg/dose 3-4 times/day
  - I.M., I.V.: 4-10 μg/kg/dose every 3-4 hours
- Preoperative: I.M.:
  - <2 years: 4.4-8.8 μg/kg 30-60 minutes before procedure
  - >2 years: 4.4 μg/kg 30-60 minutes before procedure

Children and Adults: Reverse neuromuscular blockade: I.V.: 0.2 mg for each 1 mg of neostigmine or 5 mg of pyridostigmine administered

Adults:
- Peptic ulcer:
  - Oral: 1-2 mg 2-3 times/day
  - I.M., I.V.: 0.1-0.2 mg 3-4 times/day
- Preoperative: I.M.: 4.4 μg/kg 30-60 minutes before procedure

Administration Dilute to a concentration of 2 μg/mL (maximum concentration: 200 μg/mL); infuse over 15-20 minutes; may be administered direct I.V. at a maximum rate of 20 μg/minute

Monitoring Parameters Heart rate

Dosage Forms

Injection: 0.2 mg/mL (1 mL, 2 mL, 5 mL, 20 mL)

Tablet: 1 mg, 2 mg

Extemporaneous Preparation(s) A suspension of crushed tablets in syrup at 100 μg/mL is stable for 2 weeks refrigerated

Glycopyrronium Bromide *see* Glycopyrrolate *on previous page*

Glycotuss® [OTC] *see* Guaifenesin *on page 278*

Glynase Prestab® *see* Glyburide *on page 272*

Gly-Oxide® [OTC] *see* Carbamide Peroxide *on page 103*

Glyrol® *see* Glycerin *on page 273*

Glytuss® [OTC] *see* Guaifenesin *on page 278*

GM-CSF *see* Sargramostim *on page 517*

G-myticin® *see* Gentamicin *on page 268*

Gold Sodium Thiomalate

Brand Names Myochrysine®

Therapeutic Category Gold Compound

Use Treatment of progressive rheumatoid arthritis

Pregnancy Risk Factor C

Contraindications Severe hepatic or renal dysfunction; hypersensitivity to gold compounds or other heavy metals; systemic lupus erythematosus; history of blood dyscrasias; congestive heart failure, exfoliative dermatitis, or colitis; avoid concomitant use of antimalarials, immunosuppressive agents, penicillamine, or phenylbutazone

Warnings Explain the possibility of adverse reactions before initiating therapy; signs of gold toxicity include: decrease in hemoglobin, leukocytes, granulocytes and platelets; proteinuria, hematuria, pigmentation, pruritus, stomatitis or persistent diarrhea, rash, metallic taste; advise patient to report any symptoms of toxicity

Precautions Frequent monitoring of patients for signs and symptoms of toxicity will prevent serious adverse reactions; nonsteroidal anti-inflammatory drugs (NSAIDs) and corticosteroids may be discontinued after initiating gold therapy; must not be injected I.V.

Adverse Reactions

Cardiovascular: Flushing

Dermatologic: Exfoliative urticaria, dermatitis, erythema nodosum, alopecia, shedding of nails, pruritus, gray-to-blue pigmentation of skin and mucous membranes

(Continued)

Gold Sodium Thiomalate *(Continued)*

Gastrointestinal: Stomatitis, nausea, diarrhea, abdominal cramps
Hematologic: Eosinophilia, leukopenia, agranulocytosis, thrombocytopenia
Hepatic: Hepatitis
Musculoskeletal: Arthralgias
Nervous system: Peripheral neuropathy, seizures, headache
Ocular: Blurred vision, conjunctivitis, corneal ulcers, iritis
Renal & genitourinary: Hematuria, proteinuria, nephrotic syndrome, vaginitis
Respiratory: Interstitial pneumonitis and fibrosis
Miscellaneous: Hypersensitivity reactions including anaphylaxis (rarely), metallic taste

Mechanism of Action Unknown, may decrease prostaglandin synthesis or may alter cellular mechanisms by inhibiting sulfhydryl systems

Pharmacokinetics

Half-life: 3-27 days (may lengthen with multiple doses)
Peak serum levels: I.M.: Within 3-6 hours
Elimination: Majority (50% to 90%) is excreted in the urine with smaller amounts (10% to 50%) excreted in feces (via bile)

Usual Dosage I.M.:

Children: Initial: Test dose of 10 mg I.M. is recommended, followed by 1 mg/kg I.M. weekly for 20 weeks (maximum dose: 50 mg); maintenance: 1 mg/kg/dose at 2- to 4-week intervals thereafter for as long as therapy is clinically beneficial and toxicity does not develop. Administration for 2-4 months is usually required before clinical improvement is observed

Adults: 10 mg first week; 25 mg second week; then 25-50 mg/week until clinical improvement or a 1 g cumulative dose has been given. If improvement occurs without adverse reactions, give 25-50 mg every 2 weeks for 2-20 weeks; if continues stable, give 25-50 mg every 3-4 weeks indefinitely

Administration Give I.M. only, preferably intragluteally; patients should be recumbent during injection and for 10 minutes afterwards; observe closely for 15 minutes after injection

Monitoring Parameters CBC, platelets, hemoglobin, urinalysis, renal and liver function tests

Reference Range Gold: Normal: 0-0.1 μg/mL (SI: 0-0.5 μmol/L); Therapeutic: 1-3 μg/mL (SI: 5.1-15.2 μmol/L); Urine <0.1 μg/24 hours

Dosage Forms Injection: 25 mg/mL (1 mL); 50 mg/mL (1 mL, 10 mL)

GoLYTELY® *see* Polyethylene Glycol-Electrolyte Solution *on page 466*

Gonadorelin (goe nad oh rell' in)

Brand Names Factrel®; Lutrepulse®

Synonyms LRH

Therapeutic Category Diagnostic Agent, Gonadotrophic Hormone; Gonadotropin

Use Evaluation of the functional capacity and response of gonadotrophic hormones; used to evaluate abnormal gonadotropin regulation as in precocious puberty and delayed puberty

Pregnancy Risk Factor B

Contraindications Known hypersensitivity to gonadorelin

Adverse Reactions

Cardiovascular: Flushing
Central nervous system: Light headedness, headache
Dermatologic: Skin rash
Gastrointestinal: Nausea, abdominal discomfort

Drug Interactions Androgens, estrogens, progestins, glucocorticoids, spironolactone, levodopa, oral contraceptives, digoxin, phenothiazines, dopamine antagonists

Stability Prepare immediately prior to use; after reconstitution, store at room temperature and use within 1 day; discard unused portion

Mechanism of Action Stimulates the release of luteinizing hormone (LH) from the anterior pituitary gland

Pharmacodynamics

Onset of action: Following administration maximal LH release occurs within 20 minutes

Duration: 3-5 hours

Pharmacokinetics Half-life: 4 minutes

Usual Dosage

Children: I.V.: 100 μg to evaluate abnormal gonadotropin regulation

Children >12 years and Adults: I.V., S.C.: 100 μg administered in women during early phase of menstrual cycle (day 1-7)

Administration Dilute in 3 mL of normal saline; give I.V. push over 30 seconds

Monitoring Parameters LH, FSH

Dosage Forms

Injection, as acetate: 0.8 mg, 3.2 mg

Injection, as hydrochloride: 100 μg, 500 μg

References

Pescovitz OH, Comite F, Hench K, et al, "The NIH Experience With Precocious Puberty: Diagnostic Subgroups and Response to Short-Term Luteinizing Hormone-Releasing Hormone Analogue Therapy," *J Pediatr*, 1986, 108(1):47-54.

Gonic® *see* Chorionic Gonadotropin *on page 134*

Granulocyte Colony Stimulating Factor *see* Filgrastim *on page 244*

Granulocyte Macrophage Colony Stimulating Factor *see* Sargramostim *on page 517*

Grifulvin® V *see* Griseofulvin *on this page*

Grisactin® *see* Griseofulvin *on this page*

Grisactin® Ultra *see* Griseofulvin *on this page*

Griseofulvin (gri see oh ful' vin)

Brand Names Fulvicin® P/G; Fulvicin-U/F®; Grifulvin® V; Grisactin®; Grisactin® Ultra; Gris-PEG®

Synonyms Griseofulvin Microsize; Griseofulvin Ultramicrosize

Therapeutic Category Antifungal Agent, Systemic

Use Treatment of susceptible tinea infections of the skin, hair, and nails

Pregnancy Risk Factor C

Contraindications Hypersensitivity to griseofulvin or any component; severe liver disease, porphyria (interferes with porphyrin metabolism)

Precautions Avoid exposure to intense sunlight to prevent photosensitivity reactions

Adverse Reactions

Central nervous system: Fatigue, confusion, impaired judgment, insomnia, paresthesia, headache, incoordination

Dermatologic: Rash, urticaria, photosensitivity reaction

Gastrointestinal: Nausea, vomiting, diarrhea

Hematologic: Leukopenia, granulocytopenia

Hepatic: Hepatotoxicity

Renal & genitourinary: Proteinuria

Miscellaneous: Lupus-like syndrome

Drug Interactions Phenobarbital, warfarin, alcohol, oral contraceptives

Mechanism of Action Inhibits fungal cell mitosis at metaphase; binds to human keratin making it resistant to fungal invasion

Pharmacokinetics

Absorption: Ultramicrosize griseofulvin absorption is almost complete; absorption of microsize griseofulvin is variable (25% to 70% of an oral dose); absorption is enhanced by ingestion of a fatty meal

Distribution: Crosses the placenta

Metabolism: Extensively metabolized in the liver

Half-life: 9-22 hours

Elimination: <1% is excreted unchanged in the urine; also excreted in feces and perspiration

Usual Dosage Oral:

Children:

Microsize: 10-15 mg/kg/day in single or divided doses;

Ultramicrosize: >2 years: 5.5-7.3 mg/kg/day in single or divided doses

(Continued)

Griseofulvin *(Continued)*

Adults:
- Microsize: 500-1000 mg/day in single or divided doses
- Ultramicrosize: 330-375 mg/day in single or divided doses; doses up to 750 mg/day have been used for infections more difficult to eradicate such as tinea unguium

Duration of therapy depends on the site of infection:
- Tinea corporis: 2-4 weeks
- Tinea capitis: 4-6 weeks or longer
- Tinea pedis: 4-8 weeks
- Tinea unguium: 3-6 months

Monitoring Parameters Periodic renal, hepatic, and hematopoietic function tests

Test Interactions False-positive urinary VMA levels

Patient Information Avoid exposure to sunlight; take with fatty meal

Dosage Forms

Capsule, microsize: 125 mg, 250 mg
Suspension, oral, microsize: 125 mg/5 mL (120 mL)
Tablet:
- Microsize: 250 mg, 500 mg
- Ultramicrosize: 125 mg, 165 mg, 250 mg, 330 mg

References

Ginsburg CM, McCracken GH Jr, Petruska M, et al, "Effect of Feeding on Bioavailability of Griseofulvin in Children," *J Pediatr*, 1983, 102(2):309-11.

Griseofulvin Microsize *see* Griseofulvin *on previous page*

Griseofulvin Ultramicrosize *see* Griseofulvin *on previous page*

Gris-PEG® *see* Griseofulvin *on previous page*

Guaifenesin (gwye fen' e sin)

Related Information

OTC Cold Preparations, Pediatric *on page 723-726*

Formerly Known As Glyceryl Guaiacolate

Brand Names Amonidrin® [OTC]; Anti-Tuss® [OTC]; Breonesin® [OTC]; Fenesin™; Genatuss® [OTC]; GG-CEN® [OTC]; Glyate® [OTC]; Glycotuss® [OTC]; Glytuss® [OTC]; Guaituss® [OTC]; Halotussin® [OTC]; Humibid® L.A.; Humibid® Sprinkle; Hytuss-2X® [OTC]; Liquibid®; Malotuss [OTC]; Medi-Tuss® [OTC]; Mytussin® [OTC]; Naldecon® Senior EX [OTC]; Robafen® [OTC]; Robitussin® [OTC]; Uni Tussin® [OTC]

Synonyms GG

Therapeutic Category Expectorant

Use Temporary control of cough due to minor throat and bronchial irritation

Pregnancy Risk Factor C

Contraindications Hypersensitivity to guaifenesin or any component

Adverse Reactions

Central nervous system: Drowsiness
Gastrointestinal: Nausea, vomiting

Mechanism of Action Thought to act as an expectorant by irritating the gastric mucosa and stimulating respiratory tract secretions, thereby increasing respiratory fluid volumes and decreasing phlegm viscosity

Usual Dosage Oral:

Children:
- <2 years: 12 mg/kg/day in 6 divided doses
- 2-5 years: 50-100 mg every 4 hours, not to exceed 600 mg/day
- 6-11 years: 100-200 mg every 4 hours, not to exceed 1.2 g/day

Children >12 years and Adults: 200-400 mg every 4 hours to a maximum of 2.4 g/day

Dosage Forms

Capsule: 200 mg
Capsule, sustained release: 300 mg
Liquid: 200 mg/5 mL (118 mL)
Syrup: 100 mg/5 mL (30 mL, 120 mL, 240 mL, 473 mL, 946 mL)
Tablet: 100 mg, 200 mg
Tablet, sustained release: 600 mg

Guaifenesin and Codeine

Related Information

OTC Cold Preparations, Pediatric *on page 723-726*

Brand Names Cheracol®; Guaituss AC®; Medi-Tuss® AC; Mytussin® AC; Robitussin® A-C; Tolu-Sed®

Synonyms Codeine and Guaifenesin

Therapeutic Category Antitussive; Cough Preparation

Use Temporary control of cough due to minor throat and bronchial irritation

Restrictions C-V

Pregnancy Risk Factor C

Contraindications Hypersensitivity to guaifenesin, codeine or any component

Adverse Reactions

Codeine:

- Cardiovascular: Hypotension, palpitations, bradycardia, peripheral vasodilation, increased intracranial pressure
- Central nervous system: CNS depression, dizziness, drowsiness, sedation
- Endocrine & metabolic: Antidiuretic hormone release
- Gastrointestinal: Nausea, vomiting, constipation
- Ocular: Miosis
- Renal & genitourinary: Biliary or urinary tract spasm
- Respiratory: Respiratory depression
- Sensitivity reactions: Histamine release
- Miscellaneous: Physical and psychological dependence with prolonged use

Guaifenesin:

- Central nervous system: Drowsiness
- Gastrointestinal: Nausea, vomiting

Drug Interactions CNS depressant medications produce additive sedative properties

Usual Dosage Oral:

Children:

- 2-6 years: 1-1.5 mg/kg codeine/day divided into 4 doses administered every 4-6 hours (maximum: 30 mg/24 hours)
- 6-12 years: 5 mL every 4 hours, not to exceed 30 mL/24 hours
- >12 years: 10 mL every 4 hours, up to 60 mL/24 hours

Adults: 5-10 mL every 6-8 hours

Dosage Forms Syrup: Guaifenesin 100 mg and codeine phosphate 10 mg per 5 mL (60 mL, 120 mL, 480 mL)

Guaifenesin and Dextromethorphan

Related Information

OTC Cold Preparations, Pediatric *on page 723-726*

Brand Names Guaituss DM® [OTC]; Halotussin® DM [OTC]; Mytussin® DM [OTC]; Queltuss® [OTC]; Robitussin-DM® [OTC]

Synonyms Dextromethorphan and Guaifenesin

Therapeutic Category Antitussive; Antitussive, Combination

Use Temporary control of cough due to minor throat and bronchial irritation

Pregnancy Risk Factor C

Contraindications Hypersensitivity to guaifenesin, dextromethorphan or any component

Adverse Reactions

- Central nervous system: Drowsiness, dizziness
- Gastrointestinal: Nausea

Pharmacodynamics Onset of action: Exerts its antitussive effect in 15-30 minutes after oral administration

Pharmacokinetics Absorption: Dextromethorphan is rapidly absorbed from the GI tract

Usual Dosage Oral (dose expressed in mg of dextromethorphan):

Children: 1-2 mg/kg/day every 6-8 hours

Adults: 60-120 mg/day divided every 6-8 hours

(Continued)

Guaifenesin and Dextromethorphan *(Continued)*

Dosage Forms

Syrup:

Guaifenesin 67 mg and dextromethorphan hydrobromide 10 mg per 5 mL
Guaifenesin 85 mg and dextromethorphan hydrobromide 10 mg per 5 mL
Guaifenesin 100 mg and dextromethorphan hydrobromide 10 mg per 5 mL
Guaifenesin 100 mg and dextromethorphan hydrobromide 15 mg per 5 mL
Guaifenesin 150 mg and dextromethorphan hydrobromide 10 mg per 5 mL
Guaifenesin 200 mg and dextromethorphan hydrobromide 15 mg per 5 mL

Tablet:

Guaifenesin 100 mg and dextromethorphan hydrobromide 10 mg
Guaifenesin 100 mg and dextromethorphan hydrobromide 15 mg
Guaifenesin 200 mg and dextromethorphan hydrobromide 10 mg
Extended release: Guaifenesin 600 mg and dextromethorphan hydrobromide 30

Guaifenesin, Phenylpropanolamine, and Phenylephrine (fen ill ef' rin)

Brand Names Contuss®; Dura-Gest®; Enomine®; Entex®

Therapeutic Category Decongestant; Expectorant

Use Temporary relief of nasal congestion, running nose, sneezing, itching of nose and throat, and itchy, watery eyes due to common cold, hay fever, or other upper respiratory allergies

Pregnancy Risk Factor C

Contraindications Known hypersensitivity to guaifenesin, phenylephrine, or phenylpropanolamine; severe hypertension or coronary artery disease; MAO inhibitor therapy; GI or GU obstruction, narrow-angle glaucoma, peripheral vascular disease

Warnings May impair ability to perform hazardous activities requiring mental alertness and physical coordination

Adverse Reactions

Cardiovascular: Hypertension, tachycardia, arrhythmias
Central nervous system: Sedation, nervousness, insomnia, restlessness, tremor, headache
Gastrointestinal: Nausea, gastric irritation, vomiting, anorexia
Genitourinary: Urinary retention

Drug Interactions MAO inhibitors, alpha- and beta-adrenergic blocking agents, sympathomimetics, ASA, NSAIDs

Mechanism of Action Phenylephrine and phenylpropanolamine are alpha-adrenergic receptor agonists which produce vasoconstriction resulting in shrinking of swollen nasal mucous membranes and reduction of tissue hyperemia and edema; guaifenesin promotes lower respiratory tract drainage

Usual Dosage Oral (safety and efficacy in children <2 years of age have not been established):

Children:

2-4 years: 2.5 mL every 6 hours
4-6 years: 5 mL every 6 hours
6 to ≤12 years: 7.5 mL every 6 hours **or** ½ extended release tablet every 12 hours

Children >12 years and Adults: 10 mL every 6 hours **or** 1 capsule every 6 hours **or** 1 extended release tablet every 12 hours

Additional Information Extended release tablets may be cut in half and still maintain effective release properties, do not crush or chew them

Dosage Forms

Capsule: Guaifenesin 200 mg, phenylpropanolamine hydrochloride 45 mg, and phenylephrine hydrochloride 5 mg
Liquid: Guaifenesin 100 mg, phenylpropanolamine hydrochloride 20 mg, and phenylephrine hydrochloride 5 mg per 5 mL

Guaituss® [OTC] *see* Guaifenesin *on page 278*

G-well® *see* Lindane *on page 344*

Gyne-Lotrimin® [OTC] *see* Clotrimazole *on page 145*

H_2O_2 *see* Hydrogen Peroxide *on page 294*

***Haemophilus* b Oligosaccharide Conjugate Vaccine** *see* Immunization Guidelines *on page 660-667*

Halcion® *see* Triazolam *on page 581*

Haldol® *see* Haloperidol *on this page*

Haldol® Decanoate *see* Haloperidol *on this page*

Halenol® [OTC] *see* Acetaminophen *on page 16*

Haloperidol (ha loe per' i dole)

Brand Names Haldol®; Haldol® Decanoate

Therapeutic Category Antipsychotic Agent

Use Treatment of psychoses, Tourette's disorder, and severe behavioral problems in children

Pregnancy Risk Factor C

Contraindications Hypersensitivity to haloperidol or any component; narrow-angle glaucoma, bone marrow depression, CNS depression, severe liver or cardiac disease, parkinsonism

Warnings Safety and efficacy have not been established in children <3 years of age; some tablets contain tartrazine which may cause allergic reactions

Precautions Use with caution in patients with renal or hepatic dysfunction, thyrotoxicosis

Adverse Reactions

Cardiovascular: Tachycardia, hypotension

Central nervous system: Extrapyramidal reactions, neuroleptic malignant syndrome, tardive dyskinesia, drowsiness

Dermatologic: Rash, contact dermatitis

Endocrine & metabolic: Galactorrhea, gynecomastia

Gastrointestinal: Dry mouth, constipation

Hematologic: Leukopenia, leukocytosis, anemia

Hepatic: Hepatotoxicity (rarely)

Ocular: Blurred vision

Renal & genitourinary: Urinary retention

Drug Interactions CNS depressants may ↑ adverse effects; epinephrine may cause hypotension; carbamazepine and phenobarbital may ↑ metabolism and ↓ effectiveness of haloperidol; haloperidol and anticholinergic agents → ↑ intraocular pressure; concurrent use with lithium has occasionally caused acute encephalopathy-like syndrome

Mechanism of Action Competitive blockade of postsynaptic dopamine receptors in the mesolimbic dopaminergic system; depresses cerebral cortex and hypothalamus; exhibits a strong alpha-adrenergic and anticholinergic blocking activity

Usual Dosage

Children:

- 3-12 years (15-40 kg): Oral: Initial: 0.05 mg/kg/day or 0.25-0.5 mg/day given in 2-3 divided doses; ↑ by 0.25-0.5 mg every 5-7 days; maximum: 0.15 mg/kg/day; usual maintenance:
  - Agitation or hyperkinesia: 0.01-0.03 mg/kg/day once daily
  - Tourette's disorder: 0.05-0.075 mg/kg/day in 2-3 divided doses
  - Psychotic disorders: 0.05-0.15 mg/kg/day in 2-3 divided doses
- 6-12 years: I.M. (as lactate): 1-3 mg/dose every 4-8 hours to a maximum of 0.15 mg/kg/day; change over to oral therapy as soon as able

Adults:

- Oral: 0.5-5 mg 2-3 times/day; usual maximum: 30 mg/day; some patients may require 100 mg/day
- I.M.:
  - As lactate: 2-5 mg every 4-8 hours as needed
  - As decanoate: Initial: 10-15 times the individual patients' stabilized oral dose, given at 3- to 4-week intervals

Nursing Implications Do not give I.V.

Dosage Forms

Concentrate, oral, as lactate: 2 mg/mL (5 mL, 10 mL, 15 mL, 120 mL, 240 mL)

(Continued)

Haloperidol *(Continued)*

Injection, as decanoate: 50 mg/mL (1 mL, 5 mL); 100 mg/mL (1 mL, 5 mL)
Injection, as lactate: 5 mg/mL (1 mL, 2 mL, 2.5 mL, 10 mL)
Tablet: 0.5 mg, 1 mg, 2 mg, 5 mg, 10 mg, 20 mg

References

Serrano AC, "Haloperidol - Its Use in Children," *J Clin Psychiatry*, 1981, 42(4):154-6.

Haloprogin (ha loe proe' jin)

Brand Names Halotex®

Therapeutic Category Antifungal Agent, Topical

Use Topical treatment of tinea pedis, tinea cruris, tinea corporis, tinea manuum caused by *Trichophyton rubrum*, *Trichophyton tonsurans*, *Trichophyton mentagrophytes*, *Microsporum canis*, or *Epidermophyton floccosum*

Pregnancy Risk Factor C

Contraindications Hypersensitivity to haloprogin or any component

Warnings Safety and efficacy have not been established in children

Adverse Reactions

Dermatologic: Pruritus, folliculitis, vesicle formation, erythema
Local: Irritation, burning sensation

Mechanism of Action Inhibits yeast cell respiration and disrupts its cell membrane

Pharmacokinetics Absorption: Poorly absorbed through the skin (~11%)

Usual Dosage Children and Adults: Topical: Twice daily for 2-3 weeks; intertriginous areas may require up to 4 weeks of treatment

Patient Information Avoid contact with eyes, for topical use only

Dosage Forms

Cream: 1% (15 g, 30 g)
Solution, topical: 1% with alcohol 75% (10 mL, 30 mL)

Halotestin® *see* Fluoxymesterone *on page 260*

Halotex® *see* Haloprogin *on this page*

Halotussin® [OTC] *see* Guaifenesin *on page 278*

Halotussin® DM [OTC] *see* Guaifenesin and Dextromethorphan *on page 279*

Haltran® [OTC] *see* Ibuprofen *on page 300*

hCG *see* Chorionic Gonadotropin *on page 134*

HCTZ *see* Hydrochlorothiazide *on page 291*

Heavy Mineral Oil *see* Mineral Oil *on page 390*

Hemofil® M *see* Antihemophilic Factor, Human *on page 55*

Hemorrhoidal Preparations

Brand Names Anusol® [OTC]

Therapeutic Category Topical Skin Product

Use Symptomatic relief of pain and discomfort associated with hemorrhoids and anal fissures

Contraindications Known hypersensitivity to any of the components

Adverse Reactions

Dermatologic: Rash
Local: Irritation

Usual Dosage Adults: Rectal: Insert 1 suppository in the morning and at bedtime and after each bowel movement

Patient Information If anorectal symptoms do not improve in 7 days, or if bleeding, protrusion or seepage occurs, consult physician

Dosage Forms Suppository: Benzyl benzoate, Peruvian balsam, resorcinol, cod liver oil, lanolin, bismuth subgallate, zinc oxide

Heparin (hep' a rin)

Related Information

Medications Compatible With PN Solutions *on page 649-650*
Overdose and Toxicology Information *on page 696-700*

Brand Names Calciparine®; Hep-Lock®; Liquaemin®

Synonyms Heparin Calcium; Heparin Lock Flush; Heparin Sodium

Therapeutic Category Anticoagulant

Use Prophylaxis and treatment of thromboembolic disorders

Pregnancy Risk Factor C

Contraindications Hypersensitivity to heparin or any component; severe thrombocytopenia, subacute bacterial endocarditis, suspected intracranial hemorrhage, shock, severe hypotension, uncontrollable bleeding (unless secondary to disseminated intravascular coagulation)

Warnings Some preparations contain benzyl alcohol as a preservative. In neonates, large amounts of benzyl alcohol (>100 mg/kg/day) have been associated with fatal toxicity (gasping syndrome). The use of preservative free heparin is, therefore, recommended in neonates. Some preparations contain sulfite which may cause allergic reactions.

Precautions Use with caution as hemorrhage may occur; risk factors for hemorrhage include I.M. injections, peptic ulcer disease, intermittent I.V. injections (vs continuous I.V. infusion), increased capillary permeability, menstruation, severe renal, hepatic, or biliary disease, and indwelling catheters

Heparin does not possess fibrinolytic activity and, therefore, cannot lyse established thrombi; discontinue heparin if hemorrhage occurs; severe hemorrhage or overdosage may require protamine.

Adverse Reactions

Central nervous system: Fever, headache, chills

Dermatologic: Urticaria

Gastrointestinal: Nausea, vomiting

Hematologic: Hemorrhage, thrombocytopenia

Hepatic: Elevation of liver enzymes

Local: Irritation, ulceration, cutaneous necrosis has been rarely reported with deep S.C. injections

Musculoskeletal: Osteoporosis

Drug Interactions Thrombolytic agents (urokinase, streptokinase) and drugs which affect platelet function (aspirin, NSAIDs, dipyridamole) may potentiate the risk of hemorrhage; I.V. nitroglycerin may antagonize heparin's anticoagulant effect.

Mechanism of Action Potentiates the action of antithrombin III and thereby inactivates thrombin (as well as activated coagulation factors IX, X, XI, XII, and plasmin) and prevents the conversion of fibrinogen to fibrin; heparin also stimulates release of lipoprotein lipase (lipoprotein lipase hydrolyzes triglycerides to glycerol and free fatty acids)

Pharmacodynamics Onset of anticoagulation effect:

S.C.: 20-60 minutes

I.V.: Immediate

Pharmacokinetics

Absorption: Oral, rectal, S.L., I.M.: Erratic

Distribution: Does not cross the placenta; does not appear in breast milk

Metabolism: Believed to be partially metabolized in the reticuloendothelial system

Half-life: Mean: 90 minutes (range: 1-2 hours); effected by obesity, renal function, hepatic function, malignancy, presence of pulmonary embolism, and infections

Elimination: Renal excretion, small amount excreted unchanged in urine

Usual Dosage

Line flushing: When using daily flushes of heparin to maintain patency of single and double lumen central catheters, 10 units/mL is commonly used for younger infants (eg, <10 kg) while 100 units/mL is used for older infants, children, and adults. Capped PVC catheters and peripheral heparin locks require flushing more frequently (eg, every 6-8 hours). Volume of heparin flush is usually similar to volume of catheter (or slightly greater) or may be standardized according to specific hospital's policy (eg, 2-5 mL/flush). Dose of heparin flush used should not approach therapeutic unit per kg dose. Additional flushes should be given when stagnant blood is observed in catheter, after catheter is used for drug or blood administration, and after blood withdrawal from catheter.

TPN: Heparin 1 unit/mL (final concentration) may be added to TPN solutions, both central and peripheral. (Addition of heparin to peripheral TPN has been shown to increase duration of line patency.) The final concentration of heparin used for TPN solutions may need to be decreased to 0.5 units/mL in small infants receiving larger amounts of volume in order to avoid approaching therapeutic amounts.

(Continued)

Heparin *(Continued)*

Arterial lines: Heparinize with a usual final concentration of 1 unit/mL; range: 0.5-2 units/mL; in order to avoid large total doses and systemic effects, use 0.5 unit/mL in low birth weight/premature newborns and in other patients receiving multiple lines containing heparin

Children:

Intermittent I.V.: Initial: 50-100 units/kg, then 50-100 units/kg every 4 hours

I.V. infusion: Initial: 50 units/kg, then 15-25 units/kg/hour; increase dose by 2-4 units/kg/hour every 6-8 hours dependent on APTT

Adults:

Prophylaxis (low dose heparin): S.C.: 5000 units every 8-12 hours

Intermittent I.V.: Initial: 10,000 units, then 50-70 units/kg (5000-10,000 units) every 4-6 hours

I.V. infusion: Initial: 70-100 units/kg, then 15-25 units/kg/hour with dose adjusted according to APTT results; usual range: 10-30 units/kg/hour

Monitoring Parameters Platelet counts, signs of bleeding, hemoglobin, hematocrit, APTT or PTT; for full-dose heparin (ie, non-low dose), the dose should be titrated according to APTT or PTT results. For anticoagulation, an APTT or PTT 1.5-2.5 times normal is usually desired. APTT or PTT is usually measured prior to heparin therapy, 6-8 hours after initiation of a continuous infusion (following a loading dose), and 6-8 hours after changes in the infusion rate; increase or decrease infusion by 2-4 units/kg/hour dependent on APTT or PTT. Continuous I.V. infusion is preferred vs I.V. intermittent injections. For intermittent I.V. injections, APTT or PTT is measured 3.5-4 hours after I.V. injection.

Test Interactions ↑ thyroxine (S) (competitive protein binding methods)

Nursing Implications Do not administer I.M. due to pain, irritation, and hematoma formation

Dosage Forms

Heparin sodium: Injection:

Beef lung, multiple-dose vial, with preservative: 1000 units/mL (5 mL, 10 mL, 30 mL); 5000 units/mL (10 mL); 10,000 units/mL (4 mL, 5 mL, 10 mL); 20,000 units/mL (2 mL, 5 mL, 10 mL); 40,000 units/mL (5 mL)

Beef lung, single-dose vial: 1000 units/mL (1 mL); 5000 units/mL (1 mL); 10,000 units/mL (1 mL); 20,000 units/mL (1 mL); 40,000 units/mL (1 mL)

Beef lung, lock flush: 10 units/mL (1 mL, 2 mL, 2.5 mL, 3 mL, 5 mL, 10 mL, 30 mL); 100 units/mL (1 mL, 2 mL, 2.5 mL, 3 mL, 5 mL, 10 mL, 30 mL)

Porcine intestinal mucosa, lock flush: 10 units/mL (1 mL, 2 mL, 10 mL, 30 mL); 100 units/mL (1 mL, 2 mL, 10 mL, 30 mL)

Porcine intestinal mucosa, lock flush, preservative free: 10 units/mL (1 mL); 100 units/mL (1 mL)

Porcine intestinal mucosa, multiple-dose vial, with preservative: 1000 units/mL (10 mL, 30 mL); 5000 units/mL (10 mL); 10,000 units/mL (4 mL); 20,000 units/mL (2 mL, 5 mL)

Porcine intestinal mucosa, single-dose vial: 1000 units/mL (1 mL); 5000 units/mL (1 mL); 10,000 units/mL (1 mL); 20,000 units/mL (1 mL); 40,000 units/mL (1 mL)

Porcine intestinal mucosa, unit dose, with preservative: 1000 units/dose (1 mL, 2 mL); 2500 units/dose (1 mL); 5000 units/dose (0.5 mL, 1 mL); 7500 units/dose (1 mL); 10,000 units/dose (1 mL); 15,000 units/dose (1 mL); 20,000 units/dose (1 mL)

Heparin sodium in dextrose: Infusion, porcine intestinal mucosa, in D_5W: 40 units/mL (500 mL); 50 units/mL (250 mL, 500 mL); 100 units/mL (100 mL, 250 mL)

Heparin sodium in sodium chloride: Infusion:

Porcine intestinal mucosa, in 0.45% NaCl: 2 units/mL (500 mL, 1000 mL); 50 units/mL (250 mL); 100 units/mL (250 mL)

Porcine intestinal mucosa, in 0.9% NaCl: 2 units/mL (500 mL, 1000 mL); 5 units/mL (1000 mL); 50 units/mL (250 mL, 500 mL, 1000 mL)

Heparin calcium: Injection, porcine intestinal mucosa, preservative free, unit dose: 5000 units/dose (0.2 mL); 12,500 units/dose (0.5 mL); 20,000 units/dose (0.8 mL)

Heparin Calcium *see* Heparin *on page 282*

Heparin Lock Flush *see* Heparin *on page 282*

Heparin Sodium *see* Heparin *on page 282*

Hepatitis B Immune Globulin *see* Immunization Guidelines *on page 660-667*

Hepatitis B Vaccine *see* Immunization Guidelines *on page 660-667*

Hep-Lock® *see* Heparin *on page 282*

Herplex® *see* Idoxuridine *on page 303*

Hexachlorocyclohexane *see* Lindane *on page 344*

Hexachlorophene (hex a klor' oh feen)

Brand Names pHisoHex®; Septisol®

Therapeutic Category Antibacterial, Topical; Soap

Use Surgical scrub and as a bacteriostatic skin cleanser; to control an outbreak of gram-positive infection when other procedures have been unsuccessful

Pregnancy Risk Factor C

Contraindications Known hypersensitivity to halogenated phenol derivatives or hexachlorophene; use in premature infants; use on burned or denuded skin; use with an occlusive dressing; application to mucous membranes

Warnings Do not use for bathing infants; premature infants are particularly susceptible to hexachlorophene topical absorption; do not apply to mucous membranes; exposure of preterm infants or patients with extensive burns has been associated with apnea, convulsions, agitation and coma

Adverse Reactions

Central nervous system: CNS injury, seizures, irritability

Dermatologic: Dermatitis, erythema, dry skin, photosensitivity

Stability Store in nonmetallic container (incompatible with many metals)

Mechanism of Action Bacteriostatic polychlorinated biphenyl which inhibits membrane-bound enzymes and disrupts the cell membrane

Pharmacokinetics

Absorption: Absorbed percutaneously through inflamed, excoriated and intact skin

Distribution: Crosses the placenta

Half-life, infants: 6.1-44.2 hours

Usual Dosage Children and Adults: Topical: Apply 5 mL cleanser and water to area to be cleansed; lather and rinse thoroughly under running water

Patient Information For external use only; rinse thoroughly after each use; avoid prolonged contact with skin

Dosage Forms

Foam: 0.23% (180 mL, 600 mL)

Liquid, topical: 3% (8 mL, 150 mL, 500 mL, 3840 mL)

References

Lester RS, "Topical Formulary for the Pediatrician," *Pediatr Clin North Am*, 1983, 30(4):749-65.

Hexadrol® *see* Dexamethasone *on page 178*

Hexamethylenetetramine *see* Methenamine *on page 369*

Hiprex® *see* Methenamine *on page 369*

Hismanal® *see* Astemizole *on page 63*

Histaject® *see* Brompheniramine Maleate *on page 88*

Histamine Acid Phosphate *see* Histamine Phosphate *on this page*

Histamine Diphosphate *see* Histamine Phosphate *on this page*

Histamine Phosphate (hiss' ta meen)

Synonyms Histamine Acid Phosphate; Histamine Diphosphate

Therapeutic Category Diagnostic Agent, Achlorhydria and Pheochromocytoma

Use Diagnostic test for achlorhydria and pheochromocytoma

Pregnancy Risk Factor C

Contraindications Severe hypertension, hypotension, bronchial asthma, severe cardiac, pulmonary or renal disease

(Continued)

Histamine Phosphate *(Continued)*

Warnings Monitor blood pressure and pulse rate frequently during and immediately following administration

Precautions Epinephrine should be readily available to treat severe adverse effects

Adverse Reactions

Cardiovascular: Tachycardia, hypertension or hypotension, flushing, vasomotor collapse, shock, anginal pain

Central nervous system: Nervousness, dizziness, headache

Gastrointestinal: Nausea, vomiting, metallic taste

Respiratory: Dyspnea, bronchospasm

Miscellaneous: Hypersensitivity reactions

Mechanism of Action Stimulates exocrine gland secretion such as the secretion of gastric acid by the gastric parietal cells; dilates capillaries, small arteries and veins, and cerebral blood vessels; constricts all other arteries and veins; potent bronchoconstrictor in patients with bronchial asthma, emphysema

Pharmacodynamics

Onset of action: 15-30 minutes

Duration: 4-5 hours

Pharmacokinetics Metabolism: Primarily metabolized in the liver

Usual Dosage Adults:

Gastric: Function test: S.C.: 0.0275 mg/kg histamine phosphate (10 μg/kg histamine)

Augmented histamine test: After a basal secretion study is completed and an appropriate I.M. dose of an antihistamine (ie, diphenhydramine) is administered, give S.C. 0.04 mg/kg histamine phosphate (0.0145 mg/kg histamine)

Pheochromocytoma: I.V.: 10 μg (histamine), then 50 μg 5 minutes later if no response after first dose

Administration When used as a diagnostic agent for pheochromocytoma, histamine should be administered by rapid, direct I.V. push

Monitoring Parameters Heart rate, blood pressure; pH, volume and acid output of gastric contents (for achlorhydria evaluation)

Nursing Implications Patient needs to fast for at least 12 hours before the test for achlorhydria; for pheochromocytoma test, antihypertensive agents, sympathomimetic agents, sedatives and opiates should be withheld from the patient for at least 24 hours, and preferably 72 hours

Additional Information Each 1 mg histamine = 2.75 mg histamine phosphate

Dosage Forms Injection: 0.275 mg/mL [0.1 mg base] (1 mL); 0.55 mg/mL [0.2 mg base] (5 mL); 2.75 mg/mL [1 mg base] (1 mL)

Histerone® *see* Testosterone *on page 550*

Histrelin

Brand Names Supprelin™

Synonyms ORF17070; RWJ17070

Therapeutic Category Gonadotropin Releasing Hormone Analog

Use Central idiopathic precocious puberty; also used to treat estrogen-associated gynecological disorders (ie, endometriosis, intermittent porphyria, possibly premenstrual syndrome, leiomyomata uteri [uterine fibroids])

Pregnancy Risk Factor X

Contraindications Hypersensitivity to histrelin; pregnancy or expected pregnancy, breast feeding

Precautions Inadequate control of pubertal process may occur with noncompliance or changes in the dosing schedule

Adverse Reactions

Central nervous system: Anxiety, depression, irritability, insomnia, headaches, rarely ↑ in seizure frequency

Endocrine & metabolic: Prevention of ovulation and menses, inhibition of spermatogenesis, breast tenderness, amenorrhea, vaginal dryness, dyspareunia, transient testicular enlargement

Gastrointestinal: Nausea, vomiting

Renal & genitourinary: Increase in urinary calcium excretion

Local: Irritation at injection site
Musculoskeletal: Joint stiffness, possible osteoporosis
Miscellaneous: Severe hypersensitivity reactions (ie, angioedema, hives, hypotension, etc)

Stability Protect from light, store in refrigerator, discard unused portion

Mechanism of Action Central idiopathic precocious puberty: Histrelin is a synthetic long-acting gonadotropin-releasing hormone analog; with daily administration, it desensitizes the pituitary to endogenous gonadotropin-releasing hormone (ie, suppresses gonadotropin release by causing down regulation of the pituitary); this results in a decrease in gonadal sex steroid production which stops the secondary sexual development

Pharmacokinetics Hormonal response: Physical evidence of reduction in secretion of sex steroids within 3 months

Usual Dosage S.C.:
Children: Central idiopathic precocious puberty: 6-10 μg/kg/day; give as single daily dose at the same time every day
Adult women:
Acute intermittent porphyria: 5 μg/day
Endometriosis: 100 μg/day
Leiomyomata uteri: 20-50 μg/day or 4 μg/day

Administration S.C.: Vary the injection site daily

Monitoring Parameters Precocious puberty: Prior to initiating therapy: Height and weight, hand and wrist x-rays, total sex steroid levels, beta-hCG level, adrenal steroid level, gonadotropin-releasing hormone stimulation test, pelvic/adrenal/testicular ultrasound/head CT; during therapy monitor 3 months after initiation and then every 6-12 months; serial levels of sex steroids and gonadotropin-releasing hormone testing; physical exam; secondary sexual development; histrelin may be discontinued when the patient reaches the appropriate age for puberty

Additional Information Dose should be given at the same time each day; noncompliance or changing the dosage schedule may result in inadequate control

Dosage Forms 7-day kits of single use:
Injection: 120 μg/0.6 mL; 300 μg/0.6 mL; 600 μg/0.6 mL

Hi-Vegi-Lip® *see* Pancreatin *on page 430*

HMS Liquifilm® *see* Medrysone *on page 360*

HN$_2$ *see* Mechlorethamine Hydrochloride *on page 357*

Homatropine Hydrobromide (hoe ma' troe peen)

Brand Names AK-Homatropine®; Isopto® Homatropine

Therapeutic Category Anticholinergic Agent, Ophthalmic; Ophthalmic Agent, Mydriatic

Use Producing cycloplegia and mydriasis for refraction; treatment of acute inflammatory conditions of the uveal tract

Pregnancy Risk Factor C

Contraindications Hypersensitivity to homatropine or any component; narrow-angle glaucoma, acute hemorrhage

Precautions Use with caution in patients with hypertension, cardiac disease, or increased intraocular pressure

Adverse Reactions
Cardiovascular: Vascular congestion, edema
Central nervous system: Drowsiness
Dermatologic: Eczematoid dermatitis
Ocular: Follicular conjunctivitis, blurred vision, increased intraocular pressure, stinging, exudate

Mechanism of Action Blocks response of iris sphincter muscle and the accommodative muscle of the ciliary body to cholinergic stimulation resulting in dilation and loss of accommodation

Pharmacodynamics
Onset of action: Following ophthalmic instillation, the maximum mydriatic effect occurs in 10-30 minutes; the maximum cycloplegic effect occurs in 30-90 minutes
Duration:
Mydriasis: Persists for 6 hours to 4 days

(Continued)

Homatropine Hydrobromide *(Continued)*

Cycloplegia: 10-48 hours

Usual Dosage

Children:

Mydriasis and cycloplegia for refraction: 1 drop of 2% solution immediately before the procedure; repeat at 10-minute intervals as needed

Uveitis: 1 drop of 2% solution 2-3 times/day

Adults:

Mydriasis and cycloplegia for refraction: 1-2 drops of 2% solution or 1 drop of 5% solution before the procedure; repeat at 5- to 10-minute intervals as needed

Uveitis: 1-2 drops of either 2% or 5% 2-3 times/day up to every 3-4 hours as needed

Nursing Implications Finger pressure should be applied to lacrimal sac for 1-2 minutes after instillation to decrease risk of absorption and systemic reactions

Dosage Forms Solution, ophthalmic: 2% (1 mL, 5 mL, 15 mL); 5% (1 mL, 2 mL, 5 mL, 15 mL)

Horse Anti-human Thymocyte Gamma Globulin *see* Lymphocyte Immune Globulin *on page 350*

H.P. Acthar® Gel *see* Corticotropin *on page 153*

HuEPO *see* Epoetin Alfa *on page 222*

Human Growth Hormone (soe' ma trem)

Brand Names Humatrope®; Protropin®

Synonyms Somatrem; Somatropin

Therapeutic Category Growth Hormone

Use Long term treatment of growth failure from lack of adequate endogenous growth hormone secretion

Pregnancy Risk Factor B

Contraindications Closed epiphyses, known hypersensitivity to drug, benzyl alcohol (somatrem), or M-cresol or glycerin (somatropin); progression of any underlying intracranial lesion or actively growing intracranial tumor

Precautions Use with caution in patients with diabetes or family history of diabetes; somatrem contains benzyl alcohol, use with caution in neonates

Adverse Reactions

Central nervous system: Headache

Endocrine & metabolic: Reversible hypothyroidism (reported in pituitary derived growth hormone), mild hyperglycemia, glucosuria

Hematologic: Small risk for developing leukemia

Miscellaneous: Mild transient edema

Drug Interactions Stanozolol, corticosteroids

Stability Store in refrigerator; somatrem stable for 7 days after reconstitution; somatropin stable 14 days after reconstitution

Mechanism of Action Somatrem and somatropin are purified polypeptide hormones of recombinant DNA origin; somatrem contains the identical sequence of amino acids found in human growth hormone while somatropin's amino acid sequence is identical plus an additional amino acid, methionine; human growth hormone stimulates growth of linear bone, skeletal muscle, and organs; stimulates erythropoietin which increases red blood cell mass; exerts both insulin-like and diabetogenic effects

Pharmacokinetics Somatrem and somatropin have equivalent pharmacokinetic profiles

Absorption: I.M.: Well absorbed; maintains supraphysiologic levels for 18-20 hours

Metabolism: ~90% of dose is metabolized in the liver

Half-life: 15-50 minutes

Elimination: 0.1% of dose is excreted in urine unchanged

Usual Dosage Children: I.M., S.C.:

Somatrem: Up to 0.1 mg/kg (0.26 IU/kg) 3 times/week

Somatropin: Up to 0.06 mg/kg (0.15 IU/kg) 3 times/week

Note: Therapy should be discontinued when patient has reached satisfactory adult height, when epiphyses have fused, or when the patient ceases to respond

Administration Do not shake

Somatrem: Reconstitute each 5 mg vial with 1-5 mL bacteriostatic water for injection, USP (benzyl alcohol preserved) only; when using in newborns, reconstitute with preservative-free sterile water

Somatropin: Reconstitute each 5 mg vial with 1.5-5 mL diluent

Monitoring Parameters Growth curve, periodic thyroid function tests, bone age (annually), periodical urine testing for glucose, somatomedin C levels

Nursing Implications Do not shake vial when reconstituting; 1 mg = 2.6 units; a patient's booklet on mixing and administration is available; rotate injection site

Additional Information S.C. administration can cause local lipoatrophy or lipodystrophy and may enhance the development of neutralizing antibodies

Dosage Forms Injection:

Somatrem: 5 mg (~13 units)

Somatropin: 5 mg (~ 13 units)

References

Howrie DL, "Growth Hormone for the Treatment of Growth Failure in Children," *Clin Pharm*, 1987, 6(4):283-91.

Humate-P® *see* Antihemophilic Factor, Human *on page 55*

Humatrope® *see* Human Growth Hormone *on previous page*

Humibid® L.A. *see* Guaifenesin *on page 278*

Humibid® Sprinkle *see* Guaifenesin *on page 278*

Humulin® *see* Insulin Preparations *on page 311*

Hurricaine® *see* Benzocaine *on page 77*

Hyaluronidase (hye al yoor on' i dase)

Related Information

Extravasation Treatment *on page 640*

Brand Names Wydase®

Therapeutic Category Antidote, Extravasation

Use Increase the dispersion and absorption of other drugs; increase rate of absorption of parenteral fluids given by hypodermoclysis; treatment of I.V. extravasations

Pregnancy Risk Factor C

Contraindications Hypersensitivity to hyaluronidase or any component; do not inject in or around infected, inflamed, or cancerous areas

Warnings Drug infiltrates in which hyaluronidase is contraindicated are dopamine and alpha agonists

Precautions Hypersensitivity reactions may occur; a preliminary intradermal skin test should be performed utilizing 0.02 mL of a 150 units/mL solution

Adverse Reactions

Cardiovascular: Tachycardia, hypotension

Central nervous system: Dizziness, chills

Dermatologic: Urticaria, erythema

Gastrointestinal: Nausea, vomiting

Drug Interactions Salicylates, cortisone, ACTH, estrogens, antihistamines (↓ effectiveness of hyaluronidase)

Stability Reconstituted hyaluronidase solution is stable for 24 hours

Mechanism of Action Modifies the permeability of connective tissue through hydrolysis of hyaluronic acid, one of the chief ingredients of tissue cement which offers resistance to diffusion of liquids through tissues

Pharmacodynamics

Onset by the S.C. or I.D. routes for the treatment of extravasation: Immediate

Duration: 24-48 hours

Usual Dosage

Infants and Children: Management of I.V. extravasation: Reconstitute the 150 unit vial of lyophilized powder with 1 mL normal saline; take 0.1 mL of this solution and dilute with 0.9 mL normal saline to yield 15 units/mL; using a 25- or 26-gauge needle, five 0.2 mL injections are made subcutaneously or intradermally into the extravasation site at the leading edge, changing the needle after each injection

Adults: Absorption and dispersion of drugs: 150 units is added to the vehicle containing the drug

(Continued)

Hyaluronidase *(Continued)*

Hypodermoclysis: S.C.: 15 units is added to each 100 mL of I.V. fluid to be administered

Premature Infants and Neonates: Volume of a single clysis should not exceed 25 mL/kg and the rate of administration should not exceed 2 mL/minute

Children <3 years: Volume of a single clysis should not exceed 200 mL

Children ≥3 years and Adults: Rate and volume of administration should not exceed those used for I.V. infusion

Nursing Implications Administer hyaluronidase within the first few minutes to one hour after the extravasation is recognized

Dosage Forms

Injection, stabilized solution: 150 units/mL (1 mL, 10 mL)

Powder for injection, lyophilized: 150 units, 1500 units

References

Zenk KE, "Hyaluronidase: An Antidote for Intravenous Extravasations," *CSHP Voice*, 1981, 66-8.

Zenk KE, Dungy CI, and Greene GR, "Nafcillin Extravasation Injury: Use of Hyaluronidase as an Antidote," *Am J Dis Child*, 1981, 135(12):1113-4.

Hydeltrasol® *see* Prednisolone *on page 476*

Hydeltra-T.B.A.® *see* Prednisolone *on page 476*

Hydralazine Hydrochloride (hye dral' a zeen)

Brand Names Apresoline®

Therapeutic Category Antihypertensive; Vasodilator

Use Management of moderate to severe hypertension, congestive heart failure, hypertension secondary to pre-eclampsia/eclampsia; has also been used to treat primary pulmonary hypertension

Pregnancy Risk Factor C

Contraindications Hypersensitivity to hydralazine or any component, dissecting aortic aneurysm, mitral valve rheumatic heart disease, coronary artery disease

Warnings Monitor blood pressure closely with I.V. use; some formulations may contain tartrazines or sulfites

Precautions Discontinue hydralazine in patients who develop SLE-like syndrome or positive ANA. Use with caution in patients with severe renal disease or cerebral vascular accidents.

Adverse Reactions

Cardiovascular: Palpitations, flushing, tachycardia, edema, orthostatic hypotension (rarely)

Central nervous system: Malaise, peripheral neuritis, fever, headache, dizziness

Dermatologic: Rash

Gastrointestinal: Anorexia, nausea, vomiting, diarrhea

Musculoskeletal: Arthralgias, weakness

Miscellaneous: Positive ANA, positive LE cells

Drug Interactions MAO inhibitors → significant ↓ in blood pressure; indomethacin → ↓ hypotensive effects

Stability Changes color after contact with a metal filter; do not store intact ampuls in refrigerator

Mechanism of Action Direct vasodilation of arterioles (with little effect on veins) which results in decreased systemic resistance

Pharmacodynamics

Onset of action:

Oral: 20-30 minutes

I.V.: 5-20 minutes

Duration:

Oral: 2-4 hours

I.V.: 2-6 hours

Pharmacokinetics

Distribution: Crosses placenta; appears in breast milk

Protein-binding: 85% to 90%

Metabolism: Acetylated in liver

Bioavailability: 30% to 50%; large first pass effect orally

Half-life, adults: 2-8 hours; half-life varies with genetically determined acetylation rates

Elimination: 14% excreted unchanged in urine

Usual Dosage

Children:

Oral: Initial: 0.75-1 mg/kg/day in 2-4 divided doses, not to exceed 25 mg/dose; increase over 3-4 weeks to maximum of 7.5 mg/kg/day in 2-4 divided doses; maximum daily dose: 200 mg/day

I.M., I.V.: Initial: 0.1-0.2 mg/kg/dose (not to exceed 20 mg) every 4-6 hours as needed; up to 1.7-3.5 mg/kg/day divided in 4-6 doses

Adults:

Oral: Initial: 10 mg 4 times/day, ↑ by 10-25 mg/dose every 2-5 days to maximum of 300 mg/day

I.M., I.V.: Hypertension: Initial: 10-20 mg/dose every 4-6 hours as needed, may ↑ to 40 mg/dose

I.M., I.V.: Pre-eclampsia/eclampsia: 5 mg/dose then 5-10 mg every 20-30 minutes as needed

Dosing interval in renal impairment:

Cl_{cr} 10-50 mL/minute: Administer every 8 hours

Cl_{cr} <10 mL/minute: Administer every 8-16 hours in fast acetylators and every 12-24 hours in slow acetylators

Administration I.V.: Do not exceed rate of 0.2 mg/kg/minute; maximum concentration for I.V. use: 20 mg/mL

Monitoring Parameters Heart rate, blood pressure, ANA titer

Additional Information Slow acetylators, patients with ↓ renal function and patients receiving >200 mg/day (chronically) are at higher risk for SLE. Titrate dosage to patient's response. Usually administered with diuretic and a beta blocker to counteract hydralazine's side effects of sodium and water retention and reflex tachycardia.

Dosage Forms

Injection: 20 mg/mL (1 mL)

Tablet: 10 mg, 25 mg, 50 mg, 100 mg

Hydrate® *see* Dimenhydrinate *on page 193*

Hydrated Chloral *see* Chloral Hydrate *on page 122*

Hydrea® *see* Hydroxyurea *on page 297*

Hydrocet® *see* Hydrocodone and Acetaminophen *on next page*

Hydrochlorothiazide (hye droe klor oh thye' a zide)

Brand Names Diaqua®; Esidrix®; Ezide®; HydroDIURIL®; Hydro-T®; Oretic®

Synonyms HCTZ

Therapeutic Category Antihypertensive; Diuretic, Thiazide

Use Management of mild to moderate hypertension; treatment of edema in congestive heart failure and nephrotic syndrome

Pregnancy Risk Factor D

Contraindications Hypersensitivity to hydrochlorothiazide or any component; cross-sensitivity with other thiazides or sulfonamides

Precautions Use with caution in patients with severe renal disease (Cl_{cr} <10 mL/minute), impaired hepatic function

Adverse Reactions

Central nervous system: Drowsiness, paresthesias

Endocrine & metabolic: Hypokalemia, hyperglycemia, hypochloremic metabolic alkalosis, hyperlipidemia, hyperuricemia

Gastrointestinal: Nausea, vomiting, anorexia

Hematologic: Aplastic anemia, hemolytic anemia, leukopenia, agranulocytosis, thrombocytopenia

Hepatic: Hepatitis, intrahepatic cholestasis

Musculoskeletal: Muscle weakness

Renal & genitourinary: Polyuria, prerenal azotemia

Drug Interactions Digitalis glycosides, lithium, antidiabetic agents, hypotensive agents, probenecid, additive potassium losses with steroids and amphotericin B; NSAIDs ↓ natriuretic response; ↑ NSAIDs nephrotoxicity

Mechanism of Action Inhibits sodium reabsorption in the distal tubules causing increased excretion of sodium and water as well as potassium, hydrogen, magnesium, phosphate, calcium, and bicarbonate ions

Pharmacodynamics

Onset of diuretic action: Oral: Within 2 hours

Peak effects: Within 3-6 hours

(Continued)

Hydrochlorothiazide *(Continued)*

Duration: 6-12 hours

Pharmacokinetics

Absorption: Oral: ~60% to 80%

Elimination: Excreted unchanged in urine

Usual Dosage Oral:

Children (daily dosages should be decreased if used with other antihypertensives):

<6 months: 2-3.3 mg/kg/day in 2 divided doses

>6 months: 2 mg/kg/day in 2 divided doses

Adults: 25-100 mg/day in 1-2 doses; maximum: 200 mg/day

Monitoring Parameters Serum electrolytes, BUN, creatinine, blood pressure

Dosage Forms Tablet: 25 mg, 50 mg, 100 mg

Hydrocil® [OTC] *see* Psyllium *on page 498*

Hydrocodone and Acetaminophen (hye droe koe' done)

Related Information

Narcotic Analgesics Comparison Chart *on page 721-722*

Brand Names Anexia®; Bancap® HC; Dolacet®; DuoCet™; Hydrocet®; Hydrogesic®; Hy-Phen®; Lorcet®; Lortab®; Margesic H®; Norcet®; Stagesic®; T-Gesic®; Vicodin®; Zydone®

Synonyms Acetaminophen and Hydrocodone

Therapeutic Category Analgesic, Narcotic; Antitussive

Use Relief of moderate to severe pain; antitussive (hydrocodone)

Restrictions C-III

Pregnancy Risk Factor C

Contraindications CNS depression, hypersensitivity to hydrocodone, acetaminophen or any component; severe respiratory depression

Warnings Some tablets contain sulfites which may cause allergic reactions

Precautions Use with caution in patients with hypersensitivity reactions to other phenanthrene derivative opioid agonists (morphine, codeine, hydromorphone, oxycodone, oxymorphone, levorphanol)

Adverse Reactions

Cardiovascular: Hypotension, bradycardia, peripheral vasodilation, increased intracranial pressure

Central nervous system: CNS depression, drowsiness, dizziness, sedation

Endocrine & metabolic: Antidiuretic hormone release

Gastrointestinal: Nausea, vomiting, constipation

Hepatic: Biliary tract spasm

Ocular: Miosis

Renal & genitourinary: Urinary tract spasm

Respiratory: Respiratory depression

Sensitivity reactions: Histamine release

Miscellaneous: Physical and psychological dependence with prolonged use

Drug Interactions CNS depressants, phenothiazines, tricyclic antidepressants may potentiate the adverse effects of hydrocodone

Mechanism of Action Inhibits the synthesis of prostaglandins in the central nervous system and peripherally blocks pain impulse generation; produces antipyresis from inhibition of hypothalamic heat regulating center

Pharmacodynamics Narcotic analgesia: Oral:

Onset of action: Within 10-20 minutes

Duration: 3-6 hours

Usual Dosage Doses should be titrated to appropriate analgesic effect

Antitussive: Oral (hydrocodone):

Children: 0.6 mg/kg/day or 20 mg/m^2/day divided in 3-4 doses/day

<2 years: Do not exceed 1.25 mg/single dose

2-12 years: Do not exceed 5 mg/single dose

>12 years: Do not exceed 10 mg/single dose

Analgesic: Adults: 1-2 tablets or capsules every 4-6 hours as needed

Monitoring Parameters Pain relief, respiratory rate, blood pressure

Dosage Forms

Capsule: Hydrocodone bitartrate 5 mg and acetaminophen 500 mg

Solution, oral (tropical fruit punch flavor): Hydrocodone bitartrate 2.5 mg and acetaminophen 120 mg per 5 mL (480 mL)

Tablet: Hydrocodone bitartrate 2.5 mg and acetaminophen 500 mg; hydrocodone bitartrate 5 mg and acetaminophen 500 mg; hydrocodone bitartrate 7.5 mg and acetaminophen 500 mg

Hydrocortisone (hye droe kor' ti sone)

Related Information

Medications Compatible With PN Solutions *on page 649-650*
Systemic Corticosteroids Comparison Chart *on page 727*
Topical Steroids Comparison Chart *on page 728*

Brand Names Aeroseb-HC®; A-hydroCort®; CaldeCORT®; Cetacort®; Cortaid® [OTC]; Cort-Dome®; Cortef®; Cortifoam®; Dermolate® [OTC]; Hydrocortone®; Hydro-Tex®; Hytone®; Nutracort®; Orabase® HCA; Penecort®; Proctocort™; Solu-Cortef®; Synacort®; U-Cort™; Westcort®

Synonyms Compound F; Cortisol; Hydrocortisone Acetate; Hydrocortisone Cypionate; Hydrocortisone Sodium Phosphate; Hydrocortisone Sodium Succinate

Therapeutic Category Anti-inflammatory Agent; Corticosteroid, Rectal; Corticosteroid, Systemic; Corticosteroid, Topical; Glucocorticoid

Use Management of adrenocortical insufficiency; relief of inflammation of corticosteroid-responsive dermatoses; adjunctive treatment of ulcerative colitis

Pregnancy Risk Factor C

Contraindications Serious infections, except septic shock or tuberculous meningitis; known hypersensitivity to hydrocortisone; viral, fungal, or tubercular skin lesions

Warnings Acute adrenal insufficiency may occur with abrupt withdrawal after long-term therapy or with stress; infants and small children may be more susceptible to adrenal axis suppression from topical therapy

Precautions Use with caution in patients with hyperthyroidism, cirrhosis, nonspecific ulcerative colitis, hypertension, osteoporosis, thromboembolic tendencies, CHF, convulsive disorders, myasthenia gravis, thrombophlebitis, peptic ulcer, diabetes

Adverse Reactions

Cardiovascular: Hypertension, edema
Central nervous system: Euphoria, insomnia, headache
Dermatologic: Acne, dermatitis, skin atrophy
Endocrine & metabolic: Hypokalemia, hyperglycemia, Cushing's syndrome
Gastrointestinal: Peptic ulcer
Ocular: Cataracts
Miscellaneous: Immunosuppression

Drug Interactions Live virus vaccines

Mechanism of Action Decreases inflammation by suppression of migration of polymorphonuclear leukocytes and reversal of increased capillary permeability

Pharmacodynamics Anti-inflammatory effects:

Peak effect:
- Oral: 12-24 hours
- I.V.: 4-6 hours

Duration: 8-12 hours

Pharmacokinetics

Absorption: Rapid by all routes, except rectally
Metabolism: Metabolized in the liver
Elimination: Excreted renally, mainly as 17-hydroxysteroids and 17-ketosteroids

Usual Dosage

Acute adrenal insufficiency:
- Infants and young Children: I.M., I.V.: 1-2 mg/kg/dose bolus, then 25-150 mg/day in divided doses
- Older Children: I.M., I.V.: 1-2 mg/kg bolus then 150-250 mg/day in divided doses
- Adults: I.M., I.V., S.C.: 15-240 mg every 12 hours

Physiologic replacement: Children:
- Oral: 0.5-0.75 mg/kg/day or 20-25 mg/m^2/day divided every 8 hours
- I.M.: 0.25-0.35 mg/kg/day or 12-15 mg/m^2/day once daily

Anti-inflammatory or immunosuppressive:
- Infants and Children:
  - Oral: 2.5-10 mg/kg/day or 75-300 mg/m^2/day divided every 6-8 hours

(Continued)

Hydrocortisone *(Continued)*

I.M., I.V.: 1-5 mg/kg/day or 30-150 mg/m²/day divided every 12-24 hours
Adults: I.M., I.V., S.C.: 15-240 mg every 12 hours

Congenital adrenal hyperplasia: Oral: Initial: 30-36 mg/m²/day with ⅓ of dose every morning and ⅔ every evening or ¼ every morning and midday and ½ every evening; maintenance: 20-25 mg/m²/day in divided doses

Status asthmaticus: Children: Loading: 1-2 mg/kg/dose every 6 hours for 24 hours then maintenance 0.5-1 mg/kg/dose every 6 hours

Shock: I.M., I.V.:
Children: Initial: 50 mg/kg (succinate), then repeated in 4 hours and/or every 24 hours if needed
Adults: 500 mg to 2 g every 2-6 hours (succinate)

Children and Adults:
Rectal: Apply 1 application 1-2 times/day for 2-3 weeks
Topical: Apply 3-4 times/day

Administration
I.V. bolus: Dilute to 50 mg/mL and give over 3-5 minutes
I.V. intermittent infusion: Dilute to 1 mg/mL and give over 20-30 minutes

Monitoring Parameters Blood pressure, weight, serum glucose and electrolytes

Reference Range Hydrocortisone (endogenous levels) 4-30 μg/mL

Dosage Forms
Aerosol, topical: 0.53 mg/1 sec spray (58 g)
Cream, as acetate: 0.5% (15 g, 30 g); 1% (30 g, 120 g)
Cream, as butyrate: 0.1% (15 g, 45 g, 60 g)
Cream:
Rectal: 1% (30 g with applicator)
Topical: 0.25% (30 g); 0.5% (15 g, 30 g, 120 g, 454 g); 1% (15 g, 20 g, 30 g, 120 g, 454 g); 2.5% (20 g, 30 g, 60 g, 454 g)
Topical, as valerate: 0.2% (15 g, 45 g, 60 g)
Enema: 100 mg/60 mL each unit (7 units/box)
Foam, rectal, as acetate: 10% (20 g)
Injection, as acetate: 25 mg/mL (3 mL, 10 mL); 50 mg/mL (5 mL, 10 mL)
Injection, as sodium phosphate: 50 mg/mL (2 mL, 10 mL)
Injection, as succinate: 100 mg, 250 mg, 500 mg
Injection, as sodium succinate: 100 mg, 250 mg, 500 mg, 1000 mg
Lotion: 0.25% (30 mL, 120 mL); 0.5% (30 mL, 60 mL, 120 mL); 1% (30 mL, 60 mL, 120 mL); 2.5% (60 mL, 120 mL)
Lotion, as acetate: 0.5% (30 mL)
Ointment:
Topical: 0.5% (30 g)
Topical, as acetate: 0.5% (15 g); 1% (30 g)
Topical, as butyrate: 0.1% (15 g, 45 g)
Topical, as valerate: 0.2% (15 g, 45 g, 60 g)
Paste, oral topical, as acetate: 0.5%
Suppository, as acetate: 25 mg
Suspension, as cypionate, oral: 10 mg/5 mL (120 mL)
Tablet: 5 mg, 10 mg, 20 mg

Hydrocortisone Acetate *see* Hydrocortisone *on previous page*

Hydrocortisone Cypionate *see* Hydrocortisone *on previous page*

Hydrocortisone Sodium Phosphate *see* Hydrocortisone *on previous page*

Hydrocortisone Sodium Succinate *see* Hydrocortisone *on previous page*

Hydrocortone® *see* Hydrocortisone *on previous page*

HydroDIURIL® *see* Hydrochlorothiazide *on page 291*

Hydrogen Dioxide *see* Hydrogen Peroxide *on this page*

Hydrogen Peroxide (hye' droe jen per ox' ide)

Brand Names Peroxyl®

Synonyms H_2O_2; Hydrogen Dioxide; Peroxide

Therapeutic Category Antibacterial, Otic; Antibacterial, Topical; Antibiotic, Oral Rinse

Use Cleanse wounds, suppurating ulcers, and local infections; used in the treatment of inflammatory conditions of the external auditory canal and as a mouthwash or gargle

Contraindications Should not be used in abscesses

Precautions Repeat use as a mouthwash or gargle may produce irritation of the buccal mucous membrane or "hairy tongue"; bandages should not be applied too quickly after its use

Adverse Reactions

Dermatologic: Bleaching effect on hair

Gastrointestinal: Rupture of the colon, proctitis, ulcerative colitis, gas embolism

Local: Irritation of the buccal mucous membrane

Stability Protect from light and heat

Mechanism of Action Antiseptic oxidant that slowly releases oxygen and water upon contact with serum or tissue catalase

Pharmacodynamics Duration of action: Only while bubbling action occurs

Usual Dosage Children and Adults:

Mouthwash or gargle: Dilute the 3% solution with an equal volume of water; swish around in the mouth over the affected area for at least one minute and then expel; use up to 4 times/day (after meals and at bedtime)

Topical: 1.5% to 3% solution for cleansing wounds

Dosage Forms

Gel, oral: 1.5% (15 g)

Solution:

Concentrate: 30.5% (480 mL)

Topical: 3% (120 mL, 480 mL)

Hydrogesic® *see* Hydrocodone and Acetaminophen *on page 292*

Hydromorphone Hydrochloride (hye droe mor' fone)

Related Information

Narcotic Analgesics Comparison Chart *on page 721-722*

Overdose and Toxicology Information *on page 696-700*

Brand Names Dilaudid®; Dilaudid® Cough Syrup

Therapeutic Category Analgesic, Narcotic; Antitussive

Use Management of moderate to severe pain; antitussive at lower doses

Restrictions C-II

Pregnancy Risk Factor C

Contraindications Hypersensitivity to hydromorphone or any component

Warnings Injection contains benzyl alcohol

Precautions Syrup contains tartrazine which may cause allergic reactions; use with caution in patients with hypersensitivity reactions to other phenanthrene derivative opioid agonists (morphine, hydrocodone, levorphanol, oxycodone, oxymorphone, codeine) or significant respiratory disease

Adverse Reactions

Cardiovascular: Palpitations, hypotension, bradycardia, peripheral vasodilation

Central nervous system: CNS depression, increased intracranial pressure, drowsiness, dizziness, sedation

Dermatologic: Pruritus

Endocrine & metabolic: Antidiuretic hormone release

Gastrointestinal: Nausea, vomiting, constipation

Hepatic: Biliary tract spasm

Ocular: Miosis

Renal & genitourinary: Urinary tract spasm

Respiratory: Respiratory depression

Sensitivity reactions: Histamine release

Miscellaneous: Physical and psychological dependence

Drug Interactions CNS depressants, phenothiazines, tricyclic antidepressants may potentiate the adverse effects of hydromorphone

Mechanism of Action Binds to opiate receptors in the CNS, causing inhibition of ascending pain pathways, altering the perception of and response to pain; causes cough supression by direct central action in the medulla; produces generalized CNS depression

(Continued)

Hydromorphone Hydrochloride *(Continued)*

Pharmacodynamics Analgesic effects: Oral:
- Onset of action: Within 15-30 minutes
- Peak effect: Within 30-90 minutes
- Duration: 4-5 hours

Pharmacokinetics
- Metabolism: Metabolized primarily in the liver
- Bioavailability: 62%
- Half-life: 1-3 hours
- Elimination: Excreted in the urine, principally as glucuronide conjugates

Usual Dosage
- Antitussive: Oral:
  - Children 6-12 years: 0.5 mg every 3-4 hours as needed
  - Children >12 years and Adults: 1 mg every 3-4 hours as needed
- Pain (doses should be titrated to appropriate analgesic effects); when changing routes of administration, note that oral doses are less than half as effective as parenteral doses (may be only 20% as effective):
  - Young children:
    - Oral: 0.03-0.08 mg/kg/dose every 4-6 hours as needed; maximum: 5 mg/dose
    - I.V.: 0.015 mg/kg/dose every 4-6 hours as needed
  - Older Children and Adults: Oral, I.M., I.V., S.C.: 1-4 mg/dose every 4-6 hours as needed; usual adult dose: 2 mg/dose

Additional Information Equianalgesic doses: Morphine 10 mg I.M. = hydromorphone 1.5 mg I.M.

Dosage Forms
- Injection: 1 mg/mL (1 mL); 2 mg/mL (1 mL, 20 mL); 3 mg/mL (1 mL); 4 mg/mL (1 mL); 10 mg/mL (1 mL, 2 mL, 5 mL)
- Suppository, rectal: 3 mg
- Syrup: Hydromorphone hydrochloride 1 mg and guaifenesin 100 mg/5 mL (450 mL)
- Tablet: 1 mg, 2 mg, 3 mg, 4 mg

Hydro-T® *see* Hydrochlorothiazide *on page 291*

Hydro-Tex® *see* Hydrocortisone *on page 293*

Hydroxacen® *see* Hydroxyzine *on page 298*

Hydroxychloroquine Sulfate (hye drox ee klor' oh kwin)

Brand Names Plaquenil® Sulfate

Therapeutic Category Antimalarial Agent

Use Suppress and treat acute attacks of malaria; treatment of systemic lupus erythematosus and rheumatoid arthritis

Pregnancy Risk Factor C

Contraindications Retinal or visual field changes; hypersensitivity to hydroxychloroquine, 4-aminoquinoline derivatives, or any component; patients with porphyria or psoriasis

Warnings Long-term use in children is **not** recommended

Precautions Use with caution in patients with hepatic disease and G-6-PD deficiency

Adverse Reactions
- Central nervous system: Insomnia, nervousness, nightmares, psychosis, ataxia, headache, confusion, agitation
- Dermatologic: Lichenoid dermatitis, bleaching of the hair, pruritus
- Gastrointestinal: GI irritation, anorexia, nausea, vomiting
- Hematologic: Bone marrow depression
- Musculoskeletal: Muscle weakness
- Ocular: Visual field defects, blindness, retinitis

Drug Interactions ↑ digoxin serum levels

Mechanism of Action Interferes with digestive vacuole function within sensitive malarial parasites by increasing the pH and interfering with lysosomal degradation of hemoglobin; inhibits locomotion of neutrophils and chemotaxis of eosinophils; impairs complement-dependent antigen-antibody reactions

Pharmacokinetics
- Metabolism: Metabolized in the liver

Elimination: Metabolites and unchanged drug slowly excreted in the urine

Usual Dosage Oral:

Children:

Chemoprophylaxis of malaria: 5 mg/kg (base) once weekly; should not exceed the recommended adult dose; begin 1-2 weeks before exposure; continue for 6-8 weeks after leaving endemic area

Acute attack: 10 mg/kg (base) initial dose; followed by 5 mg/kg (base) in 6 hours on day 1; 5 mg/kg (base) as a single dose on day 2 and on day 3

JRA or SLE: 3-5 mg/kg/day divided 1-2 times/day to a maximum of 400 mg/day; not to exceed 7 mg/kg/day

Adults:

Chemoprophylaxis of malaria: 2 tablets weekly on same day each week; begin 1-2 weeks before exposure; continue for 6-8 weeks after leaving endemic area

Acute attack: 4 tablets first dose day 1; 2 tablets in 6 hours day 1; 2 tablets as a single dose day 2; and 2 tablets as a single dose on day 3

Rheumatoid arthritis: 400-600 mg/day once daily to start, taken with food or milk; increase dose until optimum response level is reached; usually after 4-12 weeks dose should be reduced by 50% and a maintenance dose of 200-400 mg/day given once daily

Lupus erythematosus: 400 mg every day or twice daily for several weeks depending on response; 200-400 mg/day for prolonged maintenance therapy

Monitoring Parameters Ophthalmologic examination, CBC

Patient Information Give with food or milk; patient should wear sunglasses in bright sunlight

Dosage Forms Tablet: 200 mg [155 mg base]

References

Emery H, "Clinical Aspects of Systemic Lupus Erythematosus in Childhood," *Pediatr Clin North Am*, 1986, 33(5):1177-90.

Hydroxydaunomycin Hydrochloride *see* Doxorubicin Hydrochloride *on page 208*

Hydroxyurea (hye drox' ee yoo ree ah)

Brand Names Hydrea®

Therapeutic Category Antineoplastic Agent

Use Treatment of malignant neoplasms including melanoma, granulocytic leukemia, and ovarian carcinomas; also used with radiation in treatment of tumors of the head and neck

Pregnancy Risk Factor D

Contraindications Severe anemia, severe bone marrow depression; WBC $<2500/mm^3$ or platelet count $<100,000/mm^3$; hypersensitivity to hydroxyurea

Warnings The US Food and Drug Administration (FDA) currently recommends that procedures for proper handling and disposal of antineoplastic agents be considered

Precautions Use with caution in patients with renal impairment

Adverse Reactions

Central nervous system: Dizziness, disorientation, hallucinations, seizures, headache

Dermatologic: Maculopapular rash, facial erythema

Endocrine & metabolic: Hyperuricemia

Gastrointestinal: Nausea, vomiting, diarrhea, constipation, anorexia, stomatitis

Hematologic: Myelosuppression, megaloblastic anemia

Hepatic: Elevation of hepatic enzymes

Renal & genitourinary: Dysuria, renal tubular function impairment

Drug Interactions Fluorouracil

Mechanism of Action Interferes with synthesis of DNA, during the S phase of cell division, without interfering with RNA synthesis; inhibits ribonucleoside diphosphate reductase preventing conversion of ribonucleotides to deoxyribonucleotides

Pharmacokinetics

Absorption: Readily absorbed from the GI tract

Distribution: Readily crosses the blood-brain barrier, excreted in breast milk

(Continued)

Hydroxyurea *(Continued)*

Metabolism: Metabolized in the liver with renal excretion of urea (metabolite) and respiratory excretion of CO_2 (metabolic end product)
Half-life: 3-4 hours
Peak serum levels: Within 2 hours
Elimination: 50% of the drug is excreted unchanged in urine

Usual Dosage Oral (refer to individual protocols):

Children: No FDA approved dosage regimens have been established. Dosages of 1500-3000 mg/m^2 as a single dose in combination with other agents every 4-6 weeks have been used in the treatment of pediatric astrocytoma, medulloblastoma and primitive neuroectodermal tumors

Adults:
- Solid tumors:
  - Intermittent therapy: 80 mg/kg as a single dose every third day
  - Continuous therapy: 20-30 mg/kg/day given as a single dose/day
- Concomitant therapy with irradiation: 80 mg/kg as a single dose every third day starting at least 7 days before initiation of irradiation
- Resistant chronic myelocytic leukemia: 20-30 mg/kg/day divided daily

Dosing adjustment in renal impairment: Dose should be reduced 50% in patients with a GFR <10 mL/minute

Monitoring Parameters CBC with differential and platelet count, hemoglobin, renal function and liver function tests, serum uric acid

Patient Information Contents of capsule may be emptied into a glass of water if taken immediately; inform the physician if you develop fever, sore throat, bruising, or bleeding

Additional Information Myelosuppressive effects:
WBC: Moderate
Platelets: Moderate
Onset (days): 7
Nadir (days): 10
Recovery (days): 21

Dosage Forms Capsule: 500 mg

References

Bennett WM, Aronoff GR, Morrison G, et al, "Drug Prescribing in Renal Failure: Dosing Guidelines for Adults," *Am J Kidney Dis*, 1983, 3(3):155-93.
Geyer JR, Pendergrass TW, Milstein JM, et al, "Eight Drugs in One Day Chemotherapy in Children With Brain Tumors: A Critical Toxicity Appraisal," *J Clin Oncol*, 1988, 6(6):996-1000.

Hydroxyzine (hye drox' i zeen)

Related Information

Compatibility of Medications Mixed in a Syringe *on page 717*

Brand Names Anxanil®; Atarax®; E-Vista®; Hydroxacen®; Quiess®; Rezine®; Vistaril®; Vistazine®

Therapeutic Category Antianxiety Agent; Antiemetic; Antihistamine; Sedative

Use Treatment of anxiety; preoperative sedative; an antipruritic; an antiemetic

Pregnancy Risk Factor C

Contraindications Hypersensitivity to hydroxyzine or any component

Warnings Subcutaneous, intra-arterial and I.V. administration **not** recommended since thrombosis and digital gangrene can occur; extravasation can result in sterile abscess and marked tissue induration

Precautions Injection may contain benzyl alcohol

Adverse Reactions
Cardiovascular: Hypotension
Central nervous system: Drowsiness, dizziness, headache, ataxia, weakness
Gastrointestinal: Dry mouth
Local: Pain at injection site

Drug Interactions Hydroxyzine may potentiate other CNS depressants or anticholinergics, and can antagonize the vasopressor effects of epinephrine

Stability Protect from light

Mechanism of Action Competes with histamine for H_1-receptor sites on effector cells in the gastrointestinal tract, blood vessels, and respiratory tract

Pharmacodynamics
Onset of effects: Within 15-30 minutes
Duration: 4-6 hours

Usual Dosage
Children:
Oral: 2 mg/kg/day divided every 6-8 hours
I.M.: 0.5-1 mg/kg/dose every 4-6 hours as needed

Adults:
Antiemetic: I.M.: 25-100 mg/dose every 4-6 hours as needed
Anxiety: Oral: 25-100 mg 4 times/day; maximum dose: 600 mg/day
Preoperative sedation:
Oral: 50-100 mg
I.M.: 25-100 mg
Management of pruritus: Oral: 25 mg 3-4 times/day

Administration For I.M. administration in children, injections should be made into the midlateral muscles of the thigh; hydroxyzine has been given slowly I.V. to oncology patients via central venous lines without problems

Dosage Forms
Capsule, as pamoate: 25 mg, 50 mg, 100 mg
Injection, as hydrochloride: 25 mg/mL (1 mL, 2 mL, 10 mL); 50 mg/mL (1 mL, 2 mL, 10 mL)
Suspension, oral, as pamoate: 25 mg/5 mL (120 mL, 480 mL)
Syrup, as hydrochloride: 10 mg/5 mL (120 mL, 480 mL, 4000 mL)
Tablet, as hydrochloride: 10 mg, 25 mg, 50 mg, 100 mg

Hyoscine Hydrobromide *see* Scopolamine *on page 519*

Hyoscyamine, Atropine, Scopolamine and Phenobarbital

Brand Names Barophen®; Donnatal®; Hyosophen®; Kinesed®; Relaxadon®; Spasmolin; Spasquid®

Therapeutic Category Anticholinergic Agent; Antispasmodic Agent, Gastrointestinal

Use As an adjunct in treatment of peptic ulcer disease, irritable bowel, spastic colitis, spastic bladder, and renal colic

Pregnancy Risk Factor C

Contraindications Hypersensitivity to hyoscyamine, atropine, scopolamine, phenobarbital, or any component; narrow-angle glaucoma, tachycardia, GI and GU obstruction, myasthenia gravis

Warnings Swallow extended release tablets whole, do not crush or chew

Precautions Use with caution in patients with hepatic or renal disease, hyperthyroidism, cardiovascular disease, hypertension, prostatic hypertrophy, autonomic neuropathy. Observe caution while driving or performing other tasks requiring alertness, as may cause drowsiness, dizziness, or blurred vision.

Adverse Reactions
Cardiovascular: Tachycardia
Central nervous system: Headache, drowsiness
Gastrointestinal: Dry mouth, nausea, vomiting, constipation
Ocular: Blurred vision
Renal & genitourinary: Urinary retention

Drug Interactions CNS depressants, coumarin anticoagulants, amantadine, antihistamines, phenothiazines, antidiarrheal suspensions, corticosteroids, digitalis, griseofulvin, tetracyclines, anticonvulsants, MAO inhibitors, tricyclic antidepressants

Pharmacokinetics Absorption: Well absorbed from the GI tract

Usual Dosage Oral:
Children 2-12 years: Kinesed® dose: 0.5-1 tablet 3-4 times/day

Children: Donnatal®: 0.1 mL/kg/dose every 4 hours; maximum dose: 5 mL **or** see table for alternative.

Adults:
Kinesed®: 1-2 tablets 3-4 times/day
Donnatal®: 1-2 tablets 3-4 times/day **or** 5-10 mL 3-4 times/day **or** 1 sustained release tablet every 12 hours

(Continued)

Hyoscyamine, Atropine, Scopolamine and Phenobarbital *(Continued)*

Weight (kg)	Dose (mL)	
	q4h	q6h
4.5	0.5	0.75
10	1	1.5
14	1.5	2
23	2.5	3.8
34	3.8	5
≥45	5	7.5

Patient Information Maintain good oral hygiene habits, because lack of saliva may increase chance of cavities. Notify physician if skin rash, flushing or eye pain occurs; or if difficulty in urinating, constipation or sensitivity to light becomes severe or persists. Do not attempt tasks requiring mental alertness or physical coordination until you know the effects of the drug.

Dosage Forms

Elixir: Hyoscyamine sulfate 0.1037 mg, atropine sulfate 0.0194 mg, scopolamine hydrobromide 0.0065 mg, and phenobarbital 16.2 mg per 5 mL (120 mL, 480 mL, 4000 mL)

Tablet: Hyoscyamine sulfate 0.1037 mg, atropine sulfate 0.0194 mg, scopolamine hydrobromide 0.0065 mg, and phenobarbital 16.2 mg

Tablet:

Chewable: Hyoscyamine hydrobromide 0.12 mg, atropine sulfate 0.12 mg, scopolamine hydrobromide 0.007 mg, and phenobarbital 16 mg

Long acting: Hyoscyamine sulfate 0.3111 mg, atropine sulfate 0.0582 mg, scopolamine hydrobromide 0.0195 mg, and phenobarbital 48.6 mg

Hyosophen® *see* Hyoscyamine, Atropine, Scopolamine and Phenobarbital *on previous page*

Hyperstat® I.V. *see* Diazoxide *on page 184*

Hy-Phen® *see* Hydrocodone and Acetaminophen *on page 292*

HypRho®-D *see* Rh_o(D) Immune Globulin *on page 510*

HypRho®-D Mini-Dose *see* Rh_o(D) Immune Globulin *on page 510*

Hytakerol® *see* Dihydrotachysterol *on page 192*

Hytone® *see* Hydrocortisone *on page 293*

Hytuss-2X® [OTC] *see* Guaifenesin *on page 278*

Ibenzmethyzin *see* Procarbazine Hydrochloride *on page 483*

Ibidomide Hydrochloride *see* Labetalol Hydrochloride *on page 331*

Ibuprin® [OTC] *see* Ibuprofen *on this page*

Ibuprofen (eye byoo proe' fen)

Related Information

Overdose and Toxicology Information *on page 696-700*

Brand Names Advil® [OTC]; Genpril® [OTC]; Haltran® [OTC]; Ibuprin® [OTC]; Ibu-Tab®; Medipren® [OTC]; Menadol® [OTC]; Midol® 200 [OTC]; Motrin®; Motrin® IB [OTC]; Nuprin® [OTC]; Pamprin IB® [OTC]; Pedia-Profen™; Rufen®; Saleto-200® [OTC]; Saleto-400®; Trendar® [OTC]

Synonyms *p*-Isobutylhydratropic Acid

Therapeutic Category Analgesic, Non-Narcotic; Anti-inflammatory Agent; Antipyretic; Nonsteroidal Anti-Inflammatory Agent (NSAID), Oral

Use Inflammatory diseases and rheumatoid disorders including juvenile rheumatoid arthritis; mild to moderate pain; fever; dysmenorrhea; gout

Pregnancy Risk Factor B (D if used in the 3rd trimester)

Contraindications Hypersensitivity to ibuprofen, any component, aspirin or other nonsteroidal anti-inflammatory drugs (NSAIDs)

Precautions Use with caution in patients with congestive heart failure, hypertension, ↓ renal or hepatic function, history of GI disease (bleeding or ulcers), or those receiving anticoagulants

Adverse Reactions

Cardiovascular: Edema

Central nervous system: Dizziness, drowsiness, fatigue, headache

Dermatologic: Rash, urticaria

Gastrointestinal: Dyspepsia, heartburn, nausea, vomiting, abdominal pain, peptic ulcer, GI bleed, GI perforation

Hematologic: Neutropenia, anemia, agranulocytosis, inhibition of platelet aggregation

Hepatic: Hepatitis

Ocular: Vision changes

Otic: Tinnitus

Renal & genitourinary: Acute renal failure

Drug Interactions May ↑ digoxin, methotrexate and lithium serum concentrations; aspirin may ↓ ibuprofen serum concentrations; other nonsteroidal anti-inflammatories may ↑ adverse GI effects

Mechanism of Action Inhibits prostaglandin synthesis by decreasing the activity of the enzyme, cyclo-oxygenase, which results in decreased formation of prostaglandin precursors

Usual Dosage Oral:

Children:

Antipyretic: 6 months to 12 years: Temperature <102.5°F (39°C): 5 mg/kg/dose; temperature >102.5°F: 10 mg/kg/dose given every 6-8 hours; maximum daily dose: 40 mg/kg/day

Juvenile rheumatoid arthritis: 30-50 mg/kg/day in 4 divided doses; start at lower end of dosing range and titrate; maximum: 2.4 g/day

Analgesic: 4-10 mg/kg/dose every 6-8 hours

Adults:

Inflammatory disease: 400-800 mg/dose 3-4 times/day; maximum dose: 3.2 g/day

Pain/fever/dysmenorrhea: 200-400 mg/dose every 4-6 hours; maximum daily dose: 1.2 g

Monitoring Parameters CBC, occult blood loss, liver enzymes; urine output, serum BUN, and creatinine in patients receiving diuretics, those with ↓ renal function, or in patients on chronic therapy; patients receiving long term therapy for JRA should receive periodic ophthalmological exams

Reference Range Plasma concentrations >200 μg/mL may be associated with severe toxicity

Nursing Implications Administer with food or milk to ↓ GI adverse effects

Additional Information Each 5 mL of suspension contains 2.5 g of sucrose; nystagmus, dizziness, hypotension, apnea and coma have been reported with overdose

Dosage Forms

Suspension, oral: 100 mg/5 mL (120 mL, 480 mL)

Tablet: 200 mg, 300 mg, 400 mg, 600 mg, 800 mg

References

Berde C, Ablin A, Glazer J, et al, "American Academy of Pediatrics Report of the Subcommittee on Disease-Related Pain in Childhood Cancer," *Pediatrics*, 1990, 86(5 Pt 2):818-25.

Brewer EJ, "Nonsteroidal Anti-inflammatory Agents," *Arthritis Rheum*, 1977, 20(2):513-25.

Ibu-Tab® *see* Ibuprofen *on previous page*

Idamycin® *see* Idarubicin Hydrochloride *on this page*

Idarubicin Hydrochloride (eye da rue' bi sin)

Brand Names Idamycin®

Synonyms 4-Demethoxydaunorubicin; 4-DMDR; IDR

Therapeutic Category Antineoplastic Agent

Use Used in combination with other antineoplastic agents for treatment of acute myeloid leukemia (AML) in adults and acute lymphocytic leukemia (ALL) in children

Pregnancy Risk Factor D

Contraindications Hypersensitivity to idarubicin or any component; pa-

(Continued)

Idarubicin Hydrochloride *(Continued)*

tients with pre-existing bone marrow suppression unless the benefit warrants the risk; severe congestive heart failure, cardiomyopathy

Warnings The US Food and Drug Administration (FDA) currently recommends that procedures for proper handling and disposal of antineoplastic agents be considered; I.V. use only, severe local tissue necrosis will result if extravasation occurs; pre-existing heart disease and previous therapy with anthracyclines at high cumulative doses increase risk of idarubicin-induced cardiac toxicity (manifested by potentially fatal congestive heart failure, life-threatening arrhythmias, or cardiomyopathies); the maximum lifetime anthracycline dose for idarubicin is approximately 137.5 mg/m^2; severe myelosuppression occurs in all patients given a therapeutic dose and is the dose-limiting adverse effect associated with idarubicin

Precautions Reduce dose in patients with impaired hepatic or renal function

Adverse Reactions

Cardiovascular: Arrhythmias, EKG changes, cardiomyopathy, congestive heart failure

Dermatologic: Alopecia; rash, urticaria

Endocrine & metabolic: Hyperuricemia

Gastrointestinal: Nausea, vomiting, diarrhea, stomatitis

Hematologic: Leukopenia (nadir: 8-29 days), thrombocytopenia (nadir: 10-15 days), anemia

Hepatic: Elevations in liver enzymes or bilirubin

Local: Tissue necrosis upon extravasation, erythematous streaking

Stability Store vials at room temperature; reconstituted solutions are stable for 7 days when refrigerated or 72 hours at room temperature; incompatible with heparin; inactivated by alkaline solutions

Mechanism of Action Intercalates with DNA causing strand breakage and affecting topoisomerase II activity resulting in inhibition of chain elongation and inhibition of DNA and RNA synthesis

Pharmacokinetics

Distribution: V_d: Large volume of distribution due to extensive tissue binding, distributes into CSF

Protein binding:

Idarubicin: 97%

Idarubicinol: 94%

Metabolism: Metabolized in the liver to idarubicinol (active metabolite)

Half-life:

Children: 18.7 hours (range: 2.5-22.4 hours)

Adults: 19 hours (range: 10.5-34.7 hours)

Idarubicinol: 45 hours

Elimination: Eliminated primarily by biliary excretion; 2.3% to 6.5% of a dose is eliminated renally

Usual Dosage I.V. (refer to individual protocols):

Children:

Leukemia: 10 mg/m^2 once daily for 3 days, repeat every 3 weeks

Solid tumors: 5 mg/m^2 once daily for 3 days, repeat every 3 weeks

Adults: 12 mg/m^2 once daily for 3 days

Dosing adjustment in hepatic and/or renal impairment: Reduce dose by 25%

Bilirubin >2.5 mg/dL: Reduce dose by 50%

Bilirubin >5 mg/dL: **Do not administer**

Administration Administer by intermittent infusion over 10-30 minutes into a free flowing I.V. solution of NS or D_5W; administer at a final concentration of 1 mg/mL

Monitoring Parameters CBC with differential, platelet count, ECHO, EKG, serum electrolytes, creatinine, uric acid, ALT, AST, bilirubin, signs of extravasation

Patient Information Notify physician if fever, sore throat, bleeding, or bruising occur

Nursing Implications Local erythematous streaking along the vein may indicate too rapid a rate of administration

Dosage Forms Powder for injection, lyophilized: 5 mg, 10 mg

References

Reid JM, Pendergrass TW, Krailo MD, et al, "Plasma Pharmacokinetics and

Cerebrospinal Fluid Concentrations of Idarubicin and Idarubicinol in Pediatric Leukemia Patients: A Children's Cancer Study Group Report," *Cancer Res*, 1990, 50(20):6525-8.

Idoxuridine (eye dox yoor' i deen)

Brand Names Herplex®

Synonyms IDU; IUDR

Therapeutic Category Antiviral Agent, Ophthalmic

Use Treatment of herpes simplex keratitis

Pregnancy Risk Factor C

Contraindications Hypersensitivity to idoxuridine or any component; concurrent use in patients receiving corticosteroids with superficial dendritic keratitis

Warnings Recurrence of infection may occur if idoxuridine is not continued for 5-7 days after healing appears complete

Precautions Use with caution in patients with corneal ulceration or patients receiving corticosteroid applications

Adverse Reactions

Local: Irritation, pruritus, pain, inflammation

Ocular: Corneal clouding, photophobia, small punctate defects on the corneal epithelium, mild edema of the eyelids and cornea, follicular conjunctivitis; ointment may produce a temporary visual haze

Drug Interactions Boric acid (increased local irritation)

Stability Refrigerate ophthalmic solution

Mechanism of Action Incorporated into viral DNA in place of thymidine resulting in mutations and inhibition of viral replication

Pharmacokinetics

Absorption: Ophthalmic: Poorly absorbed; absorption decreases as the concentration of drug increases

Distribution: Tissue uptake is a function of cellular metabolism which is inhibited by high concentrations of the drug; crosses the placenta

Metabolism: Metabolized to iodouracil, uracil and iodide

Elimination: Unchanged drug and metabolites excreted in the urine

Usual Dosage Children and Adults: Ophthalmic:

Solution: 1 drop in eye(s) every hour during day and every 2 hours at night, continue until definite improvement is noted, then reduce daytime dose to 1 drop every 2 hours and every 4 hours at night; continue for 5-7 days after healing appears complete

Ointment: Instill 5 times/day (every 4 hours) in the conjunctival sac with last dose at bedtime; continue therapy for 5-7 days after healing appears complete

Patient Information May cause sensitivity to bright light; minimize by wearing sunglasses; notify physician if condition worsens or does not improve in 7-8 days, or if pain, decreased vision, itching, or eye swelling occurs

Nursing Implications Idoxuridine solution should not be mixed with other medications

Dosage Forms Ophthalmic:

Ointment: 0.5% (4 g)

Solution: 0.1% (15 mL)

IDR *see* Idarubicin Hydrochloride *on page 301*

IDU *see* Idoxuridine *on this page*

Ifex® *see* Ifosfamide *on this page*

IFLrA *see* Interferon Alfa-2a *on page 314*

IFN *see* Interferon Alfa-2a *on page 314*

IFN-α-2 *see* Interferon Alfa-2b *on page 315*

Ifosfamide (eye foss' fa mide)

Brand Names Ifex®

Therapeutic Category Antineoplastic Agent

Use In combination with other antineoplastics in treatment of lung cancer, Hodgkin's and non-Hodgkin's lymphoma, breast cancer, acute and chronic lymphocytic leukemia, ovarian cancer, testicular cancer, and sarcomas

(Continued)

Ifosfamide *(Continued)*

Pregnancy Risk Factor D

Contraindications Patients who have demonstrated a previous hypersensitivity to ifosfamide; patients with severely depressed bone marrow function

Warnings The US Food and Drug Administration (FDA) currently recommends that procedures for proper handling and disposal of antineoplastic agents be considered. May require therapy cessation if confusion or coma occurs; be aware of hemorrhagic cystitis and severe myelosuppression; carcinogenic in rats

Precautions Use with caution in patients with impaired renal function or those with compromised bone marrow reserve

Adverse Reactions

Cardiovascular: Cardiotoxicity

Central nervous system: Somnolence, confusion, depressive psychoses, hallucinations, dizziness, seizures, fever, polyneuropathy

Dermatologic: Alopecia

Gastrointestinal: Nausea, vomiting, stomatitis

Hematologic: Myelosuppression (leukocyte nadir: 7-14 days)

Hepatic: Elevated liver enzymes

Local: Phlebitis

Renal & genitourinary: Hemorrhagic cystitis, dysuria, renal tubular acidosis

Drug Interactions Phenobarbital, phenytoin, chloral hydrate → ↑ conversion of ifosfamide to active metabolites and increased toxicity

Stability Reconstituted solution is stable for 7 days at room temperature and 21 days when refrigerated

Mechanism of Action Causes cross-linking of DNA strands by binding with nucleic acids and other intracellular structures; inhibits protein synthesis and DNA synthesis

Pharmacokinetics

Requires biotransformation in the liver before it can act as an alkylating agent

Dose-dependent pharmacokinetics: Beta phase half-life: 11-15 hours with high-dose (3800-5000 mg/m^2) or 4-7 hours with lower doses (1800 mg/m^2)

Metabolism: Metabolized in the liver to active species

Elimination: Metabolites and unchanged drug (15%) excreted in the urine

Usual Dosage I.V. (refer to individual protocols):

Children: 1800 mg/m^2/day for 3-5 days every 21-28 days or 5000 mg/m^2 as a single 24-hour infusion or 3 g/m^2/day for 2 days

Adults: 700-2000 mg/m^2/day for 5 days or 2400 mg/m^2/day for 3 days every 21-28 days; 5000 mg/m^2 as a single dose over 24 hours

Administration Administer as a slow I.V. intermittent infusion over at least 30 minutes at a final concentration for administration not to exceed 40 mg/mL (usual concentration for administration is between 0.6-20 mg/mL) or administer as a 24-hour infusion

Monitoring Parameters CBC with differential and platelet count, urine output, urinalysis, liver function and renal function tests

Nursing Implications Maintain adequate patient hydration

Additional Information Usually used in combination with mesna, a prophylactic agent for hemorrhagic cystitis

Dosage Forms Powder for injection: 1 g, 3 g

References

Ninane J, Baurain R, and de Kraker J, "Alkylating Activity in Serum, Urine, and CSF Following High-Dose Ifosfamide in Children," *Cancer Chemother Pharmacol*, 1989, 24(Suppl 1):S2-6.

Pinkerton CR, Rogers H, James C, et al, "A Phase II Study of Ifosfamide in Children With Recurrent Solid Tumors," *Cancer Chemother Pharmacol*, 1985, 15(3):258-62.

Ilosone® *see* Erythromycin *on page 226*

Ilosone® Pulvules® *see* Erythromycin *on page 226*

Ilotycin® *see* Erythromycin *on page 226*

Ilozyme® *see* Pancrelipase *on page 431*

I-Methasone® *see* Dexamethasone *on page 178*

Imidazole Carboxamide *see* Dacarbazine *on page 168*

Imipemide *see* Imipenem/Cilastatin *on this page*

Imipenem/Cilastatin (i mi pen' em)

Brand Names Primaxin®

Synonyms Imipemide

Therapeutic Category Antibiotic, Miscellaneous

Use Treatment of documented multidrug resistant gram-negative infection due to organisms proven or suspected to be susceptible to imipenem/cilastatin; treatment of multiple organism infection in which other agents have an insufficient spectrum of activity or are contraindicated due to toxic potential

Pregnancy Risk Factor C

Contraindications Hypersensitivity to imipenem/cilastatin or any component

Warnings Safety and efficacy in children <12 years of age have not yet been established; has been used in a limited number of children 3 months to 13 years of age without serious adverse effects; prolonged use may result in superinfection

Precautions Dosage adjustment required in patients with impaired renal function; use with caution in patients with history of seizures or who are predisposed and in patients with a history of hypersensitivity to penicillins

Adverse Reactions

Cardiovascular: Hypotension

Central nervous system: Seizures, hallucinations, altered effect, confusion

Dermatologic: Rash

Gastrointestinal: Nausea, vomiting, diarrhea, pseudomembranous colitis

Hematologic: Neutropenia, eosinophilia, positive Coombs' test

Hepatic: Transient elevation in liver enzymes

Local: Phlebitis

Miscellaneous: Emergence of resistant strains of *P. aeruginosa*

Drug Interactions Beta-lactam antibiotics, probenecid; ganciclovir (increased risk of seizures)

Stability When reconstituted suspension is further diluted with normal saline, it is stable for 10 hours at room temperature or 48 hours under refrigeration; when reconstituted suspension is further diluted with a compatible solution other than normal saline, it is stable for 4 hours at room temperature and 24 hours under refrigeration; incompatible with TPN; inactivated at alkaline or acidic pH

Mechanism of Action Inhibits cell wall synthesis by binding to penicillin-binding proteins on the bacterial outer membrane; cilastatin prevents renal metabolism of imipenem by competitive inhibition of dehydropeptidase along the brush border of the proximal renal tubules

Pharmacokinetics

Distribution: Imipenem appears in breast milk; crosses the placenta; only low concentrations penetrate into CSF

Protein binding:

- Imipenem: 13% to 21%
- Cilastatin: 40%

Metabolism: Imipenem is metabolized in the kidney by dehydropeptidase; cilastatin is partially metabolized in the kidneys

Half-life, both: 60 minutes, prolonged with renal insufficiency

Elimination: When imipenem is given with cilastatin, urinary excretion of unchanged imipenem increases to 70%; 70% to 80% of a cilastatin dose is excreted unchanged in the urine

Moderately dialyzable (20% to 50%)

Usual Dosage I.V. infusion, I.M. is limited to mild-moderate infections **(dosage recommendation based on imipenem component)**:

Neonates:

- 0-4 weeks, <1200 g: 20 mg/kg/dose every 18-24 hours
- Postnatal age:
  - ≤7 days, ≥1200 g: 40 mg/kg/day divided every 12 hours
  - >7 days, 1200-2000 g: 40 mg/kg/day divided every 12 hours
  - >7 days, >2000 g: 60 mg/kg/day divided every 8 hours

Children: 60-100 mg/kg/day divided every 6 hours; maximum: 4 g/day

(Continued)

Imipenem/Cilastatin *(Continued)*

Adults:

Serious infections: 2-4 g/day in 3-4 divided doses
Mild to moderate infections: 1-2 g/day in 3-4 divided doses

Dosing adjustment in renal impairment: Cl_{cr} <30-70 mL/minute/1.73 m^2: Reduce dose; see table.

Creatinine Clearance mL/min/1.73 m²	Frequency	% Decrease in Daily Maximum Dose
30–70	q6h	50
20–30	q8h	63
5–20	q12h	75

Administration Administer by I.V. intermittent infusion; final concentration for administration should not exceed 5 mg/mL; in fluid-restricted patients, a final concentration of 7 mg/mL has been administered; infuse over 20-60 minutes

Monitoring Parameters Periodic renal, hepatic, and hematologic function tests

Test Interactions Interferes with urinary glucose determination using Clinitest®

Nursing Implications If nausea and/or vomiting occur during administration, decrease the rate of I.V. infusion

Additional Information Sodium content of 1 g: 3.2 mEq

Dosage Forms Powder for injection:

I.V.:

Imipenem 250 mg and cilastatin 250 mg
Imipenem 500 mg and cilastatin 500 mg

I.M.:

Imipenem 500 mg and cilastatin 500 mg
Imipenem 750 mg and cilastatin 750 mg

References

Ahonkhai VI, Cyhan GM, Wilson SE, et al, "Imipenem-Cilastatin in Pediatric Patients: An Overview of Safety and Efficacy in Studies Conducted in the United States," *Pediatr Infect Dis J*, 1989, 8(11):740-4.

Overturf GD, "Use of Imipenem-Cilastatin in Pediatrics," *Pediatr Infect Dis J*, 1989, 8(11):792-4.

Wong VK, Wright HT Jr, Ross LA, et al, "Imipenem/Cilastatin Treatment of Bacterial Meningitis in Children," *Pediatr Infect Dis J*, 1991, 10(2):122-5.

Imipramine (im ip' ra meen)

Related Information

Overdose and Toxicology Information *on page 696-700*

Brand Names Janimine®; Tofranil®; Tofranil-PM®

Synonyms Imipramine Hydrochloride; Imipramine Pamoate

Therapeutic Category Antidepressant, Tricyclic

Use Treatment of various forms of depression, often in conjunction with psychotherapy; enuresis in children; analgesic for certain chronic and neuropathic pain

Pregnancy Risk Factor B

Contraindications Hypersensitivity to imipramine (cross-sensitivity with other tricyclics may occur); patients receiving MAO inhibitors within past 14 days; narrow-angle glaucoma

Warnings Do not discontinue abruptly in patients receiving long term high dose therapy; some oral preparations contain tartrazine and injection contains sulfites both of which can cause allergic reactions

Precautions Use with caution in patients with cardiovascular disease, conduction disturbances, seizure disorders, urinary retention, hyperthyroidism or those receiving thyroid replacement

Adverse Reactions Less sedation and anticholinergic effects than amitriptyline

Cardiovascular: Arrhythmias, hypotension

Central nervous system: Drowsiness, sedation, confusion, dizziness, weakness, fatigue, anxiety, nervousness, sleep disorders, seizures

Dermatologic: Rash, photosensitivity
Gastrointestinal: Nausea, vomiting, constipation, dry mouth
Hematologic: Blood dyscrasias
Hepatic: Hepatitis
Ocular: Blurred vision, increases intraocular pressure
Renal & genitourinary: Urinary retention
Miscellaneous: Hypersensitivity reactions

Drug Interactions May ↓ or reverse effects of guanethidine and clonidine; may ↑ effects of CNS depressants, adrenergic agents, anticholinergic agents; with MAO inhibitors, hyperpyrexia, tachycardia, hypertension, seizures and death may occur; similar interactions as with other tricyclics may occur

Mechanism of Action Increases the synaptic concentration of serotonin and/or norepinephrine in the central nervous system by inhibition of their reuptake by the presynaptic neuronal membrane

Pharmacodynamics Maximum antidepressant effects usually occur after ≥2 weeks

Usual Dosage

Children: Oral:

Depression: 1.5 mg/kg/day with dosage increments of 1 mg/kg every 3-4 days to a maximum dose of 5 mg/kg/day in 1-4 divided doses; monitor carefully especially with doses ≥3.5 mg/kg/day

Enuresis: ≥6 years: Initial: 10-25 mg at bedtime, if inadequate response still seen after 1 week of therapy, increase by 25 mg/day; dose should not exceed 2.5 mg/kg/day or 50 mg at bedtime if 6-12 years of age or 75 mg at bedtime if ≥12 years of age

Adjunct in the treatment of cancer pain: Initial: 0.2-0.4 mg/kg at bedtime; dose may be increased by 50% every 2-3 days up to 1-3 mg/kg/dose at bedtime

Adolescents: Oral: Initial: 25-50 mg/day; increase gradually; maximum: 100 mg/day in single or divided doses

Adults:

Oral: Initial: 25 mg 3-4 times/day, increase dose gradually, total dose may be given at bedtime; maximum: 300 mg/day

I.M.: Initial: Up to 100 mg/day in divided doses; change to oral as soon as possible

Monitoring Parameters EKG, CBC, supine and standing blood pressure (especially in children)

Reference Range Therapeutic: Imipramine and desipramine 150-250 ng/mL (SI: 530-890 nmol/L); desipramine 150-300 ng/mL (SI: 560-1125 nmol/L); Potentially toxic: >300 ng/mL (SI: >1070 nmol/L); Toxic: >1000 ng/mL (SI: >3570 nmol/L)

Dosage Forms

Capsule, as pamoate: 75 mg, 100 mg, 125 mg, 150 mg
Injection, as hydrochloride: 12.5 mg/mL (2 mL)
Tablet, as hydrochloride: 10 mg, 25 mg, 50 mg

References

Berde C, Ablin A, Glazer J, et al, "American Academy of Pediatrics Report of the Subcommittee on Disease-Related Pain in Childhood Cancer," *Pediatrics*, 1990, 86(5 Pt 2):818-25.

Imipramine Hydrochloride *see* Imipramine *on previous page*

Imipramine Pamoate *see* Imipramine *on previous page*

Immune Globulin, Intramuscular *see* Immunization Guidelines *on page 660-667*

Immune Globulin, Intravenous

Brand Names Gamimune® N; Gammagard®; Iveegam®; Polygam®; Sandoglobulin®; Venoglobulin®-I

Synonyms IVIG

Therapeutic Category Immune Globulin

Use Immunodeficiency syndrome, idiopathic thrombocytopenic purpura; used in conjunction with appropriate anti-infective therapy to prevent or modify acute bacterial or viral infections in patients with iatrogenically-induced or disease-associated immunodepression; autoimmune neutrope-

(Continued)

INTRAVENOUS IMMUNE GLOBULIN PRODUCT COMPARISON

	Gamimune® N	Gammagard®	Gammar®–IV	Iveegam®	Polygam®	Sandoglobulin®	Venoglobulin®–I
FDA indication	Primary immunodeficiency, ITP	Primary immunodeficiency, ITP, CLL prophylaxis	Primary immunodeficiency	Primary immunodeficiency, Kawasaki syndrome	Primary immunodeficiency, ITP, CLL	Primary immunodeficiency, ITP	Primary immunodeficiency, ITP
Contraindication	IgA deficiency	None (caution with IgA deficiency)	IgA deficiency	IgA deficiency	None (caution with IgA deficiency)	IgA deficiency	IgA deficiency
IgA content	270 μg/mL	0.92–1.6 μg/mL	<20 μg/mL	10 μg/mL	0.74 ± 0.33 μg/mL	720 μg/mL	20–24 μg/mL
Adverse reactions (%)	5.2	6	15	1	6	2.5–6.6	6
Plasma source	>2000 paid donors	4000–5000 paid donors	>8000 paid donors	>6000 paid donors	50,000 voluntary donors	8000–15,000 voluntary donors	6000–9000 paid donors
Half-life	21 d	24 d	21–24 d	26–29 d	21–25 d	21–23 d	29 d
IgG subclass (%) IgG_1 (60–70) IgG_2 (19–31) IgG_3 (5–8.4) IgG_4 (0.7–4)	 60 29.4 6.5 4.1	 67 (66.8)[1] 25 (25.4) 5 (7.4) 3 (0.3)	 69 23 6 2	 64.1[2] 30.3 4 1.5	 67 25 5 3	 60.5 (55.3)[1] 30.2 (35.7) 6.6 (6.3) 2.6 (2.6)	 62.3[2] 32.8 2.9 2
Monomers (%)	>95	>95	>98	93.8	>95	>92	>98
Gammaglobulin (%)	>98	>90	>98	100	>90	>96	>98
Storage	Refrigerate	Room temp	Room temp	Refrigerate	Room temp	Room temp	Room temp
Recommendations for **initial** infusion rate	0.01–0.02 mL/kg/min	0.5 mL/kg/h	0.01–0.02 mL/kg/min	1 mL/min	0.5 mL/kg/h	0.01–0.03 mL/kg/min	0.01–0.02 mL/kg/min
Maximum infusion rate	0.08 mL/kg/min	4 mL/kg/h	0.06 mL/kg/min	2 mL/min	4 mL/kg/h	2.5 mL/min	0.04 mL/kg/min
Maximum concentration for infusion (%)	10	5	5	5	10	12	10

[1]Skvaril F and Gardi A, "Differences Among Available Immunoglobulin Preparations for Intravenous Use," *Pediatr Infect Dis J,* 1988, 7:543–48.
[2]Roomer J, Morgenthaler JJ, Scherz R, et al, "Characterization of Various Immunoglobulin Preparations for Intravenous Application', *Vox Sang,* 1982, 42:62–73.
[3]ASHP Commission on Therapeutics, ASHP Therapeutic Guidelines for Intravenous Immune Globulin, *Clin Pharm,* 1992, 11:117–36.
[4]Manufacturer's Product Information/Personal Communication.

nia, bone marrow transplantation patients, Kawasaki disease, Guillain-Barré syndrome, demyelinating polyneuropathies

Pregnancy Risk Factor C

Contraindications Hypersensitivity to immune globulin, blood products, or any component, IgA deficiency (except with the use of Gammagard® or Polygam®)

Adverse Reactions

Cardiovascular: Flushing of the face, hypotension

Central nervous system: Dizziness, fever, headache

Gastrointestinal: Nausea

Miscellaneous: Chills, diaphoresis, tightness in the chest, hypersensitivity reactions

Drug Interactions Live virus vaccines (measles, mumps, rubella)

Stability Do not mix with other drugs

Mechanism of Action Replacement therapy for primary and secondary immunodeficiencies; interference with F_c receptors on the cells of the reticuloendothelial system for autoimmune cytopenias and ITP

Pharmacokinetics Half-life: 21-24 days

Usual Dosage Children and Adults: I.V.:

Immunodeficiency syndrome: 100-400 mg/kg/dose every 2-4 weeks

Idiopathic thrombocytopenic purpura: 400-1000 mg/kg/day for 2-5 consecutive days; maintenance dose: 400-1000 mg/kg/dose every 3-6 weeks based on clinical response and platelet count

Kawasaki disease: 400 mg/kg/day for 4 days or 2 g/kg as a single dose

Congenital and acquired antibody deficiency syndrome: 100-400 mg/kg/dose every 3-4 weeks

Bone marrow transplant: 400-500 mg/kg/dose every week

Severe systemic viral and bacterial infections:

- Neonates: 500 mg/kg/day for 2-6 days then once weekly
- Children: 500-1000 mg/kg/week

Prevention of gastroenteritis: Infants and Children: Oral: 50 mg/kg/day divided every 6 hours

Administration See table for administration information.

Monitoring Parameters Platelet count, vital signs, QUIGS

Nursing Implications I.V. use only; for initial treatment, a lower concentration and/or a slower rate of infusion should be used

Dosage Forms

Injection: Gamimune® N: 50 mg/mL with maltose 10% (10 mL, 50 mL, 100 mL); 100 mg/mL (50 mL, 100 mL, 200 mL)

Powder for injection, lyophilized:

- Gammagard®, Polygam®: 0.5 g, 2.5 g, 5 g, 10 g
- Gammar®-IV: 2.5 g
- Iveegam®: 0.5 g, 1 g, 2.5 g, 5 g
- Polygam®: 5 g, 10 g
- Sandoglobulin®: 1 g, 3 g, 6 g
- Venoglobulin®-I: 2.5 g, 5 g

References

ASHP Commission on Therapeutics, "ASHP Therapeutic Guidelines for Intravenous Immune Globulin," *Am J Hosp Pharm*, 1992, 49(3):652-4.

NIH Consensus Conference, "Intravenous Immunoglobulin, Prevention and Treatment of Disease," *JAMA*, 1990, 264(24):3189-93.

Imodium® *see* Loperamide Hydrochloride *on page 348*

Imodium® A-D [OTC] *see* Loperamide Hydrochloride *on page 348*

Imuran® *see* Azathioprine *on page 68*

I-Naphline® *see* Naphazoline Hydrochloride *on page 403*

Inapsine® *see* Droperidol *on page 212*

Inderal® *see* Propranolol Hydrochloride *on page 493*

Inderal® LA *see* Propranolol Hydrochloride *on page 493*

Indocin® *see* Indomethacin *on next page*

Indocin® I.V. *see* Indomethacin *on this page*

Indocin® SR *see* Indomethacin *on this page*

Indo-Lemmon® *see* Indomethacin *on this page*

Indomethacin (in doe meth' a sin)

Related Information

Overdose and Toxicology Information *on page 696-700*

Brand Names Indocin®; Indocin® I.V.; Indocin® SR; Indo-Lemmon®

Therapeutic Category Analgesic, Non-Narcotic; Anti-inflammatory Agent; Antipyretic; Nonsteroidal Anti-Inflammatory Agent (NSAID), Oral; Nonsteroidal Anti-Inflammatory Agent (NSAID), Parenteral

Use Management of inflammatory diseases and rheumatoid disorders; moderate pain; acute gouty arthritis; I.V. form used as alternative to surgery for closure of patent ductus arteriosus in neonates

Pregnancy Risk Factor B (D if used longer than 48 hours or after 34 weeks gestation)

Contraindications Hypersensitivity to indomethacin, any component, aspirin, or other nonsteroidal anti-inflammatory drugs (NSAIDs); active GI bleeding, ulcer disease; premature neonates with necrotizing enterocolitis, impaired renal function, IVH, active bleeding, thrombocytopenia

Precautions Use with caution in patients with cardiac dysfunction, hypertension, renal or hepatic impairment, epilepsy, patients receiving anticoagulants and for treatment of JRA in children (fatal hepatitis has been reported)

Adverse Reactions

Cardiovascular: Hypertension, edema

Central nervous system: Somnolence, fatigue, depression, confusion, dizziness, headache

Dermatologic: Rash

Endocrine & metabolic: Hyperkalemia, dilutional hyponatremia (I.V.), hypoglycemia (I.V.)

Gastrointestinal: Nausea, vomiting, epigastric pain, abdominal pain, anorexia, GI bleeding, ulcers, perforation

Hematologic: Hemolytic anemia, bone marrow depression, agranulocytosis, thrombocytopenia, inhibition of platelet aggregation

Hepatic: Hepatitis

Ocular: Corneal opacities

Otic: Tinnitus

Renal & genitourinary: Renal failure, oliguria

Miscellaneous: Hypersensitivity reactions

Drug Interactions Indomethacin may ↑ serum concentrations of digoxin, methotrexate, lithium, and aminoglycosides (reported with I.V. use in neonates); may ↑ nephrotoxicity of cyclosporin; may ↓ antihypertensive and diuretic effects of furosemide and thiazides; may ↑ serum potassium with potassium sparing diuretics; may ↓ antihypertensive effects of beta blockers, hydralazine and captopril; aspirin may ↓ and probenecid may ↑ indomethacin serum concentrations; other NSAIDs may ↑ GI adverse effects

Stability Protect from light; not stable in alkaline solution; reconstitute just prior to administration; discard any unused portion; do not use preservative containing diluents for reconstitution

Mechanism of Action Inhibits prostaglandin synthesis by decreasing the activity of the enzyme, cyclo-oxygenase, which results in decreased formation of prostaglandin precursors

Usual Dosage

Neonates: I.V.: Initial: 0.2 mg/kg, followed by 2 doses depending on postnatal age (PNA) **at time of first dose:**

- PNA <48 hours: 0.1 mg/kg at 12- to 24-hour intervals
- PNA 2-7 days: 0.2 mg/kg at 12- to 24-hour intervals
- PNA >7 days: 0.25 mg/kg at 12- to 24-hour intervals

Children: Oral: 1-2 mg/kg/day in 2-4 divided doses; maximum: 4 mg/kg/day; not to exceed 150-200 mg/day

Adults: 25-50 mg/dose 2-3 times/day; maximum dose: 200 mg/day; extended release capsule should be given on a 1-2 times/day schedule

Administration I.V.: Administer over 20-30 minutes at a concentration of 0.5-1 mg/mL in preservative free sterile water for injection or normal saline

Monitoring Parameters BUN, serum creatinine, liver enzymes, CBC; periodic ophthalmic exams with chronic use

Nursing Implications Avoid I.V. bolus administration or infusion via an umbilical catheter into vessels near the superior mesenteric artery as these may cause vasoconstriction and can compromise blood flow to the intestines. Do not give intra-arterially. Administer orally with food, milk, or antacids to decrease GI adverse effects; extended release capsules must be swallowed intact.

Additional Information Indomethacin may mask signs and symptoms of infections; fatalities in children have been reported, due to unrecognized overwhelming sepsis; drowsiness, lethargy, nausea, vomiting, seizures, paresthesia, headache, dizziness, tinnitus, GI bleeding, cerebral edema, and cardiac arrest have been reported with overdoses

Dosage Forms

Capsule: 25 mg, 50 mg
Capsule, sustained release: 75 mg
Powder for injection, as sodium trihydrate: 1 mg
Suppository, rectal: 50 mg
Suspension, oral: 25 mg/5 mL (5 mL, 10 mL, 237 mL, 500 mL)

References

Coombs RC, Morgan MEI, Durbin GM, et al, "Gut Blood Flow Velocities in the Newborn, Effects of Patent Ductus Arteriosus and Parenteral Indomethacin," *Arch Dis Child*, 1990, 65:1067-71.

Gersony WM, Peckham GJ, Ellison RC, et al, "Effects of Indomethacin in Premature Infants With Patent Ductus Arteriosus: Results of a National Collaborative Study," *J Pediatr*, 1983, 102(6):895-906.

Infectrol® *see* Dexamethasone, Neomycin and Polymyxin B *on page 180*

InFed™ *see* Iron Dextran Complex *on page 320*

Inflamase® *see* Prednisolone *on page 476*

Inflamase® Mild *see* Prednisolone *on page 476*

Influenza Virus Vaccine *see* Immunization Guidelines *on page 660-667*

INH *see* Isoniazid *on page 322*

Innovar® *see* Droperidol and Fentanyl *on page 212*

Inocor® *see* Amrinone Lactate *on page 51*

Insulatard® NPH *see* Insulin Preparations *on this page*

Insulin Preparations (in' su lin)

Related Information

Medications Compatible With PN Solutions *on page 649-650*

Brand Names Beef NPH Iletin® II; Beef Regular Iletin® II; Humulin®; Insulatard® NPH; Lente® Iletin® I; Lente® Iletin® II; Lente® Purified Pork Insulin; Mixtard®; Novolin®; NPH Iletin® I; Pork NPH Iletin® II; Pork Regular Iletin® II; Regular [Concentrated] Iletin® II U-500; Regular Iletin® I; Semilente® Iletin® I; Ultralente® Iletin® I; Velosulin®

Therapeutic Category Antidiabetic Agent

Use Treatment of insulin-dependent diabetes mellitus, also noninsulin-dependent diabetes mellitus unresponsive to treatment with diet and/or oral hypoglycemics; to assure proper utilization of glucose and reduce glucosuria in nondiabetic patients receiving parenteral nutrition whose glucosuria cannot be adequately controlled with infusion rate adjustments or those who require assistance in achieving optimal caloric intakes

Pregnancy Risk Factor B

Warnings Any change of insulin should be made cautiously; changing manufacturers, type and/or method of manufacture, may result in the need for a change of dosage; human insulin differs from animal-source insulin

Adverse Reactions Primarily symptoms of hypoglycemia

Cardiovascular: Palpitations, tachycardia, pallor
Central nervous system: Fatigue, tingling of fingers, tremors, mental confusion, loss of consciousness, headache, hypothermia
Endocrine & metabolic: Hypoglycemia, hypokalemia
Gastrointestinal: Hunger, nausea, numbness of mouth
Hypersensitivity: Urticaria, anaphylaxis
Local: Itching, redness, swelling, stinging, or warmth at injection site, atrophy or hypertrophy of S.C. fat tissue

(Continued)

Insulin Preparations *(Continued)*

Musculoskeletal: Muscle weakness
Ocular: Transient presbyopia or blurred vision
Miscellaneous: Perspiration

Drug Interactions Anabolic steroids, alcohol, MAO inhibitors, and salicylates may increase the hypoglycemic response to insulin; diazoxide, epinephrine, oral contraceptives, phenytoin, thiazide diuretics, furosemide, ethacrynic acid, oral antidiabetic agents, and corticosteroids may antagonize hypoglycemic effect; beta blockers may mask symptoms of hypoglycemia (ie, tachycardia)

Stability Bottle in use is stable at room temperature up to 1 month and 3 months refrigerated; cold (freezing) causes more damage to insulin than room temperatures up to 100°F; avoid direct sunlight; cold injections should be avoided

Pharmacodynamics Onset and duration of hypoglycemic effects depend upon the route of administration, site of injection, volume and concentration of injection, and the preparation administered. See table.

Insulin

Insulin Preparations	Onset (h)	Peak (h)	Duration (h)	Compatible Mixed With
Rapid Acting				
Insulin injection (regular)	0.5–1	2–3	5–7	All
Prompt insulin zinc suspension (Semilente®)	0.5–1	4–7	12–16	Lente®
Intermediate Acting				
Isophane insulin suspension (NPH)	1–2	4–12	18–24	Regular
Insulin zinc suspension (Lente®)	1–2	8–12	18–24	Regular, Semilente®
Long Acting				
Protamine zinc insulin suspension (PZI)	4–8	14–20	36	Regular
Extended insulin zinc suspension (Ultralente®)	4–8	16–18	36	Regular, Semilente®

Usual Dosage Dose requires continuous medical supervision; only regular insulin may be given I.V. The daily dose should be divided up depending upon the product used and the patient's response (see table), (eg, regular insulin every 4-6 hours; NPH insulin every 8-12 hours).

Children and Adults: S.C.: 0.5-1 unit/kg/day

Adolescents (during growth spurt) S.C.: 0.8-1.2 units/kg/day

Diabetic ketoacidosis: Children: I.V. loading dose: 0.1 unit/kg, then maintenance continuous infusion: 0.1 unit/kg/hour (range: 0.05-0.2 unit/kg/hour depending upon the rate of decrease of serum glucose). **Note:** Too rapid decrease of serum glucose may lead to cerebral edema.

Optimum rate of decrease (serum glucose): 80-100 mg/dL/hour

Note: Newly diagnosed patients with JODM presenting in DKA and patients with blood sugars <800 mg/dL may be relatively "sensitive" to insulin and should receive loading and initial maintenance doses approximately ½ of those indicated above.

Sliding scale: Use only for brief transitional periods of treatment; newly diagnosed patients with juvenile onset diabetes may be "sensitive" to exogenous insulin and should be treated with the lower end of these ranges. See table.

Dosage adjustment in renal impairment: Children and Adults:

Cl_{cr} 10-50 mL/minute: Administer 75% of recommended dose

Cl_{cr} <10 mL/minute: Administer 25% to 50% of recommended dose (follow blood sugar closely)

Monitoring Parameters Urine sugar and acetone, blood sugar, serum electrolytes

Insulin Sliding Scale

Urine Glucose	Insulin Dose (units/kg)	
	Urine Ketones (–)	Urine Ketones (+)
0–½%	0	0
¾%	0.03–0.10	0.05–0.12
1%	0.07–0.20	0.10–0.25
2%	0.15–0.40	0.20–0.50

Patient Information Do not change insulins without physician's approval

Nursing Implications When mixing regular insulin with other insulin preparations, regular insulin should be drawn into the syringe first

Additional Information The term "purified" refers to insulin preparations containing no more than 10 ppm proinsulin (purified and human insulins are less immunogenic)

Dosage Forms

All insulins are 100 units per mL (10 mL) except where indicated:

Rapid-acting:
- Regular beef and pork (Regular Iletin® I)
- Regular beef (purified) (Beef Regular Iletin® II)
- Regular human (rDNA) (Humulin® R)
- Regular human (rDNA, buffered) (Humulin® BR)
- Regular human (semisynthetic) (Humulin® R, Velosulin®)
- Regular human (semisynthetic) (Humulin® R PenFil®): 1.5 mL
- Regular pork (purified) (Pork Regular Iletin® II, Velosulin®)
- Regular pork (purified, concentrated) (Regular [Concentrated] Iletin® II U-500): 500 units/mL (20 mL)
- Regular pork (Regular Insulin)
- Zinc suspension, prompt beef (Semilente® Insulin)
- Zinc suspension, prompt beef and pork (Semilente® Iletin® I)

Intermediate-acting:
- Isophane suspension beef (NPH Insulin)
- Isophane suspension beef and pork (NPH Iletin® I)
- Isophane suspension beef (purified) (Beef NPH Iletin® II)
- Isophane suspension pork (purified) (NPH Purified, Pork NPH Iletin® II, Insulatard® NPH)
- Isophane suspension human (rDNA) (Humulin® N)
- Isophane suspension human (semisynthetic) (Insulatard® NPH, Humulin® N)
- Isophane suspension human (semisynthetic) (Humulin® N PenFil®): 1.5 mL
- Zinc suspension beef (Lente® Insulin)
- Zinc suspension beef and pork (Lente® Iletin® I)
- Zinc suspension beef (purified) (Lente® Iletin® II)
- Zinc suspension pork (purified) (Lente® Iletin® II, Lente® Purified Pork Insulin)
- Zinc suspension human (rDNA) (Humulin® L)
- Zinc suspension human (semisynthetic) (Humulin® L)

Long-acting:
- Zinc suspension, extended beef (Ultralente® Insulin)
- Zinc suspension, extended beef and pork (Ultralente® Iletin® I)
- Zinc suspension, extended human (rDNA) (Humulin® U)
- Ultralente® beef (standard)

Combinations:
- Isophane insulin suspension (50%) and insulin injection (50%) human (rDNA) (Humulin® 50/50)
- Isophane insulin suspension (70%) and insulin injection (30%) human (rDNA) (Humulin® 70/30)
- Isophane insulin suspension (70%) and insulin injection (30%) human (semisynthetic) (Mixtard® Human 70/30, Novolin® 70/30)

(Continued)

Insulin Preparations *(Continued)*

Isophane insulin suspension (70%) and insulin injection (30%) human (semisynthetic) (Novolin® 70/30 PenFil®): 1.5 mL

Isophane insulin suspension (70%) and insulin injection (30%) pork (purified) (Mixtard®)

Intal® *see* Cromolyn Sodium *on page 158*

α-2-interferon *see* Interferon Alfa-2b *on next page*

Interferon Alfa-2a (in ter feer' on)

Brand Names Roferon-A®

Synonyms IFLrA; IFN; rIFN-α

Therapeutic Category Interferon

Use Hairy cell leukemia, AIDS-related Kaposi's sarcoma in patients >18 years of age, multiple unlabeled uses

Pregnancy Risk Factor C

Contraindications Hypersensitivity to alpha interferon or any component of the product

Warnings The US Food and Drug Administration (FDA) currently recommends that procedures for proper handling and disposal of antineoplastic agents be considered; safety and efficacy in children <18 years of age have not been established

Precautions Use with caution in patients with seizure disorders, brain metastases, multiple sclerosis, compromised CNS, and patients with pre-existing cardiac disease, myelosuppression, or severe renal/hepatic impairment

Adverse Reactions Flu-like symptoms (fever, fatigue/malaise, myalgia, chills, headache, arthralgia, rigors) begin about 2-6 hours after the dose is given and may persist as long as 24 hours; usually patient can build up a tolerance to side effects

Cardiovascular: Tachycardia, sweating, arrhythmias, hypotension, edema, nasal congestion

Central nervous system: Fatigue/malaise, dizziness, depression, confusion, sensory neuropathy, psychiatric effects, fever, headache, EEG abnormalities, chills

Dermatologic: Partial alopecia, rash

Endocrine & metabolic: Increased uric acid level

Gastrointestinal: Anorexia, dry mouth, nausea, vomiting, diarrhea, abdominal cramps, weight loss, change in taste

Hematologic: Leukopenia (mainly neutropenia), anemia, thrombocytopenia; decreased hemoglobin, hematocrit, platelets; neutralizing antibodies

Hepatic: Increased ALT and AST

Musculoskeletal: Myalgia, arthralgia, rigors

Ocular: Blurred vision

Renal & genitourinary: Proteinuria, increased Cr, increased BUN

Respiratory: Coughing, chest pain

Miscellaneous: Thyroid dysfunction

Drug Interactions

Interferon Alfa-2b: Possible competitive binding to same receptors

AZT: Possible additive myelosuppression; vidarabine: may increase neurotoxicity

Acyclovir: Possible synergistic effects

Theophylline: Clearance is reduced

Stability Store in refrigerator; do not shake; after reconstitution stable at room temperature for 24 hours; do not store in syringes for prolonged periods

Mechanism of Action Inhibits cellular growth, alters the state of cellular differentiation, interferes with oncogene expression, alters cell surface antigen expression, increases phagocytic activity of macrophages and augments cytotoxicity of lymphocytes for target cells

Pharmacokinetics

Absorption: I.M., S.C.: >80% of dose is absorbed

Metabolism: Metabolized in the kidney, filtered, and absorbed at the renal tubule

Half-life: 3.7-8.5 hours

Peak serum concentrations: Within 3-8 hours

Usual Dosage Refer to individual protocols

Infants and Children: Hemangiomas of infancy, pulmonary hemangiomatosis: S.C.: 1-3 million units/m²/day once daily

Children >18 years and Adults: I.M., S.C.:

Hairy cell leukemia: Induction dose is 3 million units/day for 16-24 weeks; maintenance: 3 million units 3 times/week

AIDS-related Kaposi's sarcoma: Induction dose: 36 million units/day for 10-12 weeks; maintenance: 36 million units 3 times/week (may begin with dose escalation from 3-9-18 million units each day over 3 consecutive days followed by 36 million units/day for the remainder of the 10-12 weeks of induction)

Chronic hepatitis B: 5 million units/m² given once daily or 3 times/week

Monitoring Parameters Baseline EKG, CBC with differential and platelet count, electrolytes, liver and renal function tests, weight

Patient Information Do not change brands as changes in dosage may result; possible mental status changes may occur while on therapy

Nursing Implications S.C. administration is suggested for those who are at risk for bleeding or are thrombocytopenic; rotate S.C. injection site; patient should be well hydrated; pretreatment with nonsteroidal anti-inflammatory drug (NSAID) or acetaminophen can decrease fever and its severity and alleviate headache

Additional Information Indications and dosage regimens are specific for a particular brand of interferon; other brands of interferon (ie, Intron® A) have different indications and dosage guidelines; do not change brands of interferon as changes in dosage may result

Dosage Forms

Injection: 3 million units/mL (1 mL); 6 million units/mL (3 mL); 36 million units/mL (1 mL)

Powder for injection: 6 million units/mL when reconstituted

References

Ezekowitz RAB, Mulliken JB, and Folkman J, "Interferon Alfa-2a Therapy for Life-Threatening Hemangiomas of Infancy," *N Engl J Med*, 1992, 326(22):1456-63.

Hoofnagle JH, "Alpha-Inteferon Therapy of Chronic Hepatitis B, Current Status and Recommendations," *J Hepatol*, 1990, 11(Suppl 1):S100-7.

White CW, Sondheimer HM, Crouch EC, et al, "Treatment of Pulmonary Hemangiomatosis With Recombinant Interferon Alfa-2a," *N Engl J Med*, 1989, 320(18):1197-200.

Interferon Alfa-2b (in ter feer' on)

Brand Names Intron® A

Synonyms IFN-α-2; α-2-interferon; rIFN-α2

Therapeutic Category Interferon

Use Induce hairy-cell leukemia remission; treatment of AIDS-related Kaposi's sarcoma; condylomata acuminata; chronic hepatitis C

Pregnancy Risk Factor C

Contraindications Known hypersensitivity to interferon alfa-2b or any component

Warnings The US Food and Drug Administration (FDA) currently recommends that procedures for proper handling and disposal of antineoplastic agents be considered; safety and efficacy in children <18 years of age has not been established

Precautions Use with caution in patients with seizure disorders, brain metastases, compromised CNS, multiple sclerosis, and patients with pre-existing cardiac disease, severe renal or hepatic impairment, or myelosuppression

Adverse Reactions Flu-like symptoms (fever, fatigue/malaise, myalgia, chills, headache, arthralgia, rigors) begin about 2-6 hours after the dose is given and may persist as long as 24 hours; usually patient can build up a tolerance to side effects

Cardiovascular: Tachycardia, sweating, arrhythmias, hypotension, edema, nasal congestion

Central nervous system: Fatigue/malaise, dizziness, depression, confusion, sensory neuropathy, psychiatric effects, fever, headache, EEG abnormalities, chills

(Continued)

Interferon Alfa-2b *(Continued)*

Dermatologic: Partial alopecia, rash
Endocrine & metabolic: Increased uric acid level
Gastrointestinal: Anorexia, dry mouth, nausea, vomiting, diarrhea, abdominal cramps, weight loss, change in taste
Hematologic: Leukopenia (mainly neutropenia), anemia, thrombocytopenia; decreased hemoglobin, hematocrit, platelets; neutralizing antibodies
Hepatic: Increased ALT and AST
Musculoskeletal: Myalgia, arthralgia, rigors
Ocular: Blurred vision
Renal & genitourinary: Proteinuria, increased Cr, increased BUN
Respiratory: Coughing, chest pain
Miscellaneous: Thyroid dysfunction

Drug Interactions

Interferon Alfa-2a: May competitively bind to same receptors
AZT: Possible additive myelosuppression
Vidarabine: May increase neurotoxicity
Acyclovir: Possible synergistic effect
Theophylline: Clearance is reduced

Stability Refrigerate; reconstituted solution is stable for 1 month when refrigerated

Mechanism of Action Inhibits cellular growth, alters the state of cellular differentiation, interferes with oncogene expression, alters cell surface antigen expression, increases phagocytic activity of macrophages, and augments cytotoxicity of lymphocytes for target cells

Pharmacokinetics

Metabolism: Majority of dose is thought to be metabolized in the kidney, filtered and absorbed at the renal tubule
Half-life, elimination:
I.M., I.V.: 2 hours
S.C.: 3 hours
Peak serum levels: I.M., S.C.: Achieved in ~6-8 hours

Usual Dosage Adults (refer to individual protocols):

Hairy-cell leukemia: I.M., S.C.: 2 million units/m^2 3 times/week

AIDS-related Kaposi's sarcoma: I.M., S.C.: 30 million units/m^2 3 times/week or 50 million units/m^2 I.V. 5 days/week every other week

Condylomata acuminata: Intralesionally: 1 million units/lesion 3 times/week for 3 weeks; not to exceed 5 million units per treatment (maximum: 5 lesions at one time)

Chronic hepatitis C: I.M., S.C.: 3 million units 3 times/week for approximately a 6-month course; relapse of hepatitis has occurred after treatment was stopped

Monitoring Parameters Baseline EKG, CBC with differential and platelet count, liver function tests, electrolytes, weight, chest x-ray

Patient Information Do not change brands of interferon as changes in dosage may result; do not operate heavy machinery while on therapy since changes in mental status may occur

Nursing Implications S.C. administration is suggested for those patients who are at risk for bleeding or are thrombocytopenic; rotate S.C. injection site; patient should be well hydrated; may pretreat with nonsteroidal anti-inflammatory drug (NSAID) or acetaminophen to decrease fever and its severity and to alleviate headache

Additional Information Myelosuppressive effects:

WBC: Mild
Platelets: Mild
Onset (days): 7-10
Nadir (days): 14
Recovery (days): 21

Dosage Forms Powder for injection, lyophilized: 3 million units, 5 million units, 10 million units, 18 million units, 25 million units, 50 million units

References

Davis GL, Balart LA, Schiff ER, et al, "Treatment of Chronic Hepatitis C With Recombinant Interferon Alfa. A Multicenter Randomized, Controlled Trial. Hepatitis Interventional Therapy Group," *N Engl J Med*, 1989, 321(22):1501-6.

Intralipid® *see* Fat Emulsion *on page 239*

Intravenous Fat Emulsion *see* Fat Emulsion *on page 239*

Intron® A *see* Interferon Alfa-2b *on page 315*

Intropin® *see* Dopamine Hydrochloride *on page 204*

Iodinated Glycerol (eye' oh di nay ted gli' ser ole)

Brand Names Iophen®; Organidin®; R-Gen®

Therapeutic Category Expectorant

Use As a mucolytic expectorant in adjunctive treatment of bronchitis, bronchial asthma, pulmonary emphysema, cystic fibrosis, or chronic sinusitis

Pregnancy Risk Factor X

Contraindications Hypersensitivity to inorganic iodides, iodinated glycerol, or any component; pregnancy, newborns

Precautions Use with caution in patients with thyroid disease

Adverse Reactions

Central nervous system: Headache

Dermatologic: Acne, dermatitis

Endocrine & metabolic: Thyroid gland enlargement, acute parotitis

Gastrointestinal: GI irritation, burning of mouth and throat

Ocular: Swelling of the eyelids

Respiratory: Pulmonary edema

Miscellaneous: Hypersensitivity, allergic reactions

Mechanism of Action Increases respiratory tract secretions by decreasing surface tension and thereby decreases the viscosity of mucus, which aids in removal of the mucus

Pharmacokinetics

Absorption: Absorbed from the GI tract and accumulates in the thyroid gland

Metabolism: Unknown; however it is postulated that it is secreted into GI tract from bloodstream

Usual Dosage Oral (as iodinated glycerol):

Children: 30 mg 4 times/day

Adults: 60 mg 4 times/day

Dosage Forms

Elixir: 60 mg/5 mL [organically bound iodine 30 mg per 5 mL] (120 mL, 480 mL)

Solution, oral: 50 mg/mL [organically bound iodine 25 mg per mL] (30 mL)

Tablet: 30 mg [organically bound iodine 15 mg]

Iodine (eye' oh din)

Therapeutic Category Topical Skin Product

Use Used topically as an antiseptic in the management of minor, superficial skin wounds and has been used to disinfect the skin preoperatively

Pregnancy Risk Factor D

Contraindications Hypersensitivity to iodide preparations; neonates

Warnings May be highly toxic if ingested

Adverse Reactions

Dermatologic: Skin irritation and burns

Miscellaneous: Hypersensitivity, allergic reactions

Mechanism of Action Free iodine oxidizes microbial protoplasm making it effective against bacteria, fungi, yeasts, protozoa, and viruses; complexes with amino groups in tissue compounds to form iodophors from which the iodine is slowly released causing a sustained action

Usual Dosage Apply topically as necessary to affected areas of skin

Patient Information May stain skin and clothing

Nursing Implications Avoid tight bandages because iodine may cause burns on occluded skin

Additional Information Sodium thiosulfate inactivates iodine and is an effective chemical antidote for codeine poisoning; solutions of sodium thiosulfate may be used to remove iodine stains from skin and clothing

Dosage Forms

Solution: 2%

Tincture: 2%

Iodine *see* Trace Metals *on page 574*

Iodochlorhydroxyquin (eye oh doe klor' hye drox ee kwin)

Brand Names Vioform® [OTC]

Synonyms Clioquinol

Therapeutic Category Antifungal Agent, Topical

Use Used topically in the treatment of tinea pedis, tinea cruris, and skin infections caused by dermatophytic fungi (ring worm)

Contraindications Not effective in the treatment of scalp or nail fungal infections; children <2 years of age

Warnings Topical application poses a potential risk of toxicity to infants and children; known to cause serious and irreversible optic atrophy and peripheral neuropathy with muscular weakness, sensory loss, spastic paraparesis, and blindness

Precautions Routine use is not recommended, may irritate sensitized skin; use with caution in patients with iodine intolerance

Adverse Reactions

Central nervous system: Peripheral neuropathy

Dermatologic: Skin irritation, rash

Ocular: Optic atrophy

Mechanism of Action Chelates bacterial surface and trace metals needed for bacterial growth

Pharmacokinetics

Absorption: With an occlusive dressing up to 40% of a dose can be absorbed systemically during a 12-hour period; drug absorption is enhanced when applied under diapers

Half-life: 11-14 hours

Elimination: Conjugated and excreted in the urine

Usual Dosage Children and Adults: Topical: Apply 2-4 times/day; do not use for >7 days

Test Interactions Thyroid function tests (↓ ^{131}I uptake); false-positive ferric chloride test for phenylketonuria

Patient Information Can stain skin and fabrics; for external use only; avoid contact with eyes and mucous membranes

Dosage Forms

Cream: 3% (30 g)

Ointment, topical: 3% (30 g)

References

American Academy of Pediatrics Committee on Drugs, "Clioquinol (Iodochlorhydroxyquin, Vioform®) and Iodoquinol (Diiodohydroxyquin): Blindness and Neuropathy," *Pediatrics*, 1990, 86(5):797-8.

Iodopen® *see* Trace Metals *on page 574*

Iodoquinol (eye oh doe kwin' ole)

Brand Names Yodoxin®

Synonyms Diiodohydroxyquin

Therapeutic Category Amebicide

Use Treatment of acute and chronic intestinal amebiasis; asymptomatic cyst passers; *Blastocystis hominis* infections

Pregnancy Risk Factor C

Contraindications Known hypersensitivity to iodine or iodoquinol; hepatic or renal damage; pre-existing optic neuropathy

Precautions Use with caution in patients with thyroid disease or neurological disorders

Adverse Reactions

Central nervous system: Peripheral neuropathy, agitation, retrograde amnesia, fever, headache

Dermatologic: Anal pruritus, rash, acne

Endocrine & metabolic: Enlargement of the thyroid

Gastrointestinal: Nausea, vomiting, diarrhea, gastritis

Musculoskeletal: Weakness

Ocular: Optic neuritis, optic atrophy, visual impairment

Mechanism of Action Contact amebicide that works in the lumen of the intestine by an unknown mechanism

Pharmacokinetics
Absorption: Poor and irregular oral absorption
Metabolism: Metabolized in the liver
Elimination: Excreted in feces and urine

Usual Dosage Oral:
Children: 30-40 mg/kg/day in 3 divided doses for 20 days; not to exceed 1.95 g/day
Adults: 650 mg 3 times/day after meals for 20 days; not to exceed 2 g/day

Monitoring Parameters Ophthalmologic exam

Test Interactions May increase protein-bound serum iodine concentrations reflecting a decrease in iodine 131 uptake; false-positive ferric chloride test for phenylketonuria

Patient Information Take medication after meals

Nursing Implications Tablets may be crushed and mixed with applesauce or chocolate syrup

Dosage Forms
Powder: 25 g
Tablet: 210 mg, 650 mg

Iophen® *see* Iodinated Glycerol *on page 317*

I-Paracaine® *see* Proparacaine Hydrochloride *on page 490*

Ipecac Syrup (ip' e kak)

Therapeutic Category Antidote, Emetic

Use Treatment of acute oral drug overdosage and certain poisonings

Pregnancy Risk Factor C

Contraindications Do not use in unconscious patients, patients with absent gag reflex; ingestion of strong bases or acids, volatile oils; seizures

Warnings Do not confuse ipecac syrup with ipecac fluid extract; fluid extract is 14 times more potent than syrup

Precautions Use with caution in patients with cardiovascular disease and bulimics

Adverse Reactions
Cardiovascular: Cardiotoxicity
Central nervous system: Lethargy
Gastrointestinal: Protracted vomiting, diarrhea
Musculoskeletal: Myopathy

Drug Interactions Activated charcoal, milk, carbonated beverages → ↓ effectiveness

Mechanism of Action Irritates the gastric mucosa and stimulates the medullary chemoreceptor trigger zone to induce vomiting

Pharmacodynamics
Onset of vomiting after oral dose: Within 15-30 minutes
Duration: 20-25 minutes; can last longer, up to 60 minutes

Usual Dosage Oral:
Children:
- 6-12 months: 5-10 mL followed by 10-20 mL/kg of water; repeat dose one time if vomiting does not occur within 20 minutes
- 1-12 years: 15 mL followed by 10-20 mL/kg of water; repeat dose one time if vomiting does not occur within 20 minutes

Adults: 30 mL followed by 200-300 mL of water; repeat dose one time if vomiting does not occur within 20 minutes

Additional Information Patients should be kept active and moving following administration of ipecac; if vomiting does not occur after second dose, gastric lavage may be considered to remove ingested substance

Dosage Forms Syrup: 70 mg/mL (15 mL, 30 mL, 473 mL, 4000 mL)

I-Pentolate® *see* Cyclopentolate Hydrochloride *on page 161*

I-Phrine® Ophthalmic Solution *see* Phenylephrine Hydrochloride *on page 453*

I-Picamide® *see* Tropicamide *on page 588*

Ipratropium Bromide (i pra troe' pee um)

Brand Names Atrovent®

Therapeutic Category Anticholinergic Agent; Bronchodilator

Use A bronchodilator used in bronchospasm associated with COPD, bronchitis, and emphysema

(Continued)

Ipratropium Bromide *(Continued)*

Pregnancy Risk Factor B

Contraindications Hypersensitivity to atropine or its derivatives

Warnings Not indicated for the initial treatment of acute episodes of bronchospasm

Precautions Use with caution in patients with narrow-angle glaucoma, bladder neck obstruction, or prostatic hypertrophy

Adverse Reactions

Cardiovascular: Palpitations
Central nervous system: Nervousness, dizziness, headache, fatigue
Dermatologic: Rash
Gastrointestinal: Nausea, dry mouth
Ocular: Blurred vision
Respiratory: Cough

Mechanism of Action Blocks the action of acetylcholine at parasympathetic sites in bronchial smooth muscle causing bronchodilation

Pharmacodynamics

Onset of bronchodilation: 1-3 minutes after administration
Peak effect: Maximal effect within 1.5-2 hours
Duration: Bronchodilation persists for up to 4-6 hours

Pharmacokinetics

Absorption: Not readily absorbed into the systemic circulation from the surface of the lung or from the GI tract
Distribution: Following inhalation 15% of a dose reaches the lower airways

Usual Dosage

Children:
- <2 years: Nebulization of 250 μg 3 times/day
- 3-14 years: 1-2 inhalations (metered dose inhaler) 3 times/day; up to 6 inhalations/24 hours

Children >14 years and Adults: 2 inhalations 4 times/day; up to 12 inhalations/24 hours

Dosage Forms Solution, inhalation: 18 μg/actuation (14 g)

References

Henry RI, Hiller EG, Milner AD, et al, "Nebulised Ipratropium Bromide and Sodium Cromoglycate in the First 2 Years of Life," *Arch Dis Child*, 1984, 59(1):54-7.

Mann NP and Hiller RG, "Ipratropium Bromide in Children With Asthma," *Thorax*, 1982, 37(1):72-4.

Iproveratril Hydrochloride *see* Verapamil Hydrochloride *on page 597*

Iron Dextran Complex

Brand Names InFed™

Therapeutic Category Iron Salt

Use Treatment of microcytic, hypochromic anemia resulting from iron deficiency when oral iron administration is infeasible or ineffective

Pregnancy Risk Factor C

Contraindications Hypersensitivity to iron dextran; anemias that are not involved with iron deficiency

Warnings Deaths associated with parenteral administration following anaphylactic-type reactions have been reported; use only in patients where the iron deficient state is not amenable to oral iron therapy

Precautions Use with caution in patients with a history of asthma, hepatic impairment, rheumatoid arthritis; not recommended in infants <4 months of age

Adverse Reactions

Anaphylactoid reactions: Respiratory difficulties and cardiovascular collapse have been reported and occur most frequently within the first several minutes of administration
Cardiovascular: Hypotension, flushing
Central nervous system: Dizziness, fever, headache
Dermatologic: Urticaria
Gastrointestinal: Nausea
Genitourinary: Hematuria
Hematologic: Leukocytosis

Local: Pain, staining of skin at the site of I.M. injection, phlebitis

Musculoskeletal: Arthralgia

Miscellaneous: Chills, lymphadenopathy, metallic taste, sweating

Note: Sweating, urticaria, arthralgia, fever, chills, dizziness, headache, and nausea may be delayed 24-48 hours after I.V. administration or 3-4 days after I.M. administration

Mechanism of Action The released iron, from the plasma, eventually replenishes the depleted iron stores in the bone marrow where it is incorporated into hemoglobin

Pharmacokinetics

Absorption: I.M.: 60% absorbed after 3 days; 90% after 1-3 weeks, the balance is slowly absorbed over months

Following I.V. doses, the uptake of iron by the reticuloendothial system appears to be constant at about 10-20 mg/hour

Elimination: Eliminated by the reticuloendothelial system and excreted in the urine and feces (via bile)

Usual Dosage I.M., I.V.:

A 0.5 mL test dose (0.25 mL in infants) should be given 1 hour prior to starting iron dextran therapy

Total replacement dosage of iron dextran (mL) = 0.0476 x weight (kg) x (Hb_n-Hb_o) + 1 mL/per 5 kg body weight (up to maximum of 14 mL)

Hb_n = desired hemoglobin (g/dL) = 12 if <15 kg or 14.8 if >15 kg

Hb_o = measured hemoglobin (g/dL)

Note: Total dose infusions have been used safely and are the preferred method of administration

Maximum daily dose: I.M.:

Infants and Children: 5 mg/kg or maximum of 100 mg

Adults >50 kg: 100 mg iron

Administration

I.M.: Use Z-track technique for I.M. administration (deep into the upper outer quadrant of buttock)

I.V.: Direct I.V. push administration is **not** recommended; dilute in normal saline (250-1000 mL) and infuse over 1-6 hours at a maximum rate of 50 mg/minute; avoid dilution in dextrose due to an increased incidence of local pain and phlebitis

Monitoring Parameters Reticulocyte count, serum ferritin, hemoglobin, serum iron concentrations and TIBC may not be meaningful for 3 weeks after administration, especially after large I.V. doses

Test Interactions May cause falsely elevated values of serum bilirubin and falsely decreased values of serum calcium

Dosage Forms Injection:

I.M.: 50 mg/mL with phenol 0.5% (**for I.M. administration only**)

I.V., I.M.: 50 mg/mL with sodium chloride 0.9%

References

Auerbach M, Witt D, and Toler W, "Clinical Use of the Total Dose Intravenous Infusion of Iron Dextran," *J Lab Clin Med*, 1988, 111(5):566-70.

Benito RR and Guerrero TC, "Response to a Single Intravenous Dose Versus Multiple Intramuscular Administration of Iron Dextran Complex: A Comparative Study," *Curr Ther Res*, 1973, 15:373-82.

Iron Sulfate *see* Ferrous Sulfate *on page 243*

Isoetharine (eye soe eth' a reen)

Brand Names Arm-a-Med® Isoetharine; Beta-2®; Bronkometer®; Bronkosol®; Dey-Lute® Isoetharine

Synonyms Isoetharine Hydrochloride; Isoetharine Mesylate

Therapeutic Category Adrenergic Agonist Agent; Bronchodilator; Sympathomimetic

Use Bronchodilator used in asthma and for the reversible bronchospasm occurring with bronchitis and emphysema

Pregnancy Risk Factor C

Contraindications Known hypersensitivity to isoetharine or other sympathomimetics

Warnings Isoetharine hydrochloride solution contains sulfites which may cause allergic reactions in some patients; use with caution in patients with

(Continued)

Isoetharine *(Continued)*

hyperthyroidism, hypertension, acute coronary artery disease, cerebral arteriosclerosis

Precautions Excessive, prolonged use may lead to decreased effectiveness

Adverse Reactions

Cardiovascular: Tachycardia

Central nervous system: Tremor, weakness, anxiety, dizziness, restlessness, excitement, headache

Gastrointestinal: Nausea

Mechanism of Action Relaxes bronchial smooth muscle and peripheral vasculature by action on $beta_2$ receptors with little effect on heart rate

Pharmacodynamics

Peak effect: Following inhaler administration, within 5-15 minutes

Duration: 1-4 hours

Pharmacokinetics Metabolism: Primarily metabolized (90%) in many tissues including the liver and lungs

Usual Dosage Treatments are usually not repeated more often than every 4 hours, except in severe cases

Nebulizer:

Children: 0.01 mL/kg of 1% solution; minimum dose 0.1 mL; maximum dose: 0.5 mL diluted in 2-3 mL normal saline

Adults: 0.5-1 mL of a 0.5% solution (or 0.5 mL of a 1% solution) diluted with 2 mL normal saline; equivalent dosages using 0.125%, 0.20% and 0.25% solutions may be used undiluted

Inhalation: Adults: 1-2 inhalations every 4 hours as needed

Monitoring Parameters Heart rate, blood pressure, respiratory rate

Dosage Forms

Aerosol, oral, as mesylate: 340 μg per metered spray

Solution, inhalation, as hydrochloride: 0.062% (4 mL); 0.08% (3.5 mL); 0.1% (2.5 mL, 5 mL); 0.125% (4 mL); 0.167% (3 mL); 0.17% (3 mL); 0.2% (2.5 mL); 0.25% (2 mL, 3.5 mL); 0.5% (0.5 mL); 1% (0.5 mL, 0.25 mL, 10 mL, 14 mL, 30 mL)

References

Rachelefsky GS and Siegel SC, "Asthma in Infants and Children - Treatment of Childhood Asthma: Part 11," *J Allergy Clin Immunol*, 1985, 76(3):409-25.

Isoetharine Hydrochloride *see* Isoetharine *on previous page*

Isoetharine Mesylate *see* Isoetharine *on previous page*

Isoniazid (eye soe nye' a zid)

Related Information

Overdose and Toxicology Information *on page 696-700*

Brand Names Laniazid®; Nydrazid®

Synonyms INH; Isonicotinic Acid Hydrazide

Therapeutic Category Antitubercular Agent

Use In treatment of susceptible tuberculosis infections and prophylactically to those individuals exposed to tuberculosis

Pregnancy Risk Factor C

Contraindications Acute liver disease; hypersensitivity to isoniazid or any component; previous history of hepatic damage during isoniazid therapy

Warnings Severe and sometimes fatal hepatitis may occur or develop even after many months of treatment; the administration of isoniazid in combination with rifampin is associated with an increased incidence of hepatotoxicity if the isoniazid dose >10 mg/kg/day; patients must report any prodromal symptoms of hepatitis such as fatigue, weakness, malaise, anorexia, nausea, vomiting, dark urine, or yellowing of eyes

Precautions Use with caution in patients with renal impairment and chronic liver disease

Adverse Reactions

Central nervous system: Peripheral neuritis, seizure, stupor, dizziness, agitation, psychosis, fever, ataxia

Dermatologic: Skin eruptions

Endocrine & metabolic: Hyperglycemia

Gastrointestinal: Nausea, vomiting, epigastric distress
Hematologic: Agranulocytosis, hemolytic anemia, aplastic anemia, thrombocytopenia, eosinophilia
Hepatic: Hepatitis, 3% to 10% of children experience transient elevated liver transaminase levels
Ocular: Optic neuritis
Otic: Tinnitus

Drug Interactions May increase serum concentrations of phenytoin, carbamazepine, diazepam; prednisone, disulfiram; aluminum salts may decrease isoniazid absorption

Mechanism of Action Inhibits mycolic acid synthesis resulting in disruption of the bacterial cell wall

Pharmacokinetics

Absorption: Oral, I.M.: Rapid and complete; rate and extent of absorption may be reduced when administered with food
Distribution: Crosses the placenta; appears in breast milk; distributes into all body tissues and fluids including the CSF
Protein binding: 10% to 15%
Metabolism: Metabolized by the liver with decay rate determined genetically by acetylation phenotype
Half-life: May be prolonged in patients with impaired hepatic function or severe renal impairment
Fast acetylators: 30-100 minutes
Slow acetylators: 2-5 hours
Peak serum levels: Oral: Within 1-2 hours
Elimination: Excreted in the urine (75% to 95%), feces, and saliva
Dialyzable (50% to 100%)

Usual Dosage Oral, I.M.:

Infants and Children:
Treatment: 10-20 mg/kg/day in 1-2 divided doses
Prophylaxis: 10 mg/kg/day given once daily, not to exceed 300 mg/day

Adults:
Treatment: 5 mg/kg/day given daily (usual dose: 300 mg)
Disseminated disease: 10 mg/kg/day in 1-2 divided doses
Prophylaxis: 300 mg/day given daily

American Thoracic Society and CDC currently recommend twice weekly therapy as part of a short-course regimen which follows 1-2 months of daily treatment for uncomplicated pulmonary tuberculosis in **compliant** patients
Children: 20-40 mg/kg/dose (up to 900 mg/dose) twice weekly
Adults: 15 mg/kg/dose (up to 900 mg/dose) twice weekly

Duration of therapy:
Asymptomatic infection (positive skin test):
Isoniazid susceptible: 9 months of isoniazid
Isoniazid resistant: 9 months of rifampin
Pulmonary, hilar adenopathy, and extrapulmonary infection other than meningitis, bone/joint, or disseminated infection:
6 months which includes 2-month therapy of isoniazid, rifampin, and pyrazinamide daily followed by 4 months of isoniazid and rifampin daily **or** 2 months of isoniazid, rifampin, and pyrazinamide daily, followed by 4 months of isoniazid and rifampin twice weekly under direct observation
9 months of isoniazid and rifampin daily **or** 1 month of isoniazid and rifampin daily followed by 8 months of isoniazid and rifampin twice weekly under direct observation.
Note: If drug resistance is possible, ethambutol or streptomycin should be added to the initial therapy regimen until susceptibility is determined
Meningitis, bone/joint, and disseminated infection:
2 months of isoniazid, rifampin, pyrazinamide, and streptomycin daily followed by 10 months of isoniazid and rifampin daily **or** 2 months of isoniazid, rifampin, pyrazinamide, and streptomycin daily followed by 10 months of isoniazid and rifampin twice weekly under direct observation

Monitoring Parameters Periodic liver function tests; monitoring for prodromal signs of hepatitis

(Continued)

Isoniazid *(Continued)*

Test Interactions False-positive urinary glucose with Clinitest®

Patient Information Report any prodromal symptoms of hepatitis (fatigue, weakness, nausea, vomiting, dark urine, or yellowing of eyes) or any burning, tingling, or numbness in the extremities

Nursing Implications The American Academy of Pediatrics recommends that pyridoxine supplementation (1-2 mg/kg/day) should be administered to malnourished patients, children or adolescents on meat or milk-deficient diets, breast feeding infants, and those predisposed to neuritis to prevent peripheral neuropathy; administration of isoniazid syrup has been associated with diarrhea

Dosage Forms

Injection: 100 mg/mL (10 mL)

Syrup (orange flavor): 50 mg/5 mL (473 mL)

Tablet: 50 mg, 100 mg, 300 mg

References

American Academy of Pediatrics, Committee on Infectious Diseases, "Chemotherapy for Tuberculosis in Infants and Children," *Pediatrics*, 1992, 89(1):161-5.

Starke JR, "Modern Approach to the Diagnosis and Treatment of Tuberculosis in Children," *Pediatr Clin North Am*, 1988, 35(3):441-64.

Starke JR, "Multidrug Therapy for Tuberculosis in Children," *Pediatr Infect Dis J*, 1990, 9(11):785-93.

Van Scoy RE and Wilkowske CJ, "Antituberculous Agents: Isoniazid, Rifampin, Streptomycin, Ethambutol, and Pyrazinamide," *Mayo Clin Proc*, 1983, 58(4):233-40.

Isonicotinic Acid Hydrazide *see* Isoniazid *on page 322*

Isonipecaine Hydrochloride *see* Meperidine Hydrochloride *on page 362*

Isoprenaline Hydrochloride *see* Isoproterenol *on this page*

Isoproterenol (eye soe proe ter' e nole)

Related Information

Emergency Pediatric Drip Calculations *on page 615*

Medications Compatible With PN Solutions *on page 649-650*

Brand Names Arm-a-Med® Isoproterenol; Dey-Dose® Isoproterenol; Dispos-a-Med® Isoproterenol; Isuprel®; Medihaler-Iso®; Norisodrine®

Synonyms Isoprenaline Hydrochloride; Isoproterenol Hydrochloride; Isoproterenol Sulfate

Therapeutic Category Adrenergic Agonist Agent; Bronchodilator; Sympathomimetic

Use Asthma or COPD (reversible airway obstruction); ventricular arrhythmias due to A-V nodal block; hemodynamically compromised bradyarrhythmias or atropine-resistant bradyarrhythmias, temporary use in 3rd degree A-V block until pacemaker insertion; low cardiac output or vasoconstrictive shock states

Pregnancy Risk Factor C

Contraindications Angina, pre-existing cardiac arrhythmias (ventricular); tachycardia or A-V block caused by cardiac glycoside intoxication; allergy to sulfites or isoproterenol or other sympathomimetic amines

Precautions Geriatric patients, diabetics, renal or cardiovascular disease, hyperthyroidism

Adverse Reactions

Cardiovascular: Flushing of the face or skin, ventricular arrhythmias, tachycardias, or profound hypotension

Central nervous system: Nervousness, restlessness, anxiety, dizziness, tremors, headache

Miscellaneous: Sweating

Drug Interactions Additive effects and increased cardiotoxicity when administered concomitantly with other sympathomimetic amines; beta-adrenergic blocking agents; may increase theophylline elimination

Mechanism of Action Stimulates $beta_1$ and $beta_2$ receptors resulting in relaxation of bronchial, GI, and uterine smooth muscle, increased heart rate and contractility, vasodilation of peripheral vasculature

Pharmacodynamics

Onset of action: Oral inhalation: Bronchodilation occurs immediately

Duration:

Oral inhalation: 1 hour

S.L. or S.C.: Up to 2 hours

Pharmacokinetics

Metabolism: Metabolized by conjugation in many tissues including the liver and lungs

Half-life: 2.5-5 minutes

Elimination: Excreted in the urine principally as sulfate conjugates

Usual Dosage

Children:

Oral inhalation: 1-2 metered doses up to 6 times/day

Nebulization: 0.01 mL/kg of 1% solution; minimum dose: 0.1 mL; maximum dose: 0.5 mL diluted in 2-3 mL normal saline; equivalent doses using 0.25% and 0.5% solutions may be used undiluted

S.L.: 5-10 mg every 3-4 hours (maximum: 30 mg/day)

I.V. infusion: 0.05-2 μg/kg/minute; rate (mL/hour) = dose (μg/kg/minute) x weight (kg) x 60 minutes/hour divided by concentration (μg/mL)

Adults:

Oral inhalation: 1-2 metered doses 4-6 times/day

Nebulization: 0.25-0.5 mL of a 1% solution diluted in 2-3 mL normal saline; equivalent doses using 0.25% and 0.5% solutions may be used undiluted

S.L.: 10-20 mg every 3-4 hours (maximum: 60 mg/day)

I.V. infusion: 2-20 μg/minute

Administration May be given undiluted by direct I.V. injection; for continuous infusions, dilute in dextrose or normal saline to a maximum concentration of 64 μg/mL

Monitoring Parameters Heart rate, blood pressure, respiratory rate, arterial blood gases, central venous pressure

Additional Information When discontinuing an isoproterenol continuous infusion used for bronchodilation, the infusion **must** be gradually tapered over a 24- to 48-hour period; hypotension is more common in hypovolemic patients

Dosage Forms

Inhalation:

Aerosol: 0.2% [1:500] (15 mL, 22.5 mL); 0.25% [1:400] (15 mL)

Injection: 0.2 mg/mL [1:5000] (1 mL, 5 mL, 10 mL)

Solution for nebulization: 0.031% (4 mL); 0.062% (4 mL); 0.25% (0.5 mL, 30 mL); 0.5% (0.5 mL, 10 mL, 60 mL); 1% (10 mL)

Tablet, sublingual: 10 mg, 15 mg

References

Rachelefsky GS and Siegel SC, "Asthma in Infants and Children - Treatment of Childhood Asthma: Part II," *J Allergy Clin Immunol*, 1985, 76(3):409-25.

Isoproterenol Hydrochloride *see* Isoproterenol *on previous page*

Isoproterenol Sulfate *see* Isoproterenol *on previous page*

Isoptin® *see* Verapamil Hydrochloride *on page 597*

Isopto® Atropine *see* Atropine Sulfate *on page 65*

Isopto® Carpine *see* Pilocarpine *on page 459*

Isopto® Eserine *see* Physostigmine Salicylate *on page 457*

Isopto® Frin Ophthalmic Solution *see* Phenylephrine Hydrochloride *on page 453*

Isopto® Homatropine *see* Homatropine Hydrobromide *on page 287*

Isopto® Hyoscine *see* Scopolamine *on page 519*

Isotretinoin (eye soe tret' i noyn)

Brand Names Accutane®

Synonyms 13-*cis*-Retinoic Acid

Therapeutic Category Acne Product; Retinoic Acid Derivative; Vitamin, Fat Soluble

(Continued)

Isotretinoin *(Continued)*

Use Treatment of severe recalcitrant cystic and/or conglobate acne unresponsive to conventional therapy; used investigationally for the treatment of children with metastatic neuroblastoma or leukemia that does not respond to conventional therapy

Pregnancy Risk Factor X

Contraindications Sensitivity to parabens, vitamin A or other retinoids; patients who are pregnant or intend to become pregnant during treatment

Warnings Risk of isotretinoin teratogenesis is ~20%; it can cause fetal defects in the CNS, ears, and cardiovascular system; not to be used in women of childbearing potential unless woman is capable of complying with effective contraceptive measures; therapy is normally begun on the second or third day of next normal menstrual period; effective contraception must be used for at least one month before beginning therapy, during therapy, and for one month after discontinuation of therapy

Precautions Use with caution in patients with diabetes mellitus

Adverse Reactions

Cardiovascular: Epistaxis

Central nervous system: Fatigue, headache

Dermatologic: Pruritus, hair loss, cheilitis, photosensitivity

Endocrine & metabolic: Hypertriglyceridemia, hyperuricemia

Gastrointestinal: Xerostomia, anorexia, nausea, vomiting, inflammatory bowel syndrome

Hematologic: Increase in erythrocyte sedimentation rate, decrease in hemoglobin and hematocrit

Hepatic: Hepatitis

Musculoskeletal: Bone or joint pain, muscle aches

Ocular: Conjunctivitis, corneal opacities

Drug Interactions ↑ clearance of carbamazepine; vitamin A supplements increase toxic effects

Mechanism of Action Reduces sebaceous gland size and reduces sebum production; regulates cell proliferation and differentiation

Pharmacokinetics

Absorption: Following oral administration, drug demonstrates biphasic absorption

Distribution: Crosses the placenta; appears in breast milk

Protein binding: 99% to 100%

Metabolism: Metabolized in the liver; major metabolite: 4-oxo-isotretinoin (active)

Half-life, terminal: 10-20 hours for isotretinoin, and 11-50 hours for its metabolite

Peak serum levels: Within 3 hours

Elimination: Excreted equally in the urine and feces

Usual Dosage Oral:

Children and Adults: 0.5-2 mg/kg/day in 2 divided doses (dosages as low as 0.05 mg/kg/day have been reported to be beneficial) for 15-20 weeks or until the total cyst count decreases by 70%, whichever is sooner

Children: Maintenance therapy for neuroblastoma: 100-250 mg/m^2/day in 2 divided doses has been used investigationally

Monitoring Parameters CBC with differential, platelet count, baseline sed rate, serum triglyceride, liver enzymes

Patient Information Do not take vitamin supplements containing vitamin A

Nursing Implications Capsules can be swallowed or chewed and swallowed; the capsule may be opened with a large needle and the contents placed on apple sauce or ice cream for patients unable to swallow the capsule

Dosage Forms Capsule: 10 mg, 20 mg, 40 mg

References

American Academy of Pediatrics Committee on Drugs, "Retinoid Therapy for Severe Dermatological Disorders," *Pediatrics*, 1992, 90(1 Pt 1):119-20.

DiGiovanna JJ and Peck GL, "Oral Synthetic Retinoid Treatment in Children," *Pediatr Dermatol*, 1983, 1(1):77-88.

Isoxazolyl Penicillin *see* Oxacillin Sodium *on page 425*

I-Sulfacet® *see* Sulfacetamide Sodium *on page 539*

Isuprel® *see* Isoproterenol *on page 324*

I-Tropine® *see* Atropine Sulfate *on page 65*

IUDR *see* Idoxuridine *on page 303*

Iveegam® *see* Immune Globulin, Intravenous *on page 307*

IVIG *see* Immune Globulin, Intravenous *on page 307*

Janimine® *see* Imipramine *on page 306*

Jenamicin® *see* Gentamicin *on page 268*

Kabikinase® *see* Streptokinase *on page 534*

K Acetate *see* Potassium Acetate *on page 468*

Kaochlor® S-F *see* Potassium Chloride *on page 469*

Kaon® *see* Potassium Gluconate *on page 470*

Kaon-CL® *see* Potassium Chloride *on page 469*

Kaopectate® II [OTC] *see* Loperamide Hydrochloride *on page 348*

Karidium® *see* Fluoride *on page 255*

Karigel® *see* Fluoride *on page 255*

Kasof® [OTC] *see* Docusate *on page 202*

Kato® *see* Potassium Chloride *on page 469*

Kayexalate® *see* Sodium Polystyrene Sulfonate *on page 531*

KCl *see* Potassium Chloride *on page 469*

K-Dur® 20 *see* Potassium Chloride *on page 469*

Keflex® *see* Cephalexin Monohydrate *on page 120*

Keftab® *see* Cephalexin Monohydrate *on page 120*

Kefurox® *see* Cefuroxime *on page 118*

Kefzol® *see* Cefazolin Sodium *on page 110*

Kenacort® Syrup *see* Triamcinolone *on page 579*

Kenacort® Tablet *see* Triamcinolone *on page 579*

Kenalog® Injection *see* Triamcinolone *on page 579*

Keralyt® *see* Salicylic Acid *on page 516*

Ketalar® *see* Ketamine *on this page*

Ketamine (keet' a meen)

Related Information

Preprocedure Sedatives in Children *on page 687-689*

Brand Names Ketalar®

Therapeutic Category General Anesthetic

Use Anesthesia, short surgical procedures, dressing changes

Restrictions C-III

Pregnancy Risk Factor D

Contraindications Elevated intracranial pressure; patients with hypertension, aneurysms, thyrotoxicosis, congestive heart failure, angina, psychotic disorders; hypersensitivity to ketamine or any component

Warnings Use only by or under the direct supervision of physicians experienced in administering general anesthetics. Resuscitative equipment should be available for use. Postanesthetic emergence reactions which can manifest as vivid dreams, hallucinations and/or frank delirium occur in 12% of patients; these reactions are less common in pediatric patients; emergence reactions may occur up to 24 hours postoperatively and may be reduced by minimization of verbal, tactile and visual patient stimulation during recovery, or by pretreatment with a benzodiazepine

Adverse Reactions

Cardiovascular: Hypertension, tachycardia, increased cardiac output, paradoxical direct myocardial depression, hypotension, bradycardia, increases cerebral blood flow

Central nervous system: Tremors, tonic-clonic movements, fasciculations, increased intracranial pressure

(Continued)

Ketamine *(Continued)*

Endocrine & metabolic: Increased metabolic rate
Gastrointestinal: Hypersalivation, vomiting, postoperative nausea
Musculoskeletal: Increased skeletal muscle tone
Ocular: Diplopia, nystagmus, increased intraocular pressure
Respiratory: Increased airway resistance, cough reflex may be depressed, decreased bronchospasm, respiratory depression or apnea with large doses or rapid infusions, laryngospasm
Miscellaneous: Emergence reactions

Drug Interactions Barbiturates, narcotics, hydroxyzine prolong recovery from anesthesia

Stability Do not mix with barbiturates or diazepam → precipitation may occur

Mechanism of Action Produces dissociative anesthesia by direct action on the cortex and limbic system

Pharmacodynamics Following single dose, unconsciousness lasts for 10-15 minutes and analgesia persists for 30-40 minutes, amnesia may persist for 1-2 hours

Usual Dosage

Children:
- Oral: 6-10 mg/kg for 1 dose (mixed in 0.2-0.3 mL/kg of cola or other beverage) given 30 minutes before the procedure
- I.M.: 3-7 mg/kg
- I.V.: Range: 0.5-2 mg/kg, use smaller doses (0.5-1 mg/kg) for sedation for minor procedures; usual induction dosage: 1-2 mg/kg
- Continuous I.V. infusion: Sedation: 5-20 μg/kg/minute

Adults:
- I.M.: 3-8 mg/kg
- I.V.: Range: 1-4.5 mg/kg; usual induction dosage: 1-2 mg/kg

Children and Adults: Maintenance: Supplemental doses of ⅓ to ½ of initial dose

Administration I.V.: Do not exceed 0.5 mg/kg/minute or give faster than 60 seconds; do not exceed final concentration of 2 mg/mL

Monitoring Parameters Cardiovascular effects, heart rate, blood pressure, respiratory rate, transcutaneous O_2 saturation

Additional Information Used in combination with anticholinergic agents to ↓ hypersalivation

Dosage Forms Injection: 10 mg/mL (20 mL, 25 mL, 50 mL); 50 mg/mL (10 mL); 100 mg/mL (5 mL)

References

Gutstein HB, Johnson KL, Heard MN, et al, "Oral Ketamine Premedication in Children," *Anesthesiology*, 1992, 76(1):28-33.
Tobias JD, Phipps S, Smith B, et al, "Oral Ketamine Premedication to Alleviate the Distress of Invasive Procedures in Pediatric Oncology Patients," *Pediatrics*, 1992, 90(4):537-41.

Ketoconazole (kee toe koe' na zole)

Brand Names Nizoral®

Therapeutic Category Antifungal Agent, Systemic; Antifungal Agent, Topical

Use Treatment of susceptible fungal infections, including candidiasis, oral thrush, blastomycosis, histoplasmosis, coccidioidomycosis, paracoccidioidomycosis, chronic mucocutaneous candidiasis, as well as certain recalcitrant cutaneous dermatophytoses; used topically for treatment of tinea corporis, tinea cruris, tinea versicolor, and cutaneous candidiasis

Pregnancy Risk Factor C

Contraindications Hypersensitivity to ketoconazole or any component; CNS fungal infections (due to poor CNS penetration); concomitant administration of astemizole or terfenadine

Warnings Has been associated with hepatotoxicity, including some fatalities; perform periodic liver function tests; high doses of ketoconazole may depress adrenocortical function; risk of serious cardiac arrhythmias in patients receiving ketoconazole and astemizole or ketoconazole and terfenadine

Precautions Gastric acidity is necessary for the dissolution and absorption of ketoconazole; avoid concomitant (within 2 hours) administration of antacids, H_2-blockers, anticholinergics; use with caution in patients with impaired hepatic function

Adverse Reactions

Central nervous system: Lethargy, nervousness, headache, dizziness
Dermatologic: Pruritus, rash
Endocrine & metabolic: Adrenocortical insufficiency, gynecomastia
Gastrointestinal: Nausea, vomiting, abdominal discomfort, GI bleeding
Hepatic: Hepatotoxicity
Local: Irritation, stinging
Renal & genitourinary: Oligospermia

Drug Interactions Drugs that affect absorption (raise gastric pH) such as antacids, H_2 receptor blockers; drugs that ↓ serum concentrations of ketoconazole (rifampin, isoniazid); drug concentrations that are ↑ by ketoconazole (phenytoin, astemizole, cyclosporine, theophylline, terfenadine, warfarin); drugs that cause hepatotoxicity

Mechanism of Action Alters the permeability of the cell wall; inhibits fungal biosynthesis of triglycerides and phospholipids; inhibits several fungal enzymes that results in a build-up of toxic concentrations of hydrogen peroxide

Pharmacokinetics

Absorption: Oral: Rapid (~75%)
Distribution: Minimal into the CNS
Protein binding: 93% to 96%
Metabolism: Partially metabolized in the liver by enzymes to inactive compounds
Bioavailability: Decreases as pH of the gastric contents increase
Half-life, biphasic:
 Initial: 2 hours
 Terminal: 8 hours
Peak serum levels: Within 1-2 hours
Elimination: Excreted primarily in the feces (57%) with smaller amounts excreted in the urine (13%)
Not dialyzable (0% to 5%)

Usual Dosage

Children: Oral: 5-10 mg/kg/day divided every 12-24 hours until lesions clear; not to exceed 800 mg/day

Adults:
 Oral: 200-400 mg/day as a single daily dose
 Topical: Rub gently into the affected area once daily to twice daily

Monitoring Parameters Liver function tests, signs of adrenal dysfunction

Patient Information Cream is for topical application to the skin only; avoid contact with the eye; avoid taking antacids or H_2 antagonists at the same time as oral ketoconazole

Nursing Implications Administer 2 hours prior to antacids or H_2 receptor antagonists to prevent decreased ketoconazole absorption

Additional Information Cream contains sodium sulfite

Dosage Forms

Cream: 2% (15 g, 30 g, 60 g)
Shampoo: 2% (120 mL)
Suspension, oral: 100 mg/5 mL (120 mL)
Tablet: 200 mg

References

Ginsburg AM, McCracken GH Jr, and Olsen K, "Pharmacology of Ketoconazole Suspension in Infants and Children," *Antimicrob Agents Chemother*, 1983, 23(5):787-9.

Herrod HG, "Chronic Mucocutaneous Candidiasis in Childhood and Complications of non-Candida Infection: A Report of the Pediatric Immunodeficiency Collaborative Study Group," *J Pediatr*, 1990, 116(3):377-82.

Ketorolac Tromethamine (kee' toe role ak)

Brand Names Toradol®

Therapeutic Category Analgesic, Non-Narcotic; Anti-inflammatory Agent; Antipyretic; Nonsteroidal Anti-Inflammatory Agent (NSAID), Oral; Nonsteroidal Anti-Inflammatory Agent (NSAID), Parenteral

Use Short-term management of moderate to severe pain, including postoperative pain, visceral pain associated with cancer, pain associated with trauma, renal colic

(Continued)

Ketorolac Tromethamine *(Continued)*

Pregnancy Risk Factor C

Contraindications Hypersensitivity to ketorolac or in patients with nasal polyps, angioedema or bronchospastic reactions to aspirin or other NSAIDs

Precautions Use with caution and reduce dose in patients with decreased renal function; hepatic impairment; CHF; patients in whom prolongation of bleeding time would cause adverse effects; not recommended after plastic or neurosurgery due to increased risk of bleeding

Adverse Reactions Total incidence: 39%

Cardiovascular: Edema (<1%)

Central nervous system: Somnolence or drowsiness (3% to 14%); dizziness and headache (1% to 3%); insomnia, euphoria, hallucinations, malaise (<1%)

Dermatologic: Purpura

Gastrointestinal: Dyspepsia, nausea, diarrhea, GI pain (3% to 9%); peptic ulcer, melena, rectal bleeding, constipation (<1%)

Hematologic: Inhibits platelet aggregation, may prolong bleeding time

Hepatic: Elevation of liver enzyme tests

Ocular: Blurred vision

Renal: Oliguria, urinary frequency; interstitial nephritis, acute renal failure (rare)

Sensitivity reactions: Urticaria, dyspnea, wheezing, chills

Miscellaneous: Pain at injection site (2% to 4%)

Drug Interactions Warfarin, lithium, methotrexate, salicylates

Stability Protect from light; color change indicates degradation

Mechanism of Action Inhibits prostaglandin synthesis by decreasing the activity of the enzyme, cyclo-oxygenase, which results in decreased formation of prostaglandin precursors

Pharmacodynamics Analgesia:

Onset of effect: Within 10 minutes

Peak: 75-150 minutes

Duration: 6-8 hours

Pharmacokinetics

Distribution: Crosses placenta; crosses into breast milk, poor penetration into CSF; follows two-compartment model

Protein binding: 99%

Metabolism: Metabolized in the liver; undergoes hydroxylation and glucuronide conjugation; in children 4-8 years, V_{dss} and plasma clearance were twice as high as adults, but terminal half-life was similar

Half-life, terminal:

- Children 1-7 years: 5.6 hours
- Adults: 4-6 hours
- With renal impairment: 9-10 hours

Peak concentrations: I.M.: 30-60 minutes

Elimination: Renal excretion, 58% to 61% appears in urine as unchanged drug

Usual Dosage Note: The use of ketorolac in children and the I.V. route of administration is outside of product labeling

Children <18 years: Dosing guidelines not established; doses of 0.5 mg/kg/dose (range: 0.2-0.9 mg/kg/dose) have been used in studies in children 3-15 years of age; most studies are single-dose studies, every 6-hour dosing appears reasonable based on pharmacokinetics, however, further studies with multiple doses are needed; do not exceed adult doses

Adults:

- Oral: 10 mg every 4-6 hours; maximum: 40 mg/day
- I.M.:
  - <50 kg: 30 mg loading dose then 15 mg every 6 hours; maximum dose in the first 24 hours: 150 mg; maximum dose after 24 hours: 120 mg/24 hours
  - >50 kg: 30-60 mg loading dose then 15-30 mg every 6 hours

Monitoring Parameters Signs of pain relief, such as increased appetite and activity; BUN, serum creatinine, liver enzymes, occult blood loss, U/A

Reference Range Serum concentration: Therapeutic: 0.3-5 μg/mL; Toxic: >5 μg/mL

Additional Information First parenteral NSAID for analgesia; 30 mg provides the analgesia comparable to 12 mg of morphine or 100 mg of meperidine; diarrhea, pallor, vomiting, and labored breathing may occur with overdose

Dosage Forms

Injection, single-dose syringes: 15 mg/mL (1 mL); 30 mg/mL (1 mL, 2 mL)

Tablet: 10 mg

References

Maunuksela E, Kokki H, and Bullingham RES, "Comparison of Intravenous Ketorolac With Morphine for Postoperative Pain in Children," *Clin Pharmacol Ther*, 1992, 52(4):436-43.

Watcha MF, Jones MB, Lagueruela RG, et al, "Comparison of Ketorolac and Morphine as Adjuvants During Pediatric Surgery," *Anesthesiology*, 1992, 76(3):368-72.

Key-Pred® *see* Prednisolone *on page 476*

Key-Pred-SP® *see* Prednisolone *on page 476*

KI *see* Potassium Iodide *on page 471*

Kinesed® *see* Hyoscyamine, Atropine, Scopolamine and Phenobarbital *on page 299*

Klonopin™ *see* Clonazepam *on page 142*

K-Lor™ *see* Potassium Chloride *on page 469*

Klor-con® *see* Potassium Chloride *on page 469*

Klorvess® *see* Potassium Chloride *on page 469*

Klotrix® *see* Potassium Chloride *on page 469*

K-Lyte/CL® *see* Potassium Chloride *on page 469*

Kōate®-HP *see* Antihemophilic Factor, Human *on page 55*

Kōate®-HS *see* Antihemophilic Factor, Human *on page 55*

KoGENate® *see* Antihemophilic Factor, Human *on page 55*

Kolyum® *see* Potassium Gluconate *on page 470*

Konakion® *see* Phytonadione *on page 458*

Kondremul® [OTC] *see* Mineral Oil *on page 390*

Konsyl® [OTC] *see* Psyllium *on page 498*

Konsyl-D® [OTC] *see* Psyllium *on page 498*

Konȳne® 80 *see* Factor IX Complex (Human) *on page 239*

K-PHOS® Neutral *see* Potassium Phosphate *on page 472*

K-Tab® *see* Potassium Chloride *on page 469*

Ku-Zyme® HP *see* Pancrelipase *on page 431*

Kwell® *see* Lindane *on page 344*

***L*-3-Hydroxytyramine** *see* Levodopa *on page 338*

Labetalol Hydrochloride (la bet' a lole)

Related Information

Overdose and Toxicology Information *on page 696-700*

Brand Names Normodyne®; Trandate®

Synonyms Ibidomide Hydrochloride

Therapeutic Category Alpha-/Beta- Adrenergic Blocker; Antihypertensive

Use Treatment of mild to severe hypertension; I.V. for hypertensive emergencies

Pregnancy Risk Factor C

Contraindications Asthma, cardiogenic shock, uncompensated congestive heart failure, bradycardia, pulmonary edema, or heart block

Warnings Orthostatic hypotension may occur with I.V. administration; patient should remain supine during and for up to three hours after I.V. administration

Precautions Paradoxical increase in blood pressure has been reported with treatment of pheochromocytoma or clonidine withdrawal syndrome; use with extreme caution in patients with hyper-reactive airway disease, congestive heart failure, diabetes mellitus, hepatic dysfunction

(Continued)

Labetalol Hydrochloride *(Continued)*

Adverse Reactions

Cardiovascular: Orthostatic hypotension especially with I.V. administration, edema, congestive heart failure, A-V conduction disturbances (but less than with propranolol), bradycardia

Central nervous system: Drowsiness, fatigue, paresthesia, dizziness, behavior disorders, headache, reversible myopathy has been reported in 2 children

Dermatologic: Tingling in scalp or skin (transient with initiation of therapy), rash

Gastrointestinal: Nausea, dry mouth

Renal & genitourinary: Sexual dysfunction, urinary problems

Respiratory: Bronchospasm, nasal congestion

Drug Interactions Cimetidine may potentiate labetalol action; additive hypotensive effects with other hypotensive drugs; halothane → synergistic hypotension

Stability Stable in D_5W, saline for 24 hours; incompatible with $NaHCO_3$; most stable in pH of 2-4

Mechanism of Action Blocks alpha, $beta_1$- and $beta_2$-adrenergic receptor sites; elevated renins are reduced

Pharmacodynamics

Onset of action:

- Oral: 20 minutes to 2 hours
- I.V.: 2-5 minutes

Peak effect:

- Oral: 1-4 hours
- I.V.: 5-15 minutes

Duration:

- Oral: 8-24 hours (dose dependent)
- I.V.: 2-4 hours

Pharmacokinetics

Distribution: Crosses the placenta; small amounts in breast milk

V_d:

- Adults: 3-16 L/kg
- Mean: 9.4 L/kg

Protein-binding: 50%

Metabolism: Metabolized in liver primarily via glucuronide conjugation; extensive first pass effect

Bioavailability: Oral: 25%; increased bioavailability with liver disease, elderly and concurrent cimetidine

Half-life: 6-8 hours

Elimination: Possible ↓ clearance in neonates/infants; <5% excreted in urine unchanged

Usual Dosage

Children: Limited information regarding labetalol use in pediatric patients is currently available in the literature.

Oral: Some centers recommend initial oral doses of 4 mg/kg/day in 2 divided doses. (Reported oral doses have started at 3 mg/kg/day and 20 mg/kg/day and have increased up to 40 mg/kg/day.)

I.V., intermittent bolus doses of 0.3-1 mg/kg/dose have been reported

Treatment of pediatric hypertensive emergencies: Initial continuous infusions of 0.4-1 mg/kg/hour with a maximum of 3 mg/kg/hour have been used; one study used initial bolus dose of 0.2-1 mg/kg (maximum: 20 mg, mean: 0.5 mg/kg) followed by a continuous infusion of 0.25-1.5 mg/kg/hour (mean: 0.78 mg/kg/hour)

Due to limited documentation of its use, labetalol should be initiated cautiously in pediatric patients with careful dosage adjustment and blood pressure monitoring.

Adults:

Oral: Initial: 100 mg twice daily, may increase as needed every 2-3 days by 100 mg until desired response is obtained; usual dose: 200-400 mg twice daily; not to exceed 2.4 g/day

I.V.: 20 mg or 1-2 mg/kg whichever is lower; may give 40-80 mg at 10-minute intervals, up to 300 mg total dose

I.V. infusion: Initial: 2 mg/minute; titrate to response

Administration IVP: Give over 2-3 minutes

Monitoring Parameters Blood pressure, heart rate

Test Interactions False-positive urine catecholamines, VMA if measured by fluorometric or photometric methods; use HPLC or specific catecholamine radioenzymatic technique

Nursing Implications Instruct patient regarding compliance; do **not** abruptly withdraw medication in patients with ischemic heart disease

Dosage Forms

Injection: 5 mg/mL (20 mL, 40 mL, 60 mL)

Tablet: 100 mg, 200 mg, 300 mg

References

Bunchman TE, Lynch RE, and Wood EG, "Intravenously Administered Labetalol for Treatment of Hypertension in Children," *J Pediatr*, 1992, 120(1):140-4.

Farine M, and Arbus GS, "Management of Hypertensive Emergencies in Children," *Pediatr Emerg Care*, 1989, 5(1):51-5.

Ishisaka DY, Yonan CD, Housel BF, "Labetalol for Treatment of Hypertension in a Child," *Clin Pharm*, 1991, 10(7):500-1 (case report).

Jones SE, "Coarctation in Children. Controlled Hypotension Using Labetalol and Halothane," *Anaesthesia*, 1979, 34(10):1052-5.

Jureidini KF, "Oral Labetalol in a Child With Phaeochromocytoma and Five Children With Renal Hypertension," *J Med*, Aust NZ, 1980, 10:479 (abstract).

Mueller JB and Solhaug MJ, "Labetalol in Pediatric Hypertensive Emergencies," *Pediatr Res*, 1988, 23(Pt 2):543A (abstract).

Wesley AG, Hariparsad D, Pather M, et al, "Labetalol in Tetanus. The Treatment of Sympathetic Nervous System Overactivity," *Anaesthesia*, 1983, 38(3):243-9.

Lacri-Lube® [OTC] *see* Ocular Lubricant *on page 423*

Lactinex® [OTC] *see Lactobacillus acidophilus* and *Lactobacillus bulgaricus on this page*

Lactobacillus acidophilus and *Lactobacillus bulgaricus*

Brand Names Bacid® [OTC]; Lactinex® [OTC]; More-Dophilus® [OTC]

Therapeutic Category Antidiarrheal

Use Uncomplicated diarrhea particularly that caused by antibiotic therapy; re-establish normal physiologic and bacterial flora of the intestinal tract

Pregnancy Risk Factor NR

Contraindications Allergy to milk or lactose

Warnings Discontinue if high fever present

Adverse Reactions Gastrointestinal: Intestinal flatus

Stability Store in the refrigerator

Mechanism of Action Creates an environment unfavorable to potentially pathogenic fungi or bacteria through the production of lactic acid, and favors establishment of an aciduric flora, thereby suppressing the growth of pathogenic microorganisms; helps re-establish normal intestinal flora

Pharmacokinetics

Absorption: Not orally absorbed

Distribution: Locally, primarily in the colon

Elimination: Excreted in the feces

Usual Dosage Children and Adults: Oral:

Granules: 1 packet added to or taken with cereal, food, milk, fruit juice, or water, 3-4 times/day

Tablet, chewable: 4 tablets 3-4 times/day; may follow each dose with a small amount of milk, fruit juice, or water

Recontamination protocol for BMT unit: 1 packet 3 times/day for 6 doses for those patients who refuse yogurt.

Nursing Implications Granules or contents of capsules may be added to or given with cereal, food, milk, fruit juice, or water

Dosage Forms

Capsule: 50's, 100's

Granules: 1 g/packet (12 packets/box)

Powder: 12 oz

Tablet, chewable: 50's

Lactoflavin *see* Riboflavin *on page 512*

Lactulose (lak' tyoo lose)

Brand Names Cephulac®; Cholac®; Chronulac®; Constilac®; Constulose®; Duphalac®; Enulose®; Lactulose PSE®

Therapeutic Category Ammonium Detoxicant; Laxative, Miscellaneous

Use Adjunct in the prevention and treatment of portal-systemic encephalopathy (PSE); treatment of chronic constipation

Pregnancy Risk Factor C

Contraindications Patients with galactosemia

Precautions Use with caution in patients with diabetes mellitus

Adverse Reactions Gastrointestinal: Flatulence, abdominal discomfort, diarrhea, nausea, vomiting

Drug Interactions Oral antibiotics, laxatives, nonabsorbable antacids

Mechanism of Action The bacterial degradation of lactulose resulting in an acidic pH inhibits the diffusion of NH_3 into the blood by causing the conversion of NH_3 to NH_4+; also enhances the diffusion of NH_3 from the blood into the gut where conversion to NH_4+ occurs; produces an osmotic effect in the colon with resultant distention promoting peristalsis

Pharmacokinetics

- Absorption: Oral: Not absorbed appreciably; this is desirable since the intended site of action is within the colon; requires colonic flora for primary drug activation
- Metabolism: Metabolized by colonic flora to lactic acid and acetic acid
- Elimination: Excreted primarily in the feces and urine (~3%)

Usual Dosage

Prevention and treatment of portal systemic encephalopathy (PSE): Oral:
- Infants: 2.5-10 mL/day divided 3-4 times/day, adjust dosage to produce 2-3 soft stools per day
- Children: 40-90 mL/day divided 3-4 times/day, adjust dosage to produce 2-3 soft stools per day

Acute episodes of PSE: Adults: Oral: 30-45 mL at 1- to 2-hour intervals until laxative effect observed, then adjust dosage to produce 2-3 soft stools per day
- Chronic therapy: 30-45 mL/dose 3-4 times/day; titrate dose every 1-2 days to produce 2-3 soft stools per day
- Rectal: 300 mL diluted with 700 mL of water or normal saline, and given via a rectal balloon catheter and retained for 30-60 minutes; may give every 4-6 hours

Constipation: Oral:
- Children: 7.5 mL/day after breakfast
- Adults: 15-30 mL/day; increase to a maximum of 60 mL/day if needed

Monitoring Parameters Serum ammonia

Additional Information Upon discontinuation of therapy, allow 24-48 hours for resumption of normal bowel movements

Dosage Forms Syrup: 3.3 g/5 mL (15 mL, 30 mL, 237 mL, 473 mL, 946 mL, 1890 mL)

Lactulose PSE® *see* Lactulose *on this page*

Lamprene® *see* Clofazimine *on page 141*

Laniazid® *see* Isoniazid *on page 322*

Lanoxicaps® *see* Digoxin *on page 189*

Lanoxin® *see* Digoxin *on page 189*

Larodopa® *see* Levodopa *on page 338*

Lasix® *see* Furosemide *on page 265*

Lassar's Zinc Paste *see* Zinc Oxide *on page 609*

***L*-Bunolol Hydrochloride** *see* Levobunolol Hydrochloride *on page 337*

L-Carnitine *see* Levocarnitine *on page 338*

LCD *see* Coal Tar *on page 147*

LCR *see* Vincristine Sulfate *on page 602*

***L*-Dopa** *see* Levodopa *on page 338*

Ledercillin® VK *see* Penicillin V Potassium *on page 442*

Legatrin® [OTC] *see* Quinine Sulfate *on page 507*

Lente® Iletin® I *see* Insulin Preparations *on page 311*

Lente® Iletin® II *see* Insulin Preparations *on page 311*

Lente® Purified Pork Insulin *see* Insulin Preparations *on page 311*

Leucovorin Calcium (loo koe vor' in)

Brand Names Wellcovorin®

Synonyms Calcium Leucovorin; Citrovorum Factor; Folinic Acid; 5-Formyl Tetrahydrofolate

Therapeutic Category Antidote, Folic Acid Antagonist; Vitamin, Water Soluble

Use Antidote for folic acid antagonists; treatment of folate deficient megaloblastic anemias of infancy, sprue, pregnancy; nutritional deficiency when oral folate therapy is not possible

Pregnancy Risk Factor C

Contraindications Pernicious anemia

Adverse Reactions Dermatologic: Rash, pruritus, erythema

Drug Interactions Fluorouracil

Stability When powder for injection is reconstituted with bacteriostatic water for injection, stability is 7 days at room temperature

Mechanism of Action A derivative of tetrahydrofolic acid, a reduced form of folic acid; does not require a reduction reaction by an enzyme for activation, allows for purine and thymidine synthesis, a necessity for normal erythropoiesis

Pharmacodynamics Onset of action:

Oral: Within 30 minutes

I.V.: Within 5 minutes

Pharmacokinetics

Absorption: Oral, I.M.: Rapid

Distribution: Rapidly converted to (5MTHF) 5-methyl-tetrahydrofolate (active) in the intestinal mucosa and by the liver

Half-life:

Leucovorin: 15 minutes

5MTHF: 33-35 minutes

Elimination: Excreted primarily in the urine (80% to 90%) with small losses appearing in the feces (5% to 8%)

Usual Dosage Children and Adults:

Adjunctive therapy with antimicrobial agents (pyrimethamine): Oral: 2-15 mg/day for 3 days or until blood counts are normal or 5 mg every 3 days; doses of 6 mg/day are needed for patients with platelet counts $<100,000/mm^3$

Folate deficient megaloblastic anemia: I.M.: 1 mg/day

Megaloblastic anemia secondary to congenital deficiency of dihydrofolate reductase: I.M.: 3-6 mg/day

Rescue dose: I.V.: 10 mg/m^2 to start, then 10 mg/m^2 every 6 hours orally for 72 hours; if serum creatinine 24 hours after methotrexate is elevated 50% or more **or** the serum MTX concentration is $>5 \times 10^{-6}M$ (see table), increase dose to 100 mg/m^2/dose every 3 hours until serum methotrexate level is less than $1 \times 10^{-8}M$

Investigational: Post I.T. methotrexate: Oral, I.V.: 12 mg/m^2 as a single dose; post high-dose methotrexate: 100-1000 mg/m^2/dose until the serum methotrexate level is less than 1×10^{-7} molar

Administration Reconstitute 50 mg or 100 mg powder for injection vials with 5-10 mL concentration (350 mg vial requires 17 mL diluent resulting in 20 mg/mL); infuse at a maximum rate of 160 mg/minute

Monitoring Parameters Plasma MTX concentration as a therapeutic guide to high-dose MTX therapy with leucovorin factor rescue. Leucovorin is continued until the plasma MTX level is less than 1×10^{-7} molar. Each dose of leucovorin is increased if the plasma MTX concentration is excessively high (see table). With 4- to 6-hour high-dose MTX infusions, plasma drug values

(Continued)

Leucovorin Calcium *(Continued)*

in excess of 5 x 10^{-5} and 10^{-6} molar at 24 and 48 hours after starting the infusion, respectively, are often predictive of delayed MTX clearance. See table.

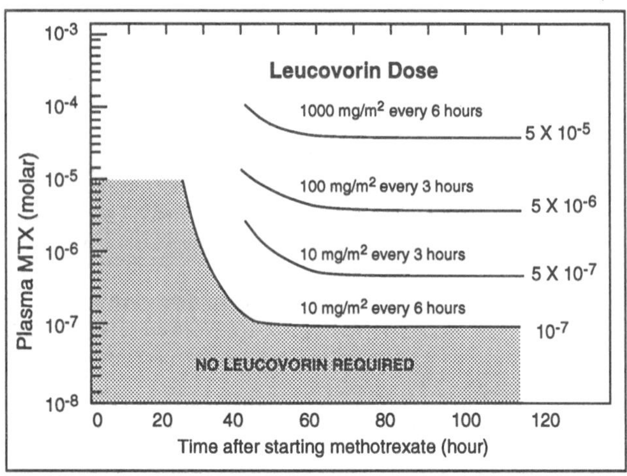

Additional Information The drug should be given parenterally instead of orally in patients with GI toxicity, nausea, vomiting, and when individual doses are >25 mg

Dosage Forms

Injection: 3 mg/mL (1 mL)

Powder for injection: 25 mg, 50 mg, 100 mg, 350 mg (10 mL)

Powder for oral solution: 1 mg/mL (60 mL)

Tablet: 5 mg, 10 mg, 15 mg, 25 mg

Leukeran® *see* Chlorambucil *on page 123*

Leukine™ *see* Sargramostim *on page 517*

Leuprolide Acetate (loo proe' lide)

Brand Names Lupron®

Synonyms Leuprorelin Acetate

Therapeutic Category Gonadotropin Releasing Hormone Analog

Use Palliative treatment of advanced prostate carcinoma; treatment of precocious puberty

Pregnancy Risk Factor X

Contraindications Pernicious anemia; hypersensitivity to leuprolide

Warnings The US Food and Drug Administration (FDA) currently recommends that procedures for proper handling and disposal of antineoplastic agents be considered; urinary tract obstruction may occur upon initiation of therapy

Precautions Use with caution in patients hypersensitive to benzyl alcohol; long-term safety of leuprolide in children has not been established

Adverse Reactions

Cardiovascular: Hot flashes, edema, cardiac arrhythmias

Central nervous system: Dizziness, paresthesia, lethargy, insomnia, headache, pain

Dermatologic: Rash

Endocrine & metabolic: Estrogenic effects (gynecomastia, breast tenderness)

Gastrointestinal: Nausea, vomiting, diarrhea, GI bleed

Hematologic: Decreased hemoglobin and hematocrit

Musculoskeletal: Myalgia

Ocular: Blurred vision

Stability Refrigerate leuprolide acetate injection; leuprolide (Depot®) powder for suspension and its diluent may be stored at room temperature; upon reconstitution, the suspension is stable for 24 hours

Mechanism of Action Continuous daily administration results in suppression of ovarian and testicular steroidogenesis due to decreased levels of LH and FSH

Pharmacokinetics

Serum testosterone levels first increase within 3 days of therapy, then decrease after 2-4 weeks with continued therapy; requires parenteral administration since it is rapidly destroyed within the GI tract

Bioavailability: Not bioavailable if given orally; bioavailability of S.C. and I.V. doses is comparable

Half-life: 3-4.25 hours

Elimination: Not well defined

Usual Dosage Refer to individual protocol

Children: Precocious puberty:

S.C.: 20-45 μg/kg/day

I.M. (Depot®) formulation: 0.15-0.3 mg/kg/dose given every 28 days; maximum dose: 7.5 mg

Adults: Advanced prostatic carcinoma:

S.C.: 1 mg/day **or**

I.M. (suspension): 7.5 mg/dose given monthly

Monitoring Parameters Serum estradiol, FSH, LH levels; closely monitor patients with prostatic carcinoma for weakness, paresthesias, and urinary tract obstruction in first few weeks of therapy

Nursing Implications Rotate S.C. injection sites frequently

Dosage Forms

Injection: 5 mg/mL (2.8 mL)

Suspension, Depot®: 3.75 mg/mL; 7.5 mg/mL

References

Kappy MS, Stuart T, and Perelman A, "Efficacy of Leuprolide Therapy in Children With Central Precocious Puberty," *Am J Dis Child*, 1988, 142(10):1061-4.

Lee PA and Page JG, "Effects of Leuprolide in the Treatment of Central Precocious Puberty," *J Pediatr*, 1989, 114(2):321-4.

Leuprorelin Acetate *see* Leuprolide Acetate *on previous page*

Leurocristine *see* Vincristine Sulfate *on page 602*

Levarterenol Bitartrate *see* Norepinephrine Bitartrate *on page 418*

Levobunolol Hydrochloride (lee voe byoo' noe lole)

Brand Names Betagan® Liquifilm®

Synonyms *L*-Bunolol Hydrochloride

Therapeutic Category Beta-Adrenergic Blocker, Ophthalmic

Use To lower intraocular pressure in chronic open-angle glaucoma or ocular hypertension

Pregnancy Risk Factor C

Contraindications Known hypersensitivity to levobunolol; bronchial asthma, severe COPD, sinus bradycardia, second or third degree A-V block

Precautions Use with caution in patients with congestive heart failure, diabetes mellitus, hyperthyroidism; contains metabisulfite

Adverse Reactions

Cardiovascular: Bradycardia, arrhythmias, hypotension

Central nervous system: Dizziness, headache

Ocular: Stinging, burning, erythema, itching, blepharoconjunctivitis, decreased visual acuity, conjunctivitis

Respiratory: Bronchospasm

Drug Interactions Systemic beta-adrenergic blocking drugs → additive toxicity

Mechanism of Action A nonselective beta-adrenergic blocking agent that lowers intraocular pressure by reducing aqueous humor production and possibly increases the outflow of aqueous humor

Pharmacodynamics

Onset of action: Following ophthalmic instillation decreases in intraocular pressure (IOP) can be noted within 1 hour

Peak effect: Within 2-6 hours

Duration: Reductions in IOP can last from 1-7 days

(Continued)

Levobunolol Hydrochloride *(Continued)*

Pharmacokinetics Elimination: Not well defined

Usual Dosage Adults: 1 drop of 0.5% solution in eye(s) once daily or 2 drops of 0.25% solution twice daily

Dosage Forms Solution: 0.25% (2 mL, 5 mL, 10 mL, 15 mL); 0.5% (2 mL, 5 mL, 10 mL, 15 mL)

Levocarnitine (lee voe kar' ni teen)

Brand Names Carnitor®; Vitacarn®

Synonyms L-Carnitine

Therapeutic Category Dietary Supplement

Use Treatment of primary carnitine deficiency

Pregnancy Risk Factor B

Adverse Reactions

Gastrointestinal: Nausea, vomiting, abdominal cramps, diarrhea

Musculoskeletal: Myasthenia (in uremic patients)

Miscellaneous: Body odor (dose related)

Drug Interactions Valproic acid, sodium benzoate

Stability Protect from light

Mechanism of Action Endogenous substance required in energy metabolism; facilitates long-chain fatty acid entry into the mitochondria; secondary carnitine deficiency may be a consequence of inborn errors of metabolism

Pharmacokinetics

Absorption: 16%

Metabolism: Major metabolites: Trimyethylamine-N-oxide and acylcarnitine

Half-life, terminal: Adults: 17.4 hours

Elimination: Renal excretion of free and conjugated metabolites (acylcarnitine)

Usual Dosage

Oral:

Children: 50-100 mg/kg/day divided 2-3 times/day, maximum 3 g/day; dosage must be individualized based upon patient response; higher dosages have been used

Adults: 330 mg to 1 g/dose 2-3 times/day

I.V.: Children and Adults: 50 mg/kg as a loading dose, followed (in severe cases) by 50 mg/kg/day infusion; maintenance: 50 mg/kg/day given every 4-6 hours, increase as needed to a maximum of 300 mg/kg/day

Administration May be given by direct I.V. infusion over 2-3 minutes or as continuous infusion

Monitoring Parameters Serum triglycerides, fatty acids, and carnitine levels

Reference Range Plasma free carnitine level: 35-60 μmol/L

Patient Information Dilute in drinks or liquid food; take with meals; consume slowly

Additional Information Levocarnitine has been used investigationally in doses of 8-16 mg/kg/day I.V. to improve utilization of I.V. fat emulsion in premature infants

Dosage Forms

Capsule: 250 mg

Injection: 1 g/5 mL (5 mL)

Liquid (cherry flavor): 100 mg/mL (10 mL)

Tablet: 330 mg

References

Helms RA, Mauer EC, and Hay WW Jr, "Effect of Intravenous L-Carnitine on Growth Parameters and Fat Metabolism During Parenteral Nutrition in Neonates," *J Parenter Enteral Nutr*, 1990, 14(5):448-53.

Levodopa (lee voe doe' pa)

Brand Names Dopar®; Larodopa®

Synonyms *L*-3-Hydroxytyramine; *L*-Dopa

Therapeutic Category Antiparkinson Agent

Use Used as a diagnostic agent for growth hormone deficiency

Pregnancy Risk Factor C

Contraindications Hypersensitivity to levodopa or any component; narrow-angle glaucoma, MAO inhibitor therapy, melanomas or any undiagnosed skin lesions

Adverse Reactions

Cardiovascular: Orthostatic hypotension, palpitations, cardiac arrhythmias

Central nervous system: Memory loss, nervousness, anxiety, insomnia, fatigue, hallucinations, dystonic movements, ataxia

Gastrointestinal: Nausea, vomiting, GI bleeding

Ocular: Blurred vision

Drug Interactions Monoamine oxidase inhibitors, pyridoxine

Mechanism of Action Increases dopamine levels in the brain; stimulates dopaminergic receptors in the basal ganglia to improve the balance between cholinergic and dopaminergic activity

Pharmacokinetics

Peak serum levels: Oral: Within 1-2 hours

Metabolism: Majority of drug is peripherally decarboxylated to dopamine; small amounts of levodopa reach the brain where it is also decarboxylated to active dopamine

Half-life: 1.2-2.3 hours

Elimination: Excreted primarily in the urine (80%) as dopamine, norepinephrine, and homovanillic acid

Usual Dosage Children: Oral (given as a single dose to evaluate growth hormone deficiency)

0.5 g/m^2 **or**

<30 lbs: 125 mg

30-70 lbs: 250 mg

>70 lbs: 500 mg

Monitoring Parameters Growth hormone level

Test Interactions False-positive reaction for urinary glucose with Clinitest®; false-negative reaction using Clinistix®; false-positive urine ketones with Acetest®, Ketostix®, Labstix®

Dosage Forms

Capsule: 100 mg, 250 mg, 500 mg

Tablet: 100 mg, 250 mg, 500 mg

References

Cara JF and Johanson HJ, "Growth Hormone for Short Stature Not Due to Classic Growth Hormone Deficiency," *Pediatr Clin North Am*, 1990, 37(6):1229-54.

Levophed® *see* Norepinephrine Bitartrate *on page 418*

Levo-T® *see* Levothyroxine Sodium *on this page*

Levothroid® *see* Levothyroxine Sodium *on this page*

Levothyroxine Sodium (lee voe thye rox' een)

Brand Names Levo-T®; Levothroid®; Levoxine®; Synthroid®

Synonyms *L*-Thyroxine Sodium; T_4 Thyroxine Sodium

Therapeutic Category Thyroid Product

Use Replacement or supplemental therapy in hypothyroidism

Pregnancy Risk Factor A

Contraindications Hypersensitivity to levothyroxine sodium or any component; recent myocardial infarction or thyrotoxicosis; uncorrected adrenal insufficiency

Warnings High doses may produce serious or even life threatening toxic effects particularly when used with some anorectic drugs

Adverse Reactions

Cardiovascular: Palpitations, tachycardia, cardiac arrhythmias

Central nervous system: Nervousness, tremors, insomnia, fever, headache

Dermatologic: Hair loss

Gastrointestinal: Diarrhea, abdominal cramps

Miscellaneous: Weight loss, increased appetite, sweating

Drug Interactions Warfarin, sympathomimetics, cholestyramine resin

Pharmacodynamics

Onset of action:

Oral: 3-5 days for therapeutic effects

I.V.: Within 6-8 hours

Pharmacokinetics

Absorption: Oral: Erratic

(Continued)

Levothyroxine Sodium *(Continued)*

Metabolism: Metabolized in the liver to tri-iodothyronine (active)
Peak serum levels: Within 2-4 hours
Elimination: Excreted in the feces and the urine

Usual Dosage

Children: Daily dosage:
Oral:
0-6 months: 8-10 μg/kg or 25-50 μg
6-12 months: 6-8 μg/kg or 50-75 μg
1-5 years: 5-6 μg/kg or 75-100 μg
6-12 years: 4-5 μg/kg or 100-150 μg
>12 years: 2-3 μg/kg or ≥150 μg
I.V., I.M.: 50% to 75% of the oral dose

Adults:
Oral: 12.5-50 μg/day to start, then increase by 25-50 μg/day at intervals of 2-4 weeks; average adult dose: 100-200 μg/day
I.V., I.M.: 50% of the oral dose

Myxedema coma or stupor: I.V.: 200-500 μg one time, then 100-300 μg the next day if necessary

Administration Dilute vial with 5 mL normal saline; use immediately after reconstitution; give by direct I.V. infusion over 2- to 3-minute period

Monitoring Parameters Serum thyroxine, resin tri-iodothyronine uptake (RT_3U), free thyroxine index (FTI)

Additional Information Levothroid® tablets contain lactose

Dosage Forms

Injection: 0.2 mg/vial (6 mL, 10 mL); 0.5 mg/vial (6 mL, 10 mL)
Tablet: 0.0125 mg, 0.025 mg, 0.05 mg, 0.075 mg, 0.088 mg, 0.1 mg, 0.112 mg, 0.125 mg, 0.15 mg, 0.175 mg, 0.2 mg, 0.3 mg

Levoxine® *see* Levothyroxine Sodium *on previous page*

Lidex® *see* Fluocinonide *on page 255*

Lidex-E® *see* Fluocinonide *on page 255*

Lidocaine and Epinephrine

Brand Names Xylocaine® With Epinephrine

Therapeutic Category Local Anesthetic, Injectable; Local Anesthetic, Topical

Use Local infiltration anesthesia

Pregnancy Risk Factor B

Contraindications Hypersensitivity to local anesthetics of the amide type

Warnings Some products contain sulfites which may cause allergic reactions

Precautions Do not use solutions in distal portions of the body (digits, nose, ears, penis); do not use large doses in patients with conduction defects (ie, heart block)

Adverse Reactions

Cardiovascular: Hypotension, bradycardia
Central nervous system: Lightheadedness, nervousness, confusion, dizziness, drowsiness, tremors, convulsions
Dermatologic: Urticaria
Ocular: Blurred vision
Otic: Tinnitus

Mechanism of Action Lidocaine blocks both the initiation and conduction of nerve impulses via decreased permeability of sodium ions; epinephrine increases the duration of action of lidocaine by causing vasoconstriction (via alpha effects) which slows the vascular absorption of lidocaine

Pharmacodynamics

Peak effect: Within 5 minutes
Duration: 2-6 hours, dependent on dose and anesthetic procedure

Usual Dosage Dosage varies with the anesthetic procedure

Children: Use lidocaine concentrations of 0.5% or 1% (or even more dilute) to decrease possibility of toxicity; lidocaine dose should not exceed 7 mg/kg/dose; do not repeat within 2 hours

Additional Information Use preservative free solutions for epidural or caudal use

Dosage Forms Injection, with epinephrine:

1:200,000: Lidocaine hydrochloride 0.5% (50 mL)
1:200,000: Lidocaine hydrochloride 1% (30 mL)
1:100,000: Lidocaine hydrochloride 1% (20 mL, 50 mL)
1:200,000: Lidocaine hydrochloride 1.5% (5 mL, 10 mL, 30 mL)
1:50,000: Lidocaine hydrochloride 2% (1.8 mL)
1:100,000: Lidocaine hydrochloride 2% (1.8 mL, 20 mL, 50 mL)
1:200,000: Lidocaine hydrochloride 2% (20 mL)

Lidocaine and Prilocaine

Brand Names EMLA®

Synonyms Eutectic Mixture of Lidocaine and Prilocaine

Therapeutic Category Local Anesthetic, Topical

Use Topical anesthetic for use on normal intact skin to provide local analgesia for minor procedures such as I.V. cannulation or venipuncture; has also been used for painful procedures such as lumbar puncture and skin graft harvesting

Pregnancy Risk Factor B

Contraindications Known hypersensitivity to lidocaine, prilocaine, any component or local anesthetics of the amide type; patients with congenital or idiopathic methemoglobinemia, infants <1 month of age, infants <12 months of age who are receiving concurrent treatment with methemoglobin-inducing agents (ie, sulfas, acetaminophen, benzocaine, chloroquine, dapsone, nitrofurantoin, nitroglycerin, nitroprusside, phenobarbital, phenytoin)

Precautions Use with caution in patients with severe hepatic disease; use with caution in patients with G-6-PD deficiency and patients taking drugs associated with drug-induced methemoglobinemia; adjust dosage by using smaller areas for application in small children or patients with impaired renal or hepatic function

Adverse Reactions

Cardiovascular: Bradycardia, angioedema, hypotension, shock

Central nervous system: Nervousness, euphoria, confusion, dizziness, drowsiness, tremors, convulsions, CNS excitation

Hematologic: Methemoglobinemia

Local: Erythema, edema, blanching, itching, rash, alteration in temperature sensation, urticaria

Ocular: Blurred vision

Otic: Tinnitus

Respiratory: Respiratory depression, bronchospasm

Drug Interactions Class I antiarrhythmic drugs (tocainide, mexiletine): toxic effects are additive; drugs known to induce methemoglobinemia

Stability Store at room temperature

Mechanism of Action Local anesthetic action occurs by stabilization of neuronal membranes and inhibiting the ionic fluxes required for the initiation and conduction of impulses

Pharmacodynamics

Onset of action: 1 hour for sufficient dermal analgesia

Peak effect: 2-3 hours

Duration: 1-2 hours after removal of the cream

Pharmacokinetics

Absorption: Related to the duration of application and to the area over which it is applied

3-hour application: 3.6% lidocaine and 6.1% prilocaine were absorbed

24-hour application: 16.2% lidocaine and 33.5% prilocaine were absorbed

Distribution: Both cross the blood-brain barrier; V_d:

Lidocaine: 1.1-2.1 L/kg

Prilocaine: 0.7-4.4 L/kg

Protein binding:

Lidocaine: 70%

Prilocaine: 55%

Metabolism:

Lidocaine: Metabolized by the liver to inactive and active metabolites

Prilocaine: Metabolized in both the liver and kidneys

Half-life:

Lidocaine: 65-150 minutes, prolonged with cardiac or hepatic dysfunction

Prilocaine: 10-150 minutes, prolonged in hepatic or renal dysfunction

Usual Dosage Children and Adults: Topical: Apply a thick layer of cream to intact skin and cover with an occlusive dressing; for minor procedures,

(Continued)

Lidocaine and Prilocaine *(Continued)*

apply 2.5 g/site for at least 60 minutes; for painful procedures, apply 2 g/10 cm^2 of skin and leave on for at least 2 hours; see table.

EMLA® Cream Maximum Recommended Application Area*
For Infants and Children
Based on Application to Intact Skin

Body Weight (kg)	Maximum Application Area (cm^2)†
<10 kg	100
10–20 kg	600
>20 kg	2000

*These are broad guidelines for avoiding systemic toxicity in applying EMLA® to patients with normal intact skin and with normal renal and hepatic function.
†For more individualized calculation of how much lidocaine and prilocaine may be absorbed, physicians can use the following estimates of lidocaine and prilocaine absorption for children and adults:
Estimated mean (±SD) absorption of lidocaine: 0.045 (±0.016) $mg/cm^2/h$.
Estimated mean (±SD) absorption of prilocaine: 0.077 (±0.036) $mg/cm^2/h$.

Patient Information Not for ophthalmic use; for external use only. EMLA® may block sensation in the treated skin.

Nursing Implications In small infants and children, an occlusive bandage should be placed over the EMLA® cream to prevent the child from placing the cream in his mouth

Additional Information Do not use on mucous membranes

Dosage Forms Cream: Lidocaine 2.5% and prilocaine 2.5% [2 Tegaderm® dressings] (5 g, 30 g)

References

Broadman LM, Soliman IE, Hannallah RG, et al, "Analgesic Efficacy of Eutectic Mixture of Local Anesthetics (EMLA®) vs Intradermal Infiltration Prior to Venous Cannulation in Children," *Am J Anaesth*, 1987, 34:S56.

Halperin DL, Koren G, Attias D, et al, "Topical Skin Anesthesia for Venous Subcutaneous Drug Reservoir and Lumbar Puncture in Children," *Pediatrics*, 1989, 84(2):281-4.

Robieux I, Kumar R, Radhakrishnan S, et al, "Assessing Pain and Analgesia With a Lidocaine-Prilocaine Emulsion in Infants and Toddlers During Venipuncture," *J Pediatr*, 1991, 118(6):971-3.

Lidocaine Hydrochloride (lye' doe kane)

Related Information

CPR Pediatric Drug Dosages *on page 614*
Emergency Pediatric Drip Calculations *on page 615*
Medications Compatible With PN Solutions *on page 649-650*

Brand Names Anestacon®; Dalcaine®; Dilocaine®; Duo-Trach®; LidoPen®; Nervocaine®; Oçtocaine®; Xylocaine®

Synonyms Lignocaine Hydrochloride

Therapeutic Category Antiarrhythmic Agent, Class Ib; Local Anesthetic, Injectable; Local Anesthetic, Topical

Use Drug of choice for ventricular ectopy, ventricular tachycardia, ventricular fibrillation; for pulseless VT or VF preferably give **after** defibrillation and epinephrine; control of premature ventricular contractions, wide-complex PSVT

Pregnancy Risk Factor B

Contraindications Known hypersensitivity to amide-type local anesthetics; patients with Adams-Stokes syndrome or with severe degree of S-A, A-V, or intraventricular heart block (without a pacemaker)

Warnings Decrease dose in patients with decreased cardiac output or hepatic disease; do not use lidocaine solutions containing epinephrine for treatment of arrhythmias; do not use preservative containing solution for I.V. use

Precautions Hepatic disease, heart failure, marked hypoxia, severe respiratory depression, hypovolemia or shock; incomplete heart block or bradycardia, atrial fibrillation

Adverse Reactions

Cardiovascular: Bradycardia, hypotension, heart block, arrhythmias, cardiovascular collapse

Central nervous system: Lethargy, coma, paresthesias, agitation, slurred speech, muscle twitching, seizures, anxiety, euphoria, hallucinations

Gastrointestinal: Nausea, vomiting

Ocular: Blurred or double vision

Respiratory: Depression or arrest

Drug Interactions Cimetidine or beta blocker → ↑ lidocaine serum concentration and toxicity

Mechanism of Action Class IB antiarrhythmic; suppresses automaticity of conduction tissue, by increasing electrical stimulation threshold of ventricle, HIS-Purkinje system, and spontaneous depolarization of the ventricles during diastole by a direct action on the tissues; blocks both the initiation and conduction of nerve impulses by decreasing the neuronal membrane's permeability to sodium ions, which results in inhibition of depolarization with resultant blockade of conduction

Pharmacodynamics

Onset of action (single bolus dose): 45-90 seconds

Duration: 10-20 minutes

Pharmacokinetics

Distribution: V_d alterable by many patient factors; ↓ V_d in CHF and liver disease

Protein binding: 60% to 80%; binds to $alpha_1$ acid glycoprotein

Metabolism: 90% metabolized in liver; active metabolites monoethylglycinexylidide (MEGX) and glycinexylidide (GX) can accumulate and may cause CNS toxicity

Half-life, biphasic:

- Alpha: 7-30 minutes
- Beta, terminal:
  - Infants, premature: 3.2 hours
  - Adults: 1.5-2 hours
- CHF, liver disease, shock, severe renal disease: Prolonged half-life

Usual Dosage

Topical: Apply to affected area as needed; maximum: 3 mg/kg/dose; do not repeat within 2 hours

Injectable local anesthetic: Varies with procedure, degree of anesthesia needed, vascularity of tissue, duration of anesthesia required, and physical condition of patient; maximum: 4.5 mg/kg/dose; do not repeat within 2 hours

Children: I.V., I.O., E.T.: Loading dose: 1 mg/kg; may repeat if needed in 10-15 minutes times 2 doses; after loading dose, start I.V. continuous infusion 20-50 μg/kg/minute. Use 20 μg/kg/minute in patients with shock, hepatic disease, cardiac arrest, mild congestive heart failure (CHF); moderate to severe CHF may require ½ loading dose and lower infusion rates to avoid toxicity.

Adults: I.V.:

- Initial bolus: 1-1.5 mg/kg; may repeat doses of 0.5-1.5 mg/kg every 5-10 minutes if needed to a total of 3 mg/kg
- Continuous infusion: 2-4 mg/minute
- Ventricular fibrillation (after defibrillation and epinephrine): Initial dose: 1.5 mg/kg, may repeat boluses as above; follow with continuous infusion after return of perfusion
- Prevention of ventricular fibrillation: I.V.: Initial bolus: 0.5 mg/kg; repeat every 5-10 minutes to a total dose of 2 mg/kg
- Refractory ventricular fibrillation: Repeat 1.5 mg/kg bolus may be given 3-5 minutes after initial dose
- E.T.: 2-2.5 times the I.V. dose
- Decrease the dose in patients with CHF, acute myocardial infarction, shock, or hepatic disease

Administration

Endotracheal doses should be diluted to 1-2 mL with normal saline prior to E.T. administration

I.V.: Solutions of 40-200 mg/mL must be diluted for I.V. use; final concentration not to exceed 20 mg/mL for I.V. push or 8 mg/mL for I.V. infusion; I.V. push rate of administration should not exceed 0.7 mg/kg/minute or 50 mg/minute, whichever is less

(Continued)

Lidocaine Hydrochloride *(Continued)*

Monitoring Parameters Monitor EKG continuously; serum concentrations with continuous infusion; I.V. site (local thrombophlebitis may occur with prolonged infusions)

Reference Range Therapeutic: 1.5-5.0 μg/mL (SI: 6-21 μmol/L); potentially toxic: >6 μg/mL (SI: >26 μmol/L); toxic: >9 μg/mL (SI: >38 μmol/L)

Nursing Implications Multiple products and concentrations exist

Dosage Forms

Injection: 0.5% (50 mL); 1% (2 mL, 5 mL, 10 mL, 20 mL, 30 mL, 50 mL); 1.5% (20 mL); 2% (2 mL, 5 mL, 10 mL, 20 mL, 30 mL, 50 mL); 4% (5 mL); 10% (10 mL); 20% (10 mL, 20 mL)

Injection:

- I.M. use: 100 mg/mL (3 mL, 5 mL)
- Direct I.V.: 10 mg/mL (5 mL, 10 mL); 20 mg/mL (5 mL)
- I.V. admixture, preservative free: 40 mg/mL (25 mL, 30 mL); 100 mg/mL (10 mL); 200 mg/mL (5 mL, 10 mL)
- I.V. infusion, D_5W: 2 mg/mL (500 mL); 4 mg/mL (250 mL, 500 mL, 1000 mL); 8 mg/mL (250 mL, 500 mL)

Jelly, topical: 2% (30 mL)

Liquid, viscous: 2% (20 mL, 100 mL)

Ointment, topical: 2.5% [OTC], 5% (35 g)

Solution, topical: 2% (15 mL, 240 mL); 4% (50 mL)

References

Emergency Cardiac Care Committee and Subcommittees, American Heart Association, "Guidelines for Cardiopulmonary Resuscitation and Emergency Cardiac Care, III: Adult Advanced Cardiac Life Support" and "VI: Pediatric Advanced Life Support," *JAMA*, 1992, 268(16):2199-241 and 2262-75.

LidoPen® *see* Lidocaine Hydrochloride *on page 342*

Lignocaine Hydrochloride *see* Lidocaine Hydrochloride *on page 342*

Lindane (lin' dane)

Brand Names G-well®; Kwell®; Scabene®

Synonyms Benzene Hexachloride; Gamma Benzene Hexachloride; Hexachlorocyclohexane

Therapeutic Category Antiparasitic Agent, Topical; Scabicidal Agent; Shampoos

Use Treatment of scabies (*Sarcoptes scabiei*), *Pediculus capitis* (head lice), and *Pediculus pubis* (crab lice)

Pregnancy Risk Factor B

Contraindications Hypersensitivity to lindane or any component; premature neonates; acutely inflamed skin or raw, weeping surfaces

Warnings Avoid contact with the face, eyes, mucous membranes, and urethral meatus

Precautions Use with caution in infants and small children and patients with pre-existing seizure disorders due to its greater potential for neurologic toxicity; consider alternative therapies for the treatment of scabies in infants and children (ie, crotamiton, permethrin, or precipitated sulfur)

Adverse Reactions

Cardiovascular: Cardiac arrhythmia

Central nervous system: Dizziness, restlessness, ataxia, seizures, headache

Dermatologic: Eczematous eruptions, contact dermatitis

Gastrointestinal: Nausea, vomiting

Hematologic: Aplastic anemia

Hepatic: Hepatitis

Local: Burning and stinging

Renal & genitourinary: Hematuria

Respiratory: Pulmonary edema

Mechanism of Action Directly absorbed by parasites and ova through the exoskeleton; stimulates the nervous system resulting in seizures and death of parasitic arthropods

Pharmacokinetics

Absorption: Topical: Up to 13% is absorbed systemically

Distribution: Stored in body fat and accumulates in the brain; skin and adipose tissue may act as repositories

Metabolism: Metabolized by the liver

Half-life, children: 17-22 hours

Time to peak serum concentration: Children: Occurs 6 hours after topical application

Elimination: Excreted in urine and feces

Usual Dosage Children and Adults: Topical:

Scabies: Apply a thin layer of lotion and massage it on skin from the neck to the toes (head to toe in infants). For adults, bathe and remove the drug after 8-12 hours; for children, wash off 6-8 hours after application; for infants, wash off 6 hours after application. Do not reapply sooner than 1 week later if live mites appear.

Pediculosis: 15-30 mL of shampoo is applied and lathered for 4-5 minutes; rinse hair thoroughly and comb with a fine tooth comb to remove nits; repeat treatment in 7 days if lice or nits are still present

Patient Information For topical use only; do not apply to face; avoid getting in eyes; do **not** apply lotion immediately after a hot, soapy bath. Clothing and bedding should be washed in hot water or by dry cleaning to kill the scabies mite. Combs and brushes may be washed with lindane shampoo then thoroughly rinsed with water.

Nursing Implications Lindane lotion should be applied to dry, cool skin

Dosage Forms

Cream: 1% (60 g, 454 g)

Lotion: 1% (60 mL, 473 mL, 4000 mL)

Shampoo: 1% (60 mL, 473 mL, 4000 mL)

References

Eichenfield LF, Honig PJ, "Blistering Disorders in Childhood," *Pediatr Clin North Am*, 1991, 38(4):959-76.

Hogan DJ, Schachner L, Tanglertsampan C, "Diagnosis and Treatment of Childhood Scabies and Pediculosis," *Pediatr Clin North Am*, 1991, 38(4):941-57.

Pramanik AK and Hansen RC, "Transcutaneous Gamma Benzene Hexachloride Absorption and Toxicity in Infants and Children," *Arch Dermatol*, 1979, 115(10):1224-5.

Lioresal® *see* Baclofen *on page 74*

Lipancreatin *see* Pancrelipase *on page 431*

Liposyn® *see* Fat Emulsion *on page 239*

Liquaemin® *see* Heparin *on page 282*

Liquibid® *see* Guaifenesin *on page 278*

Liqui-Char® [OTC] *see* Charcoal *on page 121*

Liquid Antidote *see* Charcoal *on page 121*

Liquid Paraffin *see* Mineral Oil *on page 390*

Liquid Pred® *see* Prednisone *on page 477*

Lithane® *see* Lithium *on this page*

Lithium (lith' ee um)

Brand Names Cibalith-S®; Eskalith®; Lithane®; Lithobid®; Lithonate®; Lithotabs®

Therapeutic Category Antimanic Agent

Use Management of acute manic episodes, bipolar disorders, and depression

Pregnancy Risk Factor D

Contraindications Hypersensitivity to lithium or any component; severe cardiovascular or renal disease

Warnings Lithium toxicity is closely related to serum levels and can occur at therapeutic doses; serum lithium determinations are required to monitor therapy

Precautions Use with caution in patients with cardiovascular or thyroid disease; some preparations may contain tartrazine

(Continued)

Lithium *(Continued)*

Adverse Reactions

Cardiovascular: Arrhythmias, sinus node dysfunction

Central nervous system: Sedation, tremor, confusion, somnolence, seizures, fatigue, muscle weakness, headache, vertigo

Dermatologic: Rash

Endocrine & metabolic: Nephrogenic diabetes insipidus, (thirst, polyuria, polydipsia), goiter, hypothyroidism

Gastrointestinal: Nausea, diarrhea, vomiting, dry mouth

Hematologic: Leukocytosis

Musculoskeletal: Muscle hyperirritability

Drug Interactions Concomitant use of lithium with thiazide diuretics or nonsteroidal anti-inflammatory drugs (NSAIDs) may decrease renal excretion and enhance lithium toxicity; lithium and iodide salts (or iodine) → ↑ hypothyroid effects

Mechanism of Action Alters cation transport across cell membrane in nerve and muscle cells and influences reuptake of serotonin and/or norepinephrine

Pharmacokinetics

Distribution: Crosses the placenta; appears in breast milk at 35% to 50% the concentrations in serum

Adults:

V_d: Initial: 0.3-0.4 L/kg

V_{dss}: 0.7-1 L/kg

Half-life, terminal: Adults: 18-24 hours, can increase to more than 36 hours in elderly or patients with renal impairment

Peak serum levels (nonsustained release product): Within 0.5-2 hours

Elimination: 90% to 98% of a dose is excreted in the urine as unchanged drug; other excretory routes include feces (1%) and sweat (4% to 5%)

Dialyzable (50% to 100%)

Usual Dosage Oral: Monitor serum concentrations and clinical response (efficacy and toxicity) to determine proper dose

Children: 15-60 mg/kg/day in 3-4 divided doses; dose not to exceed usual adult dosage

Adults: 300 mg 3-4 times/day; usual maximum maintenance dose: 2.4 g/day

Dosing adjustment in renal impairment:

Cl_{cr} 10-50 mL/minute: Administer 50% to 75% of normal dose

Cl_{cr} <10 mL/minute: Administer 25% to 50% of normal dose

Monitoring Parameters Serum lithium every 3-4 days during initial therapy; draw lithium serum concentrations 8-12 hours postdose; renal, hepatic, thyroid and cardiovascular function; CBC with differential, urinalysis

Reference Range Therapeutic: Acute mania: 0.6-1.5 mEq/L (SI: 0.6-1.5 mmol/L); protection against future episodes in most patients with bipolar disorder: 0.8-1 (SI: 0.8-1 mmol/L). A higher rate of relapse is described in subjects who are maintained below 0.4 mEq/L (SI: 0.4 mmol/L); Toxic: >2 mEq/L (SI: >2 mmol/L)

Nursing Implications Avoid dehydration; give with meals to avoid GI upset

Additional Information Do not crush or chew slow or extended release dosage form; swallow whole; avoid changes in sodium content of diet

Dosage Forms

Capsule, as carbonate: 150 mg, 300 mg, 600 mg

Syrup, as citrate: 300 mg/5 mL (5 mL, 10 mL, 480 mL)

Tablet, as carbonate: 300 mg

Tablet:

Controlled release, as carbonate: 450 mg

Slow release, as carbonate: 300 mg

Lithobid® *see* Lithium *on previous page*

Lithonate® *see* Lithium *on previous page*

Lithotabs® *see* Lithium *on previous page*

Lofene® *see* Diphenoxylate and Atropine *on page 196*

Logen® *see* Diphenoxylate and Atropine *on page 196*

Lomanate® *see* Diphenoxylate and Atropine *on page 196*

Lomodix® *see* Diphenoxylate and Atropine *on page 196*

Lomotil® *see* Diphenoxylate and Atropine *on page 196*

Lomustine (loe mus' teen)

Related Information

Emetogenic Potential of Single Chemotherapeutic Agents *on page 655*

Brand Names CeeNU®

Synonyms CCNU

Therapeutic Category Antineoplastic Agent

Use Treatment of brain tumors, Hodgkin's and non-Hodgkin's lymphomas

Pregnancy Risk Factor D

Contraindications Hypersensitivity to lomustine or any component

Warnings The US Food and Drug Administration (FDA) currently recommends that procedures for proper handling and disposal for antineoplastic agents be considered. Bone marrow depression, notably thrombocytopenia and leukopenia, may lead to bleeding and overwhelming infections in an already compromised patient; nadir: ~6 weeks; do not give courses more frequently than every 6 weeks because the toxicity is cumulative

Precautions Use with caution in patients with depressed platelet, leukocyte or erythrocyte counts

Adverse Reactions

Central nervous system: Disorientation, lethargy, ataxia

Dermatologic: Alopecia

Gastrointestinal: Nausea, vomiting

Hematologic: Anemia, thrombocytopenia, myelosuppression (occurs 4-6 weeks after a dose and may persist 1-2 weeks)

Hepatic: Hepatotoxicity

Musculoskeletal: Dysarthria

Renal & genitourinary: Renal failure

Respiratory: Pulmonary fibrosis with cumulative doses >600 mg

Mechanism of Action Inhibits DNA and RNA synthesis via carbamylation of DNA polymerase, alkylation of DNA, and alteration of RNA, proteins, and enzymes

Pharmacokinetics

Absorption: Completely absorbed from the GI tract with rapid conversion to its metabolites; enterohepatically recycled

Protein binding: 50%

Metabolism: Metabolized in the liver by hydroxylation producing at least 2 active metabolites

Half-life, terminal (active metabolite): 1.3-2 days

Peak serum levels (of active metabolite): Within 3 hours

Elimination: Excreted in the urine, feces (<5%) and in the expired air (<10%)

Usual Dosage Oral (refer to individual protocol):

Children: 75-150 mg/m^2 as a single dose every 6 weeks; subsequent doses are readjusted after initial treatment according to platelet and leukocyte counts

Adults: 100-130 mg/m^2 as a single dose every 6 weeks; readjust after initial treatment according to platelet and leukocyte counts

Monitoring Parameters CBC with differential and platelet count, hepatic and renal function tests, pulmonary function tests

Patient Information Take with fluids on an empty stomach, no food or drink for 2 hours after administration; notify physician if fever, sore throat, bleeding, or bruising occur

Dosage Forms

Capsule: 10 mg, 40 mg, 100 mg

Dose Pack: 10 mg (2s); 100 mg (2s); 40 mg (2s)

References

Berg SL, Grisell DL, DeLaney TF, et al, "Principles of Treatment of Pediatric Solid Tumors," *Pediatr Clin North Am*, 1991, 38(2):249-67.

Loniten® *see* Minoxidil *on page 390*

Lonox® *see* Diphenoxylate and Atropine *on page 196*

Loperamide Hydrochloride (loe per' a mide)

Brand Names Imodium®; Imodium® A-D [OTC]; Kaopectate® II [OTC]; Pepto® Diarrhea Control [OTC

Therapeutic Category Antidiarrheal

Use Treatment of acute diarrhea and chronic diarrhea associated with inflammatory bowel disease; chronic functional diarrhea (idiopathic), chronic diarrhea caused by bowel resection or organic lesions; to decrease the volume of ileostomy discharge

Pregnancy Risk Factor B

Contraindications Hypersensitivity to loperamide or any component; patients who must avoid constipation; diarrhea resulting from some infections; patients with pseudomembranous colitis

Adverse Reactions

Central nervous system: Sedation, fatigue, dizziness

Dermatologic: Rash

Gastrointestinal: Nausea, vomiting, constipation, abdominal cramping, dry mouth

Mechanism of Action Acts directly on intestinal muscles to inhibit peristalsis and prolong transit time

Pharmacodynamics Onset of action: Within 30-60 minutes

Pharmacokinetics

Absorption: Oral: <1%

Protein binding: 97%

Metabolism: Hepatic (>50%) to inactive compounds

Half-life: 9-14 hours

Elimination: Fecal and urinary (1%) excretion of metabolites and unchanged drug (30% to 40%)

Usual Dosage Oral:

Children:

- Acute diarrhea: Initial doses (in first 24 hours):
  - 2-6 years: 1 mg 3 times/day
  - 6-8 years: 2 mg twice daily
  - 8-12 years: 2 mg 3 times/day
  - After initial dosing, 0.1 mg/kg doses after each loose stool but not exceeding initial dosage
- Chronic diarrhea: 0.08-0.24 mg/kg/day divided 2-3 times/day, maximum: 2 mg/dose

Adults: 4 mg (2 capsules) initially, followed by 2 mg after each loose stool, up to 16 mg/day (8 capsules)

Dosage Forms

Capsule: 2 mg

Liquid, oral: 1 mg/5 mL (60 mL, 90 mL, 120 mL)

Tablet: 2 mg

Lopremone *see* Protirelin *on page 496*

Lorazepam (lor a' ze pam)

Related Information

Overdose and Toxicology Information *on page 696-700*

Preprocedure Sedatives in Children *on page 687-689*

Brand Names Ativan®

Therapeutic Category Antianxiety Agent; Anticonvulsant; Benzodiazepine; Sedative

Use Management of anxiety, status epilepticus, preoperative sedation, and amnesia

Restrictions C-IV

Pregnancy Risk Factor D

Contraindications Hypersensitivity to lorazepam or any component; there may be a cross sensitivity with other benzodiazepines; do not use in a comatose patient, those with pre-existing CNS depression, narrow-angle glaucoma, severe uncontrolled pain, severe hypotensive

Warnings Dilute injection prior to I.V. use with equal volume of compatible diluent; do **not** inject intra-arterially, arteriospasm and gangrene may occur; injection contains benzyl alcohol 2%, polyethylene glycol and propylene glycol, which may be toxic to newborns in high doses

Precautions Use caution in patients with renal or hepatic impairment, compromised pulmonary function, or those receiving other CNS depressants

Adverse Reactions

Cardiovascular: Bradycardia, circulatory collapse, hypertension, or hypotension

Central nervous system: Confusion, CNS depression, sedation, drowsiness, lethargy, hangover effect, dizziness, transitory hallucinations, ataxia

Gastrointestinal: Constipation, dry mouth, nausea, vomiting

Ocular: Diplopia, nystagmus

Renal & genitourinary: Urinary incontinence or retention

Respiratory: Respiratory depression

Miscellaneous: Physical and psychological dependence

Drug Interactions Other CNS or respiratory depressants may ↑ adverse effects

Stability Do not use if injection is discolored or contains precipitate; protect from light; refrigerate injectable form

Mechanism of Action Depresses all levels of the CNS, including the limbic and reticular formation, probably through the increased action of gamma-aminobutyric acid (GABA), which is a major inhibitory neurotransmitter in the brain

Pharmacodynamics Hypnosis:

Onset of effect: I.M.: ~20-30 minutes

Duration: 6-8 hours

Pharmacokinetics

Distribution: V_d:

- Neonates: 0.76 L/kg
- Adults: 1.3 L/kg

Metabolism: Metabolized primarily by glucuronide conjugation

Half-life:

- Neonates: 40.2 hours
- Older Children: 10.5 hours
- Adults: 12.9 hours

Elimination: Excreted in urine

Usual Dosage

Anxiety and sedation:

- Infants and Children: Oral, I.V.: Usual: 0.05 mg/kg/dose every 4-8 hours; range: 0.02-0.09 mg/kg given 1 hour before procedure
- Adults: Oral: 1-10 mg/day in 2-3 divided doses; usual dose: 2-6 mg/day in divided doses

Insomnia: Adults: Oral: 2-4 mg at bedtime

Preoperative: Adults: I.M.: 0.05 mg/kg administered 2 hours before surgery; maximum: 4 mg/dose; I.V.: 0.044 mg/kg 15-20 minutes before surgery; usual maximum: 2 mg/dose

Operative amnesia: Adults: I.V.: up to 0.05 mg/kg; maximum: 4 mg/dose

Status epilepticus: I.V.:

- Neonates: 0.05 mg/kg over 2-5 minutes; may repeat in 10-15 minutes (see warning regarding benzyl alcohol)
- Infants and Children: 0.1 mg/kg slow I.V. over 2-5 minutes, do not exceed 4 mg/single dose; may repeat second dose of 0.05 mg/kg slow I.V. in 10-15 minutes if needed
- Adolescents: 0.07 mg/kg slow I.V. over 2-5 minutes; maximum: 4 mg/dose; may repeat in 10-15 minutes
- Adults: 4 mg/dose given slowly over 2-5 minutes; may repeat in 10-15 minutes; usual maximum dose: 8 mg

Adjunct to antiemetic therapy: Children: I.V.: 0.04-0.08 mg/kg/dose every 6 hours as needed

Administration I.V.: Do not exceed 2 mg/minute or 0.05 mg/kg over 2-5 minutes; dilute I.V. dose with equal volume of compatible diluent (D_5W, NS, SWI)

Monitoring Parameters Respiratory rate, blood pressure, heart rate

Additional Information Oral doses >0.09 mg/kg produced ↑ ataxia without ↑ sedative benefit vs lower doses

Dosage Forms

Injection: 2 mg/mL (1 mL, 10 mL); 4 mg/mL (1 mL, 10 mL)

Solution, oral concentrated: 2 mg/mL (30 mL)

Tablet: 0.5 mg, 1 mg, 2 mg

References

Crawford TO, Mitchell WG, and Snodgrass SR, "Lorazepam in Childhood

(Continued)

Lorazepam *(Continued)*

Status Epilepticus and Serial Seizures: Effectiveness and Tachyphylaxis," *Neurology*, 1987, 37(2):190-5.

Deshmukh A, Wittert W, Schnitzler E, et al, "Lorazepam in the Treatment of Refractory Neonatal Seizures: A Pilot Study," *Am J Dis Child*, 1986, 140(10):1042-4.

Henry DW, Burwinkle JW, and Klutman NE, "Determination of Sedative and Amnestic Doses of Lorazepam in Children," *Clin Pharm*, 1991, 10(8):625-9.

McDermott CA, Kowalczyk AL, Schnitzler ER, et al, "Pharmacokinetics of Lorazepam in Critically Ill Neonates With Seizures," *J Pediatr*, 1992, 120(3):479-83.

Lorcet® *see* Hydrocodone and Acetaminophen *on page 292*

Loroxide® [OTC] *see* Benzoyl Peroxide *on page 78*

Lortab® *see* Hydrocodone and Acetaminophen *on page 292*

Lotrimin® *see* Clotrimazole *on page 145*

Lotrimin AF® [OTC] *see* Clotrimazole *on page 145*

Low-Quel® *see* Diphenoxylate and Atropine *on page 196*

L-PAM *see* Melphalan *on page 360*

LRH *see* Gonadorelin *on page 276*

L-Sarcolysin *see* Melphalan *on page 360*

***L*-Thyroxine Sodium** *see* Levothyroxine Sodium *on page 339*

Lugol's Solution *see* Potassium Iodide *on page 471*

Luminal® *see* Phenobarbital *on page 450*

Lupron® *see* Leuprolide Acetate *on page 336*

Luramide® *see* Furosemide *on page 265*

Luride® *see* Fluoride *on page 255*

Luride®-SF F Lozi-Tabs® *see* Fluoride *on page 255*

Lutrepulse® *see* Gonadorelin *on page 276*

Lymphocyte Immune Globulin

Brand Names Atgam®

Synonyms Antithymocyte Globulin (equine); ATG; Horse Anti-human Thymocyte Gamma Globulin

Therapeutic Category Immunosuppressant Agent

Use Prevention and treatment of acute allograft rejection; treatment of moderate to severe aplastic anemia in patients not considered suitable candidates for bone marrow transplantation; prevention of graft-vs-host disease following bone marrow transplantation

Pregnancy Risk Factor C

Contraindications Known hypersensitivity to ATG, thimerosal, or other equine gamma globulins; severe, unremitting leukopenia and/or thrombocytopenia

Warnings Should only be used by physicians experienced in immunosuppressive therapy or management of renal transplant patients; adequate laboratory and supportive medical resources must be readily available in the facility for patient management

Adverse Reactions

Cardiovascular: Hypotension, hypertension, tachycardia, edema
Central nervous system: Seizures, weakness, fever, headache, chills
Dermatologic: Rash, pruritus, urticaria
Gastrointestinal: Diarrhea, nausea, stomatitis
Hematologic: Leukopenia, thrombocytopenia, hemolysis, anemia
Local: Thrombophlebitis
Musculoskeletal: Arthralgia, pain in the chest, flank, or back
Renal & genitourinary: Acute renal failure
Respiratory: Dyspnea
Miscellaneous: Night sweats, lymphadenopathy, serum sickness, anaphylaxis may be indicated by hypotension, respiratory distress

Stability Store in refrigerator; dilute in 0.45% or 0.9% sodium chloride; when diluted to concentrations up to 4 mg/mL, ATG infusion solution is stable for

24 hours; use of dextrose solutions is not recommended; precipitation can occur in solutions with a low salt concentration (ie, D_5W)

Mechanism of Action May involve elimination of antigen-reactive T-lymphocytes (killer cells) in peripheral blood or alteration of T-cell function

Pharmacokinetics

Distribution: Poorly distributed into lymphoid tissues

Binds to circulating lymphocytes, granulocytes, platelets, bone marrow cells

Half-life, plasma: 1.5-12 days

Elimination: ~1% of dose is excreted in the urine

Usual Dosage Intradermal skin test is recommended prior to administration of the initial dose of ATG. Use 0.1 mL of a 1:1000 dilution of ATG in normal saline.

I.V.:

Children:

Aplastic anemia protocol: 10-20 mg/kg/day for 8-14 days, then give every other day for 7 more doses

Cardiac allograft: 10 mg/kg/day for 7 days

Renal allograft: 5-25 mg/kg/day

Children and Adults:

Rejection prevention: 15 mg/kg/day for 14 days, then give every other day for 7 more doses; initial dose should be administered within 24 hours before or after transplantation

Rejection treatment: 10-15 mg/kg/day for 14 days, then give every other day for 7 more doses

Administration Administer via central line; use of high flow veins will minimize the occurrence of phlebitis and thrombosis; administer by slow I.V. infusion through an inline filter with pore size of 0.2-1 micrometer over 4-8 hours at a final concentration not to exceed 4 mg ATG/mL

Monitoring Parameters Lymphocyte profile; CBC with differential and platelet count, vital signs during administration, renal function test

Nursing Implications Patient may need to be pretreated with an antipyretic, antihistamine, and/or corticosteroid to prevent chills and fever

Dosage Forms Injection: 50 mg/mL (5 mL)

References

Whitehead B, James I, Helms P, et al, "Intensive Care Management of Children Following Heart and Heart-Lung Transplantation," *Intensive Care Med*, 1990, 16(7):426-30.

Lyphocin® *see* Vancomycin Hydrochloride *on page 593*

Maalox® [OTC] *see* Antacid Preparations *on page 53*

Maalox® Plus Extra Strength [OTC] *see* Antacid Preparations *on page 53*

Macrobid® *see* Nitrofurantoin *on page 414*

Macrodantin® *see* Nitrofurantoin *on page 414*

Mafenide Acetate (ma' fe nide)

Brand Names Sulfamylon®

Therapeutic Category Antibacterial, Topical; Antibiotic, Topical

Use Adjunct in the treatment of second and third degree burns to prevent septicemia caused by susceptible organisms such as *Pseudomonas aeruginosa*

Pregnancy Risk Factor C

Contraindications Hypersensitivity to mafenide, sulfites, or any component

Precautions Use with caution in patients with renal impairment and in patients with G-6-PD deficiency

Adverse Reactions

Dermatologic: Erythema

Endocrine & metabolic: Hyperchloremia, metabolic acidosis

Hematologic: Bone marrow suppression, hemolytic anemia, bleeding, porphyria

Local: Burning sensation, excoriation, pain

Respiratory: Hyperventilation, tachypnea

Miscellaneous: Hypersensitivity reactions

Mechanism of Action Interferes with bacterial folic acid synthesis through competitive inhibition of para-aminobenzoic acid

(Continued)

Mafenide Acetate *(Continued)*

Pharmacokinetics

Absorption: Diffuses through devascularized areas and is rapidly absorbed from burned surface

Metabolism: Metabolized to para-carboxybenzene sulfonamide which is a carbonic anhydrase inhibitor

Peak serum levels: Attained 2-4 hours after topical application

Elimination: Excreted in the urine as metabolites

Usual Dosage Children and Adults: Topical: Apply once or twice daily with a sterile gloved hand; apply to a thickness of approximately 16 mm; the burned area should be covered with cream at all times

Monitoring Parameters Acid base balance

Patient Information Inform physician if rash, blisters, or swelling appear

Nursing Implications For external use only

Dosage Forms Cream, topical: 85 mg/g (60 g, 120 g, 435 g)

Magnesia Magma *see* Magnesium Hydroxide *on this page*

Magnesium Citrate

Brand Names Citro-Nesia™ [OTC]; Evac-Q-Mag® [OTC]

Synonyms Citrate of Magnesia

Therapeutic Category Laxative, Saline

Use To evacuate bowel prior to certain surgical and diagnostic procedures

Pregnancy Risk Factor B

Contraindications Renal failure, appendicitis, abdominal pain, intestinal impaction, obstruction or perforation

Precautions Use with caution in patients with impaired renal function

Adverse Reactions

Cardiovascular: Hypotension

Endocrine & metabolic: Hypermagnesemia

Gastrointestinal: Abdominal cramps, diarrhea, gas formation

Musculoskeletal: Muscle weakness

Respiratory: Respiratory depression

Mechanism of Action Promotes bowel evacuation by causing osmotic retention of fluid which distends the colon and produces increased peristaltic activity

Pharmacokinetics

Absorption: Oral: 15% to 30%

Elimination: Renally eliminated

Usual Dosage Cathartic: Oral:

Children:

- <6 years: 2-4 mL/kg given as a single daily dose or in divided doses
- 6-12 years: 100-150 mL

Children ≥12 years and Adults: 150-300 mL

Additional Information Magnesium content of 5 mL: 3.85-4.71 mEq

Dosage Forms Solution: 300 mL

Magnesium Hydroxide

Brand Names Phillips'® Milk of Magnesia [OTC]

Synonyms Magnesia Magma; Milk of Magnesia; MOM

Therapeutic Category Antacid; Laxative, Saline; Magnesium Salt

Use Short-term treatment of occasional constipation and symptoms of hyperacidity

Pregnancy Risk Factor B

Contraindications Patients with colostomy or an ileostomy, intestinal obstruction, fecal impaction, renal failure, appendicitis, abdominal pain

Precautions Use with caution in patients with impaired renal function

Adverse Reactions

Cardiovascular: Hypotension

Endocrine & metabolic: Hypermagnesemia

Gastrointestinal: Diarrhea, abdominal cramps

Musculoskeletal: Muscle weakness

Respiratory: Respiratory depression

Mechanism of Action Promotes bowel evacuation by causing osmotic retention of fluid which distends the colon and produces increased peristaltic activity; reacts with hydrochloric acid in stomach to form magnesium chloride

Pharmacodynamics Onset of action: Laxative action occurs in 4-8 hours

Pharmacokinetics Elimination: Absorbed magnesium ions (up to 30%) are usually excreted by kidneys, unabsorbed drug is excreted in feces

Usual Dosage Oral:

Laxative (milk of magnesia):
- $<$2 years: 0.5 mL/kg/dose
- 2-5 years: 5-15 mL/day or in divided doses
- 6-12 years: 15-30 mL/day or in divided doses
- $\geq$12 years: 30-60 mL/day or in divided doses

Antacid:
- Children: 2.5-5 mL as needed
- Adults: 5-15 mL as needed

Dosage Forms

Liquid: 390 mg/5 mL (10 mL, 15 mL, 20 mL, 30 mL, 100 mL, 120 mL, 180 mL, 360 mL, 720 mL)

Liquid, concentrate: 10 mL equivalent to 30 mL milk of magnesia USP

Suspension, oral: 2.5 g/30 mL (10 mL, 15 mL, 30 mL)

Tablet: 300 mg, 600 mg

Magnesium Sulfate

Synonyms Epsom Salts

Therapeutic Category Antacid; Anticonvulsant; Electrolyte Supplement, Parenteral; Laxative, Saline; Magnesium Salt

Use Treatment and prevention of hypomagnesemia; hypertension; encephalopathy and seizures associated with acute nephritis in children; also used as a cathartic

Pregnancy Risk Factor B

Contraindications Serious renal impairment, myocardial damage, heart block

Precautions Use with caution in patients with impaired renal function (accumulation of magnesium may lead to magnesium intoxication); use with caution in digitalized patients (may alter cardiac conduction leading to heart block)

Adverse Reactions Adverse effects with parenteral $MgSO_4$ therapy are related to the magnesium serum level; serum magnesium levels $>$3 mg/dL are associated with depressed CNS, blocked peripheral neuromuscular transmission leading to anticonvulsant effects; serum magnesium $>$5 mg/dL: depressed deep tendon reflexes, flushing, somnolence; magnesium $>$12 mg/dL: respiratory paralysis, complete heart block; $MgSO_4$ infusion can cause diarrhea

Drug Interactions Use with caution with neuromuscular blocking agents; with CNS depressants, may see additive central depressant effects

Mechanism of Action Promotes bowel evacuation by causing osmotic retention of fluid which distends the colon and produces increased peristaltic activity when taken orally; parenterally, decreases acetylcholine in motor nerve terminals and acts on myocardium by slowing rate of S-A node impulse formation and prolonging conduction time

Pharmacodynamics

Onset of action:
- Oral: Within 1-2 hours
- I.M.: 60 minutes
- I.V.: Immediately

Duration:
- I.M.: 3-4 hours
- I.V.: 30 minutes

Pharmacokinetics Elimination: Primarily excreted in the feces after oral administration; parenterally administered magnesium is rapidly eliminated by the kidneys

Usual Dosage Dose represented as $MgSO_4$ unless stated otherwise

Hypomagnesemia:
- Neonates: I.V.: 25-50 mg/kg/dose (0.2-0.4 mEq/kg/dose) every 8-12 hours for 2-3 doses
- Children:
  - Oral: 100-200 mg/kg/dose 4 times/day

(Continued)

Magnesium Sulfate *(Continued)*

I.M., I.V.: 25-50 mg/kg/dose (0.2-0.4 mEq/kg/dose) every 4-6 hours for 3-4 doses, maximum single dose: 2000 mg (16 mEq), may repeat if hypomagnesemia persists (higher dosage up to 100 mg/kg/dose $MgSO_4$ I.V. has been used)

Daily maintenance magnesium: I.V.: 30-60 mg/kg/day (0.25-0.5 mEq/kg/day)

Adults:

Oral: 3 g every 6 hours for 4 doses as needed

I.M., I.V.: 1 g every 6 hours for 4 doses or 250 mg/kg over a 4-hour period; for severe hypomagnesemia: 8-12 g $MgSO_4$/day in divided doses has been used

Daily maintenance magnesium: I.V.: 4-24 mEq (0.5-3 g)

Management of seizures and hypertension: Children: I.M., I.V.: 20-100 mg/kg/dose every 4-6 hours as needed; in severe cases doses as high as 200 mg/kg/dose have been used

Cathartic: Oral:

Children: 0.25 g/kg/dose

Adults: 10-30 g

Administration Dilute to a maximum concentration of 100 mg/mL and infuse over 2-4 hours; do not exceed 125 mg/kg/hour (1 mEq/kg/hour)

Monitoring Parameters Serum magnesium, deep tendon reflexes, respiratory rate, renal function, blood pressure

Reference Range

Children: 1.5-1.9 mg/dL ~1.2-1.6 mEq/L

Adults: 2.2-2.8 mg/dL ~1.8-2.3 mEq/L

Additional Information 500 mg $MgSO_4$ = 4.06 mEq magnesium = 49.3 mg elemental magnesium

Dosage Forms

Granules: Approximately 40 mEq magnesium/5 g (240 g)

Injection: 100 mg/mL (20 mL); 125 mg/mL (8 mL); 250 mg/mL (150 mL) 500 mg/mL (2 mL, 5 mL, 10 mL, 30 mL, 50 mL)

Solution, oral: 50% (30 mL)

References

Chernow B, Smith J, Rainey TG, et al, "Hypomagnesemia: Implications for the Critical Care Specialist," *Crit Care Med*, 1982, 10(3):193-6.

Engel J, "Normal Laboratory Values," *Pocket Guide to Pediatric Assessment*, St Louis, MO: CV Mosby, 1989, 259.

Ford DC, Leist ER and Phelps SJ, *Guidelines for Administration of Intravenous Medications to Pediatric Patients*, 3rd ed, Bethesda, MD: American Society of Hospital Pharmacists, 1988, 49.

Nichols B, "Minerals," *Pediatrics*, Norwalk, CT: Appleton & Lange, 1987, 176-7.

Mallergan-VC® With Codeine *see* Promethazine, Phenylephrine and Codeine *on page 489*

Malotuss [OTC] *see* Guaifenesin *on page 278*

Malt Soup Extract

Brand Names Maltsupex® [OTC]

Therapeutic Category Laxative, Bulk-Producing

Use Short-term treatment of constipation

Warnings Do not use when abdominal pain, nausea, or vomiting are present

Adverse Reactions Gastrointestinal: Abdominal cramps, diarrhea, rectal obstruction

Mechanism of Action Holds water in stool, reduces fecal pH

Pharmacodynamics Onset of action: Effect is usually apparent in 12-24 hours

Pharmacokinetics Hydrolyzed in the colon, metabolized by the liver

Usual Dosage Oral:

Infants >1 month:

Breast fed: 1-2 teaspoonfuls in 2-4 oz of water or fruit juice 1-2 times/day

Bottle fed: ½ to 2 tablespoonfuls/day in formula for 3-4 days, then 1-2 teaspoonfuls/day

Children 2-11 years: 1-2 tablespoonfuls 1-2 times/day

Adults ≥12 years: 2 tablespoonfuls twice daily for 3-4 days, then 1-2 tablespoonfuls every evening

Patient Information Add to warm water and stir; then add milk, water, or fruit juice until dissolved

Dosage Forms

Liquid: Nondiastatic barley malt extract 16 g/15 mL
Powder: Nondiastatic barley malt extract 16 g/heaping tablespoonful
Tablet: Nondiastatic barley malt extract 750 mg

Maltsupex® [OTC] *see* Malt Soup Extract *on previous page*

Mandelamine® *see* Methenamine *on page 369*

Manganese *see* Trace Metals *on page 574*

Mannitol (man' i tole)

Brand Names Osmitrol®; Resectisol®

Synonyms *D*-Mannitol

Therapeutic Category Diuretic, Osmotic

Use Reduction of increased intracranial pressure associated with cerebral edema; promotion of diuresis in the prevention and/or treatment of oliguria or anuria due to acute renal failure; reduction of increased intraocular pressure; promotion of urinary excretion of toxic substances

Pregnancy Risk Factor C

Contraindications Hypersensitivity to mannitol or any component; severe renal disease, dehydration, active intracranial bleeding, severe pulmonary edema, or congestion

Adverse Reactions

Cardiovascular: Circulatory overload, congestive heart failure (due to inadequate urine output and overexpansion of extracellular fluid)
Central nervous system: Convulsions, headache
Endocrine & metabolic: Fluid and electrolyte imbalance, hyponatremia or hypernatremia, hypokalemia or hyperkalemia, water intoxication, dehydration and hypovolemia secondary to rapid diuresis
Gastrointestinal: Dry mouth
Local: Tissue necrosis
Respiratory: Pulmonary edema
Sensitivity reactions: Allergic reactions

Drug Interactions Lithium

Stability Store at room temperature (15°C to 30°C); protect from freezing; crystallization may occur at low temperatures; do not use solutions that contain crystals; heating in a hot water bath and vigorous shaking may be utilized for resolubilization of crystals; cool solutions to body temperature before using; incompatible with strongly acidic or alkaline solutions; potassium chloride or sodium chloride may cause precipitation of mannitol 20% or 25% solution

Mechanism of Action Increases the osmotic pressure of glomerular filtrate, which inhibits tubular reabsorption of water and electrolytes and increases urinary output

Pharmacodynamics

After I.V. injection:
Diuresis: Onset of action: Within 1-3 hours
Reduction in ICP:
Onset of action: Within 15 minutes
Duration: 3-6 hours

Pharmacokinetics

Distribution: Remains confined to extracellular space; does not penetrate blood-brain barrier (except in very high concentrations or with acidosis)
Metabolism: Minimal amounts metabolized in the liver to glycogen
Half-life: 1.1-1.6 hours
Elimination: Primarily excreted unchanged in the urine by glomerular filtration

Usual Dosage I.V.:

Children:
Test dose (to assess adequate renal function): 200 mg/kg (maximum: 12.5 g) over 3-5 minutes to produce a urine flow of at least 1 mL/kg/hour for 1-3 hours

(Continued)

Mannitol *(Continued)*

Initial: 0.5-1 g/kg
Maintenance: 0.25-0.5 g/kg every 4-6 hours

Adults:
Test dose: 12.5 g (200 mg/kg) over 3-5 minutes to produce a urine flow of at least 30-50 mL of urine per hour over the next 2-3 hours
Initial: 0.5-1 g/kg
Maintenance: 0.25-0.5 g/kg every 4-6 hours

Administration In-line 5 micron filter set should always be used for mannitol infusion with concentrations of 20% or greater; administer test dose (for oliguria) I.V. push over 3-5 minutes; for cerebral edema or elevated ICP, administer over 20-30 minutes

Monitoring Parameters Renal function, daily fluid I & O, serum electrolytes, serum and urine osmolality. For treatment of elevated intracranial pressure, maintain serum osmolality 310-320 mOsm/kg.

Nursing Implications Avoid extravasation; crenation and agglutination of red blood cells may occur if administered with whole blood

Additional Information Mannitol 20% has an approximate osmolarity of 1100 mOsm/L and mannitol 25% has an approximate osmolarity of 1375 mOsm/L

Dosage Forms
Injection: 5% (1000 mL); 10% (500 mL, 1000 mL); 15% (150 mL, 500 mL); 20% (150 mL, 250 mL, 500 mL); 25% (50 mL, 500 mL)
Solution, urogenital: 0.54% (2000 mL)

Marbaxin® *see* Methocarbamol *on page 372*

Marcaine® *see* Bupivacaine Hydrochloride *on page 90*

Marcillin® *see* Ampicillin *on page 48*

Margesic H® *see* Hydrocodone and Acetaminophen *on page 292*

Marinol® *see* Dronabinol *on page 211*

Marmine® [OTC] *see* Dimenhydrinate *on page 193*

Matulane® *see* Procarbazine Hydrochloride *on page 483*

Maxidex® *see* Dexamethasone *on page 178*

Maxitrol® *see* Dexamethasone, Neomycin and Polymyxin B *on page 180*

Maxivate® *see* Betamethasone *on page 81*

Maxolon® *see* Metoclopramide Hydrochloride *on page 381*

Mazicon™ *see* Flumazenil *on page 252*

Measles and Rubella Vaccines, Combined *see* Immunization Guidelines *on page 660-667*

Measles, Mumps and Rubella Vaccines, Combined *see* Immunization Guidelines *on page 660-667*

Measles Virus Vaccine, Live, Attenuated *see* Immunization Guidelines *on page 660-667*

Measurin® [OTC] *see* Aspirin *on page 61*

Mebaral® *see* Mephobarbital *on page 364*

Mebendazole (me ben' da zole)

Brand Names Vermox®

Therapeutic Category Anthelmintic

Use Treatment of pinworms, whipworms, roundworms, and hookworms

Pregnancy Risk Factor C

Contraindications Hypersensitivity to mebendazole or any component

Warnings Pregnancy and children <2 years of age are relative contraindications since safety has not been established

Adverse Reactions
Central nervous system: Dizziness, fever, headache
Dermatologic: Rash, pruritus
Gastrointestinal: Diarrhea, abdominal pain, nausea, vomiting

Hematologic: Neutropenia, anemia, leukopenia
Hepatic: Transient abnormalities in liver function tests
Otic: Tinnitus
Renal & genitourinary: Hematuria

Drug Interactions Anticonvulsants such as carbamazepine and phenytoin may ↑ metabolism of mebendazole

Mechanism of Action Selectively and irreversibly blocks glucose uptake and other nutrients in susceptible adult intestine-dwelling helminths

Pharmacokinetics
Absorption: Oral: 2% to 10% of a dose is absorbed
Protein binding: 95%
Metabolism: Extensively metabolized in the liver
Half-life: 1-11.5 hours
Peak serum levels: Within 2-4 hours
Elimination: Primarily excreted in the feces as inactive metabolites with 5% to 10% eliminated in the urine
Not dialyzable

Usual Dosage Children and Adults: Oral:
Pinworms: Single chewable tablet; may need to repeat after 2 weeks

Whipworms, roundworms, hookworms: 1 tablet twice daily, morning and evening on 3 consecutive days; if patient is not cured within 3-4 weeks, a second course of treatment may be administered

Capillariasis: 200 mg twice daily for 20 days

Monitoring Parameters For treatment of trichuriasis, ascariasis, hookworm, or mixed infections, check for helminth ova in the feces within 3-4 weeks following the initial therapy

Nursing Implications Tablet can be crushed and mixed with food, swallowed whole, or chewed

Dosage Forms Tablet, chewable: 100 mg

Mechlorethamine Hydrochloride (me klor eth' a meen)

Related Information
Emetogenic Potential of Single Chemotherapeutic Agents *on page 655*
Extravasation Treatment *on page 640*

Brand Names Mustargen® Hydrochloride

Synonyms HN_2; Mustine; Nitrogen Mustard

Therapeutic Category Antineoplastic Agent

Use Combination therapy of Hodgkin's disease, brain tumors, non-Hodgkin's lymphoma, and malignant lymphomas; palliative treatment of bronchogenic, breast and ovarian carcinoma; may be used by intracavitary injection for treatment of metastatic tumors, pleural and other malignant effusions

Pregnancy Risk Factor D

Contraindications Hypersensitivity to mechlorethamine or any component; pre-existing profound myelosuppression

Warnings The US Food and Drug Administration (FDA) currently recommends that procedures for proper handling and disposal of antineoplastic agents be considered. Mechlorethamine is potentially carcinogenic and mutagenic. It may cause permanent sterility and birth defects. Extravasation of the drug into subcutaneous tissues results in painful inflammation and induration; sloughing may occur; promptly infiltrate the area with sterile isotonic sodium thiosulfate ($^1/_6$ molar) and apply a cold compress for 6-12 hours.

Precautions Use with caution in patients with myelosuppression; patients with lymphoma should receive adequate hydration, alkalinization of the urine and/or prophylactic allopurinol to prevent complications such as uric acid nephropathy

Adverse Reactions
Cardiovascular: Thrombosis
Central nervous system: Vertigo
Dermatologic: Rash, alopecia
Gastrointestinal: Nausea, vomiting
Hematologic: Myelosuppression, hemolytic anemia
Local: Thrombophlebitis
Musculoskeletal: Weakness

(Continued)

Mechlorethamine Hydrochloride *(Continued)*

Otic: Tinnitus

Miscellaneous: Hypersensitivity reactions

Stability Highly unstable in neutral or alkaline solutions; use immediately after reconstitution; discard any unused drug after 15 minutes

Mechanism of Action Alkylating agent that inhibits DNA and RNA synthesis via formation of carbonium ions; cross-links strands of DNA causing miscoding, breakage, and failure of replication

Pharmacokinetics

Absorption: Incomplete after intracavitary administration secondary to rapid deactivation by body fluids

Distribution: Following I.V. administration, the drug undergoes rapid chemical transformation and unchanged drug is undetectable in the blood within a few minutes

Half-life: <1 minute

Elimination: <0.01% of unchanged drug is recovered in the urine

Usual Dosage Refer to individual protocols

Children: MOPP: I.V.: 6 mg/m^2 on days 1 and 8 of a 28-day cycle

Adults:

I.V.: 0.4 mg/kg or 12-16 mg/m^2 for one dose or divided into 0.1 mg/kg/day for 4 days

Intracavitary: 10-20 mg or 0.2-0.4 mg/kg

Administration Administer I.V. push through a free flowing I.V. over 1-3 minutes at a concentration not to exceed 1 mg/mL

Monitoring Parameters CBC with differential and platelet count, hemoglobin

Patient Information Report to physician any pain or irritation at the site of injection, fever, sore throat, bruising, bleeding, shortness of breath, itching, or wheezing

Nursing Implications Avoid extravasation or contact with skin and eyes since mechlorethamine is a potent vesicant; sodium thiosulfate is the specific antidote for nitrogen mustard extravasations

Additional Information Myelosuppressive effects:

WBC: Severe

Platelets: Severe

Onset (days): 4-7

Nadir (days): 14

Recovery (days): 21

Dosage Forms Powder for injection: 10 mg

References

Berg SL, Grisell DL, DeLaney TF, et al, "Principles of Treatment of Pediatric Solid Tumors," *Pediatr Clin North Am*, 1991, 38(2):249-67.

Meclizine Hydrochloride (mek' li zeen)

Related Information

Overdose and Toxicology Information *on page 696-700*

Brand Names Antivert®; Antrizine®; Bonine® [OTC]; Dizmiss® [OTC]; Meni-D®; Ru-Vert-M®; Vergon® [OTC]

Synonyms Meclozine Hydrochloride

Therapeutic Category Antihistamine

Use Prevention and treatment of motion sickness; management of vertigo with diseases affecting the vestibular system

Pregnancy Risk Factor B

Contraindications Hypersensitivity to meclizine or any component; pregnancy

Precautions Use with caution in patients with angle-closure glaucoma; may impair ability to perform hazardous activities requiring mental alertness or physical coordination

Adverse Reactions

Central nervous system: Drowsiness, fatigue

Gastrointestinal: Dry mouth

Ocular: Blurred vision

Drug Interactions Additive sedation with central nervous system depressants (eg, sedative, alcohol, antihistamines)

Mechanism of Action Has central anticholinergic action and central nervous system depressant activity; decreases excitability of the middle ear labyrinth and blocks conduction in the middle ear vestibular-cerebellar pathways

Pharmacodynamics

Onset of action: Oral: Within 1-2 hours

Duration: 8-24 hours

Pharmacokinetics

Metabolism: Metabolized in the liver

Half-life: 6 hours

Elimination: Excreted as metabolites in the urine and as unchanged drug in the feces

Usual Dosage Children >12 years and Adults: Oral:

Motion sickness: 25-50 mg 1 hour before travel, repeat dose every 24 hours if needed

Vertigo: 25-100 mg/day in divided doses

Patient Information May cause drowsiness

Dosage Forms

Capsule: 15 mg, 25 mg, 30 mg

Tablet: 12.5 mg, 25 mg, 50 mg

Tablet:

Chewable: 25 mg

Film coated: 25 mg

Meclozine Hydrochloride *see* Meclizine Hydrochloride *on previous page*

Medications Compatible With PN Solutions *see page 649*

Medicinal Carbon *see* Charcoal *on page 121*

Medicinal Charcoal *see* Charcoal *on page 121*

Medihaler-Epi® *see* Epinephrine *on page 220*

Medihaler Ergotamine™ *see* Ergotamine *on page 225*

Medihaler-Iso® *see* Isoproterenol *on page 324*

Mediplast® [OTC] *see* Salicylic Acid *on page 516*

Medipren® [OTC] *see* Ibuprofen *on page 300*

Medi-Quick® Ointment [OTC] *see* Neomycin, Polymyxin B, and Bacitracin *on page 407*

Medi-Tuss® [OTC] *see* Guaifenesin *on page 278*

Medi-Tuss® AC *see* Guaifenesin and Codeine *on page 279*

Medralone® *see* Methylprednisolone *on page 379*

Medrol® *see* Methylprednisolone *on page 379*

Medroxyprogesterone Acetate

(me drox' ee proe jess' te rone)

Brand Names Amen®; Curretab®; Cycrin®; Depo-Provera®; Provera®

Synonyms Acetoxymethylprogesterone; Methylacetoxyprogesterone

Therapeutic Category Progestin

Use Secondary amenorrhea or abnormal uterine bleeding due to hormonal imbalance

Pregnancy Risk Factor D

Contraindications Thrombophlebitis; hypersensitivity to medroxyprogesterone or any component; cerebral apoplexy, undiagnosed vaginal bleeding, liver dysfunction

Precautions Use with caution in patients with mental depression, diabetes, epilepsy, asthma, migraines, renal or cardiac dysfunction

Adverse Reactions

Cardiovascular: Edema, thromboembolic disorders

Central nervous system: Depression, dizziness, nervousness

Dermatologic: Melasma, chloasma, urticaria, acne

Endocrine & metabolic: Menstrual irregularities, amenorrhea, breakthrough bleeding, breast tenderness

Hepatic: Cholestatic jaundice

Miscellaneous: Weight gain

Mechanism of Action Inhibits secretion of pituitary gonadotropins, which prevents follicular maturation and ovulation, transforms a proliferative endometrium into a secretory one

(Continued)

Medroxyprogesterone Acetate *(Continued)*

Usual Dosage Adolescents and Adults: Oral:

Amenorrhea: 5-10 mg/day for 5-10 days

Abnormal uterine bleeding: 5-10 mg for 5-10 days starting on day 16 or 21 of menstrual cycle

Test Interactions Altered thyroid and liver function tests

Additional Information I.M. dosing is recommended only for contraceptive purposes or in the treatment of endometrial or renal carcinoma

Dosage Forms

Injection, suspension: 100 mg/mL (5 mL); 150 mg/mL (1 mL); 400 mg/mL (1 mL, 2.5 mL, 10 mL)

Tablet: 2.5 mg, 5 mg, 10 mg

Medrysone (me' dri sone)

Brand Names HMS Liquifilm®

Therapeutic Category Anti-inflammatory Agent; Corticosteroid, Ophthalmic

Use Treatment of allergic conjunctivitis, vernal conjunctivitis, episcleritis, ophthalmic epinephrine sensitivity reaction

Pregnancy Risk Factor C

Contraindications Known hypersensitivity to medrysone; ocular fungal, viral, or tuberculosis infections; acute superficial herpes simplex

Warnings Effectiveness and safety has not been established in children

Precautions Prolonged use has been associated with the development of corneal or scleral perforation and posterior subcapsular cataracts; may mask or enhance the establishment of acute purulent untreated infections of the eye

Adverse Reactions

Local: Stinging, burning

Ocular: Corneal thinning, increased intraocular pressure, glaucoma, damage to the optic nerve, defects in visual activity, cataracts

Miscellaneous: Hypersensitivity reactions

Mechanism of Action Inhibits inflammatory response by suppression of migration of polymorphonuclear leukocytes and reversal of increased capillary permeability

Pharmacokinetics

Absorption: Through aqueous humor

Metabolism: Metabolized in the liver

Elimination: Excreted by the kidneys and feces

Usual Dosage Ophthalmic: Children and Adults: 1 drop in conjunctival sac 2-4 times/day up to every 4 hours; may use every 1-2 hours during first 1-2 days

Monitoring Parameters With prolonged use monitor intraocular pressure and periodic examination of lens

Nursing Implications Shake well before using; do not touch dropper to the eye

Additional Information Medrysone is a synthetic corticosteroid; structurally related to progesterone; if no improvement after several days of treatment, discontinue medrysone and institute other therapy; duration of therapy: 3-4 days to several weeks dependent on type and severity of disease; taper dose to avoid disease exacerbation

Dosage Forms Solution, ophthalmic: 1% (5 mL)

Mefoxin® *see* Cefoxitin Sodium *on page 113*

Mellaril® *see* Thioridazine Hydrochloride *on page 562*

Mellaril-S® *see* Thioridazine Hydrochloride *on page 562*

Melphalan (mel' fa lan)

Brand Names Alkeran®

Synonyms L-PAM; L-Sarcolysin; Phenylalanine Mustard

Therapeutic Category Antineoplastic Agent

Use Palliative treatment of multiple myeloma and nonresectable epithelial ovarian carcinoma; neuroblastoma, rhabdomyosarcoma, sarcomas

Pregnancy Risk Factor D

Contraindications Hypersensitivity to melphalan or any component; severe bone marrow depression; patients whose disease was resistant to prior therapy

Warnings The US Food and Drug Administration (FDA) currently recommends that procedures for proper handling and disposal of antineoplastic agents be considered; potentially mutagenic, carcinogenic, and teratogenic; produces amenorrhea

Precautions Reduce dosage or discontinue therapy if leukocyte count $<3000/mm^3$ or platelet count $<100,000/mm^3$; use with caution in patients with bone marrow suppression and impaired renal function; dosage reduction may be necessary in patients with impaired renal function

Adverse Reactions

Cardiovascular: Vasculitis

Dermatologic: Alopecia, rash, pruritus, vesiculation of skin

Endocrine & metabolic: Amenorrhea

Gastrointestinal: Nausea, vomiting, diarrhea, stomatitis

Hematologic: Leukopenia, thrombocytopenia, anemia, agranulocytosis, hemolytic anemia

Local: Burning and discomfort at injection site

Renal & genitourinary: Bladder irritation, hemorrhagic cystitis

Respiratory: Pulmonary fibrosis

Drug Interactions Cyclosporine

Stability Do not refrigerate, store at room temperature; protect from light; use within 1 hour of reconstitution

Mechanism of Action Alkylating agent that inhibits DNA and RNA synthesis via formation of carbonium ions; cross-links strands of DNA

Pharmacokinetics

Absorption: Oral: Variable and incomplete; food interferes with absorption

Distribution: Distributes throughout total body water

Half-life, terminal: 90 minutes

Peak serum levels: Oral: Within 2 hours

Elimination: 10% to 15% of a dose is excreted unchanged in the urine; after oral administration, 20% to 50% is excreted in the stool

Usual Dosage Refer to individual protocols

Children:

- I.V.: (Investigational, distributed under the auspices of the NCI for authorized studies):
  - Pediatric rhabdomyosarcoma: 10-35 mg/m^2 bolus every 21-28 days
  - Chemoradiotherapy supported by marrow infusions for neuroblastoma: 70-140 mg/m^2 on day 7 and 6 before BMT or 140-220 mg/m^2 single dose before BMT
- Oral: 4-20 mg/m^2/day for 1-21 days

Adults: Oral:

- Multiple myeloma: 6 mg/day or 10 mg/day for 7-10 days, or 0.15 mg/kg/day for 7 days
- Ovarian carcinoma: 0.2 mg/kg/day for 5 days, repeat in 4-5 weeks

Administration Reconstitute injection with special diluent 50 mg vial with special diluent to yield a 5 mg/mL solution; filter through a 0.45 μM Millex-HV filter; dilute the reconstituted solution with normal saline to a final concentration not to exceed 2 mg/mL; administer by I.V. infusion at a rate not to exceed 10 mg/minute but total infusion should be given within 1 hour

Monitoring Parameters CBC with differential and platelet count, serum electrolytes, serum uric acid

Test Interactions False-positive Coombs' test [direct]

Patient Information Notify physician if fever, shortness of breath, sore throat, bleeding, or bruising occurs

Additional Information Myelosuppressive effects:

WBC: Moderate

Platelets: Moderate

Onset (days): 7

Nadir (days): 14-21

Recovery (days): 42-50

Dosage Forms Tablet: 2 mg

References

Berg SL, Grisell DL, DeLaney TF, et al, "Principles of Treatment of Pediatric Solid Tumors," *Pediatr Clin North Am*, 1991, 38(2):249-67.

(Continued)

Melphalan *(Continued)*

Pole JG, Casper J, Elfenbein G, et al, "High-Dose Chemoradiotherapy Supported by Marrow Infusions for Advanced Neuroblastoma: A Pediatric Oncology Group Study," *J Clin Oncol*, 1991, 9(1):152-8.

Schroeder H, Pinkerton CR, Powles RL, et al, "High-Dose Melphalan and Total Body Irradiation With Autologous Marrow Rescue in Childhood Acute Lymphoblastic Leukemia After Relapse," *Bone Marrow Transplant*, 1991, 7(1):11-15.

Menadol® [OTC] *see* Ibuprofen *on page 300*

Meni-D® *see* Meclizine Hydrochloride *on page 358*

Meningococcal Polysaccharide Vaccine, Groups A, C, Y, and W-135 *see* Immunization Guidelines *on page 660-667*

Mepacrine Hydrochloride *see* Quinacrine Hydrochloride *on page 504*

Meperidine Hydrochloride (me per' i deen)

Related Information

Compatibility of Medications Mixed in a Syringe *on page 717*
Medications Compatible With PN Solutions *on page 649-650*
Narcotic Analgesics Comparison Chart *on page 721-722*
Overdose and Toxicology Information *on page 696-700*
Preprocedure Sedatives in Children *on page 687-689*

Brand Names Demerol®

Synonyms Isonipecaine Hydrochloride; Pethidine Hydrochloride

Therapeutic Category Analgesic, Narcotic

Use Management of moderate to severe pain; adjunct to anesthesia and preoperative sedation

Restrictions C-II

Pregnancy Risk Factor B (D if used for prolonged periods or in high doses at term)

Contraindications Hypersensitivity to meperidine or any component; patients receiving MAO inhibitors presently or in the past 14 days

Warnings Some preparations contain sulfites which may cause allergic reaction; use with caution in patients with renal failure or seizure disorders or those receiving high dose meperidine: normeperidine (an active metabolite and CNS stimulant) may accumulate and precipitate twitches, tremors, or seizures

Precautions Use with caution in patients with pulmonary, hepatic, or renal disorders; patients with tachycardias, biliary, colic, or increased intracranial pressure

Adverse Reactions

Cardiovascular: Palpitations, hypotension, bradycardia, peripheral vasodilation, tachycardia
Central nervous system: CNS depression, dizziness, drowsiness, sedation, increased intracranial pressure
Dermatologic: Pruritus
Endocrine & metabolic: Antidiuretic hormone release
Gastrointestinal: Nausea, vomiting, constipation
Hepatic: Biliary tract spasm
Ocular: Miosis
Renal & genitourinary: Urinary tract spasm
Respiratory: Respiratory depression
Sensitivity reactions: Histamine release
Miscellaneous: Physical and psychological dependence

Drug Interactions May aggravate the adverse effects of isoniazid; MAO inhibitors greatly potentiate the effects of meperidine: acute opioid overdosage symptoms can be seen, including severe toxic reactions; CNS depressants, tricyclic antidepressants, phenothiazines may potentiate the effects of meperidine; phenytoin may ↓ the analgesic effects

Stability Incompatible with aminophylline, heparin, phenobarbital, phenytoin, and sodium bicarbonate

Mechanism of Action Binds to opiate receptors in the CNS, causing inhibition of ascending pain pathways, altering the perception of and response to pain; produces generalized CNS depression

Pharmacodynamics Analgesia:
- Onset of action:
  - Oral, I.M., S.C.: Within 10-15 minutes
  - I.V.: Within 5 minutes
- Peak effect: Oral, I.M., S.C.: Within 1 hour
- Duration: Oral, I.M., S.C.: 2-4 hours

Pharmacokinetics
- Distribution: Crosses the placenta; appears in breast milk
- Protein binding: 65% to 75%
- Metabolism: Metabolized in liver
- Bioavailability: ~50% to 60%, ↑ bioavailability with liver disease
- Half-life, terminal:
  - Preterm infants 3.6-65 days of age: 11.9 hours (range: 3.3-59.4 hours)
  - Term infants:
    - 0.3-4 days of age: 10.7 hours (range: 4.9-16.8)
    - 26-73 days of age: 8.2 hours (range: 5.7-31.7 hours)
  - Neonates: 23 hours (range: 12-39 hours)
  - Adults: 2.5-4 hours
  - Adults with liver disease: 7-11 hours
  - Normeperidine (active metabolite): 15-30 hours; normeperidine half-life is dependent on renal function and can accumulate with high doses or in patients with ↓ renal function; normeperidine may precipitate tremors or seizures
- Elimination: ~5% meperidine eliminated unchanged in urine

Usual Dosage Doses should be titrated to appropriate analgesic effect; when changing route of administration, note that oral doses are about half as effective as parenteral dose

Children:
- Oral, I.M., I.V., S.C.: 1-1.5 mg/kg/dose every 3-4 hours as needed; 1-2 mg/kg as a single dose preoperative medication may be used; maximum: 100 mg/dose
- I.V. continuous infusion: After 0.3 mg/kg bolus, initial rate: 0.3 mg/kg/hour; titrate dose to effect; may require 0.5-0.7 mg/kg/hour

Adults: Oral, I.M., I.V.: S.C.: 50-150 mg/dose every 3-4 hours as needed

Dosing adjustment in renal impairment:
- Cl_{cr} 10-50 mL/minute: Administer 75% of normal dose
- Cl_{cr} <10 mL/minute: Administer 50% of normal dose

Administration Do not administer rapid I.V., give over at least 5 minutes; intermittent infusion: dilute to 1 mg/mL and administer over 15-30 minutes; dilute to ≤10 mg/mL for intermittent I.V. use

Monitoring Parameters Respiratory and cardiovascular status

Additional Information Decrease the dose in patients with renal or hepatic impairment; equianalgesic dóses: morphine 10 mg I.M. = meperidine 75-100 mg I.M.

Dosage Forms
- Injection:
  - Single-dose: 10 mg/mL (5 mL, 10 mL, 30 mL); 25 mg/dose (0.5 mL, 1 mL); 50 mg/dose (1 mL); 75 mg/dose (1 mL, 1.5 mL); 100 mg/dose (1 mL)
  - Multiple-dose vials: 50 mg/mL (30 mL); 100 mg/mL (20 mL)
- Syrup: 50 mg/5 mL (500 mL)
- Tablet: 50 mg, 100 mg

References

Cole TB, Sprinkle RH, Smith SJ, et al, "Intravenous Narcotic Therapy for Children With Severe Sickle Cell Pain Crisis," *Am J Dis Child*, 1986, 140(12):1255-9.

Pokela ML, Olkkola KT, Koivisto ME, et al, "Pharmacokinetics and Pharmacodynamics of Intravenous Meperidine in Neonates and Infants," *Clin Pharmacol Ther*, 1992, 52(4):342-9.

Mephenytoin (me fen' i toyn)

Related Information

Overdose and Toxicology Information *on page 696-700*

Brand Names Mesantoin®

Synonyms Methoin; Methylphenylethylhydantoin; Phenantoin

(Continued)

Mephenytoin *(Continued)*

Therapeutic Category Anticonvulsant

Use Treatment of tonic-clonic and partial seizures in patients who are uncontrolled with less toxic anticonvulsants

Pregnancy Risk Factor C

Contraindications Hypersensitivity to mephenytoin or any component

Warnings Fatal irreversible aplastic anemia has occurred

Precautions Abrupt withdrawal may precipitate seizures

Adverse Reactions

Central nervous system: Insomnia, slurred speech, dizziness, lethargy, confusion, coma, tremor, ataxia, sedation, nervousness

Dermatologic: Rash, erythema multiforme, alopecia

Endocrine & metabolic: Weight gain

Gastrointestinal: Nausea, vomiting

Hematologic: Neutropenia, leukopenia, thrombocytopenia, agranulocytosis, anemia, Hodgkin's disease-like syndrome

Hepatic: Hepatitis

Ocular: Nystagmus, blurred vision, diplopia

Sensitivity reactions: Photophobia, serum sickness

Mechanism of Action Stabilizes neuronal membranes and decreases seizure activity by increasing efflux or decreasing influx of sodium ions across cell membranes in the motor cortex during generation of nerve impulses; prolongs effective refractory period and suppresses ventricular pacemaker automaticity, shortens action potential in the heart

Usual Dosage Oral:

Children: 3-15 mg/kg/day in 3 divided doses; usual maintenance dose: 100-400 mg/day in 3 divided doses

Adults: Initial dose: 50-100 mg/day given daily; increase by 50-100 mg at weekly intervals; usual maintenance dose: 200-600 mg/day in 3 divided doses; maximum: 800 mg/day

Monitoring Parameters CBC and platelet count

Reference Range Total mephenytoin (mephenytoin plus 5-ethyl - 5-phenylhydantoin) = 25-40 μg/mL

Additional Information Usually used in combination with other anticonvulsants

Dosage Forms Tablet: 100 mg

Mephobarbital (me foe bar' bi tal)

Brand Names Mebaral®

Synonyms Methylphenobarbital

Therapeutic Category Anticonvulsant; Barbiturate; Sedative

Use Treatment of generalized tonic-clonic and simple partial seizures

Restrictions C-IV

Pregnancy Risk Factor D

Contraindications Hypersensitivity to mephobarbital or any component; pre-existing CNS depression; respiratory depression; severe uncontrolled pain; history of porphyria

Precautions Use with caution in patients with hepatic or renal impairment or respiratory diseases

Adverse Reactions

Central nervous system: Drowsiness, lethargy; paradoxical excitement (especially in children)

Dermatologic: Rash, including Stevens-Johnson syndrome or erythema multiforme

Gastrointestinal: Nausea, vomiting

Hematologic: Agranulocytosis, thrombocytopenic purpura

Miscellaneous: Psychological and physical dependence

Drug Interactions Mephobarbital is expected to have similar drug interactions as phenobarbital, since mephobarbital is metabolized in the liver to phenobarbital

Mechanism of Action Increases seizure threshold in the motor cortex; depresses monosynaptic and polysynaptic transmission in the CNS

Pharmacokinetics

Absorption: Oral: ~50%

Protein binding: 58% to 68%
Metabolism: Metabolized to phenobarbital in the liver
Half-life: 30-70 hours

Usual Dosage Epilepsy: Oral:
Children: 4-10 mg/kg/day in 2-4 divided doses
Adults: 200-600 mg/day in 2-4 divided doses

Reference Range Phenobarbital level should be in the range of 15-40 μg/mL (SI: 65-172 μmol/L)

Additional Information Sometimes used in specific patients who have excessive sedation or hyperexcitability from phenobarbital; avoid abrupt discontinuation

Dosage Forms Tablet: 32 mg, 50 mg, 100 mg

Mephyton® *see* Phytonadione *on page 458*

Mercaptopurine (mer kap toe pyoor' een)

Brand Names Purinethol®

Synonyms 6-Mercaptopurine; 6-MP

Therapeutic Category Antineoplastic Agent

Use Treatment of leukemias

Pregnancy Risk Factor D

Contraindications Hypersensitivity to mercaptopurine or any component; severe liver disease; severe bone marrow depression; patients whose disease showed prior resistance to mercaptopurine or thioguanine

Warnings The US Food and Drug Administration (FDA) currently recommends that procedures for proper handling and disposal of antineoplastic agents be considered; mercaptopurine may cause birth defects; potentially carcinogenic

Precautions Adjust dosage in patients with renal impairment or hepatic failure; patients who receive allopurinol concurrently should have the mercaptopurine dose reduced 66% to 75%

Adverse Reactions
Dermatologic: Rash, hyperpigmentation
Gastrointestinal: Mild nausea or vomiting, diarrhea, stomatitis
Hematologic: Myelosuppression
Hepatic: Hepatotoxicity
Renal & genitourinary: Renal toxicity (hyperuricemia, oliguria, hematuria)
Miscellaneous: Drug fever

Drug Interactions Allopurinol may potentiate the effect of bone marrow suppression (inhibits xanthine oxidase); warfarin

Stability Intact vials and tablets should be stored at room temperature; reconstitute 500 mg vial with 49.8 mL sterile water; the 10 mg/mL solution is stable for 24 hours

Mechanism of Action Prodrug incorporated into DNA and RNA; blocks purine synthesis and inhibits DNA and RNA synthesis

Pharmacokinetics
Absorption: Oral: Variable and incomplete (16% to 50%)
Distribution: Distributed throughout total body water; penetrates into CSF at low concentrations
Protein binding: 19%
Metabolism: Undergoes first pass metabolism in the GI mucosa and liver; metabolized in the liver to sulfate conjugates, 6-thiouric acid, and other inactive compounds
Half-life: Age dependent
  Children: 21 minutes
  Adults: 47 minutes
Peak concentrations: Within 2 hours after an oral dose
Elimination: Excreted in the urine

Usual Dosage Refer to individual protocols
Children:
  Oral:
    Induction: 2.5-5 mg/kg/day given once daily or 70-100 mg/m²/day given once daily
    Maintenance: 1.5-2.5 mg/kg/day given once daily
  I.V. continuous infusion (investigational; distributed under the auspices of the NCI for authorized studies): 50 mg/m²/hour for 24-48 hours

(Continued)

Mercaptopurine *(Continued)*

Adults: Oral:

Induction: 2.5-5 mg/kg/day or 80-100 mg/m^2/day given once daily
Maintenance: 1.5-2.5 mg/kg/day

Administration Further dilute the 10 mg/mL reconstituted solution in normal saline or D_5W to a final concentration for administration of 1-2 mg/mL; administer by slow I.V. continuous infusion

Monitoring Parameters CBC with differential and platelet count, liver function tests, uric acid, urinalysis

Patient Information Do not take with meals; report to physician if fever, sore throat, bleeding, bruising, shortness of breath, or painful urination occurs

Additional Information Myelosuppressive effects:

WBC: Moderate
Platelets: Moderate
Onset (days): 7-10
Nadir (days): 14
Recovery (days): 21

Dosage Forms Tablet: 50 mg

References

Zimm S, Ettinger LJ, Holcenberg JS, et al, "Phase I and Clinical Pharmacological Study of Mercaptopurine Administered as a Prolonged Intravenous Infusion," *Cancer Res*, 1988, 45:1869-73.

6-Mercaptopurine *see* Mercaptopurine *on previous page*

Merlenate® [OTC] *see* Undecylenic Acid and Derivatives *on page 590*

Mesantoin® *see* Mephenytoin *on page 363*

Mesna

Brand Names Mesnex™

Synonyms Sodium 2-Mercaptoethane Sulfonate

Therapeutic Category Antidote, Cyclophosphamide-induced Hemorrhagic Cystitis; Antidote, Ifosfamide-induced Hemorrhagic Cystitis

Use Detoxifying agent used as a protectant against hemorrhagic cystitis induced by ifosfamide and cyclophosphamide

Pregnancy Risk Factor B

Contraindications Hypersensitivity to mesna or other thiol compounds

Precautions Examine morning urine specimen for hematuria prior to ifosfamide or cyclophosphamide treatment; if hematuria develops, reduce the ifosfamide/cyclophosphamide dose or discontinue the drug

Adverse Reactions

Cardiovascular: Hypotension
Central nervous system: Malaise, headache
Dermatologic: Skin rash
Gastrointestinal: Diarrhea, nausea, vomiting, bad taste in mouth
Musculoskeletal: Limb pain

Stability Diluted solutions are chemically and physically stable for 24 hours at room temperature; however, it is recommended that solutions be refrigerated and used within 6 hours; incompatible with cisplatin

Mechanism of Action Binds with and detoxifies acrolein and other urotoxic metabolites of ifosfamide and cyclophosphamide

Pharmacokinetics

Distribution: No tissue penetration; following glomerular filtration, mesna disulfide is reduced in the renal tubules back to mesna

Half-life: 24 minutes (mesna); after I.V. administration, mesna is rapidly oxidized intravascularly to mesna disulfide (half-life: 72 minutes)

Elimination: Unchanged drug and metabolite are excreted primarily in the urine; time for maximum urinary mesna excretion: 1 hour after I.V. and 2-3 hours after an oral mesna dose

Usual Dosage Children and Adults (refer to individual protocols):

Ifosfamide: I.V.: 20% W/W of ifosfamide dose at time of administration and 4 and 8 hours after each dose of ifosfamide; for high-dose ifosfamide, mesna has been administered at a dose of 20% W/W at time of administration and 3, 6, 9, and 12 hours after ifosfamide dose

Cyclophosphamide: I.V.: 20% W/W of cyclophosphamide dose prior to administration and 3, 6, 9, 12 hours after cyclophosphamide dose (total daily dose: 120% to 180% of cyclophosphamide dose)

Oral: 40% W/W of the antineoplastic agent dose in 3 doses at 4-hour intervals or 20 mg/kg/dose every 4 hours x 3

Administration Administer by I.V. infusion over 15-30 minutes or per protocol; mesna can be diluted in D_5W or NS to a final concentration of 1-20 mg/mL

Monitoring Parameters Urinalysis

Test Interactions False-positive urinary ketones with Multistix® or Labstix®

Nursing Implications Used concurrent with and/or following high dose ifosfamide or cyclophosphamide; mesna also has been given orally with carbonated beverages or juice (most palatable in grape juice)

Dosage Forms Injection: 100 mg/mL (2 mL, 4 mL, 10 mL)

References

Ben Yehuda A, Heyman A and Steiner Salz D, "False Positive Reaction for Urinary Ketones With Mesna," *Drug Intell Clin Pharm*, 1987, 21(6): 547-8.

Brock N and Pohl J, "The Development of Mesna for Regional Detoxification," *Cancer Treat Rev*, 1983, 10(Suppl A):33-43.

"Cancer Chemotherapy," *Med Lett Drugs Ther*, 1989, 31(793):49-56.

Schoenike SE and Dana WJ, "Ifosfamide and Mesna," *Clin Pharm*, 1990, 9(3):179-91.

Mesnex™ *see* Mesna *on previous page*

Mestinon® *see* Pyridostigmine Bromide *on page 500*

Metacortandralone *see* Prednisolone *on page 476*

Metamucil® [OTC] *see* Psyllium *on page 498*

Metamucil® Instant Mix [OTC] *see* Psyllium *on page 498*

Metaprel® *see* Metaproterenol Sulfate *on this page*

Metaproterenol Sulfate (met a proe ter' e nol)

Brand Names Alupent®; Arm-a-Med® Metaproterenol; Dey-Dose® Metaproterenol; Metaprel®; Prometa®

Synonyms Orciprenaline Sulfate

Therapeutic Category Beta-2-Adrenergic Agonist Agent; Bronchodilator; Sympathomimetic

Use Bronchodilator in reversible airway obstruction due to asthma or COPD

Pregnancy Risk Factor C

Contraindications Hypersensitivity to metaproterenol or any component; pre-existing cardiac arrhythmias associated with tachycardia

Warnings Excessive use may result in cardiac arrest and death; do not use concurrently with other sympathomimetic bronchodilators

Precautions Ischemic heart disease, hypertension, hyperthyroidism, seizure disorders, congestive heart failure, cardiac arrhythmias

Adverse Reactions

Cardiovascular: Tachycardia, palpitations, hypertension

Central nervous system: Tremor, nervousness, dizziness, headache, fatigue

Gastrointestinal: Nausea, vomiting, GI distress

Miscellaneous: Throat irritation, cough, bad taste

Drug Interactions Beta-adrenergic blockers (ie, propranolol); ↑ adverse effects if administered concomitantly with other sympathomimetics

Mechanism of Action Relaxes bronchial smooth muscle and peripheral vasculature by action on $beta_2$ receptors with little effect on heart rate

Pharmacodynamics

Onset of bronchodilation:

Oral: Within 15 minutes

Inhalation: Within 60 seconds

Peak effect: Oral: Within 1 hour

Duration: (approximately 1-5 hours) regardless of route administered

Pharmacokinetics

Absorption: Oral: Well absorbed

Metabolism: Extensive first pass in the liver (~40% of oral dose is available)

Elimination: Excreted mainly as glucuronic acid conjugates

(Continued)

Metaproterenol Sulfate *(Continued)*

Usual Dosage

Oral:

Children:

<2 years: 0.4 mg/kg/dose given 3-4 times/day; in infants, the dose can be given every 8-12 hours

2-6 years: 1-2.6 mg/kg/day divided every 6-8 hours

6-9 years: 10 mg/dose given 3-4 times/day

Children >9 years and Adults: 20 mg/dose given 3-4 times/day

Inhalation: Children >12 years and Adults: 2-3 inhalations every 3-4 hours, up to 12 inhalations in 24 hours

Nebulizer: Infants and Children: 0.01-0.02 mL/kg of 5% solution; minimum dose: 0.1 mL; maximum dose: 0.3 mL diluted in 2-3 mL normal saline every 4-6 hours (may be given more frequently according to need) (equivalent doses using more dilute solutions, eg, 0.6% may be administered without dilution)

Adolescents and Adults: 5-20 breaths of full strength 5% metaproterenol **or** 0.2 to 0.3 mL 5% metaproterenol in 2.5-3 mL normal saline until nebulized every 4-6 hours (can be given more frequently according to need)

Monitoring Parameters Heart rate, respiratory rate, blood pressure, arterial or capillary blood gases if applicable

Dosage Forms

Aerosol, oral: 0.65 mg/dose (5 mL, 10 mL)

Solution for inhalation, preservative free: 0.4% (2.5 mL); 0.6% (2.5 mL); 5% (10 mL, 30 mL)

Syrup: 10 mg/5 mL (480 mL)

Tablet: 10 mg, 20 mg

Methadone Hydrochloride (meth' a done)

Related Information

Narcotic Analgesics Comparison Chart *on page 721-722*

Overdose and Toxicology Information *on page 696-700*

Brand Names Dolophine®

Therapeutic Category Analgesic, Narcotic

Use Management of severe pain, used in narcotic detoxification maintenance programs

Restrictions C-II

Pregnancy Risk Factor B (D if used for prolonged periods or in high doses at term)

Contraindications Hypersensitivity to methadone or any component

Warnings Tablets are to be used only for oral administration and **must not** be used for injection

Precautions Due to the cumulative effects of methadone, the dose and frequency of administration need to be reduced with repeated use; use with caution in patients with respiratory diseases; methadone's effect on respiration lasts longer than analgesic effects

Adverse Reactions

Cardiovascular: Hypotension, bradycardia, peripheral vasodilation

Central nervous system: CNS depression, increased intracranial pressure, drowsiness, dizziness, sedation (marked sedation seen after repeated administration)

Endocrine & metabolic: Antidiuretic hormone release

Gastrointestinal: Nausea, vomiting, constipation, dry mouth

Hepatic: Biliary tract spasm

Ocular: Miosis

Renal & genitourinary: Urinary tract spasm

Respiratory: Respiratory depression

Miscellaneous: Histamine release, physical and psychological dependence with prolonged use

Drug Interactions CNS depressants, phenothiazines, tricyclic antidepressants may potentiate the adverse effects of methadone; phenytoin and rifampin may ↑ the metabolism of methadone and may precipitate withdrawal

Mechanism of Action Binds to opiate receptors in the CNS, causing inhibition of ascending pain pathways, altering the perception of and response to pain; produces generalized CNS depression

Pharmacodynamics Analgesia:
Onset of action:
Oral: Within 30-60 minutes
Parenteral: Within 10-20 minutes
Peak action: Parenteral: 1-2 hours
Duration: Oral: 6-8 hours; after repeated doses, duration increases to 22-48 hours

Pharmacokinetics
Distribution: Crosses the placenta; appears in breast milk
Protein binding: 80% to 85%
Metabolism: Liver metabolism (N-demethylation)
Half-life: 15-29 hours, half-life may be prolonged with alkaline pH
Elimination: Excreted in the urine (<10% as unchanged drug); increased renal excretion with urine pH <6

Usual Dosage Doses should be titrated to appropriate effects:
Children: Analgesia:
Oral, I.M., S.C.: 0.7 mg/kg/24 hours divided every 4-6 hours as needed or 0.1-0.2 mg/kg every 4-12 hours as needed; maximum: 10 mg/dose
I.V.: 0.1 mg/kg every 4 hours initially for 2-3 doses, then every 6-12 hours as needed; maximum: 10 mg/dose

Adults:
Analgesia: Oral, I.M., I.V., S.C.: 2.5-10 mg every 3-8 hours as needed, up to 5-20 mg every 6-8 hours
Detoxification: Oral: 15-40 mg/day
Maintenance of opiate dependence: Oral: 20-120 mg/day

Children and Adults: Dosing adjustment in renal impairment: Cl_{cr} <10 mL/minute: Administer 50% to 75% of normal dose

Monitoring Parameters Respiratory and cardiovascular status

Additional Information Methadone accumulates with repeated doses and dosage may need to be adjusted downward after 3-5 days to prevent toxic effects. Some patients may benefit from every 8- to 12-hour dosing interval (pain control); oral dose for detoxification and maintenance may be administered in Tang®, Kool-Aid®, apple juice, grape Crystal Light®

Dosage Forms
Injection: 10 mg/mL (1 mL, 10 mL, 20 mL)
Solution:
Oral: 5 mg/5 mL (5 mL, 500 mL); 10 mg/5 mL (500 mL)
Oral, concentrate: 10 mg/mL (30 mL)
Tablet: 5 mg, 10 mg
Tablet, dispersible: 40 mg

References

Berde C, Ablin A, Glazer J, et al, "American Academy of Pediatrics Report of the Subcommittee on Disease-Related Pain in Childhood Cancer," *Pediatrics*, 1990, 86(5 Pt 2):818-25.
Lauriault G, LeBelle MJ, Lodge BA, et al, "Stability of Methadone in Four Vehicles for Oral Administration," *Am J Hosp Pharm*, 1991, 48(6):1252-6.

Methenamine (meth en' a meen)

Brand Names Hiprex®; Mandelamine®; Urex®; Urised®

Synonyms Hexamethylenetetramine

Therapeutic Category Antibiotic, Miscellaneous

Use Prophylaxis or suppression of recurrent urinary tract infections

Pregnancy Risk Factor C

Contraindications Severe dehydration, renal insufficiency, hepatic insufficiency in patients receiving hippurate salt; hypersensitivity to methenamine or any component

Adverse Reactions
Central nervous system: Headache
Dermatologic: Rash, pruritus
Gastrointestinal: Nausea, vomiting, diarrhea, abdominal cramping, anorexia
Hepatic: Elevation in AST and ALT
Renal & genitourinary: Hematuria, bladder irritation, dysuria, crystalluria

Drug Interactions Sulfamethizole

Stability Protect from excessive heat

Mechanism of Action Methenamine is hydrolyzed to formaldehyde and ammonia in acidic urine; formaldehyde has nonspecific bactericidal action

(Continued)

Methenamine *(Continued)*

Pharmacokinetics

Absorption: Readily absorbed from the GI tract; 10% to 30% of the drug will be hydrolyzed by gastric juices unless it is protected by an enteric coating

Metabolism: ~10% to 25% is metabolized in the liver

Half-life: 3-6 hours

Elimination: Excretion occurs via glomerular filtration and tubular secretion with ~70% to 90% of a dose excreted unchanged in the urine within 24 hours

Usual Dosage Oral:

Children 6-12 years:

Hippurate: 25-50 mg/kg/day divided every 12 hours

Mandelate: 50-75 mg/kg/day divided every 6 hours

Adults:

Hippurate: 1 g twice daily

Mandelate: 1 g 4 times/day after meals and at bedtime

Monitoring Parameters Urinary pH, urinalysis, periodic liver function tests in patients receiving hippurate salt

Test Interactions ↑ catecholamines and VMA (U)

Patient Information Take with ascorbic acid to acidify urine and avoid intake of alkalinizing agents (sodium bicarbonate, antacids); take with food to minimize GI upset; drink plenty of fluids to ensure adequate urine flow

Nursing Implications Urine should be acidic, pH <5.5 for maximum effect

Additional Information Should not be used to treat infections outside of the lower urinary tract

Dosage Forms

Granules (orange flavor): 1 g (56s)

Suspension, oral, as mandelate (Mandelamine®): 250 mg/5 mL (coconut flavor), 500 mg/5 mL (cherry flavor)

Tablet, as hippurate (Hiprex®, Urex®): 1 g (Hiprex® contains tartrazine dye)

Tablet, as mandelate, enteric coated (Mandelamine®): 250 mg, 500 mg, 1 g

Methicillin Sodium (meth i sill' in)

Related Information

Medications Compatible With PN Solutions *on page 649-650*

Brand Names Staphcillin®

Synonyms Dimethoxyphenyl Penicillin Sodium; Sodium Methicillin

Therapeutic Category Antibiotic, Penicillin

Use Treatment of susceptible bacterial infections such as osteomyelitis, septicemia, endocarditis, and CNS infections due to penicillinase-producing strains of *Staphylococcus*

Pregnancy Risk Factor B

Contraindications Known hypersensitivity to methicillin or any penicillin or cephalosporin

Warnings Elimination rate will be decreased in neonates

Precautions Modify dosage in patients with renal impairment

Adverse Reactions

Central nervous system: Fever

Dermatologic: Rash

Hematologic: Eosinophilia, anemia leukopenia, neutropenia, thrombocytopenia

Hepatic: ↑ AST

Local: Phlebitis

Renal & genitourinary: Nephrotoxicity (interstitial nephritis), hemorrhagic cystitis, hematuria

Miscellaneous: Serum sickness-like reactions

Drug Interactions Probenecid

Stability Reconstituted solution containing methicillin 500 mg/mL is stable for 24 hours at room temperature and 4 days when refrigerated; incompatible with aminoglycosides and tetracyclines

Mechanism of Action Interferes with bacterial cell wall synthesis during active multiplication, causing cell wall death and resultant bactericidal activity against susceptible bacteria

Pharmacokinetics

Distribution: Crosses the placenta; distributes into milk; distributes into synovial, pleural, and pericardial fluids, bone and bile; low concentrations attained in CSF

Protein binding: 40%

Half-life:

- Neonates:
  - <2 weeks: 2-3.9 hours
  - >2 weeks: 0.9-3.3 hours
- Children 2-16 years: 0.8 hours
- Adults: 0.4-0.5 hours with normal renal function

Peak serum levels:

- I.M.: Within 30-60 minutes
- I.V. infusion: Within 5 minutes

Elimination: ~60% to 70% of a dose is eliminated unchanged in the urine within 4 hours by tubular secretion and glomerular filtration

Not dialyzable (0% to 5%)

Usual Dosage I.M., I.V.:

Neonates:

- 0-4 weeks, <1200 g: 50 mg/kg/day divided every 12 hours; meningitis: 100 mg/kg/day divided every 12 hours
- ≤7 days:
  - 1200-2000 g: 50 mg/kg/day divided every 12 hours; meningitis: 100 mg/kg/day divided every 12 hours
  - >2000 g: 75 mg/kg/day divided every 8 hours; meningitis: 150 mg/kg/day divided every 8 hours
- >7 days:
  - 1200-2000 g: 75 mg/kg/day divided every 8 hours; meningitis: 150 mg/kg/day divided every 8 hours
  - >2000 g: 100 mg/kg/day divided every 6 hours; meningitis: 200 mg/kg/day divided every 6 hours

Children: 150-200 mg/kg/day divided every 6 hours; 200-400 mg/kg/day divided every 4-6 hours has been used for treatment of severe infections; maximum dose: 12 g/day

Adults: 4-12 g/day in divided doses every 4-6 hours

Dosing interval in renal impairment: Cl_{cr} <10 mL/minute: Administer every 8-12 hours

Administration Can be administered IVP at a rate not to exceed 200 mg/minute or intermittent infusion over 15-30 minutes; final concentration for administration should not exceed 20 mg/mL; in fluid-restricted patients, a final concentration for administration of 100 mg/mL has been used

Monitoring Parameters Urinalysis, BUN, serum creatinine, CBC with differential, and periodic liver function tests

Test Interactions Positive Coombs' test [direct]

Additional Information Sodium content of 1 g: 2.9 mEq

Dosage Forms Powder for injection: 1 g, 4 g, 6 g, 10 g

References

Prober CG, Stevenson DK, and Benitz WE, "The Use of Antibiotics in Neonates Weighing Less Than 1200 Grams," *Pediatr Infect Dis J*, 1990, 9(2):111-21.

Yow MD, Taber LH, Barrett FF, et al, "A Ten-Year Assessment of Methicillin-Associated Side Effects," *Pediatrics*, 1976, 58(3):329-34.

Methimazole (meth im' a zole)

Brand Names Tapazole®

Synonyms Thiamazole

Therapeutic Category Antithyroid Agent

Use Palliative treatment of hyperthyroidism, to return the hyperthyroid patient to a normal metabolic state prior to thyroidectomy, and to control thyrotoxic crisis that may accompany thyroidectomy

Pregnancy Risk Factor D

Contraindications Hypersensitivity to methimazole or any component

Precautions Use with extreme caution in patients receiving other drugs known to cause agranulocytosis

(Continued)

Methimazole *(Continued)*

Adverse Reactions

Cardiovascular: Edema

Central nervous system: Paresthesias, drowsiness, vertigo, headache

Dermatologic: Rash, urticaria, pruritus, hair loss, skin pigmentation

Gastrointestinal: Loss of taste, nausea, vomiting

Hematologic: Agranulocytosis, hypoprothrombinemia

Hepatic: Cholestatic jaundice

Musculoskeletal: Arthralgia

Miscellaneous: Drug fever, lupus-like syndrome

Drug Interactions Iodinated glycerol, lithium, potassium iodide

Mechanism of Action Inhibits the synthesis of thyroid hormones by blocking the oxidation of iodine in the thyroid gland, blocking iodine's ability to combine with tyrosine to form thyroxine

Pharmacodynamics

Peak effect: 1 hour

Duration: 2-4 hours

Pharmacokinetics

Half-life: 5-13 hours

Elimination: Excreted in the urine

Usual Dosage Oral:

Children: Initial: 0.4 mg/kg/day in 3 divided doses; maintenance: 0.2 mg/kg/day in 3 divided doses

Adults: Initial: 15-60 mg/day divided every 8 hours; maintenance doses range 5-30 mg/day

Dosing adjustment in renal impairment: Children and Adults:

Cl_{cr} 10-50 mL/minute: Administer 75% of recommended dose

Cl_{cr} <10 mL/minute: Administer 50% of recommended dose

Monitoring Parameters CBC with differential, liver function (baseline and as needed); serum thyroxine, free thyroxine index

Patient Information Take with meals

Dosage Forms Tablet: 5 mg, 10 mg

References

Raby C, Lagorce JF, Jambut-Absil AC, et al, "The Mechanism of Action of Synthetic Antithyroid Drugs: Iodine Complexation During Oxidation of Iodide," *Endocrinology*, 1990, 126(3):1683-91.

Methocarbamol (meth oh kar' ba mole)

Brand Names Delaxin®; Marbaxin®; Robaxin®; Robaxisal®; Robomol®

Therapeutic Category Skeletal Muscle Relaxant, Central Acting

Use Treatment of muscle spasm associated with acute painful musculoskeletal conditions; supportive therapy in tetanus

Pregnancy Risk Factor C

Contraindications Hypersensitivity to methocarbamol or any component

Warnings Avoid using injection in patients with impaired renal function because the polyethylene glycol vehicle may be irritating to the kidneys

Precautions May impair ability to perform hazardous activities requiring mental alertness and physical coordination

Adverse Reactions

Cardiovascular: Syncope, bradycardia

Central nervous system: Drowsiness, dizziness, lightheadedness, headache, fever

Gastrointestinal: Nausea, metallic taste, GI upset

Local: Pain and phlebitis at injection site

Ophthalmic: Blurred vision

Miscellaneous: Hypersensitivity reactions

Stability Injection when diluted to 4 mg/mL in sterile water, 5% dextrose, or 0.9% saline is stable for 6 days at room temperature; do **not** refrigerate after dilution

Mechanism of Action Central nervous system depressant with sedative and skeletal muscle relaxant effects; exact mechanism of action is unknown

Pharmacokinetics Oral:

Peak serum levels: Occur within ~1-2 hours

Half-life: 0.9-1.8 hours

Metabolism: Extensively metabolized in the liver

Usual Dosage

Tetanus: I.V.:

Children (recommended **only** for use in tetanus): 15 mg/kg/dose or 500 mg/m^2/dose, may repeat every 6 hours if needed; maximum dose: 1.8 g/m^2/day for 3 days only

Adults: 1-2 g by direct I.V. injection followed by additional 1-2 g (maximum: 3 g total); repeat with 1-2 g every 6 hours until NG tube or oral therapy possible; total daily dose of up to 24 g may be needed

Muscle spasm: Adults:

Oral: 1.5 g 4 times/day for 2-3 days, then decrease to 4-4.5 g/day in 3-6 divided doses

I.M., I.V.: 1 g every 8 hours if oral not possible; maximum: 3 g/day for 3 consecutive days (except when treating tetanus); may be reinstituted after 2 drug-free days

Administration May be injected directly without dilution at a maximum rate of 180 mg/m^2/minute; may also be diluted in normal saline or 5% dextrose to a concentration of 4 mg/mL and infused more slowly; patient should be in the recumbent position during and for 10-15 minutes after I.V. administration

Nursing Implications Avoid infiltration, extremely irritating to tissues

Dosage Forms

Injection: 100 mg/mL in 50% polyethylene glycol (10 mL)

Tablet: 500 mg, 750 mg

Tablet (Robaxisal®): Methocarbamol 400 mg and aspirin 325 mg

Methohexital Sodium (meth oh hex' i tal)

Related Information

Preprocedure Sedatives in Children *on page 687-689*

Brand Names Brevital® Sodium

Therapeutic Category Barbiturate; General Anesthetic; Sedative

Use Induction and maintenance of general anesthesia for short procedures

Restrictions C-IV

Pregnancy Risk Factor C

Contraindications Porphyria, hypersensitivity to methohexital or any component

Precautions Use with extreme caution in patients with liver impairment, asthma, cardiovascular instability

Adverse Reactions

Cardiovascular: Hypotension, peripheral vascular collapse

Central nervous system: Seizures, tremor, headache

Gastrointestinal: Nausea, vomiting

Local: Pain on I.M. injection, thrombophlebitis

Musculoskeletal: Involuntary muscle movement, twitching, rigidity

Respiratory: Apnea, respiratory depression, laryngospasm, hiccups, coughing

Drug Interactions CNS depressants

Stability Do not dilute with solutions containing bacteriostatic agents; solutions are alkaline (pH 9.5-11) and incompatible with acids (ie, atropine sulfate, succinylcholine), also incompatible with phenol containing solutions and silicone

Mechanism of Action Ultra short-acting I.V. barbiturate anesthetic

Usual Dosage Doses must be titrated to effect

Children:

I.M.: Preop: 5-10 mg/kg/dose

I.V.: Induction: 1-2 mg/kg/dose

Rectal: Preop/induction: 20-35 mg/kg/dose; usual 25 mg/kg/dose; give as 10% aqueous solution

Adults: I.V.: Induction: 50-120 mg to start; 20-40 mg every 4-7 minutes

Administration Dilute to a maximum concentration of 1% for I.V. use

Monitoring Parameters Blood pressure, heart rate, respiratory rate

Nursing Implications Avoid extravasation or intra-arterial administration

Dosage Forms Injection: 500 mg, 2.5 g, 5 g

Methoin *see* Mephenytoin *on page 363*

Methotrexate (meth oh trex' ate)

Related Information

Emetogenic Potential of Single Chemotherapeutic Agents *on page 655*

Brand Names Folex®; Rheumatrex®

Synonyms Amethopterin; MTX

Therapeutic Category Antineoplastic Agent

Use Treatment of trophoblastic neoplasms, leukemias, osteosarcoma, non-Hodgkin's lymphoma; psoriasis, rheumatoid arthritis

Pregnancy Risk Factor D

Contraindications Hypersensitivity to methotrexate or any component; severe renal or hepatic impairment; pre-existing profound bone marrow depression

Warnings The US Food and Drug Administration (FDA) currently recommends that procedures for proper handling and disposal of antineoplastic agents be considered. Due to the possibility of severe toxic reactions, fully inform patient of the risks involved; do not use in women of child bearing age unless benefit outweighs risks; may cause hepatotoxicity, fibrosis and cirrhosis, along with marked bone marrow depression; death from intestinal perforation may occur

Precautions Use with caution in patients with peptic ulcer disease, ulcerative colitis, pre-existing bone marrow suppression; reduce dosage in patients with renal or hepatic impairment, ascites, and pleural effusion

Adverse Reactions

Cardiovascular: Vasculitis

Central nervous system: Malaise, fatigue, dizziness, encephalopathy, seizures, confusion, fever, headache, chills

Dermatologic: Alopecia, rash, depigmentation or hyperpigmentation of skin, photosensitivity

Endocrine & metabolic: Diabetes

Gastrointestinal: Nausea, vomiting, diarrhea, anorexia, stomatitis, enteritis

Hematologic: Myelosuppression, leukopenia, thrombocytopenia, anemia, hemorrhage

Hepatic: Hepatotoxicity

Musculoskeletal: Arthralgia

Ocular: Blurred vision

Renal & genitourinary: Nephropathy (azotemia, hematuria, renal failure), cystitis

Respiratory: Interstitial pneumonitis

Miscellaneous: Anaphylaxis

Drug Interactions Salicylates (may delay MTX's clearance); sulfonamides (displace MTX from protein-binding sites); live virus vaccines, pyrimethamine, phenytoin, 5-FU; nonsteroidal anti-inflammatory drugs (↑ toxicity with NSAIDs); probenecid ↓ renal elimination of MTX

Stability Protect from light

Mechanism of Action An antimetabolite that inhibits DNA synthesis and cell reproduction in cancerous cells; interferes with the conversion of folic acid to tetrahydrofolic acid by binding to the enzyme dihydrofolate reductase

Pharmacokinetics

Absorption:

Oral: Rapidly and well absorbed at low doses (<30 mg/m^2), incomplete absorption after large doses

I.M. injection: Completely absorbed

Distribution: Small amounts distributed into breast milk; crosses the placenta; does not achieve therapeutic concentrations in the CSF; sustained concentrations are retained in the kidney and liver

Protein binding: 50%

Peak serum levels:

Oral: 1-2 hours

Parenteral: 30-60 minutes

Half-life: 8-12 hours with high doses and 3-10 hours with low doses

Elimination: Small amounts excreted in the feces; primarily excreted in the urine (90%) via glomerular filtration and active transport

Usual Dosage Refer to individual protocols

Children:

Juvenile rheumatoid arthritis: Oral, I.M.: 5-15 mg/m^2/week as a single dose or in 3 divided doses given 12 hours apart

Antineoplastic dosage range: I.V.: 10-33,000 mg/m^2 bolus dosing or continuous infusion over 6-42 hours

Pediatric solid tumors: 8-12 g/m^2 <12 years: 12 g/m^2 (dosage range: 12-18 g); ≥12 years: 8 g/m^2 (maximum: 18 g)

Meningeal leukemia: 6 g/m^2 loading dose over 1 hour, followed by I.V. continuous infusion 1.2 g/m^2/hour for 23 hours

Acute lymphocytic leukemia (high dose): Loading dose: 200 mg/m^2 followed by a 24-hour infusion of 1200 mg/m^2/day

ANLL: 7.5 mg/m^2/day on days 1-5

Resistant ANLL: 100 mg/m^2/dose on day 1

Non-Hodgkin's lymphoma: 200-300 mg/m^2

Oral, I.M., I.V.:

Induction of remission in acute lymphoblastic leukemias: 3.3 mg/m^2/day for 4-6 weeks

Remission maintenance: 20-30 mg/m^2 2 times/week

I.T.: 10-15 mg/m^2 (maximum: 15 mg) by protocol **or**

≤3 months: 3 mg dose

4-11 months: 6 mg dose

1 year: 8 mg dose

2 years: 10 mg dose

≥3 years: 12 mg dose

Adults:

Trophoblastic neoplasms: Oral, I.M.: 15-30 mg/day for 5 days, repeat in 7 days for 3-5 courses

Rheumatoid arthritis: Oral: 7.5 mg once weekly or 2.5 mg every 12 hours for 3 doses/week; not to exceed 20 mg/week

Administration Methotrexate can be administered I.V. push, I.V. intermittent infusion, or I.V. continuous infusion at a concentration <25 mg/mL; doses >100-300 mg/m^2 are usually given by I.V. continuous infusion and are followed by a course of leucovorin rescue

Monitoring Parameters CBC with differential and platelet count, creatinine clearance, serum creatinine, BUN, hepatic function tests, serum electrolytes, urinalysis, serum MTX concentrations

Reference Range Serum levels >1 x 10^{-7} moles/L for more than 40 hours are toxic

Patient Information Report to physician any fever, sore throat, bleeding or bruising, shortness of breath, painful urination

Nursing Implications For intrathecal use, mix methotrexate without preservatives with normal saline or LR to a concentration no greater than 2 mg/mL

Additional Information Myelosuppressive effects:

WBC: Mild

Platelets: Moderate

Onset (days): 7

Nadir (days): 10

Recovery (days): 21

Dosage Forms

Dose Pack: 2.5 mg (4 cards with 3 tablets each)

Injection, as sodium: 2.5 mg/mL (2 mL); 25 mg/mL (2 mL, 4 mL, 8 mL, 10 mL)

Injection, as sodium, preservative free: 25 mg (2 mL, 4 mL, 8 mL, 10 mL)

Powder for injection, as sodium: 20 mg, 25 mg, 50 mg, 100 mg, 250 mg

Tablet, as sodium: 2.5 mg

References

Berg SL, Grisell DL, DeLaney TF, et al, "Principles of Treatment of Pediatric Solid Tumors," *Pediatr Clin North Am*, 1991, 38(2):249-67.

Crom WR, Glynn-Barnhart AM, Rodman JH, et al, "Pharmacokinetics of Anticancer Drugs in Children," *Clin Pharmacokinet*, 1987, 12(3):168-213.

Giannini EH, Brewer EJ, Kuzmina N, et al, "Methotrexate in Resistant Juvenile Rheumatoid Arthritis. Results of the USA-USSR Double-Blind, Placebo-Controlled Trial," *N Engl J Med*, 1992, 326(16):1043-9.

Rose CD, Singsen BH, and Eichenfield AH, "Safety and Efficacy of Methotrexate Therapy for Juvenile Rheumatoid Arthritis," *J Pediatr*, 1990, 117(4):653-9.

Methsuximide (meth sux' i mide)

Brand Names Celontin®

Therapeutic Category Anticonvulsant

Use Control of absence (petit mal) seizures; useful adjunct in refractory, partial complex (psychomotor) seizures

Pregnancy Risk Factor C

Contraindications Known hypersensitivity to methsuximide

Precautions Use with caution in patients with hepatic or renal disease; avoid abrupt withdrawal of methsuximide

Adverse Reactions

Central nervous system: Dizziness, drowsiness, lethargy, euphoria, nervousness, hallucinations, insomnia, mental confusion, ataxia, headache

Dermatologic: Rash, urticaria, Stevens-Johnson syndrome

Gastrointestinal: Nausea, vomiting, anorexia, diarrhea, abdominal pain

Hematologic: Leukopenia, thrombocytopenia, eosinophilia, pancytopenia, monocytosis

Miscellaneous: Hiccups, periorbital edema

Stability Protect from high temperature

Mechanism of Action Increases the seizure threshold and suppresses paroxysmal spike-and-wave pattern in absence seizures; depresses nerve transmission in the motor cortex

Pharmacokinetics

Distribution: Methsuximide is rapidly demethylated in the liver to N-desmethylmethsuximide (active metabolite)

Half-life: 2-4 hours

N-desmethylsuximide:

Children: 26 hours

Adults: 28-80 hours

Peak serum levels: Within 1-3 hours

Elimination: <1% excreted in urine as unchanged drug

Usual Dosage Oral:

Children: Initial: 10-15 mg/kg/day in 3-4 divided doses; increase weekly up to maximum of 30 mg/kg/day; mean dose required:

<30 kg: 20 mg/kg/day

>30 kg: 14 mg/kg/day

Adults: 300 mg/day for the first week; may increase by 300 mg/day at weekly intervals up to 1.2 g in 2-4 divided doses/day

Monitoring Parameters CBC with differential, liver enzymes, U/A; measure trough serum levels for efficacy and 3-hour postdose concentrations for toxicity

Reference Range Measure N-desmethylmethsuximide concentrations: Therapeutic: 10-40 μg/mL (SI: 53-212 μmol/L); Toxic: >40 μg/mL (SI: >212 μmol/L)

Dosage Forms Capsule: 150 mg, 300 mg

References

Miles MV, Tennison MB, Greenwood RS, et al, "Pharmacokinetics of N-desmethylmethsuximide in Pediatric Patients," *J Pediatr*, 1989, 114(4 Pt 1):647-50.

Methylacetoxyprogesterone *see* Medroxyprogesterone Acetate *on page 359*

Methyldopa (meth ill doe' pa)

Brand Names Aldomet®

Therapeutic Category Alpha-Adrenergic Inhibitors, Central; Antihypertensive

Use Management of moderate to severe hypertension

Pregnancy Risk Factor B

Contraindications Hypersensitivity to methyldopa or any component; liver disease, pheochromocytoma

Precautions Oral suspension contains benzoic acid and sodium bisulfite, injection contains sodium bisulfite

Adverse Reactions

Cardiovascular: Orthostatic hypotension, bradycardia, sodium retention, edema

Central nervous system: Drowsiness, sedation, vertigo, headache, depression, weakness, memory lapse; fever
Dermatologic: Rash
Endocrine & metabolic: Gynecomastia, sexual dysfunction
Gastrointestinal: Nausea, vomiting, diarrhea, dry mouth, "black" tongue
Hematologic: Hemolytic anemia, positive Coombs' test, leukopenia
Hepatic: Hepatitis, ↑ liver enzymes, jaundice, cirrhosis
Miscellaneous: Nasal congestion

Drug Interactions Lithium → ↑ lithium toxicity

Mechanism of Action Stimulates inhibitory alpha-adrenergic receptors via alpha-methynorepinephrine (false transmitter); this results in a decreased sympathetic outflow to the heart, kidneys, and peripheral vasculature; may decrease plasma renin activity

Pharmacodynamics Hypotensive effects:
Peak effects: Oral, parenteral: Within 3-6 hours
Duration: 12-24 hours

Pharmacokinetics
Distribution: Crosses placenta; appears in breast milk
Protein binding: <15%
Metabolism: Metabolized intestinally and in the liver
Half-life:
Neonates: 10-20 hours
Adults: 1-3 hours
Slightly dialyzable (5% to 20%)

Usual Dosage
Children:
Oral: Initial: 10 mg/kg/day in 2-4 divided doses; increase every 2 days as needed to maximum dose of 65 mg/kg/day; do not exceed 3 g/day
I.V.: Initial: 2-4 mg/kg/dose; if response is not seen within 4-6 hours, may increase to 5-10 mg/kg/dose; administer doses every 6-8 hours; maximum daily dose: 65 mg/kg or 3 g, whichever is less

Adults:
Oral: Initial: 250 mg 2-3 times/day; increase every 2 days as needed; usual dose 1-1.5 g/day in 2-4 divided doses; maximum dose: 3 g/day
I.V.: 250-1000 mg every 6-8 hours; maximum: 4 g/day

Children and Adults: Dosing interval in renal impairment:
Cl_{cr} >50 mL/minute: Administer every 8 hours
Cl_{cr} 10-50 mL/minute: Administer every 8-12 hours
Cl_{cr} <10 mL/minute: Administer every 12-24 hours

Administration Infuse I.V. dose slowly over 30-60 minutes at a concentration ≤10 mg/mL

Monitoring Parameters Blood pressure, CBC, hemoglobin, hematocrit, Coombs' test (direct), liver enzymes

Test Interactions Methyldopa interferes with the following laboratory tests: urinary uric acid, serum creatinine (alkaline picrate method), AST (colorimetric method), and urinary catecholamines (falsely high levels)

Nursing Implications May cause urine discoloration

Additional Information Most effective if used with diuretic. Titrate dose to optimal blood pressure control with minimal side effects

Dosage Forms
Injection, as methyldopate HCl: 50 mg/mL (5 mL, 10 mL)
Suspension, oral: 250 mg/5 mL (5 mL, 473 mL)
Tablet: 125 mg, 250 mg, 500 mg

Methylene Blue (meth' i leen)

Brand Names Urolene Blue®

Therapeutic Category Antidote, Cyanide; Antidote, Drug Induced Methemoglobinemia

Use Antidote for cyanide poisoning and drug-induced methemoglobinemia; an indicator dye

Pregnancy Risk Factor C (D if injected intra-amniotically)

Contraindications Renal insufficiency; hypersensitivity to methylene blue or any component

Warnings Do not inject subcutaneously or intrathecally

Precautions Use with caution in young patients and in patients with G-6-PD deficiency due to potential hemolysis

(Continued)

Methylene Blue *(Continued)*

Adverse Reactions

Cardiovascular: Hypertension, sweating, cyanosis, large I.V. doses have been associated with precordial pain

Central nervous system: Dizziness, mental confusion, headache, fever

Dermatologic: Stains skin

Gastrointestinal: Nausea, vomiting, abdominal pain

Hematologic: Formation of methemoglobin

Renal & genitourinary: Bladder irritation

Mechanism of Action In low concentrations, hastens the conversion of methemoglobin to hemoglobin; has opposite effect at high concentrations by converting ferrous iron of reduced hemoglobin to ferric iron to form methemoglobin; in cyanide toxicity, it combines with cyanide to form cyanmethemoglobin preventing the interference of cyanide with the cytochrome system

Pharmacokinetics

Absorption: Well absorbed from GI tract

Elimination: Excreted in bile, feces, and urine

Usual Dosage

Methemoglobinemia: Children and Adults: I.V.: 1-2 mg/kg or 25-50 mg/m^2; may be repeated after 1 hour if necessary

NADPH-methemoglobin reductase deficiency: Children: Oral: 1-1.5 mg/kg/day (maximum: 300 mg/day) given with 5-8 mg/kg/day ascorbic acid

Genitourinary antiseptic: Adults: Oral: 65-130 mg 3 times/day; maximum: 390 mg/day

Administration Administer undiluted by direct I.V. injection over several minutes

Patient Information May discolor urine and feces blue green

Additional Information Has been used topically (0.1% solutions) in conjunction with polychromatic light to photoinactivate viruses such as herpes simplex; this is an unlabeled indication; has been used alone or in combination with vitamin C for the management of chronic urolithiasis; skin stains may be removed using a hypochlorite solution

Dosage Forms

Injection: 10 mg/mL (1 mL, 10 mL)

Tablet: 65 mg

Methylmorphine *see* Codeine *on page 149*

Methylone® *see* Methylprednisolone *on next page*

Methylphenidate Hydrochloride (meth ill fen' i date)

Brand Names Ritalin®

Therapeutic Category Central Nervous System Stimulant, Nonamphetamine

Use Attention deficit disorder with hyperactivity (ADDH); narcolepsy

Restrictions C-II

Pregnancy Risk Factor C

Contraindications Hypersensitivity to methylphenidate or any component; glaucoma; motor tics; Tourette's syndrome; patients with marked agitation, tension, and anxiety

Precautions Use with caution in patients with hypertension, seizures

Adverse Reactions

Cardiovascular: Tachycardia, hypertension, hypotension, palpitations, cardiac arrhythmias

Central nervous system: Nervousness, insomnia, dizziness, drowsiness, movement disorders, precipitation of Tourette's syndrome; toxic psychosis (rare); fever, headache

Dermatologic: Rash

Endocrine & metabolic: Growth retardation, weight loss

Gastrointestinal: Anorexia, nausea, abdominal pain

Hematologic: Thrombocytopenia

Miscellaneous: Hypersensitivity reactions

Drug Interactions May ↑ serum concentrations of tricyclic antidepressants, warfarin, phenytoin, phenobarbital and primidone; MAO inhibitors may potentiate effects of methylphenidate; effects of guanethidine, bretylium may be antagonized by methylphenidate

Mechanism of Action Blocks the reuptake mechanism of dopaminergic neurons, appears to act at the cerebral cortex and subcortical structures

Pharmacodynamics Cerebral stimulation:

Peak effects:

Immediate release tablet: Within 2 hours

Sustained release tablet: Within 4-7 hours

Duration:

Immediate release tablet: 3-6 hours

Sustained release tablet: 8 hours

Pharmacokinetics

Absorption: From the GI tract, slow and incomplete

Metabolism: Metabolized in liver via hydroxylation to ritolinic acid

Half-life: 2-4 hours

Elimination: Excreted in the urine as metabolites and unchanged drug; 45% to 50% excreted in the feces via bile

Usual Dosage Oral:

Children ≥6 years: Attention deficit disorder: Initial: 0.3 mg/kg/dose or 2.5-5 mg/dose given before breakfast and lunch; increase by 0.1 mg/kg/dose or by 5-10 mg/day at weekly intervals; usual dose: 0.5-1 mg/kg/day; maximum dose: 2 mg/kg/day or 60 mg/day

Adults: Narcolepsy: 10 mg 2-3 times/day, up to 60 mg/day

Nursing Implications Do not crush or allow patient to chew sustained release dosage form; last daily dose should be given several hours before retiring

Additional Information Treatment with methylphenidate should include "drug holidays" or periodic discontinuation in order to assess the patient's requirements and to decrease tolerance and limit suppression of linear growth and weight; specific patients may require 3 doses/day for treatment of ADDH (ie, additional dose at 4 PM)

Dosage Forms

Tablet: 5 mg, 10 mg, 20 mg

Tablet, sustained release: 20 mg

References

Bond WS, "Recognition and Treatment of Attention Deficit Disorder," *Clin Pharm*, 1987, 6(8):617-24.

Shaywitz SE and Shaywitz BA, "Diagnosis and Management of Attention Deficit Disorder: A Pediatric Perspective," *Pediatr Clin North Am*, 1984, 31(2):429-57.

Methylphenobarbital *see* Mephobarbital *on page 364*

Methylphenyl *see* Oxacillin Sodium *on page 425*

Methylphenylethylhydantoin *see* Mephenytoin *on page 363*

Methylphytyl Napthoquinone *see* Phytonadione *on page 458*

Methylprednisolone (meth ill pred niss' oh lone)

Related Information

Medications Compatible With PN Solutions *on page 649-650*

Systemic Corticosteroids Comparison Chart *on page 727*

Brand Names Adlone®; A-methaPred®; depMedalone®; Depoject®; Depo-Medrol®; Depopred®; Duralone®; Medralone®; Medrol®; Methylone®; Solu-Medrol®

Synonyms 6-α-Methylprednisolone; Methylprednisolone Acetate; Methylprednisolone Sodium Succinate

Therapeutic Category Anti-inflammatory Agent; Corticosteroid, Systemic; Corticosteroid, Topical; Glucocorticoid

Use Anti-inflammatory or immunosuppressant agent in the treatment of a variety of diseases including those of hematologic, allergic, inflammatory, neoplastic, and autoimmune origin

Pregnancy Risk Factor C

Contraindications Hypersensitivity to methylprednisolone or any component; administration of live virus vaccines; systemic fungal infections

Warnings May retard bone growth

Precautions Use with caution in patients with hypothyroidism, cirrhosis, hypertension, congestive heart failure, ulcerative colitis, thromboembolic disorders

(Continued)

Methylprednisolone *(Continued)*

Adverse Reactions

Cardiovascular: Edema, hypertension

Central nervous system: Vertigo, seizures, psychoses, pseudotumor cerebri, headache

Dermatologic: Acne, skin atrophy

Endocrine & metabolic: Cushing's syndrome, pituitary-adrenal axis suppression, growth suppression, glucose intolerance, hypokalemia, alkalosis

Gastrointestinal: Peptic ulcer, nausea, vomiting

Musculoskeletal: Muscle weakness, osteoporosis, fractures

Ocular: Cataracts, glaucoma

Drug Interactions Barbiturates, phenytoin, rifampin: ↑ clearance of methylprednisolone; salicylates; vaccines; toxoids

Mechanism of Action Decreases inflammation by suppression of migration of polymorphonuclear leukocytes and reversal of increased capillary permeability

Pharmacodynamics The time of peak effects and the duration of these effects is dependent upon the route of administration. See table.

Route	Peak Effect	Duration
Oral	1–2 h	30–36 h
I.M. (acetate)	4–8 d	1–4 wk
Intra–articular	1 wk	1–5 wk

Usual Dosage

Children:

- Anti-inflammatory or immunosuppressive: Oral, I.M., I.V.: 0.12-1.7 mg/kg/day or 5-25 mg/m^2/day in divided doses every 6-12 hours
- Status asthmaticus: I.V.: Loading dose: 2 mg/kg/dose, then 0.5-1 mg/kg/dose every 6 hours
- Lupus nephritis: I.V.: 30 mg/kg every other day for 6 doses
- Acute spinal cord injury: I.V.: 30 mg/kg over 15 minutes followed in 45 minutes by a continuous infusion of 5.4 mg/kg/hour for 23 hours

Adults:

- Oral: 2-60 mg in 1-4 divided doses
- I.M. (acetate): 10-80 mg/day once daily
- Lupus nephritis: I.V.: 1 g/day for 3 days
- Intra-articular, intralesional: 4-40 mg, up to 80 mg for large joints every 1-5 weeks

Administration Succinate: I.V. push over 1-15 minutes; intermittent infusion over 15-60 minutes; maximum concentration: IVP: 125 mg/mL; I.V. infusion: 2.5 mg/mL

Monitoring Parameters Blood pressure, serum glucose, and electrolytes

Test Interactions Interferes with skin tests

Nursing Implications Give after meals or with food or milk; do **not** give acetate form I.V.

Additional Information Sodium content of 1 g sodium succinate injection: 2.01 mEq; 53 mg of sodium succinate salt is equivalent to 40 mg of methylprednisolone base

Dosage Forms

Injection, as sodium succinate: 40 mg (1 mL, 3 mL); 125 mg (2 mL, 5 mL); 500 mg (1 mL, 4 mL, 8 mL, 20 mL); 1000 mg (1 mL, 8 mL, 50 mL); 2000 mg (30.6 mL)

Injection, as acetate: 20 mg/mL (5 mL, 10 mL); 40 mg/mL (1 mL, 5 mL, 10 mL); 80 mg/mL (1 mL, 5 mL)

Ointment, topical, as acetate: 0.25% (30 g); 1% (30 g)

Tablet: 2 mg, 4 mg, 8 mg, 16 mg, 24 mg, 32 mg

Tablet, dose pack: 4 mg (21s)

6-α-Methylprednisolone *see* Methylprednisolone *on previous page*

Methylprednisolone Acetate *see* Methylprednisolone *on previous page*

Methylprednisolone Sodium Succinate *see* Methylprednisolone *on page 379*

Methylrosaniline Chloride *see* Gentian Violet *on page 270*

Meticorten® *see* Prednisone *on page 477*

Metoclopramide Hydrochloride (met oh kloe pra' mide)

Related Information

Compatibility of Medications Mixed in a Syringe *on page 717*
Medications Compatible With PN Solutions *on page 649-650*

Brand Names Clopra®; Maxolon®; Octamide®; Reglan®

Therapeutic Category Antiemetic

Use Gastroesophageal reflux; prevention of nausea associated with chemotherapy; facilitates intubation of the small intestine and symptomatic treatment of diabetic gastric stasis

Pregnancy Risk Factor B

Contraindications Hypersensitivity to metoclopramide or any component; GI obstruction, pheochromocytoma, history of seizure disorder

Warnings May impair ability to perform hazardous activities requiring mental alertness and physical coordination

Precautions Use with caution and reduce dosage in patients with renal impairment; hypertension; some formulations contain sulfite

Adverse Reactions Extrapyramidal reactions occur most frequently in children and young adults and following I.V. administration of high doses, usually within 24-48 hours after starting therapy

Central nervous system: Drowsiness, fatigue, restlessness, anxiety, agitation, depression
Endocrine & metabolic: Gynecomastia, amenorrhea, galactorrhea
Gastrointestinal: Constipation, diarrhea
Hematologic: Methemoglobinemia
Miscellaneous: Hypersensitivity reactions

Drug Interactions Anticholinergic agents, opiate analgesics, alcohol, barbiturates, CNS depressants, phenothiazines, butyrophenones

Stability Stable for 24 hours at room temperature when admixed with ascorbic acid, cimetidine (in NS only), clindamycin (in NS only), cyclophosphamide, cytarabine, dexamethasone sodium phosphate, diphenhydramine, doxorubicin, heparin, hydrocortisone sodium phosphate, lidocaine, magnesium sulfate, mannitol, potassium acetate and chloride, and potassium phosphate

Mechanism of Action Potent dopamine receptor antagonist; blocks dopamine receptors in chemoreceptor trigger zone of the CNS, preventing emesis; accelerates gastric emptying and intestinal transit time without stimulating gastric, biliary, or pancreatic secretions

Pharmacodynamics

Onset of action:
- Oral: Within 30-60 minutes
- I.V.: Within 1-3 minutes

Duration: Therapeutic effects persist for 1-2 hours, regardless of route administered

Pharmacokinetics

Distribution: Crosses the placenta; appears in breast milk
Protein binding: 30%
Half-life: 2.5-6 hours (half-life and clearance may be dose-dependent)
Elimination: Excreted primarily as unchanged drug in the urine and feces

Usual Dosage

Intubation of small intestine to facilitate radiographic examination of upper GI tract: I.V.:
- Children:
  - <6 years: 0.1 mg/kg
  - 6-14 years: 2.5-5 mg
- Children >14 years and Adults: 10 mg

Gastroesophageal reflux: Oral, I.M., I.V.:
- Children: 0.4-0.8 mg/kg/day in 4 divided doses
- Adults: 10-15 mg 30 minutes before meals or food and at bedtime

Antiemetic (chemotherapy induced emesis): Children and Adults: Oral, I.V.: 1-2 mg/kg/dose every 2-4 hours

(Continued)

Metoclopramide Hydrochloride *(Continued)*

Dosing adjustment in renal impairment: Children and Adults:

Cl_{cr} 10-50 mL/minute: Administer 75% of recommended dose

Cl_{cr} <40 mL/minute/1.73 m^2: Administer 50% of recommended dose

Cl_{cr} <10 mL/minute: Administer 25% to 50% of recommended dose

Administration Dilute to 0.2 mg/mL (maximum concentration: 5 mg/mL) and infuse over 15-30 minutes (maximum rate of infusion: 5 mg/minute); rapid I.V. administration is associated with a transient but intense feeling of anxiety and restlessness, followed by drowsiness

Monitoring Parameters Renal function

Additional Information To prevent extrapyramidal reactions associated with antiemetic dosages, patients may be pretreated with diphenhydramine

Dosage Forms

Injection: 5 mg/mL (2 mL, 10 mL, 30 mL, 50 mL, 100 mL)

Solution, oral, concentrated: 10 mg/mL (10 mL, 30 mL)

Syrup, sugar free: 5 mg/5 mL (10 mL, 480 mL)

Tablet: 5 mg, 10 mg

Metolazone (me tole' a zone)

Brand Names Diulo®; Mykrox®; Zaroxolyn®

Therapeutic Category Antihypertensive; Diuretic, Miscellaneous

Use Management of mild to moderate hypertension; treatment of edema in congestive heart failure, nephrotic syndrome, and impaired renal function

Pregnancy Risk Factor D

Contraindications Hypersensitivity to metolazone or any component; patients with hepatic coma

Warnings Mykrox® is **not** therapeutically equivalent to Zaroxolyn® or Diulo® and should not be interchanged for one another

Adverse Reactions

Cardiovascular: Palpitations, chest pain, orthostatic hypotension

Central nervous system: Vertigo, headache

Dermatologic: Rash

Endocrine & metabolic: Hypokalemia, hyponatremia, hypochloremia, metabolic alkalosis, hyperglycemia, hyperuricemia

Gastrointestinal: Abdominal bloating, GI irritation

Miscellaneous: Chills

Drug Interactions ↑ digoxin toxicity; ↑ lithium toxicity; additive potassium losses with amphotericin B, steroids; salicylates and NSAIDs ↓ antihypertensive effects

Mechanism of Action Inhibits sodium reabsorption in the distal tubules causing increased excretion of sodium and water as well as potassium and hydrogen ions

Pharmacokinetics

Absorption: Oral: Rate and extent vary with the preparation

Protein binding: 33%

Half-life: 6-20 hours

Elimination: 70% to 95% excreted unchanged in urine

Usual Dosage Oral (dosage based on Zaroxolyn®, lower dosages may be used with Mykrox®):

Children: 0.2-0.4 mg/kg/day divided every 12-24 hours

Adults:

Edema: 5-10 mg/dose every 24 hours

Edema associated with renal disease: 5-20 mg/dose every 24 hours

Hypertension:

Zaroxolyn®: 2.5-5 mg/dose every 24 hours

Mykrox®: 0.5 mg/day; increase to a maximum of 1 mg/day, if needed

Monitoring Parameters Serum electrolytes, renal function, blood pressure

Dosage Forms

Tablet (Diulo®, Zaroxolyn®): 2.5 mg, 5 mg, 10 mg

Tablet (Mykrox®): 0.5 mg

References

Arnold WC, "Efficacy of Metolazone and Furosemide in Children With Furosemide-Resistant Edema," *Pediatrics*, 1984, 74(5):872-5.

Metreton® *see* Prednisolone *on page 476*

MetroGel® *see* Metronidazole *on this page*

Metro I.V.® *see* Metronidazole *on this page*

Metronidazole (me troe ni' da zole)

Brand Names Flagyl®; MetroGel®; Metro I.V.®; Protostat®

Therapeutic Category Amebicide; Antibiotic, Anaerobic; Antibiotic, Topical; Antiprotozoal

Use Treatment of susceptible anaerobic bacterial and protozoal infections in the following conditions: amebiasis, symptomatic and asymptomatic trichomoniasis; skin and skin structure infections; CNS infections; intra-abdominal infections; systemic anaerobic infections; topically for the treatment of acne rosacea; treatment of antibiotic-associated pseudomembranous colitis (AAPC)

Pregnancy Risk Factor B

Contraindications Hypersensitivity to metronidazole or any component

Warnings Has been shown to be carcinogenic in rodents

Precautions Use with caution in patients with liver impairment, blood dyscrasias, CNS disease; reduce dosage in patients with severe liver impairment or severe renal failure (Cl_{cr} <10 mL/minute)

Adverse Reactions

Central nervous system: Peripheral neuropathy, dizziness, confusion, seizures, headache

Dermatologic: Rash

Gastrointestinal: Metallic taste, nausea, dry mouth, diarrhea, furry tongue

Hematologic: Leukopenia

Local: Thrombophlebitis

Miscellaneous: Disulfiram-type reaction with alcohol

Drug Interactions Alcohol, warfarin, disulfiram; phenytoin, phenobarbital (may ↑ metabolism of metronidazole)

Stability Do not refrigerate neutralized solution because precipitation will occur; reconstituted vials are stable for 96 hours when stored at room temperature

Mechanism of Action Reduced to a product which interacts with DNA to cause a loss of helical DNA structure and strand breakage resulting in inhibition of protein synthesis and cell death in susceptible organisms

Pharmacokinetics

Absorption: Oral: Well absorbed

Distribution: Excreted in breast milk; widely distributed into body tissues, fluids and into erythrocytes

Protein binding: <20%

Metabolism: 30% to 60% in the liver

Half-life:

- Neonates: 25-75 hours
- Adults: 6-8 hours (half-life increases with hepatic impairment)

Peak serum levels: Within 1-2 hours; peak levels delayed when taken with food

Elimination: Excreted via the urine (20% as unchanged drug) and feces (6% to 15%)

Extensively removed by hemodialysis and peritoneal dialysis; dosage adjustment is not necessary in patients with mild to moderate renal insufficiency

Usual Dosage

Neonates: Anaerobic infections: Oral, I.V.:

- 0-4 weeks, <1200 g: 7.5 mg/kg every 48 hours
- Postnatal age ≤7 days:
  - 1200-2000 g: 7.5 mg/kg/day given every 24 hours
  - >2000 g: 15 mg/kg/day in divided doses every 12 hours
- Postnatal age >7 days:
  - 1200-2000 g: 15 mg/kg/day in divided doses every 12 hours
  - >2000 g: 30 mg/kg/day in divided doses every 12 hours

Infants and Children:

- Amebiasis: Oral: 35-50 mg/kg/day in divided doses every 8 hours
- Other parasitic infections: Oral: 15-30 mg/kg/day in divided doses every 8 hours
- Anaerobic infections: Oral, I.V.: 30 mg/kg/day in divided doses every 6 hours

(Continued)

Metronidazole *(Continued)*

Clostridium difficile (antibiotic-associated colitis): Oral: 20 mg/kg/day divided every 6 hours
Maximum dose: 4 g/day

Adults:
Amebiasis: Oral: 500-750 mg every 8 hours
Other parasitic infections: Oral: 250 mg every 8 hours or 2 g as a single dose
Anaerobic infections: Oral, I.V.: 30 mg/kg/day in divided doses every 6 hours; not to exceed 4 g/day
AAPC: Oral: 250-500 mg 3-4 times/day for 10-14 days
Topical: Apply a thin film twice daily to affected areas

Administration Administer I.V. by slow intermittent infusion over 30-60 minutes at a final concentration for administration of 5-8 mg/mL

Monitoring Parameters WBC count

Test Interactions May cause falsely decreased AST and ALT levels

Patient Information Urine may be discolored to a dark or reddish brown; do not take alcohol for at least 24 hours after the last dose

Nursing Implications Avoid contact between the drug and aluminum in the infusion set

Additional Information Sodium content of 500 mg RTU vial: 14 mEq

Dosage Forms
Gel, topical: 0.75% (30 g)
Injection, ready to use: 5 mg/mL (100 mL)
Powder for injection, as hydrochloride: 500 mg
Tablet: 250 mg, 500 mg

References

Oldenburg B and Speck WT, "Metronidazole," *Pediatr Clin North Am*, 1983, 30(1):71-5.
"Treatment of *Clostridium difficile* Diarrhea," *Med Lett Drugs Ther*, 1989, 31(803):94-5.

Mexiletine (mex' i le teen)

Brand Names Mexitil®

Therapeutic Category Antiarrhythmic Agent, Class Ib

Use Management of serious ventricular arrhythmias; suppression of PVCs

Pregnancy Risk Factor C

Contraindications Cardiogenic shock, second or third degree heart block, hypersensitivity to mexiletine or any component

Warnings Exercise extreme caution in patients with pre-existing sinus node dysfunction; mexiletine can worsen bradycardias and other arrhythmias

Precautions Use with caution in patients with seizure disorders, severe congestive heart failure, hypotension

Adverse Reactions
Cardiovascular: Palpitations, bradycardia, chest pain, syncope, hypotension, atrial or ventricular arrhythmias
Central nervous system: Tremor, dizziness, confusion, paresthesias, ataxia
Dermatologic: Rash
Gastrointestinal: Nausea, vomiting, diarrhea
Hematologic: Rarely thrombocytopenia
Hepatic: Hepatitis
Ocular: Diplopia
Otic: Tinnitus
Respiratory: Dyspnea
Miscellaneous: Positive antinuclear antibody

Drug Interactions Phenobarbital, phenytoin, rifampin, and other hepatic enzyme inducers may lower mexiletine plasma levels; cimetidine may ↑ mexiletine levels; antacids, narcotics, or anticholinergics may ↓ rate of absorption; metoclopramide may ↑ rate of absorption; drugs or diets which affect urine pH can ↑ or ↓ excretion of mexiletine

Mechanism of Action Class IB antiarrhythmic; structurally related to lidocaine; may cause ↑ in systemic vascular resistance and ↓ in cardiac output; no significant negative inotropic effect

Pharmacodynamics Onset after oral dose: 30-120 minutes

Pharmacokinetics
Distribution: V_d: 5-7 L/kg; found in breast milk in similar concentrations as plasma

Protein-binding: 50% to 70%
Metabolism: Extensive in the liver (some minor active metabolites)
Bioavailability: Oral: 88%
Half-life, adults: 10-14 hours; increase in half-life with hepatic or heart failure
Elimination: 10% to 15% excreted unchanged in urine; urinary acidification increases excretion

Usual Dosage Oral:

Children: Range: 1.4-5 mg/kg/dose (mean: 3.3 mg/kg/dose) given every 8 hours; start with lower initial dose and increase according to effects and serum concentrations

Adults: Initial: 200 mg every 8 hours (may load with 400 mg if necessary); adjust dose every 2-3 days; usual dose: 200-300 mg every 8 hours; maximum dose: 1.2 g/day

Children and Adults:

Dosing adjustment in renal impairment: Cl_{cr} <10 mL/minute: Administer 50% to 75% of normal dose

Dosing adjustment in hepatic disease: Administer 25% to 30% of normal dose; patients with severe liver disease may require even lower doses, monitor closely

Reference Range Therapeutic range: 0.5-2 μg/mL; potentially toxic: >2 μg/mL

Additional Information I.V. form under investigation

Dosage Forms Capsule: 150 mg, 200 mg, 250 mg

References

Moak JP, Smith RT, and Garson A Jr, "Mexiletine: An Effective Antiarrhythmic Drug for Treatment of Ventricular Arrhythmias in Congenital Heart Disease," *J Am Coll Cardiol*, 1987, 10(4):824-9.

Mexitil® *see* Mexiletine *on previous page*

Mezlin® *see* Mezlocillin Sodium *on this page*

Mezlocillin Sodium (mez loe sill' in)

Related Information

Medications Compatible With PN Solutions *on page 649-650*

Brand Names Mezlin®

Therapeutic Category Antibiotic, Penicillin

Use Treatment of infections caused by susceptible gram-negative aerobic bacilli (*Klebsiella*, *Proteus*, *Escherichia coli*, *Enterobacter*, *Pseudomonas aeruginosa*, *Serratia*) involving the skin and skin structure, bone and joint, respiratory tract, urinary tract, gastrointestinal tract, as well as septicemia

Pregnancy Risk Factor B

Contraindications Hypersensitivity to mezlocillin or any component or penicillins

Warnings If bleeding occurs during therapy, mezlocillin should be discontinued

Precautions Use with caution in patients with renal impairment or biliary obstruction; dosage modification required in patients with impaired renal function

Adverse Reactions

Central nervous system: Seizures, dizziness, fever, headache
Dermatologic: Rash, exfoliative dermatitis
Endocrine & metabolic: Hypokalemia, hypernatremia
Gastrointestinal: Diarrhea
Hematologic: Eosinophilia, hemolytic anemia, neutropenia, leukopenia, thrombocytopenia, prolonged bleeding time, positive direct Coombs' test
Hepatic: Elevated liver enzymes
Local: Thrombophlebitis
Renal & genitourinary: Interstitial nephritis, elevated serum creatinine and BUN
Miscellaneous: Serum sickness-like reaction

Drug Interactions Aminoglycosides, probenecid, vecuronium

Stability Reconstituted solution is stable for 48 hours at room temperature and 7 days when refrigerated; incompatible with aminoglycosides

Mechanism of Action Interferes with bacterial cell wall synthesis during active multiplication, causing cell wall death and resultant bactericidal activity against susceptible bacteria

(Continued)

Mezlocillin Sodium *(Continued)*

Pharmacokinetics

Absorption: I.M.: 63%

Distribution: Distributes into bile, heart, peritoneal fluid, sputum, bone; does not cross the blood-brain barrier well unless meninges are inflamed; crosses the placenta; distributes into breast milk at low concentrations

Protein binding: 30%

Metabolism: Minimal

Half-life:

Neonates:

<7 days: 3.7-4.4 hours

>7 days: 2.5 hours

Children 2-19 years: 0.9 hours

Adults: 50-70 minutes (dose dependent); half-life prolonged in renal impairment

Peak serum levels:

I.M.: Within 45-90 minutes

I.V. infusion: Within 5 minutes

Elimination: Principally excreted as unchanged drug in the urine, also excreted via bile

Moderately dialyzable (20% to 50%)

Usual Dosage I.M., I.V.:

Neonates:

0-4 weeks, <1200 g: 150 mg/kg/day divided every 12 hours

Postnatal age ≤7 days, ≥1200 g: 150 mg/kg/day divided every 12 hours

Postnatal age >7 days, ≥1200 g: 225 mg/kg/day divided every 8 hours

Children: 200-300 mg/kg/day divided every 4-6 hours; maximum: 24 g/day

Adults:

Uncomplicated urinary tract infection: 1.5-2 g every 6 hours; serious infections: 3-4 g every 4-6 hours

Dosing interval in renal impairment:

Cl_{cr} 10-30 mL/minute: Administer every 6-8 hours

Cl_{cr} <10 mL/minute: Administer every 8-12 hours

Administration Administer IVP over 3-5 minutes at a final concentration for administration not to exceed 100 mg/mL or give by I.V. intermittent infusion over 15-30 minutes at a concentration of 10-20 mg/mL; maximum concentration for administration in a fluid-restricted patient: 178 mg/mL

Monitoring Parameters Serum electrolytes; periodic renal, hepatic, and hematologic function tests

Test Interactions False-positive direct Coombs'; false-positive urinary protein

Additional Information Sodium content of 1 g: 1.8 mEq

Dosage Forms Powder for injection: 1 g, 2 g, 3 g, 4 g, 20 g

References

Odio C, Threlkeld N, Thomas ML, et al, "Pharmacokinetic Properties of Mezlocillin in Newborn Infants," *Antimicrob Agents Chemother*, 1984, 25(5):556-9.

Prober CG, Stevenson DK, and Benitz WE, "The Use of Antibiotics in Neonates Weighing Less Than 1200 Grams," *Pediatr Infect Dis J*, 1990, 9(2):111-21.

Miacalcin® *see* Calcitonin, Salmon *on page 93*

Micatin® [OTC] *see* Miconazole *on this page*

Miconazole (mi kon' a zole)

Related Information

Medications Compatible With PN Solutions *on page 649-650*

Brand Names Micatin® [OTC]; Monistat™; Monistat-Derm™; Monistat i.v.™

Synonyms Miconazole Nitrate

Therapeutic Category Antifungal Agent, Topical; Antifungal Agent, Vaginal

Use Topical: Treatment of vulvovaginal candidiasis and a variety of skin and mucous membrane fungal infections; I.V.: Treatment of severe systemic fungal infections and fungal meningitis that are refractory to standard treatment

Pregnancy Risk Factor C

Contraindications Hypersensitivity to miconazole or polyoxyl 35 castor oil or any component

Warnings The safety of miconazole in infants <1 year of age has not been established

Precautions I.V.: Use with caution in patients with hepatic insufficiency

Adverse Reactions

Cardiovascular: Tachycardia, arrhythmias,

Central nervous system: Arachnoiditis and 12th cranial nerve palsy (I.T.); headache, fever, dizziness

Dermatologic: Maceration, hives, rash, pruritus

Endocrine & metabolic: Hyperlipidemia (may be due to the Cremophor EL® vehicle), hyponatremia

Gastrointestinal: Nausea, vomiting, diarrhea

Hematologic: Transient anemia, thrombocytopenia, thrombocytosis

Local: Irritation, burning, itching, phlebitis

Renal & genitourinary: Pelvic cramps

Miscellaneous: Anaphylactoid reactions

Drug Interactions Warfarin, oral sulfonylureas; may be antagonistic with amphotericin B

Stability Further dilution of miconazole injection with normal saline or D_5W is stable for 24 hours at room temperature

Mechanism of Action Inhibits biosynthesis of ergosterol, damaging the fungal cell wall membrane which increases permeability causing leaking of nutrients

Pharmacokinetics

Distribution: Distributes into body tissues, joints, and fluids; poor penetration into sputum, saliva, urine, and CSF

Protein binding: 91% to 93%

Metabolism: Metabolized in the liver

Half-life: Multiphasic degradation:

- Initial: 40 minutes
- Secondary: 126 minutes
- Terminal: 24 hours

Elimination: ~50% excreted in the feces and <1% in urine as unchanged drug

Usual Dosage

Neonates: I.V.: 5-15 mg/kg/day divided every 8-24 hours

Infants and Children:

- Topical: Apply twice daily
- Vaginal: Insert contents of one applicator of vaginal cream or 100 mg suppository at bedtime for 7 days, or 200 mg suppository at bedtime for 3 days
- I.V.: 20-40 mg/kg/day divided every 8 hours

Adults:

- Topical: Apply twice daily
- Vaginal: Insert contents of one applicator of vaginal cream or 100 mg suppository at bedtime for 7 days, or 200 mg suppository at bedtime for 3 days
- I.T.: 20 mg every 1-2 days (using undiluted miconazole injection)
- I.V.: Initial: 200 mg, then 1.2-3.6 g/day divided every 8 hours
- Bladder irrigation: Dilute 200 mg in 250 mL normal saline; instill into the bladder 2-4 times/day or by continuous irrigation

Administration Administer by slow I.V. intermittent infusion over 1-2 hours at a final concentration not to exceed 6 mg/mL

Monitoring Parameters Hematocrit, hemoglobin, serum electrolytes and lipids

Patient Information Avoid contact with the eyes

Nursing Implications I.V. administration over 2 hours may minimize the potential for arrhythmias or anaphylactoid reactions; diphenhydramine may help to reduce pruritus; an antihistamine or antiemetic prior to miconazole administration, or dosage reduction, or slowing the I.V. rate and avoiding administration at mealtime may decrease nausea and vomiting

(Continued)

Miconazole *(Continued)*

Dosage Forms

Cream:

Topical, as nitrate: 2% (15 g, 30 g, 85 g)

Vaginal, as nitrate: 2% (47 g = 7 doses)

Injection: 10 mg/mL (20 mL)

Lotion, as nitrate: 2% (30 mL, 60 mL)

Powder, topical: 2% (45 g, 90 g)

Spray, topical: 2% (105 mL)

Suppository, vaginal, as nitrate: 100 mg (7s); 200 mg (3s)

MICRhoGAM™ *see* Rh_0(D) Immune Globulin *on page 510*

Micro-K® *see* Potassium Chloride *on page 469*

Micronase® *see* Glyburide *on page 272*

microNefrin® *see* Epinephrine *on page 220*

Micronor® *see* Norethindrone *on page 419*

Midazolam Hydrochloride (mid' ay zoe lam)

Related Information

Compatibility of Medications Mixed in a Syringe *on page 717*

Overdose and Toxicology Information *on page 696-700*

Preprocedure Sedatives in Children *on page 687-689*

Brand Names Versed®

Therapeutic Category Anticonvulsant; Benzodiazepine; Sedative

Use Preoperative sedation; conscious sedation prior to diagnostic or radiographic procedures

Restrictions C-IV

Pregnancy Risk Factor D

Contraindications Hypersensitivity to midazolam or any component (cross-sensitivity with other benzodiazepines may occur); uncontrolled pain; existing CNS depression; shock; narrow-angle glaucoma

Warnings Midazolam may cause respiratory depression/arrest; deaths and hypoxic encephalopathy have resulted when these were not promptly recognized and treated appropriately

Precautions Use with caution in patients with congestive heart failure, renal impairment, pulmonary disease, hepatic dysfunction

Adverse Reactions

Cardiovascular: Cardiac arrest, hypotension, bradycardia

Central nervous system: Drowsiness, ataxia, amnesia, dizziness, paradoxical excitement, sedation, headache

Gastrointestinal: Nausea, vomiting

Local: Pain and local reactions at injection site (severity less than diazepam)

Ocular: Blurred vision, diplopia

Respiratory: Respiratory depression, apnea, laryngospasm, bronchospasm, hiccups

Miscellaneous: Physical and psychological dependence with prolonged use

Drug Interactions CNS depressants, → ↑ sedation and respiratory depression; doses of anesthetic agents should be reduced when used in conjunction with midazolam; cimetidine may ↑ midazolam serum concentrations; theophylline may antagonize the sedative effects of midazolam

Mechanism of Action Depresses all levels of the CNS, including the limbic and reticular formation, probably through the increased action of gamma-aminobutyric acid (GABA), which is a major inhibitory neurotransmitter in the brain

Pharmacodynamics Sedation:

Onset:

I.M.: Within 15 minutes

I.V. within 1-5 minutes

Peak:

I.M.: 30-60 minutes

Intranasal: 10 minutes

Duration:

I.M.: Mean: 2 hours, up to 6 hours

Intranasal: 60 minutes

Pharmacokinetics

Absorption: Oral, nasal: Rapid

Distribution: V_d: 0.8-2.5 L/kg; increased V_d with congestive heart failure (CHF) and chronic renal failure

Protein binding: 95%

Metabolism: Extensively metabolized in the liver (microsomally)

Bioavailability, mean: Oral: 45%

Half-life, elimination: 1-4 hours; ↑ half-life with cirrhosis, CHF, obesity, elderly

Elimination: Excreted as glucuronide conjugated metabolites in the urine; ~2% to 10% is excreted in the feces

Usual Dosage Dosage must be individualized

Children:

Preoperative sedation:

Oral: <5 years: 0.5 mg/kg; >5 years: 0.4-0.5 mg/kg

I.M.: 0.07-0.08 mg/kg 30-60 minutes pre-surgery

Intranasal: 0.2 mg/kg administered by a 1 mL needleless syringe to the nares over 15 seconds; may repeat in 5-15 minutes

I.V.: 0.035 mg/kg/dose, repeat over several minutes as required to achieve the desired sedative effect up to a total dose of 0.1-0.2 mg/kg

Conscious sedation during mechanical ventilation: I.V.: Loading dose: 0.05-0.2 mg/kg then follow with initial continuous infusion: 1-2 μg/kg/minute; titrate to the desired effect; range: 0.4-6 μg/kg/minute

Conscious sedation for procedures:

Oral: 0.2-0.4 mg/kg (maximum: 15 mg) 30-45 minutes before the procedure

I.V.: 0.05-0.1 mg/kg 3 minutes before procedure

Adolescents >12 years: Sedation for procedure: I.V.: 0.5 mg every 3-4 minutes until effect achieved

Adults:

Preoperative sedation: I.M.: 0.07-0.08 mg/kg 30-60 minutes presurgery; usual dose: 5 mg

Conscious sedation: I.V.: Initial: 0.5-2 mg slow I.V. over at least 2 minutes; slowly titrate to effect by repeating doses every 2-3 minutes if needed; usual total dose: 2.5-5 mg; use decreased doses in elderly

Administration Infuse I.V. doses over 2-3 minutes

Monitoring Parameters Respiratory rate, heart rate, blood pressure

Additional Information Sodium content of 5 mg/mL: 0.14 mEq

Dosage Forms Injection: 1 mg/mL (2 mL, 5 mL, 10 mL); 5 mg/mL (1 mL, 2 mL, 5 mL, 10 mL)

Extemporaneous Preparation(s) A 2.5 mg/mL oral solution of injectable midazolam in a flavored, dye-free syrup (Syrpalata®) was stable for 56 days at 7°C, 20°C, or 40°C; the oral solution was made by combining the 5 mg/mL injection in a 1:1 ratio with the syrup. A liquid gelatin solution of midazolam 1 mg/mL was stable when stored for 14 days at 4°C and for 28 days at -20°C.

Bhatt-Mehta V, Johnson CE, Kostoff L, et al, "Stability of Midazolam Hydrochloride in Extemporaneously Prepared Flavored Gelatin," *Am J Hosp Pharm*, 1993, 50:472-5.

Steedman SL, Koonce JR, Wynn JE, et al, "Stability of Midazolam Hydrochloride in a Flavored Dye-Free Oral Solution," *Am J Hosp Pharm*, 1992, 49(3):615-8.

References

Booker PD, Beechey A, and Lloyd-Thomas AR, "Sedation of Children Requiring Artificial Ventilation Using an Infusion of Midazolam," *Br J Anaesth*, 1986, 58(10):1104-8.

Fraser G, "Intranasal Midazolam," *Hospital Pharmacy*, 1992, 27:73-4.

Rita L, Seleny FL, Mazurek A, et al, "Intramuscular Midazolam for Pediatric Preanesthetic Sedation: A Double-Blind Controlled Study With Morphine," *Anesthesiology*, 1985, 63(5):528-31.

Silvasi DL, Rosen DA, and Rosen KR, "Continuous Intravenous Midazolam Infusion for Sedation in the Pediatric Intensive Care Unit," *Anesth Analg*, 1988, 67(3):286-8.

Zeltzer LK, Altman A, Cohen D, et al, "American Academy of Pediatrics Report of the Subcommittee on the Management of Pain Associated With Procedures in Children With Cancer," *Pediatrics*, 1990, 86(5 Pt 2):826-31.

Midol® 200 [OTC] *see* Ibuprofen *on page 300*

Milkinol® [OTC] *see* Mineral Oil *on this page*

Milk of Magnesia *see* Magnesium Hydroxide *on page 352*

Mineral Oil

Brand Names Agoral® Plain [OTC]; Fleet® Mineral Oil Enema [OTC]; Kondremul® [OTC]; Milkinol® [OTC]; Neo-Cultol® [OTC]

Synonyms Heavy Mineral Oil; Liquid Paraffin; White Mineral Oil

Therapeutic Category Laxative, Lubricant

Use Temporary relief of constipation, to relieve fecal impaction, preparation for bowel studies or surgery

Pregnancy Risk Factor C

Contraindications Patients with colostomy or an ileostomy, appendicitis, ulcerative colitis, diverticulitis

Warnings Oral form should be avoided in children <4 years of age and bedtime doses should be avoided because of the risk of aspiration

Adverse Reactions

Gastrointestinal: Nausea, vomiting, diarrhea, abdominal cramps, anal itching, anal seepage

Respiratory: Lipid pneumonitis with aspiration

Drug Interactions May impair absorption of fat-soluble vitamins, oral contraceptives, coumarin; increased absorption with docusate

Mechanism of Action Eases passage of stool by decreasing water absorption and lubricating the intestine

Pharmacodynamics Onset of action: ~6-8 hours

Pharmacokinetics Elimination: Excreted in the feces

Usual Dosage

Children:
- Oral: 5-11 years: 5-15 mL once daily or in divided doses
- Rectal: 2-11 years: 30-60 mL as a single dose

Children ≥12 years and Adults:
- Oral: 15-45 mL/day once daily or in divided doses
- Rectal: Retention enema, contents of one enema (range 60-150 mL)/day as a single dose

Patient Information Do not take with food or meals; do not take if experiencing abdominal pain, nausea, or vomiting

Dosage Forms

Emulsion, oral: 1.4 g/5 mL (480 mL); 2.5 mL/5 mL (420 mL); 2.75 mL/5 mL (480 mL); 4.75 mL/5 mL (240 mL)

Jelly, oral: 2.75 mL/5 mL (180 mL)

Liquid:
- Oral: 500 mL, 1000 mL, 4000 mL
- Rectal: 133 mL

Mini-Gamulin® Rh *see* Rh_o(D) Immune Globulin *on page 510*

Minipress® *see* Prazosin Hydrochloride *on page 475*

Minitran® *see* Nitroglycerin *on page 415*

Minodyl® *see* Minoxidil *on this page*

Minoxidil (mi nox' i dill)

Brand Names Loniten®; Minodyl®; Rogaine®

Therapeutic Category Antihypertensive; Vasodilator

Use Management of severe hypertension; topically for management of alopecia or male pattern alopecia

Pregnancy Risk Factor C

Contraindications Pheochromocytoma, hypersensitivity to minoxidil or any component

Precautions Use with caution in patients with coronary artery disease or with recent myocardial infarction, pulmonary hypertension, significant renal dysfunction, congestive heart failure

Adverse Reactions

Cardiovascular: Edema, congestive heart failure, tachycardia, angina, pericardial effusion tamponade, EKG changes

Central nervous system: Dizziness, fatigue, headache
Dermatologic: Hypertrichosis (commonly occurs within 1-2 months of therapy), coarsening facial features, dermatologic reactions, rash, Stevens-Johnson syndrome, sunburn
Endocrine & metabolic: Sodium and water retention, weight gain
Respiratory: Pulmonary hypertension/edema

Drug Interactions Concurrent administration with guanethidine may cause profound orthostatic hypotensive effects; additive hypotensive effects with other hypotensive agents or diuretics

Mechanism of Action Produces vasodilation by directly relaxing arteriolar smooth muscle, with little effect on veins; effects may be mediated by cyclic AMP; stimulation of hair growth is secondary to vasodilation, increased cutaneous blood flow and stimulation of resting hair follicles

Pharmacodynamics Hypotensive effects:
Onset of action: Oral: Within 30 minutes
Peak effect: Within 2-8 hours
Duration: Up to 2-5 days

Pharmacokinetics
Metabolism: 88% metabolized primarily via glucuronidation
Protein-binding: None
Bioavailability: Oral: 90%
Half-life, adults: 3.5-4.2 hours
Elimination: 12% excreted unchanged in urine
Dialyzable (50% to 100%)

Usual Dosage
Children <12 years: Hypertension: Oral: Initial: 0.1-0.2 mg/kg once daily; maximum: 5 mg/day; increase gradually every 3 days; usual dosage: 0.25-1 mg/kg/day in 1-2 divided doses; maximum: 50 mg/day

Adults:
Hypertension: Oral: Initial: 5 mg once daily, increase gradually every 3 days; usual dose: 10-40 mg/day in 1-2 divided doses; maximum: 100 mg/day
Alopecia: Apply twice daily

Monitoring Parameters Fluids and electrolytes, body weight, blood pressure

Additional Information Usually used with a beta blocker (to treat minoxidil induced tachycardia) and a diuretic (for treatment of water retention/edema); may take 1-6 months for hypertrichosis to totally reverse after minoxidil therapy is discontinued.

Dosage Forms
Solution, topical: 20 mg/mL (60 mL)
Tablet: 2.5 mg, 10 mg

Mintezol® *see* Thiabendazole *on page 558*

Miochol® *see* Acetylcholine Chloride *on page 19*

Mithracin® *see* Plicamycin *on page 463*

Mithramycin *see* Plicamycin *on page 463*

Mitomycin (mye toe mye' sin)

Related Information
Emetogenic Potential of Single Chemotherapeutic Agents *on page 655*

Brand Names Mutamycin®

Synonyms Mitomycin-C; MTC

Therapeutic Category Antineoplastic Agent

Use Therapy of disseminated adenocarcinoma of stomach or pancreas in combination with other approved chemotherapeutic agents; bladder cancer

Pregnancy Risk Factor C

Contraindications Platelet counts <75,000/mm^3; leukocyte counts <3,000/mm^3 or serum creatinine of >1.7 mg/dL; coagulation disorders; hypersensitivity to mitomycin or any component

Warnings The US Food and Drug Administration (FDA) currently recommends that procedures for proper handling and disposal of antineoplastic agents be considered. Bone marrow depression, notably thrombocytopenia

(Continued)

Mitomycin *(Continued)*

and leukopenia, may contribute to the development of a secondary infection; hemolytic uremic syndrome, a serious and often fatal syndrome has occurred in patients receiving long-term therapy; the risk of renal toxicity increases with a total cumulative dose >50 mg/m^2; mitomycin is potentially carcinogenic and teratogenic

Precautions Use with caution in patients with myelosuppression, impaired renal or hepatic function; modify dosage in patients with myelosuppression

Adverse Reactions

Central nervous system: Weakness, paresthesia, fever
Dermatologic: Alopecia, pruritus
Gastrointestinal: Nausea, vomiting, mouth ulcers
Hematologic: Bone marrow suppression (leukopenia, thrombocytopenia), microangiopathic hemolytic anemia
Local: Thrombophlebitis
Renal & genitourinary: Hemolytic uremic syndrome, renal toxicity
Respiratory: Pulmonary toxicity

Drug Interactions *Vinca* alkaloids

Stability Reconstitute solution with sterile water at a concentration of 0.5 mg/mL; stable for 7 days at room temperature and 14 days when refrigerated; for I.V. infusion in D_5W, solution is stable for 3 hours at room temperature; in NS solution is stable for 12 hours at room temperature

Mechanism of Action Inhibits DNA and RNA synthesis by alkylation and cross-linking the strands of DNA

Pharmacokinetics

Half-life, terminal: 50 minutes
Elimination: Primarily by hepatic metabolism followed by urinary excretion (<10% as unchanged drug) and to a small extent biliary excretion

Usual Dosage Children and Adults: I.V. (refer to individual protocols): 10-20 mg/m^2/dose every 6-8 weeks, or 2 mg/m^2/day for 5 days, stop for 2 days then repeat; subsequent doses should be adjusted to platelet and leukocyte response. See table.

Nadir After Prior Dose per mm^3		% of Prior Dose to Be Given
Leukocytes	Platelets	
4000	>100,000	100
3000–3999	75,000–99,999	100
2000–2999	25,000–74,999	70
2000	<25,000	50

Dosing adjustment in renal impairment: Cl_{cr} <10 mL/minute: Administer 75% of normal dose

Administration Administer by short I.V. infusion over 30-60 minutes or by slow I.V. push over 5-10 minutes via a running I.V.; short I.V. infusions are usually administered at a final concentration of 20-40 μg/mL (in 50-250 mL of D_5W or NS) or I.V. slow push can be administered at a concentration not to exceed 0.5 mg/mL

Monitoring Parameters Platelet count, CBC with differential, hemoglobin, prothrombin time, renal and pulmonary function tests

Patient Information Notify physician if fever, sore throat, bruising, bleeding, shortness of breath, or painful urination occur

Nursing Implications Care should be taken to avoid extravasation since ulceration and tissue sloughing can occur

Additional Information Myelosuppressive effects:

WBC: Moderate
Platelets: Severe
Onset (days): 21
Nadir (days): 36
Recovery (days): 42-56

Dosage Forms Powder for injection: 5 mg, 20 mg, 40 mg

Mitomycin-C *see* Mitomycin *on page 391*

Mitoxantrone Hydrochloride (mye toe zan' trone)

Brand Names Novantrone®

Synonyms DHAD

Therapeutic Category Antineoplastic Agent

Use FDA approved for the treatment of acute nonlymphocytic leukemia (ANLL) in adults; mitoxantrone is also found to be very active against various leukemias, lymphoma, and breast cancer, and moderately active against pediatric sarcoma

Pregnancy Risk Factor D

Contraindications Hypersensitivity to mitoxantrone or any component

Warnings Avoid in patients with pre-existing myelosuppression; mitoxantrone is less cardiotoxic than anthracyclines. The predisposing factors for mitoxantrone-induced cardiotoxicity include prior anthracycline therapy, prior cardiovascular disease, and mediastinal irradiation. The risk of developing cardiotoxicity is <3% when the cumulative dose is <100-120 mg/m^2 in patients with predisposing factors and <160 mg/m^2 in patients with no predisposing factors; the FDA currently recommends that procedures for proper handling and disposal of antineoplastic agents be considered.

Precautions Dosage should be reduced in patients with pre-existing bone marrow suppression and patients with impaired hepatobiliary function

Adverse Reactions

Cardiovascular: Cardiotoxicity (arrhythmias, congestive heart failure), hypotension

Central nervous system: Seizures, headache

Dermatologic: Alopecia, pruritus, skin desquamation

Gastrointestinal: Nausea, diarrhea, vomiting, stomatitis

Hematologic: Myelosuppression

Hepatic: Transient elevation of liver enzymes, jaundice

Stability After penetration of the stopper, undiluted mitoxantrone solution is stable for 7 days at room temperature or 14 days when refrigerated; incompatible with heparin

Mechanism of Action Inhibits DNA and RNA synthesis by template disordering and steric obstruction; replication is decreased by binding to DNA topoisomerase II (enzyme responsible for DNA helix supercoiling); active throughout entire cell cycle

Pharmacokinetics

Distribution: Distributes into thyroid, liver, heart, and red blood cells

Albumin binding: 76%

Half-life, terminal: 43-215 hours and may be prolonged with liver impairment

Elimination: Slowly excreted in urine (6% to 11%) and bile as unchanged drug and metabolites

Usual Dosage I.V. (refer to individual protocols):

Leukemias:

Children ≤2 years: 0.4 mg/kg/day once daily for 3-5 days

Children >2 years and Adults: 8-12 mg/m^2/day once daily for 5 days or 12 mg/m^2/day once daily for 3 days

Solid tumors:

Children: 18-20 mg/m^2 every 3-4 weeks

Adults: 12-14 mg/m^2 every 3-4 weeks

Administration **Do not** give I.V. bolus over <3 minutes; can be administered I.V. intermittent infusion over 15-30 minutes at a concentration of 0.02 to 0.5 mg/mL in D_5W or normal saline

Monitoring Parameters CBC, serum uric acid, liver function tests, echocardiogram

Patient Information May discolor skin, sclera, and urine to a blue-green color

Nursing Implications Mitoxantrone is a nonvesicant; if extravasation occurs, the drug should be discontinued and restarted in another vein

Additional Information Myelosuppression (leukocyte nadir: 10-14 days; recovery: 21 days)

Dosage Forms Injection, as base: 2 mg/mL (10 mL, 12.5 mL, 15 mL)

References

Koeller J and Eble M, "Mitoxantrone: A Novel Anthracycline Derivative," *Clin Pharm*, 1988, 7(8):574-81.

(Continued)

Mitoxantrone Hydrochloride *(Continued)*

LeMaistre CF and Herzig R, "Mitoxantrone: Potential for Use in Intensive Therapy," *Semin Oncol*, 1990, 17(1 Suppl 3):43-8.

Nathanson L, "Mitoxantrone," *Cancer Treat Rev*, 1984, 11(4):289-93.

Pratt CB, Vietti TJ, Etcubanas E, et al, "Novantrone® for Childhood Malignant Solid Tumors. A Pediatric Oncology Group Phase II Study," *Invest New Drugs*, 1986, 4(1):43-8.

Mixtard® *see* Insulin Preparations *on page 311*

Modane® Bulk [OTC] *see* Psyllium *on page 498*

Modane® Soft [OTC] *see* Docusate *on page 202*

Mol-Iron® [OTC] *see* Ferrous Sulfate *on page 243*

Molybdenum *see* Trace Metals *on page 574*

Molypen® *see* Trace Metals *on page 574*

MOM *see* Magnesium Hydroxide *on page 352*

Monistat™ *see* Miconazole *on page 386*

Monistat-Derm™ *see* Miconazole *on page 386*

Monistat i.v.™ *see* Miconazole *on page 386*

Monoclate-P® *see* Antihemophilic Factor, Human *on page 55*

Monoclonal Antibody *see* Muromonab-CD3 *on page 397*

Monodox® *see* Doxycycline *on page 210*

Mononine® *see* Factor IX Complex (Human) *on page 239*

More-Dophilus® [OTC] *see* *Lactobacillus acidophilus* and *Lactobacillus bulgaricus* *on page 333*

Morphine Sulfate (mor' feen)

Related Information

Compatibility of Medications Mixed in a Syringe *on page 717*
Medications Compatible With PN Solutions *on page 649-650*
Narcotic Analgesics Comparison Chart *on page 721-722*
Overdose and Toxicology Information *on page 696-700*
Preprocedure Sedatives in Children *on page 687-689*

Brand Names Astramorph™ PF; Duramorph®; MS Contin®; MSIR®; OMS®; Oramorph SR®; RMS®; Roxanol™; Roxanol SR™

Synonyms MS

Therapeutic Category Analgesic, Narcotic

Use Relief of moderate to severe acute and chronic pain; pain of myocardial infarction; relieves dyspnea of acute left ventricular failure and pulmonary edema; preanesthetic medication

Restrictions C-II

Pregnancy Risk Factor B (D if used for prolonged periods or in high doses at term)

Contraindications Known hypersensitivity to morphine sulfate; increased intracranial pressure; severe respiratory depression; severe liver or renal insufficiency

Warnings Some preparations contain sulfites which may cause allergic reactions; infants <3 months of age are more susceptible to respiratory depression, use with caution and in reduced doses in this age group

Precautions Use with caution in patients with hypersensitivity reactions to other phenanthrene derivative opioid agonists (codeine, hydrocodone, hydromorphone, levorphanol, oxycodone, oxymorphone)

Adverse Reactions

Cardiovascular: Palpitations, hypotension, bradycardia, peripheral vasodilation

Central nervous system: CNS depression, drowsiness, dizziness, sedation, increased intracranial pressure

Dermatologic: Pruritus (more common with epidural or intrathecal administration)

Endocrine & metabolic: Antidiuretic hormone release

Gastrointestinal: Nausea, vomiting, constipation

Hepatic: Biliary tract spasm
Ocular: Miosis
Renal & genitourinary: Urinary tract spasm, urinary retention,
Respiratory: Respiratory depression
Sensitivity reactions: Histamine release
Miscellaneous: Physical and psychological dependence

Drug Interactions CNS depressants, phenothiazines, tricyclic antidepressants may potentiate the adverse effects of morphine

Stability Refrigerate suppositories; do not freeze; degradation depends on pH and presence of oxygen; relatively stable in pH 4 and below; darkening of solutions indicate degradation

Mechanism of Action Binds to opiate receptors in the CNS, causing inhibition of ascending pain pathways, altering the perception of and response to pain; produces generalized CNS depression

Pharmacodynamics See table.

Dosage	Analgesia	
Form/Route	Peak	Duration
Tablets	1 h	3–5 h
Oral solution	1 h	3–5 h
Extended release tablets	3–4 h	8–12 h
Suppository	20–60 min	3–7 h
Subcutaneous injection	50–90 min	3–5 h
I.M. injection	30–60 min	3–5 h
I.V. injection	20 min	3–5 h

Pharmacokinetics

Absorption: Oral: Variable
Metabolism: Metabolized in liver via glucuronide conjugation to morphine-6-glucuronide (active)
Half-life:
Neonates: 4.5-13.3 hours (mean: 7.6 hours)
Adults: 2-4 hours
Elimination: Excreted unchanged in urine; neonates: 3% to 15%, adults: 6% to 10%
Clearance:
Neonates: 5 mL/kg/minute
Children 6 months to 2.5 years: 21 mL/kg/minute

Usual Dosage Doses should be titrated to appropriate effect; when changing routes of administration in chronically treated patients, please note that oral doses are approximately one-half as effective as parenteral dose

Neonates: For select neonatal patients, continuous infusions of 0.01 mg/kg/hour (10 μg/kg/hour) have been utilized, but do **not** exceed infusion rates of 0.015-0.02 mg/kg/hour due to decreased elimination and ↑ CNS sensitivity

Infants and Children:
Oral: Tablet and solution (prompt release): 0.2-0.5 mg/kg/dose every 4-6 hours as needed; tablet (controlled release): 0.3-0.6 mg/kg/dose every 12 hours
I.M., I.V., S.C.: 0.1-0.2 mg/kg/dose every 2-4 hours as needed; may initiate at 0.05 mg/kg/dose; usual maximum: 15 mg/dose
I.V., S.C. continuous infusion: Sickle cell or cancer pain: 0.025-2 mg/kg/hour; postoperative pain: 0.01-0.04 mg/kg/hour
Sedation/analgesia for procedures: I.V.: 0.05-0.1 mg/kg 5 minutes before the procedure

Adolescents >12 years: Sedation/analgesia for procedures: I.V.: 3-4 mg; may repeat in 5 minutes if necessary

Adults:
Oral: Prompt release: 10-30 mg every 4 hours as needed; controlled release: 15-30 mg every 8-12 hours

(Continued)

Morphine Sulfate *(Continued)*

I.M., I.V., S.C.: 2.5-20 mg/dose every 2-6 hours as needed; usual: 10 mg/dose every 4 hours as needed
I.V., S.C. continuous infusion: 0.8-10 mg/hour; may ↑ depending on pain relief/adverse effects; usual range up to 80 mg/hour
Epidural: Initial: 5 mg in lumbar region; if inadequate pain relief within 1 hour, give 1-2 mg, maximum dose: 10 mg/24 hours
Intrathecal ($^1/_{10}$ of epidural dose): 0.2-1 mg/dose; repeat doses **not** recommended

Children and Adults: Dosing adjustment in renal impairment:
Cl_{cr} 10-50 mL/minute: Administer 75% of normal dose
Cl_{cr} <10 mL/minute: Administer 50% of normal dose

Administration Administer I.V. push over at least 5 minutes at a final concentration of 0.5-5 mg/mL; give intermittent infusion over 15-30 minutes; continuous I.V. infusion concentration: 0.1-1 mg/mL in D_5W

Monitoring Parameters Respiratory and cardiovascular status

Nursing Implications Do not crush controlled release drug product; do not administer rapidly I.V.

Additional Information Use only preservative free injections for epidural or intrathecal administration; less adverse effects are associated with epidural compared to intrathecal route of administration; equianalgesic doses: Codeine: 120 mg I.M. = morphine 10 mg I.M. = single dose oral morphine 60 mg **or** chronic dosing oral morphine 15-25 mg

Dosage Forms

Injection: 0.5 mg/mL (10 mL); 1 mg/mL (10 mL, 30 mL, 60 mL); 2 mg/mL (1 mL, 2 mL, 60 mL); 3 mg/mL (50 mL); 4 mg/mL (1 mL, 2 mL); 5 mg/mL (1 mL, 30 mL); 8 mg/mL (1 mL, 2 mL); 10 mg/mL (1 mL, 2 mL, 10 mL); 15 mg/mL (1 mL, 2 mL, 20 mL)
Injection:
Preservative free: 0.5 mg/mL (2 mL, 10 mL); 1 mg/mL (2 mL, 10 mL)
I.V. via PCA pump: 1 mg/mL (10 mL, 30 mL, 60 mL); 5 mg/mL (30 mL)
I.V. infusion preparation: 25 mg/mL (4 mL, 10 mL, 20 mL)
Solution, oral: 10 mg/5 mL (5 mL, 10 mL, 100 mL, 120 mL, 500 mL); 20 mg/5 mL (5 mL, 100 mL, 120 mL, 500 mL); 20 mg/mL (30 mL)
Suppository, rectal: 5 mg, 10 mg, 20 mg, 30 mg
Tablet: 15 mg, 30 mg
Tablet:
Controlled release: 15 mg, 30 mg, 60 mg, 100 mg
Soluble: 10 mg, 15 mg, 30 mg
Sustained release: 30 mg, 60 mg, 100 mg

References

Berde C, Ablin A, Glazer J, et al, "American Academy of Pediatrics Report of the Subcommittee on Disease-Related Pain in Childhood Cancer," *Pediatrics*, 1990, 86(5 Pt 2):818-25.
McRorie TI, Lynn AM, Nespeca MK, et al, "The Maturation of Morphine Clearance and Metabolism," *Am J Dis Child*, 1992, 147(8):972-6.

Motrin® *see* Ibuprofen *on page 300*

Motrin® IB [OTC] *see* Ibuprofen *on page 300*

6-MP *see* Mercaptopurine *on page 365*

MS *see* Morphine Sulfate *on page 394*

MS Contin® *see* Morphine Sulfate *on page 394*

MSIR® *see* Morphine Sulfate *on page 394*

MTC *see* Mitomycin *on page 391*

M.T.E.-4® *see* Trace Metals *on page 574*

M.T.E.-5® *see* Trace Metals *on page 574*

M.T.E.-6® *see* Trace Metals *on page 574*

MTX *see* Methotrexate *on page 374*

Mucomyst® *see* Acetylcysteine *on page 20*

Mucosol® *see* Acetylcysteine *on page 20*

Multe-Pak-4® *see* Trace Metals *on page 574*

Mumps Virus Vaccine, Live, Attenuated *see* Immunization Guidelines *on page 660-667*

Mupirocin (myoo peer' oh sin)

Brand Names Bactroban®

Synonyms Pseudomonic Acid A

Therapeutic Category Antibiotic, Topical

Use Topical treatment of impetigo caused by *Staphylococcus aureus* and *Streptococcus pyrogenes*; used for eradication of *S. aureus* from nasal and perineal carriage sites

Pregnancy Risk Factor B

Contraindications Known hypersensitivity to mupirocin or polyethylene glycol

Warnings Potentially toxic amounts of polyethylene glycol contained in the vehicle may be absorbed percutaneously in patients with extensive burns or open wounds; prolonged use may result in overgrowth of nonsusceptible organisms

Precautions Use with caution in patients with impaired renal function

Adverse Reactions

Cardiovascular: Swelling

Dermatologic: Pruritus, rash, erythema, dry skin

Local: Burning, stinging, pain, tenderness

Stability Do not mix with Aquaphor®, coal tar solution, or salicylic acid

Mechanism of Action Binds to bacterial isoleucyl transfer-RNA synthetase resulting in the inhibition of protein and RNA synthesis

Pharmacokinetics

Absorption: Following topical administration, penetrates the outer layers of the skin; systemic absorption is minimal through intact skin

Protein binding: 95%

Metabolism: Extensively metabolized in the liver and skin to monic acid

Half-life: 17-36 minutes

Elimination: Metabolite is excreted in the urine

Usual Dosage Children and Adults: Topical: Apply small amount 2-5 times/day for 5-14 days

Patient Information For topical use only; do not apply into the eye

Additional Information Contains polyethylene glycol vehicle

Dosage Forms Ointment: 2% (15 g)

References

Blumer JL, Lemon E, O'Horo J, et al, "Changing Therapy for Skin and Soft Tissue Infections in Children: Have We Come Full Circle?," *Pediatr Infect Dis J*, 1987, 6(1):117-22.

Britton JW, Fajardo JE, and Krafte-Jacobs B, "Comparison of Mupirocin and Erythromycin in the Treatment of Impetigo," *J Pediatr*, 1990, 117(5):827-9.

Goldfarb J, Crenshaw D, O'Horo J, et al, "Randomized Clinical Trial of Topical Mupirocin Versus Oral Erythromycin for Impetigo," *Antimicrob Agents Chemother*, 1988, 32(12):1780-3.

Murine® Ear Drops [OTC] *see* Carbamide Peroxide *on page 103*

Muro 128® Ophthalmic [OTC] *see* Sodium Chloride *on page 527*

Muromonab-CD3 (myoo roe moe' nab)

Brand Names Orthoclone® OKT_3

Synonyms Monoclonal Antibody; OKT_3

Therapeutic Category Immunosuppressant Agent

Use Treatment of acute allograft rejection in renal transplant patients; effective in reversing acute hepatic, cardiac, and bone marrow transplant rejection episodes resistant to conventional treatment

Pregnancy Risk Factor C

Contraindications Patients with known hypersensitivity to OKT_3 or any Murine® product; patients in fluid overload or those with >3% weight gain within 1 week prior to start of OKT_3

Warnings May result in an increased susceptibility to infection; severe pulmonary edema has occurred in patients with fluid overload; first dose effect

(Continued)

Muromonab-CD3 *(Continued)*

(flu-like symptoms, anaphylactic-type reaction) may occur within 30 minutes to 6 hours, up to 24 hours after the first dose. Cardiopulmonary resuscitation may be needed.

Precautions Dosage of concomitant immunosuppressants should be reduced by 50% and cyclosporine discontinued during OKT_3 therapy; maintenance immunosuppression and cyclosporine should be resumed about 3 days before stopping OKT_3

Adverse Reactions

Cardiovascular: Tachycardia, hypertension, hypotension, perioral and peripheral cyanosis, pulmonary edema

Central nervous system: Tremor, aseptic meningitis, seizures, headache, pyrexia

Dermatologic: Pruritus, rash

Gastrointestinal: Diarrhea, nausea, vomiting

Musculoskeletal: Joint pain

Ocular: Photophobia

Renal & genitourinary: Increased BUN and creatinine

Respiratory: Dyspnea, chest pain, tightness, wheezing

Miscellaneous: Flu-like symptoms (ie, fever, chills), anaphylactic-type reactions

Stability Store in refrigerator; do not freeze or shake; OKT_3 left out of the refrigerator for more than 4 hours must not be used

Mechanism of Action Reverses graft rejection by binding to T cells and interfering with their function

Usual Dosage I.V. (refer to individual protocols):

Children <12 years: 0.1 mg/kg/day once daily for 10-14 days

Children ≥12 years and Adults: 5 mg/day once daily for 10-14 days

Children and Adults: Methylprednisolone sodium succinate 1 mg/kg I.V. given prior to first muromonab-CD3 administration and I.V. hydrocortisone sodium succinate 50-100 mg given 30 minutes after administration are strongly recommended to decrease the incidence of reactions to the first dose; patient temperature should not exceed 37.8°C (100°F) at time of administration

Administration Filter each dose through a low protein-binding 0.22 micron filter (Millex GV) before administration; give I.V. push over <1 minute at a final concentration of 1 mg/mL

Monitoring Parameters Chest x-ray, weight gain, CBC with differential, vital signs (blood pressure, temperature, pulse, respiration) and immunologic monitoring of T cells, serum levels of OKT_3

Reference Range Mean serum trough levels rise during the first 3 days, then average 0.9 μg/mL on days 3-14

Nursing Implications Inform patient of expected first dose effects which are markedly reduced with subsequent doses; monitor patient closely for 48 hours after the first dose; acetaminophen and antihistamines can be given concomitantly with OKT_3 to reduce early reactions

Additional Information Recommend decreasing dose of prednisone to 0.5 mg/kg, azathioprine to 0.5 mg/kg (approximate 50% decrease in dose), and discontinuing cyclosporine while patient is receiving OKT_3

Dosage Forms Injection: 5 mg/5 mL

References

Ettenger RB, Marik JL, Rosenthal JT, et al, "OKT_3 for Rejection Reversal in Pediatric Renal Transplantation," *Clin Transpl*, 1988, 2:180-4.

Niaudet P, Murcia I, Jean G, et al, "A Comparative Trial of OKT_3 and Antilymphocyte Serum in the Preventive Treatment of Rejection After Kidney Transplantation in Children," *Ann Pediatr Paris*, 1990, 37(2):83-5.

Todd PA and Brogden RN, "Muromonab CD3 A Review of its Pharmacology and Therapeutic Potential," *Drugs*, 1989, 37(6):871-99.

Mustargen® Hydrochloride *see* Mechlorethamine Hydrochloride *on page 357*

Mustine *see* Mechlorethamine Hydrochloride *on page 357*

Mutamycin® *see* Mitomycin *on page 391*

Myambutol® *see* Ethambutol Hydrochloride *on page 234*

Myapap® Drops [OTC] *see* Acetaminophen *on page 16*

Mycelex® *see* Clotrimazole *on page 145*

Mycelex®-G *see* Clotrimazole *on page 145*

Mycifradin® Sulfate *see* Neomycin Sulfate *on page 408*

Mycitracin® [OTC] *see* Neomycin, Polymyxin B, and Bacitracin *on page 407*

Mycobutin® *see* Rifabutin *on page 513*

Mycostatin® *see* Nystatin *on page 421*

Mydfrin® Ophthalmic Solution *see* Phenylephrine Hydrochloride *on page 453*

Mydriacyl® *see* Tropicamide *on page 588*

Mykrox® *see* Metolazone *on page 382*

Mylanta® [OTC] *see* Antacid Preparations *on page 53*

Mylanta Gas® [OTC] *see* Simethicone *on page 524*

Mylanta®-II [OTC] *see* Antacid Preparations *on page 53*

Myleran® *see* Busulfan *on page 91*

Mylicon® [OTC] *see* Simethicone *on page 524*

Myochrysine® *see* Gold Sodium Thiomalate *on page 275*

Myotonachol™ *see* Bethanechol Chloride *on page 82*

Myphetapp® [OTC] *see* Brompheniramine and Phenylpropanolamine *on page 87*

Mysoline® *see* Primidone *on page 479*

Mytussin® [OTC] *see* Guaifenesin *on page 278*

Mytussin® AC *see* Guaifenesin and Codeine *on page 279*

Mytussin® DM [OTC] *see* Guaifenesin and Dextromethorphan *on page 279*

***N*-Acetylcysteine** *see* Acetylcysteine *on page 20*

***N*-Acetyl-L-cysteine** *see* Acetylcysteine *on page 20*

N-Acetyl-P-Aminophenol *see* Acetaminophen *on page 16*

NaCl *see* Sodium Chloride *on page 527*

Nadolol (nay doe' lole)

Related Information

Overdose and Toxicology Information *on page 696-700*

Brand Names Corgard®

Therapeutic Category Antianginal Agent; Antiarrhythmic Agent, Class II; Beta-Adrenergic Blocker

Use Treatment of hypertension and angina pectoris; prophylaxis of migraine headaches

Pregnancy Risk Factor C

Contraindications Uncompensated congestive heart failure, cardiogenic shock, bradycardia or heart block, bronchial asthma, bronchospasms

Precautions Therapy should not be discontinued abruptly; reduce dosage gradually over a period of 1-2 weeks; increase dosing interval in patients with renal dysfunction

Adverse Reactions

Cardiovascular: Persistent bradycardia, orthostatic hypotension, Raynaud's syndrome, congestive heart failure, edema

Central nervous system: Fatigue, dizziness

Dermatological: Rash

Gastrointestinal: GI discomfort

Respiratory: Bronchospasm

Drug Interactions Other hypotensive agents, diuretics and phenothiazines may ↑ hypotensive effects of nadolol; nadolol may enhance neuromuscular blocking agents and will antagonize beta-sympathomimetic drugs; other drug interactions similar to propranolol may occur

Mechanism of Action Competitively blocks response to beta-adrenergic stimulation; nonselective beta blocker

(Continued)

Nadolol *(Continued)*

Pharmacodynamics Duration of effect: 24 hours

Pharmacokinetics

Absorption: Oral: 30% to 40%

Distribution: Concentration in human breast milk is 4.6 times higher than serum

Protein-binding: 28%

Half-life, adults: 10-24 hours; increased half-life with decreased renal function

Usual Dosage

Children: No information regarding pediatric dosage currently available in literature

Adults: Initial: 40 mg once daily; increase gradually; usual dosage: 40-80 mg/day; may need up to 240-320 mg/day; doses as high as 640 mg/day have been used

Monitoring Parameters Blood pressure, heart rate, fluid I&O, weight

Dosage Forms Tablet: 20 mg, 40 mg, 80 mg, 120 mg, 160 mg

References

Devlin RG and Duchin KL, "Nadolol in Human Serum and Breast Milk," *Br J Clin Pharmacol*, 1981, 12(3):393-6.

Nafazair® *see* Naphazoline Hydrochloride *on page 403*

Nafcil™ *see* Nafcillin Sodium *on this page*

Nafcillin Sodium (naf sill' in)

Related Information

Extravasation Treatment *on page 640*

Medications Compatible With PN Solutions *on page 649-650*

Brand Names Nafcil™; Nallpen®; Unipen®

Synonyms Ethoxynaphthamido Penicillin Sodium; Sodium Nafcillin

Therapeutic Category Antibiotic, Penicillin

Use Treatment of susceptible bacterial infections such as osteomyelitis, septicemia, endocarditis, and CNS infections due to penicillinase-producing strains of *Staphylococcus*

Pregnancy Risk Factor B

Contraindications Hypersensitivity to nafcillin or any component or penicillins or cephalosporins

Warnings Elimination rate will be decreased in neonates; avoid using in neonates during the first 2 weeks of life

Precautions Extravasation of I.V. infusions should be avoided; modification of dosage is necessary in patients with both severe renal and hepatic impairment

Adverse Reactions

Central nervous system: Fever

Dermatologic: Skin rash

Endocrine & metabolic: Hypokalemia

Gastrointestinal: Nausea, diarrhea

Hematologic: Neutropenia, anemia, eosinophilia

Hepatic: Elevations in AST

Local: Pain, thrombophlebitis

Renal & genitourinary: Rare acute interstitial nephritis

Miscellaneous: Hypersensitivity reactions

Drug Interactions Probenecid, oral anticoagulants (monitor PT in patients receiving nafcillin and oral anticoagulants concurrently)

Stability Refrigerate oral suspension after reconstitution, discard after 7 days. Reconstituted nafcillin 250 mg/mL solution for injection is stable for 3 days at room temperature and 7 days when refrigerated

Mechanism of Action Interferes with bacterial cell wall synthesis during active multiplication, causing cell wall death and resultant bactericidal activity against susceptible bacteria

Pharmacokinetics

Absorption: Oral: Poor and erratic

Distribution: Crosses the placenta

Protein binding: 90%

Half-life:
- Neonates:
  - <3 weeks: 2.2-5.5 hours
  - 4-9 weeks: 1.2-2.3 hours
- Children 1 month to 14 years: 0.75-1.9 hours
- Adults with normal renal and hepatic function: 0.5-1.5 hours

Peak serum levels:
- Oral: Within 2 hours
- I.M.: Within 30-60 minutes

Elimination: Primarily in the bile and 10% to 30% in the urine as unchanged drug; undergoes enterohepatic recycling

Not dialyzable (0% to 5%)

Usual Dosage

Neonates: I.M., I.V.:
- 0-4 weeks, <1200 g: 50 mg/kg/day in divided doses every 12 hours
- ≤7 days:
  - 1200-2000 g: 50 mg/kg/day in divided doses every 12 hours
  - >2000 g: 75 mg/kg/day in divided doses every 8 hours
- >7 days:
  - 1200-2000 g: 75 mg/kg/day in divided doses every 8 hours
  - >2000 g: 100 mg/kg/day in divided doses every 6 hours

Children: I.M., I.V.:
- Mild to moderate infections: 50-100 mg/kg/day in divided doses every 6 hours
- Severe infections: 100-200 mg/kg/day in divided doses every 4-6 hours
- Maximum dose: 12 g/day
- Oral: 50-100 mg/kg/day divided every 6 hours

Adults:
- Oral: 250-500 mg every 4-6 hours, up to 1 g every 4-6 hours for more severe infections
- I.M.: 500 mg every 4-6 hours
- I.V.: 500-2000 mg every 4-6 hours

Administration Nafcillin can be administered by I.V. push over 5-10 minutes or by I.V. intermittent infusion over 15-60 minutes at a final concentration not to exceed 40 mg/mL; in fluid-restricted patients, a maximum concentration of 100 mg/mL can be administered

Monitoring Parameters Periodic CBC, urinalysis, BUN, serum creatinine, AST and ALT

Test Interactions False-positive urinary and serum proteins

Nursing Implications Extravasation may cause tissue sloughing and necrosis; hyaluronidase infiltration may help avoid injury

Additional Information Sodium content of 1 g: 2.9 mEq

Dosage Forms
- Capsule: 250 mg
- Powder for injection: 500 mg, 1 g, 2 g, 4 g, 10 g
- Tablet: 500 mg

References

Banner W Jr, Gooch WM 3d, Burckart G, et al, "Pharmacokinetics of Nafcillin in Infants With Low Birth Weights," *Antimicrob Agents Chemother*, 1980, 17(4):691-4.

Zenk KE, Dungy CL, and Greene CR, "Nafcillin Extravasation Injury: Use of Hyaluronidase as an Antidote," *Am J Dis Child*, 1981, 135(12):1113-4.

$NaHCO_3$ *see* Sodium Bicarbonate *on page 525*

Naldecon® Senior EX [OTC] *see* Guaifenesin *on page 278*

Nalidixic Acid (nal i dix' ik)

Brand Names NegGram®

Synonyms Nalidixinic Acid

Therapeutic Category Antibiotic, Quinolone

Use Lower urinary tract infections due to susceptible *E. coli*, *Enterobacter*, *Klebsiella*, and *Proteus*

Pregnancy Risk Factor B

Contraindications History of convulsive disorders, hypersensitivity to nalidixic acid or any component; infants <3 months of age

(Continued)

Nalidixic Acid *(Continued)*

Warnings Has been shown to cause cartilage degeneration in immature animals; usefulness may be limited by the emergence of bacterial resistance

Precautions Use with caution in patients with impaired hepatic or renal function, prepubertal children, and patients with G-6-PD deficiency

Adverse Reactions

Central nervous system: Malaise, drowsiness, vertigo, confusion, toxic psychosis, convulsions, fever, headache, increased intracranial pressure, chills

Dermatologic: Rash, urticaria, pruritus, photosensitivity

Endocrine & metabolic: Metabolic acidosis

Gastrointestinal: Nausea, vomiting

Hematologic: Leukopenia, thrombocytopenia, eosinophilia

Hepatic: Hepatotoxicity

Ocular: Visual disturbances

Drug Interactions Warfarin (↑ anticoagulant effect due to displacement from albumin binding sites), antacids (↓ nalidixic acid absorption)

Mechanism of Action Inhibits DNA polymerization in late stages of chromosomal replication

Pharmacokinetics

Absorption: Rapid and complete absorption from the GI tract

Distribution: Crosses the placenta; appears in breast milk; achieves significant antibacterial concentrations only in the urinary tract

Protein binding: 90%

Metabolism: Partial in the liver

Half-life: 6-7 hours (increases significantly with renal impairment)

Elimination: Excreted in the urine as unchanged drug and 80% as metabolites; small amounts appear in the feces

Usual Dosage Oral:

Children: 55 mg/kg/day divided every 6 hours; suppressive therapy is 33 mg/kg/day divided every 6 hours

Adults: 1 g 4 times/day for 2 weeks; then suppressive therapy of 500 mg 4 times/day

Monitoring Parameters Urinalysis, urine culture; CBC, renal and hepatic function tests

Test Interactions False-positive urine glucose with Clinitest®, false ↑ in urinary VMA

Patient Information Avoid undue exposure to direct sunlight; take 1 hour before meals

Dosage Forms

Suspension, oral (raspberry flavor): 250 mg/5 mL (473 mL)

Tablet: 250 mg, 500 mg, 1 g

References

Stutman HR and Marks MI, "Review of Pediatric Antimicrobial Therapies," *Semin Pediatr Infect Dis*, 1991, 2:3-17.

Nalidixinic Acid *see* Nalidixic Acid *on previous page*

Nallpen® *see* Nafcillin Sodium *on page 400*

***N*-allylnoroxymorphine Hydrochloride** *see* Naloxone Hydrochloride *on this page*

Naloxone Hydrochloride (nal ox' one)

Related Information

CPR Pediatric Drug Dosages *on page 614*

Brand Names Narcan®

Synonyms *N*-allylnoroxymorphine Hydrochloride

Therapeutic Category Antidote, Narcotic Agonist

Use Reverses CNS and respiratory depression in suspected narcotic overdose; neonatal opiate depression; coma of unknown etiology; used investigationally for shock, PCP and alcohol ingestion

Pregnancy Risk Factor B

Contraindications Hypersensitivity to naloxone or any component

Warnings May precipitate withdrawal symptoms (hypertension, sweating, agitation, irritability, shrill cry, failure to feed) in patients addicted to opiates

Precautions Use with caution in patients with coronary artery disease; following the use of narcotics during surgery, naloxone may reverse analgesia and increase blood pressure; use with caution in patients suspected to be opioid dependent

Adverse Reactions

Cardiovascular: Hypertension, hypotension, tachycardia, ventricular arrhythmias, cardiac arrest

Endocrine & metabolic: Sweating

Gastrointestinal: Nausea, vomiting

Stability Protect from light; stable in 0.9% NaCl and D_5W at 4 µg/mL for 24 hours; do not mix with alkaline solutions

Mechanism of Action Competes and displaces narcotics at narcotic receptor sites

Pharmacodynamics

Onset of action:

I.V.: Within 2 minutes

Endotracheal, I.M., S.C.: Within 2-5 minutes

Duration: (20-60 minutes) is shorter than that of most opioids, therefore, repeated doses are usually needed

Pharmacokinetics

Distribution: Crosses the placenta

Metabolism: Metabolized primarily by glucuronidation in the liver

Half-life:

Neonates: 1.2-3 hours

Adults: 1-1.5 hours

Elimination: Excreted in the urine as metabolites

Usual Dosage I.M., I.V. (preferred), intratracheal, S.C.:

Neonates: Narcotic-induced asphyxia: 0.01-0.1 mg/kg every 2-3 minutes as needed; may need to repeat every 1-2 hours

Infants and Children: Postanesthesia narcotic reversal: 0.01 mg/kg; may repeat every 2-3 minutes as needed based on response

Opiate intoxication: Birth (including premature infants) to 5 years or <20 kg: 0.1 mg/kg; repeat every 2-3 minutes if needed; may need to repeat doses every 20-60 minutes

>5 years or ≥20 kg: 2 mg/dose; if no response, repeat every 2-3 minutes; may need to repeat doses every 20-60 minutes

Children and Adults: I.V. continuous infusion: If continuous infusion is required, calculate dosage/hour based on effective intermittent dose used and duration of adequate response seen, titrate dose; 2.5-33 µg/kg/hour has been used

Adults: Opiate intoxication: 0.4-2 mg every 2-3 minutes as needed; may need to repeat doses every 20-60 minutes; **Note:** Use 0.1-0.2 mg increments in patients who are opioid dependent and in postoperative patients to avoid large cardiovascular changes

Administration

Endotracheal: Dilute to 1-2 mL with normal saline

I.V. push: Administer over 30 seconds as undiluted preparation

I.V. continuous infusion: Dilute to 4 µg/mL in D_5W or normal saline

Monitoring Parameters Respiratory rate, heart rate, blood pressure

Nursing Implications Use of neonatal naloxone (0.02 mg/mL) is no longer recommended because unacceptable fluid volumes may result, especially in small neonates; the 0.4 mg/mL preparation is available and can be accurately dosed with appropriately sized syringes (1 mL)

Additional Information May contain methyl and propylparabens

Dosage Forms

Injection: 0.4 mg/mL (1 mL, 2 mL, 10 mL); 1 mg/mL (2 mL, 10 mL)

Injection, neonatal: 0.02 mg/mL (2 mL)

References

American Academy of Pediatrics Committee on Drugs, "Naloxone Dosage and Route of Administration for Infants and Children: Addendum to Emergency Drug Doses for Infants and Children," *Pediatrics*, 1990, 86(3):484-5.

Naphazoline Hydrochloride (naf az' oh leen)

Brand Names AK-Con®; Albalon® Liquifilm®; Allerest® Eye Drops [OTC]; Clear Eyes® [OTC]; Comfort® [OTC]; Degest® 2 [OTC]; Estivin® II [OTC]; I-Naphline®; Nafazair®; Naphcon® [OTC]; Naphcon Forte®; Opcon®; Privine® [OTC]; VasoClear® [OTC]; Vasocon Regular®

(Continued)

Naphazoline Hydrochloride *(Continued)*

Therapeutic Category Adrenergic Agonist Agent, Ophthalmic; Nasal Agent, Vasoconstrictor; Ophthalmic Agent, Vasoconstrictor

Use Topical ocular vasoconstrictor (to soothe, refresh, moisturize, and relieve redness due to minor eye irritation); temporarily relieves nasal congestion associated with rhinitis, sinusitis, hay fever, or the common cold

Pregnancy Risk Factor C

Contraindications Hypersensitivity to naphazoline or any component, narrow-angle glaucoma, prior to peripheral iridectomy (in patients susceptible to angle block)

Warnings Excessive dosage may cause marked sedation in children, particularly infants

Precautions Rebound congestion may occur with extended use; use with caution in the presence of hypertension, diabetes, hyperthyroidism, heart disease, coronary artery disease, cerebral arteriosclerosis, or long-standing bronchial asthma

Adverse Reactions

Cardiovascular: Systemic cardiovascular stimulation (rarely)

Central nervous system: Dizziness, headache, nervousness

Gastrointestinal: Nausea

Local: Transient stinging, nasal mucosa irritation, dryness, sneezing, rebound congestion

Ocular: Mydriasis, increased intraocular pressure, blurring of vision

Drug Interactions Anesthetics (discontinue mydriatic prior to use of anesthetics that sensitize the myocardium to sympathomimetics, ie, cyclopropane, halothane); MAO inhibitors; tricyclic antidepressants

Mechanism of Action Stimulates alpha-adrenergic receptors in the arterioles of the conjunctiva and the nasal mucosa to produce vasoconstriction

Pharmacodynamics

Onset of action: Following topical administration, decongestion occurs within 10 minutes

Duration: 2-6 hours

Pharmacokinetics Elimination: Not well defined

Usual Dosage

Nasal: Intranasal not recommended for use in children <6 years of age (especially in infants) due to CNS depression; therapy should not exceed 3-5 days

- Children 6-12 years: 0.05%, one (1) drop every 6 hours if needed
- Children >12 years to Adults: 0.05%, 1-2 drops or sprays every 3-6 hours if needed

Ophthalmic: Therapy should generally not exceed 3-4 days; not recommended for use in children <6 years of age due to CNS depression (especially in infants)

- Children >6 years and Adults (0.01% to 0.1%): 1-3 drops into conjunctival sac of affected eye(s) every 3-4 hours

Patient Information Discontinue eye drops if visual changes or ocular pain occur

Dosage Forms

Solution, nasal:

- Drops: 0.05% (20 mL)
- Spray: 0.05% (15 mL)

Ophthalmic: 0.012% (7.5 mL, 30 mL); 0.02% (15 mL); 0.03% (15 mL); 0.1% (15 mL)

Naphcon® [OTC] *see* Naphazoline Hydrochloride *on previous page*

Naphcon Forte® *see* Naphazoline Hydrochloride *on previous page*

Naprosyn® *see* Naproxen *on this page*

Naproxen (na prox' en)

Related Information

Overdose and Toxicology Information *on page 696-700*

Brand Names Anaprox®; Naprosyn®

Therapeutic Category Analgesic, Non-Narcotic; Anti-inflammatory Agent; Antipyretic; Nonsteroidal Anti-Inflammatory Agent (NSAID), Oral

Use Management of inflammatory disease and rheumatoid disorders (including juvenile rheumatoid arthritis); acute gout; mild to moderate pain; dysmenorrhea; fever

Pregnancy Risk Factor B

Contraindications Hypersensitivity to naproxen, aspirin, or other nonsteroidal anti-inflammatory drugs (NSAIDs)

Precautions Use with caution in patients with GI disease, cardiac disease, renal or hepatic impairment, and patients receiving anticoagulants

Adverse Reactions

Cardiovascular: Edema

Central nervous system: Fatigue, drowsiness, vertigo, headache

Dermatologic: Pruritus, rash

Gastrointestinal: Abdominal discomfort, nausea, heartburn, constipation, vomiting, GI bleed, ulcers, perforation

Hematologic: Thrombocytopenia, inhibits platelet aggregation, prolongs bleeding time, agranulocytosis

Hepatic: Hepatitis

Otic: Tinnitus

Renal & genitourinary: Renal dysfunction

Drug Interactions Naproxen may ↑ serum concentrations of methotrexate and ↓ the effects of furosemide; aspirin may ↓ and probenecid may ↑ naproxen serum concentrations; drug interactions similar to other NSAIDs may also occur

Mechanism of Action Inhibits prostaglandin synthesis by decreasing the activity of the enzyme, cyclo-oxygenase, which results in decreased formation of prostaglandin precursors

Pharmacokinetics

Absorption: Oral: Almost 100%

Peak serum levels: Within 1-2 hours and persisting for up to 12 hours

Usual Dosage Oral as naproxen:

Children >2 years:

- Analgesia: 5-7 mg/kg/dose every 8-12 hours
- Inflammatory disease: 10-15 mg/kg/day in 2 divided doses

Adults:

- Rheumatoid arthritis, osteoarthritis, and ankylosing spondylitis: 500-1000 mg/day in 2 divided doses
- Acute gout: 250 mg every 8 hours
- Mild to moderate pain or dysmenorrhea: Initial: 500 mg, then 250 mg every 6-8 hours; maximum: 1250 mg/day

Monitoring Parameters CBC, BUN, serum creatinine, liver enzymes, occult blood loss, periodic ophthalmologic exams

Nursing Implications Administer with food, milk, or antacids to ↓ GI adverse effects

Additional Information Naproxen sodium 275 mg = naproxen 250 mg

Dosage Forms

Suspension, oral: 125 mg/5 mL (480 mL)

Tablet, as sodium: 275 mg, 500 mg

Tablet: 250 mg, 375 mg, 500 mg

References

Berde C, Ablin A, Glazer J, et al, "American Academy of Pediatrics Report of the Subcommittee on Disease-Related Pain in Childhood Cancer," *Pediatrics*, 1990, 86(5 Pt 2):818-25.

Narcan® *see* Naloxone Hydrochloride *on page 402*

Narcotic Analgesics Comparison Chart *see page 721*

Nasahist B® *see* Brompheniramine Maleate *on page 88*

Nasalcrom® *see* Cromolyn Sodium *on page 158*

Nasalide® *see* Flunisolide *on page 253*

Natural Lung Surfactant *see* Beractant *on page 80*

Navane® *see* Thiothixene *on page 564*

ND-Stat® *see* Brompheniramine Maleate *on page 88*

Nebcin® *see* Tobramycin Sulfate *on page 570*

NebuPent™ *see* Pentamidine Isethionate *on page 443*

NegGram® *see* Nalidixic Acid *on page 401*

Nembutal® *see* Pentobarbital *on page 446*

Neo-Calglucon® [OTC] *see* Calcium Glubionate *on page 96*

Neo-Cultol® [OTC] *see* Mineral Oil *on page 390*

Neofed® [OTC] *see* Pseudoephedrine *on page 497*

Neo-fradin® *see* Neomycin Sulfate *on page 408*

Neoloid® [OTC] *see* Castor Oil *on page 109*

Neomixin® *see* Neomycin, Polymyxin B, and Bacitracin *on next page*

Neomycin and Polymyxin B

Brand Names Neosporin® Cream [OTC]; Neosporin® G.U. Irrigant

Synonyms Polymyxin B and Neomycin

Therapeutic Category Antibiotic, Irrigation; Antibiotic, Topical

Use Short-term use as a continuous irrigant or rinse in the urinary bladder to prevent bacteriuria and gram-negative rod septicemia associated with the use of indwelling catheters; to help prevent infection in minor cuts, scrapes, and burns

Pregnancy Risk Factor C (D G.U. irrigant)

Contraindications Known hypersensitivity to neomycin or polymyxin B; ophthalmic use

Warnings Topical neomycin is a contact sensitizer

Precautions Use with caution in patients with impaired renal function, dehydrated patients, burn patients, and patients receiving a high dose for prolonged treatment; use topical cream with caution in infants with diaper rash involving large area of abraded skin

Adverse Reactions

Dermatologic: Contact dermatitis, erythema, rash, urticaria

Local: Burning

Musculoskeletal: Neuromuscular blockade

Otic: Ototoxicity

Renal & genitourinary: Nephrotoxicity, bladder irritation

Stability Store irrigant solution in the refrigerator

Pharmacokinetics Absorption: Not absorbed following topical application to intact skin; absorbed through denuded or abraded skin, peritoneum, wounds, or ulcers

Usual Dosage Children and Adults:

Topical: Apply cream 1-4 times/day

Bladder irrigation: Continuous irrigant or rinse in the urinary bladder for up to 10 days where 1 mL is added to 1 L of normal saline with administration rate adjusted to patient's urine output; usually administered via a 3-way catheter (approximately 40 mL/hour)

Monitoring Parameters Urinalysis

Patient Information Notify physician if condition worsens or if rash/irritation develops

Nursing Implications Do not inject irrigant solution; connect irrigation container to the inflow lumen of a 3-way catheter to permit continuous irrigation of the urinary bladder

Additional Information GU irrigant contains methylparaben

Dosage Forms

Cream: Neomycin sulfate 3.5 mg and polymyxin B sulfate 10,000 units per g (0.94 g, 15 g)

Solution, irrigant: Neomycin sulfate 40 mg and polymyxin B sulfate 200,000 units per mL (1 mL, 20 mL)

Neomycin, (Bacitracin) Polymyxin B and Hydrocortisone

Brand Names AK-Spore H.C.®; Cortatrigen®; Cortisporin® Cream; Cortisporin® Ophthalmic Suspension; Cortisporin® Otic; Drotic®; Octicair®; Ocutricin® HC; Otomycin-HPN®; PediOtic®

Therapeutic Category Antibiotic, Ophthalmic; Antibiotic, Otic; Antibiotic, Topical; Corticosteroid, Ophthalmic; Corticosteroid, Otic; Corticosteroid, Topical

Use Steroid-responsive inflammatory condition for which a corticosteroid is indicated and where bacterial infection or a risk of bacterial infection exists

Pregnancy Risk Factor C

Contraindications Known hypersensitivity to hydrocortisone, polymyxin B sulfate, bacitracin, or neomycin sulfate; in herpes simplex, vaccinia and varicella; otic use: perforated tympanic membrane

Warnings Neomycin may cause cutaneous and conjunctival sensitization; children are more susceptible to topical corticosteroid-induced hypothalamic - pituitary - adrenal axis suppression and Cushing's syndrome

Precautions Use with caution in patients with chronic otitis media and when the integrity of the tympanic membrane is in question

Adverse Reactions

Dermatologic: Contact dermatitis

Local: Itching, swelling, pain, stinging, burning

Ocular: Elevation of intraocular pressure, glaucoma, cataracts, conjunctival erythema

Otic: Ototoxicity

Miscellaneous: Sensitization to neomycin, secondary infections

Usual Dosage

Children: Otic: Solution and suspension: 3 drops into affected ear 3-4 times/day

Adults: Otic: Solution and suspension: 4 drops into affected ear 3-4 times/day

Children and Adults:

Topical ointment: Apply thin layer to affected area 2-4 times/day

Ophthalmic:

Suspension: 1-2 drops in the affected eye every 3-4 hours

Ointment: Instill $\frac{1}{2}$" ribbon to inside of lower lid every 3-4 hours until improvement occurs then 1-3 times/day

Patient Information

Ophthalmic: May cause sensitivity to bright light; may cause temporary blurring of vision or stinging following administration

Otic: Drops can be instilled directly into the affected ear, or a cotton wick may be saturated with suspension and inserted in ear canal. Keep wick moist with suspension every 4 hours; wick should be replaced every 24 hours.

Additional Information Otic suspension is the preferred otic preparation; otic suspension can be used for the treatment of infections of mastoidectomy and fenestration cavities caused by susceptible organisms; otic solution is used **only** for superficial infections of the external auditory canal (ie, swimmer's ear)

Dosage Forms

Ointment: Neomycin sulfate 5 mg, bacitracin 400 units, polymyxin B sulfate 5000 units and hydrocortisone 10 mg per g (15 g)

Ointment, ophthalmic: Neomycin sulfate 5 mg, bacitracin 400 units, polymyxin B sulfate and hydrocortisone 10 mg per g (3.5 g)

Solution, otic: Neomycin sulfate 5 mg, polymyxin B sulfate 10,000 units, and hydrocortisone 10 mg per mL (10 mL)

Suspension:

Ophthalmic: Neomycin sulfate 5 mg, polymyxin B sulfate 10,000 units and hydrocortisone 10 mg per mL (7.5 mL)

Otic: Neomycin sulfate 5 mg, polymyxin B sulfate 10,000 units and hydrocortisone 10 mg per mL (10 mL)

Neomycin, Polymyxin B, and Bacitracin

Brand Names Medi-Quick® Ointment [OTC]; Mycitracin® [OTC]; Neomixin®; Neosporin® Ophthalmic Ointment; Neosporin® Topical Ointment [OTC]; Ocutricin®; Septa® Ointment [OTC]; Triple Antibiotic®

Therapeutic Category Antibiotic, Ophthalmic; Antibiotic, Topical

Use To help prevent infection in minor cuts, scrapes and burns; short-term treatment of superficial external ocular infections caused by susceptible organisms

Pregnancy Risk Factor C

Contraindications Known hypersensitivity to neomycin, polymyxin B or zinc bacitracin

(Continued)

Neomycin, Polymyxin B, and Bacitracin *(Continued)*

Warnings Symptoms of neomycin sensitization include itching, reddening, edema, failure to heal; ophthalmic ointments may retard corneal healing

Precautions Prolonged use may result in overgrowth of nonsusceptible organisms

Adverse Reactions

Local: Rash and hypersensitivity reactions ranging from generalized itching, swelling, and erythema have been reported

Ocular: Conjunctival sensitization

Usual Dosage Children and Adults:

Ophthalmic ointment: Instill into the conjunctival sac 1 or more times daily every 3-4 hours for 7-10 days

Topical: Apply 1-3 times/day

Patient Information Ophthalmic: May cause sensitivity to bright light; may cause temporary blurring of vision or stinging following administration

Dosage Forms Ointment:

Ophthalmic: Neomycin sulfate 3.5 mg, polymyxin B sulfate 10,000 units and bacitracin 400 units per g

Topical: Neomycin sulfate 3.5 mg, polymyxin B sulfate 5000 units and bacitracin 400 units per g

Neomycin, Polymyxin B and Prednisolone

Brand Names Poly-Pred® Liquifilm®

Therapeutic Category Antibiotic, Ophthalmic; Corticosteroid, Ophthalmic

Use Used for steroid-responsive inflammatory ocular condition in which bacterial infection or a risk of bacterial ocular infection exists

Pregnancy Risk Factor C

Contraindications Known hypersensitivity to neomycin, polymyxin B, or prednisolone; dendritic keratitis, viral disease of the cornea and conjunctiva, mycobacterial infection of the eye, fungal disease of the ocular structure, or after uncomplicated removal of a corneal foreign body

Warnings Symptoms of neomycin sensitization include itching, reddening, edema, or failure to heal

Precautions Prolonged use may result in overgrowth of nonsusceptible organisms, glaucoma, damage to the optic nerve, defects in visual acuity, and cataract formation

Adverse Reactions

Dermatologic: Cutaneous sensitization, skin rash, delayed wound healing

Ocular: Increased intraocular pressure, glaucoma, optic nerve damage, cataracts, conjunctival sensitization

Usual Dosage Children and Adults: Ophthalmic: Instill 1-2 drops every 3-4 hours; acute infections may require every 30-minute instillation initially with frequency of administration reduced as the infection is brought under control. To treat the lids: Instill 1-2 drops every 3-4 hours, close the eye and rub the excess on the lids and lid margins.

Patient Information Ophthalmic: May cause sensitivity to bright light; may cause temporary blurring of vision or stinging following administration

Nursing Implications Shake suspension before using

Dosage Forms Suspension: Neomycin sulfate 0.35%, polymyxin B sulfate 10,000 units and prednisolone acetate 0.5% per mL (5 mL, 10 mL)

Neomycin Sulfate (nee oh mye' sin)

Related Information

Overdose and Toxicology Information *on page 696-700*

Brand Names Mycifradin® Sulfate; Neo-fradin®; Neo-Tabs®

Therapeutic Category Ammonium Detoxicant; Antibiotic, Aminoglycoside; Antibiotic, Irrigation; Antibiotic, Topical

Use Given orally to prepare GI tract for surgery; treat minor skin infections; treat diarrhea caused by *E. coli*; adjunct in the treatment of hepatic encephalopathy

Pregnancy Risk Factor C

Contraindications Hypersensitivity to neomycin or any component; patients with intestinal obstruction

Warnings Neomycin is more toxic than other aminoglycosides when given parenterally; **do not administer parenterally**; topical neomycin is a contact sensitizer with sensitivity occurring in 5% to 15% of patients treated with the drug

Precautions Use with caution in patients with renal impairment, pre-existing hearing impairment, neuromuscular disorders; modify dosage in patients with renal impairment

Adverse Reactions

Dermatologic: Contact dermatitis, burning, erythema, rash, urticaria
Gastrointestinal: Nausea, vomiting, diarrhea, colitis, malabsorption
Musculoskeletal: Neuromuscular blockade
Otic: Ototoxicity
Renal & genitourinary: Nephrotoxicity
Miscellaneous: Candidiasis, contact conjunctivitis

Drug Interactions Oral neomycin may potentiate the effects of oral anticoagulants; may decrease GI absorption of digoxin and methotrexate; synergistic effects seen with penicillins; increase adverse effects with other neurotoxic, ototoxic or nephrotoxic drugs

Stability Reconstituted neomycin solution is stable for 7 days when refrigerated

Mechanism of Action Interferes with bacterial protein synthesis by binding to 30S ribosomal subunits

Pharmacokinetics

Absorption: Poorly absorbed orally (3%) or percutaneously
Distribution: V_d: 0.36 L/kg
Metabolism: Slight hepatic metabolism
Half-life: 3 hours (age and renal function dependent)
Peak serum levels:
- I.M.: Within 2 hours
- Oral: 1-4 hours

Elimination: Excreted in the urine (30% to 50% as unchanged drug); 97% of an oral dose is eliminated unchanged in feces

Usual Dosage

Neonates: Oral: Diarrhea: 50 mg/kg/day divided every 6 hours

Children: Oral: 50-100 mg/kg/day in divided doses every 6-8 hours
- Preoperative intestinal antisepsis: 90 mg/kg/day divided every 4 hours for 2 days; or 25 mg/kg at 1, 2, and 11 PM on the day preceding surgery as an adjunct to mechanical cleansing of the intestine and in combination with erythromycin base
- Hepatic coma: 2.5-7 g/m^2/day divided every 4-6 hours for 5-6 days not to exceed 12 g/day

Children and Adults: Topical: Apply ointment 1-3 times/day; topical solutions containing 0.1% to 1% neomycin have been used for irrigation

Adults: Oral: 500-2000 mg every 6-8 hours
- Preoperative intestinal antisepsis: 1 g each hour for 4 doses then 1 g every 4 hours for 5 doses; or 1 g at 1 PM, 2 PM, and 11 PM on day preceding surgery as an adjunct to mechanical cleansing of the bowel and oral erythromycin; or 6 g/day divided every 4 hours for 2-3 days
- Hepatic coma: 4-12 g/day divided every 4-6 hours

Monitoring Parameters Renal function tests

Patient Information Notify physician if ringing in the ears, hearing impairment, or dizziness occurs

Dosage Forms

Cream: 0.5% (15 g)
Ointment, topical: 0.5% (15 g, 30 g, 120 g)
Solution, oral: 125 mg/5 mL (480 mL)
Tablet: 500 mg

References

Feigin RD and Cherry JD, *Textbook of Pediatric Infectious Disease*, 2nd ed, Vol 1, Philadelphia, PA: WB Saunders Co, 1987.

Neonatal Trace Metals *see* Trace Metals *on page 574*

Neopap® [OTC] *see* Acetaminophen *on page 16*

Neoquess® *see* Dicyclomine Hydrochloride *on page 187*

Neosar® *see* Cyclophosphamide *on page 162*

Neosporin® Cream [OTC] *see* Neomycin and Polymyxin B *on page 406*

Neosporin® G.U. Irrigant *see* Neomycin and Polymyxin B *on page 406*

Neosporin® Ophthalmic Ointment *see* Neomycin, Polymyxin B, and Bacitracin *on page 407*

Neosporin® Topical Ointment [OTC] *see* Neomycin, Polymyxin B, and Bacitracin *on page 407*

Neostigmine (nee oh stig' meen)

Related Information

Overdose and Toxicology Information *on page 696-700*

Brand Names Prostigmin®

Synonyms Neostigmine Bromide; Neostigmine Methylsulfate

Therapeutic Category Antidote, Neuromuscular Blocking Agent; Cholinergic Agent; Diagnostic Agent, Myasthenia Gravis

Use Treatment of myasthenia gravis and to prevent and treat postoperative bladder distention and urinary retention; reversal of the effects of nondepolarizing neuromuscular blocking agents after surgery

Pregnancy Risk Factor C

Contraindications Hypersensitivity to neostigmine, bromides or any component; GI or GU obstruction, peritonitis

Warnings Does **not** antagonize, and may prolong the phase I block of depolarizing muscle relaxants (eg, succinylcholine)

Precautions Use with caution in patients with epilepsy, asthma, bradycardia, hyperthyroidism, cardiac arrhythmias, peptic ulcer, vagotonia, or recent coronary occlusion

Adverse Reactions

Cardiovascular: Bradycardia, hypotension, asystole

Central nervous system: Restlessness, agitation, seizures, tremor, fasciculations, weakness

Gastrointestinal: Hyperperistalsis, nausea, vomiting, diarrhea, salivation, abdominal cramps

Ocular: Miosis

Respiratory: Bronchoconstriction

Drug Interactions Antagonizes effects of nondepolarizing muscle relaxants (eg, pancuronium, tubocurarine); atropine antagonizes the muscarinic effects of neostigmine

Mechanism of Action Competitively inhibits the hydrolysis of acetylcholine by acetylcholinesterase facilitating the transmission of impulses across myoneural junction and producing cholinergic activity

Pharmacodynamics

Onset of action:

- I.M.: Within 20-30 minutes
- I.V.: Within 1-20 minutes

Duration:

- I.M.: 2.5-4 hours
- I.V.: 1-2 hours

Pharmacokinetics

Absorption: Oral: Poorly absorbed (~1% to 2%)

Metabolism: Metabolized in the liver

Half-life: 40-60 minutes

Elimination: 50% excreted renally as unchanged drug

Usual Dosage

Myasthenia gravis:

Diagnosis: I.M. (all cholinesterase medications should be discontinued at least 8 hours before; atropine should be administered I.V. immediately prior to or I.M. 30 minutes before neostigmine):

- Children: 0.025-0.04 mg/kg as a single dose
- Adults: 0.022 mg/kg as a single dose

Treatment (dosage requirements are variable; adjust dosage so patient takes larger doses at times of greatest fatigue):

- Children: I.M., I.V., S.C.: 0.01-.04 mg/kg every 2-4 hours; Oral: 0.333 mg/kg or 10 mg/m^2 6 times/day

Adults: I.M., I.V., S.C.: 0.5-2.5 mg every 1-3 hours; Oral: Initial: 15 mg/dose 3 times/day, gradually increase every 1-2 days; usual daily range: 15-375 mg

Reversal of nondepolarizing neuromuscular blockade after surgery in conjunction with atropine or glycopyrrolate: I.V.:
Infants: 0.025-0.1 mg/kg/dose
Children: 0.025-0.08 mg/kg/dose
Adults: 0.5-2.5 mg; total dose not to exceed 5 mg

Bladder atony: Adults: I.M., S.C.:
Prevention: 0.25 mg every 4-6 hours for 2-3 days
Treatment: 0.5-1 mg every 3 hours for 5 doses after bladder has emptied

Administration May be given undiluted by slow I.V. injection over several minutes

Monitoring Parameters Muscle strength, heart rate, respiratory rate

Patient Information The side effects are generally due to exaggerated pharmacologic effects; the most common side effects are salivation and muscle fasiculations; notify physician if nausea, vomiting, muscle weakness, severe abdominal pain, or difficulty breathing occurs

Dosage Forms

Injection, as methylsulfate: 0.25 mg/mL (1 mL); 0.5 mg/mL (1 mL, 10 mL); 1 mg/mL (10 mL)
Tablet, as bromide: 15 mg

Neostigmine Bromide *see* Neostigmine *on previous page*

Neostigmine Methylsulfate *see* Neostigmine *on previous page*

Neo-Synephrine® 12 Hour Nasal Solution [OTC] *see* Oxymetazoline Hydrochloride *on page 429*

Neo-Synephrine® Nasal Solution [OTC] *see* Phenylephrine Hydrochloride *on page 453*

Neo-Synephrine® Ophthalmic Solution *see* Phenylephrine Hydrochloride *on page 453*

Neo-Tabs® *see* Neomycin Sulfate *on page 408*

Neotrace-4® *see* Trace Metals *on page 574*

Nervocaine® *see* Lidocaine Hydrochloride *on page 342*

Nestrex® *see* Pyridoxine Hydrochloride *on page 501*

Neupogen® *see* Filgrastim *on page 244*

Neut® *see* Sodium Bicarbonate *on page 525*

Neutra-Phos®-K *see* Potassium Phosphate *on page 472*

Neutrogena® T/Derm *see* Coal Tar *on page 147*

Niac® [OTC] *see* Niacin *on this page*

Niacels™ [OTC] *see* Niacin *on this page*

Niacin (nye' a sin)

Brand Names Niac® [OTC]; Niacels™ [OTC]; Nicobid® [OTC]; Nicolar® [OTC]; Nicotinex [OTC]; Slo-Niacin® [OTC]

Synonyms Nicotinic Acid; Vitamin B_3

Therapeutic Category Antilipemic Agent; Vitamin, Water Soluble

Use Adjunctive treatment of hyperlipidemias; peripheral vascular disease and circulatory disorders; treatment of pellagra; dietary supplement

Pregnancy Risk Factor A (C if used in doses greater than RDA suggested doses)

Contraindications Liver disease, peptic ulcer, severe hypotension, arterial hemorrhaging, hypersensitivity to niacin

Precautions May elevate uric acid levels, use with caution in patients predisposed to gout; large doses should be administered with caution to patients with gallbladder disease, jaundice, liver disease, or diabetes; some products may contain tartrazine

Adverse Reactions

Cardiovascular: Hypotension, tachycardia, syncope, vasovagal attacks
Central nervous system: Dizziness, headache
Dermatologic: Flushing and pruritus; burning, tingling skin, increased sebaceous gland activity

(Continued)

Niacin *(Continued)*

Endocrine & metabolic: Hyperuricemia
Gastrointestinal: GI upset, nausea, vomiting, heartburn, diarrhea
Hepatic: Abnormal liver function tests, jaundice, and chronic liver damage
Ocular: Blurred vision

Drug Interactions May inhibit uricosuric effects of sulfinpyrazone and probenecid; adrenergic blocking agents → additive vasodilating effect and postural hypotension

Mechanism of Action Component of two coenzymes necessary for tissue respiration, lipid metabolism, and glycogenolysis; inhibits the synthesis of very low density lipoproteins

Pharmacodynamics Vasodilation:
Onset of action: Within 20 minutes
Extended release: Within 1 hour
Duration: 20-60 minutes
Extended release: 8-10 hours

Pharmacokinetics
Distribution: Crosses into breast milk
Metabolism: Niacin in smaller doses is converted to niacinamide which is metabolized in the liver
Half-life: 45 minutes
Elimination: Excreted in the urine; with larger doses, a greater percentage is excreted unchanged in the urine

Usual Dosage
Children: Pellagra: Oral: 50-100 mg/dose 3 times/day
Oral: Recommended daily allowances:
0-0.5 years: 5 mg/day
0.5-1 year: 6 mg/day
1-3 years: 9 mg/day
4-6 years: 12 mg/day
7-10 years: 13 mg/day
Males:
11-14 years: 17 mg/day
15-18 years: 20 mg/day
19-24 years: 19 mg/day
Females: 11-24 years: 15 mg/day

Adults: Oral:
Recommended daily allowances:
Males: 25-50 years: 19 mg/day; >51 years: 15 mg/day
Females: 25-50 years: 15 mg/day; >51 years: 13 mg/day
Hyperlipidemia: 1.5-6 g/day in 3 divided doses with or after meals
Pellagra: 50-100 mg 3-4 times/day, maximum: 500 mg/day
Niacin deficiency: 10-20 mg/day, maximum: 100 mg/day

Monitoring Parameters Blood glucose; periodic liver function tests (with large doses or prolonged therapy)

Test Interactions False elevations in some fluorometric determinations of urinary catecholamines; false-positive urine glucose (Benedict's reagent)

Nursing Implications If dizziness occurs, avoid sudden changes in posture; give with food

Dosage Forms
Capsule, timed release: 125 mg, 250 mg, 300 mg, 400 mg, 500 mg
Elixir: 50 mg/5 mL (473 mL, 4000 mL)
Tablet: 25 mg, 50 mg, 100 mg, 250 mg, 500 mg
Tablet, timed release: 150 mg, 250 mg, 500 mg, 750 mg

Niclocide® *see* Niclosamide *on this page*

Niclosamide (ni kloe' sa mide)

Brand Names Niclocide®

Therapeutic Category Anthelmintic

Use Treatment of intestinal beef and fish tapeworm infections and dwarf tapeworm infections

Pregnancy Risk Factor B

Contraindications Known hypersensitivity to niclosamide; treatment of cysticercosis

Adverse Reactions
Central nervous system: Drowsiness, dizziness, fever, headache
Dermatologic: Rash, pruritus
Gastrointestinal: Mild abdominal pain, bloating, nausea, vomiting, diarrhea

Mechanism of Action Inhibits the synthesis of ATP through inhibition of oxidative phosphorylation in the mitochondria of cestodes

Pharmacokinetics
Absorption: Oral: Not significantly absorbed
Elimination: Excreted in feces

Usual Dosage Oral:
Beef and fish tapeworm:
Children: 40 mg/kg as a single dose one time
Adults: 2 g (4 tablets) in a single dose

Dwarf tapeworm:
Children: 40 mg/kg/day once every 24 hours for 7 days, maximum: 2 g/day
Adults: 2 g (4 tablets) in a single dose daily for 7 days

Monitoring Parameters Stool cultures

Patient Information Chew tablets thoroughly; tablets can be pulverized and mixed with water to form a paste for administration to children

Nursing Implications Administer laxative 2-3 hours after the niclosamide dose if treating *Taenia solium* infections to prevent the development of cysticercosis

Dosage Forms Tablet, chewable (vanilla flavor): 500 mg

Nicobid® [OTC] *see* Niacin *on page 411*

Nicolar® [OTC] *see* Niacin *on page 411*

Nicotinex [OTC] *see* Niacin *on page 411*

Nicotinic Acid *see* Niacin *on page 411*

Nico-Vert® *see* Dimenhydrinate *on page 193*

Nidryl® [OTC] *see* Diphenhydramine Hydrochloride *on page 195*

Nifedipine (nye fed' i peen)

Brand Names Adalat®; Procardia®; Procardia XL®

Therapeutic Category Antianginal Agent; Antihypertensive; Calcium Channel Blocker

Use Angina, hypertrophic cardiomyopathy, hypertension

Pregnancy Risk Factor C

Contraindications Hypersensitivity to nifedipine

Precautions May increase frequency, duration, and severity of angina during initiation of therapy; use with caution in patients with congestive heart failure or aortic stenosis (especially with concomitant beta blocker)

Adverse Reactions
Cardiovascular: Flushing, hypotension, tachycardia, palpitations, syncope, peripheral edema
Central nervous system: Dizziness, fever, headache, chills
Dermatologic: Dermatitis, urticaria, purpura
Endocrine & metabolic: Sweating
Gastrointestinal: Nausea, diarrhea, constipation, gingival hyperplasia
Hematologic: Thrombocytopenia, leukopenia, anemia
Musculoskeletal: Joint stiffness, arthritis with increased ANA
Ocular: Blurred vision, transient blindness
Respiratory: Shortness of breath

Drug Interactions Beta blockers may ↑ cardiovascular adverse effects; anesthetic doses of fentanyl → hypotension; cimetidine may ↑ nifedipine serum concentration; nifedipine may ↑ phenytoin and possibly digoxin serum concentrations

Mechanism of Action Inhibits calcium ion from entering the "slow channels" or select voltage-sensitive areas of vascular smooth muscle and myocardium during depolarization, producing a relaxation of coronary vascular smooth muscle and coronary vasodilation; increases myocardial oxygen delivery in patients with vasospastic angina

Pharmacodynamics Onset:
S.L.: Within 1-5 minutes

(Continued)

Nifedipine *(Continued)*

Oral: Within 20 minutes

Pharmacokinetics

Protein-binding: 92% to 98% (concentration-dependent)
Metabolism: Metabolized in liver to inactive metabolites
Bioavailability:
Capsules: 45% to 75%
Sustained release: 65% to 86%
Half-life:
Normal adults: 2-5 hours
Cirrhosis: 7 hours
Elimination: Excreted in urine

Usual Dosage Oral, S.L. (doses are usually titrated upward at 7- to 14-day intervals; may increase every 3 days if clinically necessary):

Children:
Hypertensive emergencies: 0.25-0.5 mg/kg/dose
Hypertrophic cardiomyopathy: 0.6-0.9 mg/kg/24 hours in 3-4 divided doses

Adults: Initial: 10 mg 3 times/day (capsules) or 30-60 mg once daily (sustained release tablet); maintenance: 10-30 mg 3-4 times/day (capsules); maximum: 180 mg/24 hours (capsules) or 120 mg/day (sustained release)

Monitoring Parameters Blood pressure

Nursing Implications Do not crush or break sustained release tablets

Additional Information Capsule may be punctured and drug solution administered sublingually or orally; when measuring smaller doses from the liquid-filled capsules, consider the following concentrations (for Adalat® and Procardia®) 10 mg capsule = 10 mg/0.34 mL; 20 mg capsule = 20 mg/0.45 mL

Dosage Forms

Capsule, liquid-filled: 10 mg, 20 mg
Tablet, sustained release: 30 mg, 60 mg, 90 mg

References

Dilmen U, Çağlar MK, Şenses A, et al, "Nifedipine in Hypertensive Emergencies of Children," *Am J Dis Child*, 1983, 137(12):1162-5.

Lopez-Herce J, Albajara L, Cagigas P, et al, "Treatment of Hypertensive Crisis in Children With Nifedipine," *Intensive Care Med*, 1988, 14(5):519-21.

Rosen WJ and Johnson CE, "Evaluation of Five Procedures for Measuring Nonstandard Doses of Nifedipine Liquid," *Am J Hosp Pharm*, 1989, 46(11):2313-7.

Nilstat® *see* Nystatin *on page 421*

Nipride® *see* Nitroprusside Sodium *on page 417*

Nitro-Bid® *see* Nitroglycerin *on next page*

Nitrocine® *see* Nitroglycerin *on next page*

Nitrodisc® *see* Nitroglycerin *on next page*

Nitro-Dur® *see* Nitroglycerin *on next page*

Nitrofurantoin (nye troe fyoor an' toyn)

Brand Names Furadantin®; Furalan®; Furan®; Furanite®; Macrobid®; Macrodantin®

Therapeutic Category Antibiotic, Miscellaneous

Use Prevention and treatment of urinary tract infections caused by susceptible gram-negative and some gram-positive organisms; *Pseudomonas*, *Serratia*, and most species of *Proteus* are generally resistant to nitrofurantoin

Pregnancy Risk Factor B

Contraindications Hypersensitivity to nitrofurantoin or any component; renal impairment; infants <1 month of age (due to the possibility of hemolytic anemia); pregnant patients at term

Warnings Therapeutic concentrations of nitrofurantoin are not attained in the urine of patients with renal insufficiency (Cl_{cr} <40 mL/minute, anuria, or oliguria)

Precautions Use with caution in patients with G-6-PD deficiency, patients with anemia, vitamin B deficiency, diabetes mellitus, or electrolyte abnormalities

Adverse Reactions

Central nervous system: Peripheral neuropathy, dizziness, headache, chills, fever

Dermatologic: Rash, exfoliative dermatitis, urticaria

Gastrointestinal: Nausea, vomiting, anorexia, pancreatitis

Hematologic: Hemolytic anemia, eosinophilia

Hepatic: Hepatotoxicity

Musculoskeletal: Arthralgia

Respiratory: Interstitial pneumonitis and/or fibrosis

Drug Interactions Probenecid (↓ renal excretion of nitrofurantoin), antacids (↓ absorption of nitrofurantoin)

Mechanism of Action Inhibits several bacterial enzyme systems including acetyl coenzyme A

Pharmacokinetics

Absorption: Well absorbed from the GI tract; macrocrystalline form is absorbed more slowly due to slower dissolution, but causes less GI distress

Distribution: V_d: 0.8 L/kg; crosses the placenta; appears in breast milk

Protein binding: ~40%

Metabolism: Partially metabolized in the liver

Bioavailability: Presence of food increases bioavailability

Half-life: 20-60 minutes and is prolonged with renal impairment

Elimination: Excreted as metabolites and unchanged drug (40%) in the urine and small amounts in the bile; renal excretion is via glomerular filtration and tubular secretion

Usual Dosage Oral:

Children: 5-7 mg/kg/day divided every 6 hours; maximum: 400 mg/day

Chronic therapy: 1-2.5 mg/kg/day in divided doses every 12-24 hours; maximum dose: 400 mg/day

Adults: 50-100 mg/dose every 6 hours

Prophylaxis: 50-100 mg/dose at bedtime

Monitoring Parameters Signs of pulmonary reaction; signs of numbness or tingling of the extremities; periodic liver function tests

Test Interactions Causes false-positive urine glucose with Clinitest®

Patient Information Take with food or milk; may discolor urine to a dark yellow or brown color

Nursing Implications Suspension may be mixed with water, milk, fruit juice, or infant formula

Dosage Forms

Capsule: 50 mg, 100 mg

Capsule, macrocrystal: 25 mg, 50 mg, 100 mg

Capsule, macrocrystal/monohydrate: 100 mg

Suspension, oral: 25 mg/5 mL (470 mL)

Tablet: 50 mg, 100 mg

References

Coraggio MJ, Gross TP, and Roscelli JD, "Nitrofurantoin Toxicity in Children," *Pediatr Infect Dis J*, 1989, 8(3):163-6.

Nitrogard® *see* Nitroglycerin *on this page*

Nitrogen Mustard *see* Mechlorethamine Hydrochloride *on page 357*

Nitroglycerin (nye troe gli' ser in)

Brand Names Deponit®; Minitran®; Nitro-Bid®; Nitrocine®; Nitrodisc®; Nitro-Dur®; Nitrogard®; Nitroglyn®; Nitrol®; Nitrolingual®; Nitrong®; Nitrostat®; Transdermal-NTG®; Transderm-Nitro®; Tridil®

Synonyms Glyceryl Trinitrate; Nitroglycerol; NTG

Therapeutic Category Antianginal Agent; Antihypertensive; Nitrate; Vasodilator; Vasodilator, Coronary

Use Angina pectoris; I.V. for congestive heart failure (especially when associated with acute myocardial infarction); pulmonary hypertension; hypertensive emergencies occurring perioperatively (especially during cardiovascular surgery)

Pregnancy Risk Factor C

Contraindications Hypersensitivity to nitroglycerin or any component; glaucoma; severe anemia

(Continued)

Nitroglycerin *(Continued)*

Warnings Do not chew or swallow sublingual dosage form.

Precautions Use with caution in patients with increased intracranial pressure, hypovolemia, hypotension, or constrictive pericarditis

Adverse Reactions

Cardiovascular: Flushing, hypotension, reflex tachycardia, perspiration and collapse, severe hypotension, bradycardia, coronary vascular insufficiency with abrupt withdrawal

Central nervous system: Dizziness, restlessness, headache

Dermatologic: Allergic contact dermatitis, exfoliative dermatitis, pallor

Endocrine & metabolic: Alcohol intoxication from one I.V. formulation

Gastrointestinal: Nausea, vomiting

Drug Interactions I.V. nitroglycerin may antagonize the anticoagulant effect of heparin, monitor closely, may need to ↓ heparin dosage when nitroglycerin is discontinued; alcohol, beta blockers, calcium channel blockers may enhance nitroglycerin's hypotensive effect

Stability Do not mix with other drugs; store sublingual tablets and ointment in tightly closed container; store at 15°C to 30°C

Mechanism of Action Reduces cardiac oxygen demand by decreasing left ventricular and diastolic pressure and systemic vascular resistance; dilates coronary arteries and improves collateral flow to ischemic regions; vasodilates veins >arteries

Pharmacodynamics Onset and duration of action is dependent upon dosage form administered; see table.

Nitroglycerin*

Dosage Form	Onset (min)	Duration
I.V.	1–2	3–5 min
Sublingual	1–3	30–60 min
Translingual spray	2	30–60 min
Buccal (extended release)	2–3	3–5 hours
Oral, sustained release	40	4–8 h
Topical ointment	20–60	2–12 h
Transdermal	40–60	18–24 h

Adapted from Corwin S and Reiffel, JA, "Nitrate Therapy for Angina Pectoris," *Arch Intern Med,* 1985, 145:538–43 and Franciosa JA, "Nitroglycerin and Nitrates in Congestive Heart Failure," *Heart and Lung,* 1980, 9(5):873–82.

* Hemodynamic and antianginal tolerance often develops within 24–48 h of continuous nitrate administration.

Pharmacokinetics

Protein binding: 60%

Metabolism: Extensive first-pass

Half-life: 1-4 minutes

Elimination: Excretion of inactive metabolites in the urine

Usual Dosage Tolerance to the hemodynamic and antianginal effects can develop within 24-48 hours of continuous use

Children: Continuous infusion: Start 0.25-0.5 μg/kg/minute and titrate by 0.5-1 μg/kg/minute every 3-5 minutes as needed; usual dose: 1-3 μg/kg/minute; usual maximum: 5 μg/kg/minute; doses up to 20 μg/kg/minute may be used

Adults:

Oral: 2.5-9 mg every 8-12 hours

I.V.: 5 μg/minute, increase by 5 μg/minute every 3-5 minutes to 20 μg/minute, then increase by 10 μg/minute every 3-5 minutes, up to 200 μg/minute

Sublingual: 0.2-0.6 mg every 5 minutes for maximum of 3 doses in 15 minutes

Ointment: 1" to 2" every 8 hours

Patch, transdermal: 2.5-15 mg/24 hours

Lingual: 1-2 sprays into mouth under tongue every 3-5 minutes for maximum of 3 doses in 15 minutes

Buccal: Initial: 1 mg every 5 hours while awake (3 times/day); titrate dosage upward if angina occurs with tablet in place

Administration I.V. continuous infusion: Dilute in D_5W or normal saline to 50-100 μg/mL; maximum concentration not to exceed 400 μg/mL

Monitoring Parameters Blood pressure and heart rate continuously with I.V. use

Nursing Implications I.V. must be prepared in glass bottles and special sets intended for nitroglycerin must be used; transdermal patches labeled as mg/hour; do not crush sublingual or buccal drug product

Additional Information I.V. preparations contain alcohol and/or propylene glycol; may need to use nitrate-free interval (10-12 hours/day) to avoid tolerance development; tolerance may possibly be reversed with acetylcysteine; gradually decrease dose in patients receiving NTG for prolonged period to avoid withdrawal reaction

Dosage Forms

Capsule, sustained release: 2.5 mg, 6.5 mg, 9 mg

Injection: 0.5 mg/mL (10 mL); 0.8 mg/mL (10 mL); 5 mg/mL (1 mL, 5 mL, 10 mL, 20 mL); 10 mg/mL (5 mL, 10 mL)

Ointment, topical (Nitrol®): 2% (30 g, 60 g)

Patch, transdermal, topical: Systems designed to deliver 2.5, 5, 7.5, 10, or 15 mg NTG over 24 hours

Spray, translingual: 0.4 mg/metered spray (13.8 g)

Tablet:

- Buccal, controlled release: 1 mg, 2 mg, 3 mg
- Sublingual (Nitrostat®): 0.15 mg, 0.3 mg, 0.4 mg, 0.6 mg
- Sustained release: 2.6 mg, 6.5 mg, 9 mg

References

Elkayam U, "Tolerance to Organic Nitrates: Evidence, Mechanisms, Clinical Relevance, and Strategies for Prevention," *Ann Intern Med*, 1991, 114(8):667-77.

Nitroglycerol *see* Nitroglycerin *on page 415*

Nitroglyn® *see* Nitroglycerin *on page 415*

Nitrol® *see* Nitroglycerin *on page 415*

Nitrolingual® *see* Nitroglycerin *on page 415*

Nitrong® *see* Nitroglycerin *on page 415*

Nitropress® *see* Nitroprusside Sodium *on this page*

Nitroprusside Sodium (nye troe pruss' ide)

Brand Names Nipride®; Nitropress®

Synonyms Sodium Nitroferricyanide; Sodium Nitroprusside

Therapeutic Category Antihypertensive; Vasodilator

Use Management of hypertensive crises; congestive heart failure; used for controlled hypotension during anesthesia

Pregnancy Risk Factor C

Contraindications Hypersensitivity to nitroprusside or components; decreased cerebral perfusion; arteriovenous shunt or coarctation of the aorta (ie, compensatory hypertension)

Warnings Use only as an infusion with 5% dextrose in water; continuously monitor patient's blood pressure; excessive amounts of nitroprusside can cause cyanide toxicity (usually in patients with ↓ liver function) or thiocyanate toxicity (usually in patients with ↓ renal function, or in patients with normal renal function but prolonged nitroprusside use)

Precautions Severe renal impairment, hepatic failure, hypothyroidism, hyponatremia, patients with ↑ intracranial pressure

Adverse Reactions

Cardiovascular: Excessive hypotensive response, palpitations, substernal distress

Central nervous system: Restlessness, weakness, disorientation, psychosis, headache, increased intracranial pressure

Endocrine & metabolic: Sweating, thyroid suppression, thiocyanate toxicity, cyanide toxicity

(Continued)

Nitroprusside Sodium *(Continued)*

Gastrointestinal: Nausea, vomiting

Stability Discard solution 24 hours after reconstitution and dilution

Mechanism of Action Causes peripheral vasodilation by direct action on venous and arteriolar smooth muscle, thus reducing peripheral resistance; will increase cardiac output by decreasing afterload; reduces aortal and left ventricular impedance

Pharmacodynamics Hypotensive effects:

Onset of action: Within 2 minutes

Duration: 1-10 minutes

Pharmacokinetics

Half-life: <10 minutes

Thiocyanate: 2.7-7 days

Metabolism: Converted to cyanide by erythrocyte and tissue sulfhydryl group interactions; cyanide is converted in the liver by rhodanese to thiocyanate

Elimination: Thiocyanate is excreted in the urine

Usual Dosage Children and Adults: I.V. continuous infusion: Start 0.3-0.5 μg/kg/minute, titrate to effect; usual dose: 3 μg/kg/minute; rarely need >4 μg/kg/minute; maximum: 10 μg/kg/minute

Monitoring Parameters Blood pressure, heart rate; monitor for cyanide and thiocyanate toxicity; monitor acid-base status as acidosis can be the earliest sign of cyanide toxicity; monitor thiocyanate levels if requiring prolonged infusion (>3 days) or dose ≥4 μg/kg/minute or patient has renal dysfunction; monitor cyanide blood levels in patients with decreased hepatic function

Reference Range Thiocyanate serum levels of 35-100 μg/mL are considered toxic; >200 μg/mL fatal

Cyanide: Normal <0.2 μg/mL; normal (smoker): <0.4 μg/mL; toxic: >2 μg/mL, potentially lethal: >3 μg/mL

Nursing Implications I.V. continuous infusion only via controlled infusion device; not for direct injection; solution should be protected from light, but not necessary to wrap administration set or I.V. tubing. Discard highly colored solutions. Do not add other medications to nitroprusside solutions.

Additional Information Thiocyanate toxicity includes psychoses, blurred vision, confusion, weakness, tinnitus, seizures; cyanide toxicity includes metabolic acidosis, tachycardia, pink skin, ↓ pulse, ↓ reflexes, altered consciousness, coma, almond smell on breath, methemoglobinemia, dilated pupils

Dosage Forms Injection: 10 mg/mL (5 mL); 25 mg/mL (2 mL)

Nitrostat® *see* Nitroglycerin *on page 415*

Nix™ *see* Permethrin *on page 448*

Nizoral® *see* Ketoconazole *on page 328*

Noctec® *see* Chloral Hydrate *on page 122*

Noradrenaline Acid Tartrate *see* Norepinephrine Bitartrate *on this page*

Norcet® *see* Hydrocodone and Acetaminophen *on page 292*

Norcuron® *see* Vecuronium Bromide *on page 596*

Nordeoxyguanosine *see* Ganciclovir *on page 267*

Nordryl® *see* Diphenhydramine Hydrochloride *on page 195*

Norepinephrine Bitartrate (nor ep i nef' rin)

Related Information

Extravasation Treatment *on page 640*

Brand Names Levophed®

Synonyms Levarterenol Bitartrate; Noradrenaline Acid Tartrate

Therapeutic Category Alpha-Adrenergic Agonist; Sympathomimetic

Use Treatment of shock which persists after adequate fluid volume replacement; severe hypotension; cardiogenic shock

Pregnancy Risk Factor C

Contraindications Hypersensitivity to norepinephrine or sulfites

Warnings Potent drug; must be diluted prior to use; monitor hemodynamic status

Precautions Blood/volume depletion should be corrected, if possible, before norepinephrine therapy; extravasation may cause severe tissue necrosis; do **not** give to patients with peripheral or mesenteric vascular thrombosis because ischemia may be increased and the area of infarct extended; use with caution during cyclopropane or halothane anesthesia and in patients with occlusive vascular disease

Adverse Reactions

Cardiovascular: Cardiac arrhythmias, palpitations, bradycardia, tachycardia, hypertension, chest pain, diaphoresis

Central nervous system: Anxiety, headache

Dermatologic: Pallor

Endocrine & metabolic: Uterine contractions

Gastrointestinal: Vomiting

Local: Organ ischemia (due to vasoconstriction of renal and mesenteric arteries); ischemic necrosis and sloughing of superficial tissue after extravasation

Ocular: Photophobia

Respiratory: Respiratory distress

Drug Interactions Atropine sulfate may block the reflex bradycardia caused by norepinephrine and enhance the pressor response; tricyclic antidepressants, MAO inhibitors, antihistamines (diphenhydramine, tripelennamine), guanethidine, ergot alkaloids, and methyldopa may potentiate the effect of norepinephrine

Stability Readily oxidized, do not use if brown coloration; dilute with D_5W or D_5W/NS, but not recommended to dilute in normal saline; not stable with alkaline solutions

Mechanism of Action Stimulates beta$_1$-adrenergic receptors and alpha-adrenergic receptors causing increased contractility and heart rate as well as vasoconstriction, thereby increasing systemic blood pressure and coronary blood flow; clinically alpha effects (vasoconstriction) are greater than beta effects (inotropic and chronotropic effects)

Pharmacodynamics Very rapid acting but of limited duration following I.V. injection

Pharmacokinetics

Metabolism: Metabolized by catechol-o-methyltransferase (COMT) and monoamine oxidase (MAO)

Elimination: Excreted in the urine (84% to 96% as inactive metabolites)

Usual Dosage I.V. (dose stated in terms of norepinephrine base):

Children: Initial: 0.05-0.1 μg/kg/minute, titrate to desired effect; maximum dose: 1-2 μg/kg/minute; rate (mL/hour) = dose (μg/kg/minute) x weight (kg) x 60 minutes/hour divided by concentration (μg/mL)

Adults: 8-12 μg/minute as an infusion; initiate at 4 μg/minute and titrate to desired response; ACLS dosing range: 0.5-30 μg/minute

Administration Administer into large vein to avoid the potential for extravasation; standard concentration: 4 mg/500 mL but 8 mg/500 mL has been used

Monitoring Parameters Blood pressure, heart rate, urine output, peripheral perfusion

Additional Information Treat extravasations with local injections of phentolamine

Dosage Forms Injection: 1 mg/mL (4 mL)

Norethindrone (nor eth in' drone)

Brand Names Aygestin®; Micronor®; Norlutate®; Norlutin®; NOR-Q.D.®

Synonyms Norethindrone Acetate; Norethisterone

Therapeutic Category Contraceptive, Oral; Progestin

Use Treatment of amenorrhea; abnormal uterine bleeding; endometriosis

Pregnancy Risk Factor X

Contraindications Known hypersensitivity to norethindrone; thromboembolic disorders, severe hepatic disease, breast cancer, undiagnosed vaginal bleeding

Warnings Use of any progestin during the first four months of pregnancy is not recommended

Precautions Use with caution in patients with asthma, diabetes, seizure disorder, migraine, cardiac or renal dysfunction

(Continued)

Norethindrone *(Continued)*

Adverse Reactions

Cardiovascular: Edema, thromboembolic disorders, hypertension

Central nervous system: Mental depression, nervousness, dizziness, fatigue, headache

Dermatologic: Hirsutism, rash, melasma or chloasma

Endocrine & metabolic: Breakthrough bleeding, spotting, changes in menstrual flow

Hepatic: Cholestatic jaundice

Miscellaneous: Weight gain or loss

Mechanism of Action Inhibits secretion of pituitary gonadotropin (LH) which prevents follicular maturation and ovulation; in the presence of adequate endogenous estrogen, transforms a proliferative endometrium to a secretory one

Pharmacokinetics

Protein binding: 80%

Metabolism: Metabolized in the liver

Half-life: 10 hours

Usual Dosage Adolescents and Adults: Oral:

Amenorrhea and abnormal uterine bleeding: Norethindrone 5-20 mg or norethindrone acetate 2.5-10 mg on days 5-25 of menstrual **or** to induce optimum secretory transformation of the endometrium, administer norethindrone acetate 2.5-10 mg/day for 5-10 days beginning during the latter half of the menstrual cycle

Endometriosis: Norethindrone 10 mg/day for 14 days; increase at increments of 5 mg/day every 2 weeks up to 30 mg/day **or** using norethindrone acetate 5 mg/day for 14 days; increase at increments of 2.5 mg/day every 2 weeks up to 15 mg/day

Test Interactions Thyroid function test, metyrapone test, liver function tests

Patient Information Progestin-induced withdrawal bleeding occurs within 3-7 days after discontinuation of the drug

Dosage Forms

Tablet: 5 mg

Tablet, as acetate: 5 mg

Norethindrone Acetate *see* Norethindrone *on previous page*

Norethisterone *see* Norethindrone *on previous page*

Norisodrine® *see* Isoproterenol *on page 324*

Norlutate® *see* Norethindrone *on previous page*

Norlutin® *see* Norethindrone *on previous page*

Normal Human Serum Albumin *see* Albumin Human *on page 25*

Normal Saline *see* Sodium Chloride *on page 527*

Normal Serum Albumin (Human) *see* Albumin Human *on page 25*

Normodyne® *see* Labetalol Hydrochloride *on page 331*

Norpace® *see* Disopyramide Phosphate *on page 199*

Norpramin® *see* Desipramine Hydrochloride *on page 176*

NOR-Q.D.® *see* Norethindrone *on previous page*

Nor-tet® *see* Tetracycline Hydrochloride *on page 552*

North and South American Antisnake-bite Serum *see* Antivenin (Crotalidae) Polyvalent *on page 56*

Nōstrilla® Long Acting Nasal Solution [OTC] *see* Oxymetazoline Hydrochloride *on page 429*

Nostril® Nasal Solution [OTC] *see* Phenylephrine Hydrochloride *on page 453*

Novafed® *see* Pseudoephedrine *on page 497*

Novantrone® *see* Mitoxantrone Hydrochloride *on page 393*

Novolin® *see* Insulin Preparations *on page 311*

NP-27® [OTC] *see* Tolnaftate *on page 573*

NPH Iletin® I *see* Insulin Preparations *on page 311*

NS *see* Sodium Chloride *on page 527*

½NS *see* Sodium Chloride *on page 527*

NTG *see* Nitroglycerin *on page 415*

NTZ® Nasal Solution [OTC] *see* Oxymetazoline Hydrochloride *on page 429*

NuLytely® *see* Polyethylene Glycol-Electrolyte Solution *on page 466*

Nupercainal® [OTC] *see* Dibucaine *on page 185*

Nuprin® [OTC] *see* Ibuprofen *on page 300*

Nuromax® Injection *see* Doxacurium Chloride *on page 205*

Nutracort® *see* Hydrocortisone *on page 293*

Nydrazid® *see* Isoniazid *on page 322*

Nystatin (nye stat' in)

Brand Names Mycostatin®; Nilstat®; Nystat-Rx®; Nystex®; O-V Staticin®

Therapeutic Category Antifungal Agent, Oral Nonabsorbed; Antifungal Agent, Topical; Antifungal Agent, Vaginal

Use Treatment of susceptible cutaneous, mucocutaneous, and oral cavity fungal infections normally caused by the *Candida* species

Pregnancy Risk Factor B

Contraindications Hypersensitivity to nystatin or any component

Adverse Reactions

Dermatologic: Contact dermatitis, Stevens-Johnson syndrome

Gastrointestinal: Nausea, vomiting, diarrhea

Local: Irritation

Stability Keep vaginal inserts in refrigerator

Mechanism of Action Binds to sterols in fungal cell membrane, changing the cell wall permeability allowing for leakage of cellular contents

Pharmacodynamics Onset of symptomatic relief from candidiasis: Within 24-72 hours

Pharmacokinetics

Absorption: Not absorbed through mucous membranes or intact skin; poorly absorbed from the GI tract

Elimination: Excreted in the feces as unchanged drug

Usual Dosage

Oral candidiasis:

- Neonates: 100,000 units 4 times/day or 50,000 units to each side of mouth 4 times/day
- Infants: 200,000 units 4 times/day or 100,000 units to each side of mouth 4 times/day
- Children and Adults: 400,000-600,000 units 4 times/day; troche: 200,000-400,000 units 4-5 times/day

Cutaneous candidal infections: Children and Adults: Topical: Apply 3-4 times/day

Intestinal infections: Adults: Oral: 500,000-1,000,000 units every 8 hours

Vaginal infections: Children and Adults: Vaginal tablets: Insert 1-2 tablets/day at bedtime for 2 weeks

Patient Information The oral suspension should be swished about the mouth and retained in the mouth for as long as possible (several minutes) before swallowing. For neonates and infants, paint nystatin suspension into recesses of the mouth. Troches must be allowed to dissolve slowly and should not be chewed or swallowed whole.

Dosage Forms

Cream: 100,000 units/g (15 g, 30 g)

Ointment, topical: 100,000 units/g (15 g, 30 g)

Powder, for preparation of oral suspension: 50 million units, 1 billion units, 2 billion units, 5 billion units

Powder, topical: 100,000 units/g (15 g)

Suspension, oral: 100,000 units/mL (5 mL, 60 mL, 480 mL)

(Continued)

Nystatin *(Continued)*

Tablet:
- Oral: 500,000 units
- Vaginal: 100,000 units (15 and 30/box with applicator)

Troche: 200,000 units

References

Dismukes WE, Wade JS, Lee JY, et al, "A Randomized, Double-Blind Trial of Nystatin Therapy for the Candidiasis Hypersensitivity Syndrome," *N Engl J Med*, 1990, 323(25):1717-23.

Nystat-Rx® *see* Nystatin *on previous page*

Nystex® *see* Nystatin *on previous page*

Nytol® [OTC] *see* Diphenhydramine Hydrochloride *on page 195*

Ocean Nasal Mist *see* Sodium Chloride *on page 527*

OCL® *see* Polyethylene Glycol-Electrolyte Solution *on page 466*

Octamide® *see* Metoclopramide Hydrochloride *on page 381*

Octicair® *see* Neomycin, (Bacitracin) Polymyxin B and Hydrocortisone *on page 406*

Octocaine® *see* Lidocaine Hydrochloride *on page 342*

Octreotide Acetate (ok tree' oh tide)

Brand Names Sandostatin®

Therapeutic Category Antisecretory Agent; Somatostatin Analog

Use Control of symptoms in patients with metastatic carcinoid, vasoactive intestinal peptide-secreting tumors (VIPomas), and secretory diarrhea

Pregnancy Risk Factor B

Contraindications Known hypersensitivity to octreotide or any components

Warnings Dosage adjustment may be required to maintain symptomatic control; insulin requirements may be reduced as well as sulfonylurea requirements; use with caution in patients with renal impairment

Adverse Reactions

Cardiovascular: Flushing, edema, chest pain, hypertension, palpitations

Central nervous system: Dizziness, fatigue, anxiety, headache, anorexia, depression, insomnia, numbness, fever

Dermatologic: Erythema, hair loss

Endocrine & metabolic: Hypoglycemia, hyperglycemia, galactorrhea

Gastrointestinal: Nausea, diarrhea, abdominal pain, vomiting, constipation, flatulence, fat malabsorption, GI bleeding (rare), dry mouth

Hepatic: Hepatitis, jaundice

Local: Injection site pain, thrombophlebitis

Musculoskeletal: Weakness, ↑ CPK

Renal & genitourinary: Oliguria, prostatitis

Respiratory: Shortness of breath, rhinorrhea

Miscellaneous: Chills

Drug Interactions Cyclosporine

Stability For prolonged storage keep in refrigerator; stable 14 days at room temperature; stable in D_5W or NS for 4 days at room temperature, not compatible in TPN solutions

Mechanism of Action Mimics natural somatostatin by inhibiting serotonin release, and the secretion of gastrin, VIP (vasoactive intestinal peptide), insulin, glucagon, secretin, motilin, and pancreatic polypeptide; in animals, also a potent inhibitor of growth hormone

Pharmacodynamics Duration of action: 6-12 hours

Pharmacokinetics

Absorption: S.C.: Rapid

Distribution: V_d (adults): 13.6 L/kg

Metabolism: Extensively metabolized by the liver

Half-life: 60-110 minutes

Elimination: 32% excreted unchanged in urine

Usual Dosage Adults: S.C.: Initial: 50 μg 1-2 times/day and titrate dose based on patient tolerance and response

Carcinoid: 100-600 μg/day in 2-4 divided doses

VIPomas: 200-300 μg/day in 2-4 divided doses

Diarrhea: Initial: I.V.: 50-100 μg every 8 hours; increase by 100 μg/dose at 48-hour intervals; maximum dose: 500 μg every 8 hours

Administration For I.V. infusion, dilute in 50-100 mL NS or D_5W and infuse over 20-30 minutes; in emergency situations, may be given by direct I.V. push over 3 minutes; see Stability for compatibility information

Monitoring Parameters Baseline and periodic ultrasound evaluations for cholelithiasis, blood sugar, baseline and periodic thyroid function tests, fluid and electrolyte balance; for carcinoid, monitor 5-HIAA, plasma serotonin, plasma substance P; for VIPoma, monitor VIP

Reference Range Vasoactive Intestinal Peptide: <75 ng/L. Levels vary considerably between laboratories.

Additional Information Doses of 1-10 μg/kg every 12 hours have been used in children beginning at the low end of the range and increasing by 0.3 μg/kg/dose at 3-day intervals; suppression of growth hormone (animal data) is of concern when used as long-term therapy

Dosage Forms Injection: 0.05 mg (1 mL); 0.1 mg (1 mL); 0.5 mg (1 mL)

References

Couper RT, Berzen A, Berall G, et al, "Clinical Response to the Long-Acting Somatostatin Analogue SMS 201-995 in a Child With Congenital Microvillus Atrophy," *Gut*, 1989, 30(7):1020-4.

Jaros W, Greer J, O'Dorisio T, et al, "Successful Treatment of Idiopathic Secretory Diarrhea of Infancy With the Somatostatin Analogue SMS 201-995," *Gastroent*, 1988, 94:189-93.

Katz MD and Erstad BL, "Octreotide, A New Somatostatin Analogue," *Clin Pharm*, 1989, 8(4):255-73.

OcuClear® [OTC] *see* Oxymetazoline Hydrochloride *on page 429*

Ocufen® *see* Flurbiprofen Sodium *on page 261*

Ocular Lubricant

Brand Names Duratears® [OTC]; Lacri-Lube® [OTC]

Therapeutic Category Ophthalmic Agent, Miscellaneous

Use Ocular lubricant

Contraindications Known hypersensitivity to any of the components

Warnings Discontinue if eye pain, vision change, redness or eye irritation occurs or if condition worsens or persists >72 hours

Adverse Reactions Ocular: Temporary blurring of vision, irritation

Stability Store away from heat

Usual Dosage Children and Adults: Ophthalmic: Instill $^1/_4$" of ointment to the inside of the lower lid as needed

Patient Information Do not use with contact lenses

Additional Information Contains petrolatum and mineral oil

Dosage Forms Ointment, ophthalmic: 3.5 g

Ocusert® Pilo *see* Pilocarpine *on page 459*

Ocutricin® *see* Neomycin, Polymyxin B, and Bacitracin *on page 407*

Ocutricin® HC *see* Neomycin, (Bacitracin) Polymyxin B and Hydrocortisone *on page 406*

Ocu-Trol® *see* Dexamethasone, Neomycin and Polymyxin B *on page 180*

OKT_3 *see* Muromonab-CD3 *on page 397*

Oleovitamin A *see* Vitamin A *on page 603*

Oleum Ricini *see* Castor Oil *on page 109*

Omnipen® *see* Ampicillin *on page 48*

Omnipen®-N *see* Ampicillin *on page 48*

OMS® *see* Morphine Sulfate *on page 394*

Oncovin® *see* Vincristine Sulfate *on page 602*

Ondansetron (on dan' se tron)

Brand Names Zofran®

Therapeutic Category Antiemetic

Use Prevention of nausea and vomiting associated with initial and repeat courses of emetogenic cancer chemotherapy

(Continued)

Ondansetron *(Continued)*

Pregnancy Risk Factor B

Contraindications Hypersensitivity to ondansetron or any component

Precautions There is no information on dosage in children ≤3 years of age

Adverse Reactions

Cardiovascular: Tachycardia, bradycardia, angina, syncope

Central nervous system: Lightheadedness, seizures, headache

Dermatologic: Rash

Endocrine & metabolic: Hypokalemia

Gastrointestinal: Constipation, diarrhea

Hepatic: Transient elevations in liver enzymes

Ocular: Blurred vision

Respiratory: Bronchospasm

Miscellaneous: Hypersensitivity reactions

Drug Interactions No documented drug interactions; however, it does contain the same imidazole nucleus as cimetidine and omeprazole; patients receiving concurrent theophylline, phenytoin, or warfarin should be followed closely; ondansetron is metabolized by the cytochrome P450 enzyme system, inducers or inhibitors of this system may affect ondansetron's elimination

Stability Compatible for 7 days at room temperature when diluted in saline or dextrose I.V. solution; Y-site injection compatibility with bleomycin, carboplatin, carmustine, chlorpromazine, cisplatin, cyclophosphamide, cytarabine, dacarbazine, dactinomycin, daunorubicin, dexamethasone, diphenhydramine, doxorubicin, droperidol, etoposide, fludarabine, ifosfamide, methchlorethamine, methotrexate, mesna, metoclopramide, mitoxantrone, prochlorperazine, promethazine, teniposide, vinblastine, and vincristine

Mechanism of Action Selective 5-HT_3 receptor antagonist, blocking serotonin, both peripherally on vagal nerve terminals and centrally in the chemoreceptor trigger zone

Pharmacokinetics

Absorption: Oral bioavailability 60%

Protein binding, plasma: 70% to 76%

Metabolism: Extensively metabolized by hydroxylation, followed by glucuronide or sulfate conjugation

Half-life:

- Children <15 years: 2-3 hours
- Adults: 4-5 hours

Elimination: Excreted in urine and feces; 5% to 10% of the parent drug is recovered unchanged in the urine

Usual Dosage

Oral:

- Children 4-11 years: 4 mg 30 minutes before chemotherapy; repeat 4 and 8 hours after initial dose
- Children >11 years and Adults: 8 mg 30 minutes before chemotherapy; repeat 4 and 8 hours after initial dose

I.V.:

- Children >3 years: 0.15 mg/kg/dose infused 30 minutes before the start of emetogenic chemotherapy, with subsequent doses administered 4 and 8 hours after the first dose; decreased effectiveness has been reported when administered for prolonged therapy (eg, more than 3 doses)
- Adults: 0.15 mg/kg/dose infused 30 minutes before the start of emetogenic chemotherapy with subsequent doses administered 4 and 8 hours after the first dose **or** a single 32 mg dose beginning 30 minutes prior to emetogenic chemotherapy

Administration Dilute in 50 mL I.V. fluid (maximum concentration: 0.64 mg/mL) and infuse over 15 minutes

Additional Information The I.V. product has been successful when used orally

Dosage Forms

Injection: 2 mg/mL (20 mL); 32 mg (single dose vials)

Tablet: 4 mg, 8 mg

References

Carden PA, Mitchell SL, Waters KD, et al, "Prevention of Cyclophosphamide/Cytarabine-Induced Emesis With Ondansetron in Children With Leukemia," *J Clin Oncol*, 1990, 8(9):1531-5.

Marty M, Pouillart P, Scholl S, et al, "Comparison of the 5-hydroxytryptamine 3 (Serotonin) Antagonist Ondansetron (GR 38032F) With High Dose Metoclopramide in the Control of Cisplatin-Induced Emesis," *N Engl J Med*, 1990, 322(12):816-21.

Pinkerton CR, Williams D, Wootton C, et al, "5-HT_3 Antagonist Ondansetron - An Effective Outpatient Antiemetic in Cancer Treatment," *Arch Dis Child*, 1990, 65(8):822-5.

Opcon® *see* Naphazoline Hydrochloride *on page 403*

Ophthacet® *see* Sulfacetamide Sodium *on page 539*

Ophthaine® *see* Proparacaine Hydrochloride *on page 490*

Ophthalgan® *see* Glycerin *on page 273*

Ophthetic® *see* Proparacaine Hydrochloride *on page 490*

Ophthochlor® *see* Chloramphenicol *on page 124*

Opticrom® *see* Cromolyn Sodium *on page 158*

Orabase®-B [OTC] *see* Benzocaine *on page 77*

Orabase® HCA *see* Hydrocortisone *on page 293*

Orabase®-O [OTC] *see* Benzocaine *on page 77*

Oracit® *see* Sodium Citrate and Citric Acid *on page 528*

Orajel® Brace-Aid Oral Anesthetic [OTC] *see* Benzocaine *on page 77*

Orajel® Brace-Aid Rinse [OTC] *see* Carbamide Peroxide *on page 103*

Orajel® Maximum Strength [OTC] *see* Benzocaine *on page 77*

Orajel® Mouth-Aid [OTC] *see* Benzocaine *on page 77*

Oraminic® II *see* Brompheniramine Maleate *on page 88*

Oramorph SR® *see* Morphine Sulfate *on page 394*

Orasone® *see* Prednisone *on page 477*

Orciprenaline Sulfate *see* Metaproterenol Sulfate *on page 367*

Oretic® *see* Hydrochlorothiazide *on page 291*

ORF17070 *see* Histrelin *on page 286*

Organidin® *see* Iodinated Glycerol *on page 317*

ORG NC 45 *see* Vecuronium Bromide *on page 596*

Ormazine® *see* Chlorpromazine Hydrochloride *on page 129*

Orthoclone® OKT_3 *see* Muromonab-CD3 *on page 397*

Osmitrol® *see* Mannitol *on page 355*

Osmoglyn® *see* Glycerin *on page 273*

OTC Cold Preparations, Pediatric *see page 723*

Otocalm® Ear *see* Antipyrine and Benzocaine *on page 56*

Otomycin-HPN® *see* Neomycin, (Bacitracin) Polymyxin B and Hydrocortisone *on page 406*

Overdose and Toxicology Information *see page 696*

O-V Staticin® *see* Nystatin *on page 421*

Oxacillin Sodium (ox a sill' in)

Related Information

Medications Compatible With PN Solutions *on page 649-650*

Brand Names Bactocill®; Prostaphlin®

Synonyms Isoxazolyl Penicillin; Methylphenyl

Therapeutic Category Antibiotic, Penicillin

Use Treatment of susceptible bacterial infections such as osteomyelitis, septicemia, endocarditis, and CNS infections due to penicillinase-producing strains of *Staphylococcus*

Pregnancy Risk Factor B

Contraindications Hypersensitivity to oxacillin, other penicillins, any component, or cephalosporins

(Continued)

Oxacillin Sodium *(Continued)*

Warnings Elimination rate will be decreased in neonates

Precautions Use with caution in patients with severe renal impairment; dosage modification required in patients with renal impairment

Adverse Reactions

Dermatologic: Rash

Gastrointestinal: Diarrhea, nausea, vomiting, *C. difficile* colitis

Hematologic: Mild leukopenia, agranulocytosis

Hepatic: Elevated AST, hepatotoxicity

Local: Thrombophlebitis

Renal & genitourinary: Acute interstitial nephritis

Miscellaneous: Hypersensitivity reactions

Drug Interactions Probenecid

Stability Reconstituted parenteral oxacillin injection is stable for 3 days at room temperature or 7 days when refrigerated; reconstituted oxacillin oral solution is stable for 3 days at room temperature or 14 days when refrigerated

Mechanism of Action Interferes with bacterial cell wall synthesis during active multiplication, causing cell wall death and resultant bactericidal activity against susceptible bacteria

Pharmacokinetics

Absorption: Oral: ~35% to 67% of a dose is absorbed

Distribution: Penetrates the blood-brain barrier only when meninges are inflamed; crosses the placenta; appears in breast milk

Protein binding: 90% to 95%

Metabolism: Metabolized in the liver to active and inactive metabolites

Half-life:

- Children 1 week to 2 years: 0.9-1.8 hours
- Adults: 23-60 minutes (prolonged with reduced renal function and in neonates)

Peak serum levels:

- Oral: Within 120 minutes
- I.M.: Within 30-60 minutes

Elimination: Excreted by kidneys and to small degree via the bile as parent drug and metabolites

Not dialyzable (0% to 5%)

Usual Dosage

Neonates: I.M., I.V.:

- Postnatal age ≤7 days:
  - ≤2000 g: 50 mg/kg/day in divided doses every 12 hours
  - >2000 g: 75 mg/kg/day in divided doses every 8 hours
- Postnatal age >7 days:
  - <1200 g: 50 mg/kg/day in divided doses every 12 hours
  - 1200-2000 g: 75 mg/kg/day in divided doses every 8 hours
  - >2000 g: 100 mg/kg/day in divided doses every 6 hours

Infants and Children: I.M., I.V.: 100-200 mg/kg/day in divided doses every 6 hours; maximum dose: 12 g/day

Children: Oral: 50-100 mg/kg/day divided every 6 hours

Adults:

- I.M., I.V.: 250 mg to 2 g/dose every 4-6 hours
- Oral: 500-1000 mg every 4-6 hours

Dosing interval in renal impairment: Cl_{cr} <10 mL/minute: Use lower range of the usual dosage

Administration Oxacillin can be administered by I.V. push over 10 minutes at a maximum concentration of 100 mg/mL or by I.V. intermittent infusion over 15-30 minutes at a final concentration ≤40 mg/mL

Monitoring Parameters Periodic CBC, urinalysis, BUN, serum creatinine, AST and ALT

Test Interactions False-positive urinary and serum proteins

Patient Information Take orally on an empty stomach 1 hour before meals or 2 hours after meals

Additional Information Sodium content of 1 g: 2.8-3.1 mEq

Dosage Forms

Capsule: 250 mg, 500 mg

Powder for injection: 250 mg, 500 mg, 1 g, 2 g, 4 g, 10 g
Powder for oral solution: 250 mg/5 mL (100 mL)

References

Olans RN and Weiner LB, "Reversible Oxacillin Hepatotoxicity," *J Pediatr*, 1976, 89:835-8.

Prober CG, Stevenson DK, and Benitz WE, "The Use of Antibiotics in Neonates Weighing Less Than 1200 Grams," *Pediatr Infect Dis J*, 1990, 9(2):111-21.

Oxy-5® [OTC] *see* Benzoyl Peroxide *on page 78*

Oxybutynin Chloride (ox i byoo' ti nin)

Brand Names Ditropan®

Therapeutic Category Antispasmodic Agent, Urinary

Use Antispasmodic for neurogenic bladder

Pregnancy Risk Factor B

Contraindications Glaucoma, myasthenia gravis, partial or complete GI obstruction, GU obstruction, ulcerative colitis; patients hypersensitive to the drug

Warnings May impair ability to perform hazardous activities requiring mental alertness or physical coordination

Precautions Use with caution in patients with hepatic or renal disease, heart disease, hyperthyroidism, reflux esophagitis, hypertension, prostatic hypertrophy, autonomic neuropathy

Adverse Reactions

Cardiovascular: Decreased sweating, hot flashes, tachycardia, palpitations, vasodilation
Central nervous system: Drowsiness, weakness, dizziness, insomnia, fever
Dermatologic: Rash
Gastrointestinal: Dry mouth, nausea, vomiting, constipation
Ocular: Blurred vision, mydriasis, decreased lacrimation
Renal & genitourinary: Urinary hesitancy or retention
Miscellaneous: Hypersensitivity reactions

Drug Interactions Additive sedation with CNS depressants and alcohol; additive anticholinergic effects with antihistamines and anticholinergic agents

Mechanism of Action Direct antispasmodic effect on smooth muscle, also inhibits the action of acetylcholine on smooth muscle; does not block effects at skeletal muscle or at autonomic ganglia

Pharmacodynamics

Onset of action: Oral: Within 30-60 minutes
Peak effect: 3-6 hours
Duration: 6-10 hours

Pharmacokinetics

Absorption: Oral: Rapidly and well absorbed
Metabolism: Metabolized in the liver
Peak serum levels: Within 60 minutes

Usual Dosage Oral:

Children:
- 1-5 years: 0.2 mg/kg/dose 2-4 times/day
- >5 years: 5 mg twice daily, up to 5 mg 3 times/day

Adults: 5 mg 2-3 times/day up to 5 mg 4 times/day maximum

Dosage Forms

Syrup: 5 mg/5 mL (473 mL)
Tablet: 5 mg

Oxycodone Hydrochloride and Acetaminophen

Related Information

Narcotic Analgesics Comparison Chart *on page 721-722*
Overdose and Toxicology Information *on page 696-700*

Brand Names Percocet®; Tylox®

Synonyms Acetaminophen and Oxycodone Hydrochloride

Therapeutic Category Analgesic, Narcotic

Use Management of moderate to severe pain

Restrictions C-II

Pregnancy Risk Factor C

(Continued)

Oxycodone Hydrochloride and Acetaminophen *(Continued)*

Contraindications Hypersensitivity to oxycodone, acetaminophen or any component; severe respiratory depression, severe liver or renal insufficiency

Warnings Some preparations may contain bisulfites which may cause allergies

Precautions Use with caution in patients with hypersensitivity to other phenanthrene derivative opioid agonists (morphine, codeine, hydrocodone, hydromorphone, oxymorphone, levorphanol)

Adverse Reactions

Cardiovascular: Hypotension, bradycardia, peripheral vasodilation

Central nervous system: CNS depression, increased intracranial pressure, drowsiness, sedation

Dermatologic: Pruritus

Endocrine & metabolic: Antidiuretic hormone release

Gastrointestinal: Nausea, vomiting, constipation

Hepatic: Biliary tract spasm

Ocular: Miosis

Renal & genitourinary: Urinary tract spasm

Respiratory: Respiratory depression

Sensitivity reactions: Histamine release

Miscellaneous: Physical and psychological dependence

Drug Interactions CNS depressants, phenothiazines, tricyclic antidepressants may potentiate the effects of oxycodone

Usual Dosage Oral (doses should be titrated to appropriate analgesic effects):

Children: Based on oxycodone component: 0.05-0.15 mg/kg/dose to 5 mg/dose every 4-6 hours as needed

Adults: 1-2 tablets every 4-6 hours as needed for pain

Dosage Forms

Capsule: Oxycodone hydrochloride 5 mg and acetaminophen 500 mg

Solution, oral: Oxycodone hydrochloride 5 mg and acetaminophen 325 mg per 5 mL (5 mL, 500 mL)

Tablet: Oxycodone hydrochloride 5 mg and acetaminophen 325 mg

Oxycodone Hydrochloride, Oxycodone Terephthalate and Aspirin

Related Information

Overdose and Toxicology Information *on page 696-700*

Brand Names Percodan®; Percodan®-Demi

Therapeutic Category Analgesic, Narcotic

Use Relief of moderate to moderately severe pain

Restrictions C-II

Pregnancy Risk Factor D

Contraindications Hypersensitivity to oxycodone or aspirin; severe respiratory depression, severe liver or renal insufficiency

Precautions Use with caution in patients with hypersensitivity to other phenanthrene derivative opioid agonists (morphine, codeine, hydrocodone, hydromorphone, oxymorphone, levorphanol)

Adverse Reactions

Cardiovascular: Hypotension, bradycardia, peripheral vasodilation

Central nervous system: CNS depression, increased intracranial pressure, drowsiness, sedation

Dermatologic: Pruritus

Endocrine & metabolic: Antidiuretic hormone release

Gastrointestinal: Nausea, vomiting, constipation

Hepatic: Biliary tract spasm

Ocular: Miosis

Renal & genitourinary: Urinary tract spasm

Respiratory: Respiratory depression

Sensitivity reactions: Histamine release

Miscellaneous: Physical and psychological dependence

Drug Interactions CNS depressants, phenothiazines, tricyclic antidepressants may potentiate the effects of oxycodone

Usual Dosage Oral: Based on oxycodone combined salt component:

Children: 0.05-0.15 mg/kg/dose every 4-6 hours as needed; maximum: 5 mg/dose (1 tablet Percodan® or 2 tablets Percodan®-Demi/dose)

or alternatively:

Percodan®-Demi:

6-12 years: ¼ tablet every 6 hours as needed for pain

>12 years: ½ tablet every 6 hours as needed for pain

Adults: Percodan®: 1 tablet every 6 hours as needed for pain or Percodan®-Demi: 1-2 tablets every 6 hours as needed for pain

Additional Information One tablet (Percodan®) contains ~5 mg oxycodone as combined salt

Dosage Forms Tablet:

Percodan®: Oxycodone hydrochloride 4.5 mg, oxycodone terephthalate 0.38 mg, and aspirin 325 mg

Percodan®-Demi: Oxycodone hydrochloride 2.25 mg, oxycodone terephthalate 0.19 mg, and aspirin 325 mg

Oxymetazoline Hydrochloride (ox i met az' oh leen)

Related Information

OTC Cold Preparations, Pediatric *on page 723-726*

Brand Names Afrin® Nasal Solution [OTC]; Allerest® 12 Hours Nasal Solution [OTC]; Chlorphed®-LA Nasal Solution [OTC]; Dristan® Long Lasting Nasal Solution [OTC]; Duration® Nasal Solution [OTC]; Neo-Synephrine® 12 Hour Nasal Solution [OTC]; Nōstrilla® Long Acting Nasal Solution [OTC]; NTZ® Nasal Solution [OTC]; OcuClear® [OTC]; Sinarest® 12 Hour Nasal Solution; Vicks® Sinex® Long-Acting Nasal Solution [OTC]; 4-Way® Long Acting Nasal Solution [OTC]

Therapeutic Category Adrenergic Agonist Agent; Nasal Agent, Vasoconstrictor

Use Symptomatic relief of nasal mucosal congestion associated with acute or chronic rhinitis, the common cold, sinusitis, hay fever, or other allergies

Pregnancy Risk Factor C

Contraindications Hypersensitivity to oxymetazoline or any component

Warnings Use for periods exceeding 3 days may result in severe rebound nasal congestion; excessive dosage in children may cause profound CNS depression

Precautions Use with caution in patients with hyperthyroidism, heart disease, hypertension or diabetes mellitus

Adverse Reactions

Cardiovascular: Hypertension, palpitations, reflex bradycardia

Central nervous system: Nervousness, dizziness, insomnia, headache

Gastrointestinal: Nausea

Local: Transient burning, stinging, dryness of nasal mucosa, rebound congestion with prolonged use

Respiratory: Sneezing

Drug Interactions MAO inhibitors

Mechanism of Action Stimulates alpha-adrenergic receptors in the arterioles of the nasal mucosa to produce vasoconstriction

Pharmacodynamics

Onset of action: Following intranasal administration effects occur within 5-10 minutes

Duration: 5-6 hours

Pharmacokinetics Metabolic fate is unknown

Usual Dosage Therapy should not exceed 3-5 days; avoid use of 0.05% solution in children <6 years of age

Children 2-5 years: 0.025% solution, 2-3 drops in each nostril twice daily

Children ≥6 years and Adults: 0.05% solution: 2-3 drops or 2-3 sprays or 1-2 metered sprays (Nostrilla®) into each nostril twice daily

Dosage Forms Solution, nasal:

Drops: 0.05% (20 mL)

Drops, pediatric: 0.025% (20 mL)

Spray: 0.05% (15 mL, 20 mL, 30 mL)

2-PAM *see* Pralidoxime Chloride *on page 473*

Pamidronate Disodium

Brand Names Aredia™

Therapeutic Category Biphosphonate

Use Symptomatic treatment of Paget's disease and heterotopic ossification due to spinal cord injury or after total hip replacement, hypercalcemia associated with malignancy

Pregnancy Risk Factor B

Precautions Use with caution in patients with renal impairment

Adverse Reactions

Central nervous system: Malaise, fever
Endocrine & metabolic: Hypocalcemia, hypophosphatemia
Gastrointestinal: Nausea, anorexia, constipation, GI hemorrhage
Hematologic: Leukopenia
Local: Vein irritation, thrombophlebitis

Drug Interactions Incompatible with calcium-containing I.V. fluids (ie, Ringer's solution)

Mechanism of Action Pamidronate (aminohydroxypropylidene diphosphonate; APD) is a biphosphonate. Biphosphonates inhibit bone resorption via actions on osteoclasts or on osteoclast precursors. These agents do not appear to produce any significant effects on renal tubular calcium handling.

Usual Dosage Safety and efficacy in children have not been established

Adults: I.V.: Dosage based upon serum calcium measurement:
- Serum calcium 12-13 mg/dL: 60-90 mg
- Serum calcium >13 mg/dL: 90 mg

Administration Dilute in 1000 mL 5% dextrose, infuse over 24 hours

Monitoring Parameters CBC with differential, serum calcium, phosphate, potassium, sodium, creatinine, hemoglobin, hematocrit

Dosage Forms Powder for injection, lyophilized: 30 mg

Pamprin IB® [OTC] *see* Ibuprofen *on page 300*

Panadol® [OTC] *see* Acetaminophen *on page 16*

Pancrease® *see* Pancrelipase *on next page*

Pancrease® MT *see* Pancrelipase *on next page*

Pancreatin (pan' kree a tin)

See Also Pancrelipase

Brand Names Creon®; Dizymes®; Donnazyme®; Entozyme®; Hi-Vegi-Lip®; Pancreatin Enseals® [OTC]

Therapeutic Category Pancreatic Enzyme

Use Replacement therapy in symptomatic treatment of malabsorption syndrome caused by pancreatic insufficiency

Pregnancy Risk Factor C

Contraindications Hypersensitivity to pancreatin or any component or to pork protein

Warnings These products are not bioequivalent; do not substitute without consulting a physician or pharmacist

Adverse Reactions

Dermatologic: Rash
Endocrine & metabolic: Hyperuricemia
Gastrointestinal: Nausea, cramps, constipation, diarrhea
Ocular: Lacrimation
Renal & genitourinary: Hyperuricosuria
Respiratory: Sneezing, bronchospasm
Miscellaneous: Hypersensitivity reactions

Mechanism of Action Replaces endogenous pancreatic enzymes to assist in digestion of protein, starch and fats

Pharmacokinetics

Absorption: Not absorbed, acts locally in the GI tract
Elimination: Excreted in the feces

Usual Dosage Oral: Enteric coated microspheres: The following dosage recommendations are only an approximation for initial dosages. The actual dosage will depend on the digestive requirements of the individual patient.

Children:
- <1 year: 2000 units of lipase with meals/feedings
- 1-6 years: 4000-8000 units of lipase with meals and 4000 units with snacks

7-12 years: 4000-12,000 units of lipase with meals and snacks

Adults: 4000-16,000 units of lipase with meals and with snacks

Monitoring Parameters Stool fat content

Patient Information Retention in the mouth before swallowing may cause mucosal irritation and stomatitis; avoid inhaling powder dosage form

Additional Information Concomitant administration of conventional pancreatin enzymes with an H_2 receptor antagonist has been used to decrease the inactivation of enzyme activity

Dosage Forms See table.

Pancreatin

Product	Dosage Form	Lipase USP Units	Amylase USP Units	Protease USP Units	Pancreatin mg
Creon®	Capsule, delayed release	8000	30,000	13,000	Strength not known
Dizymes®	Tablet, enteric coated	6750	43,750	41,250	250
Pancreatin 4X	Tablet	12,000	60,000	60,000	2400
Pancreatin 8X	Tablet	22,500	180,000	180,000	7200
Donnazyme®	Tablet	1000	12,500	12,500	500
Entozyme®	Tablet	600	7500	7500	300
Hi-Vegi-Lip®	Tablet	4800	60,000	60,000	2400

Pancreatin Enseals® [OTC] *see* Pancreatin *on previous page*

Pancrelipase (pan kre li' pase)

Brand Names Cotazym®; Cotazym-S®; Ilozyme®; Ku-Zyme® HP; Pancrease®; Pancrease® MT; Protilase®; Viokase®; Zymase®

Synonyms Lipancreatin

Therapeutic Category Pancreatic Enzyme

Use Replacement therapy in symptomatic treatment of malabsorption syndrome caused by pancreatic insufficiency

Pregnancy Risk Factor C

Contraindications Hypersensitivity to pancrelipase or any component or to pork protein

Warnings Pancrelipase is inactivated by acids; use microencapsulated products whenever possible, since these products permit better dissolution of enzymes in the duodenum and protect the enzyme preparations from acid degradation in the stomach; these products are not bioequivalent, do not substitute without consulting a physician or pharmacist

Adverse Reactions

Dermatologic: Rash

Endocrine & metabolic: Hyperuricemia

Gastrointestinal: Nausea, cramps, constipation, diarrhea

Ocular: Lacrimation

Renal & genitourinary: Hyperuricosuria

Respiratory: Sneezing, bronchospasm

Miscellaneous: Hypersensitivity reactions

Mechanism of Action Replaces endogenous pancreatic enzymes to assist in digestion of protein, starch and fats

Pharmacokinetics

Absorption: Not absorbed, acts locally in the GI tract

Elimination: Excreted in the feces

Usual Dosage The following dosage recommendations are only an approximation for initial dosages. The actual dosage will depend on the digestive requirements of the individual patient. Oral:

Powder: Children <1 year: Start with $\frac{1}{8}$ teaspoonful with feedings

(Continued)

Pancrelipase *(Continued)*

Enteric coated microspheres and microtablets:

Children:

<1 year: 2000 units of lipase with meals/feedings

1-6 years: 4000-8000 units of lipase with meals and 4,000 units with snacks

7-12 years: 4000-12,000 units of lipase with meals and snacks

Adults: 4000-16,000 units of lipase with meals and with snacks

Monitoring Parameters Stool fat content

Patient Information Do not chew the microspheres or microtablets

Additional Information Concomitant administration of conventional pancreatin enzymes with an H_2 receptor antagonist has been used to decrease the inactivation of enzyme activity

Dosage Forms See table.

Pancrelipase

Product	Dosage Form	Lipase USP Units	Amylase USP Units	Protease USP Units
Cotazym® Ku-Zyme® HP	Capsule	8000	30,000	30,000
Cotazym®-S	Capsule, enteric coated spheres	5000	20,000	20,000
Entolase® Pancrease® Protilase®	Capsule, delayed release	4000	20,000	25,000
Ilozyme®	Tablet	11,000	30,000	30,000
Pancrease® MT 4	Capsule, enteric coated microtablets	4000	12,000	12,000
10		10,000	30,000	30,000
16		16,000	48,000	48,000
25		25,000	75,000	75,000
Ultrase® MT 12	Capsule	12,000	39,000	39,000
20		20,000	65,000	65,000
24		24,000	78,000	78,000
Viokase®	Powder	16,800 per 0.7 g	70,000 per 0.7 g	70,000 per 0.7 g
	Tablet	8000	30,000	30,000
Zymase®	Capsule, enteric coated spheres	12,000	24,000	24,000

Pancuronium Bromide (pan kyoo roe' nee um)

Brand Names Pavulon®

Therapeutic Category Neuromuscular Blocker Agent, Nondepolarizing

Use Produces skeletal muscle relaxation during surgery after induction of general anesthesia, increases pulmonary compliance during assisted mechanical respiration, facilitates endotracheal intubation

Pregnancy Risk Factor C

Contraindications Hypersensitivity to pancuronium, bromide, or any component; pre-existing tachycardia

Warnings Ventilation must be supported during neuromuscular blockade

Precautions Use with caution in patients with poor renal function

Adverse Reactions

Cardiovascular: Tachycardia, hypertension

Dermatologic: Rash

Local: Burning sensation along the vein

Respiratory: Wheezes

Miscellaneous: Excessive salivation

Drug Interactions Aminoglycosides, clindamycin, potassium depleting drugs such as diuretics, amphotericin B, and steroids; quinidine, magnesium sulfate, verapamil, lidocaine; succinylcholine (may prolong intensity and duration of effect)

Stability Refrigerate; however, stable for up to 6 months at room temperature

Mechanism of Action Blocks neural transmission at the myoneural junction by binding with cholinergic receptor sites

Pharmacodynamics

Peak effect: Following I.V. injection, within 2-3 minutes

Duration: 40-60 minutes (dose dependent)

Pharmacokinetics

Half-life: 110 minutes

Metabolism: Some (30% to 40%) liver metabolism

Elimination: Primarily excreted in the urine (55% to 70%) as unchanged drug

Usual Dosage Infants, Children, and Adults: I.V.: 0.04-0.1 mg/kg every 30-60 minutes as needed

Administration May be administered undiluted by rapid I.V. injection

Monitoring Parameters Heart rate, blood pressure, assisted ventilation status

Nursing Implications Does not alter the patient's state of consciousness; addition of sedation and analgesia are recommended

Additional Information Neuromuscular blockade will be prolonged in patients with decreased renal function

Dosage Forms Injection: 1 mg/mL (10 mL); 2 mg/mL (2 mL, 5 mL)

Panmycin® *see* Tetracycline Hydrochloride *on page 552*

PanOxyl® [OTC] *see* Benzoyl Peroxide *on page 78*

PanOxyl®-AQ *see* Benzoyl Peroxide *on page 78*

Panscol® [OTC] *see* Salicylic Acid *on page 516*

Panwarfin® *see* Warfarin Sodium *on page 607*

Papaverine Hydrochloride (pa pav' er een)

Brand Names Cerespan®; Genabid®; Pavabid®; Pavased®; Pavatine®; Paverolan®

Therapeutic Category Vasodilator

Use Relief of peripheral and cerebral ischemia associated with arterial spasm; investigationally for prophylaxis of migraine headache

Pregnancy Risk Factor C

Contraindications Complete atrioventricular block; Parkinson's disease

Precautions Use with caution in patients with glaucoma

Adverse Reactions

Cardiovascular: Flushing of the face, sweating, tachycardia, hypotension, arrhythmias with rapid I.V. use

Central nervous system: Depression, dizziness, vertigo, drowsiness, sedation, lethargy, headache

Dermatologic: Pruritus

Gastrointestinal: Dry mouth, nausea, constipation

Hepatic: Hepatic hypersensitivity

Local: Thrombosis at the I.V. administration site

Respiratory: Apnea with rapid I.V. use

Drug Interactions Additive effects with CNS depressants or morphine; papaverine decreases the effects of levodopa

Stability Protect from heat or freezing; not do refrigerate injection; solutions should be clear to pale yellow; precipitates with lactated Ringer's

Mechanism of Action Smooth muscle spasmolytic producing a generalized smooth muscle relaxation including: vasodilatation, gastrointestinal sphincter relaxation, bronchiolar muscle relaxation and potentially a depressed myocardium

Pharmacodynamics Onset of action: Rapid onset orally

Pharmacokinetics

Protein binding: 90%

Metabolism: Rapidly metabolized in the liver

Half-life: 30-120 minutes

(Continued)

Papaverine Hydrochloride *(Continued)*

Elimination: Excreted primarily as metabolites in the urine

Usual Dosage

Children: I.M., I.V.: 1.5 mg/kg 4 times/day

Migraine prophylaxis: 6-15 years: Oral: Initial: 5 mg/kg/day given once daily; range: 5-10 mg/kg/day divided into 2-3 doses/day

Adults:

Oral: 75-300 mg 3-5 times/day

Oral, sustained release: 150-300 mg every 12 hours

I.M., I.V.: 30-120 mg every 3 hours as needed

Administration Rapid I.V. administration may result in arrhythmias and fatal apnea; administer slow I.V. over 1-2 minutes

Additional Information Evidence of therapeutic value is lacking

Dosage Forms

Capsule, sustained release: 150 mg

Injection: 30 mg/mL (2 mL, 10 mL)

Tablet: 30 mg, 60 mg, 100 mg, 150 mg, 200 mg, 300 mg

Tablet, timed release: 200 mg

References

Sillanpää M and Koponen M, "Papaverine in the Prophylaxis of Migraine and Other Vascular Headache in Children," *Acta Paediatr Scand*, 1978, 67(2):209-12.

Paplex® *see* Salicylic Acid *on page 516*

Parabromdylamine *see* Brompheniramine Maleate *on page 88*

Paracetaldehyde *see* Paraldehyde *on this page*

Paracetamol *see* Acetaminophen *on page 16*

Paraflex® *see* Chlorzoxazone *on page 132*

Parafon Forte™ DSC *see* Chlorzoxazone *on page 132*

Paral® *see* Paraldehyde *on this page*

Paraldehyde (par al' de hyde)

Brand Names Paral®

Synonyms Paracetaldehyde

Therapeutic Category Anticonvulsant; Hypnotic; Sedative

Use Treatment of status epilepticus and tetanus induced seizures; has been used as a sedative/hypnotic and in the treatment of alcohol withdrawal symptoms

Restrictions C-IV

Pregnancy Risk Factor C

Contraindications Severe hepatic insufficiency, respiratory disease, GI inflammation or ulceration

Precautions May need to decrease dose in patients with liver disease

Adverse Reactions

Dermatologic: Erythematous rash

Endocrine & metabolic: Metabolic acidosis

Gastrointestinal: Gastric irritation, corrosion of the stomach or rectum

Hepatic: Hepatitis

Respiratory: Coughing, strong and unpleasant breath, pulmonary edema

Miscellaneous: Psychological and physical dependence with prolonged use

Drug Interactions Barbiturates and alcohol may enhance CNS depression

Stability Decomposes with exposure to air and light to acetaldehyde which then oxidizes to acetic acid; store in tightly closed containers; protect from light

Mechanism of Action Unknown mechanism of action; causes depression of CNS, including the ascending reticular activating system to provide sedation/hypnosis and anticonvulsant activity

Pharmacodynamics Hypnosis: Oral:

Onset of action: Within 10-15 minutes

Duration: 6-8 hours

Pharmacokinetics

Distribution: Crosses the placenta

Metabolism: ~70% to 80% metabolized in the liver
Half-life:
Neonates: 10 hours
Adults: 3.5-10 hours
Elimination: 30% excreted as unchanged drug in expired air via the lungs; trace amounts are excreted in the urine unchanged

Usual Dosage See table.

Paraldehyde

	Sedative	Hypnotic	Seizures
Children Oral, rectal	0.15 mL/kg	0.3 mL/kg	0.3 mL/kg every 2-4 h maximum dose is 5 mL
Adults Oral, rectal	5-10 mL	10-30 mL	

Administration
Oral: Dilute in milk or iced fruit juice
Rectal: Mix paraldehyde 2:1 with oil (cottonseed or olive)

Do **not** use any plastic equipment for administration, use glass syringes and rubber tubing

Nursing Implications Discard unused contents of any container which has been opened for more than 24 hours; do **not** use discolored solution or solutions with strong smell of acetic acid (vinegar); outdated preparations can be toxic

Additional Information Do not abruptly discontinue in patients receiving chronic therapy

Dosage Forms Liquid, oral or rectal: 1 g/mL (30 mL)

Paraplatin® *see* Carboplatin *on page 106*

Paregoric

Synonyms Camphorated Tincture of Opium

Therapeutic Category Analgesic, Narcotic; Antidiarrheal

Use Treatment of diarrhea or relief of pain; neonatal opiate withdrawal

Restrictions C-III

Pregnancy Risk Factor B (D when used for long term or in high doses)

Contraindications Hypersensitivity to opium or any component; diarrhea caused by poisoning until the toxic material has been removed

Precautions Use with caution in patients with respiratory, hepatic or renal dysfunction, severe prostatic hypertrophy, or history of narcotic abuse; opium shares the toxic potential of opiate agonists, usual precautions of opiate agonist therapy should be observed; some commercial preparations may contain sulfites which may cause allergic reactions; infants <3 months of age are more susceptible to respiratory depression, use with caution and generally in reduced doses in this age group

Adverse Reactions
Cardiovascular: Hypotension, bradycardia, vasodilation
Central nervous system: CNS depression, increased intracranial pressure, drowsiness, dizziness, sedation
Endocrine & metabolic: Antidiuretic hormone release
Gastrointestinal: Nausea, vomiting, constipation
Hepatic: Biliary tract spasm
Ocular: Miosis
Renal & genitourinary: Urinary tract spasm, urinary retention
Respiratory: Respiratory depression
Sensitivity reaction: Histamine release
Miscellaneous: Physical and psychological dependence

Drug Interactions CNS depressants may potentiate effects

Stability Store in light-resistant, tightly closed container

Mechanism of Action Increases smooth muscle tone in GI tract, decreases motility and peristalsis, diminishes digestive secretions

Pharmacokinetics
Metabolism: Opium is metabolized in the liver

(Continued)

Paregoric *(Continued)*

Elimination: Excreted in the urine, primarily as morphine glucuronide conjugates and as parent compound (morphine, codeine, papaverine, etc)

Usual Dosage Oral:

Neonates: Opiate withdrawal: 3-6 drops every 3-6 hours as needed, or initially 0.2 mL every 3 hours; increase dosage by approximately 0.05 mL every 3 hours until withdrawal symptoms are controlled; it is rare to exceed 0.7 mL/dose. Stabilize withdrawal symptoms for 3-5 days, then gradually decrease dosage over a 2- to 4-week period.

Children: 0.25-0.5 mL/kg 1-4 times/day

Adults: 5-10 mL 1-4 times/day

Monitoring Parameters Respiratory rate, blood pressure, heart rate, level of sedation

Additional Information Do **not** confuse this product with opium tincture which is 25 times **more** potent; each 5 mL of paregoric contains 2 mg morphine equivalent, 0.02 mL anise oil, 20 mg benzoic acid, 20 mg camphor, 0.2 mL glycerin and alcohol; final alcohol content 45%

Dosage Forms Liquid: 2 mg morphine equivalent/5 mL (equivalent to 20 mg opium powder) (5 mL, 60 mL, 473 mL, 4000 mL)

Parenteral Nutrition (PN) *see page 642*

Pathocil® *see* Dicloxacillin Sodium *on page 186*

Pavabid® *see* Papaverine Hydrochloride *on page 433*

Pavased® *see* Papaverine Hydrochloride *on page 433*

Pavatine® *see* Papaverine Hydrochloride *on page 433*

Paverolan® *see* Papaverine Hydrochloride *on page 433*

Pavulon® *see* Pancuronium Bromide *on page 432*

PCA *see* Procainamide Hydrochloride *on page 481*

PCE® *see* Erythromycin *on page 226*

PediaCare® Oral *see* Pseudoephedrine *on page 497*

Pediaflor® *see* Fluoride *on page 255*

Pediapred® *see* Prednisolone *on page 476*

PediaProfen™ *see* Ibuprofen *on page 300*

Pediazole® *see* Erythromycin and Sulfisoxazole *on page 228*

Pedi-Boro® [OTC] *see* Aluminum Acetate *on page 33*

Pedi-Dri *see* Undecylenic Acid and Derivatives *on page 590*

PediOtic® *see* Neomycin, (Bacitracin) Polymyxin B and Hydrocortisone *on page 406*

Pedi-Pro [OTC] *see* Undecylenic Acid and Derivatives *on page 590*

Pedte-Pak-5® *see* Trace Metals *on page 574*

Pedtrace-4® *see* Trace Metals *on page 574*

Pemoline (pem' oh leen)

Brand Names Cylert®

Synonyms Phenylisohydantoin

Therapeutic Category Central Nervous System Stimulant, Nonamphetamine

Use Attention deficit disorder with hyperactivity (ADDH); narcolepsy

Restrictions C-IV

Pregnancy Risk Factor B

Contraindications Liver disease; hypersensitivity to pemoline or any component; children <6 years of age; Tourette's syndrome

Precautions Use with caution in patients with renal dysfunction; hypertension or history of drug abuse; may cause growth suppression in children

Adverse Reactions

Central nervous system: Insomnia, anorexia, seizures, precipitation of Tourette's syndrome, dizziness, hallucinations, headache

Dermatologic: Skin rashes
Endocrine & metabolic: Weight loss, growth reaction
Gastrointestinal: Stomach ache, nausea, diarrhea
Hepatic: Increased liver enzymes (usually reversible upon discontinuation), hepatitis and jaundice
Musculoskeletal: Movement disorders

Drug Interactions CNS stimulants, CNS depressants, sympathomimetics; may alter insulin requirements in diabetics

Mechanism of Action Blocks the reuptake mechanism of dopaminergic neurons, appears to act at the cerebral cortex and subcortical structures; CNS and respiratory stimulant with weak sympathomimetic effects

Pharmacodynamics
Peak effect: 4 hours
Significant benefit on hyperactivity may not be evident until 3rd or 4th week of administration
Duration: 8 hours

Pharmacokinetics
Protein binding: 50%
Metabolism: Metabolized by liver
Half-life:
Children: 7-8.6 hours
Adults: 12 hours
Elimination: Excreted in urine

Usual Dosage Children ≥6 years: Oral: Initial: 37.5 mg given once daily in the morning, increase by 18.75 mg/day at weekly intervals; effective dose range: 56.25-75 mg/day; maximum: 112.5 mg/day; dosage range: 0.5-3 mg/kg/24 hours

Monitoring Parameters Liver enzymes

Nursing Implications Administer medication in the morning

Additional Information Treatment of ADDH should include "Drug Holidays" or periodic discontinuation of stimulant medication in order to assess the patient's requirements and to decrease tolerance and limit suppression of linear growth and weight

Dosage Forms
Tablet: 18.75 mg, 37.5 mg, 75 mg
Tablet, chewable: 37.5 mg

Penecort® *see* Hydrocortisone *on page 293*

Pen G *see* Penicillin G Potassium or Sodium Salts *on page 440*

Penicillamine (pen i sill' a meen)

Related Information
Overdose and Toxicology Information *on page 696-700*

Brand Names Cuprimine®; Depen®

Synonyms D-3-Mercaptovaline; β,β-Dimethylcysteine; D-Penicillamine

Therapeutic Category Antidote, Copper Toxicity; Antidote, Lead Toxicity

Use Treatment of Wilson's disease, cystinuria, adjunct in the treatment of rheumatoid arthritis; lead poisoning, primary biliary cirrhosis

Pregnancy Risk Factor D

Contraindications Hypersensitivity to penicillamine and possibly penicillin; rheumatoid arthritis patients with renal insufficiency; patients with previous penicillamine-related aplastic anemia or agranulocytosis

Warnings Patients should be warned to promptly report any symptoms suggesting toxicity

Precautions Patients on penicillamine for Wilson's disease or cystinuria should receive pyridoxine supplementation 25-50 mg/day; when treating rheumatoid arthritis, daily pyridoxine supplementation is also recommended

Adverse Reactions
Central nervous system: Fever, peripheral sensory and motor neuropathies, myasthenic syndrome
Dermatologic: Rash, pruritus, pemphigus, increased friability of the skin; hirsutism
Endocrine & metabolic: Iron deficiency
Gastrointestinal: Oral lesions, nausea, vomiting, hypogeusia

(Continued)

Penicillamine *(Continued)*

Hematologic: Leukopenia, thrombocytopenia, eosinophilia, aplastic anemia
Hepatic: Hepatic dysfunction
Musculoskeletal: Arthralgia, dermatomyositis
Ocular: Optic neuritis
Renal & genitourinary: Nephrotic syndrome, renal vasculitis
Respiratory: Obliterative bronchiolitis, pulmonary fibrosis, interstitial pneumonitis
Miscellaneous: Lymphadenopathy, allergic reactions, SLE-like syndrome

Drug Interactions Gold, antimalarials, immunosuppressants, phenylbutazone

Mechanism of Action Chelates with lead, copper, mercury, iron, and other heavy metals to form stable, soluble complexes that are excreted in the urine; depresses circulating IgM rheumatoid factor levels and *in vitro*, depresses T-cell but not B-cell activity; combines with cystine to form a more soluble compound which prevents the formation of cystine calculi

Pharmacokinetics

Absorption: Readily from the GI tract
Metabolism: Metabolized in the liver
Peak serum levels: Within 1-2 hours

Usual Dosage Oral:

Rheumatoid arthritis:
- Children: Initial: 3 mg/kg/day (≤250 mg/day) for 3 months, then 6 mg/kg/day (≤500 mg/day) in 2 divided doses for 3 months to a maximum of 10 mg/kg/day in 3-4 divided doses
- Adults: 125-250 mg/day, may increase dose at 1- to 3-month intervals up to 1-1.5 g/day; doses >500 mg/day should be given in divided doses

Wilson's disease (doses titrated to maintain urinary copper excretion >1 mg/day):
- Infants and Children: 20 mg/kg/day in 2-4 doses; maximum: 1 g/day
- Adults: 1 g/day in 4 divided doses

Cystinuria (doses titrated to maintain urinary cystine excretion at <100-200 mg/day):
- Children: 30 mg/kg/day in 4 divided doses; maximum: 4 g/day
- Adults: Initial: 2 g/day divided every 6 hours (range: 1-4 g/day)

Lead poisoning:
- Children: 25-40 mg/kg/day in 2-3 divided doses; maximum: 1.5 g/day
- Adults: 1-1.5 g/day divided every 8-12 hours

Primary biliary cirrhosis: Adults: 250 mg/day to start, increase by 250 mg every 2 weeks up to a maintenance dose of 1 g/day, as 250 mg 4 times/day

Monitoring Parameters Urinalysis, CBC with differential, hemoglobin, platelet count, liver function tests

Patient Information Take at least 1 hour before a meal; possible severe allergic reaction if patient allergic to penicillin, patients with cystinuria should drink copious amounts of water; notify physician if unusual bleeding or bruising, or persistent fever, sore throat, or fatigue occur. Report any unexplained cough, shortness of breath, or rash. Loss of taste may occur; do not skip or miss doses or discontinue without notifying physician

Dosage Forms

Capsule: 125 mg, 250 mg
Tablet: 250 mg

Extemporaneous Preparation(s) A 50 mg/mL suspension may be made by mixing 20 (250 mg capsules) with 1 g carboxymethylcellulose, 50 g sucrose, 100 mg citric acid parabens, and purified water to a total volume of 100 mL; cherry flavor may be added; stability is 30 days in refrigerator

Nahata MC and Hipple TF, *Pediatric Drug Formulations*, 1st ed, Harvey Whitney Books Co, 1990.

Penicillin G Benzathine

Brand Names Bicillin® L-A; Permapen®

Synonyms Benzathine Benzylpenicillin; Benzathine Penicillin G; Benzylpenicillin Benzathine

Therapeutic Category Antibiotic, Penicillin

Use Active against most gram-positive organisms; some gram-negative organisms such as *Neisseria gonorrhoeae* and some anaerobes and spirochetes; used only for the treatment of mild to moderately severe infections caused by organisms susceptible to low concentrations of penicillin G, or for prophylaxis of infections caused by these organisms such as rheumatic fever prophylaxis

Pregnancy Risk Factor B

Contraindications Known hypersensitivity to penicillin or any component

Warnings CDC and AAP do not currently recommend the use of penicillin G benzathine to treat congenital syphilis or neurosyphilis due to reported treatment failures and lack of published clinical data on its efficacy

Precautions Use with caution in patients with impaired renal function, impaired cardiac function, or pre-existing seizure disorder

Adverse Reactions

Central nervous system: Convulsions, confusion, drowsiness, fever

Dermatologic: Rash

Hematologic: Hemolytic anemia, positive Coombs' reaction

Musculoskeletal: Myoclonus

Renal & genitourinary: Interstitial nephritis

Miscellaneous: Jarisch-Herxheimer reaction, hypersensitivity reactions, anaphylaxis

Drug Interactions Probenecid, tetracyclines, aminoglycosides

Stability Store in the refrigerator

Mechanism of Action Interferes with bacterial cell wall synthesis during active multiplication, causing cell wall death and resultant bactericidal activity against susceptible bacteria

Pharmacokinetics

Absorption: I.M.: Slowly absorbed

Peak serum levels: Within 12-24 hours; serum levels are usually detectable for 1-4 weeks depending on the dose; larger doses result in more sustained levels rather than higher levels

Usual Dosage I.M. (dosage frequency depends on infection being treated):

Neonates >1200 g: 50,000 units/kg for 1 dose

Infants and Children:

- Group A streptococcal upper respiratory infection: 25,000-50,000 units/kg as a single dose; maximum: 1.2 million units
- Prophylaxis of recurrent rheumatic fever: 25,000-50,000 units/kg every 3-4 weeks; maximum: 1.2 million units/dose
- Early syphilis: 50,000 units/kg as a single dose; maximum: 2.4 million units/dose
- Syphilis of more than 1-year duration: 50,000 units/kg every week for 3 doses; maximum: 2.4 million units/dose

Adults:

- Group A streptococcal upper respiratory infection: 1.2 million units as a single dose
- Prophylaxis of recurrent rheumatic fever: 1.2 million units every 3-4 weeks or 600,000 units twice monthly
- Early syphilis: 2.4 million units as a single dose in 2 injection sites
- Syphilis of more than 1-year duration: 2.4 million units (in 2 injection sites) once weekly for 3 doses

Monitoring Parameters CBC, urinalysis, renal function tests

Test Interactions Positive Coombs' [direct], false-positive urinary and/or serum proteins

Nursing Implications Give undiluted injection; administer by deep I.M. injection in the upper outer quadrant of the buttock; do **not** give I.V., intra-arterially or S.C.; inadvertent I.V. administration has resulted in thrombosis, severe neurovascular damage, cardiac arrest, and death; in infants and children, I.M. injections should be made into the midlateral muscle of the thigh

Dosage Forms Injection: 300,000 units/mL (10 mL); 600,000 units/mL (1 mL, 2 mL, 4 mL)

References

Kaplan EL, Berrios X, Speth J, et al, "Pharmacokinetics of Benzathine Penicillin G: Serum Levels During the 28 Days After Intramuscular Injection of 1,200,000 Units," *J Pediatr*, 1989, 115(1):146-50.

WHO Study Group, "Rheumatic Fever and Rheumatic Heart Disease," *World Health Organ Tech Rep Ser*, 1988, 764:1-58.

Penicillin G Potassium or Sodium Salts

Related Information

Medications Compatible With PN Solutions *on page 649-650*

Brand Names Pentids®; Pfizerpen®

Synonyms Crystalline Penicillin; Pen G

Therapeutic Category Antibiotic, Penicillin

Use Treatment of susceptible bacterial infections including most gram-positive organisms (except *Staphylococcus aureus*), some gram-negative organisms such as *Neisseria gonorrhoeae*, and some anaerobes and spirochetes

Pregnancy Risk Factor B

Contraindications Known hypersensitivity to penicillin or any component

Precautions Use with caution in patients with renal impairment or pre-existing seizure disorder; dosage modification required in patients with renal impairment; further dosage reduction recommended in patients with impaired hepatic and renal function

Adverse Reactions

- Central nervous system: Convulsions, confusion, drowsiness, fever
- Dermatologic: Rash, urticaria
- Endocrine & metabolic: Electrolyte imbalance
- Gastrointestinal: Diarrhea
- Hematologic: Hemolytic anemia, neutropenia, positive Coombs' reaction
- Local: Thrombophlebitis
- Musculoskeletal: Myoclonus
- Renal & genitourinary: Acute interstitial nephritis
- Miscellaneous: Jarisch-Herxheimer reaction, hypersensitivity reactions, anaphylaxis

Drug Interactions Probenecid, tetracyclines, aminoglycosides

Stability Reconstituted parenteral solution is stable for 7 days when refrigerated; incompatible with aminoglycosides; inactivated in acidic or alkaline solutions; reconstituted oral solution is stable for 14 days when refrigerated

Mechanism of Action Interferes with bacterial cell wall synthesis during active multiplication, causing cell wall death and resultant bactericidal activity against susceptible bacteria

Pharmacokinetics

- Absorption: Oral: <30% of a dose is absorbed
- Distribution: Penetration across the blood-brain barrier is poor with uninflamed meninges; crosses the placenta; appears in breast milk
- Protein binding: 65%
- Metabolism: Metabolized in the liver (30%) to penicilloic acid
- Half-life:
  - Neonates:
    - <6 days: 3.2-3.4 hours
    - 7-13 days: 1.2-2.2 hours
    - >14 days: 0.9-1.9 hours
  - Children and adults: 20-50 minutes with normal renal function
- Peak serum levels:
  - Oral: Within 30-60 minutes
  - I.M.: Within 30 minutes
- Elimination: Penicillin G and its metabolites are excreted in urine mainly by tubular secretion
- Moderately dialyzable (20% to 50%)

Usual Dosage

- Neonates: I.M., I.V.:
  - Postnatal age ≤7 days:
    - ≤2000 g: 50,000 units/kg/day in divided doses every 12 hours; meningitis: 100,000 units/kg/day in divided doses every 12 hours
    - >2000 g: 75,000 units/kg/day in divided doses every 8 hours; meningitis: 150,000 units/kg/day in divided doses every 8 hours
    - Congenital syphilis: 100,000 units/kg/day in divided doses every 12 hours
  - Postnatal age >7 days:
    - <1200 g: 50,000 units/kg/day in divided doses every 12 hours; meningitis: 100,000 units/kg/day in divided doses every 12 hours
    - 1200-2000 g: 75,000 units/kg/day in divided doses every 8 hours; meningitis: 225,000 units/kg/day in divided doses every 8 hours

>2000 g: 100,000 units/kg/day in divided doses every 6 hours; meningitis: 200,000 units/kg/day in divided doses every 6 hours

Congenital syphilis: 150,000 units/kg/day in divided doses every 8 hours

Infants and Children:

Oral: 25-50 mg/kg/day divided every 6-8 hours

I.M., I.V.: 100,000 to 250,000 units/kg/day in divided doses every 4-6 hours

Severe infections: Up to 400,000 units/kg/day in divided doses every 4-6 hours; maximum dose: 24 million units/day

Adults:

Oral: 125-500 mg every 6-8 hours

I.M., I.V.: 2-24 million units/day in divided doses every 4-6 hours

Dosing interval in renal impairment:

Cl_{cr} 10-30 mL/minute: Administer every 8-12 hours

Cl_{cr} <10 mL/minute: Administer every 12-18 hours

Administration Administer by I.V. intermittent infusion over 15-60 minutes at a final concentration for administration of 100,000-500,000 units/mL. A final concentration of 50,000 units/mL infused over 15-30 minutes is recommended for neonates and infants.

Monitoring Parameters Periodic serum electrolytes, renal and hematologic function tests

Test Interactions False-positive or negative urinary glucose determination using Clinitest®; positive Coombs' [direct]; false-positive urinary and/or serum proteins

Additional Information

Penicillin G potassium: 1.7 mEq of potassium and 0.3 mEq of sodium per 1 million units of penicillin G

Penicillin G sodium: 2 mEq of sodium per 1 million units of penicillin G

Dosage Forms

Injection, premixed (frozen): 1 million units (50 mL); 2 million units (50 mL); 3 million units (50 mL)

Powder for injection, as potassium: 1 million units, 5 million units, 10 million units, 20 million units

Powder for injection, as sodium: 5 million units

Powder for oral solution, as potassium (fruit flavor): 200,000 units/5 mL (100 mL); 400,000 units/5 mL (100 mL, 200 mL)

Tablet, as potassium: 200,000 units, 250,000 units, 400,000 units, 500,000 units, 800,000 units

References

American Academy of Pediatrics Committee on Infectious Diseases, "Treatment of Bacterial Meningitis," *Pediatrics*, 1988, 81(6):904-7.

Prober CG, Stevenson DK, and Benitz WE, "The Use of Antibiotics in Neonates Weighing Less Than 1200 Grams," *Pediatr Infect Dis J*, 1990, 9(2):111-21.

Penicillin G Procaine

Brand Names Crysticillin® A.S.; Pfizerpen®-AS; Wycillin®

Synonyms APPG; Aqueous Procaine Penicillin G; Procaine Benzylpenicillin; Procaine Penicillin G

Therapeutic Category Antibiotic, Penicillin

Use Moderately severe infections due to *Neisseria gonorrhoeae*, *Treponema pallidum*, and other penicillin G-sensitive microorganisms that are susceptible to low but prolonged serum penicillin concentrations

Pregnancy Risk Factor B

Contraindications Known hypersensitivity to penicillin, procaine, or any component

Precautions Modify dosage in patients with severe renal impairment

Adverse Reactions

Cardiovascular: Myocardial depression, vasodilation, conduction disturbances

Central nervous system: Seizures, confusion, drowsiness, disorientation, agitation, hallucinations

Hematologic: Hemolytic anemia, positive Coombs' reaction

Local: Sterile abscess at injection site

Musculoskeletal: Myoclonus

Renal & genitourinary: Interstitial nephritis

(Continued)

Penicillin G Procaine *(Continued)*

Miscellaneous: Pseudoanaphylactic reactions, Jarisch-Herxheimer reaction, hypersensitivity reactions

Drug Interactions Probenecid, tetracycline, aminoglycosides

Stability Store in refrigerator

Mechanism of Action Interferes with bacterial cell wall synthesis during active multiplication causing cell wall death and resultant bactericidal activity against susceptible bacteria

Pharmacokinetics

Absorption: I.M.: Slowly absorbed

Distribution: Penetration across the blood-brain barrier is poor, despite inflamed meninges; appears in breast milk

Peak serum levels: Within 1-4 hours and can persist within the therapeutic range for 15-24 hours

Elimination: Renal clearance is delayed in neonates, young infants, and patients with impaired renal function

Moderately dialyzable (20% to 50%)

Usual Dosage I.M.:

Newborns ≥1200 g: 50,000 units/kg/day given once daily (avoid using in this age group since sterile abscesses and procaine toxicity occur more frequently with neonates than older patients)

Children: 25,000-50,000 units/kg/day in divided doses every 12-24 hours; not to exceed 4.8 million units/24 hours

Gonorrhea: 100,00 units/kg (maximum: 4.8 million units) one time (in 2 injection sites) along with probenecid 25 mg/kg (maximum: 1 g) orally 30 minutes prior to procaine penicillin

Adults: 0.6-4.8 million units/day in divided doses every 12-24 hours

Uncomplicated gonorrhea: 1 g probenecid orally, then 4.8 million units procaine penicillin divided into 2 injection sites 30 minutes later

When used in conjunction with an aminoglycoside for the treatment of endocarditis caused by susceptible *S. viridans*: 1.2 million units every 6 hours for 2-4 weeks

Administration Procaine suspension for deep I.M. injection only; inadvertent I.V. administration has resulted in neurovascular damage. Administer into the gluteus maximus or into the midlateral muscles of the thigh; in infants and children it is preferable to give I.M. into the midlateral muscles of the thigh.

Monitoring Parameters Periodic renal and hematologic function tests with prolonged therapy

Test Interactions Positive Coombs' [direct], false-positive urinary and/or serum proteins

Dosage Forms Injection, suspension: 300,000 units/mL (10 mL); 500,000 units/mL (1.2 mL); 600,000 units/mL (1 mL, 2 mL, 4 mL)

Penicillin V Potassium

Brand Names Beepen-VK®; Betapen®-VK; Ledercillin® VK; Pen.Vee® K; Robicillin® VK; V-Cillin K®; Veetids®

Synonyms Phenoxymethyl Penicillin

Therapeutic Category Antibiotic, Penicillin

Use Treatment of mild to moderately severe susceptible bacterial infections involving the upper respiratory tract, skin, and urinary tract; prophylaxis of pneumococcal infections and rheumatic fever

Pregnancy Risk Factor B

Contraindications Known hypersensitivity to penicillin or any component

Precautions Use with caution in patients with renal impairment; dosage adjustment may be necessary in patients with renal impairment

Adverse Reactions

Central nervous system: Convulsions, fever

Dermatologic: Rash

Gastrointestinal: Nausea, diarrhea

Hematologic: Hemolytic anemia, positive Coombs' reaction

Renal & genitourinary: Acute interstitial nephritis

Miscellaneous: Hypersensitivity reactions, anaphylaxis

Drug Interactions Probenecid, tetracycline

Stability Refrigerate suspension after reconstitution; discard after 14 days

Mechanism of Action Interferes with bacterial cell wall synthesis during active multiplication causing cell wall death and resultant bactericidal activity against susceptible bacteria

Pharmacokinetics

Absorption: 60% to 73% of an oral dose is absorbed from the GI tract
Distribution: Appears in breast milk
Protein binding: 80%
Half-life: 30 minutes and is prolonged in patients with renal impairment
Peak serum levels: Within 30-60 minutes
Elimination: Penicillin V and its metabolites are excreted in urine mainly by tubular secretion

Usual Dosage Oral:

Systemic infections:
- Children <12 years: 25-50 mg/kg/day in divided doses every 6-8 hours; maximum dose: 3 g/day
- Children ≥12 years and Adults: 125-500 mg every 6-8 hours

Prophylaxis of pneumococcal infections:
- Children <5 years: 125 mg twice daily
- Children ≥5 years and Adults: 250 mg twice daily

Prophylaxis of recurrent rheumatic fever:
- Children <5 years: 125 mg twice daily
- Children ≥5 years and Adults: 250 mg twice daily

Monitoring Parameters Periodic renal and hematologic function tests during prolonged therapy

Test Interactions False-positive or negative urinary glucose determination using Clinitest®; positive Coombs' [direct]; false-positive urinary and/or serum proteins

Patient Information Take on an empty stomach 1 hour before or 2 hours after meals

Additional Information 0.7 mEq of potassium/250 mg penicillin V; 250 mg = 400,000 units of penicillin

Dosage Forms

Powder for oral solution: 125 mg/5 mL (3 mL, 100 mL, 150 mL, 200 mL); 250 mg/5 mL (100 mL, 150 mL, 200 mL)
Tablet: 125 mg, 250 mg, 500 mg

References

Dajani AS, Bisno AL, Chung KJ, et al, "Prevention of Rheumatic Fever. A Statement for Health Professionals by the Committee on Rheumatic Fever, Endocarditis, and Kawasaki Disease of the Council on Cardiovascular Disease in the Young, The American Heart Association," *Pediatr Infect Dis J*, 1989, 8(5):263-6.

Penicilloyl-polylysine *see* Benzylpenicilloyl-polylysine *on page 80*

Pentacef® *see* Ceftazidime *on page 116*

Pentam-300® *see* Pentamidine Isethionate *on this page*

Pentamidine Isethionate (pen tam' i deen)

Brand Names NebuPent™; Pentam-300®

Therapeutic Category Antibiotic, Miscellaneous

Use Treatment and prevention of pneumonia caused by *Pneumocystis carinii*; treatment of trypanosomiasis

Pregnancy Risk Factor C

Contraindications Hypersensitivity to pentamidine isethionate or any component (inhalation and injection)

Warnings Health care personnel who administer aerosolized pentamidine inhalation therapy, a cough-producing procedure, should be aware of the possibility of secondary exposure to tuberculosis from patients with undiagnosed pulmonary disease

Precautions Use with caution in patients with diabetes mellitus, renal or hepatic dysfunction; hypertension or hypotension

Adverse Reactions

Cardiovascular: Hypotension, tachycardia, cardiac arrhythmias
Central nervous system: Dizziness, fever, fatigue
Dermatologic: Rash, itching

(Continued)

Pentamidine Isethionate *(Continued)*

Endocrine & metabolic: Hypoglycemia, hyperglycemia, hypocalcemia, hyperkalemia
Gastrointestinal: Nausea, vomiting, metallic taste, pancreatitis
Hematologic: Megaloblastic anemia, granulocytopenia, leukopenia, thrombocytopenia
Hepatic: Mild hepatic injury
Local: Pain at injection site, thrombophlebitis
Renal & genitourinary: Mild renal injury
With aerosolized pentamidine: Irritation of the airway, cough, bronchospasm, fatigue, conjunctivitis
Miscellaneous: Jarisch-Herxheimer-like reaction

Stability Reconstituted solution is stable for 24 hours at room temperature; do not refrigerate due to the possibility of crystallization

Mechanism of Action Interferes with RNA/DNA, phospholipids and protein synthesis, through inhibition of oxidative phosphorylation and/or interference with incorporation of nucleotides and nucleic acids into RNA and DNA, in protozoa

Pharmacokinetics

Absorption: I.M.: Well absorbed; significant systemic absorption following inhalation therapy of pentamidine does not appear to occur
Half-life, terminal: 6.4-9.4 hours; half-life may be prolonged in patients with severe renal impairment
Elimination: 33% to 66% excreted in urine as unchanged drug

Usual Dosage

Children:
- Treatment: I.M., I.V. (I.V. preferred): 4 mg/kg/day once daily for 10-14 days
- Prevention:
  - I.M., I.V.: 4 mg/kg monthly or biweekly
  - Inhalation (aerosolized pentamidine in children ≥5 years): 300 mg/dose given every 3 weeks or monthly via Respirgard® II inhaler (8 mg/kg dose has also been used in children <5 years)
- Treatment of trypanosomiasis: I.V.: 4 mg/kg/day once daily for 10 days

Adults:
- Treatment: I.M., I.V. (I.V. preferred): 4 mg/kg/day once daily for 14 days
- Prevention: Inhalation: 300 mg every 4 weeks via Respirgard® II nebulizer

Administration May administer deep I.M. or by slow I.V. infusion; rapid I.V. administration can cause severe hypotension; infuse I.V. slowly over a period of at least 60 minutes at a final concentration for administration not to exceed 6 mg/mL

Monitoring Parameters Liver function tests, renal function tests, blood glucose, serum potassium and calcium, CBC with differential and platelet count, EKG, blood pressure

Patient Information Maintain adequate fluid intake

Nursing Implications Patients should receive parenteral pentamidine while lying down and blood pressure should be monitored closely

Dosage Forms

Inhalation: 300 mg
Injection: 300 mg

References

Centers for Disease Control,"Guidelines for Prophylaxis Against *Pneumocystis carinii* Pneumonia for Children Infected With Human Immunodeficiency Virus," *JAMA*, 1991, 265(13):1637-40, 1643-4.
Hughes WT, "*Pneumocystis carinii* Pneumonia: New Approaches to Diagnosis, Treatment, and Prevention," *Pediatr Infect Dis J*, 1991, 10(5):391-9.

Pentazocine (pen taz' oh seen)

Related Information

Compatibility of Medications Mixed in a Syringe *on page 717*
Narcotic Analgesics Comparison Chart *on page 721-722*

Brand Names Talwin®; Talwin® NX

Therapeutic Category Analgesic, Narcotic; Sedative

Use Relief of moderate to severe pain; a sedative prior to surgery and as a supplement to surgical anesthesia

Restrictions C-II; C-IV

Pregnancy Risk Factor B (D if used for prolonged periods or in high doses at term)

Contraindications Hypersensitivity to pentazocine or any component

Warnings Pentazocine may precipitate opiate withdrawal symptoms in patients who have been receiving opiates regularly; injection contains sulfites which may cause allergic reaction

Precautions Use with caution in seizure-prone patients, acute MI, patients undergoing biliary tract surgery, patients with renal and hepatic dysfunction, and patients with a history of prior opioid dependence or abuse; decrease dosage in patients with ↓ hepatic function

Adverse Reactions

Cardiovascular: Palpitations, hypotension, tachycardia, peripheral vasodilation

Central nervous system: CNS depression, drowsiness, sedation, dizziness, euphoria, lightheadedness (more frequently than morphine), hallucinations, confusion, disorientation, increased intracranial pressure, seizures may occur in seizure-prone patients especially with large I.V. doses

Dermatologic: Pruritus, rash

Endocrine & metabolic: Antidiuretic hormone release

Gastrointestinal: Nausea (more frequently than morphine), vomiting, constipation

Hepatic: Biliary tract spasm

Local: Tissue damage and irritation with I.M./S.C. use

Ocular: Miosis

Renal & genitourinary: Urinary tract spasm

Respiratory: Respiratory depression, laryngospasm

Sensitivity reactions: Histamine release

Miscellaneous: Physical and psychological dependence

Drug Interactions May potentiate or reduce analgesic effect of opiate agonist (ie, morphine), depending on patient's tolerance to opiates; additive effects seen with other CNS depressants; tripelennamine potentiates pentazocine effects and lethality and the two have been abused in combination (Ts and blues) I.V. to provide effects similar to heroin

Mechanism of Action Binds to opiate receptors in the CNS, causing inhibition of ascending pain pathways, altering the perception of and response to pain; produces generalized CNS depression

Pharmacodynamics

Onset:

Oral, I.M., S.C.: Within 15-30 minutes

I.V.: Within 2-3 minutes

Duration:

Oral: 4-5 hours

Parenteral: 2-3 hours

Pharmacokinetics

Protein binding: 60%

Metabolism: Metabolized in liver via oxidative and glucuronide conjugation pathways

Bioavailability: Oral: ~20% due to large first pass effect; ↑ oral bioavailability to 60% to 70% in patients with cirrhosis

Half-life: Adults: 2-3 hours; increased half-life with decreased hepatic function

Elimination: Small amounts excreted unchanged in urine

Usual Dosage

Children <14 years: Limited information available: I.M. doses of 15 mg for children 5-8 years of age and 30 mg for children 9-14 years of age to treat postoperative pain have been used (n=30); in 300 children (1-14 years) I.M. doses ranging from approximately 0.45-1.5 mg/kg in children <27 kg to 0.65-1.9 mg/kg in children >27 kg were used preoperatively

Children >14 years and Adults: Oral: 50 mg every 3-4 hours; may increase to 100 mg/dose if needed; oral dose should not exceed 600 mg/day

Adults:

I.M., S.C.: 30-60 mg every 3-4 hours

I.V.: 30 mg every 3-4 hours

Children and Adults: Dosing adjustment in renal impairment:

Cl_{cr} 10-50 mL/minute: Administer 75% of normal dose

Cl_{cr} <10 mL/minute: Administer 50% of normal dose

Administration S.C. route not advised due to tissue damage; rotate injection site for I.M., S.C. use; avoid intra-arterial injection

(Continued)

Pentazocine *(Continued)*

Monitoring Parameters Respiratory and cardiovascular status; level of pain relief and sedation

Additional Information Use only in patients who are not tolerant to or physically dependent upon narcotics

Talwin® NX tablet (pentazocine hydrochloride with naloxone) was formulated to ↓ abuse potential of dissolving tablets in water and using as injection

Dosage Forms

Injection, as lactate: 30 mg/mL (1 mL, 1.5 mL, 2 mL, 10 mL)

Tablet, scored: Pentazocine hydrochloride 50 mg and naloxone hydrochloride 0.5 mg

References

Rita L, Seleny FL, and Levin RM, "A Comparison of Pentazocine and Morphine for Pediatric Premedication," *Anesth Analg*, 1970, 49(3):377-82.

Waterworth TA, "Pentazocine (Fortal) as Postoperative Analgesic in Children," *Arch Dis Child*, 1974, 49(6):488-90.

Pentids® *see* Penicillin G Potassium or Sodium Salts *on page 440*

Pentobarbital (pen toe bar' bi tal)

Related Information

Compatibility of Medications Mixed in a Syringe *on page 717*

Overdose and Toxicology Information *on page 696-700*

Preprocedure Sedatives in Children *on page 687-689*

Brand Names Nembutal®

Synonyms Pentobarbital Sodium

Therapeutic Category Anticonvulsant; Barbiturate; General Anesthetic; Sedative

Use Short-term treatment of insomnia; preoperative sedation; high dose barbiturate coma for treatment of increased intracranial pressure or status epilepticus unresponsive to other therapy

Restrictions C-II; C-III (suppositories)

Pregnancy Risk Factor D

Contraindications Marked liver function impairment or latent porphyria; chronic or acute pain; hypersensitivity to barbiturates or any component

Precautions Use with caution in patients with hypovolemic shock, congestive heart failure, or hepatic impairment; capsules may contain tartrazine, which may cause allergic reactions

Adverse Reactions

Cardiovascular: Arrhythmias, bradycardia, hypotension

Central nervous system: Drowsiness, lethargy, CNS excitation or depression, impaired judgment, hypothermia

Dermatologic: Rash

Gastrointestinal: Nausea, vomiting

Local: Arterial spasm, gangrene with inadvertent intra-arterial injection, thrombophlebitis

Renal & genitourinary: Oliguria

Respiratory: Laryngospasm, respiratory depression, apnea (especially with rapid I.V. use)

Miscellaneous: Physical and psychological dependency with chronic use

Drug Interactions Chloramphenicol, cimetidine, CNS depressants, doxycycline

Stability Protect from light; aqueous solutions are not stable; commercially available vehicle contains propylene glycol; low pH may cause precipitate; use only clear solution

Mechanism of Action Short-acting barbiturate with sedative, hypnotic, and anticonvulsant properties

Pharmacodynamics

Onset:

Oral or rectal: 15-60 minutes

I.M.: Within 10-15 minutes

I.V.: Within 1 minute

Duration:
Oral, rectal: 1-4 hours
I.V.: 15 minutes

Pharmacokinetics
Distribution: V_d:
Children: 0.8 L/kg
Adults: 1 L/kg
Protein binding: 35% to 55%
Metabolism: Metabolized extensively in liver via hydroxylation and oxidation pathways
Half-life, terminal:
Children: 25 hours
Normal adults: 22 hours; range: 35-50 hours
Elimination: <1% excreted unchanged renally

Usual Dosage
Children:
Sedative: Oral: 2-6 mg/kg/day divided in 3 doses; maximum: 100 mg/day
Hypnotic: I.M.: 2-6 mg/kg; maximum: 100 mg/dose
Rectal:
2 months to 1 year (10-20 lbs): 30 mg
1-4 years (20-40 lbs): 30-60 mg
5-12 years (40-80 lbs): 60 mg
12-14 years (80-110 lbs): 60-120 mg **or**
<4 years: 3-6 mg/kg/dose
>4 years: 1.5-3 mg/kg/dose
Preoperative/preprocedure sedation: ≥6 months:
Oral, I.M., rectal: 2-6 mg/kg; maximum: 100 mg/dose
I.V.: 1-3 mg/kg to a maximum of 100 mg until asleep
Conscious sedation prior to a procedure: 5-12 years: I.V.: 2 mg/kg 5-10 minutes before procedures, may repeat one time
Adolescents: Conscious sedation: Oral, I.V.: 100 mg prior to a procedure
Children and Adults: Pentobarbital coma: I.V.:
Loading dose: 10-15 mg/kg given slowly over 1-2 hours; monitor blood pressure and respiratory rate
Maintenance infusion: Initial: 1 mg/kg/hour; may increase to 2-3 mg/kg/hour; maintain burst suppression on EEG
Adults:
Hypnotic:
Oral: 100-200 mg at bedtime
I.M.: 150-200 mg
I.V.: Initial: 100 mg, may repeat every 1-3 minutes up to 200-500 mg total
Rectal: 120-200 mg at bedtime
Preoperative sedation: I.M.: 150-200 mg

Administration Do not inject >50 mg/minute; rapid I.V. injection may cause respiratory depression, apnea, laryngospasm, bronchospasm, and hypotension, administer over 10-30 minutes; maximum concentration: 50 mg/mL for slow I.V. push

Monitoring Parameters Vital signs; respiratory status, pulse oximetry, cardiovascular status, CNS status

Reference Range Therapeutic: Sedation: 1-5 μg/mL (SI: 4-22 μmol/L); sleep: 5-15 μg/mL (SI: 22-66 μmol/L); coma: 20-40 μg/mL (SI: 88-177 μmol/L)

Nursing Implications Suppositories should not be divided; parenteral solutions are very alkaline; avoid extravasation; avoid intra-arterial injection

Additional Information Tolerance to hypnotic effect can occur; do not use for >2 weeks to treat insomnia; taper dose to prevent withdrawal; loading doses of 15-35 mg/kg (given over 1-2 hours) have been utilized in pediatric patients for pentobarbital coma but these higher loading doses often cause hypotension requiring vasopressor therapy

Dosage Forms
Capsule, as sodium: 50 mg, 100 mg
Elixir: 18.2 mg/5 mL (473 mL, 4000 mL)
Injection, as sodium: 50 mg/mL (1 mL, 2 mL, 20 mL, 50 mL)
Suppository, rectal (C-III): 30 mg, 60 mg, 120 mg, 200 mg

References

Fischer JH and Raineri DL, "Pentobarbital Anesthesia for Status Epilepticus," *Clin Pharm*, 1987, 6(8):601-2.

(Continued)

Pentobarbital *(Continued)*

Schaible DH, Cupit GC, Swedlow DB, et al, "High-Dose Pentobarbital Pharmacokinetics in Hypothermic Brain-Injured Children," *J Pediatr*, 1982, 100(4):655-60.

Zeltzer LK, Altman A, Cohen D, et al, "American Academy of Pediatrics Report of the Subcommittee on the Management of Pain Associated With Procedures in Children With Cancer," *Pediatrics*, 1990, 86(5 Pt 2):826-31.

Pentobarbital Sodium *see* Pentobarbital *on page 446*

Pentothal® Sodium *see* Thiopental *on page 561*

Pentrax® [OTC] *see* Coal Tar *on page 147*

Pen.Vee® K *see* Penicillin V Potassium *on page 442*

Pepto® Diarrhea Control [OTC *see* Loperamide Hydrochloride *on page 348*

Percocet® *see* Oxycodone Hydrochloride and Acetaminophen *on page 427*

Percodan® *see* Oxycodone Hydrochloride, Oxycodone Terephthalate and Aspirin *on page 428*

Percodan®-Demi *see* Oxycodone Hydrochloride, Oxycodone Terephthalate and Aspirin *on page 428*

Perdiem® Plain [OTC] *see* Psyllium *on page 498*

Periactin® *see* Cyproheptadine Hydrochloride *on page 166*

Peri-Colace® [OTC] *see* Docusate and Casanthranol *on page 203*

Peri-DOS® [OTC] *see* Docusate and Casanthranol *on page 203*

Permapen® *see* Penicillin G Benzathine *on page 438*

Permethrin (per meth' rin)

Brand Names Elimite™; Nix™

Therapeutic Category Antiparasitic Agent, Topical; Scabicidal Agent; Shampoos

Use Single application treatment of infestation with *Pediculus humanus capitis* (head louse) and its nits, or *Sarcoptes scabiei* (scabies)

Pregnancy Risk Factor B

Contraindications Known hypersensitivity to pyrethyroid, pyrethrin or to chrysanthemums

Precautions For external use only

Adverse Reactions

Dermatologic: Pruritus, erythema, rash of the scalp

Local: Burning, stinging, tingling, numbness or scalp discomfort, edema

Mechanism of Action Inhibits sodium ion influx through nerve cell membrane channels in parasites resulting in delayed repolarization, paralysis, and death of organism

Pharmacokinetics

Absorption: Topical: Absorption is minimal (<2%)

Metabolism: Metabolized by ester hydrolysis to inactive metabolites

Usual Dosage Topical:

Head lice: Children >2 months and Adults: After hair has been washed with shampoo, rinsed with water and towel dried, apply a sufficient volume to saturate the hair and scalp. Leave on hair for 10 minutes before rinsing off with water; remove remaining nits. May repeat in 1 week if lice or nits still present.

Scabies: Apply cream from head to toe; leave on for 8-14 hours before washing off with water; for infants, also apply on the hairline, neck, scalp, temple, and forehead; may reapply in 1 week if live mites appear

Patient Information Avoid contact with eyes during application; shake well before using; clothing and bedding should be washed in hot water or by dry cleaning to kill the scabies mite

Additional Information Formulation contains formaldehyde which is a contact allergen

Dosage Forms

Cream: 5% (60 g)

Creme rinse: 1% (60 mL with comb)

References

Hogan DJ, Schachner L, Tanglertsampan C, "Diagnosis and Treatment of Childhood Scabies and Pediculosis," *Pediatr Clin North Am*, 1991, 38(4):941-57.

Krowchuk DP, Tunnessen WW Jr, and Hurwitz S, "Pediatric Dermatology Update," *Pediatrics*, 1992, 90(2 Pt 1):259-64.

Pernox® [OTC] *see* Sulfur and Salicylic Acid *on page 545*

Peroxide *see* Hydrogen Peroxide *on page 294*

Peroxyl® *see* Hydrogen Peroxide *on page 294*

Persa-Gel® *see* Benzoyl Peroxide *on page 78*

Persantine® *see* Dipyridamole *on page 198*

Pertofrane® *see* Desipramine Hydrochloride *on page 176*

Pethidine Hydrochloride *see* Meperidine Hydrochloride *on page 362*

PFA *see* Foscarnet *on page 263*

Pfizerpen® *see* Penicillin G Potassium or Sodium Salts *on page 440*

Pfizerpen®-AS *see* Penicillin G Procaine *on page 441*

PGE_1 *see* Alprostadil *on page 32*

Phazyme® [OTC] *see* Simethicone *on page 524*

Phenantoin *see* Mephenytoin *on page 363*

Phenaphen® With Codeine *see* Acetaminophen and Codeine Phosphate *on page 17*

Phenazine® *see* Promethazine Hydrochloride *on page 488*

Phenazopyridine Hydrochloride (fen az oh peer' i deen)

Brand Names Azo-Standard®; Geridium®; Pyridiate®; Pyridium®; Urodine®

Synonyms Phenylazo Diamino Pyridine Hydrochloride

Therapeutic Category Local Anesthetic, Urinary

Use Symptomatic relief of urinary burning, itching, frequency and urgency in association with urinary tract infection, or following urologic procedures

Pregnancy Risk Factor B

Contraindications Hypersensitivity to phenazopyridine or any component; kidney or liver disease

Adverse Reactions

Central nervous system: Vertigo, headache

Dermatologic: Skin pigmentation, rash, pruritus

Hematologic: Methemoglobinemia, hemolytic anemia

Hepatic: Hepatitis

Renal & genitourinary: Transient acute renal failure

Mechanism of Action Exerts local anesthetic or analgesic action on urinary tract mucosa through an unknown mechanism

Pharmacokinetics

Metabolism: Metabolized in the liver and other tissues

Elimination: Excreted in the urine (where it exerts its action); renal excretion (as unchanged drug) is rapid and accounts for 65% of the drug's elimination

Usual Dosage Oral:

Children: 12 mg/kg/day in 3 divided doses administered after meals

Adults: 100-200 mg 3-4 times/day

Test Interactions False-negative Clinistix®, Tes-Tape®, Ictotest®, Acetest®, Ketostix®

Patient Information May discolor urine orange or red; may stain contact lenses and fabric

Dosage Forms Tablet: 100 mg, 200 mg

Phencen® *see* Promethazine Hydrochloride *on page 488*

Phenergan® *see* Promethazine Hydrochloride *on page 488*

Phenergan® VC *see* Promethazine and Phenylephrine *on page 487*

Phenergan® VC With Codeine *see* Promethazine, Phenylephrine and Codeine *on page 489*

Phenergan® with Codeine *see* Promethazine and Codeine *on page 486*

Phenetron® *see* Chlorpheniramine Maleate *on page 128*

Phenobarbital (fee noe bar' bi tal)

Related Information

Blood Level Sampling Time Guidelines *on page 694-695*

Overdose and Toxicology Information *on page 696-700*

Brand Names Barbita®; Luminal®; Solfoton®

Synonyms Phenobarbitone; Phenylethylmalonylurea

Therapeutic Category Anticonvulsant; Barbiturate; Hypnotic; Sedative

Use Management of generalized tonic-clonic (grand mal) and partial seizures; neonatal seizures; febrile seizures in children; sedation; may also be used for prevention and treatment of neonatal hyperbilirubinemia and lowering of bilirubin in chronic cholestasis

Restrictions C-IV

Pregnancy Risk Factor D

Contraindications Hypersensitivity to phenobarbital or any component; preexisting CNS depression, severe uncontrolled pain, porphyria, severe respiratory disease with dyspnea or obstruction

Warnings Abrupt withdrawal may precipitate status epilepticus

Precautions Use with caution in patients with renal or hepatic impairment

Adverse Reactions

Cardiovascular: Hypotension, circulatory collapse

Central nervous system: Drowsiness, paradoxical excitement, hyperkinetic activity, cognitive impairment, defects in general comprehension, short-term memory deficits, decreased attention span, ataxia

Dermatologic: Skin eruptions, skin rash, exfoliative dermatitis

Hematologic: Megaloblastic anemia

Hepatic: Hepatitis

Respiratory: Respiratory depression, apnea (especially with rapid I.V. use)

Miscellaneous: Psychological and physical dependence

Drug Interactions Phenobarbital may ↓ the serum concentration or effect of ethosuximide, warfarin, oral contraceptives, chloramphenicol, griseofulvin, doxycycline, beta blockers, theophylline, corticosteroids, tricyclic antidepressants, cyclosporin, quinidine, haloperidol, and phenothiazines; valproic acid, methylphenidate, chloramphenicol and propoxyphene may inhibit the metabolism of phenobarbital with resultant ↑ in phenobarbital serum concentration; phenobarbital and benzodiazepines or other CNS depressants → ↑ CNS and respiratory depression (especially with I.V. loading doses of phenobarbital)

Stability Protect elixir from light; not stable in aqueous solutions; use only clear solutions; do not add to acidic solutions, precipitation may occur

Mechanism of Action Interferes with transmission of impulses from the thalamus to the cortex of the brain resulting in an imbalance in central inhibitory and facilitatory mechanisms

Pharmacodynamics Hypnosis:

Onset of action:

- Oral: Within 20-60 minutes
- I.V.: Within 5 minutes

Peak effect: I.V.: Within 30 minutes

Duration:

- Oral: 6-10 hours
- I.V.: 4-10 hours

Pharmacokinetics

Absorption: Oral: 70% to 90%

Distribution: V_d:

- Neonates: 0.8-1 L/kg
- Infants: 0.7-0.8 L/kg
- Children: 0.6-0.7 L/kg

Protein binding: 20% to 45%, ↓ protein binding in neonates
Metabolism: Metabolized in liver via hydroxylation and glucuronide conjugation
Half-life:
Neonates: 45-500 hours
Infants: 20-133 hours
Children: 37-73 hours
Adults: 53-140 hours
Peak serum levels: Oral: Within 1-6 hours
Elimination: 20% to 50% excreted unchanged in the urine; clearance can be ↑ with alkalinization of urine or with oral multiple-dose activated charcoal

Usual Dosage
Anticonvulsant: Status epilepticus: **Loading dose:** I.V.:
Neonates: 15-20 mg/kg in a single or divided dose
Infants, Children, and Adults: 15-18 mg/kg in a single or divided dose; usual maximum loading dose: 20 mg/kg
Note: In select patients, may give additional 5 mg/kg/dose every 15-30 minutes until seizure is controlled or a total dose of 30 mg/kg is reached; be prepared to support respirations

Anticonvulsant maintenance dose: Oral, I.V.:
Neonates: 3-4 mg/kg/day in 1-2 divided doses; assess serum concentrations; increase to 5 mg/kg/day if needed (usually by second week of therapy)
Infants: 5-6 mg/kg/day in 1-2 divided doses
Children 1-5 years: 6-8 mg/kg/day in 1-2 divided doses; 5-12 years: 4-6 mg/kg/day in 1-2 divided doses; >12 years and adults: 1-3 mg/kg/day in divided doses

Children:
Sedation: Oral: 2 mg/kg 3 times/day
Hypnotic: I.M., I.V., S.C.: 3-5 mg/kg at bedtime
Hyperbilirubinemia: <12 years: Oral: 3-8 mg/kg/day in 2-3 divided doses; doses up to 12 mg/kg/day have been used
Preoperative sedation: Oral, I.M., I.V.: 1-3 mg/kg 1-1½ hours before procedure

Adults:
Sedation: Oral, I.M.: 30-120 mg/day in 2-3 divided doses
Hypnotic: Oral, I.M., I.V., S.C.: 100-320 mg at bedtime
Hyperbilirubinemia: Oral: 90-180 mg/day in 2-3 divided doses
Preoperative sedation: I.M.: 100-200 mg 1-1½ hours before procedure

Administration Do not inject I.V. faster than 1 mg/kg/minute (50 mg/minute for patients >60 kg); do not administer intra-arterially; avoid extravasation; use only powder for injection for S.C. use, not solutions for injection

Monitoring Parameters CNS status, liver enzymes, CBC, serum concentrations; I.V. use: Respiratory rate, heart rate, blood pressure

Reference Range Therapeutic: 15-40 μg/mL (SI: 65-172 μmol/L); potentially toxic: >40 μg/mL (SI: >172 μmol/L); coma: >50 μg/mL (SI: >215 μmol/L); potentially lethal: >80 μg/mL (SI: >344 μmol/L)

Nursing Implications Parenteral solutions are very alkaline

Additional Information Injectable solutions contain propylene glycol

Dosage Forms
Capsule: 16 mg
Elixir: 15 mg/5 mL (5 mL, 10 mL, 20 mL); 20 mg/5 mL (3.75 mL, 5 mL, 7.5 mL, 120 mL, 473 mL, 946 mL, 4000 mL)
Injection, as sodium: 30 mg/mL (1 mL); 60 mg/mL (1 mL); 65 mg/mL (1 mL); 130 mg/mL (1 mL)
Powder for injection: 120 mg
Tablet: 8 mg, 15 mg, 16 mg, 30 mg, 32 mg, 60 mg, 65 mg, 100 mg

Phenobarbitone *see* Phenobarbital *on previous page*

Phenoxybenzamine Hydrochloride (fen ox ee ben' za meen)

Related Information
Overdose and Toxicology Information *on page 696-700*

Brand Names Dibenzyline®

Therapeutic Category Alpha-Adrenergic Blocking Agent, Oral; Antihypertensive; Vasodilator, Coronary

(Continued)

Phenoxybenzamine Hydrochloride *(Continued)*

Use Symptomatic management of hypertension and sweating in patients with pheochromocytoma

Pregnancy Risk Factor C

Contraindications Shock

Precautions Use with caution in patients with renal damage, cerebral or coronary arteriosclerosis

Adverse Reactions

Cardiovascular: Postural hypotension, tachycardia, syncope, shock, nasal congestion

Central nervous system: Lethargy, weakness, headache, dizziness

Gastrointestinal: Vomiting, nausea, diarrhea

Ocular: Miosis

Drug Interactions Antagonizes effects of alpha-adrenergic stimulating sympathomimetic agents

Mechanism of Action Produces long-lasting noncompetitive alpha-adrenergic blockade of postganglionic synapses in exocrine glands and smooth muscle

Pharmacodynamics Oral:

Onset of action: Within 2 hours

Peak effect: Within 4-6 hours

Duration: Effects can continue for up to 4 days

Pharmacokinetics

Distribution: Distributes to and may accumulate in adipose tissues

Half-life: Adults: 24 hours

Elimination: Excreted primarily in the urine and bile

Usual Dosage Oral:

Children: Initial: 0.2 mg/kg once daily; maximum: 10 mg/dose; increase by 0.2 mg/kg/day increments; usual maintenance dose: 0.4-1.2 mg/kg/day every 6-8 hours; higher doses may be needed

Adults: Initial: 10 mg twice daily; increase dose every other day to usual dose of 10-40 mg every 8-12 hours; higher doses may be needed

Monitoring Parameters Blood pressure, orthostasis, heart rate

Dosage Forms Capsule: 10 mg

Phenoxymethyl Penicillin *see* Penicillin V Potassium *on page 442*

Phentolamine Mesylate (fen tole' a meen)

Related Information

Extravasation Treatment *on page 640*

Overdose and Toxicology Information *on page 696-700*

Brand Names Regitine®

Therapeutic Category Alpha-Adrenergic Blocking Agent, Parenteral; Alpha-Adrenergic Inhibitors, Central; Antidote, Extravasation; Antihypertensive; Diagnostic Agent, Pheochromocytoma; Vasodilator, Coronary

Use Diagnosis of pheochromocytoma; treatment of hypertension associated with pheochromocytoma or other causes of excess sympathomimetic amines; local treatment of dermal necrosis after extravasation of drugs with alpha-adrenergic effects (norepinephrine, dopamine, epinephrine, dobutamine)

Pregnancy Risk Factor C

Contraindications Hypersensitivity to phentolamine or any component; renal impairment; coronary or cerebral arteriosclerosis; myocardial infarction

Precautions Use with caution in patients with gastritis, peptic ulcer; history of cardiac arrhythmias; myocardial infarction, cerebrovascular spasm, and cerebrovascular occlusion may occur

Adverse Reactions

Cardiovascular: Hypotension, tachycardia, angina, arrhythmias, nasal congestion

Central nervous system: Weakness, dizziness

Gastrointestinal: Nausea, vomiting, diarrhea, exacerbation of peptic ulcer

Stability Reconstituted solution is stable for 48 hours at room temperature and 1 week when refrigerated

Mechanism of Action Competitively blocks alpha-adrenergic receptors to produce brief antagonism of circulating epinephrine and norepinephrine; reduces hypertension caused by alpha effects of catecholamines; also has positive inotropic and chronotropic effects on the heart

Pharmacodynamics

Onset of action:
- I.M.: Within 15-20 minutes
- I.V.: Immediate

Peak effect:
- I.M.: Within 20 minutes
- I.V.: Within 2 minutes

Duration:
- I.M.: 30-45 minutes
- I.V.: Within 15-30 minutes

Pharmacokinetics

Metabolism: Metabolized in liver

Half-life: Adults: 19 minutes

Elimination: 10% of dose excreted in urine as unchanged drug

Usual Dosage

Treatment of extravasation: Infants, Children, and Adults: S.C.: Infiltrate area with small amount of solution (made by diluting 5-10 mg in 10 mL 0.9% sodium chloride) within 12 hours of extravasation; do not exceed 0.1-0.2 mg/kg or 5 mg total

Diagnosis of pheochromocytoma: I.M., I.V.:
- Children: 0.05-0.1 mg/kg/dose, maximum single dose: 5 mg
- Adults: 5 mg

Hypertension: I.M., I.V.:
- Children: 0.05-0.1 mg/kg/dose given 1-2 hours before pheochromocytomectomy; repeat as needed; maximum single dose: 5 mg
- Adults: 5 mg given 1-2 hours before pheochromocytomectomy

Administration Treatment of extravasation: Infiltrate area of extravasation with multiple small injections; use 27- or 30-gauge needles and change needle between each skin entry

Monitoring Parameters Blood pressure, heart rate, orthostasis

Additional Information Injection contains mannitol 25 mg/vial

Dosage Forms Injection: 5 mg/mL (1 mL)

Phenylalanine Mustard *see* Melphalan *on page 360*

Phenylazo Diamino Pyridine Hydrochloride *see* Phenazopyridine Hydrochloride *on page 449*

Phenylephrine Hydrochloride (fen ill ef' rin)

Related Information

Extravasation Treatment *on page 640*

OTC Cold Preparations, Pediatric *on page 723-726*

Brand Names AK-Dilate® Ophthalmic Solution; AK-Nefrin® Ophthalmic Solution; Alconefrin® Nasal Solution [OTC]; Doktors® Nasal Solution [OTC]; I-Phrine® Ophthalmic Solution; Isopto® Frin Ophthalmic Solution; Mydfrin® Ophthalmic Solution; Neo-Synephrine® Nasal Solution [OTC]; Neo-Synephrine® Ophthalmic Solution; Nostril® Nasal Solution [OTC]; Prefrin™ Ophthalmic Solution; Relief® Ophthalmic Solution; Rhinall® Nasal Solution [OTC]; Sinarest® Nasal Solution [OTC]; St. Joseph® Measured Dose Nasal Solution [OTC]; Vicks® Sinex® Nasal Solution [OTC]

Therapeutic Category Adrenergic Agonist Agent; Adrenergic Agonist Agent, Ophthalmic; Alpha-Adrenergic Blocking Agent, Ophthalmic; Nasal Agent, Vasoconstrictor; Ophthalmic Agent, Mydriatic; Sympathomimetic

Use Treatment of hypotension and vascular failure in shock; as a vasoconstrictor in regional analgesia; symptomatic relief of nasal and nasopharyngeal mucosal congestion; as a mydriatic in ophthalmic procedures and treatment of wide-angle glaucoma; supraventricular tachycardia

Pregnancy Risk Factor C

Contraindications Pheochromocytoma, severe hypertension, bradycardia, ventricular tachycardia, hypersensitivity to phenylephrine or any component, acute pancreatitis, hepatitis; peripheral or mesenteric vascular thrombosis, myocardial disease, severe coronary disease

(Continued)

Phenylephrine Hydrochloride *(Continued)*

Warnings Injection may contain sulfites which may cause allergic reactions in some patients; do not use if solution turns brown or contains a precipitate

Precautions Pressor therapy is **not** a substitute for replacement of blood, plasma, and body fluids in shock

Adverse Reactions

Cardiovascular: Hypertension, angina, reflex severe bradycardia, arrhythmias

Central nervous system: Restlessness, excitability, headache, anxiety, nervousness, dizziness, tremor

Dermatologic: Pilomotor response, skin blanching

Local: Necrosis if extravasation occurs

Respiratory: Respiratory distress, rebound nasal stuffiness

Drug Interactions With alpha- and beta-adrenergic blocking agents, may see decreased actions; with oxytocic drugs, may see increased actions; with sympathomimetics, tachycardia or arrhythmias may occur; with MAO inhibitors, actions may be potentiated

Mechanism of Action Potent, direct acting alpha-adrenergic stimulator with weak beta-adrenergic activity; causes vasoconstriction of the arterioles of the nasal mucosa and conjunctiva; activates the dilator muscle of the pupil to cause contraction; produces systemic arterial vasoconstriction

Pharmacodynamics

Onset of action:

- I.M.: Within 10-15 minutes
- I.V.: Following parenteral injection, effects occur immediately
- S.C.: 10-15 minutes

Duration:

- I.M.: 30 minutes to 2 hours
- I.V.: 15-20 minutes
- S.C.: 1 hour

Pharmacokinetics

Metabolism: Metabolized in the liver and intestine by the enzyme monamine oxidase

Elimination: Metabolites, routes, and rates of excretion have not been identified

Usual Dosage

Ophthalmic procedures:

- Infants <1 year: 1 drop of 2.5% 15-30 minutes before procedures
- Children and Adults: 1 drop of 2.5% or 10% solution, may repeat in 10-60 minutes as needed

Nasal decongestant (therapy should not exceed 3-5 days):

- Children:
  - <6 years: 2-3 drops every 4 hours of 0.125% solution as needed
  - 6-12 years: 2-3 drops every 4 hours of 0.25% solution as needed
- Children >12 years and Adults: 2-3 drops or 1-2 sprays every 4 hours of 0.25% to 0.5% solution as needed; 1% solution may be used in adults in cases of extreme nasal congestion

Hypotension/shock:

- Children:
  - I.M., S.C.: 0.1 mg/kg/dose every 1-2 hours as needed (maximum: 5 mg)
  - I.V. bolus: 5-20 μg/kg/dose every 10-15 minutes as needed; I.V. infusion: 0.1-0.5 μg/kg/minute, titrate to desired effect
- Adults:
  - I.M., S.C.: 2-5 mg/dose every 1-2 hours as needed (initial dose should not exceed 5 mg)
  - I.V. bolus: 0.1-0.5 mg/dose every 10-15 minutes as needed (initial dose should not exceed 0.5 mg)
  - I.V. infusion: 40-180 μg/minute, titrate to desired effect; usual dose: 20-200 μg/minute

Administration For direct I.V. administration, dilute to 1 mg/mL by adding 1-9 mL of sterile water; the specific dosage may be administered by direct I.V. injection over 20-30 seconds; continuous infusion concentrations are usually 20-60 μg/mL by adding 5 mg to 250 mL I.V. solution (20 μg/mL) or 15 mg to 250 mL (60 μg/mL)

Monitoring Parameters Heart rate, blood pressure, central venous pressure, arterial blood gases

Nursing Implications Extravasant; avoid I.V. infiltration

Dosage Forms

Jelly, nasal: 0.5% (18.75 g)
Injection: 10 mg/mL (1 mL)
Solution:
Nasal:
Drops: 0.125% (15 mL, 30 mL); 0.16% (30 mL); 0.2% (30 mL); 0.25% (15 mL, 30 mL, 473 mL)
Spray: 0.25% (15 mL, 30 mL); 0.5% (15 mL, 30 mL); 1% (15 mL)
Ophthalmic: 0.12% (15 mL); 2.5% (2 mL, 3 mL, 5 mL, 15 mL); 10% (1 mL, 2 mL, 5 mL)

Phenylethylmalonylurea *see* Phenobarbital *on page 450*

Phenylisohydantoin *see* Pemoline *on page 436*

Phenylpropanolamine and Brompheniramine *see* Brompheniramine and Phenylpropanolamine *on page 87*

Phenytoin (fen' i toyn)

Related Information

Blood Level Sampling Time Guidelines *on page 694-695*
Overdose and Toxicology Information *on page 696-700*

Brand Names Dilantin®; Diphenylan Sodium®

Synonyms Diphenylhydantoin; DPH; Phenytoin Sodium, Extended; Phenytoin Sodium, Prompt

Therapeutic Category Antiarrhythmic Agent, Class Ib; Anticonvulsant

Use Management of generalized tonic-clonic (grand mal), simple partial and complex partial seizures; prevention of seizures following head trauma/neurosurgery; ventricular arrhythmias, including those associated with digitalis intoxication, prolonged QT interval and surgical repair of congenital heart diseases in children; also used for epidermolysis bullosa

Pregnancy Risk Factor D

Contraindications Hypersensitivity to phenytoin or any component; heart block, sinus bradycardia

Precautions Use with caution in patients with porphyria; discontinue if rash or lymphadenopathy occurs

Adverse Reactions

Dose related:
Central nervous system: Ataxia, slurred speech, dizziness, drowsiness, lethargy, coma
Ocular: Nystagmus, blurred vision, diplopia

Cardiovascular: I.V.: Hypotension, bradycardia, arrhythmias, cardiovascular collapse (especially with rapid I.V. use),
Central nervous system: Fever, mood changes
Dermatologic: Hirsutism, coarsening of facial features, Stevens-Johnson syndrome, rash, exfoliative dermatitis
Endocrine & metabolic: Folic acid depletion, osteomalacia, hyperglycemia
Gastrointestinal: Nausea, vomiting, gingival hyperplasia, gum tenderness
Hematologic: Blood dyscrasias, pseudolymphoma, lymphoma
Hepatic: Hepatitis
Local: Venous irritation and pain, thrombophlebitis
Musculoskeletal: Dyskinesias
Miscellaneous: Lymphadenopathy, peripheral neuropathy, SLE-like syndrome

Drug Interactions Phenytoin may decrease the serum concentration or effectiveness of valproic acid, ethosuximide, primidone, warfarin, oral contraceptives, corticosteroids, cyclosporin, theophylline, chloramphenicol, rifampin, doxycycline, quinidine, mexiletine, disopyramide, dopamine, or nondepolarizing skeletal muscle relaxants; protein binding of phenytoin can be effected by VPA or salicylates; serum phenytoin concentrations may be ↑ by cimetidine, chloramphenicol, INH, trimethoprim, or sulfonamides and ↓ by rifampin, cisplatin, vinblastine, bleomycin, folic acid, or continuous NG feeds

Stability Parenteral solution may be used as long as there is no precipitate and it is not hazy; slightly yellowed solution may be used; refrigeration may cause precipitate, sometimes the precipitate is resolved by allowing the so-

(Continued)

Phenytoin *(Continued)*

lution to reach room temperature again; drug may precipitate with pH ≤11.5; do not mix with other medications; may dilute with normal saline for I.V. infusion, but must be diluted to concentration <6 mg/mL

Mechanism of Action Stabilizes neuronal membranes and decreases seizure activity by increasing efflux or decreasing influx of sodium ions across cell membranes in the motor cortex during generation of nerve impulses; prolongs effective refractory period and suppresses ventricular pacemaker automaticity, shortens action potential in the heart

Pharmacokinetics

Absorption: Oral: Slow

Distribution: V_d:

- Neonates:
  - Premature: 1-1.2 L/kg
  - Full-term: 0.8-0.9 L/kg
- Infants: 0.7-0.8 L/kg
- Children: 0.7 L/kg
- Adults: 0.6-0.7 L/kg

Protein binding, adults: 90% to 95%, increased free fraction (↓ protein binding) in neonates (up to 20% free), infants (up to 15% free), and patients with hyperbilirubinemia, hypoalbuminemia, uremia

Metabolism: Follows dose-dependent (Michaelis-Menten) pharmacokinetics with ↑ Vmax in infants >6 months and children vs adults; major metabolite (via oxidation) HPPA undergoes enterohepatic recycling and elimination in urine as glucuronides

Bioavailability: Formulation dependent

Peak serum levels: Dependent upon formulation administered

- Extended release capsule: Within 4-12 hours
- Immediate release preparation: Within 2-3 hours

Elimination: <5% excreted unchanged in urine; ↑ clearance and ↓ serum concentrations with febrile illness; highly variable clearance, dependent upon intrinsic hepatic function and dose administered

Usual Dosage

Status epilepticus: I.V.:

- Loading dose:
  - Neonates: 15-20 mg/kg in a single or divided dose;
  - Infants, Children, and Adults: 15-18 mg/kg in a single or divided dose
- Maintenance, anticonvulsant:
  - Neonates: Initial: 5 mg/kg/day in 2 divided doses; usual: 5-8 mg/kg/day in 2 divided doses; some patients may require dosing every 8 hours
  - Infants and Children: Initial: 5 mg/kg/day in 2 divided doses, usual doses 0.5-3 years: 8-10 mg/kg/day, 4-6 years: 7.5-9 mg/kg/day, 7-9 years: 7-8 mg/kg/day, 10-16 years: 6-7 mg/kg/day, some patients may require every 8 hours dosing
  - Adults: Usual: 300 mg/day or 5-6 mg/kg/day in 3 divided doses or 1-2 divided doses using extended release

Anticonvulsant: Children and Adults: Oral:

- Loading dose: 15-20 mg/kg; based on phenytoin serum concentrations and recent dosing history; administer oral loading dose in 3 divided doses given every 2-4 hours to ↓ GI adverse effects and to ensure complete oral absorption
- Maintenance dose: Same as I.V. listed above

Arrhythmias:

- Children and Adults: Loading dose: I.V.: 1.25 mg/kg IVP every 5 minutes may repeat up to total loading dose: 15 mg/kg
- Children: Maintenance dose: Oral, I.V.: 5-10 mg/kg/day in 2 divided doses
- Adults: Loading dose: Oral: 250 mg 4 times/day for 1 day, 250 mg twice daily for 2 days, then maintenance at 300-400 mg/day in divided doses 1-4 times/day

Administration Do not exceed I.V. infusion rate of 1-3 mg/kg/minute or 50 mg/minute; I.V. injections should be followed by normal saline flushes through the same needle or I.V. catheter to avoid local irritation of the vein; avoid extravasation; avoid I.M. use due to erratic absorption, pain on injection, and precipitation of drug at injection site

Monitoring Parameters Monitor blood pressure with I.V. use; monitor serum concentrations, CBC, liver enzymes; monitor free and total serum concentrations in patients with hyperbilirubinemia, hypoalbuminemia, or uremia

Reference Range

Neonates: Therapeutic: 8-15 μg/mL

Children and Adults: Therapeutic: 10-20 μg/mL (SI: 40-79 μmol/L). Toxicity is measured clinically, some patients require levels outside the suggested therapeutic range; toxic: >20 μg/mL (SI: >79 μmol/L); lethal: >100 μg/mL (SI: >400 μmol/L). Commonly accepted therapeutic free (unbound) concentration: 1-2 mg/mL

Nursing Implications Maintenance doses usually start 12 hours after loading dose; shake oral suspension well prior to each dose; to avoid ↓ serum levels with continuous NG feeds, hold feedings for 2 hours prior to and 2 hours after phenytoin administration if possible

Additional Information Injection contains propylene glycol; possible permanent cerebellum damage may occur with chronic toxic serum concentrations

Dosage Forms

Capsule, as sodium:
- Extended: 30 mg, 100 mg
- Prompt: 30 mg, 100 mg

Injection, as sodium: 50 mg/mL (2 mL, 5 mL)

Suspension, oral: 30 mg/5 mL (5 mL, 240 mL); 125 mg/5 mL (5 mL, 240 mL)

Tablet, chewable: 50 mg

References

Bauer LA and Blouin RA, "Phenytoin Michaelis-Menten Pharmacokinetics in Caucasian Pediatric Patients," *Clin Pharmacokinet*, 1983, 8(6):545-9.

Chiba K, Ishizaki T, Miura H, et al, "Michaelis-Menten Pharmacokinetics of Diphenylhydantoin and Application in the Pediatric Age Patient," *J Pediatr*, 1980, 96(3):479-84.

Phenytoin Sodium, Extended *see* Phenytoin *on page 455*

Phenytoin Sodium, Prompt *see* Phenytoin *on page 455*

Pherazine® VC *see* Promethazine and Phenylephrine *on page 487*

Pherazine® With Codeine *see* Promethazine and Codeine *on page 486*

Phillips'® Milk of Magnesia [OTC] *see* Magnesium Hydroxide *on page 352*

pHisoAc- BP® [OTC] *see* Benzoyl Peroxide *on page 78*

pHisoHex® *see* Hexachlorophene *on page 285*

Phos-Flur® *see* Fluoride *on page 255*

Phosphonoformate *see* Foscarnet *on page 263*

***p*-Hydroxyampicillin** *see* Amoxicillin *on page 44*

Phyllocontin® *see* Aminophylline *on page 37*

Phylloquinone *see* Phytonadione *on next page*

Physostigmine Salicylate (fye zoe stig' meen)

Related Information

Overdose and Toxicology Information *on page 696-700*

Brand Names Antilirium®; Isopto® Eserine

Synonyms Eserine Salicylate

Therapeutic Category Antidote, Anticholinergic Agent; Antidote, Belladonna Alkaloids; Cholinergic Agent; Cholinergic Agent, Ophthalmic

Use Reverse toxic CNS and cardiac effects caused by anticholinergics and tricyclic antidepressants; ophthalmic solution is used to treat open-angle glaucoma

Pregnancy Risk Factor C

Contraindications Hypersensitivity to physostigmine or any component; GI or GU obstruction, asthma, diabetes, gangrene, cardiovascular disease

Warnings Because physostigmine has the potential for producing severe adverse effects, (ie, seizures, bradycardia), routine use as an antidote is controversial; atropine should be readily available to treat severe adverse effects

(Continued)

Physostigmine Salicylate *(Continued)*

Precautions Use with caution in patients with epilepsy, bradycardia; injectable contains bisulfites, avoid in sensitive individuals

Adverse Reactions

Cardiovascular: Sweating, palpitations, bradycardia
Central nervous system: Restlessness, hallucinations, seizures
Gastrointestinal: Nausea, vomiting, epigastric pain, salivation
Musculoskeletal: Muscle twitching, weakness
Ocular: Miosis, lacrimation, stinging, burning
Respiratory: Dyspnea, bronchospasm, respiratory paralysis, pulmonary edema

Drug Interactions Bethanechol, methacholine, succinylcholine

Mechanism of Action Inhibits destruction of acetylcholine by acetylcholinesterase which prolongs the central and peripheral effects of acetylcholine

Pharmacodynamics

Onset of action:
- Ophthalmic: Within 10-30 minutes
- Parenteral: Within 3-8 minutes

Duration:
- Ophthalmic: 12-48 hours
- Parenteral: 30 minutes to 5 hours

Pharmacokinetics

Distribution: Widely distributed throughout the body; crosses into the CNS
Half-life: 15-40 minutes
Elimination: Eliminated via hydrolysis by cholinesterases

Usual Dosage

Reversal of toxic anticholinergic effects:
- Children: Reserve for life-threatening situations only: I.V.: 0.01-0.03 mg/kg/dose; may repeat after 15-20 minutes to a maximum total dose of 2 mg
- Adults: I.M., I.V., S.C.: 0.5-2 mg initially, repeat every 20 minutes until response occurs or adverse effect occurs

Preanesthetic reversal: Children and Adults:
- I.M., I.V.: Give twice the dose, on a weight basis, of the anticholinergic drug (atropine, scopolamine)

Ophthalmic: 1-2 drops of 0.25% or 0.5% solution every 4-8 hours (up to 4 times/day). The ointment may be instilled at night.

Administration Infuse slowly I.V. at a maximum rate of 0.5 mg/minute in children or 1 mg/minute in adults

Monitoring Parameters Heart rate, respiratory rate

Dosage Forms

Injection, as salicylate: 1 mg/mL (2 mL)
Ointment, ophthalmic: 0.25% (3.5 g, 3.7 g)
Solution, ophthalmic: 0.25% (15 mL); 0.5% (2 mL, 15 mL)

Phytomenadione *see* Phytonadione *on this page*

Phytonadione (fye toe na dye' one)

Brand Names AquaMEPHYTON®; Konakion®; Mephyton®

Synonyms Methylphytyl Napthoquinone; Phylloquinone; Phytomenadione; Vitamin K_1

Therapeutic Category Vitamin, Water Soluble

Use Prevention and treatment of hypoprothrombinemia caused by vitamin K deficiency or anticoagulant-induced hypoprothrombinemia; hemorrhagic disease of the newborn

Pregnancy Risk Factor C (X if used in third trimester or near term)

Contraindications Hypersensitivity to phytonadione or any component

Warnings Ineffective in hereditary hypoprothrombinemia and hypoprothrombinemia caused by severe liver disease; severe hemolytic anemia and hyperbilirubinemia has been reported rarely in neonates following large doses (10-20 mg) of phytonadione

Precautions Severe reactions resembling anaphylaxis or hypersensitivity have occurred rarely during or immediately after I.V. administration (even with proper dilution and rate of administration); restrict I.V. administration for emergency use only

Adverse Reactions See Warnings and Precautions
Gastrointestinal: GI upset
Local: Pain, swelling, tenderness at injection site

Drug Interactions Antagonizes action of warfarin

Mechanism of Action Cofactor in the liver synthesis of clotting factors (II, VII, IX, X)

Pharmacodynamics Onset of action: Blood coagulation factors increase within 6-12 hours after oral doses and within 1-2 hours following parenteral administration; after parenteral administration prothrombin time may become normal after 12-14 hours

Pharmacokinetics
Absorption: Oral: From the intestines in the presence of bile
Metabolism: Metabolized in the liver rapidly
Elimination: Excreted in the bile and the urine

Usual Dosage I.V. route should be restricted for emergency use only
Hemorrhagic disease of the newborn: I.M., S.C.:
- Prophylaxis: 0.5-1 mg within one hour of birth; may repeat if necessary 6-8 hours later
- Treatment: 1-2 mg/dose/day

Oral anticoagulant overdose:
- Infants: I.M., I.V., S.C.: 1-2 mg/dose every 4-8 hours
- Children and Adults: Oral, I.M., I.V., S.C.: 2.5-10 mg/dose (rarely up to 25-50 mg has been used); may repeat in 6-8 hours if given by I.M., I.V., S.C. route; may repeat 12-48 hours after oral route

Vitamin K deficiency: Due to drugs, malabsorption or decreased synthesis of vitamin K
- Infants and Children:
  - Oral: 2.5-5 mg/24 hours
  - I.M., I.V.: 1-2 mg/dose as a single dose
- Adults:
  - Oral: 5-25 mg/24 hours
  - I.M., I.V.: 10 mg

Minimum daily requirement: Not well established
- Infants: 1-5 μg/kg/day
- Adults: 0.03 μg/kg/day

Administration Dilute in 5-10 mL I.V. fluid (D_5W or normal saline) (maximum concentration: 10 mg/mL); infuse over 15-30 minutes; maximum rate of infusion: 1 mg/minute

Monitoring Parameters PT and PTT

Additional Information Phytonadione is more effective and is preferred to other vitamin K preparations in the presence of impending hemorrhage; oral absorption depends on the presence of bile salts; injection contains benzyl alcohol 0.9% as preservative; safe in neonates when used in appropriate doses

Dosage Forms
Injection:
- Aqueous colloidal: 2 mg/mL (0.5 mL); 10 mg/mL (1 mL, 2.5 mL, 5 mL)
- Aqueous (I.M. only): 2 mg/mL (0.5 mL); 10 mg/mL (1 mL)

Tablet: 5 mg

Pilagan® *see* Pilocarpine *on this page*

Pilocar® *see* Pilocarpine *on this page*

Pilocarpine (pye loe kar' peen)

Brand Names Adsorbocarpine®; Akarpine®; Isopto® Carpine; Ocusert® Pilo; Pilagan®; Pilocar®; Pilopine HS®; Piloptic®; Pilostat®

Therapeutic Category Cholinergic Agent, Ophthalmic; Ophthalmic Agent, Miotic

Use Management of chronic simple glaucoma, chronic and acute angle-closure glaucoma; counter effects of cycloplegics

Pregnancy Risk Factor C

Contraindications Hypersensitivity to pilocarpine or any component; acute inflammatory disease of anterior chamber

(Continued)

Pilocarpine *(Continued)*

Precautions Use with caution in patients with corneal abrasion

Adverse Reactions

Central nervous system: Headache

Ocular: Miosis, ciliary spasm, blurred vision, retinal detachment, photophobia, acute iritis, keratitis, corneal opacities, stinging, burning, lacrimation

Miscellaneous: Hypersensitivity reactions

Mechanism of Action Directly stimulates cholinergic receptors in the eye causing miosis (by contraction of the iris sphincter), loss of accommodation (by constriction of ciliary muscle), and lowering of intraocular pressure (with decreased resistance to aqueous humor outflow)

Pharmacodynamics

Onset of action: Ophthalmic solution instillation: Miosis occurs within 10-30 minutes

Duration: 4-14 hours

Ocusert® Pilo application: Maximal effects occur in 90-120 minutes; duration: 7 days

Pilocarpine

Dosage Form	Strength %	1 mL	2 mL	15 mL	30 mL	5 g
Gel	4					x
Solution as hydrochloride	0.25			x		
	0.5			x	x	
	1	x		x	x	
	2	x	x	x	x	
	3			x	x	
	4	x		x	x	
	5			x		
	6			x	x	
	8		x	x		
	10			x		
Solution as nitrate	1			x		
	2			x		
	4			x		

Usual Dosage

Ophthalmic:

Solution:

Instill 1-2 drops up to 6 times/day; adjust the concentration and frequency as required to control elevated intraocular pressure

To counteract the mydriatic effects of sympathomimetic agents: Instill 1 drop of a 1% solution in the affected eye

Gel: 0.5" (1.3 cm) ribbon applied to lower conjunctival sac once daily at bedtime; adjust dosage as required to control elevated intraocular pressure

Ocular systems: Systems are labeled in terms of the mean rate of release of pilocarpine over 7 days; begin with 20 μg/hour at night; adjust based upon response

Monitoring Parameters Intraocular pressure

Nursing Implications Following topical administration, finger pressure should be applied on the lacrimal sac for 1-2 minutes

Dosage Forms Ophthalmic ocular system: 20 μg/hour, 40 μg/hour; see table.

Pilopine HS® *see* Pilocarpine *on previous page*

Piloptic® *see* Pilocarpine *on previous page*

Pilostat® *see* Pilocarpine *on previous page*

Pima® *see* Potassium Iodide *on page 471*

Pin-Rid® [OTC] *see* Pyrantel Pamoate *on page 499*

Pin-X® [OTC] *see* Pyrantel Pamoate *on page 499*

Piperacillin Sodium (pi per' a sill in)

Related Information

Medications Compatible With PN Solutions *on page 649-650*

Brand Names Pipracil®

Therapeutic Category Antibiotic, Penicillin

Use Treatment of serious infections caused by susceptible strains of gram-positive, gram-negative, and anaerobic bacilli; mixed aerobic-anaerobic bacterial infections or empiric antibiotic therapy in granulocytopenic patients. Its primary use is in the treatment of serious carbenicillin-resistant or ticarcillin-resistant *Pseudomonas aeruginosa* infections susceptible to piperacillin.

Pregnancy Risk Factor B

Contraindications Hypersensitivity to piperacillin or any component or penicillins

Warnings Superinfection has been reported in up to 6% to 8% of patients receiving an extended spectrum penicillin

Precautions Dosage modification required in patients with impaired renal function

Adverse Reactions

Central nervous system: Seizures, fever, headache, dizziness, confusion, drowsiness

Dermatologic: Rash, exfoliative dermatitis

Endocrine & metabolic: Hypokalemia

Gastrointestinal: Diarrhea, vomiting

Hematologic: Hemolytic anemia, eosinophilia, neutropenia, prolonged bleeding time, thrombocytopenia, positive Coombs' reaction

Hepatic: Elevated liver enzymes, cholestatic hepatitis

Local: Thrombophlebitis

Musculoskeletal: Myoclonus

Renal & genitourinary: Acute interstitial nephritis

Miscellaneous: Hypersensitivity reactions, anaphylaxis, serum sickness-like reaction

Drug Interactions Aminoglycosides, probenecid, vecuronium

Stability Reconstituted piperacillin solution is stable for 24 hours at room temperature and 7 days when refrigerated; incompatible with aminoglycosides

Mechanism of Action Interferes with bacterial cell wall synthesis during active multiplication, causing cell wall death and resultant bactericidal activity against susceptible bacteria

Pharmacokinetics

Absorption: I.M.: 70% to 80%

Distribution: Crosses the placenta; distributes into milk at low concentrations; penetration across the blood-brain barrier is poor when meninges are uninflamed; good biliary concentration (30-60 times higher than serum concentration)

Protein binding: 22%

Half-life:

- Neonates:
  - 1-5 days: 3.6 hours
  - >6 days: 2.1-2.7 hours
- Children:
  - 1-6 months: 0.79 hours
  - 6 months to 12 years: 0.39-0.5 hours
- Adults: 36-80 minutes (dose-dependent), prolonged with moderately severe renal or hepatic impairment

Peak serum levels: I.M.: Within 30-50 minutes

Elimination: Excreted principally in the urine and partially in the feces (via bile)

Dialyzable (20% to 50%)

Usual Dosage Not FDA approved for children <12 years of age. I.M., I.V.:

Neonates:

- ≤7 days: 150 mg/kg/day divided every 8 hours
- >7 days: 200 mg/kg/day divided every 6 hours

Infants and Children: 200-300 mg/kg/day in divided doses every 4-6 hours; maximum dose: 24 g/day

(Continued)

Piperacillin Sodium *(Continued)*

Higher doses have been used in cystic fibrosis: 350-500 mg/kg/day in divided doses every 4 hours

Adults: 2-4 g/dose every 4-8 hours

Dosing interval in renal impairment:
Cl_{cr} 20-40 mL/minute: Administer every 8 hours
Cl_{cr} <20 mL/minute: Administer every 12 hours

Administration Piperacillin can be administered I.V. push over 3-5 minutes at a maximum concentration of 200 mg/mL or I.V. intermittent infusion over 30-60 minutes at a final concentration ≤20 mg/mL

Monitoring Parameters Serum electrolytes, bleeding time especially in patients with renal impairment; periodic tests of renal, hepatic and hematologic function

Test Interactions False-positive urinary and serum proteins, positive Coombs' test [direct]

Additional Information Sodium content of 1 g: 1.85 mEq

Dosage Forms Powder for injection: 2 g, 3 g, 4 g, 40 g

References

Placzek M, Whitelaw A, Want S, et al, "Piperacillin in Early Neonatal Infection," *Arch Dis Child*, 1983, 58(12):1006-9.

Prince AS and Neu HC, "Use of Piperacillin, A Semisynthetic Penicillin, in the Therapy of Acute Exacerbations of Pulmonary Disease in Patients With Cystic Fibrosis," *J Pediatr*, 1980, 97(1):148-51.

Thirumoorthi MC, Asmar BI, Buckley JA, et al, "Pharmacokinetics of Intravenously Administered Piperacillin in Preadolescent Children," *J Pediatr*, 1983, 102(6):941-6.

Piperazine Citrate (pi' per a zeen)

Therapeutic Category Anthelmintic

Use Treatment of pinworm and roundworm infections (used as an alternative to first-line agents, mebendazole, or pyrantel pamoate)

Pregnancy Risk Factor B

Contraindications Seizure disorders, liver or kidney impairment, hypersensitivity to piperazine or any component

Precautions Use with caution in patients with anemia or malnutrition or patients also receiving chlorpromazine; avoid prolonged or repeated piperazine use in children due to potential neurotoxicity

Adverse Reactions

Central nervous system: Dizziness, vertigo, weakness, seizures, EEG changes, headache, tremors
Gastrointestinal: Nausea, vomiting, diarrhea
Hematologic: Hemolytic anemia
Ocular: Visual impairment, nystagmus
Respiratory: Cough
Miscellaneous: Hypersensitivity reactions (urticaria, erythema multiforme, photodermatitis)

Drug Interactions Pyrantel pamoate (antagonistic mode of action)

Mechanism of Action Causes muscle paralysis of the roundworm by blocking the effects of acetylcholine at the neuromuscular junction

Pharmacokinetics

Absorption: Well absorbed from the GI tract
Peak plasma levels: 1 hour
Elimination: Excreted in the urine as metabolites and unchanged drug

Usual Dosage Oral:

Pinworms: Children and Adults: 65 mg/kg/day as a single daily dose for 7 days; in severe infections, repeat course after a 1-week interval; not to exceed 2.5 g/day

Roundworms:
Children: 75 mg/kg/day as a single daily dose for 2 days; maximum: 3.5 g/day;
Adults: 3.5 g/day for 2 days (in severe infections, repeat course, after a 1-week interval)

Monitoring Parameters Stool exam for worms and ova

Nursing Implications Cure rates may be decreased with massive infections or in patients with hypermotility of the GI tract

Dosage Forms
Syrup: 500 mg/5 mL (473 mL, 4000 mL)
Tablet: 250 mg

Pipracil® *see* Piperacillin Sodium *on page 461*

Piroxicam (peer ox' i kam)

Related Information
Overdose and Toxicology Information *on page 696-700*

Brand Names Feldene®

Therapeutic Category Analgesic, Non-Narcotic; Anti-inflammatory Agent; Nonsteroidal Anti-Inflammatory Agent (NSAID), Oral

Use Management of inflammatory diseases and rheumatoid disorders; dysmenorrhea

Pregnancy Risk Factor D

Contraindications Hypersensitivity to piroxicam, any component, aspirin or other nonsteroidal anti-inflammatory drugs (NSAIDs); active GI bleeding

Precautions Use with caution in patients with impaired cardiac function, hypertension, impaired renal function, GI disease and patients receiving anticoagulants

Adverse Reactions
Cardiovascular: Edema
Central nervous system: Dizziness, headache
Dermatologic: Rash
Gastrointestinal: Nausea, epigastric distress, anorexia, abdominal discomfort, vomiting, GI bleeding, ulcers, perforation
Hematologic: Reduction in hemoglobin and hematocrit, inhibition of platelet aggregation
Hepatic: Hepatitis
Renal & genitourinary: Acute renal failure, elevation of BUN and serum creatinine

Drug Interactions May ↑ serum concentrations of lithium; aspirin may ↓ piroxicam serum concentrations; drug interactions similar to other NSAIDs may also occur

Mechanism of Action Inhibits prostaglandin synthesis by decreasing the activity of the enzyme, cyclo-oxygenase, which results in decreased formation of prostaglandin precursors

Pharmacodynamics Analgesia:
Onset of action: Oral: Within 1 hour
Peak effect: 3-5 hours

Usual Dosage Oral:
Children: 0.2-0.3 mg/kg/day once daily; maximum dose: 15 mg/day
Adults: 10-20 mg/day once daily; although associated with ↑ in GI adverse effects, doses >20 mg/day have been used (ie, 30-40 mg/day)

Monitoring Parameters CBC, BUN, serum creatinine, liver enzymes; periodic ophthalmologic exams with chronic use

Nursing Implications Administer with food to decrease GI adverse effect

Dosage Forms Capsule: 10 mg, 20 mg

***p*-Isobutylhydratropic Acid** *see* Ibuprofen *on page 300*

Pitressin® *see* Vasopressin *on page 595*

Plantago Seed *see* Psyllium *on page 498*

Plantain Seed *see* Psyllium *on page 498*

Plaquenil® Sulfate *see* Hydroxychloroquine Sulfate *on page 296*

Plasbumin® *see* Albumin Human *on page 25*

Platinol® *see* Cisplatin *on page 137*

Platinol®-AQ *see* Cisplatin *on page 137*

Plicamycin (plye kay mye' sin)

Brand Names Mithracin®

Synonyms Mithramycin

Therapeutic Category Antidote, Hypercalcemia; Antineoplastic Agent

(Continued)

Plicamycin *(Continued)*

Use Malignant testicular tumors; treatment of hypercalcemia and hypercalciuria of malignancy not responsive to conventional treatment; chronic myelogenous leukemia in blast phase; Paget's disease

Pregnancy Risk Factor D

Contraindications Thrombocytopenia, bleeding diatheses, coagulation disorders, bone marrow function impairment, or hypocalcemia

Warnings The US Food and Drug Administration (FDA) currently recommends that procedures for proper handling and disposal of antineoplastic agents be considered. Discontinue therapy if bleeding or epistaxis occurs; plicamycin may cause permanent sterility and may cause birth defects

Precautions Use with caution in patients with hepatic or renal impairment; reduce dosage in patients with renal impairment

Adverse Reactions

Cardiovascular: Facial flushing

Central nervous system: Fever, headache

Endocrine & metabolic: Decreased serum calcium, phosphorus, and potassium

Gastrointestinal: Anorexia, stomatitis, nausea, vomiting, diarrhea

Hematologic: Thrombocytopenia, hemorrhagic diathesis (epistaxis, hematemesis, hemoptysis), leukopenia

Hepatic: Elevation in liver enzymes

Local: Phlebitis

Renal & genitourinary: Nephrotoxicity

Drug Interactions Calcitonin, etidronate, glucagon, aspirin

Stability Refrigeration is recommended but drug remains stable for up to 3 months unrefrigerated; drug is unstable at a pH <4; reconstituted solution is stable for 24 hours at room temperature and 48 hours when refrigerated

Mechanism of Action Forms a complex with DNA in the presence of magnesium or other divalent cations inhibiting DNA-directed RNA synthesis; may inhibit parathyroid hormone effect on osteoclasts; inhibits bone resorption

Pharmacodynamics

Onset of action for decreasing serum calcium: Within 24 hours

Peak effect on calcium levels: 48-72 hours

Duration: 5-15 days

Pharmacokinetics

Distribution: Drug crosses the blood-brain barrier in low concentrations

Protein-binding: 0%

Half-life, plasma: 1 hour

Elimination: 90% of the dose is excreted in the urine within the first 24 hours

Usual Dosage Adults (dose based on ideal weight): I.V. (refer to individual protocols):

Testicular cancer: 25-50 μg/kg/day or every other day for 5-10 days

Blastic chronic granulocytic leukemia: 25 μg/kg over 2-4 hours every other day for 3 weeks

Hypercalcemia: 15-25 μg/kg/day once daily for 3-4 days or 25 μg/kg every 48-72 hours; additional courses of therapy may be given at intervals of 1 week or more if the initial course is unsuccessful. Reduce dose to 12.5 μg/kg in patients with pre-existing hepatic or renal impairment

Paget's disease: 15 μg/kg/day once daily for 10 days

Dosing adjustment in renal impairment:

Cl_{cr} 10-50 mL/minute: Decrease dosage by 25%

Cl_{cr} <10 mL/minute: Decrease dosage by 50%

Administration For adults, the dose should be diluted in 1 L of D_5W or NS and administered as an I.V. infusion over 4-6 hours; bolus or short infusion over 30-60 minutes in 100-150 mL D_5W is an alternative method of administration

Monitoring Parameters Hepatic and renal function tests, CBC, platelet count, prothrombin time, serum electrolytes

Patient Information Notify physician if fever, sore throat, bleeding, bruising, shortness of breath, or painful urination occur

Nursing Implications Rapid I.V. infusion has been associated with an increased incidence of nausea and vomiting; an antiemetic given prior to and during plicamycin infusion may be helpful. Avoid extravasation since plicamycin is a strong vesicant.

Additional Information Treatment of hemorrhagic episodes should include transfusion of fresh whole blood or packed red blood cells and fresh frozen plasma, vitamin K, and corticosteroids

Myelosuppressive effects:
- WBC: Moderate
- Platelets: Moderate
- Onset (days): 7-10
- Nadir (days): 14
- Recovery (days): 21

Dosage Forms Powder for Injection: 2.5 mg

References

Mutch RS, Hutson PR, and Lewinsky DB, "Plicamycin: Bolus or Infusion?" *DICP*, 1990, 24(9):885-6.

Ritch PS, "Treatment of Cancer-Related Hypercalcemia," *Semin Oncol*, 1990, 17(2 Suppl 5):26-33.

Stumpf JL, "Pharmacologic Management of Paget's Disease," *Clin Pharm*, 1989, 8(7):485-95.

Pneumococcal Polysaccharide Vaccine, Polyvalent *see* Immunization Guidelines *on page 660-667*

Pod-Ben-25® *see* Podophyllum Resin *on this page*

Podocon-25® *see* Podophyllum Resin *on this page*

Podofin® *see* Podophyllum Resin *on this page*

Podophyllum Resin

Brand Names Pod-Ben-25®; Podocon-25®; Podofin®

Therapeutic Category Keratolytic Agent

Use Topical treatment of benign growths including external genital and perianal warts, papillomas, fibroids

Pregnancy Risk Factor X

Contraindications Not to be used on birthmarks, moles, or warts with hair growth; cervical, urethral, oral warts; not to be used by diabetic patients or patients with poor circulation; pregnant women

Warnings Avoid contact with the eyes as it can cause severe corneal damage; 25% solution should not be applied to or near mucous membranes

Precautions Use of large amounts of drug should be avoided

Adverse Reactions

Central nervous system: Confusion, lethargy, hallucinations, peripheral neuropathy

Dermatologic: Pruritus, erythema, scarring

Gastrointestinal: Nausea, vomiting, abdominal pain, diarrhea

Hematologic: Leukopenia, thrombocytopenia

Hepatic: Hepatotoxicity

Local: Pain, swelling

Renal & genitourinary: Renal failure

Mechanism of Action Directly affects epithelial cell metabolism by arresting mitosis through binding to a protein subunit of spindle microtubules (tubulin)

Usual Dosage Children and Adults: Topical: 10% to 25% solution in compound benzoin tincture; apply drug to dry surface of affected area, use 1 drop at a time allowing drying between drops until area is covered; total volume should be limited to <0.5 mL per treatment session; therapy may be repeated once daily to weekly for up to 4 applications for the treatment of genital or perianal warts; use 10% solution when applied to or near mucous membranes

Verrucae: 25% solution is applied 3-5 times/day directly to the wart

Patient Information Notify physician if undue skin irritation develops

Nursing Implications Shake well before using; solution should be washed off within 1-4 hours for genital and perianal warts and within 1-2 hours for accessible meatal warts; use protective occlusive dressing around warts to prevent contact with unaffected skin

Dosage Forms Liquid, topical: 25% in benzoin (5 mL, 7.5 mL, 30 mL)

(Continued)

Podophyllum Resin *(Continued)*

References

Goldfarb MT, Gupta AK, Gupta MA, et al, "Office Therapy for Human Papillomavirus Infection in Nongenital Sites," *Dermatol Clin,* 1991, 9(2):287-96.

Poliovirus Vaccine, Live, Inactivated *see* Immunization Guidelines *on page 660-667*

Poliovirus Vaccine, Live, Trivalent, Oral *see* Immunization Guidelines *on page 660-667*

Polycillin® *see* Ampicillin *on page 48*

Polycitra® *see* Sodium Citrate and Citric Acid *on page 528*

Polyethylene Glycol-Electrolyte Solution

(pol ee eth' i leen)

Brand Names Colovage®; CoLyte®; GoLYTELY®; NuLytely®; OCL®

Synonyms Colonic Lavage Solution; Electrolyte Lavage Solution

Therapeutic Category Cathartic; Laxative, Bowel Evacuant

Use For bowel cleansing prior to GI examination

Pregnancy Risk Factor C

Contraindications Gastrointestinal obstruction, gastric retention, bowel perforation, toxic colitis, megacolon

Warnings Do not add flavorings as additional ingredients before use

Adverse Reactions

Dermatologic: Irritative perineal rashes

Endocrine & metabolic: Mild metabolic acidosis with prolonged irrigation periods

Gastrointestinal: Nausea, cramps, vomiting, abdominal distention

Mechanism of Action Induces catharsis by strong electrolyte and osmotic effects

Pharmacodynamics Onset of action: Within 1-2 hours

Usual Dosage Patient should fast 3-4 hours prior to ingestion:

Children:

Oral: 25-40 mL/kg/hour until rectal effluent is clear (usually in 4-10 hours)

Nasogastric: 20-30 mL/minute (1.2-1.8 L/hour) until 4 L are administered

Adults: Drink 240 mL every 10 minutes until 4 L are consumed or the rectal effluent is clear

Monitoring Parameters Electrolytes, BUN, serum glucose, urine osmolality

Patient Information Chilled solution is often more palatable

Nursing Implications Rapid drinking of each portion is preferred over small amounts continuously; first bowel movement should occur in one hour

Dosage Forms Powder, for oral solution: PEG 3350 236 g, sodium sulfate 22.74 g, sodium bicarbonate 6.74 g, sodium chloride 5.86 g and potassium chloride 2.97 g (2000 mL, 4000 mL, 4800 mL, 6000 mL)

References

Sondheimer JM, Sokol RJ, Taylor SF, et al, "Safety, Efficacy and Tolerance of Intestinal Lavage in Pediatric Patients Undergoing Diagnostic Colonoscopy," *J Pediatr*, 1991, 119(1):148-52.

Tuggle DW, Hoelzer DJ, Tunell WP, et al, "The Safety and Cost-Effectiveness of Polyethylene Glycol Electrolyte Solution Bowel: Preparation in Infants and Children," *J Pediatr Surg*, 1987, 22(6):513-5.

Polygam® *see* Immune Globulin, Intravenous *on page 307*

Polymox® *see* Amoxicillin *on page 44*

Polymyxin B and Neomycin *see* Neomycin and Polymyxin B *on page 406*

Polymyxin B Sulfate (pol i mix' in)

Brand Names Aerosporin®

Therapeutic Category Antibiotic, Irrigation; Antibiotic, Miscellaneous

Use Used topically for wound irrigation and bladder instillation against *Pseudomonas aeruginosa*; used occasionally for gut decontamination. Parenteral use of polymyxin B has mainly been replaced by less toxic antibiotics. It is reserved for life-threatening infections caused by organisms resistant to the preferred drugs.

Pregnancy Risk Factor B

Contraindications Known hypersensitivity to polymyxin; concurrent use with skeletal muscle relaxants, ether or sodium citrate

Warnings Neurotoxic reactions may be manifested by irritability, weakness, drowsiness, ataxia, perioral paresthesia, numbness of the extremities and blurring of vision. These reactions are usually associated with high serum levels found in patients with impaired renal function or nephrotoxicity. Avoid concurrent or sequential use of other nephrotoxic and neurotoxic drugs, particularly bacitracin, kanamycin, streptomycin, paromomycin, colistin, tobramycin, neomycin, gentamicin, and amikacin. The drug's neurotoxicity can result in respiratory paralysis from neuromuscular blockade, especially when the drug is given soon after anesthesia or muscle relaxants. Polymyxin B sulfate is toxic when given parenterally; avoid parenteral use whenever possible.

Precautions Use with caution in patients with myasthenia gravis, patients receiving neuromuscular blocking agents or anesthetics, and in patients with impaired renal function; modify dosage in patients with renal impairment; I.M. use is not recommended in infants and children due to severe pain at injection site

Adverse Reactions

Central nervous system: Neurotoxicity (paresthesia, facial flushing, drowsiness, ataxia), fever

Dermatologic: Rash

Endocrine & metabolic: Hypocalcemia, hyponatremia, hypokalemia, hypochloremia

Local: Pain at injection site

Musculoskeletal: Neuromuscular blockade

Renal & genitourinary: Nephrotoxicity (hematuria, proteinuria, azotemia)

Respiratory: Respiratory arrest

Miscellaneous: Hypersensitivity reactions

Drug Interactions Neuromuscular blocking agents, aminoglycosides, colistin, sodium citrate

Stability Incompatible with calcium, magnesium, cephalothin, chloramphenicol, heparin, penicillins; inactivated by acidic or alkaline solutions

Mechanism of Action Binds to phospholipids, alters permeability and damages the bacterial cytoplasmic membrane permitting leakage of intracellular constituents

Pharmacokinetics

Absorption: Well absorbed from the peritoneum; minimal absorption (<10%) from the GI tract (except in neonates), from mucous membranes or intact skin

Distribution: Minimal distribution into the CSF; crosses the placenta; widely distributed into body tissues

Half-life: 4.5-6 hours, increased with reduced renal function

Peak serum levels: I.M.: Within 2 hours

Elimination: Excreted primarily as unchanged drug (>60%) in the urine via glomerular filtration

Usual Dosage

Infants <2 years:

- I.M.: 25,000-40,000 units/kg/day divided every 6 hours
- I.V.: 15,000-45,000 units/kg/day by continuous I.V. infusion or divided every 12 hours

Children ≥2 years and Adults: I.M., I.V.: 30,000-45,000 units/kg/day divided every 6-8 hours (I.M.) or continuous infusion (I.V.)

- Total daily dose should not exceed 2,000,000 units/day
- Bladder irrigation: Continuous irrigant or rinse in the urinary bladder for up to 10 days using 20 mg (equal to 200,000 units) added to 1 L of normal saline; usually no more than 1 L of irrigant is used per day unless urine flow rate is high; administration rate is adjusted to patient's urine output
- Topical irrigation or topical solution: 0.1% to 0.3% solution used to irrigate infected wounds; should not exceed 2 million units/day in adults
- Gut sterilization: Oral: 100,000-200,000 units/kg/day divided every 6-8 hours
- Ophthalmic: A concentration of 0.1% to 0.25% is administered as 1-3 drops every hour, then increasing the interval as response indicates

Administration I.V.: Infuse drug slowly over 60-90 minutes or by continuous infusion at a concentration of 1000-1667 units/mL in D_5W

(Continued)

Polymyxin B Sulfate *(Continued)*

Monitoring Parameters WBC, serum electrolytes, renal function tests, serum drug concentration, urine output

Reference Range Serum concentration >5 μg/mL are toxic in adults

Additional Information 1 mg = 10,000 units; neuromuscular blockade may be reversed with calcium chloride

Dosage Forms

Injection: 500,000 units

Powder for ophthalmic solution: 500,000 units

Poly-Pred® Liquifilm® *see* Neomycin, Polymyxin B and Prednisolone *on page 408*

Polysporin® *see* Bacitracin and Polymyxin B Sulfate *on page 74*

Polytar® [OTC] *see* Coal Tar *on page 147*

Pontocaine® *see* Tetracaine Hydrochloride *on page 551*

Pork NPH Iletin® II *see* Insulin Preparations *on page 311*

Pork Regular Iletin® II *see* Insulin Preparations *on page 311*

Potasalan® *see* Potassium Chloride *on next page*

Potassium Acetate

Synonyms K Acetate

Therapeutic Category Electrolyte Supplement, Parenteral; Potassium Salt

Use Potassium deficiency, treatment of hypokalemia

Pregnancy Risk Factor C

Contraindications Severe renal impairment, untreated Addison's disease, heat cramps, hyperkalemia, severe tissue trauma

Warnings Potassium injections should be administered only in patients with adequate urine flow; injection must be diluted before I.V. use and infused slowly (see Drug Administration)

Precautions Use with caution in patients with cardiac disease, patients receiving potassium-sparing drugs; patients must be on a cardiac monitor during intermittent infusions

Adverse Reactions

Cardiovascular: With rapid I.V. administration: Cardiac arrhythmias and cardiac arrest; heart block, hypotension

Central nervous system: Parethesias, mental confusion

Local: Pain at the site of injection, phlebitis

Musculoskeletal: Flaccid paralysis

Drug Interactions Potassium-sparing diuretics, salt substitutes, digitalis, captopril, and enalapril

Mechanism of Action Potassium is the major cation of intracellular fluid and is essential for the conduction of nerve impulses in heart, brain, and skeletal muscle; contraction of cardiac, skeletal and smooth muscles; maintenance of normal renal function, acid-base balance, carbohydrate metabolism, and gastric secretion

Pharmacokinetics Elimination: Largely excreted by the kidneys

Usual Dosage I.V. doses should be incorporated into the patient's maintenance I.V. fluids, intermittent I.V. potassium administration should be reserved for severe depletion situations and requires EKG monitoring. Doses listed as mEq of potassium.

Treatment of hypokalemia: I.V.:

Children: 2-5 mEq/kg/day

Adults: 40-100 mEq/day

I.V. intermittent infusion (must be diluted prior to administration):

Children: 0.5-1 mEq/kg/dose (maximum: 30 mEq) to infuse at 0.3-0.5 mEq/kg/hour (maximum: 1 mEq/kg/hour)

Adults: 10-20 mEq/dose (maximum: 40 mEq/dose) to infuse over 2-3 hours (maximum: 40 mEq over 1 hour)

Administration Potassium must be diluted prior to parenteral administration; maximum recommended concentration (peripheral line): 80 mEq/L; maximum recommended concentration (central line): 150 mEq/L or 15 mEq/100 mL; in severely fluid-restricted patients (with central lines): 200 mEq/L or 20 mEq/100 mL has been used; maximum rate of infusion, see Usual Dosage, I.V. intermittent infusion

Monitoring Parameters Serum potassium, glucose, bicarbonate, pH, urine output (if indicated), cardiac monitor (if intermittent infusion or potassium infusion rates of >0.25 mEq/kg/hour)

Dosage Forms Injection: 2 mEq/mL (20 mL, 50 mL, 100 mL); 4 mEq/mL (50 mL)

References

Hamill RJ, Robinson LM, Wexler HR, et al, "Efficacy and Safety of Potassium Infusion Therapy in Hypokalemic Critically Ill Patients," *Crit Care Med*, 1991, 19(5):694-9.

Khilnani P, "Electrolyte Abnormalities in Critically Ill Children," *Crit Care Med*, 1992, 20(2):241-50.

Potassium Chloride

Brand Names Cena-K®; Gen-K®; Kaochlor® S-F; Kaon-CL®; Kato®; K-Dur® 20; K-Lor™; Klor-con®; Klorvess®; Klotrix®; K-Lyte/CL®; K-Tab®; Micro-K®; Potasalan®; Rum-K®; Slow-K®

Synonyms KCl

Therapeutic Category Electrolyte Supplement, Oral; Electrolyte Supplement, Parenteral; Potassium Salt

Use Potassium deficiency, treatment or prevention of hypokalemia

Pregnancy Risk Factor C

Contraindications Severe renal impairment, untreated Addison's disease, heat cramps, hyperkalemia, severe tissue trauma; solid oral dosage forms are contraindicated in patients in whom there is a structural, pathological, and/or pharmacologic cause for delay or arrest in passage through the GI tract; an oral liquid potassium preparation should be used in patients with esophageal compression or delayed gastric emptying time

Warnings Potassium injections should be administered only in patients with adequate urine flow; injection must be diluted before I.V. use and infused slowly (see Drug Administration)

Precautions Use with caution in patients with cardiac disease, patients receiving potassium-sparing drugs; patients must be on a cardiac monitor during intermittent infusions; some oral products contain the dye tartrazine (avoid use in sensitive individuals)

Adverse Reactions

Oral administration: Gastrointestinal: Nausea, vomiting, diarrhea, abdominal pain, GI lesions, flatulence

I.V. administration:

- Cardiovascular: Arrhythmias and cardiac arrest; heart block, hypotension
- Central nervous system: Parethesias, mental confusion
- Local: Pain at the site of injection, phlebitis
- Musculoskeletal: Flaccid paralysis

Drug Interactions Potassium-sparing diuretics, salt substitutes, digitalis, captopril and enalapril

Mechanism of Action Potassium is the major cation of intracellular fluid and is essential for the conduction of nerve impulses in heart, brain, and skeletal muscle; contraction of cardiac, skeletal and smooth muscles; maintenance of normal renal function, acid-base balance, carbohydrate metabolism, and gastric secretion

Pharmacokinetics

Absorption: Absorbed well from upper GI tract; enters cells via active transport from extracellular fluid

Elimination: Largely excreted by the kidneys

Usual Dosage I.V. doses should be incorporated into the patient's maintenance I.V. fluids, intermittent I.V. potassium administration should be reserved for severe depletion situations and requires EKG monitoring. Doses listed as mEq of potassium.

Normal daily requirement: Oral, I.V.:

- Newborns: 2-6 mEq/kg/day
- Children: 2-3 mEq/kg/day
- Adults: 40-80 mEq/day

Prevention of hypokalemia during diuretic therapy: Oral:

- Children: 1-2 mEq /kg/day in 1-2 divided doses

(Continued)

Potassium Chloride *(Continued)*

Adults: 20-40 mEq/day in 1-2 divided doses

Treatment of hypokalemia: Oral, I.V.:
Children: 2-5 mEq/kg/day
Adults: 40-100 mEq/day

I.V. intermittent infusion (must be diluted prior to administration):
Children: 0.5-1 mEq/kg/dose (maximum: 30 mEq) to infuse at 0.3-0.5 mEq/kg/hour (maximum: 1 mEq/kg/hour)
Adults: 10-20 mEq/dose (maximum: 40 mEq/dose) to infuse over 2-3 hours (maximum: 40 mEq over 1 hour)

Administration Potassium must be diluted prior to parenteral administration; maximum recommended concentration (peripheral line): 80 mEq/L; maximum recommended concentration (central line): 150 mEq/L or 15 mEq/100 mL; in severely fluid-restricted patients (with central lines): 200 mEq/L or 20 mEq/100 mL has been used; maximum rate of infusion, see Usual Dosage, I.V. intermittent infusion

Monitoring Parameters Serum potassium, glucose, chloride, pH, urine output (if indicated), cardiac monitor (if intermittent infusion or potassium infusion rates of >0.25 mEq/kg/hour)

Patient Information Sustained release and wax matrix tablets should be swallowed whole, do not crush or chew; effervescent tablets must be dissolved in water before use

Nursing Implications Oral liquid potassium supplements should be diluted with water or fruit juice during administration; wax matrix tablets must be swallowed and not allowed to dissolve in mouth

Dosage Forms

Capsule, controlled release, micro encapsulated (Micro-K®): 600 mg [8 mEq]; 750 mg [10 mEq]
Injection: 1.5 mEq/mL, 2 mEq/mL, 3 mEq/mL
Liquid, oral: 10 mEq/15 mL, 15 mEq/15 mL, 20 mEq/15 mL, 30 mEq/15 mL, 40 mEq/15 mL, 45 mEq/15 mL
Powder, oral: 15 mEq, 20 mEq, 25 mEq packet
Tablet:
Effervescent, as potassium chloride: 25 mEq
Effervescent, as potassium bicarbonate: 20 mEq, 25 mEq, 50 mEq
Sustained release, microcrystalloids (K-Dur®): 750 mg [10 mEq; 1500 mg [20 mEq]
Wax matrix:
Kaon-Cl®: 500 mg [6.7 mEq]
Slow-K®: 600 mg [8 mEq]; 750 mg [10 mEq]

References

Hamill RJ, Robinson LM, Wexler HR, et al, "Efficacy and Safety of Potassium Infusion Therapy in Hypokalemic Critically Ill Patients," *Crit Care Med*, 1991, 19(5):694-9.

Khilnani P, "Electrolyte Abnormalities in Critically Ill Children," *Crit Care Med*, 1992, 20(2):241-50.

Potassium Gluconate

Brand Names Kaon®; Kolyum®

Therapeutic Category Potassium Salt

Use Treatment or prevention of hypokalemia

Pregnancy Risk Factor C

Contraindications Severe renal impairment, untreated Addison's disease, heat cramps, hyperkalemia, severe tissue trauma; solid oral dosage forms are contraindicated in patients in whom there is a structural, pathological, and/or pharmacologic cause for delay or arrest in passage through the GI tract; an oral liquid potassium preparation should be used in patients with esophageal compression or delayed gastric emptying time

Warnings Potassium should be administered only in patients with adequate urine flow

Precautions Use with caution in patients with cardiac disease, patients receiving potassium-sparing drugs

Adverse Reactions

Cardiovascular: Cardiac arrhythmias, heart block, hypotension

Central nervous system: Parethesias, mental confusion
Endocrine & metabolic: Hyperkalemia
Gastrointestinal: Nausea, vomiting, diarrhea, abdominal pain, GI lesions
Musculoskeletal: Muscle weakness, flaccid paralysis

Drug Interactions Potassium-sparing diuretics, salt substitutes, digitalis, captopril and enalapril

Mechanism of Action Potassium is the major cation of intracellular fluid and is essential for the conduction of nerve impulses in heart, brain, and skeletal muscle; contraction of cardiac, skeletal and smooth muscles; maintenance of normal renal function, acid-base balance, carbohydrate metabolism, and gastric secretion

Pharmacokinetics

Absorption: Absorbed well from upper GI tract; enters cells via active transport from extracellular fluid
Elimination: Largely excreted by the kidneys

Usual Dosage Oral (doses listed as mEq of potassium):

Normal daily requirement:
Children: 2-3 mEq/kg/day
Adults: 40-80 mEq/day

Prevention of hypokalemia during diuretic therapy:
Children: 1-2 mEq/kg/day in 1-2 divided doses
Adults: 20-40 mEq/kg/day in 1-2 divided doses

Treatment of hypokalemia:
Children: 2-5 mEq/kg/day in 2-4 divided doses
Adults: 40-100 mEq/day in 2-4 divided doses

Monitoring Parameters Serum potassium, chloride, glucose, pH, urine output (if indicated)

Patient Information Take with food, water, or fruit juice; swallow tablets whole; do not crush or chew

Nursing Implications Do not administer liquid full strength, must be diluted in 2-6 parts of water or juice

Additional Information 9.4 g potassium gluconate is approximately equal to 40 mEq potassium (4.3 mEq potassium/g salt)

Dosage Forms

Liquid, sugar free (Kaon®): 20 mEq/15 mL
Powder (Kolyum®): Potassium 20 mEq and chloride 3.4 mEq (potassium gluconate and potassium chloride combination) per packet
Tablet: 500 mg, 595 mg

Potassium Iodide

Brand Names Pima®; Potassium Iodide Enseals®; SSKI®; Thyro-Block®

Synonyms KI; Lugol's Solution; Strong Iodine Solution

Therapeutic Category Antithyroid Agent; Expectorant

Use To facilitate bronchial drainage and cough; to reduce thyroid vascularity prior to thyroidectomy and management of thyrotoxic crisis; block thyroidal uptake of radioactive isotopes of iodine in a radiation emergency

Pregnancy Risk Factor D

Contraindications Known hypersensitivity to iodine; hyperkalemia, tuberculosis, bronchitis

Warnings Some commercially available products contain sulfites, avoid use in sensitive patients

Adverse Reactions

Cardiovascular: Angioedema
Central nervous system: Fever, headache
Dermatologic: Urticaria, acne
Endocrine & metabolic: Goiter with hypothyroidism
Gastrointestinal: Metallic taste, GI upset
Hematologic: Cutaneous and mucosal hemorrhage, eosinophilia
Musculoskeletal: Arthralgia
Miscellaneous: Lymph node enlargement, soreness of teeth and gums, rhinitis

Mechanism of Action Reduces viscosity of mucus by increasing respiratory tract secretions; inhibits the release and synthesis of thyroid hormone

Pharmacodynamics

Onset of action (antithyroid effects): 24-48 hours

(Continued)

Potassium Iodide *(Continued)*

Peak effect: 10-15 days after continuous therapy

Usual Dosage Oral:

Expectorant:

Children: 60-250 mg every 4 times/day; maximum single dose: 500 mg
Adults: 300-650 mg 3-4 times/day

Preoperative thyroidectomy: Children and Adults: 50-250 mg (1-5 drops, 1 g/mL SSKI®) 3 times/day or strong iodine (Lugol's solution) 0.1-0.3 mL (3-5 drops) 3 times/day; give for 10-14 days before surgery

Graves' disease in neonates: 1 drop of strong iodine (Lugol's solution) 3 times/day

Thyrotoxic crisis:

Infants <1 year: 150-250 mg (3-5 drops, 1 g/mL SSKI®) 3 times/day
Children and Adults: 300-500 mg (6-10 drops 1 g/mL SSKI®) 3 times/day or 1 mL strong iodine (Lugol's solution) 3 times/day

Monitoring Parameters Thyroid function tests

Patient Information Administer after meals with food or milk or dilute with a large quantity of water, fruit juice, milk, or broth

Dosage Forms

Solution, oral:

SSKI®: 1 g/mL (30 mL, 240 mL, 473 mL)
Lugol's solution, strong iodine: 100 mg with iodine 50 mg per mL (120 mL)

Syrup: 325 mg/5 mL
Tablet: 130 mg

Potassium Iodide Enseals® *see* Potassium Iodide *on previous page*

Potassium Phosphate

Brand Names K-PHOS® Neutral; Neutra-Phos®-K

Therapeutic Category Electrolyte Supplement, Oral; Electrolyte Supplement, Parenteral; Phosphate Salt; Potassium Salt

Use Treatment and prevention of hypophosphatemia

Pregnancy Risk Factor C

Contraindications Hyperphosphatemia, hyperkalemia, hypocalcemia, hypomagnesemia, severe renal impairment

Precautions Use with caution in patients with renal impairment; potassium injections should be administered only in patients with adequate urine flow; injection must be diluted prior to use and infused slowly (see Drug Administration)

Adverse Reactions

Cardiovascular: Hypotension
Central nervous system: Tetany
Endocrine & metabolic: Hyperphosphatemia, hyperkalemia, hypocalcemia
Gastrointestinal: Nausea, vomiting, diarrhea
Local: Phlebitis
Renal & genitourinary: Acute renal failure

Drug Interactions Do not give orally at the same time as aluminum and magnesium containing antacids or sucralfate which can act as phosphate binders; use of potassium phosphate with potassium sparing diuretics or ACE-inhibitors may result in hyperkalemia

Stability Phosphate salts may precipitate when mixed with calcium salts; solubility is improved in amino acid parenteral nutrition solutions; check with a pharmacist to determine compatibility

Usual Dosage I.V. doses should be incorporated into the patient's maintenance I.V. fluids; intermittent I.V. infusion should be reserved for severe depletion situations and requires continuous cardiac monitoring. It is difficult to determine total body phosphorus deficit, the following dosages are empiric guidelines. **Note:** Doses listed as mmol of phosphate:

Replacement intermittent infusion: I.V.:

Children:

Low dose: 0.08 mmol/kg over 6 hours; use if recent losses and uncomplicated
Intermediate dose: 0.16-0.24 mmol/kg over 4-6 hours; use if serum PO_4 level 0.5-1 mg/dL

High dose: 0.36 mmol/kg over 6 hours; use if serum PO_4 <0.5 mg/dL

Adults: 0.15-0.3 mmol/kg/dose over 12 hours; may repeat as needed to achieve desired serum level

Maintenance:

Children: 0.5-1.5 mmol/kg/24 hours I.V. or 2-3 mmol/kg/24 hours orally in divided doses

Adults: 50-70 mmol/24 hours I.V. or 50-150 mmol/24 hours orally in divided doses **or**

Children <4 years: Oral: 1 capsule (250 mg phosphorus/8 mmol) 4 times/day; dilute as instructed

Children >4 years and Adults: Oral: 1-2 capsules (250-500 mg phosphorus/8-16 mmol) 4 times/day; dilute as instructed

Administration For intermittent infusion, if peripheral line, dilute to a maximum concentration of 0.05 mmol/mL; if central line, dilute to a maximum concentration of 0.12 mmol/mL; maximum rate of infusion: 0.06 mmol/kg/hour; do **not** infuse with calcium containing IV. fluids (ie, TPN)

Monitoring Parameters Serum potassium, calcium, phosphate, sodium, cardiac monitor (when intermittent infusion or high-dose I.V. replacement needed)

Reference Range

Newborns: 4.2-9 mg/dL

6 weeks to 18 months: 3.8-6.7 mg/dL

18 months to 3 years: 2.9-5.9 mg/dL

3-15 years: 3.6-5.6 mg/dL

>15 years: 2.5-5 mg/dL

Patient Information Do not swallow the capsule; empty contents of capsule into 75 mL (2.5 oz) of water before taking; take with food to reduce the risk of diarrhea

Nursing Implications The contents of one capsule should be diluted in 75 mL water before administration

Dosage Forms

Capsule:

Neutra-Phos®-K: Phosphorus 250 mg [8 mmol] and potassium 556 mg [14.25 mEq] per capsule

Neutra-Phos®: Phosphorus 250 mg [8 mmol], potassium 278 mg [7.125 mEq], and sodium 7.125 mEq per capsule

Injection: Potassium phosphate monobasic anhydrous 224 mg and potassium phosphate dibasic anhydrous 236 mg per mL; [phosphorus 3 mmol and potassium 4.4 mEq per mL] (15 mL)

Tablet (K-PHOS® Neutral): Phosphorus 250 mg [8 mmol], potassium 45 mg [1.1 mEq], and sodium 298 mg [13 mEq] per tablet

PPL *see* Benzylpenicilloyl-polylysine *on page 80*

Pralidoxime Chloride (pra li dox' eem)

Brand Names Protopam®

Synonyms 2-PAM; 2-Pyridine Aldoxime Methochloride

Therapeutic Category Antidote, Anticholinesterase; Antidote, Organophosphate Poisoning

Use To reverse muscle paralysis associated with toxic exposure to organophosphate anticholinesterase pesticides and chemicals

Pregnancy Risk Factor C

Contraindications Hypersensitivity to pralidoxime or any component

Precautions Use with caution in patients with myasthenia gravis; dosage modification required in patients with impaired renal function; use with caution in patients receiving theophylline, succinylcholine, phenothiazines, respiratory depressants (eg, narcotic, barbiturates)

Adverse Reactions

Cardiovascular: Tachycardia, hypertension

Central nervous system: Dizziness, headache, drowsiness

Dermatologic: Rash

Gastrointestinal: Nausea

Local: Pain at injection site after I.M. use

Musculoskeletal: Muscular weakness, muscle rigidity

Ocular: Blurred vision, diplopia

Respiratory: Hyperventilation, laryngospasm (after rapid I.V. administration)

Mechanism of Action Reactivates cholinesterase that had been inactivat-

(Continued)

Pralidoxime Chloride *(Continued)*

ed by phosphorylation as a result of exposure to organophosphate pesticides; it removes the phosphoryl group from the active site of the inactivated enzyme

Pharmacokinetics

Half-life: 0.8-2.7 hours

Elimination: 80% to 90% excreted unchanged in the urine 12 hours after administration

Usual Dosage Poisoning: I.M., I.V. (use in conjunction with atropine):

Children: 20-50 mg/kg/dose; repeat in 1-2 hours if muscle weakness has not been relieved, then at 10- to 12-hour intervals if cholinergic signs recur

Adults: 1-2 g; repeat in 1-2 hours if muscle weakness has not been relieved, then at 10- to 12-hour intervals if cholinergic signs recur

Administration Reconstitute with 20 mL sterile water (preservative free) resulting in 50 mg/mL solution; dilute in normal saline 20 mg/mL and infuse over 15-30 minutes; if a more rapid onset of effect is desired or in a fluid restricted situation, the maximum concentration is 50 mg/mL; the maximum rate of infusion is over 5 minutes

Monitoring Parameters Heart rate, respiratory rate, blood pressure, continuous EKG

Dosage Forms Injection: 20 mL vial containing 1 g pralidoxime chloride with one 20 mL ampul diluent, disposable syringe, needle, and alcohol swab

Praziquantel (pray zi kwon' tel)

Brand Names Biltricide®

Therapeutic Category Anthelmintic

Use Treatment of all stages of schistosomiasis caused by *Schistosoma* species pathogenic to humans; also active in the treatment of clonorchiasis, opisthorchiasis, cysticercosis, and many intestinal tapeworms

Pregnancy Risk Factor B

Contraindications Ocular cysticercosis, spinal cysticercosis, and known hypersensitivity to praziquantel

Precautions Use caution in patients with severe hepatic disease and in patients with a history of seizures

Adverse Reactions

Central nervous system: Dizziness, drowsiness, vertigo, malaise, CSF reaction syndrome in patients being treated for neurocysticercosis, fever, headache

Dermatologic: Urticarial rash

Gastrointestinal: Abdominal pain, nausea, vomiting, anorexia, diarrhea

Mechanism of Action Increases the cell permeability to calcium in schistosomes, causing strong contractions and paralysis of worm musculature leading to detachment of suckers from the blood vessel walls and to dislodgment

Pharmacokinetics

Absorption: Oral: ~80%

Distribution: CSF concentration is 14% to 20% of plasma concentration; excreted in breast milk

Protein binding: ~80%

Metabolism: Extensive first-pass metabolism

Half-life: 0.8-1.5 hours

Metabolites: 4.5 hours

Peak serum levels: Within 1-3 hours

Elimination: Praziquantel and metabolites excreted mainly in urine (99% as metabolites)

Usual Dosage Children and Adults: Oral:

Schistosomiasis: 20 mg/kg/dose 2-3 times/day for 1 day at 4-6 hour intervals

Flukes: 75 mg/kg/day divided every 8 hours for 1-2 days

Cysticercosis: 50 mg/kg/day divided every 8 hours for 14 days (for neurocysticercosis, steroids should be administered prior to starting praziquantel)

Tapeworms: 10-20 mg/kg as a single dose (25 mg/kg for *H. nana*)

Patient Information Do not chew tablets due to bitter taste; take with food; caution should be used when performing tasks requiring mental alertness

Nursing Implications Tablets can be halved or quartered

Dosage Forms Tablet, tri-scored: 600 mg

References

King CH and Mahmoud AA, "Drug Five Years Later: Praziquantel," *Ann Intern Med*, 1989, 110(4):290-6.

Prazosin Hydrochloride (pra' zoe sin)

Related Information

Overdose and Toxicology Information *on page 696-700*

Brand Names Minipress®

Synonyms Furazosin

Therapeutic Category Alpha-Adrenergic Blocking Agent, Oral; Antihypertensive; Vasodilator, Coronary

Use Hypertension, severe congestive heart failure (in conjunction with diuretics and cardiac glycosides)

Pregnancy Risk Factor C

Contraindications Hypersensitivity to prazosin or any component

Precautions Marked orthostatic hypotension, syncope, and loss of consciousness may occur with first dose ("first dose phenomenon"). This reaction is more likely to occur in patients receiving beta blockers, diuretics, low sodium diets or larger first doses (ie, >1 mg/dose in adults); avoid rapid ↑ in dose; use with caution in patients with renal impairment

Adverse Reactions

Cardiovascular: Orthostatic hypotension, syncope, palpitations, nasal congestion, tachycardia, edema

Central nervous system: Dizziness, lightheadedness, nightmares, drowsiness, weakness, headache, hypothermia

Dermatologic: Rash

Endocrine & metabolic: Fluid retention, sexual dysfunction

Gastrointestinal: Nausea, dry mouth

Renal & genitourinary: Urinary frequency

Drug Interactions Diuretics and antihypertensive medications (especially beta blockers) may ↑ prazosin's hypotensive effect

Mechanism of Action Competitively inhibits postsynaptic alpha-adrenergic receptors which results in vasodilation of veins and arterioles and a decrease in total peripheral resistance and blood pressure

Pharmacodynamics Hypotensive effect:

Onset of action: Within 2 hours

Maximum decrease: 2-4 hours

Duration: 10-24 hours

Pharmacokinetics

Distribution: V_d: 0.5 L/kg (hypertensive adults)

Protein-binding: 92% to 97%

Metabolism: Metabolized extensively in the liver, metabolites may be active

Bioavailability, oral: 43% to 82%

Half-life, adults: 2-4 hours, increased half-life with congestive heart failure

Elimination: 6% to 10% excreted renally as unchanged drug

Usual Dosage Oral:

Children: Initial: 5 μg/kg/dose (to assess hypotensive effects); usual dosing interval every 6 hours; increase dosage gradually up to maximum of 25 μg/kg/dose every 6 hours

Adults: Initial: 1 mg/dose 2-3 times/day; usual maintenance dose: 3-15 mg/day in divided doses 2-4 times/day; maximum daily dose: 20 mg

Monitoring Parameters Blood pressure, standing and sitting/supine

Dosage Forms Capsule: 1 mg, 2 mg, 5 mg

References

Friedman WF and George BL, "New Concepts and Drugs in the Treatment of Congestive Heart Failure," *Pediatr Clin North Am*, 1984, 31(6):1197-227.

Predair® *see* Prednisolone *on next page*

Predaject® *see* Prednisolone *on next page*

Predalone T.B.A.® *see* Prednisolone *on next page*

Predcor® *see* Prednisolone *on next page*

Predcor-TBA® *see* Prednisolone *on this page*

Pred Forte® *see* Prednisolone *on this page*

Pred-G® *see* Prednisolone and Gentamicin *on next page*

Pred Mild® *see* Prednisolone *on this page*

Prednicen-M® *see* Prednisone *on next page*

Prednisolone (pred niss' oh lone)

Related Information

Systemic Corticosteroids Comparison Chart *on page 727*

Brand Names AK-Pred®; Delta-Cortef®; Econopred®; Econopred® Plus; Hydeltrasol®; Hydeltra-T.B.A.®; Inflamase®; Inflamase® Mild; Key-Pred®; Key-Pred-SP®; Metreton®; Pediapred®; Predair®; Predaject®; Predalone T.B.A.®; Predcor®; Predcor-TBA®; Pred Forte®; Pred Mild®; Prelone®

Synonyms Deltahydrocortisone; Metacortandralone; Prednisolone Acetate; Prednisolone Sodium Phosphate; Prednisolone Tebutate

Therapeutic Category Anti-inflammatory Agent; Corticosteroid, Ophthalmic; Corticosteroid, Systemic; Glucocorticoid

Use Treatment of palpebral and bulbar conjunctivitis; corneal injury from chemical, radiation, thermal burns, or foreign body penetration; endocrine disorders, rheumatic disorders, collagen diseases, dermatologic diseases, allergic states, ophthalmic diseases, respiratory diseases, hematologic disorders, neoplastic diseases, edematous states, and gastrointestinal diseases

Pregnancy Risk Factor C

Contraindications Acute superficial herpes simplex keratitis; systemic fungal infections; varicella; hypersensitivity to prednisolone or any component

Warnings May retard bone growth

Precautions Use with caution in patients with hypothyroidism, cirrhosis, hypertension, congestive heart failure, ulcerative colitis, thromboembolic disorders

Adverse Reactions

Cardiovascular: Edema, hypertension

Central nervous system: Vertigo, seizures, psychoses, pseudotumor cerebri, headache

Dermatologic: Acne, skin atrophy

Endocrine & metabolic: Cushing's syndrome, pituitary-adrenal axis suppression, growth suppression, glucose intolerance, hypokalemia, alkalosis

Gastrointestinal: Peptic ulcer, nausea, vomiting

Musculoskeletal: Muscle weakness, osteoporosis, fractures

Ocular: Cataracts, glaucoma

Drug Interactions Barbiturates, phenytoin, rifampin, salicylates, vaccines, toxoids

Mechanism of Action Decreases inflammation by suppression of migration of polymorphonuclear leukocytes and reversal of increased capillary permeability; suppresses the immune system by reducing activity and volume of the lymphatic system

Usual Dosage Dose depends upon condition being treated and response of patient; dosage for infants and children should be based on severity of the disease and response of the patient rather than on strict adherence to dosage indicated by age, weight, or body surface area. Consider alternate day therapy for long term therapy. Discontinuation of long term therapy requires gradual withdrawal by tapering the dose.

Children:

Acute asthma:

Oral: 1-2 mg/kg/day in divided doses 1-2 times/day for 3-5 days

I.V.: 2-4 mg/kg/day divided 3-4 times/day

Anti-inflammatory or immunosuppressive dose: Oral, I.V.: 0.1-2 mg/kg/day in divided doses 1-4 times/day

Nephrotic syndrome: Oral: Initial: 2 mg/kg/day (maximum: 80 mg/day) in divided doses 3-4 times/day until urine is protein free for 5 days (maximum: 28 days); if proteinuria persists, use 4 mg/kg/dose every other day for an additional 28 days; maintenance: 2 mg/kg/dose every other day for 28 days; then taper over 4-6 weeks

Children and Adults: Ophthalmic suspension: 1-2 drops into conjunctival sac every hour during day, every 2 hours at night until favorable response is obtained, then use 1 drop every 4 hours

Adults: Oral, I.V.: 5-60 mg/day

Test Interactions Skin tests

Nursing Implications Give after meals or with food or milk to decrease GI effects; do not give acetate or tebutate salts I.V.

Dosage Forms

Injection, as acetate: 25 mg/mL (10 mL, 30 mL); 50 mg/mL (10 mL, 30 mL); 100 mg/mL (10 mL)

Injection, as sodium phosphate: 20 mg/mL (2 mL, 5 mL, 10 mL)

Injection, as tebutate: 20 mg/mL (1 mL, 5 mL, 10 mL)

Liquid, oral, as sodium phosphate: 5 mg/5 mL (120 mL)

Solution, ophthalmic, as sodium phosphate: 0.125% (5 mL, 10 mL, 15 mL); 0.5% (5 mL)

Suspension, ophthalmic, as acetate: 0.12% (5 mL, 10 mL); 0.125% (5 mL, 10 mL); 1% (1 mL, 5 mL, 10 mL, 15 mL)

Syrup: 15 mg/5 mL (240 mL)

Tablet: 5 mg

Prednisolone Acetate *see* Prednisolone *on previous page*

Prednisolone and Gentamicin

Brand Names Pred-G®

Synonyms Gentamicin and Prednisolone

Therapeutic Category Antibiotic, Ophthalmic; Corticosteroid, Ophthalmic

Use Treatment of steroid responsive inflammatory conditions and superficial ocular infections due to strains of microorganisms susceptible to gentamicin such as *Staphylococcus*, *Streptococcus*, *E. coli*, *H. influenzae*, *Klebsiella*, *Neisseria*, *Pseudomonas*, *Proteus*, and *Serratia* species

Pregnancy Risk Factor C

Contraindications Known hypersensitivity to a drug component, dendritic keratitis, fungal diseases, vaccinia, varicella and most other viral infections, and mycobacterial infection of the eye. The product's use is contraindicated after uncomplicated removal of a corneal foreign body.

Warnings Prolonged use may result in glaucoma, damage to the optic nerve, defects in visual acuity, posterior subcapsular cataract formation, and secondary ocular infections

Adverse Reactions

Local: Burning, stinging

Ocular: Elevation of intraocular pressure, glaucoma, infrequent optic nerve damage, posterior subcapsular cataract formation, superficial punctate keratitis

Miscellaneous: Delayed wound healing, development of secondary infection, allergic sensitization

Usual Dosage Children and Adults: Ophthalmic: 1 drop 2-4 times/day; during the initial 24-48 hours, the dosing frequency may be increased if necessary

Monitoring Parameters With use >10 days, monitor intraocular pressure

Nursing Implications Shake well before using

Dosage Forms

Ointment, ophthalmic: Prednisolone acetate 0.6% and gentamicin sulfate 0.3% (3.5 g)

Suspension, ophthalmic: Prednisolone acetate 1% and gentamicin sulfate 0.3% (5 mL)

Prednisolone Sodium Phosphate *see* Prednisolone *on previous page*

Prednisolone Tebutate *see* Prednisolone *on previous page*

Prednisone (pred' ni sone)

Related Information

Systemic Corticosteroids Comparison Chart *on page 727*

Brand Names Deltasone®; Liquid Pred®; Meticorten®; Orasone®; Prednicen-M®; Sterapred®

(Continued)

Prednisone *(Continued)*

Synonyms Deltacortisone; Deltadehydrocortisone

Therapeutic Category Anti-inflammatory Agent; Corticosteroid, Systemic; Glucocorticoid

Use Management of adrenocortical insufficiency; used for its anti-inflammatory or immunosuppressant effects

Pregnancy Risk Factor C

Contraindications Serious infections, except septic shock or tuberculous meningitis; systemic fungal infections; hypersensitivity to prednisone or any component; varicella

Warnings May retard bone growth

Precautions Use with caution in patients with hypothyroidism, cirrhosis, hypertension, congestive heart failure, ulcerative colitis, thromboembolic disorders

Adverse Reactions

- Cardiovascular: Edema, hypertension
- Central nervous system: Vertigo, seizures, psychoses, pseudotumor cerebri, headache
- Dermatologic: Acne, skin atrophy
- Endocrine & metabolic: Cushing's syndrome, pituitary-adrenal axis suppression, growth suppression, glucose intolerance, hypokalemia, alkalosis
- Gastrointestinal: Peptic ulcer, nausea, vomiting
- Musculoskeletal: Muscle weakness, osteoporosis, fractures
- Ocular: Cataracts, glaucoma

Drug Interactions Barbiturates, phenytoin, rifampin, salicylates, vaccines, toxoids

Mechanism of Action Decreases inflammation by suppression of migration of polymorphonuclear leukocytes and reversal of increased capillary permeability; suppresses the immune system by reducing activity and volume of the lymphatic system

Pharmacokinetics Converted rapidly to prednisolone (active)

Usual Dosage Dose depends upon condition being treated and response of patient; dosage for infants and children should be based on severity of the disease and response of the patient rather than on strict adherence to dosage indicated by age, weight, or body surface area. Consider alternate day therapy for long term therapy. Discontinuation of long term therapy requires gradual withdrawal by tapering the dose.

Children: Oral:

- Anti-inflammatory or immunosuppressive: 0.05-2 mg/kg/day divided 1-4 times/day
- Acute asthma: 1-2 mg/kg/day in divided doses 1-2 times/day for 3-5 days
  - Alternatively (for 3-5 day "burst"):
  - <1 year: 10 mg every 12 hours
  - 1-4 years: 20 mg every 12 hours
  - 5-13 years: 30 mg every 12 hours
  - >13 years: 40 mg every 12 hours
- Asthma long-term therapy (alternative dosing by age):
  - <1 year: 10 mg every other day
  - 1-4 years: 20 mg every other day
  - 5-13 years: 30 mg every other day
  - >13 years: 40 mg every other day
- Nephrotic syndrome: Initial: 2 mg/kg/day (maximum: of 80 mg/day) in divided doses 3-4 times/day until urine is protein free for 5 days (maximum: 28 days); if proteinuria persists, use 4 mg/kg/dose every other day for an additional 28 days; maintenance: 2 mg/kg/dose every other day for 28 days; then taper over 4-6 weeks

Children and Adults: Physiologic replacement: 4-5 mg/m^2/day

Adults: Oral: 5-60 mg/day in divided doses 1-4 times/day

Test Interactions Skin tests

Nursing Implications Give after meals or with food or milk

Dosage Forms

Solution:

- Concentrate: 5 mg/mL (5 mL, 30 mL)
- Oral: 5 mg/5 mL (10 mL, 20 mL, 500 mL)

Syrup: 5 mg/5 mL (120 mL, 240 mL)
Tablet: 1 mg, 2.5 mg, 5 mg, 10 mg, 20 mg, 50 mg

References

Murphy CM, Coonce SL, and Simon PA, "Treatment of Asthma in Children," *Clin Pharm*, 1991, 10(9):685-703.

Prefrin™ Ophthalmic Solution *see* Phenylephrine Hydrochloride *on page 453*

Pregnyl® *see* Chorionic Gonadotropin *on page 134*

Prelone® *see* Prednisolone *on page 476*

Premarin® *see* Estrogens, Conjugated *on page 232*

Pre-Pen® *see* Benzylpenicilloyl-polylysine *on page 80*

Preprocedure Sedatives in Children *see page 687*

Prevident® *see* Fluoride *on page 255*

Primaquine Phosphate (prim' a kween)

Therapeutic Category Antimalarial Agent

Use Provide radical cure of *P. vivax* or *P. ovale* malaria after a clinical attack has been confirmed by blood smear or serologic titer and postexposure prophylaxis

Pregnancy Risk Factor C

Contraindications Acutely ill patients who have a tendency to develop granulocytopenia (rheumatoid arthritis, SLE); patients receiving other drugs capable of depressing the bone marrow; patients receiving quinacrine

Precautions Use with caution in patients with G-6-PD deficiency, NADH methemoglobin reductase deficiency

Adverse Reactions

Central nervous system: Headache
Dermatologic: Pruritus
Gastrointestinal: Nausea, vomiting
Hematologic: Hemolytic anemia, methemoglobinemia, leukocytosis, leukopenia
Ocular: Interference with visual accommodation

Drug Interactions Quinacrine (↑ toxicity of primaquine)

Mechanism of Action Eliminates the primary tissue exoerythrocytic forms of *P. falciparum* and interferes with plasmodial DNA

Pharmacokinetics

Absorption: Oral: Well absorbed
Metabolism: Liver metabolism to carboxyprimaquine, an active metabolite
Half-life: 3.7-9.6 hours
Peak serum levels: Within 1-2 hours
Elimination: Small amount of unchanged drug excreted in urine

Usual Dosage Oral:

Children: 0.3 mg base/kg/day once daily for 14 days not to exceed 15 mg base/day, or 0.9 mg base/kg once weekly for 8 weeks not to exceed 45 mg base/week

Adults: 15 mg/day (base) once daily for 14 days or 45 mg base once weekly for 8 weeks

Monitoring Parameters Periodic CBC, visual color check of urine, hemoglobin

Patient Information Take with meals to decrease adverse GI effects; drug has a bitter taste; notify physician if a darkening of the urine occurs

Dosage Forms Tablet: 26.3 mg [15 mg base]

References

Lynk A and Gold R, "Review of 40 Children With Imported Malaria," *Pediatr Infect Dis J*, 1989, 8(11):745-50.

Primatene® Mist [OTC] *see* Epinephrine *on page 220*

Primaxin® *see* Imipenem/Cilastatin *on page 305*

Primidone (pri' mi done)

Brand Names Mysoline®

Therapeutic Category Anticonvulsant; Barbiturate

Use Management of generalized tonic-clonic (grand mal), complex partial and simple partial (focal) seizures

(Continued)

Primidone *(Continued)*

Pregnancy Risk Factor D

Contraindications Hypersensitivity to primidone or any component; porphyria

Precautions Use with caution in patients with renal or hepatic impairment; abrupt discontinuation may precipitate status epilepticus

Adverse Reactions

Central nervous system: Drowsiness, vertigo, ataxia, lethargy, behavior change

Dermatologic: Rash

Gastrointestinal: Nausea, vomiting

Hematologic: Leukopenia, malignant lymphoma-like syndrome, megaloblastic anemia

Ocular: Diplopia, nystagmus

Miscellaneous: Systemic lupus-like syndrome

Drug Interactions Primidone may ↓ serum concentrations of ethosuximide, VPA, griseofulvin; methylphenidate may ↑ primidone serum concentrations; phenytoin may ↓ primidone serum concentrations; valproic acid may ↑ phenobarbital concentrations derived from primidone

Mechanism of Action Decreases neuron excitability, raises seizure threshold similar to phenobarbital

Pharmacokinetics

Distribution: V_d: 2-3 L/kg (adults)

Protein-binding: 99%

Metabolism: Metabolized in the liver to phenobarbital (active) and phenylethylmalonamide (PEMA)

Bioavailability: 60% to 80%

Half-life:

Primidone: 10-12 hours

PEMA: 16 hours

Phenobarbital: 52-118 hours (age-dependent)

Peak concentration: Oral: Within 4 hours

Elimination: Urinary excretion of both active metabolites and unchanged primidone (15% to 25%)

Usual Dosage Oral:

Neonates: 12-20 mg/kg/day in divided doses 2-4 times/day; start with lower dosage and titrate upward

Children <8 years: Initial: 50-125 mg/day given at bedtime; ↑ by 50-125 mg/day increments every 3-7 days; usual dose: 10-25 mg/kg/day in divided doses 3-4 times/day

Children >8 years and Adults: Initial: 125-250 mg/day at bedtime; ↑ by 125-250 mg/day every 3-7 days; usual dose: 750-1500 mg/day in divided doses 3-4 times/day with maximum dosage of 2 g/day

Monitoring Parameters Serum primidone and phenobarbital concentrations; CBC; neurological status

Reference Range Therapeutic: 5-12 μg/mL (SI: 23-55 μmol/L); toxic effects rarely present with levels below 10 μg/mL (SI: 46 μmol/L) if phenobarbital concentrations are low. Toxic: >15 μg/mL (SI: >69 μmol/L)

Dosage Forms

Suspension, oral: 250 mg/5 mL (240 mL)

Tablet: 50 mg, 250 mg

Principen® *see* Ampicillin *on page 48*

Priscoline® *see* Tolazoline Hydrochloride *on page 571*

Privine® [OTC] *see* Naphazoline Hydrochloride *on page 403*

Probalan® *see* Probenecid *on this page*

Pro-Banthine® *see* Propantheline Bromide *on page 490*

Probenecid (proe ben' e sid)

Brand Names Benemid®; Probalan®

Therapeutic Category Uric Acid Lowering Agent

Use Prevention of gouty arthritis; hyperuricemia; prolong serum levels of penicillin/cephalosporin

Pregnancy Risk Factor B

Contraindications Hypersensitivity to probenecid or any component; high dose aspirin therapy; moderate to severe renal impairment (Cl_{cr} <10 mL/minute); children <2 years of age, blood dyscrasias, uric acid kidney stones

Precautions Use with caution in patients with peptic ulcer

Adverse Reactions

Cardiovascular: Flushing

Central nervous system: Dizziness, headache

Dermatologic: Rash

Gastrointestinal: Anorexia, nausea, vomiting

Hematologic: Anemia, leukopenia, aplastic anemia, hemolytic anemia (possibly related to G-6-PD deficiency)

Hepatic: Hepatic necrosis

Renal & genitourinary: Urinary frequency, uric acid stones, nephrotic syndrome

Miscellaneous: Hypersensitivity reactions

Drug Interactions Nitrofurantoin, methotrexate, salicylates, NSAIDs, pyrazinamide, diazoxide, alcohol, furosemide, ethacrynic acid

Mechanism of Action Competitively inhibits the reabsorption of uric acid at the proximal convoluted tubule, thereby promoting its excretion and reducing serum uric acid levels; increases plasma levels of weak organic acids (penicillins, cephalosporins, or other beta-lactam antibiotics) by competitively inhibiting their renal tubular secretion

Pharmacodynamics Onset of action: Exerts its maximal effects on penicillin levels after 2 hours; produces maximal renal clearance of uric acid in 30 minutes

Pharmacokinetics

Absorption: Rapidly and completely absorbed from GI tract

Metabolism: Metabolized in the liver

Half-life: 4-17 hours

Peak serum levels: Within 2-4 hours

Usual Dosage Oral:

Prolongation of penicillin serum levels:

Children 2-14 years: Initial: 25 mg/kg/dose as a single dose; maintenance: 40 mg/kg/day in 4 divided doses (maximum single dose: 500 mg)

Adults: 500 mg 4 times/day

Hyperuricemia: Adults: 250 mg twice daily for 1 week; increase to 500 mg twice daily; increase every 4 weeks if needed to a maximum of 2-3 g/day; begin therapy 2-3 weeks after an acute gouty attack

Monitoring Parameters Uric acid, renal function

Test Interactions False-positive glucosuria with Clinitest®

Patient Information Take with food or antacids to minimize GI effects

Dosage Forms Tablet: 500 mg

Procainamide Hydrochloride (proe kane a' mide)

Brand Names Procan® SR; Pronestyl®; Pronestyl-SR®

Synonyms PCA; Procaine Amide Hydrochloride

Therapeutic Category Antiarrhythmic Agent, Class Ia

Use Ventricular tachycardia, premature ventricular contractions, paroxysmal atrial tachycardia, and atrial fibrillation; to prevent recurrence of ventricular tachycardia, paroxysmal supraventricular tachycardia, atrial fibrillation or flutter

Pregnancy Risk Factor C

Contraindications Complete heart block; second or third degree heart block without pacemaker; "torsade de pointes" (twisting of the points) an unusual ventricular tachycardia; hypersensitivity to the drug or procaine, or related drugs; myasthenia gravis; SLE

Warnings Long term administration leads to the development of a positive antinuclear antibody test in 50% of patients which may lead to a lupus erythematosus-like syndrome (in 20% to 30% of patients); assess relative benefits and risks if ANA titer becomes positive and consider alternative agent; discontinue PCA with SLE symptoms and change to alternative agent; do not chew or crush sustained release dosage form, swallow whole; do not use sustained release preparation for initial therapy

Precautions Marked A-V conduction disturbances, bundle-branch block or severe cardiac glycoside intoxication, ventricular arrhythmias in patients with organic heart disease or coronary occlusion, supraventricular tachyar-

(Continued)

Procainamide Hydrochloride *(Continued)*

rhythmias unless digitalis levels adequate to prevent marked increases in ventricular rates; drug may accumulate in patients with renal or hepatic dysfunction; some tablets contain tartrazine; injection may contain bisulfite

Adverse Reactions

Cardiovascular: Hypotension, tachycardia, arrhythmias, A-V block, Q-T prolongation, widening QRS complex

Central nervous system: Confusion, disorientation

Gastrointestinal: Nausea, vomiting, GI complaints

Hematologic: Agranulocytosis, neutropenia

Miscellaneous: Drug fever, lupus-like syndrome (arthralgia, positive Coombs' test, thrombocytopenia, rash, myalgia, fever, pericarditis, pleural effusion)

Drug Interactions Cimetidine, ranitidine, and amiodarone may ↑ plasma PCA and NAPA concentrations, PCA dosage adjustment may be required; PCA may potentiate skeletal muscle relaxants and anticholinergic drugs may have enhanced effects

Stability Use only clear or slightly yellow solutions; stability of parenteral admixture with D_5W at room temperature (25°C) is 24 hours but 7 days at refrigerated temperature (2°C to 8°C)

Mechanism of Action Class IA antiarrhythmic with anticholinergic and local anesthetic effects; decreases myocardial excitability and conduction velocity and depresses myocardial contractility, by increasing the electrical stimulation threshold of ventricle, HIS-Purkinje system and through direct cardiac effects

Pharmacodynamics Onset of action: I.M. 10-30 minutes

Pharmacokinetics

Distribution: V_d:
- Children: 2.2 L/kg
- Adults: 2 L/kg; decreased V_d with congestive heart failure or shock

Protein binding: 15% to 20%

Metabolism: Metabolized by acetylation in the liver to produce N-acetyl procainamide (NAPA) (active metabolite)

Bioavailability, oral: 75% to 95%

Half-life:
- PCA:
  - Children: 1.7 hours
  - Adults with normal renal function: 2.5-4.7 hours
  - Half-life dependent upon hepatic acetylator phenotype, cardiac function and renal function
- NAPA:
  - Children: 6 hours
  - Adults with normal renal function: 6-8 hours
  - NAPA half-life dependent upon renal function

Peak plasma concentrations:
- Capsule: Within 45 minutes to 2.5 hours
- I.M.: 15-60 minutes

Elimination: Urinary excretion (25% as NAPA)

Usual Dosage Must be titrated to patient's response

Children:
- Oral: 15-50 mg/kg/24 hours divided every 3-6 hours; maximum 4 g/24 hours
- I.M.: 20-30 mg/kg/24 hours divided every 4-6 hours in divided doses; maximum 4 g/24 hours
- I.V.: Load: 3-6 mg/kg/dose over 5 minutes, not to exceed 100 mg/dose; may repeat every 5-10 minutes to maximum of 15 mg/kg/load; maintenance as continuous I.V. infusion: 20-80 μg/kg/minute; maximum: 2 g/24 hours

Adults:
- Oral: 250-500 mg/dose every 3-6 hours or 500 mg to 1 g every 6 hours sustained release; usual dose: 50 mg/kg/24 hours or 2-4 g/24 hours
- I.V.: Load: 50-100 mg/dose, repeated every 5-10 minutes until patient controlled; or load with 15-18 mg/kg; maximum loading dose: 1-1.5 g
- Continuous infusion: Usual maintenance: 3-4 mg/minute; range: 1-6 mg/minute
- ACLS guidelines: I.V.: Infuse 20 mg/minute until arrhythmia is controlled, hypotension occurs, QRS complex widens by 50% of its original width, or total of 17 mg/kg is given

Refractory ventricular fibrillation: 30 mg/minute up to a total of 17 mg/kg; I.V. maintenance infusion: 1-4 mg/minute; monitor levels and do not exceed 3 mg/minute for >24 hours in adults with renal failure.

Administration Do not administer faster than 20-30 mg/minute; severe hypotension can occur with rapid I.V. administration; give I.V. push over at least 5 minutes; administer I.V. loading dose over 25-30 minutes, use concentration of 20-30 mg/mL for loading dose and 2-4 mg/mL for maintenance infusing

Monitoring Parameters EKG, blood pressure, CBC with differential, platelet count

Reference Range Therapeutic: Procainamide: 4-10 μg/mL (SI: 15-37 μmol/L); sum of procainamide and N-acetyl procainamide: <30 μg/mL (SI: <110 μmol/L); optimal ranges must be ascertained for individual patients, with EKG monitoring; Toxic (PCA): >10-12 μg/mL (SI: >37-44 μmol/L)

Dosage Forms

Capsule: 250 mg, 375 mg, 500 mg
Injection: 100 mg/mL (10 mL); 500 mg/mL (2 mL)
Tablet: 250 mg, 375 mg, 500 mg
Tablet, sustained release: 250 mg, 500 mg, 750 mg, 1000 mg

Extemporaneous Preparation(s) A suspension of 50 mg/mL can be made with the capsules, distilled water, and a 2:1 simple syrup/cherry syrup mixture. The pH must be adjusted to 4-6 to prevent degradation.

Handbook in Extemporaneous Formulations, Bethesda, MD: American Society of Hospital Pharmacists, 1987.

Metras JI, Swenson CF, and MacDermott MP, "Stability of Procainamide Hydrochloride in an Extemporaneously Compounded Oral Liquid," *Am J Hosp Pharm*, 1992, 49(7):1720-4.

Swenson CF, "Importance of Following Instructions When Compounding," *Am J Hosp Pharm*, 1992, 50:261.

References

American College of Cardiology, American Heart Association Task Force, "Adult Advanced Cardiac Life Support" and "Pediatric Advanced Life Support Guidelines," *JAMA*, 1992, 268(16):2199-241 and 2262-75.

Singh S, Gelband H, Mehta AV, et al, "Procainamide Elimination Kinetics in Pediatric Patients," *Clin Pharmacol Ther*, 1982, 32(5):607-11.

Procaine Amide Hydrochloride *see* Procainamide Hydrochloride *on page 481*

Procaine Benzylpenicillin *see* Penicillin G Procaine *on page 441*

Procaine Penicillin G *see* Penicillin G Procaine *on page 441*

Procan® SR *see* Procainamide Hydrochloride *on page 481*

Procarbazine Hydrochloride (proe kar' ba zeen)

Related Information

Emetogenic Potential of Single Chemotherapeutic Agents *on page 655*

Brand Names Matulane®

Synonyms Ibenzmethyzin

Therapeutic Category Antineoplastic Agent

Use Treatment of Hodgkin's disease, non-Hodgkin's lymphoma, brain tumor, bronchogenic carcinoma

Pregnancy Risk Factor D

Contraindications Hypersensitivity to procarbazine or any component, or pre-existing bone marrow aplasia

Warnings The US Food and Drug Administration (FDA) currently recommends that procedures for proper handling and disposal of antineoplastic agents be considered; procarbazine is a carcinogen which may cause acute leukemia; procarbazine may cause infertility

Precautions May potentiate CNS depression when used with phenothiazine derivatives, barbiturates, phenytoin, alcohol, tricyclic antidepressants, methyldopa; use with caution in patients with pre-existing renal or hepatic impairment; modify dosage in patients with renal or hepatic impairment, or marrow disorders; reduce dosage with serum creatinine >2 mg/dL or total bilirubin >3 mg/dL

(Continued)

Procarbazine Hydrochloride *(Continued)*

Adverse Reactions

Central nervous system: CNS depression, somnolence, confusion, cerebellar ataxia, neuropathy, nervousness, irritability

Dermatologic: Dermatitis, alopecia, hypersensitivity rash

Endocrine & metabolic: Disulfiram-like reaction, cessation of menses

Gastrointestinal: Nausea, vomiting, diarrhea, stomatitis, anorexia

Hematologic: Myelosuppression

Musculoskeletal: Arthralgia, myalgia

Ocular: Nystagmus, diplopia, photophobia

Respiratory: Flu-like syndrome

Drug Interactions Alcohol (disulfiram-like reaction); MAO inhibitors, foods with high tyramine content; phenothiazines, barbiturates, tricyclic antidepressants, methyldopa, phenytoin

Mechanism of Action Inhibits DNA, RNA, and protein synthesis; may damage DNA directly via free-radical formation and suppress mitosis

Pharmacokinetics

Absorption: Oral: Well absorbed

Distribution: Crosses the blood brain barrier and distributes into CSF

Metabolism: Metabolized in the liver

Half-life: 1 hour

Time to peak serum levels: Within 1 hour

Elimination: Excreted in the urine (<5% as unchanged drug) and 70% as metabolites

Usual Dosage Oral (refer to individual protocols):

Children: 50-100 mg/m^2/day once daily for 10-14 days every 28 days; doses as high as 100-200 mg/m^2/day once daily have been used for neuroblastoma and medulloblastoma

BMT aplastic anemia conditioning regimen: 12.5 mg/kg/dose every other day for 4 doses

Adults: Initial: 2-4 mg/kg/day in single or divided doses for 7 days then increase dose to 4-6 mg/kg/day until response is obtained or leukocyte count ↓ <4000/mm^3 or the platelet count ↓ <100,000/mm^3; maintenance: 1-2 mg/kg/day

Monitoring Parameters CBC with differential, platelet count, and reticulocyte count; urinalysis, liver function test, renal function test

Patient Information Avoid food with high tyramine content (cheese, tea, coffee, cola drinks, wine, bananas); avoid alcohol; notify physician of fever, sore throat, bleeding, or bruising

Additional Information Myelosuppressive effects:

WBC: Moderate

Platelets: Moderate

Onset (days): 14

Nadir (days): 21

Recovery (days): 28

Dosage Forms Capsule: 50 mg

References

Longo DL, Young RC, Wesley M, et al, "Twenty Years of MOPP Therapy for Hodgkin's Disease, *J Clin Oncol*, 1986, 4(9):1295-306.

Rodriguez LA, Prados M, Silver P, et al, "Re-evaluation of Procarbazine for the Treatment of Recurrent Malignant Central Nervous System Tumors," *Cancer*, 1989, 64(12):2420-3.

Procardia® *see* Nifedipine *on page 413*

Procardia XL® *see* Nifedipine *on page 413*

Prochlorperazine (proe klor per' a zeen)

See Also Chlorpromazine Hydrochloride

Related Information

Compatibility of Medications Mixed in a Syringe *on page 717*

Overdose and Toxicology Information *on page 696-700*

Brand Names Compazine®

Therapeutic Category Antiemetic; Antipsychotic Agent; Phenothiazine Derivative

Use Management of nausea and vomiting; acute and chronic psychosis

Pregnancy Risk Factor C

Contraindications Hypersensitivity to prochlorperazine or any component; cross sensitivity with other phenothiazines may exist; avoid use in patients with narrow-angle glaucoma; bone marrow depression; severe liver or cardiac disease, severe toxic CNS depression or coma

Warnings High incidence of extrapyramidal reactions especially in children, reserve use in children <5 years of age to those who are unresponsive to other antiemetics; incidence of extrapyramidal reactions is increased with acute illnesses such as chicken pox, measles, CNS infections, gastroenteritis, and dehydration; injection contains sulfites which may cause allergic reactions; lowers seizure threshold, use cautiously in patients with seizure history; may impair ability to perform hazardous tasks requiring mental alertness or physical coordination; some products contain tartrazine dye, avoid use in sensitive individuals

Precautions Safety and efficacy have not been established in children <9 kg or <2 years of age

Adverse Reactions Incidence of extrapyramidal reactions are higher with prochlorperazine than chlorpromazine

Cardiovascular: Hypotension (especially with I.V. use); orthostatic hypotension; tachycardia, arrhythmias, sudden death

Central nervous system: Sedation, drowsiness, restlessness, anxiety, extrapyramidal reactions which include dystonic reactions such as spasm of neck muscles, torticollis, extensor rigidity of back muscles, opisthotonos, trismus, and mandibular tics; pseudoparkinsonian signs and symptoms, tardive dyskinesia, neuroleptic malignant syndrome, seizures, altered central temperature regulation

Dermatologic: Hyperpigmentation, pruritus, rash, photosensitivity

Endocrine & metabolic: Amenorrhea, galactorrhea, gynecomastia, impotence, weight gain, abnormal glucose tolerance

Gastrointestinal: GI upset, dry mouth, constipation

Hematologic: Agranulocytosis, leukopenia (usually in patients with large doses for prolonged periods), thrombocytopenia, hemolytic anemia, eosinophilia

Hepatic: Cholestatic jaundice

Ocular: Retinal pigmentation, blurred vision

Renal & genitourinary: Urinary retention,

Miscellaneous: Anaphylactoid reactions

Drug Interactions Additive effects with other CNS depressants; alpha-adrenergic agonists (eg, epinephrine)

Mechanism of Action Blocks postsynaptic mesolimbic dopaminergic receptors in the brain, including the medullary chemoreceptor trigger zone; exhibits a strong alpha-adrenergic blocking effect and depresses the release of hypothalamic and hypophyseal hormones

Pharmacodynamics

Onset of action:

- Oral: 30-40 minutes
- I.M.: Within 10-20 minutes
- Rectal: Within 60 minutes

Duration:

- I.M., oral extended release: 12 hours
- Rectal, oral immediate release: 3-4 hours

Usual Dosage

Antiemetic:

Children >10 kg:

- Oral, rectal: 0.4 mg/kg/24 hours in 3-4 divided doses; **or**
- 9-14 kg: 2.5 mg every 12-24 hours as needed; maximum: 7.5 mg/day
- 14-18 kg: 2.5 mg every 8-12 hours as needed; maximum: 10 mg/day
- 18-39 kg: 2.5 mg every 8 hours or 5 mg every 12 hours as needed; maximum: 15 mg/day
- I.M.: 0.1-0.15 mg/kg/dose; usual: 0.13 mg/kg/dose; change to oral as soon as possible
- I.V.: Not recommended

Adults:

- Oral: 5-10 mg 3-4 times/day; usual maximum: 40 mg/day
- Oral, extended release: 10 mg twice daily or 15 mg once daily
- I.M.: 5-10 mg every 3-4 hours; usual maximum: 40 mg/day
- I.V.: 2.5-10 mg; maximum 10 mg/dose or 40 mg/day; may repeat dose every 3-4 hours as needed

(Continued)

Prochlorperazine *(Continued)*

Rectal: 25 mg twice daily

Treatment of psychoses:

Children 2-12 years:

Oral, rectal: 2.5 mg 2-3 times/day, increase dosage as needed to a maximum daily dose of 20 mg for 2-5 years and 25 mg for 6-12 years

I.M.: 0.13 mg/kg/dose, change to oral as soon as possible

Adults:

Oral: 5-10 mg 3-4 times/day, increase as needed to a daily maximum dose of 150 mg

I.M.: 10-20 mg every 4 hours as needed, change to oral as soon as possible

Administration Avoid I.V. administration; if necessary, may be given by direct I.V. injection at a maximum rate of 5 mg/minute

Monitoring Parameters CBC with differential and periodic ophthalmic exams (if chronically used)

Test Interactions False-positives for phenylketonuria, urinary amylase, uroporphyrins, urobilinogen

Nursing Implications Avoid skin contact with oral solution or injection, contact dermatitis has occurred; do not administer by S.C. route (tissue damage may occur)

Additional Information Use lowest possible dose in pediatric patients to try to ↓ incidence of extrapyramidal reactions; sustained action capsules should be dosed 1-2 times/day in similar daily doses as listed

Dosage Forms

Capsule, sustained action, as maleate: 10 mg, 15 mg, 30 mg
Injection, as edisylate: 5 mg/mL (2 mL, 10 mL)
Suppository, rectal: 2.5 mg, 5 mg, 25 mg (12/box)
Syrup, as edisylate: 5 mg/5 mL (120 mL)
Tablet, as maleate: 5 mg, 10 mg, 25 mg

Procrit® *see* Epoetin Alfa *on page 222*

Proctocort™ *see* Hydrocortisone *on page 293*

Profasi® HP *see* Chorionic Gonadotropin *on page 134*

Profilate® OSD *see* Antihemophilic Factor, Human *on page 55*

Profilnine® Heat-Treated *see* Factor IX Complex (Human) *on page 239*

Proglycem® *see* Diazoxide *on page 184*

Prokine™ *see* Sargramostim *on page 517*

Prometa® *see* Metaproterenol Sulfate *on page 367*

Promethazine and Codeine

Brand Names Phenergan® with Codeine; Pherazine® With Codeine; Prothazine-DC®

Therapeutic Category Antihistamine; Antitussive; Cough Preparation; Phenothiazine Derivative

Use Temporary relief of coughs and upper respiratory symptoms associated with allergy or the common cold

Restrictions C-V

Pregnancy Risk Factor C

Contraindications Known hypersensitivity to promethazine or codeine; lower respiratory tract symptoms, including asthma; concurrent use of MAO inhibitors, narrow-angle glaucoma, premature and term infants

Warnings May impair ability to perform hazardous activities which require mental alertness or physical coordination

Precautions Use with caution in patients with cardiovascular disease, impaired liver function, sleep apnea, seizures, hypertensive crisis, suspected Reye's syndrome; hypersensitivity reactions to morphine, hydrocodone, hydromorphone, levorphanol, oxycodone, oxymorphone; impaired renal function

Adverse Reactions

Promethazine:

Cardiovascular: Hypertension, hypotension, tachycardia

Central nervous system: Sedation (pronounced), confusion, drowsiness, restlessness, anxiety, extrapyramidal reactions, tardive dyskinesia, seizures
Dermatologic: Rash, photosensitivity
Gastrointestinal: GI upset, dry mouth, constipation
Hematologic: Agranulocytosis, leukopenia (rarely), thrombocytopenia
Hepatic: Cholestatic jaundice
Ocular: Blurred vision
Renal & genitourinary: Urinary retention
Miscellaneous: Allergic reactions

Codeine:
Cardiovascular: Palpitations, orthostatic hypotension, tachycardia or bradycardia, peripheral vasodilation
Central nervous system: CNS depression, dizziness, sedation, euphoria, hallucination, seizures
Dermatologic: Pruritus
Gastrointestinal: Nausea, vomiting, constipation, biliary tract spasm
Ocular: Miosis
Renal & genitourinary: Urinary tract spasm
Respiratory: Respiratory depression
Miscellaneous: Physical and psychological dependence, histamine release, allergic reactions

Drug Interactions Alpha-adrenergic agonists (eg, epinephrine), CNS depressants, alcohol

Mechanism of Action See individual monographs for Codeine and Promethazine Hydrochloride

Usual Dosage Oral (**in terms of codeine**):
Children: 1-1.5 mg/kg/day every 4 hours as needed; maximum: 30 mg/day
or
2-6 years: 1.25-2.5 mL every 4-6 hours or 2.5-5 mg/dose every 4-6 hours as needed; maximum: 30 mg codeine/day
6-12 years: 2.5-5 mL every 4-6 hours as needed or 5-10 mg/dose every 4-6 hours as needed; maximum: 60 mg codeine/day

Adults: 10-20 mg/dose every 4-6 hours as needed; maximum: 120 mg codeine/day; or 5-10 mL every 4-6 hours as needed

Test Interactions Alters the flare response in intradermal allergen tests

Patient Information May cause sedation and drowsiness

Dosage Forms Syrup: Promethazine hydrochloride 6.25 mg and codeine phosphate 10 mg per 5 mL (120 mL, 180 mL, 473 mL)

Promethazine and Phenylephrine

See Also Phenylephrine Hydrochloride; Promethazine Hydrochloride

Brand Names Phenergan® VC; Pherazine® VC

Therapeutic Category Antihistamine/Decongestant Combination

Use Temporary relief of upper respiratory symptoms associated with allergy or the common cold

Pregnancy Risk Factor C

Contraindications Known hypersensitivity to promethazine or phenylephrine; asthma, peripheral vascular disease, narrow-angle glaucoma, premature and term infants, severe hypertension, cardiovascular disease, liver disease

Warnings May impair ability to perform hazardous activities requiring mental alertness or physical coordination

Precautions Use with caution in patients with cardiovascular disease, impaired liver function, asthma, peptic ulcer, sleep apnea, seizures, hypertensive crisis; avoid in patients with suspected Reye's syndrome

Adverse Reactions
Promethazine:
Cardiovascular: Hypertension, hypotension, tachycardia
Central nervous system: Sedation (pronounced), confusion, drowsiness, restlessness, anxiety, extrapyramidal reactions, tardive dyskinesia, seizures
Dermatologic: Rash, photosensitivity
Gastrointestinal: GI upset, dry mouth, constipation

(Continued)

Promethazine and Phenylephrine *(Continued)*

Hematologic: Agranulocytosis, leukopenia (rarely), thrombocytopenia
Hepatic: Cholestatic jaundice
Ocular: Blurred vision
Renal & genitourinary: Urinary retention
Miscellaneous: Allergic reactions

Phenylephrine:
Cardiovascular: Hypertension, angina, reflex bradycardia, arrhythmias, rebound nasal stuffiness
Central nervous system: Restlessness, excitability, headache

Drug Interactions Alpha-adrenergic agonists (eg, epinephrine), beta-adrenergic blocking agents, MAO inhibitors, sympathomimetics; additive effects with other CNS depressants

Usual Dosage Oral:
Children:
2-6 years: 1.25 mL every 4-6 hours, not to exceed 7.5 mL in 24 hours
6-12 years: 2.5 mL every 4-6 hours, not to exceed 15 mL in 24 hours

Children >12 years and Adults: 5 mL every 4-6 hours, not to exceed 30 mL in 24 hours

Test Interactions Alters the flare response in intradermal allergen tests

Patient Information May cause drowsiness

Dosage Forms Liquid: Promethazine hydrochloride 6.25 mg and phenylephrine hydrochloride 5 mg per 5 mL (120 mL, 180 mL, 240 mL, 480 mL, 4000 mL)

Promethazine Hydrochloride (proe meth' a zeen)

Related Information
Compatibility of Medications Mixed in a Syringe *on page 717*
Overdose and Toxicology Information *on page 696-700*

Brand Names Anergan®; Phenazine®; Phencen®; Phenergan®; Prometh®; Prorex®; V-Gan®

Therapeutic Category Antiemetic; Antihistamine; Phenothiazine Derivative; Sedative

Use Symptomatic treatment of various allergic conditions and motion sickness; sedative and an antiemetic

Pregnancy Risk Factor C

Contraindications Hypersensitivity to promethazine or any component; narrow-angle glaucoma, severe toxic CNS depression or coma, prostatic hypertrophy, GI or GU obstruction; premature and term infants (due to association of antihistaminics with SIDS)

Warnings Do not give S.C. or intra-arterially, necrotic lesions may occur; injection may contain sulfites which may cause allergic reactions in some patients; may impair ability to perform hazardous tasks which require mental alertness or physical coordination

Precautions Use with caution in patients with cardiovascular disease, impaired liver function, asthma, peptic ulcer, sleep apnea, seizures, hypertensive crisis; avoid in patients with suspected Reye's syndrome

Adverse Reactions
Cardiovascular: Tachycardia, bradycardia, hypertension, hypotension
Central nervous system: Sedation (pronounced), confusion, fatigue, excitation, extrapyramidal reactions, dystonia, tardive dyskinesia
Dermatologic: Photosensitivity
Gastrointestinal: Dry mouth, GI upset, constipation
Hematologic: Thrombocytopenia, leukopenia, agranulocytosis (rarely)
Hepatic: Cholestatic jaundice
Ocular: Blurred vision
Renal & genitourinary: Urinary retention
Miscellaneous: Allergic reactions

Drug Interactions Alpha-adrenergic agonists (eg, epinephrine); additive effects with other CNS depressants

Stability Protect from light; compatible (when comixed in the same syringe) with atropine, chlorpromazine, diphenhydramine, droperidol, fentanyl, glycopyrrolate, hydromorphone, hydroxyzine hydrochloride, meperidine, midazolam, nalbuphine, pentazocine, prochlorperazine, scopolamine

Mechanism of Action Blocks postsynaptic mesolimbic dopaminergic receptors in the brain; exhibits a strong alpha-adrenergic blocking effect and depresses the release of hypothalamic and hypophyseal hormones; competes with histamine for the H_1-receptor

Pharmacodynamics

Onset of action:

Oral, I.M.: Within 20 minutes

I.V.: 3-5 minutes

Duration: 2-8 hours

Pharmacokinetics

Metabolism: Metabolized in the liver

Elimination: Excreted principally as inactive metabolites in the urine and in the feces

Usual Dosage

Children:

Antihistamine: Oral: 0.1 mg/kg/dose every 6 hours during the day and 0.5 mg/kg/dose at bedtime as needed

Antiemetic: Oral, I.M., I.V., rectal: 0.25-1 mg/kg 4-6 times/day as needed

Motion sickness: Oral: 0.5 mg/kg 30 minutes to 1 hour before departure, then every 12 hours as needed

Sedation: Oral, I.M., I.V., rectal: 0.5-1 mg/kg/dose every 6 hours as needed

Adults:

Antihistamine:

Oral: 25 mg at bedtime or 12.5 mg 3 times/day

I.M., I.V., rectal: 25 mg, may repeat in 2 hours

Antiemetic: Oral, I.M., I.V., rectal: 12.5-25 mg every 4 hours as needed

Motion sickness: Oral: 25 mg 30 minutes to 1 hour before departure, then every 12 hours as needed

Sedation: Oral, I.M., I.V., rectal: 25-50 mg/dose; repeat every 4-6 hours if needed

Administration Avoid I.V. use; if necessary, may dilute to a maximum concentration of 25 mg/mL and infuse at a maximum rate of 25 mg/minute

Test Interactions Alters the flare response in intradermal allergen tests

Patient Information May cause drowsiness

Nursing Implications Avoid S.C. administration, promethazine is a chemical irritation which may produce necrosis

Dosage Forms

Injection: 25 mg/mL (1 mL, 10 mL); 50 mg/mL (1 mL, 10 mL)

Suppository, rectal: 12.5 mg, 25 mg, 50 mg

Syrup: 6.25 mg/5 mL (5 mL, 120 mL, 240 mL, 480 mL, 4000 mL); 25 mg/5mL (120 mL, 480 mL, 4000 mL)

Tablet: 12.5 mg, 25 mg, 50 mg

Promethazine, Phenylephrine and Codeine

Brand Names Mallergan-VC® With Codeine; Phenergan® VC With Codeine

Therapeutic Category Antitussive; Cough Preparation

Use Temporary relief of coughs and upper respiratory symptoms including nasal congestion

Restrictions C-V

Pregnancy Risk Factor C

Contraindications Known hypersensitivity to promethazine, codeine, or phenylephrine; asthma, peripheral vascular disease; patients receiving MAO inhibitors, preterm and term infants (due to association of antihistaminics with SIDS)

Warnings See individual monographs for Promethazine Hydrochloride, Phenylephrine Hydrochloride, and Codeine

Precautions See individual monographs for Promethazine Hydrochloride, Phenylephrine Hydrochloride, and Codeine

Adverse Reactions See individual monographs for Promethazine Hydrochloride, Phenylephrine Hydrochloride, and Codeine

Drug Interactions See individual monographs for Promethazine Hydrochloride, Phenylephrine Hydrochloride, and Codeine

Usual Dosage Oral:

Not recommended for children <2 years of age

Children (dose expressed in terms of codeine): 1-1.5 mg/kg/day every 4 hours, maximum: 30 mg/day **or**

<6 years:

Weight 25 lbs: 1.25-2.5 mL every 4-6 hours, not to exceed 6 mL/24 hours

Weight 30 lbs: 1.25-2.5 mL every 4-6 hours, not to exceed 7 mL/24 hours

(Continued)

Promethazine, Phenylephrine and Codeine

(Continued)

Weight 35 lbs: 1.25-2.5 mL every 4-6 hours, not to exceed 8 mL/24 hours
Weight 40 lbs: 1.25-2.5 mL every 4-6 hours, not to exceed 9 mL/24 hours
6 to <12 years: 2.5-5 mL every 4-6 hours, not to exceed 15 mL/24 hours

Adults: 5 mL every 4-6 hours, not to exceed 30 mL/24 hours

Dosage Forms Liquid: Promethazine hydrochloride 6.25 mg, phenylephrine hydrochloride 5 mg and codeine phosphate 10 mg per 5 mL with alcohol 7% (120 mL, 240 mL, 480 mL, 4000 mL)

Pronestyl® *see* Procainamide Hydrochloride *on page 481*

Pronestyl-SR® *see* Procainamide Hydrochloride *on page 481*

Propacet® *see* Propoxyphene and Acetaminophen *on page 492*

Propantheline Bromide (proe pan' the leen)

Brand Names Pro-Banthine®

Therapeutic Category Anticholinergic Agent; Antispasmodic Agent, Gastrointestinal; Antispasmodic Agent, Urinary

Use Adjunctive treatment of peptic ulcer, irritable bowel syndrome, pancreatitis, ureteral and urinary bladder spasm; to reduce duodenal motility during diagnostic radiologic procedures

Pregnancy Risk Factor C

Contraindications Narrow-angle glaucoma, known hypersensitivity to propantheline; ulcerative colitis; toxic megacolon; obstructive disease of the GI or urinary tract

Warnings Infants, blondes, patients with Down's syndrome, and children with spastic paralysis or brain damage may be hypersensitive to antimuscarinic effects

Precautions Use with caution in febrile patients, patients with hyperthyroidism, hepatic, cardiac, or renal disease, hypertension, GI infections, diarrhea, reflux esophagitis

Adverse Reactions

Cardiovascular: Tachycardia, palpitations, diaphoresis, flushing
Central nervous system: Insomnia, drowsiness, dizziness, nervousness
Dermatologic: Rash
Endocrine & metabolic: Impotence, suppression of lactation
Gastrointestinal: Dry mouth, nausea, vomiting, constipation
Ocular: Mydriasis, blurred vision
Renal & genitourinary: Urinary retention
Miscellaneous: Allergic reactions

Drug Interactions Potassium chloride wax-matrix preparations, phenothiazines, tricyclic antidepressants, quinidine

Mechanism of Action Competitively blocks the action of acetylcholine at postganglionic parasympathetic receptor sites

Pharmacodynamics

Onset of action: Within 30-45 minutes
Duration: 4-6 hours

Pharmacokinetics

Metabolism: Metabolized in the liver and GI tract
Elimination: Excreted in urine, bile and other body fluids

Usual Dosage Oral:

Antisecretory:
Children: 1-2 mg/kg/day in 3-4 divided doses
Adults: 15 mg 3 times/day before meals or food and 30 mg at bedtime

Antispasmodic: Children: 2-3 mg/kg/day in divided doses every 4-6 hours and at bedtime

Patient Information Give 30 minutes before meals and at bedtime

Dosage Forms Tablet: 7.5 mg, 15 mg

Proparacaine Hydrochloride (proe par' a kane)

Brand Names AK-Taine®; Alcaine®; I-Paracaine®; Ophthaine®; Ophthetic®

Synonyms Proxymetacaine

Therapeutic Category Local Anesthetic, Ophthalmic

Use Local anesthesia for tonometry, gonioscopy; suture removal from cornea; removal of corneal foreign body; cataract extraction, glaucoma surgery; short operative procedure involving the cornea and conjunctiva

Pregnancy Risk Factor C

Contraindications Known hypersensitivity to proparacaine

Precautions Use with caution in patients with cardiac disease, hyperthyroidism

Adverse Reactions

Dermatologic: Allergic contact dermatitis

Ocular: Irritation, stinging, sensitization, keratitis, iritis, erosion of the corneal epithelium, conjunctival congestion and hemorrhage, corneal opacification

Mechanism of Action Local anesthetic; prevents initiation and transmission of impulse at the nerve cell membrane by decreasing ion permeability

Pharmacodynamics

Onset of action: Within 20 seconds of instillation

Duration: 15-20 minutes

Usual Dosage Children and Adults:

Ophthalmic surgery: 1 drop of 0.5% solution in eye every 5-10 minutes for 5-7 doses

Tonometry, gonioscopy, suture removal: 1-2 drops 0.5% solution in eye just prior to procedure

Patient Information Do not rub eye until anesthesia has worn off

Dosage Forms Ophthalmic, solution: 0.5% (2 mL, 15 mL)

Propine® *see* Dipivefrin Hydrochloride *on page 197*

Proplex® SX-T *see* Factor IX Complex (Human) *on page 239*

Proplex® T *see* Factor IX Complex (Human) *on page 239*

Propoxyphene (proe pox' i feen)

Related Information

Overdose and Toxicology Information *on page 696-700*

Brand Names Darvon®; Darvon-N®; Dolene®

Therapeutic Category Analgesic, Narcotic

Use Management of mild to moderate pain

Restrictions C-IV

Pregnancy Risk Factor C

Contraindications Hypersensitivity to propoxyphene or any component

Warnings Do not exceed recommended dosage

Precautions Use with caution in patients with renal or hepatic dysfunction, or when substituting propoxyphene for opiates in narcotic dependent patients

Adverse Reactions

Central nervous system: Dizziness, lightheadedness, weakness, sedation, paradoxical excitement and insomnia, headache

Dermatologic: Rashes

Gastrointestinal: GI upset, nausea, vomiting, constipation

Hepatic: Increased liver enzymes

Miscellaneous: Psychologic and physical dependence

Drug Interactions CNS depressants may potentiate pharmacologic effects; propoxyphene may inhibit the metabolism and increase the serum concentrations of carbamazepine, phenobarbital, tricyclic antidepressants, and warfarin

Mechanism of Action Binds to opiate receptors in the CNS, causing inhibition of ascending pain pathways, altering the perception of and response to pain; produces generalized CNS depression

Pharmacodynamics

Onset of effects: Oral: Within 30-60 minutes

Duration: 4-6 hours

Pharmacokinetics

Metabolism: Metabolized in the liver to an active metabolite (norpropoxyphene) and inactive metabolites

Bioavailability: Oral: 30% to 70% due to first pass effect

Half-life, adults: 8-24 hours (mean: ~15 hours)

(Continued)

Propoxyphene *(Continued)*

Norpropoxyphene, adults: 34 hours

Not dialyzable (0% to 5%)

Usual Dosage Oral:

Children: Dose not well established; doses of hydrochloride of 2-3 mg/kg/day divided every 6 hours have been used

Adults:

Hydrochloride: 65 mg every 3-4 hours as needed for pain; maximum: 390 mg/day

Napsylate: 100 mg every 4 hours as needed for pain; maximum: 600 mg/day

Additional Information Propoxyphene does not possess any anti-inflammatory or antipyretic actions; it possesses little, if any, antitussive effects; propoxyphene napsylate 100 mg is equivalent to 65 mg of propoxyphene hydrochloride; several cases utilizing propoxyphene in children for opioid detoxification have been reported (see reference)

Dosage Forms

Capsule, as hydrochloride: 32 mg, 65 mg

Suspension, oral, as napsylate: 50 mg/5 mL (480 mL)

Tablet, as napsylate: 100 mg

References

Hasday JD and Weintraub M, "Propoxyphene in Children With Iatrogenic Morphine Dependence," *Am J Dis Child*, 1983, 137(8):745-8.

Propoxyphene and Acetaminophen

Related Information

Narcotic Analgesics Comparison Chart *on page 721-722*

Overdose and Toxicology Information *on page 696-700*

Brand Names Darvocet-N®; Darvocet-N® 100; E-Lor®; Genagesic®; Propacet®; Wygesic®

Therapeutic Category Analgesic, Narcotic

Use Management of mild to moderate pain

Restrictions C-IV

Pregnancy Risk Factor C

Contraindications Hypersensitivity to propoxyphene, acetaminophen or any component

Warnings Do not exceed recommended dosage

Precautions Use with caution in patients with renal or hepatic dysfunction or when substituting propoxyphene for opiates in narcotic dependent patients

Adverse Reactions

Central nervous system: Dizziness, lightheadedness, weakness, sedation, paradoxical excitement, insomnia, headache

Dermatologic: Rashes

Gastrointestinal: GI upset, nausea, vomiting, constipation

Hepatic: Increased liver enzymes

Miscellaneous: Psychologic and physical dependence

Drug Interactions CNS depressants may potentiate pharmacologic effects; propoxyphene may inhibit the metabolism and increase the serum concentrations of carbamazepine, phenobarbital, tricyclic antidepressants and warfarin

Usual Dosage Adults: Oral:

Darvocet-N®: 1-2 tablets every 4 hours as needed; maximum: 600 mg propoxyphene napsylate/day

Darvocet-N® 100 or Wygesic®: 1 tablet every 4 hours as needed; maximum: 600 mg propoxyphene napsylate/day

Additional Information Propoxyphene napsylate 100 mg is equivalent to 65 mg of propoxyphene hydrochloride

Dosage Forms Tablet:

Darvocet-N®: Propoxyphene napsylate 50 mg and acetaminophen 325 mg

Darvocet-N® 100: Propoxyphene napsylate 100 mg and acetaminophen 650 mg

E-Lor®, Genagesic®, Wygesic®: Propoxyphene hydrochloride 65 mg and acetaminophen 650 mg

Propranolol Hydrochloride (proe pran' oh lole)

Related Information

Overdose and Toxicology Information *on page 696-700*

Brand Names Inderal®; Inderal® LA

Therapeutic Category Antianginal Agent; Antiarrhythmic Agent, Class II; Antihypertensive; Beta-Adrenergic Blocker

Use Management of hypertension, angina pectoris, pheochromocytoma, essential tremor, tetralogy of Fallot cyanotic spells, and arrhythmias (such as atrial fibrillation and flutter, A-V nodal re-entrant tachycardias, and catecholamine-induced arrhythmias); prevention of myocardial infarction, migraine headache; symptomatic treatment of hypertrophic subaortic stenosis

Pregnancy Risk Factor C

Contraindications Uncompensated congestive heart failure, cardiogenic shock, bradycardia or heart block, asthma, hyperactive airway disease, chronic obstructive lung disease, Raynaud's syndrome

Warnings In patients with angina pectoris, exacerbation of angina and, in some cases, myocardial infarction, occurred following abrupt discontinuance of therapy

Adverse Reactions

Cardiovascular: Hypotension, impaired myocardial contractility, congestive heart failure, bradycardia, worsening of A-V conduction disturbances

Central nervous system: Lightheadedness, insomnia, vivid dreams, weakness, lethargy, depression

Endocrine & metabolic: Hypoglycemia, hyperglycemia

Gastrointestinal: Nausea, vomiting, diarrhea, GI distress

Hematologic: Agranulocytosis

Respiratory: Bronchospasm

Miscellaneous: Cold extremities

Drug Interactions Phenobarbital, rifampin may increase propranolol clearance and may decrease its activity; cimetidine may reduce propranolol clearance and may increase its effects; aluminum-containing antacid may reduce GI absorption of propranolol

Stability Injection is compatible in saline, incompatible with HCO_3^-

Mechanism of Action Nonselective beta-adrenergic blocker (class II antiarrhythmic); competitively blocks response to $beta_1$ and $beta_2$ adrenergic stimulation which results in decreases in heart rate, myocardial contractility, blood pressure, and myocardial oxygen demand

Pharmacodynamics Beta blockade: Oral:

Onset of action: Within 1-2 hours

Duration: ~6 hours

Pharmacokinetics

Distribution: V_d: Adults: 3.9 L/kg; crosses the placenta; small amounts appear in breast milk

Protein-binding:

- Newborns: 68%
- Adults: 93%

Metabolism: Extensive first-pass effect, metabolized in the liver to active and inactive compounds

Bioavailability: 30% to 40%; oral bioavailability may be increased in Down's syndrome children

Half-life:

- Children: 3.9-6.4 hours, possible increased half-life in neonates and infants
- Adults: 4-6 hours

Elimination: Excreted primarily in the urine (96% to 99%)

Usual Dosage

Arrhythmias:

Oral:

- Children: Initial: 0.5-1 mg/kg/day in divided doses every 6-8 hours; titrate dosage upward every 3-7 days; usual dose: 2-4 mg/kg/day; higher doses may be needed; do not exceed 16 mg/kg/day or 60 mg/day
- Adults: 10-30 mg/dose every 6-8 hours

I.V.:

- Children: 0.01-0.1 mg/kg slow IVP over 10 minutes; maximum dose: 1 mg

(Continued)

Propranolol Hydrochloride *(Continued)*

Adults: 1 mg/dose slow IVP; repeat every 5 minutes up to a total of 5 mg

Hypertension: Oral:

Children: Initial: 0.5-1 mg/kg/day in divided doses every 6-12 hours; increase gradually every 3-7 days; usual dose: 1-5 mg/kg/day

Adults: Initial: 40 mg twice daily or 60-80 mg once daily as sustained release capsules; increase dosage every 3-7 days; usual dose: ≤320 mg divided in 2-3 doses/day or once daily as sustained release; maximum daily dose: 640 mg

Migraine headache prophylaxis: Oral:

Children: 0.6-1.5 mg/kg/day **or**

≤35 kg: 10-20 mg 3 times/day

>35 kg: 20-40 mg 3 times/day

Adults: Initial: 80 mg/day divided every 6-8 hours; increase by 20-40 mg/dose every 3-4 weeks to a maximum of 160-240 mg/day given in divided doses every 6-8 hours

Tetralogy spells: Children:

Oral: 1-2 mg/kg/dose every 6 hours as needed

I.V.: 0.15-0.25 mg/kg/dose slow IVP; may repeat in 15 minutes

Thyrotoxicosis:

Neonates: Oral: 2 mg/kg/day in divided doses every 6-12 hours; occasionally higher doses may be required

Adolescents and Adults: Oral: 10-40 mg/dose every 6 hours

Adults: I.V.: 1-3 mg/dose slow IVP as a single dose

Administration I.V. administration should not exceed 1 mg/minute for adults; administer slow I.V. over 10 minutes in children

Monitoring Parameters EKG and blood pressure

Reference Range Therapeutic: 50-100 ng/mL (SI: 190-390 nmol/L) at end of dose interval

Nursing Implications I.V. dose much smaller than oral dose; propranolol may block hypoglycemia induced tachycardia and blood pressure changes

Additional Information Not significantly removed by hemodialysis; not indicated for hypertensive emergencies; do not abruptly discontinue therapy, taper dosage gradually over 2 weeks

Dosage Forms

Capsule, sustained action: 60 mg, 80 mg, 120 mg, 160 mg

Injection: 1 mg/mL (1 mL)

Solution, oral (strawberry-mint flavor): 4 mg/mL (5 mL, 500 mL); 8 mg/mL (5 mL, 500 mL)

Solution, oral, concentrate: 80 mg/mL (30 mL)

Tablet: 10 mg, 20 mg, 40 mg, 60 mg, 80 mg, 90 mg

References

Lai CW, Ziegler DK, Lansky LL, et al, "Hemiplegic Migraine in Childhood: Diagnostic and Therapeutic Aspects," *J Pediatr*, 1982, 101(5):696-9.

Pickoff AS, Zies L, Ferrer PL, et al, "High-Dose Propranolol Therapy in the Management of Supraventricular Tachycardia," *J Pediatr*, 1979, 94(1):144-6.

2-Propylpentanoic Acid *see* Valproic Acid and Derivatives *on page 592*

Propylthiouracil (proe pill thye oh yoor' a sill)

Synonyms PTU

Therapeutic Category Antithyroid Agent

Use Treatment of hyperthyroidism

Pregnancy Risk Factor D

Contraindications Hypersensitivity to propylthiouracil or any component

Adverse Reactions

Cardiovascular: Edema, cutaneous vasculitis, periarteritis

Central nervous system: Drowsiness, neuritis, vertigo, headache

Dermatologic: Rash, urticaria, pruritus, exfoliative dermatitis, abnormal hair loss, skin pigmentation

Gastrointestinal: Nausea, vomiting, loss of taste

Hematologic: Agranulocytosis, thrombocytopenia, bleeding, hypoprothrombinemia

Hepatic: Jaundice, hepatitis
Musculoskeletal: Arthralgia
Renal & genitourinary: Nephritis
Respiratory: Interstitial pneumonitis
Miscellaneous: Drug fever

Drug Interactions Anticoagulants

Mechanism of Action Inhibits the synthesis of thyroid hormones by interfering with the incorporation of iodine

Pharmacodynamics For significant therapeutic effects 24-36 hours are required and remissions of hyperthyroidism do not usually occur before 4 months of continued therapy

Pharmacokinetics
Metabolism: Hepatic
Half-life: 1-2 hours

Usual Dosage Oral:
Neonates: 5-10 mg/kg/day in divided doses every 8 hours

Children: 5-7 mg/kg/day in divided doses every 8 hours **or**
6-10 years: 50-150 mg/day divided every 8 hours
>10 years: 150-300 mg/day divided every 8 hour
Maintenance: ⅓-⅔ of the initial dose in divided doses every 8-12 hours; this begins usually after 2 months on an effective initial dosage

Adults: Initial: 300-450 mg/day in divided doses every 8 hours (doses of 600-1200 mg/day are sometimes needed); maintenance: 100-150 mg/day in divided doses every 8-12 hours

Dosing adjustment in renal impairment: Children and Adults:
Cl_{cr} 10-50 mL/minute: Decrease recommended dosage by 25%
Cl_{cr} <10 mL/minute: Decrease recommended dosage by 50%

Monitoring Parameters CBC with differential, liver function tests, platelets, thyroid function tests

Test Interactions ↑ prothrombin time (S)

Dosage Forms Tablet: 50 mg

References

Raby C, Lagorce JF, Jambut-Absil AC, et al, "The Mechanism of Action of Synthetic Antithyroid Drugs: Iodine Complexation During Oxidation of Iodide," *Endocrinology*, 1990, 126(3):1683-91.

2-Propylvaleric Acid *see* Valproic Acid and Derivatives *on page 592*

Prorex® *see* Promethazine Hydrochloride *on page 488*

Pro-Sof® [OTC] *see* Docusate *on page 202*

Prostaglandin E_1 *see* Alprostadil *on page 32*

Prostaphlin® *see* Oxacillin Sodium *on page 425*

Prostigmin® *see* Neostigmine *on page 410*

Prostin VR Pediatric® *see* Alprostadil *on page 32*

Protamine Sulfate (proe' ta meen)

Therapeutic Category Antidote, Heparin

Use Treatment of heparin overdosage; neutralize heparin during surgery or dialysis procedures

Pregnancy Risk Factor C

Contraindications Hypersensitivity to protamine or any component

Precautions Use with caution in patients allergic to fish, with prior history of vasectomy, or receiving protamine-containing insulin or previous protamine therapy

Adverse Reactions
Cardiovascular: Hypotension, bradycardia, flushing
Central nervous system: Lassitude
Gastrointestinal: Nausea, vomiting
Respiratory: Pulmonary hypertension, dyspnea
Miscellaneous: Hypersensitivity reactions

Stability Refrigerate

Mechanism of Action Combines with strongly acidic heparin to form a stable complex (salt) neutralizing the anticoagulant activity of both drugs

(Continued)

Protamine Sulfate *(Continued)*

Pharmacodynamics Onset of action: Heparin neutralization occurs within 5 minutes following I.V. injection

Pharmacokinetics Elimination: Unknown

Usual Dosage Protamine dosage is determined by the dosage of heparin; 1 mg of protamine neutralizes 90 USP units of heparin (lung) and 115 USP units of heparin (intestinal); maximum dose: 50 mg

In the situation of heparin overdosage, since blood heparin concentrations decrease rapidly **after** heparin administration, adjust the protamine dosage depending upon the duration of time since heparin administration as follows (see table):

Protamine Sulfate

Time Elapsed	Dose of Protamine (mg) to Neutralize 100 units of Heparin
Immediate	1–1.5
30–60 min	0.5–0.75
>2 h	0.25–0.375

If heparin administered by deep S.C. injection, use 1-1.5 mg protamine per 100 units heparin; this may be done by a portion of the dose (eg, 25-50 mg) given slowly I.V. followed by the remaining portion as a continuous infusion over 8-16 hours (the expected absorption time of the S.C. heparin dose)

Administration Reconstitute vial with 5 mL sterile water; if using protamine in neonates, reconstitute with preservative-free sterile water for injection; resulting solution equals 10 mg/mL; inject without further dilution over 1-3 minutes; maximum of 50 mg in any 10-minute period

Monitoring Parameters APTT or ACT

Additional Information Heparin rebound associated with anticoagulation and bleeding has been reported to occur occasionally; symptoms typically occur 8-9 hours after protamine administration, but may occur as long as 18 hours later

Dosage Forms Injection: 10 mg/mL (5 mL, 10 mL, 25 mL)

Prothazine-DC® *see* Promethazine and Codeine *on page 486*

Protilase® *see* Pancrelipase *on page 431*

Protirelin (proe tye' re lin)

Brand Names Relefact® TRH; Thypinone®

Synonyms Lopremone

Therapeutic Category Diagnostic Agent, Thyroid Function

Use Adjunct in the diagnostic assessment of thyroid function, and an adjunct to other diagnostic procedures in assessment of patients with pituitary or hypothalamic dysfunction; also causes release of prolactin from the pituitary and is used to detect defective control of prolactin secretion.

Pregnancy Risk Factor C

Contraindications Hypersensitivity to protirelin additives

Warnings Monitor blood pressure frequently during and 15 minutes after administration

Adverse Reactions

Cardiovascular: Marked changes in blood pressure – hypotension or hypertension, sweating, chest tightness

Central nervous system: Lightheadedness, anxiety, seizures (rare)

Gastrointestinal: Nausea, bad taste in mouth, abdominal discomfort, dry mouth

Renal & genitourinary: Urge to urinate

Drug Interactions Aspirin, levodopa, T_3, T_4, pharmacologic doses of steroids

Mechanism of Action Increase release of thyroid stimulating hormone from the anterior pituitary

Pharmacodynamics Peak TSH levels occur in 20-30 minutes; TSH returns to baseline after about 3 hours

Pharmacokinetics Mean plasma half-life: 5 minutes

Usual Dosage I.V.:

Children: 7 μg/kg to a maximum dose of 500 μg

Adults: 500 μg (range 200-500 μg)

Administration Administer undiluted direct I.V. over 15-30 seconds with the patient remaining supine for an additional 15 minutes

Monitoring Parameters Blood pressure, prolactin, TSH, T_4 and T_3

Nursing Implications Keep patient supine during drug administration

Dosage Forms Injection: 500 μg/mL (1 mL)

Protopam® *see* Pralidoxime Chloride *on page 473*

Protostat® *see* Metronidazole *on page 383*

Protropin® *see* Human Growth Hormone *on page 288*

Proventil® *see* Albuterol *on page 26*

Provera® *see* Medroxyprogesterone Acetate *on page 359*

Proxigel® [OTC] *see* Carbamide Peroxide *on page 103*

Proxymetacaine *see* Proparacaine Hydrochloride *on page 490*

Prozac® *see* Fluoxetine Hydrochloride *on page 259*

Pseudoephedrine (soo doe e fed' rin)

Related Information

OTC Cold Preparations, Pediatric *on page 723-726*

Brand Names Afrinol® [OTC]; Cenafed® [OTC]; Decofed® Syrup [OTC]; Drixoral® Non-Drowsy [OTC]'; Neofed® [OTC]; Novafed®; PediaCare® Oral; Sudafed® [OTC]; Sudafed® 12 Hour [OTC]; Sufedrin® [OTC]

Synonyms *d*-Isoephedrine Hydrochloride; Pseudoephedrine Hydrochloride; Pseudoephedrine Sulfate

Therapeutic Category Adrenergic Agonist Agent; Decongestant; Sympathomimetic

Use Temporary symptomatic relief of nasal congestion due to common cold, upper respiratory allergies, and sinusitis; also promotes nasal or sinus drainage

Pregnancy Risk Factor C

Contraindications Hypersensitivity to pseudoephedrine or any component; MAO inhibitor therapy, severe hypertension, severe coronary artery disease

Precautions Use with caution in patients with hyperthyroidism, diabetes mellitus, prostatic hypertrophy, mild-moderate hypertension, arrhythmias

Adverse Reactions

Cardiovascular: Tachycardia, palpitations, arrhythmias

Central nervous system: Nervousness, excitability, dizziness, insomnia, tremor, drowsiness, headache

Gastrointestinal: Nausea, vomiting

Drug Interactions MAO inhibitors, alpha and beta blocking agents, other sympathomimetics, methyldopa, reserpine

Mechanism of Action Directly stimulates alpha-adrenergic receptors of respiratory mucosa causing vasoconstriction; directly stimulates beta-adrenergic receptors causing bronchial relaxation, increased heart rate and contractility

Pharmacodynamics

Onset of action: Oral: Decongestant effects occur within 15-30 minutes

Duration: 4-6 hours (up to 12 hours with extended release formulation administration)

Pharmacokinetics

Metabolism: Incompletely metabolized in liver to inactive metabolite

Elimination: 55% to 75% of a dose excreted unchanged in urine

Usual Dosage Oral:

Children:

<2 years: 4 mg/kg/day in divided doses every 6 hours

2-5 years: 15 mg every 6 hours; maximum: 60 mg/24 hours

6-12 years: 30 mg every 6 hours; maximum: 120 mg/24 hours

Children >12 years and Adults: 60 mg every 6 hours; maximum: 240 mg/24 hours **or** extended release product: 120 mg every 12 hours

(Continued)

Pseudoephedrine *(Continued)*

Dosage Forms

Capsule: 60 mg

Capsule, timed release, as hydrochloride: 120 mg

Drops, oral, as hydrochloride: 7.5 mg/0.8 mL (15 mL)

Liquid, as hydrochloride: 15 mg/5 mL (120 mL); 30 mg/5 mL (120 mL, 240 mL, 473 mL)

Tablet, as hydrochloride: 30 mg, 60 mg

Tablet, timed release, as hydrochloride: 120 mg

Tablet, extended release, as sulfate: 120 mg

Pseudoephedrine and Triprolidine *see* Triprolidine and Pseudoephedrine *on page 586*

Pseudoephedrine Hydrochloride *see* Pseudoephedrine *on previous page*

Pseudoephedrine Sulfate *see* Pseudoephedrine *on previous page*

Pseudomonic Acid A *see* Mupirocin *on page 397*

psoriGel® [OTC] *see* Coal Tar *on page 147*

P&S® Shampoo [OTC] *see* Salicylic Acid *on page 516*

Psyllium (sill' i yum)

Brand Names Effer-Syllium® [OTC]; Fiberall® [OTC]; Hydrocil® [OTC]; Konsyl® [OTC]; Konsyl-D® [OTC]; Metamucil® [OTC]; Metamucil® Instant Mix [OTC]; Modane® Bulk [OTC]; Perdiem® Plain [OTC]; Reguloid® [OTC]; Serutan® [OTC]; Siblin® [OTC]; Syllact® [OTC]; V-Lax® [OTC]

Synonyms Plantago Seed; Plantain Seed; Psyllium Hydrophilic Mucilloid

Therapeutic Category Laxative, Bulk-Producing

Use Treatment of chronic atonic or spastic constipation and in constipation associated with rectal disorders; management of irritable bowel syndrome

Pregnancy Risk Factor C

Contraindications Fecal impaction, GI obstruction; hypersensitivity to psyllium

Warnings Drink a full glass of liquid with each dose; for phenylketonurics, products may contain aspartame

Adverse Reactions

Gastrointestinal: Esophageal or bowel obstruction, diarrhea, constipation, abdominal cramps

Respiratory: Bronchospasm

Miscellaneous: Rhinoconjunctivitis, anaphylaxis upon inhalation in susceptible individuals

Mechanism of Action Adsorbs water in the intestine to form a viscous liquid which promotes peristalsis and reduces transit time

Pharmacodynamics

Onset of action: 12-24 hours

Peak effect: May take 2-3 days

Pharmacokinetics Absorption: Oral: Generally not absorbed, small amounts of grain extracts present in the preparation have been reportedly absorbed following colonic hydrolysis

Usual Dosage Oral:

Children 6-11 years: Approximately ½ the adult dose; ½-1 rounded teaspoonful in 4 oz glass of liquid 1-3 times/day

Adults: 1-2 rounded teaspoonfuls or 1-2 packets or 1-2 wafers in 8 oz glass of liquid 1-4 times/day

Patient Information Must be mixed in a glass of water or juice; drink a full glass of liquid with each dose

Nursing Implications Inhalation of psyllium dust may cause sensitivity to psyllium (runny nose, watery eyes, wheezing)

Additional Information 3.4 g psyllium hydrophilic mucilloid/7 g powder is equivalent to a rounded teaspoonful or 1 packet

Dosage Forms

Granules: 4.03 g per rounded teaspoon (100 g, 250 g); 2.5 g per rounded teaspoon

Powder: Psyllium 50% and dextrose 50% (6.5 g, 325 g, 420 g, 480 g, 500 g)

Powder:

Effervescent: 3 g per dose (270 g, 480 g); 3.4 g per dose (single-dose packets)
Psyllium hydrophilic: 3.4 g/per rounded teaspoon (210 g, 300 g, 420 g, 630 g)
Squares, chewable: 1.7 g, 3.4 g
Wafers: 3.4 g

Psyllium Hydrophilic Mucilloid *see* Psyllium *on previous page*

P.T.E.-4® *see* Trace Metals *on page 574*

P.T.E.-5® *see* Trace Metals *on page 574*

Pteroylglutamic Acid *see* Folic Acid *on page 262*

PTU *see* Propylthiouracil *on page 494*

Purge® [OTC] *see* Castor Oil *on page 109*

Purinethol® *see* Mercaptopurine *on page 365*

Pyrantel Pamoate (pi ran' tel)

Brand Names Antiminth® [OTC]; Pin-Rid® [OTC]; Pin-X® [OTC]; Reese's® Pinworm Medicine [OTC]

Therapeutic Category Anthelmintic

Use Roundworm, pinworm, and hookworm infestations, and trichostrongyliasis

Pregnancy Risk Factor C

Contraindications Known hypersensitivity to pyrantel pamoate

Precautions Use with caution in patients with liver impairment, anemia, malnutrition

Adverse Reactions

Central nervous system: Dizziness, weakness, drowsiness, insomnia, headache, fever
Dermatologic: Rash
Gastrointestinal: Nausea, vomiting, anorexia, diarrhea, abdominal cramps, tenesmus
Hepatic: Elevated liver enzymes

Drug Interactions Piperazine (antagonist)

Stability Protect from light

Mechanism of Action Causes neuromuscular paralysis of susceptible helminths

Pharmacokinetics

Absorption: Oral: Poorly absorbed
Metabolism: Undergoes partial hepatic metabolism
Peak serum levels: Within 1-3 hours
Elimination: Excreted in the feces (50% as unchanged drug) and the urine (7% as unchanged drug)

Usual Dosage Children and Adults: Oral:

Roundworm, pinworm, or trichostrongyliasis: 11 mg/kg administered as a single dose; maximum dose is 1 g; dosage should be repeated in 2 weeks for pinworm infection
Hookworm: 11 mg/kg/day once daily for 3 days

Monitoring Parameters Stool for presence of eggs, worms, and occult blood; serum AST and ALT

Patient Information May mix drug with milk or fruit juice

Nursing Implications Shake well before pouring to assure accurate dosage

Additional Information Purgation is not required prior to use

Dosage Forms

Capsule: 180 mg
Liquid: 50 mg/mL (30 mL); 144 mg/mL (30 mL)
Suspension, oral (caramel-currant flavor): 50 mg/mL (60 mL)

Pyrazinamide (peer a zin' a mide)

Synonyms Pyrazinoic Acid Amide

Therapeutic Category Antitubercular Agent

Use Used in combination with other antituberculosis agents in the treatment of tuberculosis

Pregnancy Risk Factor C

Contraindications Severe hepatic damage; hypersensitivity to pyrazinamide or any component

(Continued)

Pyrazinamide *(Continued)*

Precautions Use with caution in patients with renal failure, gout, or diabetes mellitus

Adverse Reactions

Central nervous system: Malaise, fever
Dermatologic: Urticaria, rash, photosensitivity
Endocrine & metabolic: Gout, hyperuricemia
Gastrointestinal: Nausea, vomiting, anorexia
Hepatic: Hepatotoxicity (increased incidence with doses >30 mg/kg/day), jaundice
Musculoskeletal: Arthralgia

Drug Interactions Isoniazid (↓ INH serum levels)

Mechanism of Action Converted to pyrazinoic acid in susceptible strains of *Mycobacterium* which lowers the pH of the environment

Pharmacokinetics

Absorption: Oral: Well absorbed
Distribution: Widely distributed into body tissues and fluids including the liver, lung, and CSF
Metabolism: Metabolized in the liver
Protein binding: 50%
Half-life: 9-10 hours, prolonged with reduced renal or hepatic function
Peak serum levels: Within 2 hours
Elimination: Excreted in the urine (4% as unchanged drug)

Usual Dosage Oral:

Children: 15-40 mg/kg/day in divided doses every 12-24 hours; daily dose not to exceed 2 g; **or** directly observed therapy of 50-70 mg/kg/dose twice weekly to a maximum of 2 g/dose

Adults: 15-30 mg/kg/day in 3-4 divided doses; maximum daily dose: 2 g/day

Monitoring Parameters Periodic liver function tests, serum uric acid

Dosage Forms Tablet: 500 mg

References

American Academy of Pediatrics, Committee on Infectious Diseases, "Chemotherapy for Tuberculosis in Infants and Children," *Pediatrics*, 1992, 89(1):161-5.
Starke JR, "Modern Approach to the Diagnosis and Treatment of Tuberculosis in Children," *Pediatr Clin North Am*, 1988, 35(3):441-64.
Starke JR, "Multidrug Therapy for Tuberculosis in Children," *Pediatr Infect Dis J*, 1990, 9(11):785-93.

Pyrazinoic Acid Amide *see* Pyrazinamide *on previous page*

Pyridiate® *see* Phenazopyridine Hydrochloride *on page 449*

2-Pyridine Aldoxime Methochloride *see* Pralidoxime Chloride *on page 473*

Pyridium® *see* Phenazopyridine Hydrochloride *on page 449*

Pyridostigmine Bromide (peer id oh stig' meen)

Related Information

Overdose and Toxicology Information *on page 696-700*

Brand Names Mestinon®; Regonol®

Therapeutic Category Antidote, Neuromuscular Blocking Agent; Cholinergic Agent

Use Symptomatic treatment of myasthenia gravis by improving muscle strength; reversal of effects of nondepolarizing neuromuscular blocking agents

Pregnancy Risk Factor C

Contraindications Hypersensitivity to pyridostigmine, bromides, or any component; GI or GU obstruction

Precautions Use with caution in patients with epilepsy, asthma, bradycardia, hyperthyroidism, arrhythmias, recent coronary occlusion, vagotonia, or peptic ulcer

Adverse Reactions

Cardiovascular: Sweating, bradycardia, hypotension
Central nervous system: Headache
Dermatologic: Rash

Gastrointestinal: Nausea, vomiting, diarrhea, increased peristalsis, abdominal cramps, salivation
Local: Thrombophlebitis (after I.V. administration)
Musculoskeletal: Muscle cramps, weakness
Ocular: Miosis
Respiratory: Increased bronchial secretions, bronchospasm

Drug Interactions Succinylcholine or other depolarizing neuromuscular blockers, atropine (direct antagonist)

Stability Protect oral solution from light

Mechanism of Action Competitively inhibits destruction of acetylcholine by acetylcholinesterase which facilitates transmission of impulses across myoneural junction producing generalized cholinergic responses such as miosis, increase tonus of skeletal and intestinal musculature, bronchial and ureteral constriction, bradycardia, and increased salivary and sweat gland production

Pharmacodynamics
Onset of action:
- Oral: 30-45 minutes
- I.M.: 15 minutes
- I.V.: Within 2-5 minutes

Duration:
- Oral: 3-6 hours
- I.V.: 2-3 hours

Pharmacokinetics
Absorption: Oral: Very poor (10% to 20%) from the GI tract; sustained release products may release up to $\frac{1}{3}$ of a dose immediately after ingestion and the remainder over 8-12 hours
Metabolism: Metabolized in the liver and at tissue site by cholinesterases

Usual Dosage Myasthenia gravis (dosage should be adjusted so patient takes larger doses prior to time of greatest fatigue):
Oral:
- Neonates: 5 mg every 4-6 hours
- Children: 7 mg/kg/day in 5-6 divided doses
- Adults: Initial: 60 mg 3 times/day with maintenance dose ranging from 60 mg to 1.5 g/day (incremental increases every 48 hours or more if needed)

I.M., I.V.:
- Neonates and Children: 0.05-0.15 mg/kg/dose (maximum single dose: 10 mg)
- Adults: 2 mg every 2-3 hours (or 1/30th of oral dose)

Reversal of nondepolarizing neuromuscular blocker: I.V.:
- Children: 0.1-0.25 mg/kg/dose preceded by atropine or glycopyrrolate
- Adults: 10-20 mg preceded by atropine or glycopyrrolate

Administration Give direct I.V. slowly over 2-4 minutes; patients receiving large parenteral doses should be pretreated with atropine

Monitoring Parameters Muscle strength, heart rate, vital capacity

Additional Information Atropine should be readily available during dosage adjustments; large parenteral doses should be accompanied by parenteral atropine; ephedrine sulfate and potassium chloride have been used orally (in adult patients) to improve response; extended release products are preferred for use **only** at bedtime for patients who are very weak upon arising

Dosage Forms
Injection: 5 mg/mL (2 mL, 5 mL)
Syrup (raspberry flavor): 60 mg/5 mL (480 mL)
Tablet: 60 mg
Tablet, sustained release: 180 mg

Pyridoxine Hydrochloride (peer i dox' een)

Brand Names Beesix®; Nestrex®

Synonyms Vitamin B_6

Therapeutic Category Antidote, Cycloserine Toxicity; Antidote, Hydralazine Toxicity; Antidote, Isoniazid Toxicity; Vitamin, Water Soluble

Use Prevent and treat vitamin B_6 deficiency, pyridoxine-dependent seizures in infants, treatment of drug-induced deficiency (eg, isoniazid or hydralazine)

(Continued)

Pyridoxine Hydrochloride *(Continued)*

Pregnancy Risk Factor A (C if dose exceeds RDA recommendation)

Contraindications Hypersensitivity to pyridoxine or any component

Adverse Reactions

Central nervous system: Paresthesia, sensory neuropathy (after chronic administration of large doses), seizures (following I.V. administration of very large doses), headache

Gastrointestinal: Nausea

Hematologic: Decreased serum folic acid concentration

Hepatic: Increased AST

Local: Burning or stinging at injection site

Respiratory: Respiratory distress

Miscellaneous: Allergic reactions have been reported

Drug Interactions Levodopa (when used without carbidopa), phenobarbital, phenytoin

Mechanism of Action Precursor to pyridoxal, which functions as a cofactor in the metabolism of proteins, carbohydrates, and fats; pyridoxal also aids in the release of liver and muscle stored glycogen and in the synthesis of GABA (within the CNS) and heme

Pharmacokinetics

Absorption: Readily absorbed from GI tract

Metabolism: Converted to pyridoxal (active form in liver)

Half-life, biologic: 15-20 days

Elimination: Excretion by liver metabolism

Usual Dosage

Pyridoxine-dependent infants:

- Oral: 2-100 mg/day
- I.M., I.V., S.C.: 10-100 mg

Dietary deficiency: Oral:

- Children: 5-25 mg/24 hours for 3 weeks, then 1.5-2.5 mg/day in multivitamin product
- Adults: 10-20 mg/day for 3 weeks

Drug induced neuritis (eg, isoniazid, hydralazine, penicillamine, cycloserine): Oral:

- Children: 10-50 mg/24 hours; prophylaxis: 1-2 mg/kg/24 hours
- Adults: 100-200 mg/24 hours; prophylaxis: 25-100 mg/24 hours

Recommended daily allowance:

- Children:
  - 1-3 years: 0.9 mg
  - 4-6 years: 1.3 mg
  - 7-10 years: 1.6 mg
- Children >10 years and Adults: 1.6-2 mg

Administration Give slow I.V.

Monitoring Parameters When administering large I.V. doses, monitor respiratory rate, heart rate, and blood pressure

Additional Information

For the treatment of seizures and/or coma from acute isoniazid toxicity, a dose of pyridoxine hydrochloride equal to the amount of INH ingested can be given I.M./I.V. in divided doses together with other anticonvulsants

For the treatment of acute hydrazine toxicity, pyridoxine 25 mg/kg/dose I.M./I.V. has been used

Dosage Forms

Injection: 100 mg/mL (10 mL, 30 mL)

Tablet: 25 mg, 50 mg, 100 mg

Tablet, extended release: 100 mg

Pyrimethamine (peer i meth' a meen)

Brand Names Daraprim®

Therapeutic Category Antimalarial Agent

Use Prophylaxis of malaria due to susceptible strains of plasmodia; used in conjunction with quinine and sulfadiazine for the treatment of uncomplicated attacks of chloroquine-resistant *P. falciparum* malaria; used in conjunction with fast-acting schizonticide to initiate transmission control and suppression cure; synergistic combination with sulfonamide in treatment of toxoplasmosis

Pregnancy Risk Factor C

Contraindications Megaloblastic anemia; known hypersensitivity to pyrimethamine, chloroguanide; resistant malaria and patients with seizure disorders

Precautions Use with caution in patients with impaired renal or hepatic function, in patients with possible folate deficiency

Adverse Reactions

Cardiovascular: Shock

Central nervous system: Ataxia, tremor, seizures, fever, fatigue

Dermatologic: Rash, photosensitivity

Gastrointestinal: Anorexia, abdominal cramps, vomiting, atrophic glossitis

Hematologic: Megaloblastic anemia, leukopenia, thrombocytopenia, agranulocytosis, pancytopenia

Renal & genitourinary: Hematuria

Respiratory: Respiratory failure

Miscellaneous: Pulmonary eosinophilia, folic acid deficiency

Drug Interactions Para-aminobenzoic acid, sulfonamides

Mechanism of Action Inhibits parasitic dihydrofolate reductase resulting in inhibition of tetrahydrofolic acid synthesis

Pharmacokinetics

Absorption: Oral: Well absorbed

Distribution: V_d: Adults: 2.9 L/kg; appears in breast milk

Protein binding: 80%

Half-life: 54-148 hours

Peak serum levels: Within 1.5-8 hours

Usual Dosage Oral:

Malaria chemoprophylaxis (for areas where chloroquine-resistant *P. falciparum* exists): Begin prophylaxis 2 weeks before entering endemic area:

Children: 0.5 mg/kg once weekly; not to exceed 25 mg/dose

or

Children:

<4 years: 6.25 mg once weekly

4-10 years: 12.5 mg once weekly

Children >10 years and Adults: 25 mg once weekly

Dosage should be continued for all age groups for at least 6-10 weeks after leaving endemic areas

Chloroquine-resistant *P. falciparum* malaria (when used in conjunction with quinine and sulfadiazine):

Children:

<10 kg: 6.25 mg/day once daily for 3 days

10-20 kg: 12.5 mg/day once daily for 3 days

20-40 kg: 25 mg/day once daily for 3 days

Adults: 25 mg twice daily for 3 days

Toxoplasmosis (with sulfadiazine or trisulfapyrimidines):

Children: 2 mg/kg/day divided every 12 hours for 3 days followed by 1 mg/kg/day once daily or divided twice daily for 4 weeks given with trisulfapyrimidines or sulfadiazine

Adults: 50-75 mg/day together with 1-4 g of a sulfonamide for 1-3 weeks depending on patient's tolerance and response, then reduce dose by 50% and continue for 4-5 weeks **or** 25-50 mg/day for 3-4 weeks

Monitoring Parameters CBC including platelet counts

Patient Information Take with meals to minimize vomiting; notify physician if rash, sore throat, pallor, or glossitis occurs

Additional Information Leucovorin may be given in a dosage of 3-9 mg/day for 3 days, or 5 mg every 3 days, or as required to reverse symptoms or to prevent hematologic problems due to folic acid deficiency

Dosage Forms Tablet: 25 mg

Extemporaneous Preparation(s) Pyrimethamine tablets may be crushed to prepare oral suspensions of the drug in water, cherry syrup or sucrose-containing solutions at a concentration of 1 mg/mL; stable at room temperature for 5-7 days

References

Van Voorhis WC, "Therapy and Prophylaxis of Systemic Protozoan Infections," *Drugs*, 1990, 40(2):176-202.

Quelicin® *see* Succinylcholine Chloride *on page 537*

Queltuss® [OTC] *see* Guaifenesin and Dextromethorphan *on page 279*

Questran® *see* Cholestyramine Resin *on page 132*

Questran® Light *see* Cholestyramine Resin *on page 132*

Quibron®-T *see* Theophylline *on page 554*

Quibron®-T/SR *see* Theophylline *on page 554*

Quiess® *see* Hydroxyzine *on page 298*

Quinacrine Hydrochloride (kwin' a kreen)

Brand Names Atabrine® Hydrochloride

Synonyms Mepacrine Hydrochloride

Therapeutic Category Anthelmintic; Antimalarial Agent

Use Treatment of giardiasis; alternative treatment of cestodiasis (tapeworm); reserve agent for suppression and chemoprophylaxis of malaria

Pregnancy Risk Factor C

Contraindications Hypersensitivity to quinacrine or any component; patients receiving primaquine

Precautions Use with caution in patients with renal, cardiac, hepatic disease; patients with a history of psychosis; patients with psoriasis or porphyria; hemolysis may occur in patients with G-6-PD deficiency

Adverse Reactions

Central nervous system: Dizziness, psychosis, restlessness, confusion, seizures, headache

Dermatologic: Urticaria, black skin and nail pigmentation, exfoliative dermatitis

Gastrointestinal: Nausea, vomiting, diarrhea, abdominal cramps

Hematologic: Blood dyscrasias

Hepatic: Hepatitis

Ocular: Retinopathy, corneal deposits

Renal & genitourinary: Brown coloring of urine

Drug Interactions Quinacrine ↑ serum primaquine concentrations (↑ toxicity), alcohol (disulfiram-like reaction), hepatotoxic drugs

Mechanism of Action Binds to parasite's DNA by intercalation between adjacent base pairs inhibiting replication and protein synthesis

Pharmacokinetics

Absorption: Oral: Well absorbed

Distribution: Crosses the placenta; appears in breast milk; distributes into pancreas, lungs, muscle; extremely high concentrations achieved in the liver

Protein binding: 90%

Metabolism: Slowly metabolized

Half-life: 120 hours

Peak serum levels: Within 1-3 hours

Elimination: Excreted principally in the urine with secondary elimination in saliva, bile, sweat and milk; 11% of a dose is excreted unchanged in urine

Usual Dosage Oral:

Children:

Dwarf tapeworm: Take ½ tablespoon (15 g) of sodium or magnesium sulfate the night before administration of quinacrine

4-8 years: 200 mg stat, 100 mg before breakfast for 3 days

8-10 years: 300 mg stat, 100 mg twice daily for 3 days

11-14 years: 400 mg stat, 100 mg 3 times/day for 3 days

Tapeworm (beef, pork, or fish): Take 300 mg of sodium bicarbonate with each dose to reduce nausea and vomiting

5-10 years: 100 mg every 10 minutes for 4 doses

11-14 years: 200 mg every 10 minutes for 3 doses

Giardiasis: 6 mg/kg/day in 3 divided doses for 5-7 days; maximum dose: 300 mg/day

Suppression of malaria: ≤8 years: 50 mg/day, continue for 1-3 months; for endemic areas, drug therapy should be started 2 weeks before arrival and continued for 3-4 weeks after departure

Adults:

Dwarf tapeworm: Take 1 tablespoon (30 g) of sodium or magnesium sulfate the night before administration of quinacrine; 900 mg in 3 divided doses 20 minutes apart followed by a saline cathartic $1\frac{1}{2}$ hours later, then 100 mg 3 times/day for 3 days.

Tapeworm (beef, pork, or fish): 200 mg every 10 minutes for 4 doses; take 600 mg of sodium bicarbonate with each dose to reduce nausea and vomiting

Giardiasis: 100 mg 3 times/day for 5-7 days

Suppression of malaria: >8 years: 100 mg/day, continue for 1-3 months; for endemic areas, drug therapy should be started 2 weeks before arrival and continued for 3-4 weeks after departure

Monitoring Parameters CBC, periodic ophthalmologic examinations, liver function tests, stool for worm segments

Patient Information May discolor urine and skin; for treatment of giardiasis or malaria, take after meals with a full glass of water or fruit juice; report to physician any visual disturbances, skin rash, or mental aberrations during therapy

Nursing Implications Pulverized tablets are bitter tasting; for treatment of tapeworms, restrict patient to a bland, nonfat diet 1-2 days before treatment; patient should fast the evening before; a saline cathartic should be given 1-2 hours after quinacrine use for cestodiasis to expel the worms for examination

Dosage Forms Tablet: 100 mg

Quinaglute® Dura-Tabs® *see* Quinidine *on this page*

Quinalan® *see* Quinidine *on this page*

Quinamm® *see* Quinine Sulfate *on page 507*

Quinidex® Extentabs® *see* Quinidine *on this page*

Quinidine (kwin' i deen)

Brand Names Cardioquin®; Quinaglute® Dura-Tabs®; Quinalan®; Quinidex® Extentabs®; Quinora®

Synonyms Quinidine Gluconate; Quinidine Polygalacturonate; Quinidine Sulfate

Therapeutic Category Antiarrhythmic Agent, Class Ia

Use Prophylaxis after cardioversion of atrial fibrillation and/or flutter to maintain normal sinus rhythm; also used to prevent reoccurrence of paroxysmal supraventricular tachycardia, paroxysmal A-V junctional rhythm, paroxysmal ventricular tachycardia, paroxysmal atrial fibrillation, and atrial or ventricular premature contractions; also has activity against *Plasmodium falciparum* malaria

Pregnancy Risk Factor C

Contraindications Patients with complete A-V block with an A-V junctional or idioventricular pacemaker; patients with intraventricular conduction defects (marked widening of QRS complex); patients with cardiac-glycoside induced A-V conduction disorders; hypersensitivity to the drug or cinchona derivatives

Warnings May cause syncope, most likely due to ventricular tachycardia or fibrillation; syncope may subside spontaneously, but occasionally may be fatal; discontinue quinidine if syncope occurs

Precautions Myocardial depression, sick-sinus syndrome, incomplete A-V block, cardiac glycoside intoxication, hepatic and/or renal insufficiency, myasthenia gravis; hemolysis may occur in patients with G-6-PD (glucose-6-phosphate dehydrogenase) deficiency; quinidine-induced hepatotoxicity, including granulomatous hepatitis, increased serum AST and alkaline phosphatase concentrations, and jaundice may occur; use with caution in nursing women

Adverse Reactions

Cardiovascular: Syncope, hypotension, tachycardia, heart block, ventricular fibrillation, vascular collapse, severe hypotension with rapid I.V. administration

Central nervous system: Fever, headache

Dermatologic: Angioedema, rash

Gastrointestinal: GI disturbances, nausea, vomiting, cramps

Hematologic: Blood dyscrasias, thrombotic thrombocytopenic purpura

Respiratory: Respiratory depression

Miscellaneous: Cinchonism (nausea, tinnitus, headache, impaired hearing or vision, vomiting, abdominal pain, vertigo, confusion, delirium, syncope)

(Continued)

Quinidine *(Continued)*

Drug Interactions Quinidine potentiates nondepolarizing and depolarizing muscle relaxants; verapamil, amiodarone, alkalinizing agents, and cimetidine may ↑ quinidine serum concentrations; phenobarbital, phenytoin, and rifampin may decrease quinidine serum concentrations; quinidine may increase plasma concentration of digoxin, closely monitor digoxin concentrations, digoxin dosage may need to be reduced (by one-half) when quinidine is initiated, new steady-state digoxin plasma concentrations occur in 5-7 days; beta blockers + quinidine → ↑ bradycardia; quinidine may enhance coumarin anticoagulants.

Stability Do not use discolored parenteral solution

Mechanism of Action Class IA antiarrhythmic with anticholinergic, local anesthetic, and mild negative inotropic effects; depresses phase O of the action potential; decreases myocardial excitability, conduction velocity, and myocardial contractility by decreasing sodium influx during depolarization and potassium efflux in repolarization; also reduces calcium transport across cell membrane

Pharmacokinetics

Distribution: V_d: Adults: 2-3.5 L/kg, decreased V_d with congestive heart failure, malaria; increased V_d with cirrhosis; crosses the placenta; appears in breast milk

Protein-binding:
- Newborns: 60% to 70%
- Adults: 80% to 90%
- Decreased protein-binding with cyanotic congenital heart disease, cirrhosis, or acute myocardial infarction

Metabolism: Extensive in the liver (50% to 90%) to inactive compounds

Bioavailability:
- Sulfate: 80%
- Gluconate: 70%

Half-life, plasma:
- Children: 2.5-6.7 hours
- Adults: 6-8 hours; increased half-life with elderly, cirrhosis, and congestive heart failure

Elimination: Excretion in the urine (15% to 25% as unchanged drug)

Usual Dosage Note: Dose expressed in terms of the salt: 267 mg of quinidine gluconate = 275 mg of quinidine polygalacturonate = 200 mg of quinidine sulfate

Children: Test dose for idiosyncratic reaction (sulfate, oral or gluconate, I.M.): 2 mg/kg or 60 mg/m^2
- Oral (quinidine sulfate): 15-60 mg/kg/day in 4-5 divided doses or 6 mg/kg every 4-6 hours (AMA 1991); usual: 30 mg/kg/day or 900 mg/m^2/day given in 5 daily doses
- I.V. **not** recommended (quinidine gluconate): 2-10 mg/kg/dose every 3-6 hours as needed

Adults: Test dose: 200 mg administered several hours before full dosage (to determine possibility of idiosyncratic reaction)
- Oral (sulfate): 100-600 mg/dose every 4-6 hours; begin at 200 mg/dose and titrate to desired effect
- Oral (gluconate): 324-972 mg every 8-12 hours
- Oral (polygalacturonate): 275 mg every 8-12 hours
- I.M.: 400 mg/dose every 4-6 hours
- I.V.: 200-400 mg/dose diluted and given at a rate ≤10 mg/minute

Children and Adults: Dosing adjustment in renal impairment: Cl_{cr} <10 mL/minute: Administer 75% of normal dose

Administration I.V.: Maximum rate of infusion: 10 mg/minute

Monitoring Parameters Complete blood counts, liver and renal function tests, and serum concentrations should be routinely performed during long-term administration

Reference Range Optimal therapeutic level is method dependent; Therapeutic: 2-7 μg/mL (SI: 6.2-15.4 μmol/L); Toxic: >8 μg/mL (SI: >18 μmol/L).

Nursing Implications Do not crush sustained release product; patients should notify their physician if fever, rash, unusual bruising or bleeding, visual disturbances, or ringing in the ears occur

Dosage Forms

Injection, as gluconate: 80 mg/mL (10 mL)

Tablet, as polygalacturonate: 275 mg

Tablet, as sulfate: 200 mg, 300 mg
Tablet:
Sustained action, as sulfate: 300 mg
Sustained release, as gluconate: 324 mg

Extemporaneous Preparation(s) A 10 mg/mL quinidine sulfate solution can be made with six (6) 200 mg capsules, 12-15 mL ethanol, and citric acid syrup USP to a total amount of 120 mL

Handbook in Extemporaneous Formulations, Bethesda, MD: American Society of Hospital Pharmacists, 1987.

References

Pickoff AS, Singh S and Gelband H, *The Medical Management of Cardiac Arrhythmias in Cardiac Arrhythmias in the Neonate, Infant and Child*, Roberts NK and Gelbard H, ed, Norwalk, CT: Appleton-Century-Crofts, 1983.

Szefler SJ, Pieroni DR, Gingell RL, et al, "Rapid Elimination of Quinidine in Pediatric Patients," *Pediatrics*, 1982, 70(3):370-5.

Quinidine Gluconate *see* Quinidine *on page 505*

Quinidine Polygalacturonate *see* Quinidine *on page 505*

Quinidine Sulfate *see* Quinidine *on page 505*

Quinine Sulfate (kwye' nine)

Brand Names Legatrin® [OTC]; Quinamm®; Quiphile®; Q-vel®

Therapeutic Category Antimalarial Agent

Use Suppression or treatment of chloroquine-resistant *P. falciparum* malaria; treatment of *Babesia microti* infection; prevention and treatment of nocturnal recumbency leg muscle cramps

Pregnancy Risk Factor D

Contraindications Tinnitus, optic neuritis, G-6-PD deficiency, hypersensitivity to quinine or any component, history of black water fever, pregnancy

Precautions Use with caution in patients with cardiac arrhythmias (quinine has quinidine-like activity), in patients with myasthenia gravis, and in patients with impaired liver function

Adverse Reactions

Cardiovascular: Flushing of the skin, anginal symptoms
Central nervous system: Fever
Dermatologic: Rash, pruritus
Endocrine & metabolic: Hypoglycemia
Gastrointestinal: Nausea, vomiting, epigastric pain
Hematologic: Hemolysis, thrombocytopenia
Hepatic: Hepatitis
Ocular: Visual disturbances,
Otic: Tinnitus, impaired hearing
Miscellaneous: Hypersensitivity reactions, cinchonism

Drug Interactions Cardiac glycosides, cimetidine (prolongs half-life of quinine), aluminum-containing antacids (decreases quinine absorption), neuromuscular blocking agents, oral anticoagulants, urinary alkalinizers (may increase quinine toxicity)

Stability Protect from light

Mechanism of Action Depresses oxygen uptake and carbohydrate metabolism; intercalates into DNA, disrupting the parasite's replication and transcription; affects calcium distribution within muscle fibers and decreases the excitability of the motor end-plate region

Pharmacokinetics

Absorption: Oral: Readily absorbed, mainly from the upper small intestine
Metabolism: Metabolized primarily in the liver
Protein binding: 70% to 90%
Half-life:
Children: 6-12 hours
Adults: 8-14 hours
Peak serum levels: Within 1-3 hours after a dose
Elimination: Excreted in the bile and saliva with <5% excreted unchanged in the urine
Not effectively removed by peritoneal dialysis, removed by hemodialysis

(Continued)

Quinine Sulfate *(Continued)*

Usual Dosage Oral:

Children:

Treatment of chloroquine-resistant malaria: 25 mg/kg/day in divided doses every 8 hours for 3-7 days in conjunction with another agent

Babesiosis: 25 mg/kg/day, (up to a maximum of 650 mg/dose) divided every 8 hours for 7 days

Adults:

Treatment of chloroquine-resistant malaria: 650 mg every 8 hours for 3-7 days in conjunction with another agent

Suppression of malaria: 325 mg twice daily and continued for 6 weeks after exposure

Babesiosis: 650 mg every 6-8 hours for 7 days

Leg cramps: 200-300 mg at bedtime

Monitoring Parameters CBC with platelet count, liver function tests, blood glucose, ophthalmologic examination

Patient Information Report to physician if tinnitus, hearing loss, rash, or visual disturbances occur during therapy

Nursing Implications Do not crush tablets or capsule to avoid bitter taste

Additional Information Parenteral form of quinine (dihydrochloride) is no longer available from the CDC; quinidine gluconate should be used instead

Dosage Forms

Capsule: 64.8 mg, 65 mg, 200 mg, 300 mg, 325 mg

Tablet: 162.5 mg, 260 mg

Quinora® *see* Quinidine *on page 505*

Quinsana® Plus [OTC] *see* Undecylenic Acid and Derivatives *on page 590*

Quiphile® *see* Quinine Sulfate *on previous page*

Q-vel® *see* Quinine Sulfate *on previous page*

Rabies Immune Globulin, Human *see* Immunization Guidelines *on page 660-667*

Rabies Virus Vaccine, Human Diploid *see* Immunization Guidelines *on page 660-667*

Racemic Epinephrine *see* Epinephrine *on page 220*

Ranitidine Hydrochloride (ra nye' te deen)

Related Information

Medications Compatible With PN Solutions *on page 649-650*

Brand Names Zantac®

Therapeutic Category Histamine-2 Antagonist

Use Short-term treatment of active duodenal ulcers and benign gastric ulcers; long-term prophylaxis of duodenal ulcer and gastric hypersecretory states; gastroesophageal reflux (GER)

Pregnancy Risk Factor B

Contraindications Hypersensitivity to ranitidine or any component

Precautions Use with caution in patients with liver and renal impairment; dosage modification required in patients with renal impairment

Adverse Reactions

Cardiovascular: Bradycardia, tachycardia

Central nervous system: Dizziness, sedation, malaise, mental confusion, headache

Dermatologic: Rash

Endocrine & metabolic: Gynecomastia

Gastrointestinal: Constipation, nausea, vomiting

Hematologic: Thrombocytopenia, aplastic anemia (rare)

Hepatic: Hepatitis

Musculoskeletal: Arthralgias

Renal & genitourinary: Increase in serum creatinine

Drug Interactions Warfarin, procainamide, tricyclic antidepressants, theophylline, oral midazolam, ketoconazole, antacids

Stability Stable for 48 hours at room temperature or 30 days when frozen in D_5W or NS; stable for 24 hours in TPN solutions; stable for 12 hours in TPN with lipids

Mechanism of Action Competitive inhibition of histamine at H_2 receptors of the gastric parietal cells, which inhibits gastric acid secretion

Pharmacokinetics

Distribution: Minimally penetrates the blood-brain barrier, appears in breast milk

Protein binding: 15%

Metabolism: Metabolized in the liver

Bioavailability: Oral: ~50%

Half-life:

- Children 3.5-16 years: 1.8-2 hours
- Adults:
  - Normal renal and hepatic function: 2-2.5 hours
  - Decreased renal function: 8.7 hours

Time to peak serum levels: Oral: 1-3 hours

Elimination: Excreted primarily in the urine (35% of oral dose or 70% of I.V. dose as unchanged drug) and in bile

Slightly dialyzable (5% to 20%)

Usual Dosage

Children:

- Oral: 1.25-2.5 mg/kg/dose every 12 hours; maximum: 300 mg/day
- I.M., I.V.: 0.75-1.5 mg/kg/dose every 6-8 hours; usual dose: 0.8-3.2 mg/kg/day divided every 6-8 hours; maximum: 6 mg/kg/day or 300 mg/day
- Continuous infusion: 0.1-0.25 mg/kg/hour (preferred for stress ulcer prophylaxis in patients with concurrent maintenance I.V.s or TPNs)

Adults:

- Treatment of duodenal or gastric ulcers, GER: Oral: 150 mg/dose twice daily or 300 mg at bedtime
- Prophylaxis of recurrent duodenal ulcer: Oral: 150 mg at bedtime
- Gastric hypersecretory conditions: Oral: 150 mg twice daily, up to 6 g/day
- I.M., I.V.: 50 mg/dose every 6-8 hours (dose not to exceed 400 mg/day)
- Continuous I.V. infusion: 150 mg over 24 hours or 6.25 mg/hour titrated to gastric pH
  - Gastric hypersecretory conditions: Doses up to 2.5 mg/kg/hour (220 mg/hour) have been used

Dosing interval in renal impairment:

- Oral: Cl_{cr} <50 mL/minute: Administer every 24 hours
- I.V.: Cl_{cr} <50 mL/minute: Administer every 18-24 hours

Administration Intermittent infusion preferred over direct injection to decrease risk of bradycardia; for intermittent infusion, infuse over 15-30 minutes, at a usual concentration of 0.5 mg/mL; for direct I.V. injection, administer over a period not less than 5 minutes at a final concentration not to exceed 2.5 mg/mL

Monitoring Parameters AST, ALT, serum creatinine; when used to prevent stress-related GI bleeding, measure the intragastric pH and try to maintain pH >4

Test Interactions False-positive urine protein using Multistix®

Additional Information Causes fewer CNS adverse reactions and drug interactions compared to cimetidine; safety and efficacy of full-dose therapy extending beyond 8 weeks have not been determined

Dosage Forms

Infusion, preservative free: 0.5 mg/mL in ½ NS (100 mL)

Injection: 25 mg/mL (2 mL, 10 mL, 40 mL)

Syrup (peppermint flavor): 15 mg/mL (473 mL)

Tablet: 150 mg, 300 mg

References

Blumer JL, Rothstein FC, Kaplan BS, et al, "Pharmacokinetic Determination of Ranitidine Pharmacodynamics in Pediatric Ulcer Disease," *J Pediatr*, 1985, 107(2):301-6.

Eddleston JM, Booker PD, and Green JR, "Use of Ranitidine in Children Undergoing Cardiopulmonary Bypass," *Crit Care Med*, 1989, 17(1):26-9.

Lopez-Herce J, Albajara L, Codoceo R, et al, "Ranitidine Prophylaxis in Acute Gastric Mucosal Damage in Critically Ill Pediatric Patients," *Crit Care Med*, 1988, 16(6):591-93.

Morris DL, Markham SJ, Beechey A, et al, "Ranitidine-Bolus or Infusion Prophylaxis for Stress Ulcer," *Crit Care Med*, 1988, 16(3):229-32.

Roberts CJ, "Clinical Pharmacokinetics of Ranitidine," *Clin Pharmacokinet*, 1984, 9(3):211-21.

Redisol® *see* Cyanocobalamin *on page 160*

Reese's® Pinworm Medicine [OTC] *see* Pyrantel Pamoate *on page 499*

Regitine® *see* Phentolamine Mesylate *on page 452*

Reglan® *see* Metoclopramide Hydrochloride *on page 381*

Regonol® *see* Pyridostigmine Bromide *on page 500*

Regular [Concentrated] Iletin® II U-500 *see* Insulin Preparations *on page 311*

Regular Iletin® I *see* Insulin Preparations *on page 311*

Reguloid® [OTC] *see* Psyllium *on page 498*

Relaxadon® *see* Hyoscyamine, Atropine, Scopolamine and Phenobarbital *on page 299*

Relefact® TRH *see* Protirelin *on page 496*

Relief® Ophthalmic Solution *see* Phenylephrine Hydrochloride *on page 453*

Remular-S® *see* Chlorzoxazone *on page 132*

Resectisol® *see* Mannitol *on page 355*

Respbid® *see* Theophylline *on page 554*

Retin-A™ *see* Tretinoin *on page 578*

Retinoic Acid *see* Tretinoin *on page 578*

Retrovir® *see* Zidovudine *on page 608*

Reversol® *see* Edrophonium Chloride *on page 217*

Rezine® *see* Hydroxyzine *on page 298*

R-Gen® *see* Iodinated Glycerol *on page 317*

R-Gene® *see* Arginine Hydrochloride *on page 57*

rGM-CSF *see* Sargramostim *on page 517*

Rhesonativ® *see* Rh_o(D) Immune Globulin *on this page*

Rheumatrex® *see* Methotrexate *on page 374*

Rhinall® Nasal Solution [OTC] *see* Phenylephrine Hydrochloride *on page 453*

Rh_o(D) Immune Globulin

Brand Names HypRho®-D; HypRho®-D Mini-Dose; MICRhoGAM™; Mini-Gamulin® Rh; Rhesonativ®; RhoGAM™

Therapeutic Category Immune Globulin

Use To prevent isoimmunization in Rh-negative individuals exposed to Rh-positive blood during delivery of an Rh-positive infant, as a result of an abortion, following amniocentesis or abdominal trauma, or following a transfusion accident; to prevent hemolytic disease of the newborn if there is a subsequent pregnancy with an Rh-positive fetus

Pregnancy Risk Factor C

Contraindications Rh_o(D)-positive patient; known hypersensitivity to immune globulins or to thimerosal; transfusion of Rh_o(D)-positive blood in previous 3 months; prior sensitization to Rh_o(D)

Warnings Do not inject I.V.; do not administer to the neonate

Precautions Use with caution in patients with thrombocytopenia or bleeding disorders, patients with IgA deficiency

Adverse Reactions

Central nervous system: Lethargy, fever
Gastrointestinal: Splenomegaly
Hepatic: Elevated bilirubin
Local: Pain at the injection site
Musculoskeletal: Myalgia

Drug Interactions Live virus vaccines (Rh_o(D) may interfere with immune response to measles, mumps, rubella)

Stability Refrigerate; may be stable for up to 30 days at room temperature; avoid freezing

Mechanism of Action Suppresses the immune response and antibody formation of Rh-negative individuals to Rh-positive red blood cells

Pharmacokinetics

Distribution: Appears in breast milk, however not absorbed by the nursing infant

Half-life: 23-26 days

Usual Dosage Adults: I.M.:

Obstetrical usage: 1 vial (300 μg) prevents maternal sensitization if fetal packed red blood cell volume that has entered the circulation is <15 mL; if it is more, give additional vials. The number of vials = RBC volume of the calculated fetomaternal hemorrhage divided by 15 mL

Postpartum prophylaxis: 300 μg within 72 hours of delivery

Antepartum prophylaxis: 300 μg at approximately 26-28 weeks gestation; followed by 300 μg within 72 hours of delivery if infant is Rh-positive

Following miscarriage, abortion, or termination of ectopic pregnancy at up to 13 weeks of gestation: 50 μg ideally within 3 hours, but may be given up to 72 hours after; if pregnancy has been terminated at 13 or more weeks of gestation, administer 300 μg within 72 hours

Nursing Implications Administer I.M. preferably in the anterolateral aspects of the upper thigh or the deltoid muscle of the upper arm. The total volume can be given in divided doses at different sites at one time or may be divided and given at intervals, provided the total dosage is given within 72 hours of the fetomaternal hemorrhage or transfusion.

Dosage Forms

Injection: Each package contains one single dose 300 μg of Rh_o (D) immune globulin

Injection, microdose: Each package contains one single dose of microdose, 50 μg of Rh_o (D) immune globulin

RhoGAM™ *see* Rh_o(D) Immune Globulin *on previous page*

Rhulicaine® [OTC] *see* Benzocaine *on page 77*

Ribavirin (rye ba vye' rin)

Brand Names Virazole®

Synonyms RTCA; Tribavirin

Therapeutic Category Antiviral Agent, Inhalation Therapy

Use Treatment of patients with respiratory syncytial virus (RSV) infections; may also be used in other viral infections including influenza A and B and adenovirus; specially indicated for treatment of severe lower respiratory tract RSV infections in patients with an underlying compromising condition (prematurity, bronchopulmonary dysplasia, congenital heart disease, immunodeficiency, and immunosuppression)

Pregnancy Risk Factor X

Contraindications Females of childbearing age

Warnings Ribavirin is potentially mutagenic, tumor-promoting, and gonadotoxic; there is evidence that ribavirin is teratogenic in small animals

Precautions Use with caution in patients requiring assisted ventilation because precipitation of the drug in the respiratory equipment may interfere with safe and effective patient ventilation; also monitor carefully in patients with COPD and asthma for deterioration of respiratory function

Adverse Reactions

Cardiovascular: Hypotension, cardiac arrest

Dermatologic: Rash, skin irritation

Hematologic: Anemia

Ocular: Conjunctivitis

Respiratory: Mild bronchospasm, worsening of respiratory function

Drug Interactions Zidovudine (ribavirin antagonizes the antiviral activity of zidovudine)

Stability Reconstituted solution is stable for 24 hours at room temperature

Mechanism of Action Inhibits replication of RNA and DNA viruses; inhibits influenza virus RNA polymerase activity and inhibits the initiation and elongation of RNA fragments resulting in inhibition of viral protein synthesis

Pharmacokinetics

Absorption: Absorbed systemically from the respiratory tract following nasal and oral inhalation; absorption is dependent upon respiratory fac-

(Continued)

Ribavirin *(Continued)*

tors and method of drug delivery; maximal absorption occurs with the use of the aerosol generator via an endotracheal tube

Distribution: Highest concentrations are found in the respiratory tract and erythrocytes

Metabolism: Occurs intracellularly and may be necessary for drug action

Half-life:

Respiratory tract secretions: ~2 hours

Plasma:

Children: 6.5-11 hours

Adults: 24 hours; half-life is much longer in the erythrocyte (16-40 days), which can be used as a marker for intracellular metabolism

Peak levels: Within 60-90 minutes after administration

Elimination: Hepatic metabolism is the major route of elimination with 40% of the drug cleared renally as unchanged drug and metabolites

Usual Dosage Infants, Children, and Adults: Aerosol inhalation:

Use with Viratek® small particle aerosol generator (SPAG-2) at a concentration of 20 mg/mL (6 g reconstituted with 300 mL of sterile water without preservatives)

Aerosol only:

Continuous aerosolization: 12-18 hours/day for 3 days, or up to 7 days in length

Intermittent aerosolization (high-dose, short-duration aerosol): 2 g over 2 hours 3 times/day at a concentration of 60 mg/mL (6 g reconstituted with 100 mL of sterile water without preservatives) in **nonventilated** patients for 3-7 days has been used to permit easier accessibility for patient care and limit environmental exposure of health care workers

Monitoring Parameters Respiratory function, hemoglobin, reticulocyte count, CBC, I & O

Nursing Implications Health care workers who are pregnant or who may become pregnant should be advised of the potential risks of exposure and counseled about risk reduction strategies including alternate job responsibilities; ribavirin may adsorb to contact lenses

Additional Information RSV season is usually December to April; viral shedding period for RSV is usually 3-8 days

Dosage Forms Powder for aerosol: 6 g (100 mL)

References

American Academy of Pediatrics Committee on Infectious Diseases, "Ribavirin Therapy of Respiratory Syncytial Virus," *Pediatrics*, 1987, 79(3):475-8.

Englund JA, Piedra PA, Jefferson LS, et al, "High-Dose, Short-Duration Ribavirin Aerosol Therapy in Children With Suspected Respiratory Syncytial Virus Infection," *J Pediatr*, 1990, 117(2 Pt 1):313-20.

Janai HK, Marks MI, Zaleska M, et al, "Ribavirin: Adverse Drug Reactions 1986 to 1988," *Pediatr Infect Dis J*, 1990, 9(3):209-11.

Smith DW, Frankel LR, Mathers LH, et al, "A Controlled Trial of Aerosolized Ribavirin in Infants Receiving Mechanical Ventilation for Severe Respiratory Syncytial Virus Infection," *N Engl J Med*, 1991, 325(1):24-9.

Riboflavin (rye' boe flay vin)

Synonyms Lactoflavin; Vitamin B_2; Vitamin G

Therapeutic Category Vitamin, Water Soluble

Use Prevent riboflavin deficiency and treat ariboflavinosis

Pregnancy Risk Factor A (C if dose exceeds RDA recommendation)

Drug Interactions Probenecid

Mechanism of Action Converted to co-enzymes which act as hydrogen-carrier molecules, which are necessary for normal tissue respiration; also needed for activation of pyridoxine and conversion of tryptophan to niacin

Pharmacokinetics

Absorption: Readily absorbed via GI tract, however, food increases extent of GI absorption; GI absorption is decreased in patients with hepatitis, cirrhosis, or biliary obstruction

Metabolism: Metabolic fate is unknown

Half-life, biologic: 66-84 minutes

Elimination: 9% eliminated unchanged in urine

Usual Dosage Oral:

Riboflavin deficiency:

Children: 2.5-10 mg/day in divided doses

Adults: 5-30 mg/day in divided doses

Recommended daily allowance:

Children: 0.4-1.8 mg

Adults: 1.2-1.7 mg

Monitoring Parameters CBC and reticulocyte counts (if anemic when treating deficiency)

Test Interactions Large doses may interfere with urinalysis based on spectrometry; may cause false elevations in fluorometric determinations of catecholamines and urobilinogen

Patient Information Take with food; large doses may cause bright yellow urine

Dosage Forms Tablet: 25 mg, 50 mg, 100 mg

Rid-A-Pain® [OTC] *see* Benzocaine *on page 77*

Ridaura® *see* Auranofin *on page 67*

Rifabutin

Brand Names Mycobutin®

Synonyms Ansamycin

Therapeutic Category Antibiotic, Miscellaneous; Antitubercular Agent

Use Prevention of disseminated *Mycobacterium avium* complex (MAC) in patients with advanced HIV infection

Pregnancy Risk Factor B

Contraindications Hypersensitivity to rifabutin or any other rifamycin; rifabutin is contraindicated in patients with a WBC <1000/mm^3 or a platelet count <50,000 mm^3

Warnings Rifabutin as a single agent must not be administered to patients with active tuberculosis since its use may lead to the development of tuberculosis that is resistant to both rifabutin and rifampin; rifabutin should be discontinued in patients with AST >500 IU/L or if total bilirubin is >3 mg/dL

Precautions Use with caution in patients with liver impairment; modification of dosage should be considered in patients with renal impairment

Adverse Reactions

Central nervous system: Fever, headache, seizures, confusion

Dermatologic: Rash

Gastrointestinal: Abdominal pain, diarrhea, dyspepsia, nausea, vomiting, taste perversion

Hematologic: Thrombocytopenia, anemia, leukopenia, neutropenia

Hepatic: Elevated liver enzymes

Musculoskeletal: Arthralgia

Ocular: Uveitis

Renal & genitourinary: Discolored urine

Drug Interactions May decrease the serum concentration or effect of dapsone, narcotics, anticoagulants, corticosteroids, cyclosporine, quinidine, and oral contraceptives

Mechanism of Action Inhibits DNA-dependent RNA polymerase at the beta subunit which prevents chain initiation

Pharmacokinetics

Absorption: Oral: Readily absorbed

Distribution: Distributes to body tissues including the lungs, liver, spleen, eyes, and kidneys

Protein binding: 85%

Metabolism: Metabolized to an active and inactive metabolites

Half life, terminal: 45 hours (range: 16-69 hours)

Peak serum level: Occurs in 2-4 hours

Elimination: Renal and biliary clearance of unchanged drugs is 10%; 30% excreted in the feces

Usual Dosage Oral:

Children: Efficacy and safety of rifabutin has not been established in children; a limited number of HIV-positive children with MAC (n=22) have been given rifabutin for MAC prophylaxis; doses of 5 mg/kg/day have been useful

Adults: 300 mg once daily; for patients who experience gastrointestinal upset, rifabutin can be administered 150 mg twice daily with food

(Continued)

Rifabutin *(Continued)*

Monitoring Parameters Periodic liver function tests, CBC with differential, platelet count, hemoglobin, hematocrit

Patient Information May discolor skin, urine, tears, perspiration, or other body fluids to a brown orange color; soft contact lenses may be permanently stained

Dosage Forms Capsule: 150 mg

Extemporaneous Preparation(s) Rifabutin is insoluble in water and ethanol; prepare powder packets or compound with a suspending agent and shake well before using

References

Krause PH, Hight DW, Schwartz AN, et al, "Successful Management of *Mycobacterium* Intracellulare Pneumonia in a Child," *Pediatr Infect Dis*, 1986, 5:269-71.

Levin RH and Bolinger AM, "Treatment of Nontuberculous Mycobacterial Infections in in Pediatric Patients," *Clin Pharm*, 1988, 7:545-51.

Rifadin® *see* Rifampin *on this page*

Rifampicin *see* Rifampin *on this page*

Rifampin (rif' am pin)

Brand Names Rifadin®; Rimactane®

Synonyms Rifampicin

Therapeutic Category Antibiotic, Miscellaneous; Antitubercular Agent

Use Management of active tuberculosis; eliminate meningococci from asymptomatic carriers; prophylaxis of *Haemophilus influenzae* type B infection

Pregnancy Risk Factor C

Contraindications Hypersensitivity to rifampin or any component

Precautions Use with caution in patients with liver impairment; modification of dosage should be considered in patients with severe liver impairment

Adverse Reactions

Central nervous system: Drowsiness, fatigue, ataxia, confusion, fever, headache

Dermatologic: Rash, pruritus

Gastrointestinal: Nausea, vomiting, diarrhea, stomatitis

Hematologic: Eosinophilia, blood dyscrasias (leukopenia, thrombocytopenia)

Hepatic: Hepatitis

Local: Irritation at the I.V. site

Renal & genitourinary: Renal failure

Respiratory: Flu-like syndrome

Drug Interactions Rifampin induces liver enzymes which may ↓ the plasma concentration of the following drugs: verapamil, methadone, digoxin, cyclosporine, corticosteroids, oral anticoagulants, theophylline, barbiturates, chloramphenicol, ketoconazole, oral contraceptives, quinidine; halothane

Stability Reconstituted I.V. solution is stable for 24 hours at room temperature; once the reconstituted I.V. solution is further diluted in D_5W (preferably) or normal saline, the preparation should be used within 4 hours

Mechanism of Action Inhibits bacterial RNA synthesis by binding to the beta subunit of DNA-dependent RNA polymerase, blocking RNA transcription

Pharmacokinetics

Absorption: Oral: Well absorbed

Distribution: Highly lipophilic; crosses the blood-brain barrier and is widely distributed into body tissues and fluids

Protein binding: 80%

Metabolism: Undergoes enterohepatic recycling; metabolized in the liver

Half-life: 3-4 hours, prolonged with hepatic impairment

Peak serum levels: Within 2-4 hours after oral administration; food may delay or slightly reduce peak serum level

Elimination: Principally excreted in the feces (60% to 65%) and urine (~30%)

Plasma rifampin concentrations are not significantly affected by hemodialysis or peritoneal dialysis

Usual Dosage Oral (I.V. infusion dose is the same as for the oral route):

Tuberculosis:

Children: 10-20 mg/kg/day in divided doses every 12-24 hours

Adults: 10 mg/kg/day; maximum: 600 mg/day

American Thoracic Society and CDC currently recommend twice weekly therapy as part of a short-course regimen which follows 1-2 months of daily treatment of uncomplicated pulmonary tuberculosis in the compliant patient

Children: 10-20 mg/kg/dose (up to 600 mg) twice weekly under supervision to ensure compliance

Adults: 10 mg/kg (up to 600 mg) twice weekly

H. influenza prophylaxis:

Neonates <1 month: 10 mg/kg/day every 24 hours for 4 days

Infants and Children: 20 mg/kg/day every 24 hours for 4 days, not to exceed 600 mg/dose

Adults: 600 mg every 24 hours for 4 days

Meningococcal prophylaxis:

<1 month: 10 mg/kg/day in divided doses every 12 hours for 2 days

Infants and Children: 20 mg/kg/day in divided doses every 12 hours for 2 days

Adults: 600 mg every 12 hours for 2 days

Nasal carriers of *Staphylococcus aureus*:

Children: 15 mg/kg/day divided every 12 hours for 5-10 days in combination with other antibiotics

Adults: 600 mg every 12 hours for 5-10 days in combination with other antibiotics

Administration Administer I.V. preparation once daily by slow I.V. infusion over 30 minutes to 3 hours at a final concentration not to exceed 6 mg/mL

Monitoring Parameters Periodic monitoring of liver function (AST, ALT); bilirubin, CBC

Patient Information May discolor urine, tears, sweat, or other body fluids to a red-orange color; take one hour before or two hours after a meal on an empty stomach; soft contact lenses may be permanently stained

Nursing Implications The compounded oral suspension must be shaken well before using

Dosage Forms

Capsule: 150 mg, 300 mg

Powder for injection: 600 mg (contains a sulfite)

Extemporaneous Preparation(s) Rifampin oral suspension can be compounded with simple syrup or wild cherry syrup at a concentration of 10 mg/mL; the suspension is stable for 4 weeks at room temperature or in a refrigerator when stored in a glass amber prescription bottle. However, there are some experts who do not recommend using rifampin syrup formulated from capsules due to conflicting reports indicating that the product is unstable (30% of labeled potency after preparation).

References

American Academy of Pediatrics Committee on Infectious Diseases, "Chemotherapy for Tuberculosis in Infants and Children," *Pediatrics*, 1992, 89(1):161-5.

Starke JR, "Modern Approach to the Diagnosis and Treatment of Tuberculosis in Children," *Pediatr Clin North Am*, 1988, 35(3):441-64.

Starke JR, "Multidrug Therapy for Tuberculosis in Children," *Pediatr Infect Dis J*, 1990, 9(11):785-93.

rIFN-α *see* Interferon Alfa-2a *on page 314*

rIFN-α2 *see* Interferon Alfa-2b *on page 315*

Rimactane® *see* Rifampin *on previous page*

Riopan® [OTC] *see* Antacid Preparations *on page 53*

Ritalin® *see* Methylphenidate Hydrochloride *on page 378*

RMS® *see* Morphine Sulfate *on page 394*

Robafen® [OTC] *see* Guaifenesin *on page 278*

Robaxin® *see* Methocarbamol *on page 372*

Robaxisal® *see* Methocarbamol *on page 372*

Robicillin® VK *see* Penicillin V Potassium *on page 442*

Robinul® *see* Glycopyrrolate *on page 274*

Robitet® *see* Tetracycline Hydrochloride *on page 552*

Robitussin® [OTC] *see* Guaifenesin *on page 278*

Robitussin® A-C *see* Guaifenesin and Codeine *on page 279*

Robitussin-DM® [OTC] *see* Guaifenesin and Dextromethorphan *on page 279*

Robomol® *see* Methocarbamol *on page 372*

Rocaltrol® *see* Calcitriol *on page 93*

Rocephin® *see* Ceftriaxone Sodium *on page 117*

Roferon-A® *see* Interferon Alfa-2a *on page 314*

Rogaine® *see* Minoxidil *on page 390*

Rolaids® Calcium Rich [OTC] *see* Calcium Carbonate *on page 94*

Rondec® Drops *see* Carbinoxamine and Pseudoephedrine *on page 105*

Rondec® Filmtab® *see* Carbinoxamine and Pseudoephedrine *on page 105*

Rondec® Syrup *see* Carbinoxamine and Pseudoephedrine *on page 105*

Rondec-TR® *see* Carbinoxamine and Pseudoephedrine *on page 105*

Roxanol™ *see* Morphine Sulfate *on page 394*

Roxanol SR™ *see* Morphine Sulfate *on page 394*

RTCA *see* Ribavirin *on page 511*

Rubella Virus Vaccine, Live *see* Immunization Guidelines *on page 660-667*

Rubex® *see* Doxorubicin Hydrochloride *on page 208*

Rubidomycin Hydrochloride *see* Daunorubicin Hydrochloride *on page 172*

Rubramin-PC® *see* Cyanocobalamin *on page 160*

Rufen® *see* Ibuprofen *on page 300*

Rum-K® *see* Potassium Chloride *on page 469*

Ru-Vert-M® *see* Meclizine Hydrochloride *on page 358*

RWJ17070 *see* Histrelin *on page 286*

Sal-Acid® *see* Salicylic Acid *on this page*

Salbutamol *see* Albuterol *on page 26*

Saleto-200® [OTC] *see* Ibuprofen *on page 300*

Saleto-400® *see* Ibuprofen *on page 300*

Salicylazosulfapyridine *see* Sulfasalazine *on page 543*

Salicylic Acid (sal i sill' ik)

Brand Names Keralyt®; Mediplast® [OTC]; Panscol® [OTC]; Paplex®; P&S® Shampoo [OTC]; Sal-Acid®; Trans-Ver-Sal® [OTC]

Therapeutic Category Keratolytic Agent

Use Use topically for its keratolytic effect in controlling seborrheic dermatitis or psoriasis of body and scalp, dandruff, and other scaling dermatoses; also used to remove warts, corns, calluses

Pregnancy Risk Factor C

Contraindications Hypersensitivity to salicylic acid or any other listed ingredients; children <2 years of age

Warnings Should not be used systemically due to severe irritating effect on GI mucosa; prolonged use over large areas, especially in children, may result in salicylate toxicity; do not apply on irritated, reddened, or infected skin

Precautions For external use only; avoid contact with eyes, face, and other mucous membranes

Adverse Reactions

Dermatologic: Facial scarring, erythema, scaling

Local: Irritation, burning

Mechanism of Action Produces desquamation of hyperkeratotic epithelium; increases hydration of the stratum corneum causing the skin to swell, soften, and desquamate

Pharmacokinetics

Absorption: Percutaneous absorption

Peak serum levels: Within 5 hours when applied with an occlusive dressing

Elimination: Salicyluric acid (52%), salicylate glucuronides (42%), and salicylic acid (6%) are the major metabolites identified in urine after percutaneous absorption

Usual Dosage Children and Adults: Topical:

Lotion, cream, gel: Apply a thin layer to the affected area once or twice daily

Plaster: Cut to size that covers the corn or callus, apply and leave in place for 48 hours; do not exceed 5 applications over a 14-day period

Shampoo: Initial: Use daily or every other day; 1-2 treatments/week will usually maintain control

Solution: Apply a thin layer directly to wart using brush applicator once daily as directed for 1 week or until the wart is removed

Monitoring Parameters Signs and symptoms of salicylate toxicity: Nausea, vomiting, dizziness, tinnitus, loss of hearing, lethargy, diarrhea, psychic disturbances

Patient Information When applying in concentrations of >10%, protect surrounding normal tissue with petrolatum

Nursing Implications For warts: Before applying product, soak area in warm water for 5 minutes; dry area thoroughly, then apply medication

Dosage Forms

Cream: 2% (30 g); 2.5% (30 g); 10% (60 g)

Gel: 5% (60 g); 6% (30 g); 17% (7.5 g)

Liquid: 13.6% (9.3 mL); 17% (9.3 mL, 13.5 mL, 15 mL); 16.7% (15 mL)

Lotion: 2% (177 mL)

Ointment: 25% (60 g, 454 g); 40% (454 g); 60% (60 g)

Plaster: 15% (6 mm, 12 mm); 40%

Pledgets: 0.5%; 2%

Shampoo: 2% (120 mL, 240 mL); 4% (120 mL)

Salicylic Acid and Sulfur *see* Sulfur and Salicylic Acid *on page 545*

Salt Poor Albumin *see* Albumin Human *on page 25*

Sandimmune® *see* Cyclosporine *on page 164*

Sandoglobulin® *see* Immune Globulin, Intravenous *on page 307*

Sandostatin® *see* Octreotide Acetate *on page 422*

Sani-Supp® [OTC] *see* Glycerin *on page 273*

Sargramostim (sar gram' oh stim)

Brand Names Leukine™; Prokine™

Synonyms GM-CSF; Granulocyte Macrophage Colony Stimulating Factor; rGM-CSF

Therapeutic Category Colony Stimulating Factor

Use Myeloid reconstitution after autologous bone marrow transplantation; to accelerate myeloid recovery in patients with non-Hodgkin's lymphoma, Hodgkin's lymphoma, and acute lymphoblastic leukemia undergoing autologous BMT; to accelerate myeloid engraftment following chemotherapy

Pregnancy Risk Factor C

Contraindications Excessive leukemic myeloid blasts in bone marrow or peripheral blood ≥10%; history of idiopathic thrombocytopenic purpura; known hypersensitivity to GM-CSF, yeast derived products, or any component

Precautions Use with caution in patients with autoimmune or chronic inflammatory disease, hypertension, cardiovascular disease, pulmonary disease, or renal or hepatic impairment

(Continued)

Sargramostim *(Continued)*

Rapid increase in peripheral blood counts: If ANC >20,000/mm^3 or platelets >500,000/mm^3, decrease dose by 50% or discontinue drug (counts will fall to normal within 3-7 days after discontinuing drug)

Growth factor potential: Caution with myeloid malignancies; do **not** administer within 24 hours prior to or after chemotherapy or 12 hours prior to or after radiation therapy

Adverse Reactions

Cardiovascular: Hypotension, tachycardia, flushing, pericardial effusion, fluid retention, venous thrombosis

Central nervous system: Rigors, malaise, fever, headache, chills, asthenia

Dermatologic: Rash

Gastrointestinal: Nausea, vomiting, diarrhea, stomatitis, polydipsia, GI hemorrhage

Hepatic: Elevation in liver function tests

Musculoskeletal: Bone pain, myalgia

Respiratory: Dyspnea

"First dose" reaction (fever, hypotension, tachycardia, rigors, flushing, nausea, vomiting, dyspnea)

Drug Interactions Lithium and corticosteroids may potentiate myeloproliferative effects of sargramostim

Stability Store vial in the refrigerator; after reconstitution, it is stable for 6 hours at room temperature; use only normal saline to prepare I.V. infusion solution; GM-CSF at a concentration ≥10 μg/mL is compatible with TPN during Y-site administration

Mechanism of Action Stimulates proliferation, differentiation and functional activity of neutrophils, eosinophils, monocytes and macrophages

Pharmacodynamics

Onset of action: Increase in WBC in 7-14 days

Duration: WBC will return to baseline within 1 week after discontinuing drug

Pharmacokinetics

Half-life: 2 hours

Time to peak serum concentration: Within 1-2 hours following S.C. administration

Usual Dosage I.V., S.C.:

Children (no dosing for children has been FDA approved): 250 μg/m^2/day once daily for 21 days to begin 2-4 hours after the marrow infusion on day 0 of ABMT or not less than 24 hours after chemotherapy. If significant adverse effects or "first dose" reaction is seen at this dose, discontinue the drug until toxicity resolves, then restart at a reduced dose of 125 μg/m^2/day

Cancer chemotherapy recovery: 3-15 μg/kg/day once daily for 14-21 days

Adults: 250 μg/m^2/day once daily for 21 days to begin 2-4 hours after BMT, or not less than 24 hours after chemotherapy (to minimize first dose reaction, start with low doses and increase gradually)

Cancer chemotherapy recovery: 3-15 μg/kg/day once daily for 10 days

Administration Administer as a 2-hour I.V. infusion, 6-hour I.V. infusion, or by continuous I.V. infusion. Use normal saline for dilution of the drug. If the final concentration of GM-CSF in normal saline is ≤10 μg/mL, then add 1 mg albumin per mL of I.V. fluid. Albumin acts as a carrier molecule to prevent drug adsorption to the I.V. tubing. Albumin should be added to the saline prior to addition of GM-CSF.

Monitoring Parameters CBC with differential, platelets; renal/liver function tests, especially with previous dysfunction; vital signs, weight; pulmonary function

Reference Range Excessive leukocytosis (WBC >50,000 cells/mm^3, ANC >20,000 cells/mm^3)

Patient Information Possible bone pain

Nursing Implications Can premedicate with analgesics and antipyretics; control bone pain with non-narcotic analgesics; do not shake solution to avoid foaming. When administering GM-CSF subcutaneously, rotate injection sites.

Dosage Forms Powder for injection, lyophilized: 250 μg, 500 μg; produced by recombinant DNA technology using a yeast expression system

References

Lieschke GJ and Burgess AW, "Granulocyte Colony-Stimulating Factor and

Granulocyte-Macrophage Colony-Stimulating Factor," (1) *N Engl J Med*, 1992, 327(1):28-35.

Lieschke GJ and Burgess AW, "Granulocyte Colony-Stimulating Factor and Granulocyte-Macrophage Colony-Stimulating Factor," (2) *N Engl J Med*, 1992, 327(2):99-106.

Trissel LA, Bready BB, Kwan JW, et al, "Visual Compatibility of Sargramostim With Selected Antineoplastic Agents, Anti-Infectives, or Other Drugs During Simulated Y-Site Injection," *Am J Hosp Pharm*, 1992, 49(2):402-6.

Sastid® Plain Therapeutic Shampoo and Acne Wash [OTC] *see* Sulfur and Salicylic Acid *on page 545*

Scabene® *see* Lindane *on page 344*

Scopolamine (skoe pol' a meen)

Related Information

Overdose and Toxicology Information *on page 696-700*

Brand Names Isopto® Hyoscine; Transderm Scop®

Synonyms Hyoscine Hydrobromide; Scopolamine Hydrobromide

Therapeutic Category Anticholinergic Agent; Anticholinergic Agent, Ophthalmic; Anticholinergic Agent, Transdermal; Ophthalmic Agent, Mydriatic

Use Preoperative medication to produce amnesia and decrease salivary and respiratory secretions; to produce cycloplegia and mydriasis; treatment of iridocyclitis; prevention of motion sickness

Pregnancy Risk Factor C

Contraindications Hypersensitivity to scopolamine or any component; narrow-angle glaucoma, GI or GU obstruction, thyrotoxicosis, tachycardia secondary to cardiac insufficiency, paralytic ileus

Warnings Drug withdrawal symptoms such as nausea, vomiting, headache, dizziness, and equilibrium disturbance have been reported following removal of transdermal system, primarily in patients using the system for more than 3 days; may impair ability to perform hazardous activities requiring mental alertness or physical coordination

Precautions Use with caution with hepatic or renal dysfunction since adverse CNS effects occur more often in these patients; use with caution in infants and children since they may be more susceptible to adverse effects of scopolamine

Adverse Reactions

Cardiovascular: Tachycardia, palpitations

Central nervous system: Disorientation, drowsiness, hallucinations, confusion, psychosis, delirium

Gastrointestinal: Dry mouth, constipation

Ocular: Blurred vision, cycloplegia, mydriasis, photophobia, increased intraocular pressure

Renal & genitourinary: Urinary retention,

Miscellaneous: Anaphylaxis, allergic reactions

Note: Systemic adverse effects have been reported with both the topical and ophthalmic preparations

Drug Interactions Additive adverse effects with other anticholinergic agents; GI absorption of the following drugs may be affected: acetaminophen, levodopa, ketoconazole, digoxin, riboflavin, KCl wax-matrix preparations

Stability Physically compatible when mixed in the same syringe with atropine, butorphanol, chlorpromazine, dimenhydrinate, diphenhydramine, droperidol, fentanyl, glycopyrrolate, hydromorphone, hydroxyzine, meperidine, metoclopramide, morphine, pentazocine, pentobarbital, perphenazine, prochlorperazine, promazine, promethazine, or thiopental

Mechanism of Action Blocks the action of acetylcholine at parasympathetic sites in smooth muscle, secretory glands and the CNS; antagonizes histamine and serotonin

Pharmacodynamics

Onset of effect:

Oral, I.M.: 30 minutes to 1 hour

I.V.: 10 minutes

Transdermal: 4 hours

(Continued)

Scopolamine *(Continued)*

Duration of effect:
- Oral, I.M.: 4-6 hours
- I.V.: 2 hours
- Transdermal: 72 hours

Pharmacokinetics

Absorption: Well absorbed by all routes of administration
Metabolism: Liver metabolized

Usual Dosage

Preoperatively and antiemetic: I.M., I.V., S.C.:
- Children: 6 μg/kg/dose; may be repeated every 6-8 hours
- Adults: 0.3-0.65 mg; may be repeated 3-4 times/day

Motion sickness: Transdermal:
- Children >12 years and Adults: Apply 1 disc behind the ear at least 4 hours prior to exposure every 3 days as needed

Ophthalmic: Refraction:
- Children: 1 drop of 0.25% to eye(s) twice daily for 2 days before procedure
- Adults: 1-2 drops of 0.25% to eye(s) 1 hour before procedure

Ophthalmic: Iridocyclitis:
- Children: 1 drop of 0.25% to eye(s) up to 3 times/day
- Adults: 1-2 drops of 0.25% to eye(s) up to 3 times/day

Administration I.V.: Dilute with an equal volume of sterile water and give by direct I.V. injection over 2-3 minutes

Additional Information Disc is programmed to deliver *in vivo* 0.5 mg over 3 days; wash hands before and after applying the disc to avoid drug contact with eyes

Dosage Forms

Disc, transdermal: 1.5 mg/disc (4's)
Injection, as hydrobromide: 0.3 mg/mL (1 mL); 0.4 mg/mL (0.5 mL, 1 mL); 0.86 mg/mL (0.5 mL); 1 mg/mL (1 mL)
Solution, ophthalmic, as hydrobromide: 0.25% (5 mL, 15 mL)

Scopolamine Hydrobromide *see* Scopolamine *on previous page*

Sebulex® [OTC] *see* Sulfur and Salicylic Acid *on page 545*

Secretin

Brand Names Secretin-Ferring

Therapeutic Category Diagnostic Agent, Pancreatic Exocrine Insufficiency; Diagnostic Agent, Zollinger-Ellison Syndrome and Pancreatic Exocrine Disease

Use Diagnosis of Zollinger-Ellison syndrome, chronic pancreatic dysfunction, and some hepatobiliary diseases such as obstructive jaundice resulting from cancer or stones in the biliary tract

Contraindications Do not give to patients with acute pancreatitis

Precautions Patients with a history of hypersensitivity, allergy or asthma should receive a test dose of 0.1-1 CU; use with caution in patients who are highly nervous or have an excessive gag reflex

Adverse Reactions

Cardiovascular: Fainting, venous spasm
Miscellaneous: Hypersensitivity reactions

Stability Refrigerate; unstable; should be used immediately after reconstitution

Mechanism of Action Hormone normally secreted by duodenal mucosa and upper jejunal mucosa which increases the volume and bicarbonate content of pancreatic juice; stimulates the flow of hepatic bile with a high bicarbonate concentration, stimulates gastrin release in patients with Zollinger-Ellison syndrome

Pharmacodynamics

Peak output of pancreatic secretions: Within 30 minutes
Duration: At least 2 hours

Pharmacokinetics

Inactivated by proteolytic enzymes if administered orally
Metabolism: Metabolic fate is thought to be enzymatic inactivation in blood

Usual Dosage I.V.:
- Pancreatic function: 1 CU/kg
- Zollinger-Ellison: 2 CU/kg

Administration Reconstitute with 7.5 mL of normal saline; **do not shake**; use immediately by direct I.V. injection slowly over 1 minute

Monitoring Parameters Duodenal fluid volume and bicarbonate content; serum gastrin (Zollinger-Ellison syndrome)

Reference Range Normal adult response: Gastric volume 175-295 mL/hour, gastric bicarbonate concentration of 94-134 mEq/L and bicarbonate output of 0.295-0.577 mEq/kg/hour

Nursing Implications Patients should fast 12-15 hours before test

Additional Information Potency of secretin is expressed in terms of clinical units (CU)

Dosage Forms Powder for injection: 75 CU (10 mL)

Secretin-Ferring *see* Secretin *on previous page*

Seldane® *see* Terfenadine *on page 549*

Selenium *see* Trace Metals *on page 574*

Selenium Sulfide (se lee' nee um)

Brand Names Exsel®; Selsun®; Selsun Blue® [OTC]

Therapeutic Category Antiseborrheic Agent, Topical; Shampoos

Use To treat itching and flaking of the scalp associated with dandruff; to control scalp seborrheic dermatitis; treatment of tinea versicolor

Pregnancy Risk Factor C

Contraindications Known hypersensitivity to selenium

Warnings Safety in infants has not been established; avoid use in children <2 years of age

Precautions Do not use on damaged skin to avoid any systemic toxicity

Adverse Reactions
- Central nervous system: Tremors, lethargy
- Dermatologic: Hair loss or discoloration
- Gastrointestinal: Vomiting following long-term use on damaged skin; abdominal pain, garlic breath
- Local: Local irritation
- Miscellaneous: Perspiration

Mechanism of Action May block the enzymes involved in growth of epithelial tissue

Pharmacokinetics Absorption: Not absorbed topically through intact skin, but can be absorbed topically through damaged skin

Usual Dosage Children and Adults: Topical:
- Dandruff, seborrhea: Massage 5-10 mL into wet scalp, leave on scalp 2-3 minutes, rinse thoroughly and repeat application; shampoo twice weekly for two weeks initially, then use once every 1-4 weeks as indicated depending upon control
- Tinea versicolor: Apply the 2.5% lotion to affected area and lather with small amounts of water; leave on skin for 10 minutes, then rinse thoroughly; apply every day for 7 days

Patient Information For external use only; avoid contact with eyes or acutely inflamed skin

Dosage Forms Shampoo, as sulfide: 1% (120 mL, 210 mL, 240 mL, 330 mL); 2.5% (120 mL)

References

Lester RS, "Topical Formulary for the Pediatrician," *Pediatr Clin North Am*, 1983, 30(4):749-65.

Sele-Pak® *see* Trace Metals *on page 574*

Selepen® *see* Trace Metals *on page 574*

Selestoject® *see* Betamethasone *on page 81*

Selsun® *see* Selenium Sulfide *on this page*

Selsun Blue® [OTC] *see* Selenium Sulfide *on this page*

Semilente® Iletin® I *see* Insulin Preparations *on page 311*

Senna

Brand Names Black Draught® [OTC]; Senna-Gen® [OTC]; Senokot® [OTC]; Senolax® [OTC]; X-Prep® Liquid [OTC]

Therapeutic Category Laxative, Stimulant

Use Short-term treatment of constipation; evacuate the colon for bowel or rectal examinations

Pregnancy Risk Factor C

Contraindications Hypersensitivity to senna or any component; nausea and vomiting; undiagnosed abdominal pain, appendicitis, intestinal obstruction or perforation

Precautions Avoid prolonged use (>1 week); chronic use may lead to dependency, fluid and electrolyte imbalance, vitamin and mineral deficiencies

Adverse Reactions

Endocrine & metabolic: Electrolyte and fluid imbalance

Gastrointestinal: Nausea, vomiting, diarrhea, abdominal cramps, perianal irritation

Mechanism of Action Active metabolite (aglycone) acts as a local irritant on the colon, stimulates Auerbach's plexus to produce peristalsis

Pharmacodynamics Onset of action:

Oral: Within 6-24 hours

Rectal: Evacuation occurs in 30 minutes to 2 hours

Pharmacokinetics

Metabolism: Metabolized in the liver

Elimination: Excreted in the feces (via bile) and in the urine

Usual Dosage Oral:

Children: 10-20 mg/kg/dose at bedtime; maximum daily dose: 872 mg
- Granules: >27 kg: ½ teaspoon at bedtime to a maximum of 1 teaspoon twice daily
- Tablet: >27 kg: 1 tablet at bedtime to a maximum of 2 tablets twice daily
- Syrup:
  - 1 month to 1 year: 1.25-2.5 mL at bedtime up to a maximum of 5 mL/day
  - 1-5 years: 2.5-5 mL at bedtime to a maximum of 10 mL/day
  - 5-15 years: 5-10 mL at bedtime to a maximum of 20 mL/day
- Rectal: Children >27 kg: ½ suppository at bedtime

Adults:
- Granules: 1 teaspoonful at bedtime, not to exceed 2 teaspoonfuls twice daily
- Syrup: 2-3 teaspoonfuls at bedtime, not to exceed 3 teaspoonfuls twice daily
- Tablet: 2 tablets at bedtime, not to exceed 4 tablets twice daily
- Rectal: 1 suppository at bedtime; repeat in 2 hours if necessary

Monitoring Parameters I & O

Patient Information May discolor urine or feces; drink plenty of fluids

Dosage Forms

Granules: 326 mg/teaspoonful

Liquid: 7% (130 mL, 360 mL); 6.5% (75 mL, 150 mL)

Suppository, rectal: 652 mg

Syrup: 218 mg/5 mL (60 mL, 240 mL)

Tablet: 187 mg, 217 mg, 600 mg

References

Perkin JM, "Constipation in Childhood: A Controlled Comparison Between Lactulose and Standardized Senna," *Curr Med Res Opin*, 1977, 4:540-3.

Senna-Gen® [OTC] *see* Senna *on this page*

Senokot® [OTC] *see* Senna *on this page*

Senolax® [OTC] *see* Senna *on this page*

Sensorcaine® *see* Bupivacaine Hydrochloride *on page 90*

Septa® Ointment [OTC] *see* Neomycin, Polymyxin B, and Bacitracin *on page 407*

Septisol® *see* Hexachlorophene *on page 285*

Septra® *see* Co-trimoxazole *on page 156*

Septra® DS *see* Co-trimoxazole *on page 156*

Seromycin® Pulvules® *see* Cycloserine *on page 164*

Serutan® [OTC] *see* Psyllium *on page 498*

Shohl's Solution, Modified *see* Sodium Citrate and Citric Acid *on page 528*

Siblin® [OTC] *see* Psyllium *on page 498*

Silain® [OTC] *see* Simethicone *on next page*

Silvadene® *see* Silver Sulfadiazine *on this page*

Silver Nitrate

Therapeutic Category Topical Skin Product

Use Prevention of gonococcal ophthalmia neonatorum; cauterization of wounds and sluggish ulcers, removal of granulation tissue and warts

Pregnancy Risk Factor C

Contraindications Not for use on broken skin or cuts; hypersensitivity to silver nitrate or any component

Warnings Do not use applicator sticks on the eyes; repeated applications of the ophthalmic solution into the eye can cause cauterization of the cornea and blindness

Adverse Reactions

Dermatologic: Burning and skin irritation, staining of the skin
Hematologic: Methemoglobinemia
Ocular: Cauterization of the cornea, blindness, chemical conjunctivitis

Stability Store applicator sticks in a dry place since moisture causes the oxidized film to dissolve; protect from light

Mechanism of Action Free silver ions precipitate bacterial proteins by combining with chloride in tissue forming silver chloride; coagulates cellular protein to form an eschar

Pharmacokinetics Absorption: Not readily absorbed from mucous membranes

Usual Dosage

Neonates: Ophthalmic: 2 drops immediately after birth into conjunctival sac of each eye as a single dose; do not irrigate eyes following instillation of eye drops; silver nitrate prophylaxis should be administered immediately after delivery or no later than 1 hour after delivery

Children and Adults:
- Sticks: Apply to mucous membranes and other moist skin surfaces only on area to be treated 2-3 times/week for 2-3 weeks
- Topical solution: Apply a cotton applicator dipped in solution on the affected area 2-3 times/week for 2-3 weeks

Monitoring Parameters With prolonged use, monitor methemoglobin levels

Patient Information Discontinue topical preparation if redness or irritation develop

Nursing Implications Silver nitrate solutions stain skin and utensils

Dosage Forms

Applicator, topical: 75% with potassium nitrate 25% (6")
Ointment, topical: 10% (30 g)
Solution:
- Ophthalmic: 1% (wax ampuls)
- Topical: 10% (30 mL); 25% (30 mL); 50% (30 mL)

References

Cushing AH and Smith S, "Methemoglobinemia With Silver Nitrate Therapy of a Burn: Report of a Case," *J Pediatr*, 1969, 74:613-5.

Hammerschlag MR, Cummings C, Roblin PM, et al, "Efficacy of Neonatal Ocular Prophylaxis for the Prevention of Chlamydial and Gonococcal Conjunctivitis," *N Engl J Med*, 1989, 320(12):769-72.

Silver Sulfadiazine (sul fa dye' a zeen)

Brand Names Silvadene®; SSD® AF; SSD® Cream; Thermazene®

Therapeutic Category Antibacterial, Topical

Use Adjunct in the prevention and treatment of infection in second and third degree burns

Pregnancy Risk Factor C

Contraindications Hypersensitivity to silver sulfadiazine or any component; premature infants or neonates <2 months of age since sulfas may displace bilirubin from protein binding sites and cause kernicterus

(Continued)

Silver Sulfadiazine *(Continued)*

Precautions Use with caution in patients with G-6-PD deficiency and renal impairment; sulfadiazine may accumulate in patients with impaired hepatic or renal function

Adverse Reactions

Dermatologic: Itching, rash, erythema multiforme, skin discoloration

Hematologic: Hemolytic anemia, leukopenia, agranulocytosis, aplastic anemia, thrombocytopenia

Hepatic: Hepatitis

Local: Pain, burning

Renal & genitourinary: Interstitial nephritis

Miscellaneous: Serum hyperosmolality (due to propylene glycol component in the cream); hypersensitivity reactions to sulfas

Drug Interactions Topical proteolytic enzymes (silver may inactivate enzymes)

Stability Discard if cream is darkened (reacts with heavy metals resulting in release of silver)

Mechanism of Action Acts upon the bacterial cell wall and cell membrane

Pharmacokinetics

Absorption: Significant percutaneous absorption of sulfadiazine can occur especially when applied to extensive burns

Half-life: 10 hours and is prolonged in patients with renal insufficiency

Peak serum levels: Within 3-11 days of continuous topical therapy

Elimination: ~50% excreted unchanged in the urine

Usual Dosage Children and Adults: Topical: Apply once or twice daily with a sterile gloved hand; apply to a thickness of $^1/_{16}$"; burned area should be covered with cream at all times

Monitoring Parameters Serum electrolytes, UA, renal function test, CBC in patients with extensive burns on long-term treatment

Patient Information For external use only

Additional Information Contains methylparaben and propylene glycol

Dosage Forms Cream, topical: 1% [10 mg/g] (20 g, 50 g, 100 g, 400 g, 1000 g)

Simethicone (sye meth' i kone)

Brand Names Flatulex® [OTC]; Gas-X® [OTC]; Mylanta Gas® [OTC]; Mylicon® [OTC]; Phazyme® [OTC]; Silain® [OTC]

Synonyms Activated Dimethicone; Activated Methylpolysiloxane

Therapeutic Category Antiflatulent

Use Relieve flatulence, functional gastric bloating, and postoperative gas pains

Pregnancy Risk Factor C

Warnings Not recommended for the treatment of infant colic

Mechanism of Action Spreads on surface of aqueous liquids forming a film of low surface tension which collapses foam bubbles; allows mucous-surrounded gas bubbles to coalesce and be expelled

Pharmacokinetics Elimination: Excreted in the feces

Usual Dosage Oral:

Infants: 20 mg 4 times/day

Children <12 years: 40 mg 4 times/day

Children >12 years and Adults: 40-125 mg after meals and at bedtime as needed, not to exceed 500 mg/day

Patient Information Chew tablets thoroughly before swallowing

Nursing Implications Shake suspension before using; mix with water, infant formula or other liquids

Dosage Forms

Capsule: 125 mg

Drops, oral: 40 mg/0.6 mL (15 mL, 30 mL)

Tablet: 60 mg, 95 mg

Tablet, chewable: 40 mg, 80 mg, 125 mg

Simron® [OTC] *see* Ferrous Gluconate *on page 242*

Sinarest® 12 Hour Nasal Solution *see* Oxymetazoline Hydrochloride *on page 429*

Sinarest® Nasal Solution [OTC] *see* Phenylephrine Hydrochloride *on page 453*

Sinequan® *see* Doxepin Hydrochloride *on page 207*

Sleep-eze 3® [OTC] *see* Diphenhydramine Hydrochloride *on page 195*

Sleepinal® [OTC] *see* Diphenhydramine Hydrochloride *on page 195*

Slo-bid™ *see* Theophylline *on page 554*

Slo-Niacin® [OTC] *see* Niacin *on page 411*

Slo-Phyllin® *see* Theophylline *on page 554*

Slow-K® *see* Potassium Chloride *on page 469*

SMX-TMP *see* Co-trimoxazole *on page 156*

Snake (Pit Vipers) Antivenin *see* Antivenin (Crotalidae) Polyvalent *on page 56*

Sodium 2-Mercaptoethane Sulfonate *see* Mesna *on page 366*

Sodium Acid Carbonate *see* Sodium Bicarbonate *on this page*

Sodium Benzoate

Therapeutic Category Hyperammonemia Agent

Use Adjunctive therapy for the prevention and treatment of hyperammonemia due to suspected or proven urea cycle defects

Precautions Use with caution in patients with Reye's syndrome, propionic or methylmalonic acidemia; use with caution in neonates with hyperbilirubinemia due to potential displacement of bilirubin from albumin binding sites

Adverse Reactions

Endocrine & metabolic: Metabolic acidosis

Gastrointestinal: Nausea, vomiting

Pharmacokinetics

Half-life: 0.75-7.4 hours

Elimination: Clearance is largely attributable to metabolism with urinary excretion of hippurate, the major metabolite

Usual Dosage Investigational use (not FDA approved): Children: Oral, I.V.: 0.25 g/kg bolus followed by 0.25-0.5 g/kg/day as continuous infusion or divided every 6-8 hours

Monitoring Parameters Serum ammonia level

Additional Information Used to treat urea cycle enzyme deficiency in combination with arginine; not available commercially; oral solutions must be compounded using chemical powder form; I.V. solutions must also be compounded and tested for sterility and pyrogenicity prior to use

References

Batshaw ML, "Hyperammonemia," *Curr Probl Pediatr*, 1984, 14(11):1-69.

Batshaw ML and Brusilow SW, "Treatment of Hyperammonemic Coma Caused by Inborn Errors of Urea Synthesis," *J Pediatr*, 1980, 97(6):893-900.

Green TP, Marchessault RP, and Freese DK, "Disposition of Sodium Benzoate in Newborn Infants With Hyperammonemia," *J Pediatr*, 1983, 102(5):785-90.

Maestri NE, Hauser ER, Bartholomew D, et al, "Prospective Treatment of Urea Cycle Disorders," *J Pediatr*, 1991, 119(6):923-8.

Sodium Bicarbonate

Related Information

CPR Pediatric Drug Dosages *on page 614*

Brand Names Neut®

Synonyms Baking Soda; $NaHCO_3$; Sodium Acid Carbonate; Sodium Hydrogen Carbonate

Therapeutic Category Alkalinizing Agent Oral; Alkalinizing Agent, Parenteral; Antacid; Electrolyte Supplement, Oral; Electrolyte Supplement, Parenteral

Use Management of metabolic acidosis; antacid; alkalinize urine; stabilization of acid base status in cardiac arrest (see precautions) and treatment of life-threatening hyperkalemia

(Continued)

Sodium Bicarbonate *(Continued)*

Pregnancy Risk Factor C

Contraindications Alkalosis, hypocalcemia; unknown abdominal pain, inadequate ventilation during cardiopulmonary resuscitation; excessive chloride losses

Warnings Avoid extravasation, tissue necrosis can occur due to the hypertonicity of $NaHCO_3$

Precautions Use of I.V. $NaHCO_3$ should be reserved for documented metabolic acidosis and for life-threatening hyperkalemia. Routine use in cardiac arrest is not recommended; use with caution in patients with congestive heart failure or other sodium-retaining conditions

Adverse Reactions

Cardiovascular: Edema, cerebral hemorrhage (especially with rapid injection of the hyperosmotic $NaHCO_3$ solution in infants)

Endocrine & metabolic: Metabolic alkalosis, hypernatremia, hypokalemia, hypocalcemia, intracranial acidosis

Gastrointestinal: Gastric distention, flatulence may occur with oral administration

Local: Tissue necrosis, ulceration after I.V. extravasation

Stability Do not mix $NaHCO_3$ with calcium salts, catecholamines, atropine

Mechanism of Action Dissociates to provide bicarbonate ion which neutralizes hydrogen ion concentration and raises blood and urinary pH

Pharmacodynamics

Onset of action:
- Oral, as antacid: 15 minutes
- I.V.: Rapid

Duration:
- Oral: 1-3 hours
- I.V.: 8-10 minutes

Pharmacokinetics

Absorption: Oral: Well absorbed, reabsorbed by kidney

Elimination: <1% is excreted by urine

Usual Dosage

Cardiac arrest: See Precautions. Patient should be adequately ventilated before administering $NaHCO_3$

- Infants: 1 mEq/kg slow IVP initially; may repeat with 0.5 mEq/kg in 10 minutes one time or as indicated by the patient's acid-base status. Rate of administration should not exceed 10 mEq/minute.
- Children and Adults: IVP: 1 mEq/kg initially; may repeat with 0.5 mEq/kg in 10 minutes one time or as indicated by the patient's acid-base status

Metabolic acidosis: Dosage should be based on the following formula if blood gases and pH measurements are available:

- Infants and Children: HCO_3-(mEq) = 0.3 x weight (kg) x base deficit (mEq/L) **or** HCO_3-(mEq) = 0.5 x weight (kg) x [24 - serum HCO_3- (mEq/L)]

Adults: HCO_3-(mEq) = 0.2 x weight (kg) x base deficit (mEq/L) **or** HCO_3-(mEq) = 0.5 x weight (kg) x [24 - serum HCO_3- (mEq/L)]

- If acid-base status is not available: Dose for older Children and Adults: 2-5 mEq/kg I.V. infusion over 4-8 hours; subsequent doses should be based on patient's acid-base status

Chronic renal failure: Oral:
- Children: 1-3 mEq/kg/day
- Adults: 20-36 mEq/day in divided doses

Renal tubular acidosis: Oral:
- Distal:
  - Children: 2-3 mEq/kg/day
  - Adults: 0.5-2 mEq/kg/day given in 4-5 divided doses
- Proximal: Children and Adults: Initial: 5-10 mEq/kg/day; maintenance: Increase as required to maintain serum bicarbonate in the normal range

Urine alkalinization: Oral:
- Children: 1-10 mEq (84-840 mg)/kg/day in divided doses; dose should be titrated to desired urinary pH
- Adults: 48 mEq (4 g) initially, then 12-24 mEq (1-2 g) every 4 hours; dose should be titrated to desired urinary pH; doses up to 16 g/day have been used

Administration For I.V. administration to infants, use the 0.5 mEq/mL solution or dilute the 1 mEq/mL solution 1:1 with **sterile water**; for direct I.V. infusion in emergencies, give slowly (maximum rate in infants: 10 mEq/minute); for infusion, dilute to a maximum concentration of 0.5 mEq/mL in dextrose solution and infuse over 2 hours (maximum rate of administration: 1 mEq/kg/hour)

Monitoring Parameters Serum electrolytes including calcium, urinary pH, arterial blood gases (if indicated)

Additional Information 1 mEq $NaHCO_3$ is equivalent to 84 mg; each g of $NaHCO_3$ provides 12 mEq each of sodium and bicarbonate ions

Dosage Forms

Injection: 4% [2.4 mEq/5 mL] (5 mL); 4.2% [5 mEq/10 mL] (10 mL); 7.5% [8.92 mEq/10 mL] (10 mL, 50 mL); 8.4% [10 mEq/10 mL] (10 mL, 50 mL)

Tablet: 300 mg [3.6 mEq]; 325 mg [3.8 mEq]; 520 mg [6.3 mEq]; 600 mg [7.3 mEq]; 650 mg [7.6 mEq]

Sodium Chloride

Brand Names Adsorbonac® [OTC] Ophthalmic; Ayr®; Muro 128® Ophthalmic [OTC]; Ocean Nasal Mist

Synonyms NaCl; Normal Saline; NS; ½NS

Therapeutic Category Electrolyte Supplement, Oral; Electrolyte Supplement, Parenteral; Lubricant, Ocular; Sodium Salt

Use Prevention of muscle cramps and heat prostration; restoration of sodium ion in hyponatremia; restore moisture to nasal membranes; reduction of corneal edema

Pregnancy Risk Factor C

Contraindications Hypersensitivity to sodium chloride or any component; hypertonic uterus, hypernatremia, fluid retention

Warnings Sodium toxicity is almost exclusively related to how fast a sodium deficit is corrected; both rate and magnitude are extremely important

Precautions Use with caution in patients with congestive heart failure, renal insufficiency, cirrhosis, hypertension

Adverse Reactions

Cardiovascular: Edema

Endocrine & metabolic: Hypernatremia,

Gastrointestinal: Nausea/vomiting (oral use)

Mechanism of Action Principal extracellular cation; functions in fluid and electrolyte balance, osmotic pressure control and water distribution

Pharmacokinetics

Absorption: Oral, I.V.: Rapid

Elimination: Eliminated mainly in urine but also in sweat, tears, and saliva

Usual Dosage Dosage depends upon clinical condition, fluid, electrolyte and acid-base balance of patient; hypertonic solutions (>0.9%) should only be used for the initial treatment of acute serious symptomatic hyponatremia

Maintenance sodium requirements: Oral, I.V.:

Children: 3-4 mEq/kg/day; maximum: 100-150 mEq/day

Adults: 154 mEq/day

Nasal: Children and Adults: Use as often as needed

Heat cramps: Adults: Oral: 0.5-1 g with full glass of water, up to 10 times/day (4.8 g/day maximum)

Ophthalmic, ointment: Children and Adults: Apply once daily or more often as needed

To correct acute, serious hyponatremia: mEq sodium = [desired sodium (mEq/L) - actual sodium (mEq/L)] x 0.6 x wt (kg); for acute correction use 125 mEq/L as the desired serum sodium; acutely correct serum sodium in 5 mEq/L/dose increments; more gradual correction in increments of 10 mEq/L/day is indicated in the asymptomatic patient

Administration Infuse hypertonic solutions (>0.9% saline) via central line only; maximum rate of administration: 1 mEq/kg/hour

Monitoring Parameters Serum sodium, chloride

Reference Range Serum/plasma levels:

Premature newborns: 132-140 mEq/L

Full-term newborns: 133-142 mEq/L

Infants 2 months to Adults: 135-145 mEq/L

Nursing Implications Bacteriostatic NS should not be used for diluting or reconstituting drugs for administration in neonates

(Continued)

Sodium Chloride *(Continued)*

Additional Information Normal saline (0.9%) = 154 mEq/L; 3% NaCl = 513 mEq/L; 5% NaCl = 855 mEq/L

Dosage Forms

Drops, nasal: 0.9% with dropper

Injection: 0.45% (500 mL, 1000 mL); 0.9% (10 mL, 20 mL, 50 mL, 100 mL, 150 mL, 250 mL, 500 mL, 1000 mL); 3% (500 mL); 5% (500 mL); 14.6%, 20% (250 mL); 23.4% (30 mL, 100 mL)

Injection:

Admixtures: 50 mEq, 100 mEq, 625 mEq

Bacteriostatic: 0.9% (30 mL)

Irrigation: 0.9% (250 mL, 500 mL, 1000 mL, 3000 mL)

Ointment, ophthalmic (Muro 128®): 5% (3.5 g)

Solution:

Nasal: 0.65% (45 mL)

Ophthalmic (Adsorbonac®): 2% (15 mL); 5% (15 mL)

Tablet: 650 mg, 1 g

Tablet, enteric coated: 1 g

Sodium Citrate and Citric Acid

Brand Names Bicitra®; Oracit®; Polycitra®

Synonyms Citrate/Citric Acid; Shohl's Solution, Modified

Therapeutic Category Alkalinizing Agent Oral

Use Treatment of metabolic acidosis; alkalinizing agent in conditions where long-term maintenance of an alkaline urine is desirable

Pregnancy Risk Factor C

Contraindications Patients receiving sodium restricted diet; severe renal impairment, azotemia, oliguria

Warnings Conversion to bicarbonate may be impaired in patients with hepatic failure or in shock

Precautions Use with caution in patients with congestive heart failure, hypertension, pulmonary edema

Adverse Reactions

Endocrine & metabolic: Metabolic alkalosis, hypernatremia, hypocalcemia; hyperkalemia (if product containing potassium used)

Gastrointestinal: Laxative effect

Mechanism of Action Citrate salts are oxidized in the body to form bicarbonate

Usual Dosage Oral (dilute in water or juice):

Infants and Children: 2-3 mEq/kg/day in divided doses 3-4 times/day **or** 5-15 mL with water after meals and at bedtime

Adults: 15-30 mL with water after meals and at bedtime

Monitoring Parameters Serum sodium, bicarbonate, potassium, urine pH

Patient Information Dilute with water before administration

Additional Information 1 mL of Bicitra® contains 1 mEq of sodium and the equivalent of 1 mEq of bicarbonate; 1 mL Polycitra® contains 1 mEq each of sodium and potassium and the equivalent of 2 mEq bicarbonate

Dosage Forms Solution, oral:

Bicitra®: Sodium citrate 500 mg and citric acid 334 mg per 5 mL (15 mL unit dose, 480 mL)

Oracit®: Sodium citrate 490 mg and citric acid 640 mg per 5 mL

Polycitra®: Sodium citrate 500 mg and citric acid 334 mg with potassium citrate 550 mg per 5 mL

Sodium Etidronate *see* Etidronate Disodium *on page 236*

Sodium Fluoride *see* Fluoride *on page 255*

Sodium Hydrogen Carbonate *see* Sodium Bicarbonate *on page 525*

Sodium Methicillin *see* Methicillin Sodium *on page 370*

Sodium Nafcillin *see* Nafcillin Sodium *on page 400*

Sodium Nitroferricyanide *see* Nitroprusside Sodium *on page 417*

Sodium Nitroprusside *see* Nitroprusside Sodium *on page 417*

Sodium Phenylacetate and Sodium Benzoate

Brand Names Ucephan®

Therapeutic Category Hyperammonemia Agent

Use Adjunctive therapy to prevent/treat hyperammonemia in patients with urea cycle enzymopathy involving partial or complete deficiencies of carbamoyl-phosphate synthetase, ornithine transcarbamoylase or argininosuccinate synthetase

Pregnancy Risk Factor C

Contraindications Known hypersensitivities to sodium benzoate or sodium phenylacetate

Precautions Use with great care in patients with congestive heart failure, severe renal insufficiency, sodium retention with edema; use with caution in neonates with hyperbilirubinemia (benzoate competes for bilirubin binding sites on albumin)

Adverse Reactions

Gastrointestinal: Nausea, vomiting, possible exacerbation of peptic ulcers

Respiratory: Mild hyperventilation, mild respiratory alkalosis

Drug Interactions Penicillin, probenecid

Stability Diluting Ucephan® with an acidic solution can result in precipitation of the drug

Mechanism of Action Activates conjugation pathways to acylate amino acids which results in decreased ammonia formation

Pharmacokinetics

Metabolism: Metabolized in the liver and kidneys

Half-life, benzoate: 0.75-7.4 hours

Peak blood levels: Oral: Within 1 hour

Elimination: Excreted by the kidneys as the hippurate or phenylacetylglutamine conjugation product

Usual Dosage Infants and Children: Oral: 2.5 mL (250 mg sodium benzoate and 250 mg sodium phenylacetate)/kg/day divided 3-6 times/day; total daily dose should not exceed 100 mL

Monitoring Parameters Serum electrolytes, blood ammonia

Patient Information Must be diluted before use; due to its lingering odor, exercise care in mixing to minimize contact with skin and clothing

Nursing Implications Dilute each dose in 4-8 oz of infant formula or milk and give with meals

Additional Information Sodium content of 100 mL: 130 mEq

Dosage Forms Solution: Sodium phenylacetate 100 mg and sodium benzoate 100 mg per mL (100 mL)

References

Brusilow SW, Danney M, Waber L, et al, "Treatment of Episodic Hyperammonemia in Children With Inborn Errors of Urea Synthesis," *N Engl J Med*, 1984, 310(25):1630-4.

Sodium Phosphate

Brand Names Fleet® Enema [OTC]; Fleet® Phospho®-Soda [OTC]

Therapeutic Category Cathartic; Electrolyte Supplement, Parenteral; Phosphate Salt

Use Source of phosphate in large volume I.V. fluids; short-term treatment of constipation and to evacuate the colon for rectal and bowel exams; treatment and prevention of hypophosphatemia

Pregnancy Risk Factor C

Contraindications Hyperphosphatemia, hypernatremia, hypocalcemia, impaired renal function, congestive heart failure, abdominal pain, fecal impaction

Adverse Reactions

Cardiovascular: Edema, hypotension

Endocrine & metabolic: Hyperphosphatemia, hypocalcemia, hypernatremia, calcium phosphate precipitation

Gastrointestinal: Nausea, vomiting, and diarrhea

Renal & genitourinary: Acute renal failure

Drug Interactions Do not give with magnesium and aluminum containing antacids or sucralfate which can bind with phosphate

Stability Phosphate salts may precipitate when mixed with calcium salts; solubility is improved in amino acid parenteral nutrition solutions; check with a pharmacist to determine compatibility

(Continued)

Sodium Phosphate *(Continued)*

Mechanism of Action As a laxative, exerts osmotic effect in the small intestine by drawing water into the lumen of the gut, producing distention, promoting peristalsis, and evacuation of the bowel; phosphorous participates in bone deposition, calcium metabolism, utilization of B complex vitamins, and as a buffer in acid-base equilibrium

Pharmacodynamics Onset of action (catharsis):

Oral: 3-6 hours

Rectal: 2-5 minutes

Pharmacokinetics

Absorption: Oral: ~1% to 20%

Elimination: Oral doses excreted in the feces; I.V. doses are excreted in the urine with over 80% of dose reabsorbed by the kidney

Usual Dosage I.V. doses should be incorporated into the patient's maintenance I.V. fluids whenever possible; intermittent I.V. infusion should be reserved for severe depletion situations and requires continuous EKG monitoring. It is difficult to determine total body phosphorus deficit, the following dosages are empiric guidelines. **Note:** Doses listed as mmol of phosphate.

Severe hypophosphatemia: I.V.:

- Children:
  - Low dose: 0.08 mmol/kg over 6 hours; use if recent losses and uncomplicated
  - Intermediate dose: 0.16-0.24 mmol/kg over 4-6 hours; use if phosphorus level 0.5-1 mg/dL
  - High dose: 0.36 mmol/kg over 6 hours; use if serum phosphorus <0.5 mg/dL
- Adults: 0.15-0.3 mmol/kg/dose over 12 hours, may repeat as needed to achieve desired serum level

Maintenance:

- Children: 0.5-1.5 mmol/kg/24 hours I.V. or 2-3 mmol/kg/24 hours orally in divided doses
- Adults: 50-70 mmol/24 hours I.V. or 50-150 mmol/24 hours orally in divided doses **or**
- Children <4 years: Oral: 1 capsule (250 mg/8 mmol phosphorus) 4 times/day; dilute as instructed
- Children >4 years and Adults: Oral: 1-2 capsules (250-500 mg/8-16 mmol phosphorus) 4 times/day; dilute as instructed

Laxative (Fleet®): Rectal:

- Children 2-12 years: Contents of one 2.25 oz pediatric enema, may repeat
- Children ≥12 years and Adults: Contents of one 4.5 oz enema as a single dose, may repeat

Laxative (Fleet® Phospho®-Soda): Oral:

- Children 5-9 years: 5 mL as a single dose
- Children 10-12 years: 10 mL as a single dose
- Children ≥12 years and Adults: 20-30 mL as a single dose

Administration For intermittent I.V. infusion, dilute at a maximum concentration of 0.12 mmol/mL and infuse over 4-6 hours; maximum, rate of infusion: 0.06 mmol/kg/hour

Monitoring Parameters Serum sodium, phosphorus, calcium, renal function, EKG monitor

Reference Range

Newborns: 4.2-9 mg/dL

6 weeks to 18 months: 3.8-6.7 mg/dL

18 months to 3 years: 2.9-5.9 mg/dL

3-15 years: 3.6-5.6 mg/dL

>15 years: 2.5-5 mg/dL

Patient Information May cause diarrhea with the oral preparation

Nursing Implications The content of one capsule should be diluted in 75 mL water before administration

Additional Information Sodium content of 1 mmol PO_4 in injection: 1.3 mEq

Dosage Forms

Enema: Sodium phosphate 6 g and sodium biphosphate 16 g per 100 mL (135 mL adult enema unit, 67.5 mL pediatric enema unit)

Injection: Phosphate 3 mmol and sodium 4 mEq sodium per mL (15 mL)
Solution, oral: Sodium phosphate 18 g and sodium biphosphate 48 g per 100 mL (30 mL, 45 mL, 90 mL, 237 mL)

References

Lentz RD, Brown BM, and Kjellstrand CM, "Treatment of Severe Hypophosphatemia," *Ann Intern Med*, 1978, 89(6):941-4.
Lloyd CW and Johnson CE, "Management of Hypophosphatemia," *Clin Pharm*, 1988, 7(2):123-8.

Sodium Polystyrene Sulfonate (pol ee stye' reen)

Brand Names Kayexalate®; SPS®

Therapeutic Category Antidote, Hyperkalemia; Antidote, Potassium

Use Treatment of hyperkalemia

Pregnancy Risk Factor C

Warnings Avoid using the commercially available liquid product in neonates due to the preservative content. Enema may be prepared with powder and diluted with sorbitol 10% solution or oral solution may be made by dilution with 25% sorbitol solution. Enema will reduce the serum potassium faster than oral administration, but the oral route will result in a greater reduction over several hours.

Precautions Use with caution in patients with severe congestive heart failure, hypertension, or edema

Adverse Reactions

Endocrine & metabolic: Hypokalemia, hypocalcemia, hypomagnesemia, hypernatremia
Gastrointestinal: Anorexia, nausea, vomiting, constipation, intestinal necrosis

Drug Interactions Cation-donating antacids (such as magnesium hydroxide or calcium carbonate)

Mechanism of Action Removes potassium by exchanging sodium ions for potassium ions in the intestine before the resin is passed from the body

Pharmacodynamics Onset of action: Within 2-24 hours

Pharmacokinetics Elimination: Remains in the GI tract to be completely excreted in the feces (primarily as potassium polystyrene sulfonate)

Usual Dosage

Children:
- Oral: 1 g/kg/dose every 6 hours
- Rectal: 1 g/kg/dose every 2-6 hours

Adults:
- Oral: 15 g 1-4 times/day
- Rectal: 30-50 g every 6 hours

Monitoring Parameters Serum sodium, potassium, calcium, magnesium, EKG (if applicable)

Nursing Implications Administer oral (or NG) as ~25% sorbitol solution, never mix in orange juice; enema route is less effective than oral administration; retain enema in colon for at least 30-60 minutes and for several hours, if possible

Additional Information 1 g of resin binds ~1 mEq of potassium

Dosage Forms Oral or rectal:

Powder for suspension: 454 g
Suspension: 1.25 g/5 mL with sorbitol 33% and alcohol 0.3% (60 mL, 120 mL, 200 mL, 500 mL)

Sodium Sulamyd® *see* Sulfacetamide Sodium *on page 539*

Sodium Sulfacetamide *see* Sulfacetamide Sodium *on page 539*

Sodium Thiosulfate (thye oh sul' fate)

Brand Names Tinver® [OTC]

Therapeutic Category Antidote, Cyanide; Antifungal Agent, Topical

Use Topically in the treatment of tinea versicolor; as an adjunct in management of cyanide and nitroprusside poisoning, and to reduce the risk of nephrotoxicity associated with cisplatin therapy

Pregnancy Risk Factor C

Precautions Discontinue if irritation or sensitivity occurs; rapid I.V. infusion has caused transient hypotension and EKG changes in dogs

(Continued)

Sodium Thiosulfate *(Continued)*

Adverse Reactions

Cardiovascular: Hypotension
Dermatologic: Contact dermatitis
Local: Local irritation

Mechanism of Action

Cyanide toxicity: Increases the rate of detoxification of cyanide by the enzyme rhodanese by providing an extra sulfur

Cisplatin toxicity: Complexes with cisplatin to form a compound that is nontoxic to either normal or cancerous cells

Pharmacokinetics

Half-life: 0.65 hours
Elimination: 28.5% excreted unchanged in the urine

Usual Dosage

Cyanide and nitroprusside antidote: I.V.:

- Children <25 kg: 50 mg/kg after receiving 4.5-10 mg/kg sodium nitrite; a half dose of each may be repeated if necessary
- Children >25 kg and Adults: 12.5 g after 300 mg of sodium nitrite; a half dose of each may be repeated if necessary

Children and Adults: Topical: 20% to 25% solution: Apply a thin layer to affected areas twice daily

Cisplatin toxicity: Adults: I.V.: 12 g over 6 hours in association with cisplatin **or** 9 g/m^2 I.V. bolus then 1.2 g/m^2/hour for 6 hours; should be given before or during cisplatin administration

Antifungal: Apply thin film twice daily to affected areas for several weeks to months (thoroughly cleanse and dry affects areas prior to application)

Administration I.V.: Inject slowly, over at least 10 minutes; rapid administration may cause hypotension

Patient Information Avoid application near the eyes

Nursing Implications Do not apply topically to or near eyes

Dosage Forms

Injection: 10% (10 mL); 25% (50 mL)
Lotion, topical: 25% with salicylic acid 1%

References

Hall AH, Rumack BH, "Hydroxocobalamin/Sodium Thiosulfate as a Cyanide Antidote," *J Emerg Med*, 1987, 5(2):115-21.

Naughton M, "Acute Cyanide Poisoning," *Anaesth Intensive Care*, 1974, 4:351-6.

Sofarin® *see* Warfarin Sodium *on page 607*

Solarcaine® [OTC] *see* Benzocaine *on page 77*

Solfoton® *see* Phenobarbital *on page 450*

Solganal® *see* Aurothioglucose *on page 67*

Solu-Cortef® *see* Hydrocortisone *on page 293*

Solu-Medrol® *see* Methylprednisolone *on page 379*

Solurex L.A.® *see* Dexamethasone *on page 178*

Somatrem *see* Human Growth Hormone *on page 288*

Somatropin *see* Human Growth Hormone *on page 288*

Sominex® [OTC] *see* Diphenhydramine Hydrochloride *on page 195*

Sorbitol (sor' bi tole)

Therapeutic Category Genitourinary Irrigant

Use Humectant; sweetening agent; hyperosmotic laxative; facilitate the passage of sodium polystyrene sulfonate through the intestinal tract

Contraindications Anuria

Adverse Reactions

Endocrine & metabolic: Fluid and electrolyte losses, lactic acidosis
Gastrointestinal: Diarrhea, abdominal distress

Mechanism of Action A polyalcoholic sugar with osmotic cathartic actions

Pharmacokinetics

Absorption: Oral, rectal: Poorly absorbed
Metabolism: Metabolized mainly in the liver to fructose

Usual Dosage Hyperosmotic laxative (as single dose, at infrequent intervals):

Children 2-11 years:
- Oral: 2 mL/kg (as 70% solution)
- Rectal enema: 30-60 mL as 25% to 30% solution

Children >12 years and Adults:
- Oral: 30-150 mL (as 70% solution)
- Rectal enema: 120 mL as 25% to 30% solution
- Adjunct to sodium polystyrene sulfonate: 15 mL as 70% solution orally until diarrhea occurs (10-20 mL/2 hours) or 20-100 mL as an oral vehicle for the sodium polystyrene sulfonate resin

When administered with charcoal: Oral:
- Children: 4.3 mL/kg of 35% sorbitol with 1 g/kg of activated charcoal
- Adults: 4.3 mL/kg of 70% sorbitol with 1 g/kg of activated charcoal

Monitoring Parameters Serum electrolytes, I & O

Dosage Forms

Powder: 500 g

Solution, oral: 70% (480 mL)

References

Charney EB and Bodurtha JN, "Intractable Diarrhea Associated With the Use of Sorbitol," *J Pediatr*, 1981, 98:157-8.

Kumar A, Weatherly MR, and Beaman DC, "Sweeteners, Flavorings, and Dyes in Antibiotic Preparations," *Pediatrics*, 1991, 87(3):352-60.

Spasmolin *see* Hyoscyamine, Atropine, Scopolamine and Phenobarbital *on page 299*

Spasquid® *see* Hyoscyamine, Atropine, Scopolamine and Phenobarbital *on page 299*

Spectazole™ *see* Econazole Nitrate *on page 215*

Spectrobid® *see* Bacampicillin Hydrochloride *on page 72*

Spironolactone (speer on oh lak' tone)

Brand Names Aldactone®

Therapeutic Category Antihypertensive; Diuretic, Potassium Sparing

Use Management of edema associated with excessive aldosterone excretion; hypertension; primary hyperaldosteronism; hypokalemia; treatment of hirsutism

Pregnancy Risk Factor D

Contraindications Hypersensitivity to spironolactone or any component; renal failure, anuria, hyperkalemia

Warnings Spironolactone has been shown to be tumorigenic in toxicity studies using rats at 25 to 250 times the usual human dose

Precautions Use with caution in patients with impaired renal (Cl_{cr} <50 mL/minute) or hepatic function

Adverse Reactions

Central nervous system: Lethargy, headache, mental confusion, ataxia, fever

Dermatologic: Rash

Endocrine & metabolic: Hyperkalemia, dehydration, hyponatremia, hyperchloremic metabolic acidosis, postmenopausal bleeding, amenorrhea, gynecomastia

Gastrointestinal: Anorexia, nausea, vomiting, diarrhea, gastritis

Renal & genitourinary: Increased BUN

Drug Interactions Potassium, potassium sparing diuretics, indomethacin, angiotensin-converting enzymes inhibitors (eg, captopril)

Mechanism of Action Competes with aldosterone for receptor sites in the distal renal tubules, increasing sodium chloride and water excretion while conserving potassium and hydrogen ions; may block the effect of aldosterone on arteriolar smooth muscle as well

Pharmacokinetics

Protein binding: 91% to 98%

Metabolism: Metabolized in the liver to multiple metabolites, including canrenone (active)

(Continued)

Spironolactone *(Continued)*

Half-life:
Spironolactone: 78-84 minutes
Canrenone: 13-24 hours
Peak serum level: Within 1-3 hours (primarily as the active metabolite)
Elimination: Urinary and biliary excretion

Usual Dosage Oral:
Children:
Diuretic, hypertension: 1.5-3.5 mg/kg/day in divided doses every 6-24 hours
Diagnosis of primary aldosteronism: 125-375 mg/m^2/day in divided doses
Vaso-occlusive disease: 7.5 mg/kg/day in divided doses twice daily (non-FDA approved dose)

Adults:
Edema, hypertension, hypokalemia: 25-200 mg/day in 1-2 divided doses
Diagnosis of primary aldosteronism: 400 mg/day in 1-2 divided doses

Monitoring Parameters Serum potassium, sodium, and renal function

Test Interactions May cause false elevation in serum digoxin concentrations measured by RIA

Dosage Forms Tablet: 25 mg, 50 mg, 100 mg

Extemporaneous Preparation(s) A 5 mg/mL suspension may be made by crushing tablets, levigating with a small amount of distilled water or glycerin; dilute with 1 part Cologel® and 2 parts simple syrup and/or cherry syrup to the final concentration; stable 60 days when refrigerated

Handbook on Extemporaneous Formulations, Bethesda, MD: American Society of Hospital Pharmacists, 1987.

SPS® *see* Sodium Polystyrene Sulfonate *on page 531*

SSD® AF *see* Silver Sulfadiazine *on page 523*

SSD® Cream *see* Silver Sulfadiazine *on page 523*

SSKI® *see* Potassium Iodide *on page 471*

Stagesic® *see* Hydrocodone and Acetaminophen *on page 292*

Stannous Fluoride *see* Fluoride *on page 255*

Staphcillin® *see* Methicillin Sodium *on page 370*

Staticin® *see* Erythromycin *on page 226*

Sterapred® *see* Prednisone *on page 477*

St. Joseph® Measured Dose Nasal Solution [OTC] *see* Phenylephrine Hydrochloride *on page 453*

Streptase® *see* Streptokinase *on this page*

Streptokinase (strep toe kye' nase)

Brand Names Kabikinase®; Streptase®

Therapeutic Category Thrombolytic Agent

Use Thrombolytic agent used in treatment of recent severe or massive deep vein thrombosis, pulmonary emboli, myocardial infarction, and occluded arteriovenous cannulas

Pregnancy Risk Factor C

Contraindications Hypersensitivity to streptokinase or any component; recent strep infection; any internal bleeding, CVA (within two months); brain carcinoma, intracranial or intraspinal surgery

Warnings Avoid I.M. injections

Precautions Relative contraindications: major surgery within the last 10 days, GI bleeding, recent trauma, severe hypertension

Adverse Reactions
Cardiovascular: Hypotension, arrhythmias
Central nervous system: Fever
Dermatologic: Itching, urticaria, flushing, angioneurotic edema
Hematologic: Surface bleeding, internal bleeding, cerebral hemorrhage
Musculoskeletal: Musculoskeletal pain
Respiratory: Bronchospasm

Drug Interactions Anticoagulants, antiplatelet agents, antifibrinolytic agents

Stability Store unopened vials at room temperature; keep in refrigerator and use reconstituted solutions within 24 hours

Mechanism of Action Promotes thrombolysis; activates the conversion of plasminogen to plasmin by forming a complex, exposing plasminogen-activating site, and clearing a peptide bond that converts plasminogen to plasmin; plasmin degrades fibrin, fibrinogen and other procoagulant proteins into soluble fragments; effective both outside and within the formed thrombus/embolus

Pharmacodynamics

Onset of action: Activation of plasminogen: Almost immediate

Duration:

Fibrinolytic effects: Only a few hours

Anticoagulant effects: 12-24 hours

Pharmacokinetics

Half-life: 83 minutes

Elimination: Eliminated by circulating antibodies and via the reticuloendothelial system

Usual Dosage

Children: Safety and efficacy not established; limited studies have used: 3500-4000 units/kg over 30 minutes followed by 1000-1500 units/kg/hour

Clotted catheter: 10,000-25,000 units diluted in saline to a final volume equivalent to catheter volume; instill into catheter and leave in place for 1 hour, then aspirate contents out of catheter and flush catheter with normal saline

Adults:

Thromboses: I.V.: 250,000 units to start, then 100,000 units/hour for 24-72 hours depending on location

Cannula occlusion: 250,000 units into cannula, clamp for 2 hours, then aspirate contents out of catheter and flush with normal saline

Monitoring Parameters Blood pressure, TT, PTT, APTT, fibrinogen, platelet count, hemoglobin/hematocrit, signs of bleeding

Nursing Implications For intravenous or intracoronary use only; avoid I.M. injections

Additional Information Best results are realized if used within 5-6 hours of myocardial infarction; antibodies to streptokinase remain for 3-6 months after initial dose, use another thrombolytic enzyme (ie, urokinase) if repeat thrombolytic therapy is indicated

Dosage Forms Powder for injection: 250,000 units (5 mL, 6.5 mL); 600,000 units (5 mL); 750,000 units (6 mL, 6.5 mL); 1,500,000 units (6.5 mL, 50 mL)

Streptomycin Sulfate (strep toe mye' sin)

Related Information

Overdose and Toxicology Information *on page 696-700*

Therapeutic Category Antibiotic, Aminoglycoside; Antitubercular Agent

Use Combination therapy of active tuberculosis; used in combination with other agents for treatment of streptococcal or enterococcal endocarditis, mycobacterial infections, plague, tularemia, and brucellosis

Pregnancy Risk Factor D

Contraindications Hypersensitivity to streptomycin or any component

Warnings Aminoglycosides are associated with significant nephrotoxicity or ototoxicity; the ototoxicity is directly proportional to the amount of drug given and the duration of treatment; tinnitus or vertigo are indications of vestibular injury and impending bilateral irreversible deafness; renal damage is usually reversible

Precautions Use with caution in patients with pre-existing vertigo, tinnitus, hearing loss, neuromuscular disorders, or renal impairment; modify dosage in patients with renal impairment

Adverse Reactions

Cardiovascular: Myocarditis, cardiovascular collapse

Central nervous system: Dizziness, vertigo, ataxia, headache

Dermatologic: Toxic epidermal necrolysis

Gastrointestinal: Vomiting

Hematologic: Bone marrow depression

Musculoskeletal: Neuromuscular blockade

Otic: Ototoxicity

(Continued)

Streptomycin Sulfate *(Continued)*

Renal & genitourinary: Nephrotoxicity

Miscellaneous: Hypersensitivity reactions, serum sickness

Drug Interactions Ethacrynic acid, neuromuscular blockers

Stability Depending upon manufacturer, reconstituted solutions are stable for 2-4 weeks when refrigerated

Mechanism of Action Inhibits bacterial protein synthesis by binding directly to the 30S ribosomal subunits causing faulty peptide sequence to form in the protein chain

Pharmacokinetics

Distribution: Does not cross into the CSF; crosses the placenta; small amounts appear in breast milk

Protein binding: 34%

Half-life:

Newborns: 4-10 hours

Adults: 2-4.7 hours and is prolonged with renal impairment

Peak serum levels: I.M.: Within 1-2 hours

Elimination: 30% to 90% of a dose is excreted as unchanged drug in urine, with small amount (1%) excreted in the bile, saliva, sweat and tears

Usual Dosage I.M.:

Newborns: 10-20 mg/kg/day once daily

Infants: 20-30 mg/kg/day in divided doses every 12 hours

Children:

TB: 20-40 mg/kg/day in divided doses every 12-24 hours, not to exceed 2 g/day or 1 g/dose; **or** 20-40 mg/kg/dose twice weekly under direct observation, not to exceed 1 g/dose; usually discontinued after 2-3 months of therapy or sooner if cultures become negative

Other infections: 20-40 mg/kg/day in combination with other antibiotics divided every 6-12 hours

Adults:

TB: 15 mg/kg/day in divided doses every 12 hours, not to exceed 2 g/day

Enterococcal endocarditis: 1 g every 12 hours for 2 weeks, 500 mg every 12 hours for 4 weeks in combination with penicillin

Streptococcal endocarditis: 1 g every 12 hours for 1 week, 500 mg every 12 hours for 1 week

Tularemia: 1-2 g/day in divided doses for 7-10 days or until patient is afebrile for 5-7 days

Plague: 2-4 g/day in divided doses until the patient is afebrile for at least 3 days

Monitoring Parameters Hearing (audiogram), BUN, creatinine; serum concentration of the drug should be monitored in patients with renal impairment; eighth cranial nerve damage is usually preceded by high-pitched tinnitus, roaring noises, sense of fullness in ears, or impaired hearing and may persist for weeks after drug is discontinued

Reference Range Cp peak = 15-40 μg/mL; Cp trough <5 μg/mL

Test Interactions False-positive urine glucose with Benedict's solution

Nursing Implications Inject deep I.M. into a large muscle mass; administer at a concentration not to exceed 500 mg/mL

Additional Information Limited supplies of streptomycin are available from the Centers for Disease Control for use by patients with active tuberculosis that is resistant to isoniazid and rifampin or patients with active tuberculosis in areas where resistance is common and whose drug susceptibility is not yet known. Call CDC (TB section): 404-639-2530.

Dosage Forms Injection: 400 mg/mL (12.5 mL)

References

American Academy of Pediatrics Committee on Infectious Diseases, "Chemotherapy for Tuberculosis in Infants and Children," *Pediatrics* 1992, 89(1):161-5.

Arguedas AG and Wehrle PP, "New Concepts for Antimicrobial Use in Central Nervous System Infections," *Semin Pediatr Infect Dis*, 1991, 2(1):36-42.

Lorin MI, Hsu KH, and Jacob SC, "Treatment of Tuberculosis in Children," *Pediatr Clin North Am*, 1983, 30(2):333-48.

Strong Iodine Solution *see* Potassium Iodide *on page 471*

Sublimaze® *see* Fentanyl Citrate *on page 240*

Succimer (sux' sim mer)

Brand Names Chemet®

Therapeutic Category Antidote, Lead Toxicity; Chelating Agent, Oral

Use Treatment of lead poisoning in children with blood levels >45 μg/dL. It is not indicated for prophylaxis of lead poisoning in a lead-containing environment.

Pregnancy Risk Factor C

Contraindications Patients with known hypersensitivity to succimer

Precautions Use with caution in patients with renal or hepatic impairment; adequate hydration should be maintained during therapy

Adverse Reactions The most common events attributable to succimer have been observed in about 10% of patients treated.

Dermatologic: Rash

Gastrointestinal: Nausea, vomiting, diarrhea, appetite loss, metallic taste

Hepatic: Elevated AST, ALT, alkaline phosphatase, serum cholesterol

Renal & genitourinary: Sulfurous odor to urine, hemorrhoidal symptoms

Miscellaneous: Flu-like symptoms, sulfurous odor to breath

Drug Interactions Not recommended to be used concomitantly with edetate calcium disodium or penicillamine

Mechanism of Action Forms stable water-soluble complexes with lead resulting in increased urinary excretion; also chelates other toxic heavy metals such as arsenic and mercury

Pharmacokinetics

Absorption: Oral: Rapid, variable

Metabolism: Extensive to mixed succimer-cysteine disulfides

Elimination: Excreted renally as 10% unchanged drug and 90% metabolite

Usual Dosage Oral:

Children: 10 mg/kg/dose (or 350 mg/m^2/dose) every 8 hours for 5 days followed by 10 mg/kg/dose (or 350 mg/m^2/dose) every 12 hours for 14 days

Adults (non-FDA approved): 30 mg/kg/day every 8 hours for 5 days

Monitoring Parameters Blood lead levels, serum aminotransferases

Test Interactions Falsely elevated serum creatinine phosphokinase; false-positive urine ketones with Ketostix®, falsely decreased uric acid measurements

Patient Information Capsules may be opened and the contents sprinkled on soft foods or put on a spoon

Additional Information Concomitant iron therapy has been reported in a small number of children without the formation of a toxic complex with iron (as seen with dimercaprol); courses of therapy may be repeated if indicated by weekly monitoring of blood lead levels; lead levels should be stabilized <15 mg/dL; 2 weeks between courses is recommended unless more timely treatment is indicated by lead levels

Dosage Forms Capsule: 100 mg

References

Mann KV and Travers JF, "Succimer, An Oral Chelator," *Clin Pharm*, 1991, 10(12):914-22.

Succinylcholine Chloride (suk sin ill koe' leen)

Brand Names Anectine® Chloride; Anectine® Flo-Pack®; Quelicin®; Sucostrin®

Synonyms Suxamethonium Chloride

Therapeutic Category Cholinergic Agent; Neuromuscular Blocker Agent, Depolarizing

Use Used to produce skeletal muscle relaxation in procedures of short duration such as endotracheal intubation or endoscopic exams

Pregnancy Risk Factor C

Contraindications Hypersensitivity to succinylcholine chloride or any component; history of decreased concentrations and/or decreased activity of plasma pseudocholinesterase; malignant hyperthermia; myopathies associated with elevated serum creatinine values; narrow-angle glaucoma; penetrating eye injuries

Precautions Use with caution in patients recovering from severe trauma; in patients with pre-existing hyperkalemia, paraplegia, extensive or severe

(Continued)

Succinylcholine Chloride *(Continued)*

burns, extensive denervation of skeletal muscle because of disease or injury to the CNS or with degenerative or dystrophic neuromuscular disease

Adverse Reactions

Cardiovascular: Bradycardia, hypotension, cardiac arrhythmias
Dermatologic: Rash
Endocrine & metabolic: Hyperkalemia
Gastrointestinal: Increased intragastric pressure, salivation
Musculoskeletal: Muscle pain due to muscle fasiculations
Ocular: Increased intraocular pressure
Respiratory: Apnea, bronchospasm
Miscellaneous: Malignant hyperthermia, myoglobinuria

Drug Interactions Organophosphate cholinesterase inhibitors, procaine, cyclophosphamide, lidocaine, oral contraceptives, neostigmine, phenothiazines, thiotepa

Stability Store in refrigerator

Mechanism of Action Acts similarly to acetylcholine, produces depolarization of the motor endplate at the myoneural junction which causes sustained flaccid skeletal muscle paralysis

Pharmacodynamics

I.M.:
Onset of effect: 2-3 minutes
Duration: 10-30 minutes

I.V.:
Onset of action: Within 30-60 seconds
Duration: ~4-6 minutes

Pharmacokinetics Metabolism: Succinylcholine is rapidly hydrolyzed by plasma pseudocholinesterase

Usual Dosage

Children:
I.V.: Initial: 1-2 mg/kg; maintenance: 0.3-0.6 mg/kg every 5-10 minutes as needed; because of the risk of malignant hyperthermia, use of continuous infusions is **not** recommended in infants and children
I.M.: 2.5-4 mg/kg (maximum: 150 mg)

Adults: 0.6 mg/kg (range: 0.3-1.1 mg/kg), up to 150 mg total dose; maintenance: 0.04-0.07 mg/kg every 5-10 minutes as needed

Note: Pretreatment with atropine may reduce occurrence of bradycardia

Administration May be given by rapid I.V. injection without further dilution

Monitoring Parameters Heart rate, serum potassium, assisted ventilator status

Dosage Forms

Injection: 20 mg/mL (10 mL); 50 mg/mL (10 mL); 100 mg/mL (5 mL, 10 mL, 20 mL)
Powder for injection: 100 mg, 500 mg, 1 g

Sucostrin® *see* Succinylcholine Chloride *on previous page*

Sucralfate (soo kral' fate)

Brand Names Carafate®

Synonyms Aluminum Sucrose Sulfate, Basic

Therapeutic Category Gastrointestinal Agent, Miscellaneous

Use Short-term management of duodenal ulcers; gastric ulcers; suspension may be used topically for treatment of stomatitis due to cancer chemotherapy or other causes of esophageal and gastric erosions

Pregnancy Risk Factor B

Contraindications Hypersensitivity to sucralfate or any component

Precautions Use with caution in renal failure due to accumulation of aluminum

Adverse Reactions

Central nervous system: Dizziness, sleepiness, vertigo
Dermatologic: Rash, pruritus
Gastrointestinal: Constipation, diarrhea, nausea, gastric discomfort, indigestion, dry mouth
Musculoskeletal: Back pain

Drug Interactions Absorption of tetracycline, phenytoin, digoxin, sustained release theophylline, quinolones, cimetidine may be altered; separate administration by 2 hours; do not give antacids within 30 minutes of sucralfate

Mechanism of Action Forms a complex, a paste-like substance, when combined with gastric acid that adheres to the damaged mucosal area. This selectively forms a protective coating that protects the lining against peptic acid, pepsin, and bile salts.

Pharmacodynamics GI protection effect:

Onset of action: 1-2 hours

Duration: Up to 6 hours

Pharmacokinetics

Absorption: Oral: <5%; acts locally at ulcer sites; unbound in the GI tract to aluminum and sucrose octasulfate

Metabolism: Not metabolized

Elimination: Small amounts that are absorbed are excreted in the urine as unchanged compounds

Usual Dosage Oral:

Children: Dose not established; doses of 40-80 mg/kg/day divided every 6 hours have been used

Adults: 1 g 4 times/day, 1 hour before meals or food and at bedtime; maintenance therapy: 1 g twice daily

Stomatitis: 2.5-5 mL (1 g/5 mL extemporaneously prepared suspension), swish and spit or swish and swallow 4 times/day

Nursing Implications Give before meals or on an empty stomach

Additional Information Tablet may be broken or dissolved in water before ingestion

Dosage Forms Tablet: 1 g

Extemporaneous Preparation(s) A 200 mg/mL suspension can be made with twenty 1 g tablets and distilled water to a make total amount of 100 mL; stable for 14 days

Handbook in Extemporaneous Formulations, Bethesda, MD: American Society of Hospital Pharmacists, 1987.

Sucrets® [OTC] *see* Dyclonine Hydrochloride *on page 214*

Sudafed® [OTC] *see* Pseudoephedrine *on page 497*

Sudafed® 12 Hour [OTC] *see* Pseudoephedrine *on page 497*

Sufedrin® [OTC] *see* Pseudoephedrine *on page 497*

Sulbactam and Ampicillin *see* Ampicillin and Sulbactam *on page 50*

Sulf-10® *see* Sulfacetamide Sodium *on this page*

Sulfacetamide Sodium (sul fa see' ta mide)

Brand Names AK-Sulf®; Bleph®-10; Cetamide®; I-Sulfacet®; Ophthacet®; Sodium Sulamyd®; Sulf-10®; Sulfair®

Synonyms Sodium Sulfacetamide

Therapeutic Category Antibiotic, Ophthalmic; Antibiotic, Sulfonamide Derivative

Use Treatment and prophylaxis of conjunctivitis, corneal ulcers, and other superficial ocular infections due to susceptible organisms; adjunctive treatment with systemic sulfonamides for therapy of trachoma

Pregnancy Risk Factor C

Contraindications Hypersensitivity to sulfacetamide or any component, sulfonamides; infants <2 months of age

Warnings Inactivated by purulent exudates containing PABA; ointment may retard corneal wound healing; nonsusceptible organisms such as fungi may proliferate with the use of sulfonamide preparations

Precautions Use with caution in patients with severe dry eye

Adverse Reactions

Central nervous system: Headache, fever

Dermatologic: Stevens-Johnson syndrome, exfoliative dermatitis, toxic epidermal necrolysis, rash, photosensitivity

Hematologic: Bone marrow depression

Hepatic: Lupus-like reaction

Local: Irritation, stinging and burning (especially with 30% solution)

Ocular: Blurred vision

(Continued)

Sulfacetamide Sodium *(Continued)*

Miscellaneous: Hypersensitivity reactions

Drug Interactions Silver, gentamicin (antagonism)

Stability Protect from light; discolored or cloudy solutions should not be used; incompatible with silver and zinc sulfate; sulfacetamide is inactivated by blood or purulent exudates

Mechanism of Action Interferes with bacterial growth by inhibiting bacterial folic acid synthesis through competitive antagonism of PABA

Pharmacodynamics Onset of action: Improvement of conjunctivitis is usually seen within 3-6 days

Pharmacokinetics

Half-life: 7-13 hours

Elimination: When absorbed, excreted primarily in the urine as unchanged drug

Usual Dosage Children >2 months and Adults: Ophthalmic:

Ointment: Apply to lower conjunctival sac 1-4 times/day and at bedtime

Solution: 1-2 drops every 2-3 hours in the lower conjunctival sac during the waking hours and less frequently at night

Monitoring Parameters Response to therapy

Patient Information Eye drops may burn and sting when first instilled; may cause sensitivity to bright light

Dosage Forms Ophthalmic:

Ointment: 10% (3.5 g)

Solution: 10% (1 mL, 2 mL, 3.75 mL, 5 mL, 15 mL); 15% (2 mL, 15 mL); 30% (5 mL, 15 mL)

References

Lohr JA, Austin RD, Grossman M, et al, "Comparison of Three Topical Antimicrobials for Acute Bacterial Conjunctivitis," *Pediatr Infect Dis J*, 1988, 7(9):626-9.

Sulfadiazine (sul fa dye' a zeen)

Therapeutic Category Antibiotic, Sulfonamide Derivative

Use Adjunctive treatment in toxoplasmosis

Pregnancy Risk Factor B (D at term)

Contraindications Porphyria, hypersensitivity to any sulfa drug or any component, infants <2 months of age unless indicated for the treatment of congenital toxoplasmosis; pregnant women during third trimester

Precautions Use with caution in patients with impaired hepatic function or impaired renal function, urinary obstruction, blood dyscrasia, G-6-PD deficiency; dosage modification required in patients with renal impairment

Adverse Reactions

Cardiovascular: Vasculitis

Central nervous system: Dizziness, fever, headache

Dermatologic: Rash, exfoliative dermatitis, Stevens-Johnson syndrome, photosensitivity

Gastrointestinal: Nausea, vomiting

Hematologic: Granulocytopenia, leukopenia, thrombocytopenia, aplastic anemia, hemolytic anemia

Hepatic: Jaundice, hepatitis

Renal & genitourinary: Acute nephropathy, crystalluria

Miscellaneous: Serum sickness-like reactions

Drug Interactions PABA, paraldehyde; displaces agents from protein binding sites: coumarin anticoagulants (↑ bleeding), MTX (increased toxicity), sulfonylurea antidiabetic agents (hypoglycemia)

Mechanism of Action Interferes with bacterial growth by inhibiting bacterial folic acid synthesis through competitive antagonism of PABA

Pharmacokinetics

Absorption: Oral: Well absorbed

Distribution: Excreted in breast milk; diffuses into CSF with higher concentrations reached when meninges are inflamed

Protein binding: 32% to 56%

Metabolism: Metabolized by N-acetylation

Half-life: 10 hours

Peak serum levels: Within 3-6 hours

Elimination: Excreted in the urine as metabolites (15% to 40%) and as unchanged drug (43% to 60%)

Usual Dosage Oral:

Congenital toxoplasmosis: Newborns: 100 mg/kg/day divided every 6 hours in conjunction with pyrimethamine 1 mg/kg/day once daily and supplemental folinic acid 5 mg every 3 days for 6 months

Toxoplasmosis:

Children: 120-200 mg/kg/day divided every 6 hours in conjunction with pyrimethamine 2 mg/kg/day divided every 12 hours for 3 days followed by 1 mg/kg/day once daily (maximum: 25 mg/day) with supplemental folinic acid

Adults: 2-8 g/day divided every 6 hours in conjunction with pyrimethamine 25 mg/day and with supplemental folinic acid

Monitoring Parameters CBC, renal function tests, urinalysis

Patient Information Drink plenty of fluids; avoid prolonged exposure to sunlight

Dosage Forms Tablet: 500 mg

Extemporaneous Preparation(s) Tablets may be crushed to prepare oral suspension of the drug in water or with a sucrose-containing solution; aqueous suspension with concentrations of 100 mg/mL should be stored in the refrigerator and used within 7 days

References

Frenkel JK, "Toxoplasmosis," *Pediatr Clin North Am*, 1985, 32(4):917-32.

Sulfadoxine and Pyrimethamine (sul fa dox' een)

Brand Names Fansidar®

Therapeutic Category Antimalarial Agent

Use Treatment of *Plasmodium falciparum* malaria in patients in whom chloroquine resistance is suspected; malaria prophylaxis for travelers to areas where chloroquine-resistant malaria is endemic

Pregnancy Risk Factor C

Contraindications Known hypersensitivity to any sulfa drug, pyrimethamine, or any component; porphyria, megaloblastic anemia, severe renal insufficiency; children <2 months of age due to competition with bilirubin for protein binding sites

Warnings Fatalities associated with sulfonamides, although rare, have occurred due to severe reactions including Stevens-Johnson syndrome, toxic epidermal necrolysis, hepatic necrosis, agranulocytosis, aplastic anemia and other blood dyscrasias; discontinue use at first sign of rash or any sign of adverse reaction; hemolysis occurs in patients with G-6-PD deficiency

Precautions Use with caution in patients with renal or hepatic impairment, patients with possible folate deficiency, and patients with seizure disorders

Adverse Reactions

Cardiovascular: Vasculitis

Central nervous system: Ataxia, tremors, seizures, headache, insomnia

Dermatologic: Erythema multiforme, Stevens-Johnson syndrome, toxic epidermal necrolysis, rash, photosensitivity

Gastrointestinal: Anorexia, vomiting, gastritis, glossitis

Hematologic: Megaloblastic anemia, leukopenia, thrombocytopenia, pancytopenia, agranulocytosis

Hepatic: Hepatic necrosis

Respiratory: Respiratory failure

Drug Interactions Para-aminobenzoic acid, folic acid

Mechanism of Action Sulfadoxine interferes with bacterial folic acid synthesis and growth via competitive inhibition of para-aminiobenzoic acid; pyrimethamine inhibits microbial dihydrofolate reductase, resulting in inhibition of tetrahydrofolic acid synthesis

Pharmacokinetics

Absorption: Oral: Well absorbed

Distribution: Excreted in breast milk

Protein binding:

Pyrimethamine: 80% to 87%

Sulfadoxine: 90% to 95%

Half-life:

Pyrimethamine: 80-95 hours

Sulfadoxine: 5-8 days

Peak drug concentrations: Within 2-8 hours

(Continued)

Sulfadoxine and Pyrimethamine *(Continued)*

Elimination: Excreted in the urine as parent compounds and several unidentified metabolites

Usual Dosage Children and Adults: Oral:

Treatment of acute attack of malaria: A single dose of the following number of Fansidar® tablets is used in sequence with quinine or alone:

2-11 months: ¼ tablet
1-3 years: ½ tablet
4-8 years: 1 tablet
9-14 years: 2 tablets
>14 years: 2-3 tablets

Malaria prophylaxis (for areas where chloroquine-resistant *P. falciparum* exists):

The first dose of Fansidar® should be taken one or two days before departure to an endemic area (CDC recommends that therapy be initiated 1-2 weeks before such travel), administration should be continued during the stay and for 4-6 weeks after return. Dose = pyrimethamine 0.5 mg/kg/dose and sulfadoxine 10 mg/kg/dose up to a maximum of 25 mg pyrimethamine and 500 mg sulfadoxine/dose weekly.

2-11 months: ⅛ tablet weekly **or** ¼ tablet once every 2 weeks
1-3 years: ¼ tablet once weekly **or** ½ tablet once every 2 weeks
4-8 years: ½ tablet once weekly **or** 1 tablet once every 2 weeks
9-14 years: ¾ tablet once weekly **or** 1½ tablets once every 2 weeks
>14 years: 1 tablet once weekly **or** 2 tablets once every 2 weeks

For short-term travel (≤3 weeks): Take a single dose in the event of a febrile illness

2-11 months: ¼ tablet
1-3 years: ½ tablet
4-8 years: 1 tablet
9-14 years: 2 tablets
≥14 years: 3 tablets

Monitoring Parameters Liver function tests, CBC including platelet counts, renal function tests and urinalysis should be performed periodically

Patient Information Drink plenty of fluids; avoid prolonged exposure to the sun; notify physician if rash, sore throat, pallor, glossitis, fever, arthralgia, cough, shortness of breath, or jaundice occurs

Nursing Implications Administer with meals

Additional Information Leucovorin should be administered to reverse signs and symptoms of folic acid deficiency

Dosage Forms Tablet: Sulfadoxine 500 mg and pyrimethamine 25 mg (25s)

References

Lynk A and Gold R, "Review of 40 Children With Imported Malaria," *Pediatr Infect Dis J*, 1989, 8(11):745-50.

Randall G and Seidel JS, "Malaria," *Pediatr Clin North Am*, 1985, 32(4):893-916.

Sulfair® *see* Sulfacetamide Sodium *on page 539*

Sulfamethoprim® *see* Co-trimoxazole *on page 156*

Sulfamethoxazole (sul fa meth ox' a zole)

Brand Names Gantanol®; Urobak®

Therapeutic Category Antibiotic, Sulfonamide Derivative

Use Treatment of urinary tract infections, nocardiosis, chlamydial infections, toxoplasmosis, acute otitis media, and acute exacerbations of chronic bronchitis due to susceptible organisms

Pregnancy Risk Factor B (D at term)

Contraindications Porphyria; known hypersensitivity to sulfa drug or any component; infants <2 months of age (sulfas compete with bilirubin for protein binding sites which may result in kernicterus in newborns); pregnant women during third trimester

Warnings Should not be used for group A beta-hemolytic streptococcal infections

Precautions Maintain adequate fluid intake to prevent crystalluria; use with caution in patients with renal or hepatic impairment, patients with G-6-PD deficiency, and in patients with urinary obstruction

Adverse Reactions

Cardiovascular: Vasculitis

Central nervous system: Dizziness, fever, headache

Dermatologic: Rash, exfoliative dermatitis, Stevens-Johnson syndrome, photosensitivity

Gastrointestinal: Nausea, vomiting

Hematologic: Granulocytopenia, leukopenia, thrombocytopenia, aplastic anemia, hemolytic anemia, neutropenia

Hepatic: Jaundice

Renal & genitourinary: Acute nephropathy, crystalluria

Miscellaneous: Serum sickness-like reactions

Drug Interactions Warfarin, sulfonylurea antidiabetic agents, methotrexate, (displaces sulfonylureas, warfarin, and methotrexate from protein binding sites)

Stability Protect from light

Mechanism of Action Interferes with bacterial growth by inhibiting bacterial folic acid synthesis through competitive antagonism of PABA

Pharmacokinetics

Absorption: Oral: 90%

Distribution: Crosses the placenta

Half-life: 7-12 hours, prolonged with renal impairment

Metabolism: Metabolized primarily in the liver to a N-acetylated metabolite (inactive but contributes to nephrotoxicity) and a N-glucuronide conjugate

Protein binding: 70%

Peak serum levels: Within 3-4 hours

Elimination: Unchanged drug (20%) and its metabolites are excreted in the urine

Moderately dialyzable (20% to 50%)

Usual Dosage Oral:

Children: Initial: 50-60 mg/kg/dose one time, followed by 50-60 mg/kg/day divided every 12 hours, not to exceed 75 mg/kg/day or a maximum: 3 g/24 hours

Adults: 2 g stat, 1 g 2-3 times/day; maximum: 3 g/24 hours

Dosing interval in renal impairment: Cl_{cr} <30 mL/minute: Decrease dosage

Monitoring Parameters CBC, UA, renal function test

Patient Information Report to physician any sore throat, mouth sores, rash, unusual bleeding or fever; drink plenty of fluid; avoid aspirin and vitamin C products; avoid prolonged exposure to sunlight

Dosage Forms

Suspension, oral (cherry flavor): 500 mg/5 mL (480 mL)

Tablet: 500 mg

Sulfamethoxazole and Trimethoprim *see* Co-trimoxazole *on page 156*

Sulfamylon® *see* Mafenide Acetate *on page 351*

Sulfasalazine (sul fa sal' a zeen)

Brand Names Azulfidine®; Azulfidine® EN-tabs®

Synonyms Salicylazosulfapyridine

Therapeutic Category 5-Aminosalicylic Acid Derivative; Anti-inflammatory Agent

Use Management of ulcerative colitis

Pregnancy Risk Factor B (D at term)

Contraindications Hypersensitivity to sulfasalazine, sulfa drugs, or any component; porphyria, GI or GU obstruction; hypersensitivity to salicylates; children <2 years of age

Precautions Use with caution in patients with renal impairment; G-6-PD deficiency, blood dyscrasias

Adverse Reactions

Cardiovascular: Vasculitis

Central nervous system: Headache, fever, convulsions, vertigo, tinnitus, malaise

Dermatologic: Rash, toxic epidermal necrolysis

Endocrine & metabolic: Infertility, oligospermia

Gastrointestinal: Nausea, vomiting, diarrhea, pancreatitis

Hematologic: Hemolytic anemia, agranulocytosis

Hepatic: Hepatotoxicity

(Continued)

Sulfasalazine *(Continued)*

Renal & genitourinary: Crystalluria, nephrotoxicity
Respiratory: Fibrosing alveolitis, pulmonary eosinophilia
Miscellaneous: Serum sickness-like reaction

Drug Interactions ↓ Folic acid absorption, ↓ digoxin serum levels, iron ↓ sulfasalazine absorption

Mechanism of Action Acts locally in the colon to decrease the inflammatory response and interferes with secretion by inhibiting prostaglandin synthesis

Pharmacokinetics

Absorption: Oral: 10% to 15% absorbed as unchanged drug from the small intestine; upon administration, the drug is split into sulfapyridine and 5-aminosalicylic acid (SASA) in the colon
Metabolism: Both components are metabolized in the liver
Half-life: 5.7-10 hours
Peak levels:
Serum 5-aminosalicylic acid (active metabolite): Within 1.5-6 hours
Serum sulfapyridine (active metabolite): 6-24 hours
Elimination: Primary excretion in the urine (as unchanged drug, components, and acetylated metabolites); small amounts appear in feces and in breast milk

Usual Dosage Oral:

Children >2 years:
Severe-moderate colitis: 50-75 mg/kg/day divided every 4-6 hours, not to exceed 6 g/day
Mild colitis: 40-50 mg/kg/day divided every 6 hours
Maintenance dose: 30-50 mg/kg/day divided every 4-8 hours; not to exceed 2 g/day

Adults: 1 g 3-4 times/day divided every 4-6 hours, not to exceed 6 g/day; maintenance: 2 g/day in divided doses every 6 hours

Monitoring Parameters Stool frequency, hematocrit, reticulocyte count, CBC, urinalysis, renal function tests, liver function tests

Patient Information Maintain adequate fluid intake; may cause orange-yellow discoloration of urine and skin; take after meals or with food; do not take with antacids; may stain soft contact lenses yellow; avoid prolonged exposure to sunlight

Additional Information Since sulfasalazine impairs folate absorption, consider providing 1 mg/day folate supplement

Dosage Forms

Suspension, oral: 250 mg/5 mL (480 mL)
Tablet: 500 mg
Tablet, enteric coated: 500 mg

References

Kirschner BS, "Inflammatory Bowel Disease in Children," *Pediatr Clin North Am*, 1988, 35(1):189-208.

Sulfatrim® *see* Co-trimoxazole *on page 156*

Sulfatrim® DS *see* Co-trimoxazole *on page 156*

Sulfisoxazole (sul fi sox' a zole)

Brand Names Gantrisin®

Synonyms Sulfisoxazole Acetyl; Sulphafurazole

Therapeutic Category Antibiotic, Sulfonamide Derivative

Use Treatment of urinary tract infections, otitis media, *Chlamydia*; nocardiosis; treatment of acute pelvic inflammatory disease in prepubertal children

Pregnancy Risk Factor B (D at term)

Contraindications Hypersensitivity to any sulfa drug or any component; porphyria; infants <2 months of age (sulfas compete with bilirubin for protein binding sites which may result in kernicterus in newborns); patients with urinary obstruction; pregnant women during third trimester

Precautions Use with caution in patients with G-6-PD deficiency (hemolysis may occur), hepatic or renal impairment; dosage modification required in patients with renal impairment; risk of crystalluria should be considered in patients with impaired renal function

Adverse Reactions

Cardiovascular: Vasculitis

Central nervous system: Dizziness, headache

Dermatologic: Rash, Stevens-Johnson syndrome, photosensitivity

Gastrointestinal: Nausea, vomiting

Hematologic: Thrombocytopenia, leukopenia, agranulocytosis, aplastic anemia, hemolytic anemia, neutropenia

Hepatic: Jaundice, hepatitis

Renal & genitourinary: Crystalluria, nephrotoxicity

Miscellaneous: Hypersensitivity reactions, kernicterus

Drug Interactions Methotrexate, tolbutamide, chlorpropamide, oral anticoagulants (displaced from protein binding sites); PABA (antagonizes the antibacterial activity of sulfas); thiopental

Mechanism of Action Interferes with bacterial growth by inhibiting bacterial folic acid synthesis through competitive antagonism of PABA

Pharmacokinetics

Absorption: Sulfisoxazole acetyl is hydrolyzed in the GI tract to sulfisoxazole which is readily absorbed

Distribution: Crosses the placenta; excreted into breast milk

Protein binding: 85% to 88%

Metabolism: Metabolized in the liver by acetylation and glucuronide conjugation to inactive compounds

Half-life: 4-8 hours, prolonged with renal impairment

Peak serum levels: Within 2-4 hours

Elimination: Primarily excreted in the urine (95% within 24 hours), 40% to 60% as unchanged drug

$>$50% removed by hemodialysis

Usual Dosage

Children $>$2 months: Oral: Initial: 75 mg/kg for 1 dose, followed by 120-150 mg/kg/day in divided doses every 4-6 hours; not to exceed 6 g/day

Pelvic inflammatory disease: 100 mg/kg/day in divided doses every 6 hours; used in combination with ceftriaxone

Chlamydia trachomatis: 100 mg/kg/day divided every 6 hours

Adults: Oral: 2-4 g stat, 4-8 g/day in divided doses every 4-6 hours

Children and Adults: Ophthalmic:

Solution: 1-2 drops to affected eye every 2-3 hours

Ointment: Small amount to affected eye 1-3 times/day and at bedtime

Dosing interval in renal impairment:

Cl_{cr} 10-50 mL/minutes: Administer every 8-12 hours

Cl_{cr} $<$10 mL/minute: Administer every 12-24 hours

Monitoring Parameters CBC, urinalysis, renal function tests

Test Interactions False-positive protein in urine; false-positive urine glucose with Clinitest®

Patient Information Take with a glass of water on an empty stomach; avoid prolonged exposure to sunlight; report to physician any sore throat, mouth sores, rash, unusual bleeding, or fever

Nursing Implications Maintain adequate patient fluid intake

Dosage Forms

Ointment, ophthalmic, as diolamine: 4% (3.75 g)

Solution, ophthalmic, as diolamine: 4% (15 mL)

Suspension, oral, pediatric, as acetyl (raspberry flavor): 500 mg/5 mL (480 mL)

Syrup, as acetyl (chocolate flavor): 500 mg/5 mL (480 mL)

Tablet: 500 mg

References

Thoene DE and Johnson CE, "Pharmacotherapy of Otitis Media," *Pharmacotherapy*, 1991, 11(3):212-21.

Sulfisoxazole Acetyl *see* Sulfisoxazole *on previous page*

Sulfisoxazole and Erythromycin *see* Erythromycin and Sulfisoxazole *on page 228*

Sulfur and Salicylic Acid

Brand Names Aveeno® Cleansing Bar [OTC]; Fostex® [OTC]; Pernox® [OTC]; Sastid® Plain Therapeutic Shampoo and Acne Wash [OTC]; Sebulex® [OTC]

(Continued)

Sulfur and Salicylic Acid *(Continued)*

Synonyms Salicylic Acid and Sulfur

Therapeutic Category Antiseborrheic Agent, Topical

Use Therapeutic shampoo for dandruff and seborrheal dermatitis; acne skin cleanser

Contraindications Contraindicated in patients allergic to sulfur

Warnings For external use only; avoid contact with eyes; discontinue use if skin irritation develops

Precautions Infants are more sensitive to sulfur than adults; do not use in children <2 years of age

Adverse Reactions Topical preparations containing 2% to 5% sulfur generally are well tolerated; concentration >15% is very irritating to the skin; higher concentrations (eg, 10% or higher) may cause systemic toxicity

Cardiovascular: Collapse
Central nervous system: Dizziness, headache
Gastrointestinal: Vomiting
Local: Irritation
Musculoskeletal: Muscle cramps

Stability Preparations containing sulfur may react with metals including silver and copper, resulting in discoloration of the metal

Mechanism of Action Salicylic acid works synergistically with sulfur in its keratolytic action to break down keratin and promote skin peeling

Pharmacokinetics Absorption: 1% of topically applied sulfur is absorbed; sulfur is reduced to hydrogen sulfide

Usual Dosage Children and Adults: Topical:

Shampoo: Initial: Use daily or every other day; 1-2 treatments/week will usually maintain control
Soap: Use daily or every other day

Patient Information Avoid contact with the eyes; for external use only; contact physician if condition worsens or rash or irritation develops

Dosage Forms

Cake: Sulfur 2% and salicylic acid 2% (123 g)
Cleanser: Sulfur 2% and salicylic acid 1.5% (60 mL, 120 mL)
Shampoo: Micropulverized sulfur 2% and salicylic acid 2% (120 mL, 240 mL)
Soap: Micropulverized sulfur 2% and salicylic acid 2% (113 g)
Wash: Sulfur 1.6% and salicylic acid 1.6% (75 mL)

Sulindac (sul in' dak)

Related Information

Overdose and Toxicology Information *on page 696-700*

Brand Names Clinoril®

Therapeutic Category Analgesic, Non-Narcotic; Anti-inflammatory Agent; Nonsteroidal Anti-Inflammatory Agent (NSAID), Oral

Use Management of inflammatory disease, rheumatoid disorders; acute gouty arthritis

Pregnancy Risk Factor B (D at term)

Contraindications Hypersensitivity to sulindac, any component, aspirin or other nonsteroidal anti-inflammatory drugs (NSAIDs)

Precautions Used with caution in patients with peptic ulcer disease, GI bleeding, bleeding abnormalities, impaired renal or hepatic function, congestive heart failure, hypertension, and patients receiving anticoagulants

Adverse Reactions

Cardiovascular: Edema
Central nervous system: Dizziness, nervousness, tinnitus, headache
Dermatologic: Rash, pruritus
Gastrointestinal: Abdominal pain; GI bleeding, ulcer, perforation, nausea, vomiting, diarrhea, constipation
Hematologic: Thrombocytopenia, agranulocytosis, inhibition of platelet aggregation, bone marrow depression,
Hepatic: Hepatitis
Renal & genitourinary: Renal impairment
Respiratory: Bronchospasm

Drug Interactions Sulindac may potentiate effects of warfarin; probenecid may increase serum concentration of sulindac; DMSO or ASA may ↓ sulindac serum concentration; sulindac may ↑ methotrexate serum concentrations and may ↑ cyclosporin nephrotoxicity; drug interactions similar to other NSAIDs may also occur

Mechanism of Action Inhibits prostaglandin synthesis by decreasing the activity of the enzyme, cyclo-oxygenase, which results in decreased formation of prostaglandin precursors

Usual Dosage Oral:

Children: Dose not established; doses of 4 mg/kg/day divided in 2 doses/day have been used

Adults: 150-200 mg twice daily; not to exceed 400 mg/day

Monitoring Parameters Liver enzymes, BUN, serum creatinine, CBC; periodic ophthalmologic exams with chronic use

Nursing Implications Administer with food to decrease GI adverse effects

Dosage Forms Tablet: 150 mg, 200 mg

Sulphafurazole *see* Sulfisoxazole *on page 544*

Sumycin® *see* Tetracycline Hydrochloride *on page 552*

SuperChar® [OTC] *see* Charcoal *on page 121*

Suplical® [OTC] *see* Calcium Carbonate *on page 94*

Supprelin™ *see* Histrelin *on page 286*

Suprax® *see* Cefixime *on page 111*

Surfak® [OTC] *see* Docusate *on page 202*

Survanta® *see* Beractant *on page 80*

Sus-Phrine® *see* Epinephrine *on page 220*

Sustaire® *see* Theophylline *on page 554*

Sutilains (soo' ti lains)

Brand Names Travase®

Therapeutic Category Enzyme, Topical Debridement

Use To promote debridement of necrotic debris; as an adjunct in the treatment of second and third degree burns; decubitus ulcers

Pregnancy Risk Factor B

Contraindications Wounds communicating with major body cavities; wounds with exposed nerves; fungating neoplastic ulcers; hypersensitivity to sutilains

Warnings A topical anti-infective agent should be used with sutilains

Precautions Should not be applied to more than 10% to 15% of the burned area at one time; safety and efficacy has not been established in children

Adverse Reactions

Dermatologic: Dermatitis

Local: Pain, paresthesia, bleeding

Drug Interactions Benzalkonium chloride, hexachlorophene, iodine, thimerosal and silver nitrate decrease its activity

Stability Store in the refrigerator; activity is greatest at pH 6-6.8

Mechanism of Action Enzymatically converts denatured proteins (necrotic soft tissue, hemoglobin and purulent exudate) to peptides and amino acids

Pharmacodynamics

Onset of action: Following topical application, within 60 minutes

Peak effect: May not be seen until 5-7 days for burns or 8-12 days for decubital ulcers

Duration: 8-12 hours

Usual Dosage Children and Adults: Topical: Thoroughly cleanse and irrigate wound then apply ointment in a thin layer extending ¼" to ½" beyond the tissue being debrided; apply loose moist dressing; repeat 3-4 times/day

Patient Information Discontinue use if bleeding or dermatitis occurs

Nursing Implications Avoid contact with the eyes; keep wound area moist for optimal activity

Dosage Forms Ointment: 82,000 casein units/g (14.2 g)

Suxamethonium Chloride *see* Succinylcholine Chloride *on page 537*

Syllact® [OTC] *see* Psyllium *on page 498*

Symadine® *see* Amantadine Hydrochloride *on page 34*

Symmetrel® *see* Amantadine Hydrochloride *on page 34*

Synacort® *see* Hydrocortisone *on page 293*

Synacthen *see* Cosyntropin *on page 155*

Synalar® *see* Fluocinolone Acetonide *on page 254*

Synalgos® [OTC] *see* Aspirin *on page 61*

Synemol® *see* Fluocinolone Acetonide *on page 254*

Synthetic Lung Surfactant *see* Colfosceril Palmitate *on page 151*

Synthroid® *see* Levothyroxine Sodium *on page 339*

Systemic Corticosteroids Comparison Chart *see page 727*

T_4 Thyroxine Sodium *see* Levothyroxine Sodium *on page 339*

Tac™-3 *see* Triamcinolone *on page 579*

Tagamet® *see* Cimetidine *on page 134*

Talwin® *see* Pentazocine *on page 444*

Talwin® NX *see* Pentazocine *on page 444*

Tambocor® *see* Flecainide Acetate *on page 246*

Tamine® [OTC] *see* Brompheniramine and Phenylpropanolamine *on page 87*

Tao® *see* Troleandomycin *on page 587*

Tapazole® *see* Methimazole *on page 371*

Tazicef® *see* Ceftazidime *on page 116*

Tazidime® *see* Ceftazidime *on page 116*

TCN *see* Tetracycline Hydrochloride *on page 552*

Tebamide® *see* Trimethobenzamide Hydrochloride *on page 585*

Tegopen® *see* Cloxacillin Sodium *on page 146*

Tegretol® *see* Carbamazepine *on page 101*

Telachlor® *see* Chlorpheniramine Maleate *on page 128*

Telador® *see* Betamethasone *on page 81*

Teldrin® [OTC] *see* Chlorpheniramine Maleate *on page 128*

Teline® *see* Tetracycline Hydrochloride *on page 552*

Tempra® [OTC] *see* Acetaminophen *on page 16*

Tenormin® *see* Atenolol *on page 63*

Tensilon® *see* Edrophonium Chloride *on page 217*

Terbutaline Sulfate (ter byoo' ta leen)

Brand Names Brethaire®; Brethine®; Bricanyl®

Therapeutic Category Beta-2-Adrenergic Agonist Agent; Bronchodilator; Sympathomimetic; Toxolytic Agent

Use Bronchodilator in reversible airway obstruction and bronchial asthma

Pregnancy Risk Factor B

Contraindications Hypersensitivity to terbutaline or any component

Warnings Paradoxical bronchoconstriction may occur with excessive use; if it occurs, discontinue terbutaline immediately

Precautions Use with caution in patients with diabetes, hypertension, hyperthyroidism, history of seizures, or cardiac disease

Adverse Reactions

Cardiovascular: Tachycardia, hypertension, arrhythmias

Central nervous system: Drowsiness, tremors, headache, nervousness, seizures

Gastrointestinal: Nausea

Otic: Tinnitus

Drug Interactions Beta-receptor-blocking agents, other sympathomimetics, MAO inhibitors, tricyclic antidepressants

Mechanism of Action Relaxes bronchial smooth muscle and muscles of peripheral vasculature by action on $beta_2$ receptors with less effect on heart rate

Pharmacodynamics

Onset of action:

Oral: 30 minutes

Oral inhalation: 5-30 minutes

S.C.: 6-15 minutes

Duration:

Oral: 4-8 hours

Oral inhalation: 3-6 hours

S.C.: 1.5-4 hours

Pharmacokinetics

Absorption: 33% to 50%

Metabolism: Possible first-pass metabolism after oral use

Elimination: Primarily eliminated (60%) unchanged in urine after parenteral use

Usual Dosage

Children <12 years:

Oral: Initial: 0.05 mg/kg/dose every 8 hours, increase gradually; maximum: 0.15 mg/kg/dose or 5 mg/day

S.C.: 0.005-0.01 mg/kg/dose to a maximum of 0.4 mg/dose every 15-20 minutes for 2 doses

Children >12 years and Adults:

Oral: 2.5-5 mg/dose every 6-8 hours; maximum daily dose:

12-15 years: 7.5 mg

>15 years: 15 mg

S.C.: 0.25 mg/dose repeated in 15-30 minutes for one time only; a total dose of 0.5 mg should not be exceeded within a 4-hour period

Inhalation: Children and Adults: 1-2 puffs every 4-6 hours

Nebulization: Children and Adults: 0.01-0.03 mL/kg (1 mg = 1 mL); minimum dose: 0.1 mL; maximum dose: 2.5 mL diluted with 1-2 mL normal saline, every 4-6 hours

Monitoring Parameters Heart rate, blood pressure, respiratory rate, arterial or capillary blood gases (if applicable)

Additional Information Continuous infusion of terbutaline has been used successfully in children with asthma; a 2 μg/kg loading dose followed by a 0.08 μg/kg/minute continuous infusion; individual dosage may require titration depending upon clinical effects; doses as high as 4 μg/kg/minute have been used

Dosage Forms

Aerosol, oral: 0.2 mg/actuation (10.5 g)

Injection: 1 mg/mL (1 mL)

Tablet: 2.5 mg, 5 mg

Extemporaneous Preparation(s) A 1 mg/mL suspension made from terbutaline tablets in simple syrup NF is stable 30 days when refrigerated

Horner RK and Johnson CE, "Stability of An Extemporaneously Compounded Terbutaline Sulfate Oral Liquid," *Am J Hosp Pharm*, 1991, 48(2):293-5.

References

Bohn D, Kalloghlian A, Jenkins J, et al, "Intravenous Salbutamol in the Treatment of Status Asthmaticus in Children," *Critical Care Medicine,* 1984, 12:892-6.

Canny GJ and Levison H, "Aerosols - Therapeutic Use and Delivery in Childhood Asthma," *Ann Allergy*, 1988, 60(1):11-9.

Fuglsang G, Pedersen S, and Borgstrom L, "Dose-Response Relationships of I.V. Administered Terbutaline in Children With Asthma," *J Pediatr*, 1989, 114(2):315-20.

Goldenhersh N and Rachelefsky GS, "Childhood Asthma: Management," *Pediatr Rev*, 1989, 10(9):259-67.

Rachelefsky GS and Siegel SC, "Asthma in Infants and Children - Treatment of Childhood Asthma: Part II," *J Allergy Clin Immunol*, 1985, 76(3):409-25.

Tipton WR and Nelson HS, "Frequent Parenteral Terbutaline in the Treatment of Status Asthmaticus," *Ann Allergy*, 1987, 58:252-6.

Terfenadine (ter fen' a deen)

Related Information

Overdose and Toxicology Information *on page 696-700*

(Continued)

Terfenadine *(Continued)*

Brand Names Seldane®

Therapeutic Category Antihistamine

Use Perennial and seasonal allergic rhinitis and other allergic symptoms including urticaria

Pregnancy Risk Factor C

Contraindications Hypersensitivity to terfenadine or any component

Warnings Severe cardiovascular effects including Q-T interval prolongation, ventricular tachycardia, ventricular fibrillation, death, cardiac arrest, hypotension, palpitations, and syncope have occurred; may impair ability to perform hazardous activities requiring mental alertness or physical coordination

Precautions Safety and efficacy in children <12 years of age have not been established

Adverse Reactions

Cardiovascular: Cardiac toxicity (see Warnings)

Central nervous system: Sedation, fatigue, dizziness, nervousness, weakness, mental depression, insomnia, tremor, confusion, headache

Dermatologic: Rash

Gastrointestinal: Nausea, vomiting, weight gain, dry mouth

Hepatic: Elevation in liver enzymes, jaundice, hepatitis (rare)

Respiratory: Cough, sore throat

Miscellaneous: Hypersensitivity reactions

Drug Interactions Patients receiving ketoconazole, itraconazole, and macrolide antibiotics (eg, erythromycin, troleandomycin) are at increased risk of developing cardiac toxicity (see Warnings)

Mechanism of Action Specific, selective histamine H_1, receptor antagonist which does not readily cross the blood-brain barrier

Pharmacodynamics Oral:

Onset of antihistaminic effects: Apparent in 1-2 hours after an oral dose

Peak effects: 3-6 hours

Duration: At least 12 hours

Pharmacokinetics

Absorption: Oral: ~70%

Metabolism: Extensive first-pass metabolism in the liver

Elimination: Primarily excreted in the feces via biliary elimination and also in the urine

Usual Dosage Oral:

Children:

3-6 years: 15 mg twice daily

6-12 years: 30 mg twice daily

Children >12 years and Adults: 60 mg twice daily

Test Interactions Antigen skin testing

Dosage Forms Tablet: 60 mg

TESPA *see* Thiotepa *on page 563*

Testosterone (tess toss' ter one)

Brand Names Andro®; Andro-Cyp®; Andro-L.A.®; Andronate®; Andropository®; Delatest®; Delatestryl®; Depotest®; Depo®-Testosterone; Duratest®; Durathate®; Everone®; Histerone®

Synonyms Aqueous Testosterone; Testosterone Cypionate; Testosterone Enanthate

Therapeutic Category Androgen

Use Androgen replacement therapy in the treatment of delayed male puberty; male hypogonadism

Restrictions C-IV

Pregnancy Risk Factor X

Contraindications Severe renal or cardiac disease; male patients with prostatic or breast cancer, hypercalcemia

Warnings May accelerate bone maturation without producing compensating gain in linear growth

Precautions Use with caution in patients with hepatic, cardiac, or renal dysfunction

Adverse Reactions

Cardiovascular: Flushing, edema

Central nervous system: Excitation, aggressive behavior, sleeplessness, anxiety, mental depression, headache

Dermatologic: Acne, hirsutism, urticaria

Endocrine & metabolic: Gynecomastia, hypercalcemia, hypoglycemia

Gastrointestinal: Nausea

Hematologic: Leukopenia, suppression of clotting factors, polycythemia

Hepatic: Cholestatic hepatitis

Local: Inflammation at injection site

Renal & genitourinary: Epididymitis, priapism, bladder irritability

Drug Interactions Oral anticoagulants, cyclosporine, insulin, warfarin

Mechanism of Action Principal endogenous androgen responsible for promoting the growth and development of the male sex organs and maintaining secondary sex characteristics in androgen-deficient males

Pharmacodynamics Duration of effect: Based upon the route of administration and which testosterone ester is used; the cypionate and enanthate esters have the longest duration, up to 2-4 weeks after I.M. administration

Usual Dosage I.M.:

Children:

Male hypogonadism:

Initiation of pubertal growth: 40-50 mg/m^2/dose (cypionate or enanthate ester) monthly until the growth rate falls to prepubertal levels

Terminal growth phase: 100 mg/m^2/dose (cypionate or enanthate ester) monthly until growth ceases

Maintenance virilizing dose: 100 mg/m^2/dose (cypionate or enanthate ester) twice monthly

Delayed puberty: 40-50 mg/m^2/dose monthly (cypionate or enanthate ester) for 6 months

Adults:

Hypogonadism:

Testosterone or testosterone propionate: 10-25 mg 2-3 times/week

Testosterone cypionate or enanthate: 50-400 mg every 2-4 weeks

Postpubertal cryptorchism: Testosterone or testosterone propionate: 10-25 mg 2-3 times/week

Monitoring Parameters Periodic liver function tests, radiologic examination of wrist and hand every 6 months (when using in prepubertal children)

Reference Range Testosterone, Urine: Male: 100-1500 ng/24 hours; female: 100-500 ng/24 hours

Nursing Implications Give deep I.M.

Additional Information Topically applied 5% cream for 21 days has been effective in the treatment of microphallus

Dosage Forms Injection:

Aqueous suspension: 25 mg/mL (10 mL, 30 mL); 50 mg/mL (10 mL, 30 mL); 100 mg/mL (10 mL, 30 mL)

In oil, as cypionate: 100 mg/mL (1 mL, 10 mL); 200 mg/mL (1 mL, 10 mL)

In oil, as enanthate: 100 mg/mL (5 mL, 10 mL); 200 mg/mL (5 mL, 10 mL)

In oil, as propionate: 50 mg/mL (10 mL, 30 mL); 100 mg/mL (10 mL, 30 mL)

Testosterone Cypionate *see* Testosterone *on previous page*

Testosterone Enanthate *see* Testosterone *on previous page*

Tetanus Immune Globulin, Human *see* Immunization Guidelines *on page 660-667*

Tetanus Toxoid, Adsorbed *see* Immunization Guidelines *on page 660-667*

Tetanus Toxoid, Fluid *see* Immunization Guidelines *on page 660-667*

Tetracaine Hydrochloride (tet' ra kane)

Brand Names Pontocaine®

Synonyms Amethocaine Hydrochloride

Therapeutic Category Local Anesthetic, Injectable; Local Anesthetic, Ophthalmic; Local Anesthetic, Topical

Use Local anesthesia in the eye for various diagnostic and examination purposes; spinal anesthesia; topical anesthesia for local skin disorders; local anesthesia for mucous membranes

(Continued)

Tetracaine Hydrochloride *(Continued)*

Pregnancy Risk Factor C

Contraindications Hypersensitivity to tetracaine or any component; ophthalmic secondary bacterial infection, patients with liver disease; CNS disease, meningitis (if used for epidural or spinal anesthesia); myasthenia gravis, impaired cardiac conduction

Precautions Parenteral form may contain sulfites which may cause severe hypersensitivity reactions in sensitive individuals

Adverse Reactions

Cardiovascular: Cardiac arrest, bradycardia, myocardial depression, cardiac arrhythmias, hypotension

Central nervous system: Anxiety, apprehension, nervousness, disorientation, seizures; drowsiness, unconsciousness

Dermatologic: Urticaria, contact dermatitis with topical form

Gastrointestinal: Nausea, vomiting

Local: Stinging, burning at injection site

Ocular: Lacrimation, photophobia, corneal epithelial erosion, keratitis, corneal opacification, miosis

Otic: Tinnitus

Respiratory: Respiratory arrest

Drug Interactions Aminosalicylic acid, sulfonamides

Mechanism of Action Blocks both the generation and conduction of sensory, motor, and autonomic nerve fibers by decreasing the neuronal membrane's permeability to sodium ions, which results in decreasing the rate of depolarization of the nerve membrane

Pharmacodynamics

Onset of action:

- Ophthalmic instillation: Anesthetic effects occur within 60 seconds
- Topical: Within 3 minutes when applied to mucous membranes for spinal anesthesia

Duration: 1.5-3 hours

Pharmacokinetics

Metabolism: Metabolized by the liver

Elimination: Metabolites are renally excreted

Usual Dosage

Children: Safety and efficacy have not been established

Adults:

- Cream: Apply to affected area as needed
- Injection: Dosage varies with the anesthetic procedure, the degree of anesthesia required, and the individual patient response; it is administered by subarachnoid injection for spinal anesthesia:
  - Perineal anesthesia: 5 mg
  - Perineal and lower extremities: 10 mg
  - Anesthesia extending up to the costal margin: 15-20 mg
  - Low spinal anesthesia (saddle block): 2-5 mg
- Ointment: Apply ½" to 1" to lower conjunctival fornix
- Ophthalmic: Solution: Use 1-2 drops

Patient Information Do not touch or rub eye until anesthesia (if ophthalmic) has worn off

Nursing Implications Not for prolonged use topically

Dosage Forms

Cream: 1% (28 g)

Injection: 1% (2 mL)

Injection, with dextrose 6%: 0.2% (2 mL); 0.3% (5 mL)

Ointment:

- Ophthalmic: 0.5% (3.75 g)
- Topical: 0.5% (28 g)

Solution:

- Ophthalmic: 0.5% (1 mL, 2 mL, 15 mL, 59 mL)
- Topical: 2% (30 mL, 118 mL)

Tetracosactide *see* Cosyntropin *on page 155*

Tetracycline Hydrochloride (tet ra sye' kleen)

Brand Names Achromycin®; Achromycin® V; Ala-Tet®; Nor-tet®; Panmycin®; Robitet®; Sumycin®; Teline®; Tetracyn®; Tetralan®; Topicycline®

Synonyms TCN

Therapeutic Category Acne Product; Antibiotic, Ophthalmic; Antibiotic, Tetracycline Derivative; Antibiotic, Topical

Use Treatment of susceptible bacterial infections of both gram-positive and gram-negative organisms; some unusual organisms including *Mycoplasma*, *Chlamydia*, *Brucella*, and *Rickettsia*; may also be used for acne, exacerbations of chronic bronchitis, and treatment of gonorrhea and syphilis in patients that are allergic to penicillin

Pregnancy Risk Factor D; B (topical)

Contraindications Hypersensitivity to tetracycline or any component; in women during pregnancy; children ≤8 years of age; use of tetracyclines during tooth development may cause permanent discoloration of the teeth, enamel hypoplasia and retardation of skeletal development and bone growth with risk being greatest for children <4 years and in those receiving high doses

Warnings Photosensitivity reaction may occur with this drug; avoid prolonged exposure to sunlight or tanning equipment

Precautions Use with caution in patients with renal and liver impairment; dosage modification required in patients with renal impairment

Adverse Reactions

Cardiovascular: Angioedema
Central nervous system: Pseudotumor cerebri, fever
Dermatologic: Rash, exfoliative dermatitis, photosensitivity
Gastrointestinal: Nausea, vomiting, diarrhea, stomatitis, glossitis, antibiotic-associated pseudomembranous colitis, esophagitis
Hematologic: Fanconi-like syndrome, hemolytic anemia
Hepatic: Hepatotoxicity
Musculoskeletal: Injury to growing bones and teeth
Renal & genitourinary: Renal damage
Respiratory: Pulmonary infiltrates with eosinophilia
Miscellaneous: Hypersensitivity reactions, candidal superinfection

Drug Interactions Dairy products; calcium, magnesium or aluminum containing antacids (↓ tetracycline absorption); iron, zinc; methoxyflurane (↑ chance of nephrotoxicity)

Stability Protect from light; outdated tetracyclines have caused a Fanconi-like syndrome

Mechanism of Action Inhibits bacterial protein synthesis by binding with the 30S and possibly the 50S ribosomal subunit(s) of susceptible bacteria; may also cause alterations in the cytoplasmic membrane

Pharmacokinetics

Absorption:
 Oral: 75%
 I.M.: Poor, with less than 60% of a dose absorbed
Protein binding: 20% to 60%
Half-life: 6-12 hours with normal renal function and is prolonged with renal impairment
Peak serum levels: Within 2-4 hours
Elimination: Primary route is the kidney, with 60% of a dose excreted as unchanged drug in the urine, small amounts appear in the bile
Slightly dialyzable (5% to 20%)

Usual Dosage

Children >8 years:
 Oral: 25-50 mg/kg/day in divided doses every 6 hours; not to exceed 3 g/day
 Ophthalmic:
  Suspension: 1-2 drops 2-4 times/day
  Ointment: Instill every 2-12 hours

Adults:
 Oral: 250-500 mg/dose every 6-12 hours
 Ophthalmic:
  Suspension: 1-2 drops 2-4 times/day
  Ointment: Instill every 2-12 hours

Monitoring Parameters Renal, hepatic, and hematologic function tests

Test Interactions False-negative urine glucose with Clinistix®

Patient Information Take 1 hour before or 2 hours after meals with adequate amounts of fluid; avoid prolonged exposure to sunlight or sunlamps; avoid taking antacids, iron, or dairy products before tetracyclines

(Continued)

Tetracycline Hydrochloride *(Continued)*

Dosage Forms

Capsule: 100 mg, 250 mg, 500 mg
Ointment:
Ophthalmic: 1% (3.5 g)
Topical: 3% (14.2 g, 30 g)
Solution, topical: 2.2 mg/mL (70 mL)
Suspension:
Ophthalmic: 1% (0.5 mL, 1 mL, 4 mL)
Oral: 125 mg/5 mL (60 mL, 480 mL)
Tablet: 250 mg, 500 mg

References

Committee on Drugs, American Academy of Pediatrics, "Requiem for Tetracyclines," *Pediatrics*, 1975, 55:142.

Tetracyn® *see* Tetracycline Hydrochloride *on page 552*

Tetrahydrocannabinol, THC *see* Dronabinol *on page 211*

Tetralan® *see* Tetracycline Hydrochloride *on page 552*

TG *see* Thioguanine *on page 560*

6-TG *see* Thioguanine *on page 560*

T/Gel® [OTC] *see* Coal Tar *on page 147*

T-Gen® *see* Trimethobenzamide Hydrochloride *on page 585*

T-Gesic® *see* Hydrocodone and Acetaminophen *on page 292*

Tham® *see* Tromethamine *on page 587*

Tham-E® *see* Tromethamine *on page 587*

Theo-24® *see* Theophylline *on this page*

Theobid® *see* Theophylline *on this page*

Theochron® *see* Theophylline *on this page*

Theoclear® L.A. *see* Theophylline *on this page*

Theo-Dur® *see* Theophylline *on this page*

Theolair™ *see* Theophylline *on this page*

Theophylline (thee off' i lin)

Related Information

Blood Level Sampling Time Guidelines *on page 694-695*
Overdose and Toxicology Information *on page 696-700*

Brand Names Aerolate®; Aerolate III®; Aerolate JR®; Aerolate SR® S; Aquaphyllin®; Asmalix®; Bronkodyl®; Constant-T®; Elixicon®; Elixophyllin®; Elixophyllin® SR; Quibron®-T; Quibron®-T/SR; Respbid®; Slo-bid™; Slo-Phyllin®; Sustaire®; Theo-24®; Theobid®; Theochron®; Theoclear® L.A.; Theo-Dur®; Theolair™; Theospan®-SR; Theovent®; Theox®; Uniphyl®

Therapeutic Category Bronchodilator

Use As a bronchodilator in reversible airway obstruction due to asthma or COPD; for treatment of idiopathic apnea of prematurity in neonates

Pregnancy Risk Factor C

Serum Levels (μg/mL)*	Adverse Reactions
15–25	GI upset, GE reflux, diarrhea, nausea, vomiting, abdominal pain, nervousness, headache, insomnia, agitation, dizziness, muscle cramp, tremor
25–35	Tachycardia, occasional PVC
>35	Ventricular tachycardia, frequent PVC, seizure

*Adverse effects do not necessarily occur according to serum levels. Arrhythmia and seizure can occur without seeing the other adverse effects.

Contraindications Uncontrolled arrhythmias

Warnings Some commercial preparations may contain sulfites which may produce hypersensitivity reactions in sensitive individuals

Precautions Use with caution in patients with peptic ulcer, hyperthyroidism, hypertension, and patients with compromised cardiac function

Adverse Reactions See table on previous page.

Drug Interactions See table.

Factors Reported to Affect Theophylline Serum Levels

Decreased Theophylline Level	Increased Theophylline Level
Smoking (cigarettes, marijuana)	Hepatic cirrhosis
High protein/low carbohydrate diet	Cor pulmonale
Charcoal broiled beef	CHF
Phenytoin	Fever/viral illness
Phenobarbital	Propranolol
Carbamazepine	Allopurinol (>600 mg/d)
Rifampin	Erythromycin
I.V. isoproterenol	Cimetidine
	Troleandomycin
	Ciprofloxacin
	Oral contraceptives

Mechanism of Action Competitively inhibits the enzyme phosphodiesterase resulting in increased levels of cyclic adenine monophosphate (CAMP) which may be responsible for most of theophylline's effects; its effects on the myocardium and neuromuscular transmission may be due to the intracellular translocation of ionized calcium; overall, theophylline produces the following effects: relaxation of the smooth muscle of the respiratory tract, pulmonary, coronary, and renal artery dilation, CNS stimulation, diuresis, stimulation of catecholamine release, gastric acid secretion, and relaxation of biliary and GI smooth muscle

Pharmacokinetics

Absorption: Oral: Up to 100% depending upon the formulation used

Distribution: V_d: 0.45 L/kg; distributes into breast milk (approximates serum concentration); crosses the placenta

Metabolism: Metabolized in the liver by demethylation and oxidation; in neonates, a small portion of theophylline is metabolized to caffeine

Half-life: See table.

Patient Group	Approximate Half-Life (h)
Neonates	
Premature	30
Normal newborn	24
Infants	
4–52 weeks	4–30
Children/Adolescents	
1–9 years	2–10 (4 avg)
9–16 years	4–16
Adults	
Nonsmoker	4–16 (8.7 avg)
Smoker	4.4
Cardiac compromised, liver failure	20–30

Elimination: Excreted in the urine; adults excrete 10% in urine as unchanged drug; neonates excrete a greater percentage of the dose unchanged in the urine (up to 50%)

Usual Dosage Oral (see aminophylline for I.V. doses):

Neonates: Apnea of prematurity: Loading dose: 4 mg/kg/dose; maintenance dose: See table.

Treatment of acute bronchospasm:

Initial dosage recommendation: Loading dose (to achieve a serum level of about 10 μg/mL; loading doses should be given using a rapidly absorbed oral product **not** a sustained release product):

(Continued)

Theophylline *(Continued)*

If no theophylline has been administered in the previous 24 hours: 5 mg/kg theophylline

If theophylline has been administered in the previous 24 hours: 2.5 mg/kg theophylline can be given in emergencies when serum levels are not available

On the average, for every 1 mg/kg theophylline given, blood levels will rise 2 µg/mL

Guidelines for Drawing Theophylline Serum Levels

Dosage Form	Time to Draw Level*
I.V. bolus	30 min after end of 30 min infusion
I.V. continuous infusion	12–24 h after initiation of infusion
P.O. liquid, fast-release tab	Peak: 1 h post a dose after at least 1 day of therapy Trough: Just before a dose after at least 1 day of therapy
P.O. slow-release product	Peak: 4 h post a dose after at least 1 day of therapy Trough: Just before a dose after at least 1 day of therapy

*The time to achieve steady-state serum levels is prolonged in patients with longer half-lives (eg, premature neonates, infants, and adults with cardiac or liver failure (see theophylline half-life table). In these patients, serum theophylline levels should be drawn after 48–72 hours of therapy.

Maintenance Dose for Acute Symptoms

Population Group	Oral Theophylline (mg/kg/day)
Premature infant or newborn - 6 wk (for apnea/bradycardia)	4
6 wk - 6 mo	10
Infants 6 mo–1 y	12–18
Children 1–9 y	20–24
Children 9–12 y, and adolescent daily smokers of cigarettes or marijuana, and otherwise healthy adult smokers under 50 y	16
Adolescents 12–16 y (nonsmokers)	13
Otherwise healthy nonsmoking adults (including elderly patients)	10 (not to exceed 900 mg/day)
Cardiac decompensation, cor pulmonale and/or liver dysfunction	5 (not to exceed 400 mg/day)

These recommendations, based on mean clearance rates for age or risk factors, were calculated to achieve a serum level of 10 µg/mL (5 µg/mL for newborns with apnea/bradycardia). In newborns and infants, a fast-release oral product can be used. The total daily dose can be divided every 12 hours in newborns and every 6-8 hours in infants. In children and healthy adults, a slow-release product can be used. The total daily dose can be divided every 8-12 hours.

Use ideal body weight for obese patients

Dose should be further adjusted based on serum levels. Guidelines for drawing theophylline serum levels are shown in the table.

Monitoring Parameters Respiratory rate, heart rate, serum theophylline level, arterial or capillary blood gases (if applicable)

Reference Range Therapeutic levels: Asthma: 10-20 μg/mL; Toxic concentration: >20 μg/mL; apnea of prematurity: 6-14 μg/mL

Test Interactions May elevate uric acid levels

Patient Information Oral preparations should be taken with a full glass of water; avoid drinking or eating large quantities of caffeine containing beverages or food; take at regular intervals; take sustained release tablets whole; sustained release capsule forms may be opened and sprinkled on soft foods; do not chew beads

Nursing Implications Do not crush Theo-Dur® tablets; tablets may only be cut in half

Additional Information Due to improved theophylline clearance during the first year of life, serum concentration determinations and dosage adjustments may be needed to optimize therapy

Available also by nonproprietary name

Theophylline Immediate Release Tablet/Capsule: Bronkodyl®, Elixophyllin®, Quibron®-T, Slo-Phyllin®, Theolair™

Theophylline Liquid: Aerolate®, Aquaphyllin®, Asmalix®, Elixicon®, Elixophyllin®

Theophylline Timed Release Capsule: Aerolate III®, Aerolate JR®, Aerolate SR®, Elixophyllin® SR, Slo-bid™ Gyrocaps®, Slo-Phyllin® Gyrocaps®, Theobid®, Theoclear® L.A., Theospan®-SR, Theospan®-SR

Theophylline Timed Release Tablet: Constant-T®, Quibron®-T/S, Respbid®, Sustaire®, Theochron®, Theo-Dur®, Theolair™-SR, Uniphyl®

Dosage Forms

Capsule:

Immediate release (Bronkodyl®, Elixophyllin®): 100 mg, 200 mg

Timed release:

[8-12 hours] (Aerolate®): 65 mg [III]; 130 mg [JR], 260 mg [SR]
[8-12 hours] (Elixophyllin SR®): 125 mg, 250 mg
[8-12 hours] (Slo-bid™): 50 mg, 75 mg, 100 mg, 125 mg, 200 mg, 300 mg
[8-12 hours] (Slo-Phyllin® Gyrocaps®): 60 mg, 125 mg, 250 mg
[12 hours] (Theobid® Jr. Duracaps®): 130 mg
[12 hours] (Theobid® Duracaps®): 260 mg
[12 hours] (Theoclear® L.A.): 130 mg, 260 mg
[12 hours] (Theo-Dur® Sprinkle®): 50 mg, 75 mg, 125 mg, 200 mg
[12 hours] (Theospan®-SR): 130 mg, 260 mg
[12 hours] (Theovent®): 125 mg, 250 mg
[24 hours] (Theo-24®): 100 mg, 200 mg, 300 mg

Elixir (Asmalix®, Elixomin®, Elixophyllin®, Lanophyllin®): 80 mg/15 mL (15 mL, 30 mL, 480 mL, 4000 mL)

Solution, oral:

Theolair™: 80 mg/15 mL (15 mL, 18.75 mL, 30 mL, 480 mL)
Aerolate®: 150 mg/15 mL (480 mL)

Syrup:

Aquaphyllin®, Slo-Phyllin®, Theoclear-80®, Theostat-80®: 80 mg/15 mL (15 mL, 30 mL, 500 mL)
Accurbron®: 150 mg/15 mL (480 mL)

Tablet: Immediate release:

Slo-Phyllin®: 100 mg, 200 mg
Theolair™: 125 mg, 250 mg
Quibron®-T: 300 mg

Tablet:

Controlled release (Theox®): 100 mg, 200 mg, 300 mg

Timed release:

[12-24 hours]: 100 mg, 200 mg, 300 mg
[8-12 hours] (Constant-T®): 200 mg, 300 mg
[8-12 hours] (Quibron®-T/SR): 300 mg
[8-12 hours] (Respbid®): 250 mg, 500 mg
[8-12 hours] (Sustaire®): 100 mg, 300 mg
[8-12 hours] (T-Phyl®): 200 mg
[12-24 hours] (Theochron®): 100 mg, 200 mg, 300 mg
[8-24 hours] (Theo-Dur®): 100 mg, 200 mg, 300 mg, 450 mg
[8-24 hours] (Theo-Sav®): 100 mg, 200 mg, 300 mg
[8-24 hours] (Theolair-SR®): 200 mg, 250 mg, 300 mg, 500 mg
[24 hours] (Uniphyl®): 400 mg

References

(Continued)

Theophylline *(Continued)*

Kearney TE, Manoguerra AS, Curtis GP, et al, "Theophylline Toxicity and the Beta-Adrenergic System," *Ann Intern Med*, 1985, 102(6):766-9.

Upton RA, "Pharmacokinetic Interactions Between Theophylline and Other Medication," *Clin Pharmacokinet*, 1991, 20(1):66-80.

Theophylline Ethylenediamine *see* Aminophylline *on page 37*

Theospan®-SR *see* Theophylline *on page 554*

Theovent® *see* Theophylline *on page 554*

Theox® *see* Theophylline *on page 554*

Thera-Flur® Gel *see* Fluoride *on page 255*

Thermazene® *see* Silver Sulfadiazine *on page 523*

Thiabendazole (thye a ben' da zole)

Brand Names Mintezol®

Synonyms Tiabendazole

Therapeutic Category Anthelmintic

Use Treatment of strongyloidiasis, cutaneous larva migrans, visceral larva migrans, dracunculosis, trichinosis, and mixed helminthic infections

Pregnancy Risk Factor C

Contraindications Known hypersensitivity to thiabendazole

Precautions Use with caution in patients with renal or hepatic impairment, malnutrition or anemia, or dehydration

Adverse Reactions

Cardiovascular: Flushing

Central nervous system: Dizziness, drowsiness, vertigo, seizures, fever, headache, chills, hallucinations

Dermatologic: Rash, Stevens-Johnson syndrome, erythema multiforme

Gastrointestinal: Nausea, vomiting, diarrhea

Hematologic: Leukopenia

Hepatic: Hepatotoxicity

Otic: Tinnitus

Renal & genitourinary: Malodor of the urine, nephrotoxicity

Miscellaneous: Hypersensitivity reactions, lymphadenopathy

Drug Interactions Theophylline (↑ serum theophylline)

Mechanism of Action Inhibits helminth-specific mitochondrial fumarate reductase

Pharmacokinetics

Absorption: Absorbed from the GI tract and through the skin

Metabolism: Rapidly metabolized

Peak serum levels: Within 1-2 hours

Elimination: Excreted in the feces (5%) and urine (87%), primarily as conjugated metabolites

Usual Dosage Oral:

Children and Adults: 50 mg/kg/day divided every 12 hours (maximum dose: 3 g/day)

- Strongyloidiasis: For 2 consecutive days
- Cutaneous larva migrans: For 2-5 consecutive days; thiabendazole 10% to 15% suspension has been applied topically to lesions 4-6 times/day
- Visceral larva migrans: For 5-7 consecutive days
- Trichinosis: For 2-4 consecutive days
- Angiostrongyliasis: 50-75 mg/kg/day divided every 8-12 hours for 3 days (5 days for disseminated disease)
- Dracunculosis: 50-75 mg/kg/day divided every 12 hours for 3 days

Monitoring Parameters Periodic renal and hepatic function tests

Patient Information Take after meals, chew tablet well; may decrease alertness, avoid driving or operating machinery

Nursing Implications Purgation is not required prior to use

Dosage Forms

Suspension, oral: 500 mg/5 mL (120 mL)

Tablet, chewable (orange flavor): 500 mg

References

Walden J, "Parasitic Diseases. Other Roundworms. *Trichuris*, Hookworm, and *Strongyloides*," *Prim Care*, 1991, 18(1):53-74.

Zygmunt DJ, "*Strongyloides stearcoralis*," *Infect Control Hosp Epidemiol*, 1990, 11(9):495-7.

Thiamazole *see* Methimazole *on page 371*

Thiamine Hydrochloride (thye' a min)

Brand Names Betalin®S; Biamine®

Synonyms Aneurine Hydrochloride; Thiaminium Chloride Hydrochloride; Vitamin B_1

Therapeutic Category Vitamin, Water Soluble

Use Treatment of thiamine deficiency including beriberi, Wernicke's encephalopathy syndrome, and peripheral neuritis associated with pellagra, alcoholic patients with altered sensorium; various genetic metabolic disorders

Pregnancy Risk Factor A (C if dose exceeds RDA recommendation)

Contraindications Hypersensitivity to thiamine or any component

Warnings Large doses should be given in divided doses for better oral absorption

Precautions Use parenteral route cautiously, see Adverse Reactions

Adverse Reactions

Cardiovascular: Warmth, tingling, angioedema, cardiovascular collapse and death (primarily following repeated I.V. administration)

Dermatologic: Rash

Drug Interactions High carbohydrate diets or I.V. dextrose solutions increase thiamine requirement; may enhance the effects of neuromuscular blocking agents

Stability Unstable with alkaline solutions

Mechanism of Action An essential coenzyme in carbohydrate metabolism; combines with adenosine triphosphate to form thiamine pyrophosphate

Pharmacokinetics

Absorption:
- Oral: Poorly absorbed
- I.M.: Rapidly and completely absorbed

Metabolism: Liver metabolism

Elimination: Excreted renally as unchanged drug only after body storage sites become saturated

Usual Dosage

Recommended daily allowance:
- <6 months: 0.3 mg
- 6 months to 1 year: 0.4 mg
- 1-3 years: 0.7 mg
- 4-6 years: 0.9 mg
- 7-10 years: 1 mg
- 11-14 years: 1.1-1.3 mg
- >14 years: 1-1.5 mg

Thiamine deficiency (beriberi):
- Children: 10-25 mg/dose I.M. or I.V. daily (if critically ill), or 10-50 mg/dose orally every day for 2 weeks, then 5-10 mg/dose orally daily for 1 month
- Adults: 5-30 mg/dose I.M. or I.V. 3 times/day (if critically ill); then orally 5-30 mg/day in single or divided doses 3 times/day for 1 month

Wenicke's encephalopathy: Adults: Initial: 100 mg I.V., then 50-100 mg/day I.M. or I.V. until consuming a regular, balanced diet

Dietary supplement (depends on caloric or carbohydrate content of the diet):
- Infants: 0.3-0.5 mg/day
- Children: 0.5-1 mg/day
- Adults: 1-2 mg/day
- **Note:** The above doses can be found in multivitamin preparations

Metabolic disorders: Oral: Adults: 10-20 mg/day (dosages up to 4 g/day in divided doses have been used)

Administration Administer by slow I.V. injection

Reference Range Therapeutic: 1.6-4 mg/dL

Test Interactions False-positive for uric acid using the phosphotungstate method and for urobilinogen using the Ehrlich's reagent; large doses may interfere with the spectrophotometric determination of serum theophylline concentration

(Continued)

Thiamine Hydrochloride *(Continued)*

Dosage Forms

Injection: 100 mg/mL (1 mL, 2 mL, 10 mL, 30 mL); 200 mg/mL (30 mL)
Tablet: 50 mg, 100 mg, 250 mg, 500 mg
Tablet, enteric coated: 20 mg

Thiaminium Chloride Hydrochloride *see* Thiamine Hydrochloride *on previous page*

Thiethylperazine Maleate (thye eth il per' a zeen)

Related Information

Overdose and Toxicology Information *on page 696-700*

Brand Names Torecan®

Therapeutic Category Antiemetic; Phenothiazine Derivative

Use Relief of nausea and vomiting

Pregnancy Risk Factor X

Contraindications Comatose states, hypersensitivity to thiethylperazine or any component; pregnancy

Warnings Safety and efficacy in children <12 years of age have not been established; postural hypotension may occur after I.M. injection; the injectable form contains sulfite which may cause allergic reactions in sensitive individuals

Precautions May impair ability to perform hazardous tasks requiring mental alertness or physical coordination

Adverse Reactions

Cardiovascular: Hypotension, peripheral edema
Central nervous system: Drowsiness, extrapyramidal effects, seizures, fever, headache, trigeminal neuralgia
Gastrointestinal: Dryness of mouth
Hepatic: Cholestatic jaundice (occasional)
Ocular: Blurred vision
Respiratory: Dryness of mucous membranes

Mechanism of Action Blocks postsynaptic mesolimbic dopaminergic receptors in the brain including the medullary chemoreceptor trigger zone; exhibits a strong alpha-adrenergic blocking effect and depresses the release of hypothalamic and hypophyseal hormones

Pharmacodynamics

Onset of action: Following administration antiemetic effects occur within 30 minutes
Duration: ~4 hours

Usual Dosage Children >12 years and Adults:

Oral, I.M., rectal: 10 mg 1-3 times/day as needed
I.V. and S.C. routes of administration are not recommended

Dosage Forms

Injection: 5 mg/mL (2 mL)
Suppository, rectal: 10 mg
Tablet: 10 mg

Thioguanine (thye oh gwah' neen)

Related Information

Emetogenic Potential of Single Chemotherapeutic Agents *on page 655*

Synonyms 2-Amino-6-mercaptopurine; TG; 6-TG; 6-Thioguanine; Tioguanine

Therapeutic Category Antineoplastic Agent

Use Remission induction in acute myelogenous (nonlymphocytic) leukemia; treatment of chronic myelogenous leukemia and granulocytic leukemia

Pregnancy Risk Factor D

Contraindications History of previous therapy resistance with thioguanine and in patients resistant to mercaptopurine; hypersensitivity to thioguanine or any component

Warnings The US Food and Drug Administration (FDA) currently recommends that procedures for proper handling and disposal of antineoplastic agents be considered; thioguanine is potentially carcinogenic and teratogenic

Precautions Use with caution and reduce dose of thioguanine in patients with renal or hepatic impairment

Adverse Reactions
Central nervous system: Neurotoxicity
Dermatologic: Skin rash, photosensitivity
Endocrine & metabolic: Hyperuricemia
Gastrointestinal: Mild nausea or vomiting, anorexia, stomatitis, diarrhea
Hematologic: Myelosuppression
Hepatic: Hepatitis, jaundice, veno-occlusive hepatic disease

Drug Interactions Busulfan (↑ toxicity)

Mechanism of Action Purine analog that is incorporated into DNA and RNA resulting in the blockage of synthesis and metabolism of purine nucleotides

Pharmacokinetics
Absorption: Oral: 30%
Distribution: Crosses the placenta
Metabolism: Rapidly and extensively metabolized in the liver to 2-amino-6-methylthioguanine (active) and inactive compounds
Half-life, terminal: 11 hours
Peak serum levels: Within 8 hours
Elimination: Metabolites are excreted in the urine

Usual Dosage Oral (refer to individual protocols):
Infants <3 years: Combination drug therapy for acute nonlymphocytic leukemia: 3.3 mg/kg/day in divided doses twice daily for 4 days

Children and Adults: 2-3 mg/kg/day calculated to nearest 20 mg or 75-200 mg/m^2/day in 1-2 divided doses for 5-7 days or until remission is attained

Monitoring Parameters CBC with (differential, platelet count), liver function tests, hemoglobin, hematocrit, serum uric acid

Patient Information Notify physician if fever, sore throat, bleeding, bruising, yellow discoloration of skin or eyes, or leg swelling occurs

Additional Information Myelosuppressive effects:
WBC: Moderate
Platelets: Moderate
Onset (days): 7-10
Nadir (days): 14
Recovery (days): 21

Dosage Forms Tablet, scored: 40 mg

References

Culbert SJ, Shuster JJ, Land VJ, et al, "Remission Induction and Continuation Therapy in Children With Their First Relapse of Acute Lymphoid Leukemia: A Pediatric Oncology Group Study," *Cancer*, 1991, 67(1):37-42.
Steuber CP, Civin C, Krischer J, et al, "A Comparison of Induction and Maintenance Therapy for Acute Nonlymphocytic Leukemia in Childhood: Results of a Pediatric Oncology Group Study," *J Clin Oncol*, 1991, 9(2):247-58.

6-Thioguanine *see* Thioguanine *on previous page*

Thiopental (thye oh pen' tal)

Related Information
Preprocedure Sedatives in Children *on page 687-689*

Brand Names Pentothal® Sodium

Therapeutic Category Anticonvulsant; Barbiturate; General Anesthetic; Sedative

Use Induction of anesthesia; adjunct for intubation in head injury patients; control of convulsive states; treatment of elevated intracranial pressure

Restrictions C-III

Pregnancy Risk Factor C

Contraindications Porphyria (variegate or acute intermittent); known hypersensitivity to thiopental

Precautions Use with caution in patients with asthma or pharyngeal infections due to cough, laryngospasm or bronchospasms which can occur; hypotension; extravasation or intra-arterial injection causes necrosis due to pH of 10.6, ensure patent intravenous access

Adverse Reactions
Cardiovascular: Decreased cardiac output, hypotension
Renal & genitourinary: Decreased urine output
Respiratory: Cough, laryngospasm, bronchospasm, respiratory depression, apnea

(Continued)

Thiopental *(Continued)*

Miscellaneous: Anaphylaxis

Drug Interactions CNS depressants

Stability Solutions are alkaline and incompatible with drugs with acidic pH, such as succinylcholine, atropine sulfate, etc

Mechanism of Action Ultrashort-acting barbiturate; interferes with transmission of impulses from the thalamus to the cortex of the brain resulting in an imbalance in central inhibitory and facilitatory mechanisms

Pharmacodynamics Anesthesia effects:

Onset of action: I.V.: 30-60 seconds

Duration: 5-30 minutes

Pharmacokinetics

Distribution: V_d: 1.4 L/kg

Protein binding: 72% to 86%

Metabolism: Metabolized in liver primarily to inactive metabolites but pentobarbital is also formed

Half-life, adults: 3-11.5 hours (shorter half-life in children)

Usual Dosage

Induction anesthesia: I.V.:

Neonates: 3-4 mg/kg

Infants: 5-8 mg/kg

Children 1-12 years: 5-6 mg/kg

Children >12 years and Adults: 3-5 mg/kg

Maintenance anesthesia: I.V.:

Children: 1 mg/kg as needed

Adults: 25-100 mg as needed

Increased intracranial pressure: Children: I.V.: 1.5-5 mg/kg/dose; repeat as needed to control intracranial pressure; larger doses (30 mg/kg) to induce coma after hypoxic-ischemic injury do not appear to improve neurologic outcome

Seizures: I.V.:

Children: 2-3 mg/kg/dose, repeat as needed

Adults: 75-250 mg/dose, repeat as needed

Sedation: Rectal:

Children: 5-10 mg/kg/dose

Adults: 3-4 g/dose

Administration Rapid I.V. injection may cause hypotension or decreased cardiac output

Monitoring Parameters Respiratory rate, heart rate, blood pressure

Reference Range Therapeutic: Hypnotic: 1-5 μg/mL (SI: 4.1-20.7 μmol/L); Coma: 30-100 μg/mL (SI: 124-413 μmol/L); Anesthesia: 7-130 μg/mL (SI: 29-536 μmol/L); Toxic: >10 μg/mL (SI: >41 μmol/L)

Additional Information Accumulation may occur with chronic dosing due to lipid solubility; prolonged recovery occurs due to redistribution of thiopental from fat stores; therefore, thiopental is usually not used for procedures lasting >15-20 minutes

Dosage Forms

Injection: 250 mg, 400 mg, 500 mg, 1 g, 2.5 g, 5 g

Suspension, rectal: 400 mg/g (2 g)

Thioridazine Hydrochloride (thye oh rid' a zeen)

Related Information

Overdose and Toxicology Information *on page 696-700*

Brand Names Mellaril®; Mellaril-S®

Therapeutic Category Antipsychotic Agent; Phenothiazine Derivative

Use Management of psychotic disorders; depressive neurosis; dementia in elderly; severe behavioral problems in children

Pregnancy Risk Factor C

Contraindications Severe CNS depression, hypersensitivity to thioridazine or any component; cross-sensitivity to other phenothiazines may exist; avoid use in patients with narrow-angle glaucoma, blood dyscrasias, severe liver or cardiac disease

Precautions Use with caution in patients with severe cardiovascular disorder or seizures

Adverse Reactions Sedation and anticholinergic effects are more pronounced than extrapyramidal effects; EKG changes, retinal pigmentation are more common than with chlorpromazine

Cardiovascular: Hypotension, orthostatic hypotension; tachycardia, arrhythmias

Central nervous system: Sedation, drowsiness, restlessness, anxiety, extrapyramidal reactions, pseudoparkinsonian signs and symptoms, tardive dyskinesia, neuroleptic malignant syndrome, seizures, altered central temperature regulation

Dermatologic: Hyperpigmentation, pruritus, rash, contact dermatitis, photosensitivity (rare)

Endocrine & metabolic: Amenorrhea, galactorrhea, gynecomastia, weight gain

Gastrointestinal: GI upset, dry mouth, constipation

Hematologic: Agranulocytosis, leukopenia (usually in patients with large doses for prolonged periods)

Hepatic: Cholestatic jaundice

Ocular: Retinal pigmentation, blurred vision, decreased visual acuity (may be irreversible)

Renal & genitourinary: Urinary retention

Sensitivity reactions: Anaphylactoid reactions

Drug Interactions Additive effects with other CNS depressants; concurrent use with lithium has rarely caused acute encephalopathy-like syndrome; ↑ cardiac arrhythmias with tricyclic antidepressants; epinephrine may cause hypotension

Mechanism of Action Blocks postsynaptic mesolimbic dopaminergic receptors in the brain; exhibits a strong alpha-adrenergic blocking effect and depresses the release of hypothalamic and hypophyseal hormones

Usual Dosage Oral:

Children >2 years: Range: 0.5-3 mg/kg/day in 2-3 divided doses; usual: 1 mg/kg/day; maximum: 3 mg/kg/day

- Behavior problems: Initial: 10 mg 2-3 times/day, increase gradually
- Severe psychoses: Initial: 25 mg 2-3 times/day, increase gradually

Children >12 years and Adults:

- Psychoses: Initial: 25-100 mg 3 times/day with gradual increments as needed and tolerated; maximum daily dose: 800 mg/day in 2-4 divided doses
- Depressive disorders, dementia: Initial: 25 mg 3 times/day; maintenance dose: 20-200 mg/day

Monitoring Parameters Periodic eye exam, CBC, blood pressure, liver enzyme tests

Test Interactions False-positives for phenylketonuria, urinary amylase, uroporphyrins, urobilinogen

Nursing Implications Dilute the oral concentrate with water or juice before administration; avoid skin contact with oral suspension or solution, may cause contact dermatitis

Dosage Forms

Concentrate, oral: 30 mg/mL (120 mL); 100 mg/mL (3.4 mL, 120 mL)

Suspension, oral: 25 mg/5 mL (480 mL); 100 mg/5 mL (480 mL)

Tablet: 10 mg, 15 mg, 25 mg, 50 mg, 100 mg, 150 mg, 200 mg

References

Aman MG, Marks RE, Turbott SH, et al, "Clinical Effects of Methylphenidate and Thioridazine in Intellectually Subaverage Children," *J Am Acad Child Adolesc Psychiatry*, 1991, 30(2):246-56.

Thiotepa (thye oh tep' a)

Related Information

Emetogenic Potential of Single Chemotherapeutic Agents *on page 655*

Synonyms TESPA; Triethylenethiophosphoramide; TSPA

Therapeutic Category Antineoplastic Agent

Use Treatment of superficial tumors of the bladder; palliative treatment of adenocarcinoma of breast or ovary; lymphomas and sarcomas; meningeal neoplasms; controlling intracavitary effusions caused by metastatic tumors

Pregnancy Risk Factor D

Contraindications Hypersensitivity to thiotepa or any component; severe

(Continued)

Thiotepa *(Continued)*

myelosuppression with leukocyte count <3000/mm^3 or platelet count <150,000 mm^3

Warnings The US Food and Drug Administration (FDA) currently recommends that procedures for proper handling and disposal of antineoplastic agents be considered. The drug is potentially mutagenic, carcinogenic, and teratogenic.

Precautions Reduce dosage in patients with hepatic, renal, or bone marrow dysfunction

Adverse Reactions

Central nervous system: Dizziness, fever, headache
Dermatologic: Alopecia, rash, pruritus
Endocrine & metabolic: Amenorrhea, hyperuricemia
Gastrointestinal: Nausea, vomiting, stomatitis
Hematologic: Leukopenia, anemia, thrombocytopenia, granulocytopenia
Local: Pain at injection site
Renal & genitourinary: Rarely hemorrhagic cystitis, hematuria

Drug Interactions Succinylcholine (thiotepa inhibits pseudocholinesterase activity; prolongs muscular paralysis); other alkylating agents (intensifies toxicity)

Stability Refrigerate, protect from light; the reconstituted solution is stable for 5 days when refrigerated

Mechanism of Action Alkylating agent that reacts with DNA phosphate groups to produce cross-linking of DNA strands leading to inhibition of DNA, RNA, and protein synthesis

Pharmacokinetics

Absorption: Following intracavitary instillation, unreliably absorbed (10% to 100%) through the bladder mucosa; variable I.M. absorption
Metabolism: Extensively metabolized in the liver
Half-life, terminal: 109 minutes
Elimination: Excreted as metabolites and unchanged drug in the urine; dose-dependent clearance

Usual Dosage Refer to individual protocols

Children: Sarcomas: I.V.: 25-65 mg/m^2 as a single dose every 21 days

Adults:
I.V.: 0.3-0.4 mg/kg at 1- to 4-week intervals or 0.2 mg/kg (6 mg/m^2)/day for 4-5 days at 2- to 4-week intervals
Intracavitary: 0.6-0.8 mg/kg once weekly

Administration Can be administered slow IVP over 5 minutes at a concentration not to exceed 10 mg/mL or I.V. infusion at a final concentration for administration of 1 mg/mL

Monitoring Parameters CBC with differential and platelet count, uric acid, urinalysis

Patient Information Notify physician if fever, sore throat, bleeding, or bruising occurs

Additional Information Myelosuppressive effects:

WBC: Moderate
Platelets: Severe
Onset (days): 7-10
Nadir (days): 14-20
Recovery (days): 28

Dosage Forms Powder for injection: 15 mg

References

Heideman R, Cole D, Balis F, et al, "Phase I and Pharmacokinetic Evaluation of Thiotepa in the Cerebrospinal Fluid and Plasma of Pediatric Patients: Evidence for Dose-Dependent Plasma Clearance of Thiotepa," *Cancer Res*, 1989, 49(3):736-41.

Thiothixene (thye oh thix' een)

Related Information

Overdose and Toxicology Information *on page 696-700*

Brand Names Navane®

Therapeutic Category Antipsychotic Agent; Phenothiazine Derivative

Use Management of psychotic disorders

Pregnancy Risk Factor C

Contraindications Hypersensitivity to thiothixene or any component; cross sensitivity with other phenothiazines may exist; avoid use in patients with narrow-angle glaucoma, bone marrow depression, severe liver or cardiac disease

Precautions Use with caution in patients with cardiovascular disease or seizures

Adverse Reactions Sedation and extrapyramidal effects occur more frequently

Cardiovascular: Hypotension (especially with parenteral use); orthostatic hypotension; tachycardia, arrhythmias

Central nervous system: Sedation, drowsiness, restlessness, anxiety, insomnia, extrapyramidal reactions, tardive dyskinesia, neuroleptic malignant syndrome, seizures, altered central temperature regulation

Dermatologic: Rash

Endocrine & metabolic: Amenorrhea, galactorrhea, gynecomastia, weight gain

Gastrointestinal: GI upset, dry mouth, constipation

Hematologic: Agranulocytosis, leukopenia

Ocular: Retinal pigmentation, blurred vision

Renal & genitourinary: Urinary retention

Drug Interactions Other CNS depressants, anticholinergics, or hypotensive agents → ↑ adverse effects

Mechanism of Action Elicits antipsychotic activity by postsynaptic blockade of CNS dopamine receptors resulting in inhibition of dopamine mediated effects; also has alpha-adrenergic blocking activity

Usual Dosage

Children <12 years: Oral: Not well established; 0.25 mg/kg/24 hours in divided doses

Children >12 years and Adults:

Oral: Initial: 2 mg 3 times/day, up to 20-30 mg/day; maximum: 60 mg/day

I.M.: 4 mg 2-4 times/day, ↑ dose gradually; usual: 16-20 mg/day; maximum: 30 mg/day; change to oral dose a soon as able

Monitoring Parameters Periodic eye exam, CBC, blood pressure, liver enzyme tests

Dosage Forms

Capsule: 1 mg, 2 mg, 5 mg, 10 mg, 20 mg

Concentrate, oral, as hydrochloride: 5 mg/mL (30 mL, 120 mL)

Injection, as hydrochloride: 2 mg/mL (2 mL)

Powder for injection, as hydrochloride: 5 mg/mL (2 mL)

References

Wiener JM, "Psychopharmacology in Childhood Disorders," *Psychiatr Clin North Am*, 1984, 7(4):831-43.

Thorazine® *see* Chlorpromazine Hydrochloride *on page 129*

Thrombinar® *see* Thrombin, Topical *on this page*

Thrombin, Topical (throm' bin)

Brand Names Thrombinar®; Thrombogen®; Thrombostat®

Therapeutic Category Hemostatic Agent

Use Hemostasis whenever minor bleeding from capillaries and small venules is accessible

Pregnancy Risk Factor C

Contraindications Hypersensitivity to thrombin or any component or material of bovine origin

Warnings Do not inject - for topical use only

Adverse Reactions

Central nervous system: Fever

Miscellaneous: Allergic type reaction

Stability Following reconstitution, use within a few hours; stable frozen (reconstituted) for 48 hours

Mechanism of Action Catalyzes the conversion of fibrinogen to fibrin

Usual Dosage Topical: Apply powder directly to the site of bleeding or on oozing surfaces or use 1000-2000 units/mL of solution where bleeding is profuse; use 100 units/mL for bleeding from skin or mucosal surfaces

Administration May be applied directly as a powder or as reconstituted solution; use sterile water or 0.9% sodium chloride to reconstituted powder to

(Continued)

Thrombin, Topical *(Continued)*

desired concentration; sponge surface free of blood prior to application, if possible

Additional Information One unit is amount required to clot 1 mL of standardized fibrinogen solution in 15 seconds

Dosage Forms Powder: 1000 units, 5000 units, 10,000 units, 20,000 units, 50,000 units

Thrombogen® *see* Thrombin, Topical *on previous page*

Thrombostat® *see* Thrombin, Topical *on previous page*

Thypinone® *see* Protirelin *on page 496*

Thyro-Block® *see* Potassium Iodide *on page 471*

Tiabendazole *see* Thiabendazole *on page 558*

Ticar® *see* Ticarcillin Disodium *on next page*

Ticarcillin and Clavulanate Potassium

Brand Names Timentin®

Synonyms Ticarcillin Disodium and Clavulanate Potassium

Therapeutic Category Antibiotic, Penicillin

Use Treatment of infections caused by susceptible organisms involving the lower respiratory tract, urinary tract, skin and skin structures, bone and joint, and septicemia. Clavulanate expands activity of ticarcillin to include beta-lactamase producing strains of *S. aureus*, *H. influenzae*, *Branhamella catarrhalis*, *Enterobacteriaceae*, *Pseudomonas*, *Klebsiella*, and *Citrobacter*

Pregnancy Risk Factor B

Contraindications Known hypersensitivity to ticarcillin, clavulanate, and any penicillin

Warnings Abnormal platelet aggregation and prolonged bleeding have been reported in patients with renal impairment receiving high doses

Precautions Not approved for use in children <12 years of age; use with caution and modify dosage in patients with renal impairment

Adverse Reactions

Central nervous system: Seizures, headache, fever
Dermatologic: Rash
Endocrine & metabolic: Hypernatremia, hypokalemia
Gastrointestinal: Diarrhea, stomatitis, nausea
Hematologic: Eosinophilia, leukopenia, decreased hemoglobin and hematocrit, prolongation of bleeding time, positive Coombs' test
Hepatic: ↑ ALT and AST, hepatitis
Local: Thrombophlebitis
Renal & genitourinary: Increased serum creatinine and BUN
Miscellaneous: Hypersensitivity reactions, superinfection

Drug Interactions Aminoglycosides, probenecid

Stability Reconstituted solution is stable for 6 hours at room temperature and 72 hours when refrigerated; darkening of drug indicates loss of potency of clavulanate potassium; incompatible with sodium bicarbonate

Mechanism of Action Ticarcillin interferes with bacterial cell wall synthesis during active multiplication causing cell wall death and resultant bactericidal activity against susceptible bacteria; clavulanic acid inhibits degradation of ticarcillin by binding to beta-lactamases

Pharmacokinetics

Distribution: Low concentrations of ticarcillin distribute into the CSF but increase when meninges are inflamed
Protein binding:
  Ticarcillin: 45% to 65%
  Clavulanic acid: 9% to 30%
Metabolism: Clavulanic acid is metabolized in the liver
Half-life:
  Clavulanate: 66-90 minutes
  Ticarcillin: 66-72 minutes in patients with normal renal function
  Clavulanic acid does not affect the clearance of ticarcillin
Elimination: 45% of clavulanate is excreted unchanged in the urine, whereas 60% to 90% of ticarcillin is excreted unchanged in the urine
Removed by hemodialysis

Usual Dosage I.V.:

Children: 200-300 mg of ticarcillin component/kg/day in divided doses every 4-6 hours

Adults: 3.1 g (ticarcillin 3 g plus clavulanic acid 0.1 g) every 4-6 hours; maximum: 18-24 g/day
Urinary tract infections: 3.1 g every 6-8 hours

Dosing interval in renal impairment:
Cl_{cr} 10-30 mL/minute: Administer every 8 hours
Cl_{cr} <10 mL/minute: Administer every 12 hours

Dosing interval in hepatic impairment: Cl_{cr} <10 mL/hour: Administer every 24 hours

Administration Administer by I.V. intermittent infusion over 30 minutes; final concentration for administration should not exceed 100 mg/mL of ticarcillin; however, concentrations ≤50 mg/mL are preferred

Monitoring Parameters Serum electrolytes, periodic renal, hepatic and hematologic function tests

Test Interactions Positive Coombs' test, false-positive urinary proteins

Additional Information

Sodium content of 1 g: 4.75 mEq
Potassium content of 1 g: 0.15 mEq

Dosage Forms

Infusion, premixed (frozen): Ticarcillin disodium 3 g and clavulanic acid 0.1 (100 mL) g

Powder for injection: Ticarcillin disodium 3 g and clavulanic acid 0.1 g (3.1 g, 31 g)

References

Begue P, Quiniou F, Quinet B, "Efficacy and Pharmacokinetics of Timentin® in Paediatric Infections," *J Antimicrob Chemother*, 1986, 17(Suppl C):81-91.

Stutman HR and Marks MI, "Review of Pediatric Antimicrobial Therapies," *Semin Pediatr Infect Dis*, 1991, 2:3-17.

Ticarcillin Disodium (tye kar sill' in)

Related Information

Medications Compatible With PN Solutions *on page 649-650*

Brand Names Ticar®

Therapeutic Category Antibiotic, Penicillin

Use Treatment of infections such as septicemia, acute and chronic respiratory tract infections, skin and soft tissue infections, and urinary tract infections due to susceptible strains of *Pseudomonas*, *Proteus*, *Escherichia coli*, and *Enterobacter*

Pregnancy Risk Factor B

Contraindications Hypersensitivity to ticarcillin or any component or penicillins

Precautions Use with caution in patients with CHF due to ticarcillin's high sodium content; dosage modification required in patients with impaired renal and/or hepatic function

Adverse Reactions

Central nervous system: Seizures
Dermatologic: Rash
Endocrine & metabolic: Hypernatremia, hypokalemia, metabolic alkalosis
Gastrointestinal: Diarrhea
Hematologic: Inhibition of platelet aggregation, leukopenia, neutropenia, bleeding diathesis, hemolytic anemia
Hepatic: Elevated AST, hepatitis
Local: Phlebitis
Renal & genitourinary: Cystitis
Miscellaneous: Allergic reactions

Drug Interactions Aminoglycosides, probenecid

Stability Reconstituted ticarcillin solution 200-300 mg/mL is stable for 24 hours at room temperature or 72 hours when refrigerated; incompatible with aminoglycosides

Mechanism of Action Interferes with bacterial cell wall synthesis during active multiplication, causing cell wall death and resultant bactericidal activity against susceptible bacteria

(Continued)

Ticarcillin Disodium *(Continued)*

Pharmacokinetics

Absorption: I.M.: 86% of a dose is absorbed

Distribution: V_d: Neonates: 0.42-0.76 L/kg; distributed into milk at low concentrations; attains high concentrations in bile; minimal concentrations attained in CSF with uninflamed meninges

Protein binding: 45% to 65%

Half-life, adults: 1-1.3 hours, prolonged with renal impairment and/or hepatic impairment

Neonates:

<1 week: 3.5-5.6 hours

1-8 weeks: 1.3-2.2 hours

Children 5-13 years: 0.9 hours

Peak serum levels: I.M.: Within 30-75 minutes

Elimination: Excreted almost entirely in the urine as unchanged drug and its metabolites with small amounts excreted in the feces (3.5%)

Moderately dialyzable (20% to 50%)

Usual Dosage Ticarcillin is generally given I.M. only for the treatment of uncomplicated urinary tract infections

Neonates: I.V.:

Postnatal age ≤7 days:

≤2000 g: 150 mg/kg/day in divided doses every 12 hours

>2000 g: 225 mg/kg/day in divided doses every 8 hours

Postnatal age >7 days:

<1200 g: 150 mg/kg/day in divided doses every 12 hours

1200-2000 g: 225 mg/kg/day in divided doses every 8 hours

>2000 g: 300 mg/kg/day in divided doses every 6 hours

Infants and Children: I.V.: 200-300 mg/kg/day in divided doses every 4-6 hours; doses as high as 400 mg/kg/day divided every 4 hours have been used in acute pulmonary exacerbations of cystic fibrosis

Maximum dose: 24 g/day

Adults: I.V.: 1-4 g every 4-6 hours

Dosing interval in renal impairment:

Cl_{cr} 10-30 mL/minute: Administer every 8 hours

Cl_{cr} <10 mL/minute: Administer every 12 hours

Administration Ticarcillin can be administered I.V. push over 10-20 minutes or by I.V. intermittent infusion over 30-120 minutes at a final concentration not to exceed 100 mg/mL; concentrations of ≤50 mg/mL are preferred for peripheral intermittent infusions to avoid vein irritation

Monitoring Parameters Serum electrolytes, bleeding time, and periodic tests of renal, hepatic, and hematologic function

Test Interactions False-positive urinary or serum protein

Additional Information Sodium content of 1 g: 5.2-6.5 mEq

Dosage Forms Powder for injection: 1 g, 3 g, 6 g, 20 g, 30 g

References

Brogden RN, Heel RC, Speight TM, et al, "Ticarcillin: A Review of Its Pharmacological Properties and Therapeutic Efficacy," *Drugs*, 1980, 20(5):325-52.

Nelson JD, Kusmiesz H, Shelton S, et al, "Clinical Pharmacology and Efficacy of Ticarcillin in Infants and Children," *Pediatrics*, 1978, 61(6):858-63.

Ticarcillin Disodium and Clavulanate Potassium *see* Ticarcillin and Clavulanate Potassium *on page 566*

Ticon® *see* Trimethobenzamide Hydrochloride *on page 585*

Tigan® *see* Trimethobenzamide Hydrochloride *on page 585*

Tiject® *see* Trimethobenzamide Hydrochloride *on page 585*

Timentin® *see* Ticarcillin and Clavulanate Potassium *on page 566*

Timolol Maleate (tye' moe lole)

Related Information

Overdose and Toxicology Information *on page 696-700*

Brand Names Blocadren®; Timoptic®

Therapeutic Category Beta-Adrenergic Blocker, Ophthalmic

Use Ophthalmic dosage form used to treat elevated intraocular pressure such as glaucoma or ocular hypertension; orally for treatment of hypertension and angina and for prevention of myocardial infarction and migraine headaches

Pregnancy Risk Factor C

Contraindications Uncompensated congestive heart failure, cardiogenic shock, bradycardia or heart block, bronchial asthma, severe chronic obstructive pulmonary disease or history of asthma, congestive heart failure or bradycardia

Warnings Severe CNS, cardiovascular and respiratory adverse effects have been seen following ophthalmic use; patients with a history of asthma, congestive heart failure, or bradycardia appear to be at a higher risk

Precautions Similar to other beta blockers; use with caution in patients with ↓ renal or hepatic function (dosage adjustment required)

Adverse Reactions

Cardiovascular: Bradycardia, arrhythmia, hypotension, syncope
Central nervous system: Dizziness, headache
Dermatologic: Rash
Gastrointestinal: Diarrhea, nausea
Ocular: Irritation, conjunctivitis, keratitis, visual disturbances
Respiratory: Bronchospasm

Drug Interactions Similar to other beta blockers

Mechanism of Action Blocks both $beta_1$-adrenergic and $beta_2$-adrenergic receptors; reduces intraocular pressure by reducing aqueous humor production or possibly outflow; reduces blood pressure by blocking adrenergic receptors and decreasing sympathetic outflow; produces negative chronotropic and inotropic activity

Pharmacodynamics Hypotensive effects:

Onset of action: Oral: Within 15-45 minutes
Peak effect: 30-150 minutes
Duration:
Oral: 4 hours
Ophthalmic (intraocular effects): 24 hours

Pharmacokinetics

Protein binding: 60%
Metabolism: Extensive in the liver, extensive first pass effect
Half-life, adults: 2-2.7 hours; half-life prolonged with reduced renal function
Elimination: Urinary excretion (15% to 20% as unchanged drug)

Usual Dosage

Ophthalmic: Children and Adults: Initial: 0.25% solution, 1 drop twice daily; increase to 0.5% solution if response not adequate; decrease to 1 drop/day if controlled; do not exceed 1 drop twice daily of 0.5% solution

Oral:
Children: No information regarding pediatric dose is currently available in literature
Adults:
Hypertension: Initial: 10 mg twice daily, ↑ gradually every 7 days, usual dosage: 20-40 mg/day in 2 divided doses; maximum: 60 mg/day
Prevention of myocardial infarction: 10 mg twice daily initiated within 1-4 weeks after infarction

Additional Information Ophthalmic: Use lowest effective dose in pediatric patients. Children had higher plasma concentrations vs adults following ophthalmic use; some achieved therapeutic levels; this may result in ↑ adverse systemic effects

Dosage Forms

Solution, ophthalmic (Timoptic®): 0.25% (2.5 mL, 5 mL, 10 mL, 15 mL); 0.5% (2.5 mL, 5 mL, 10 mL, 15 mL)
Solution, ophthalmic, preservative free, single use (Timoptic® OcuDose®): 0.25%, 0.5%
Tablet (Blocadren®): 5 mg, 10 mg, 20 mg

References

Hoskins HD, Hetherington J Jr, Magee SD, et al, "Clinical Experience With Timolol in Childhood Glaucoma," *Arch Ophthalmol*, 1985, 103(8):1163-5.
Passo MS, Palmer EA and Van Buskirk EM, "Plasma Timolol in Glaucoma Patients," *Ophthalmology*, 1984, 91(11):1361-3.

Timoptic® *see* Timolol Maleate *on page 568*

Tinactin® [OTC] *see* Tolnaftate *on page 573*

Tinver® [OTC] *see* Sodium Thiosulfate *on page 531*

Tioguanine *see* Thioguanine *on page 560*

Titralac® [OTC] *see* Calcium Carbonate *on page 94*

TMP-SMX *see* Co-trimoxazole *on page 156*

Tobramycin Sulfate (toe bra mye' sin)

Related Information

Blood Level Sampling Time Guidelines *on page 694-695*
Medications Compatible With PN Solutions *on page 649-650*
Overdose and Toxicology Information *on page 696-700*

Brand Names Nebcin®; Tobrex®

Therapeutic Category Antibiotic, Aminoglycoside; Antibiotic, Ophthalmic

Use Treatment of documented or suspected *Pseudomonas aeruginosa* infection; infection with a nonpseudomonal enteric bacillus which is more sensitive to tobramycin than gentamicin based on susceptibility tests; susceptible organisms in lower respiratory tract infections, septicemia; intra-abdominal, skin, bone, and urinary tract infections; empiric therapy in cystic fibrosis and immunocompromised patients; used topically to treat superficial ophthalmic infections caused by susceptible bacteria

Pregnancy Risk Factor D

Contraindications Hypersensitivity to tobramycin, aminoglycosides, or any component

Warnings (I.M. & I.V.) Aminoglycosides are associated with significant nephrotoxicity or ototoxicity; the ototoxicity is directly proportional to the amount of drug given and the duration of treatment; tinnitus or vertigo are indications of vestibular injury and impending irreversible bilateral deafness; renal damage is usually reversible

Precautions Use with caution in patients with renal impairment, pre-existing auditory or vestibular impairment, patients receiving anesthetics or neuromuscular blocking agents, and in patients with neuromuscular disorders; dosage modification required in patients with impaired renal function

Adverse Reactions

Central nervous system: Delirium
Dermatologic: Allergic contact dermatitis, rash
Endocrine & metabolic: Hypomagnesemia
Local: Thrombophlebitis
Musculoskeletal: Neuromuscular blockade
Ocular: Ophthalmic use: Lacrimation, itching, edema of the eyelid, keratitis
Otic: Ototoxicity
Renal & genitourinary: Nephrotoxicity

Drug Interactions Extended spectrum penicillins, neuromuscular blockers, amphotericin B, cephalosporins, loop diuretics

Stability Incompatible with penicillins

Mechanism of Action Interferes with bacterial protein synthesis by binding to 30S and 50S ribosomal subunits resulting in a defective bacterial cell membrane

Pharmacokinetics

Absorption: I.M.: Rapid and complete

Distribution: Crosses the placenta; distributes primarily in the extracellular fluid volume; poor penetration into the CSF

- V_d: Increased by fever, edema, ascites, fluid overload, and in neonates
  - Children: 0.2-0.7 L/kg
  - Adults: 0.2-0.3 L/kg

Protein binding: <30%

Half-life:

- Neonates:
  - ≤1200 g: 11 hours
  - >1200 g: 2-9 hours
- Adults with normal renal function: 2-3 hours, directly dependent upon glomerular filtration rate; impaired renal function: 5-70 hours

Peak serum levels:

- I.M.: Within 30-60 minutes

30-minute I.V. infusion: Within 30 minutes

Elimination: With normal renal function, ~90% to 95% of a dose is excreted in the urine within 24 hours

Dialyzable (50% to 100%)

Usual Dosage Dosage should be based on an estimate of ideal body weight

Neonates: I.M., I.V.:

0-4 weeks, <1200 g: 2.5 mg/kg/dose every 18-24 hours

Postnatal age ≤7 days:

1200-2000 g: 2.5 mg/kg/dose every 12-18 hours

>1200 g: 2.5 mg/kg/dose every 12 hours

Postnatal age >7 days:

1200-2000 g: 2.5 mg/kg/dose every 12-18 hours

>2000 g: 2.5 mg/kg/dose every 8 hours

Infants and Children <5 years: I.M., I.V.: 2.5 mg/kg/dose every 8 hours*

Children ≥5 years: 1.5-2.5 mg/kg/dose every 8 hours

***Note:** Some patients may require larger or more frequent doses if serum levels document the need (ie, cystic fibrosis, patients with major burns, or febrile granulocytopenic patients)

Adults: I.M., I.V.: 3-6 mg/kg/day in 3 divided doses

Children and Adults: Renal dysfunction: 2.5 mg/kg (2-3 serum level measurements should be obtained after the initial dose to measure the half-life in order to determine the frequency of subsequent doses)

Children and Adults: Ophthalmic: 1-2 drops every 4 hours; apply ointment 2-3 times/day; for severe infections apply ointment every 3-4 hours, or 2 drops every 30-60 minutes initially, then reduce to less frequent intervals

Administration Administer by I.V. slow intermittent infusion over 30 minutes; final concentration for administration should not exceed 10 mg/mL

Monitoring Parameters Urinalysis, urine output, BUN, serum creatinine, peak and trough serum tobramycin levels; be alert to ototoxicity

Reference Range Peak: 4-10 μg/mL; Trough: 0.5-2 μg/mL

Test Interactions Aminoglycoside levels measured in blood taken from Silastic® central line catheters can sometimes give falsely high readings

Patient Information Report any dizziness or sensation of ringing or fullness in ears to the physician

Nursing Implications Obtain serum concentration after the third dose except in neonates and patients with rapidly changing renal function in whom levels need to be measured sooner; peak levels are drawn 30 minutes after the end of a 30-minute infusion; the trough is drawn just before the next dose; administer other antibiotics such as penicillins and cephalosporins at least one hour before or after tobramycin; provide optimal patient hydration and perfusion

Dosage Forms

Injection, as sulfate: 10 mg/mL (2 mL, 6 mL, 8 mL); 40 mg/mL (1.5 mL, 2 mL)

Ointment, ophthalmic: 0.3% (3.5 g)

Powder for injection: 30 mg/mL (1.2 g)

Solution, ophthalmic: 0.3% (5 mL)

References

Green TP, Mirkin BL, Peterson PK, et al, "Tobramycin Serum Level Monitoring in Young Patients With Normal Renal Function," *Clin Pharmacokinet*, 1984, 9(5):457-68.

Nahata MC, Powell DA, Durrell DE, et al, "Effect of Gestational Age and Birth Weight on Tobramycin Kinetics in Newborn Infants," *J Antimicrob Chemother*, 1984, 14(1):59-65.

Tobrex® *see* Tobramycin Sulfate *on previous page*

Tofranil® *see* Imipramine *on page 306*

Tofranil-PM® *see* Imipramine *on page 306*

Tolazoline Hydrochloride (tole az' oh leen)

Related Information

Overdose and Toxicology Information *on page 696-700*

Brand Names Priscoline®

Synonyms Benzazoline Hydrochloride

Therapeutic Category Alpha-Adrenergic Blocking Agent, Parenteral; Antihypertensive; Vasodilator, Coronary

(Continued)

Tolazoline Hydrochloride *(Continued)*

Use Persistent fetal circulation (PFC); persistent pulmonary hypertension of the newborn

Pregnancy Risk Factor C

Contraindications Hypersensitivity to tolazoline; known or suspected coronary artery disease

Warnings May activate stress ulcers via stimulation of gastric secretions

Precautions Use with caution in patients with mitral stenosis

Adverse Reactions

Cardiovascular: Hypotension, flushing, tachycardia, arrhythmias

Endocrine & metabolic: Hypochloremic alkalosis

Gastrointestinal: Increased secretions, nausea, vomiting, diarrhea, epigastric discomfort, GI bleeding

Hematology: Agranulocytosis, thrombocytopenia, pancytopenia

Ocular: Mydriasis

Renal & genitourinary: Oliguria

Respiratory: Pulmonary hemorrhage

Miscellaneous: Increased pilomotor activity

Drug Interactions A paradoxical ↓ in blood pressure followed by a significant rebound ↑ in blood pressure can be seen when epinephrine or norepinephrine is administered with tolazoline; a disulfiram reaction may possibly be seen with concomitant ethanol use

Stability Compatible in D_5W, $D_{10}W$ and saline solutions; do not mix with other drugs

Mechanism of Action Competitively blocks alpha-adrenergic receptors to produce brief antagonism of circulating epinephrine and norepinephrine; reduces hypertension caused by catecholamines and causes vascular smooth muscle relaxation (direct action); results in peripheral vasodilation and decreased peripheral resistance

Pharmacodynamics Peak effects: Within 30 minutes

Pharmacokinetics

Half-life, neonates: 3-10 hours; increased half-life with decreased renal function, oliguria

Elimination: Excreted rapidly in the urine primarily as unchanged drug

Usual Dosage

Neonates: Initial: I.V.: 1-2 mg/kg over 10-15 minutes via scalp vein or upper extremity; maintenance: 1-2 mg/kg/hour, little experience with infusions >48 hours

Decreased renal function: Use lower maintenance doses

Acute vasospasm "cath toes": 0.25 mg/kg/hour (no load)

Adults: Peripheral vasospastic disorder: I.M., I.V., S.C.: 10-50 mg 4 times/day

Administration I.V.: Usual maximum concentration: 0.1 mg/mL

Monitoring Parameters Vital signs, blood gases

Additional Information Acidosis may ↓ tolazoline's effects

Dosage Forms Injection: 25 mg/mL (4 mL)

Tolectin® *see* Tolmetin Sodium *on this page*

Tolmetin Sodium (tole' met in)

Related Information

Overdose and Toxicology Information *on page 696-700*

Brand Names Tolectin®

Therapeutic Category Analgesic, Non-Narcotic; Nonsteroidal Anti-Inflammatory Agent (NSAID), Oral

Use Treatment of inflammatory and rheumatoid disorders, including juvenile rheumatoid arthritis

Pregnancy Risk Factor B (D at term)

Contraindications Known hypersensitivity to tolmetin or any component, aspirin, or other nonsteroidal anti-inflammatory drugs (NSAIDs)

Precautions Use with caution in patients with upper GI disease, impaired renal function, congestive heart failure, hypertension, and patients receiving anticoagulants

Adverse Reactions

Cardiovascular: Edema

Central nervous system: Dizziness, nervousness, drowsiness, headache
Dermatologic: Rash, urticaria
Gastrointestinal: Nausea, abdominal pain, dyspepsia, diarrhea, constipation; GI bleeding, ulcer, perforation
Hematologic: Anemia, leukopenia, prolongation of bleeding time
Hepatic: Hepatitis
Otic: Tinnitus
Renal & genitourinary: Acute renal failure, renal dysfunction

Drug Interactions Tolmetin and warfarin → ↑ prothrombin time and bleeding; ASA may ↓ tolmetin serum concentration; tolmetin may ↑ serum concentrations of methotrexate; drug interactions similar to other NSAIDs may also occur

Mechanism of Action Inhibits prostaglandin synthesis by decreasing the activity of the enzyme, cyclo-oxygenase, which results in decreased formation of prostaglandin precursors

Pharmacokinetics
Absorption: Oral: Well absorbed
Peak serum levels: Within 30-60 minutes

Usual Dosage Oral:
Children ≥2 years: Anti-inflammatory: Initial: 20 mg/kg/day in 3 divided doses, then 15-30 mg/kg/day in 3 divided doses
Analgesic: 5-7 mg/kg/dose every 6-8 hours
Adults: 400 mg 3 times/day; usual dose: 600-1.8 g/day; maximum: 2 g/day

Monitoring Parameters CBC, liver enzymes, occult blood loss, BUN, serum creatinine; periodic ophthalmologic exams

Nursing Implications Administer with food, milk, or antacids to ↓ GI adverse effects

Additional Information Although rare, anaphylactoid reactions occur more commonly with tolmetin than other NSAIDs

Dosage Forms
Capsule: 400 mg
Tablet: 200 mg, 600 mg

References

Berde C, Ablin A, Glazer J, et al, "American Academy of Pediatrics Report of the Subcommittee on Disease-Related Pain in Childhood Cancer," *Pediatrics*, 1990, 86(5 Pt 2):818-25.

Tolnaftate (tole naf' tate)

Brand Names Aftate® [OTC]; Desenex® [OTC]; Genaspor® [OTC]; NP-27® [OTC]; Tinactin® [OTC]; Zeasorb-AF® [OTC]

Therapeutic Category Antifungal Agent, Topical

Use Treatment of tinea pedis, tinea cruris, tinea corporis, tinea manuum caused by *Trichophyton rubrum*, *T. mentagrophytes*, *T. tonsurans*, *M. canis*, *M. audouini*, and *E. floccosum*; also effective in the treatment of tinea versicolor infections due to *Malassezia furfur*

Pregnancy Risk Factor C

Contraindications Known hypersensitivity to tolnaftate; nail and scalp infections

Adverse Reactions
Dermatologic: Pruritus, contact dermatitis
Local: Irritation, stinging

Mechanism of Action Distorts the hyphae and stunts mycelial growth in susceptible fungi

Pharmacodynamics Onset of action: Response may be seen 24-72 hours after initiation of therapy

Usual Dosage Children and Adults: Topical: Wash and dry affected area; apply 1-3 drops of solution or a small amount of cream or powder and rub into the affected areas 2-3 times/day for 2-4 weeks

Monitoring Parameters Resolution of skin infection

Patient Information Avoid contact with the eyes; apply to clean dry area; consult the physician if a skin irritation develops or if the skin infection worsens or does not improve after 10 days of therapy

Additional Information Usually not effective alone for the treatment of infections involving hair follicles or nails

Dosage Forms
Aerosol, topical:
Liquid: 1% (120 mL)

(Continued)

Tolnaftate *(Continued)*

Powder: 1% (100 g, 105 g, 150 g)
Cream: 1% (0.7 g, 15 g, 30 g)
Gel, topical: 1% (15 g)
Powder, topical: 1% (45 g, 90 g)
Solution, topical: 1% (10 mL)

Tolu-Sed® *see* Guaifenesin and Codeine *on page 279*

Topical Steroids Comparison Chart *see page 728*

Topicycline® *see* Tetracycline Hydrochloride *on page 552*

Toradol® *see* Ketorolac Tromethamine *on page 329*

Torecan® *see* Thiethylperazine Maleate *on page 560*

Totacillin® *see* Ampicillin *on page 48*

Totacillin®-N *see* Ampicillin *on page 48*

Trace-4® *see* Trace Metals *on this page*

Trace Metals

Related Information

Parenteral Nutrition (PN) *on page 642-648*

Brand Names Chroma-Pak®; Iodopen®; Molypen®; M.T.E.-4®; M.T.E.-5®; M.T.E.-6®; Multe-Pak-4®; Neotrace-4®; Pedte-Pak-5®; Pedtrace-4®; P.T.E.-4®; P.T.E.-5®; Sele-Pak®; Selepen®; Trace-4®; Zinca-Pak®

Synonyms Chromium; Copper; Iodine; Manganese; Molybdenum; Neonatal Trace Metals; Selenium; Zinc

Therapeutic Category Trace Element, Parenteral

Use Prevent and correct trace metal deficiencies

Pregnancy Risk Factor C

Contraindications Do not give by direct injection because of potential for phlebitis, tissue irritation, and potential to increase renal loss of minerals from a bolus injection

Warnings Metals may accumulate in conditions of renal failure or biliary obstruction; consider reduction in dosage or deletion of copper and manganese in patients with biliary obstruction; avoid copper use in patients with Wilson's Disease; administration of copper in the absence of zinc or zinc in the absence of copper may cause decreases in their respective plasma levels; molybdenum promotes the utilization of copper and increases its excretion; excessive amounts of molybdenum may produce copper deficiency; multiple trace metal solutions present a risk of overdosage when the need for one trace element is appreciably higher than for others in the formulation; utilization of individual trace metal solutions may be needed

Precautions Some of these products may contain benzyl alcohol which has been associated with fatal "gasping" syndrome in premature infants

Adverse Reactions The following describe the symptomatology associated with excess trace metals

Chromium: Nausea, vomiting, GI ulcers, renal and hepatic dysfunction, convulsions, coma

Copper: Prostration, behavioral changes, diarrhea, progressive marasmus, hypotonia, photophobia, hepatic dysfunction, and peripheral edema

Manganese: Irritability, speech disturbances, abnormal gait, headache, anorexia, apathy, impotence

Molybdenum: Gout-like syndrome with increased blood levels of uric acid and xanthine oxidase

Selenium: Hair loss, weak nails, dermatitis, dental defects, GI disorders, nervousness, mental depression, metallic taste, garlic odor of breath and sweat

Zinc: Profuse sweating, decreased consciousness, blurred vision, tachycardia, hypothermia

Mechanism of Action

Chromium: Part of glucose tolerance factor, an essential activator of insulin-mediated reactions; helps maintain normal glucose metabolism and peripheral nerve function

Copper: Cofactor for serum ceruloplasmin, helps maintain normal rates of red and white cell formation

Manganese: Activator for several enzymes including manganese-dependent superoxide dismutase and pyruvate carboxylase; activates glycosyl transferases involved in mucopolysaccharide synthesis

Molybdenum: Constituent of the enzymes xanthine oxidase, sulfite oxidase, and aldehyde oxidase

Selenium: Part of glutathione peroxidase which protects cell components from oxidative damage due to peroxides produced in cellular metabolism

Zinc: A cofactor for >70 different enzymes; facilitates wound healing, helps maintain normal growth rates, normal skin hydration, and the senses of taste and smell

Pharmacokinetics

Chromium: 10% to 20% oral absorption; excretion primarily via kidneys and bile

Copper: 30% oral absorption; 80% elimination via bile; intestinal wall 16% and urine 4%

Manganese: 10% oral absorption; excretion primarily via bile; ancillary routes via pancreatic secretions or reabsorption into the intestinal lumen occur during periods of biliary obstruction

Molybdenum: 30% to 70% oral absorption; primarily renal excretion; some biliary excretion associated with an enterohepatic cycle

Selenium: Very poor oral absorption; 75% excretion via kidneys, remainder via feces, lung, and skin

Zinc: 10% to 40% oral absorption; 90% excretion in stools, remainder via urine and perspiration

Usual Dosage See table.

Recommended Daily Parenteral Dosage

	Infants	Children	Adults
Chromium[1]	0.2 μg/kg	0.2 μg/kg (max 5 μg)	10–15 μg
Copper[2]	20 μg/kg	20 μg/kg (max 300 μg)	0.5–1.5 mg
Manganese[2,3]	1 μg/kg	1 μg/kg (max 50 μg)	150–800 μg
Molybdenum[1,4]	0.25 μg/kg	0.25 μg/kg (max 5 μg)	20–120 μg
Selenium[1,4]	2 μg/kg	2 μg/kg max 30 μg	20–40 μg
Zinc preterm term <3 mo term >3 mo	 400 μg/kg 250 μg/kg 100 μg/kg	50 μg/kg (max 5 μg)	2.5–4 mg

[1]Omit in patients with renal dysfunction.
[2]Omit in patients with obstructive jaundice.
[3]Current available commercial products are not in appropriate ratios to maintain this recommendation — doses of up to 10 μg/kg have been used safely.
[4]Indicated for use in long-term parenteral nutrition patients.

Zinc deficiency: Oral:

Infants and Children: 0.5-1 mg/kg/day 3 times/day; larger doses may be needed for replacement of excessive losses

Adults: 100-220 mg (25-50 mg elemental zinc) 3 times/day

Reference Range

Chromium: 0.18-0.47 ng/mL (SI: 35-90 nmol/L). Some laboratories report much higher

*Copper: Approximately 0.7-1.5 μg/mL (SI: 11-24 μmol/L). Levels are higher in pregnant women and children.

Manganese: 18-30 μg/dL (SI: 2.3-3.8 μmol/L)

Selenium: 95-165 ng/mL (SI: 120-209 nmol/L)

Zinc: 70-120 μg/dL (SI: 10-18.4 μmol/L)

*May not be a meaningful measurement of body stores

Additional Information Persistent diarrhea or excessive gastrointestinal fluid losses from ostomy sites may grossly increase zinc losses

(Continued)

Trace Metals *(Continued)*

Multiple Trace Metal Parenteral Solutions

	(Content per mL)					
	Chromium (µg)	Copper (mg)	Iodide (µg)	Manganese (mg)	Selenium (µg)	Zinc (mg)
Pedtrace-4®	0.85	0.1	—	0.025	—	0.5
Multiple trace element neonatal; Neotrace-4®	0.85	0.1	—	0.025	—	1.5
PedTE-PAK-4®; P.T.E.-4®	1	0.1	—	0.025	—	1
Multiple trace element pediatric	1	0.1	—	0.03	—	0.5
Trace metals additive in NS	2	0.2	—	0.16	—	0.8
M.T.E.-4®; MulTE-PAK-4®; Multiple trace element	4	0.4	—	0.1	—	1
Multiple trace element conc; ConTE-PAK-4®; M.T.E.-4® conc	10	1	—	0.5	—	5
PTE-5®	1	0.1	—	0.025	15	1
M.T.E.-5®; MulTE-PAK-5®; Multiple trace element w/selenium	4	0.4	—	0.1	20	1
M.T.E.-5® conc; Multiple trace element w/selenium concentrated	10	1	—	0.5	60	5
M.T.E.-6®; M.T.E.-7®*	4	0.4	25	0.1	20	1
M.T.E.-6® conc	10	1	75	0.5	60	5

*With 25 µg molybdenum.

Dosage Forms See table.

Chromium: Injection: 4 µg/mL, 20 µg/mL
Copper: Injection: 0.4 mg/mL, 2 mg/mL
Manganese: Injection: 0.1 mg/mL (as chloride or sulfate salt)
Molybdenum: Injection: 25 µg/mL
Selenium: Injection: 40 µg/mL
Zinc:
- Capsule: 110 mg (25 mg elemental zinc); 220 mg (50 mg elemental zinc)
- Injection: 1 mg/mL (sulfate); 1 mg/mL (chloride); 5 mg/mL (sulfate)
- Liquid, as carbonate: 15 mg/mL
- Tablet, as gluconate: 10 mg (1.4 mg elemental zinc); 15 mg (2 mg elemental zinc); 50 mg (7 mg elemental zinc); 78 mg (11 mg elemental zinc)
- Tablet, as sulfate: 66 mg (15 mg elemental zinc); 200 mg (45 mg elemental zinc)

References

Dahlstrom KA, Ament ME, Medhin MG, et al, "Serum Trace Elements in Children Receiving Long-Term Parenteral Nutrition," *J Pediatr*, 1986, 109(4):625-30.

Greene HL, Hambridge KM, Schanler R, et al, "Guidelines for the Use of Vitamins, Trace Elements, Calcium, Magnesium and Phosphorus in Infants and Children Receiving Total Parenteral Nutrition: Report of the Subcommittee on Pediatric Nutrient Requirements From the Committee on Clinical Practice Issues of The American Society for Clinical Nutrition," *Am J Clin Nutr*, 1988, 48(5):1324-42.

Litov RE, and Combs GF Jr, "Selenium in Pediatric Nutrition," *Pediatrics*, 1991, 87(3):339-51.

Tracrium® *see* Atracurium Besylate *on page 65*

Trandate® *see* Labetalol Hydrochloride *on page 331*

Tranexamic Acid (tran ex am' ik)

Brand Names Cyklokapron®

Therapeutic Category Antihemophilic Agent

Use Short-term use (2-8 days) in hemophilia patients during and following tooth extraction to reduce or prevent hemorrhage

Pregnancy Risk Factor B

Contraindications Subarachnoid hemorrhage; acquired defective color vision, active intravascular clotting process

Precautions Dosage modification required in patients with renal impairment; use with caution in patients with cardiovascular, renal, cerebrovascular disease, or transurethral prostatectomy

Adverse Reactions

Cardiovascular: Hypotension, thromboembolic complications, cerebral ischemia and infarction

Central nervous system: Headache, hydrocephalus, giddiness

Gastrointestinal: Nausea, diarrhea, vomiting

Hematologic: Thrombocytopenia, coagulation defects, abnormal bleeding times

Ocular: Visual abnormalities (focal areas of retinal degeneration have been seen in animals)

Drug Interactions Chlorpromazine

Stability Incompatible with solutions containing penicillin

Mechanism of Action Competitively inhibits activation of plasminogen and directly inhibits plasmin activity

Pharmacokinetics

Bioavailability: Oral: 30% to 50%

Half-life: 2 hours

Elimination: 95% excreted as unchanged drug in urine

Usual Dosage Children and Adults: 10 mg/kg I.V. immediately before surgery, then 25 mg/kg/dose orally 3-4 times/day for 2-8 days

Administration May be given by direct I.V. injection at a maximum rate of 100 mg/minute; compatible with dextrose, saline, and electrolyte solutions

Monitoring Parameters Ophthalmologic exams (baseline and at regular intervals) of chronic therapy

Reference Range 0.13 mg/mL is required to decrease fibrinolysis

Dosage Forms

Injection: 100 mg/mL (10 mL)

Tablet: 500 mg

Transdermal-NTG® *see* Nitroglycerin *on page 415*

Transderm-Nitro® *see* Nitroglycerin *on page 415*

Transderm Scop® *see* Scopolamine *on page 519*

***trans*-Retinoic Acid** *see* Tretinoin *on next page*

Trans-Ver-Sal® [OTC] *see* Salicylic Acid *on page 516*

Tranxene® *see* Clorazepate Dipotassium *on page 144*

Travase® *see* Sutilains *on page 547*

Trazodone (traz' oh done)

Brand Names Desyrel®

Therapeutic Category Antidepressant

Use Treatment of depression

Pregnancy Risk Factor C

Contraindications Hypersensitivity to trazodone or any component

Warnings Monitor closely and use with extreme caution in patients with cardiac disease or arrhythmias

(Continued)

Trazodone *(Continued)*

Adverse Reactions Possesses fewer anticholinergic and cardiac adverse effects than tricyclic antidepressants

Cardiovascular: Postural hypotension (5%), arrhythmias

Central nervous system: Drowsiness (20% to 50%), sedation, weakness, dizziness, insomnia, confusion, agitation, seizures, extrapyramidal reactions, headache

Gastrointestinal: Dry mouth, constipation, nausea, vomiting

Hepatic: Hepatitis

Ocular: Blurred vision (15% to 30%)

Renal & genitourinary: Urinary retention (rare), prolonged priapism (1:6000)

Drug Interactions May antagonize the antihypertensive effects of clonidine and methyldopa; may increase the serum concentrations of phenytoin or digoxin; effects may be additive with other CNS depressants; fluoxetine may ↑ trazodone serum concentration

Mechanism of Action Inhibits reuptake of serotonin; minimal or no effect on reuptake of norepinephrine or dopamine; possesses little if any anticholinergic effects; alpha-adrenergic blockage thought to be responsible for orthostatic hypotension and dry mouth

Pharmacodynamics Maximum antidepressant effect usually seen around 2-6 weeks

Usual Dosage Oral:

Children 6-18 years: Initial: 1.5-2 mg/kg/day in divided doses; increase gradually every 3-4 days as needed; maximum: 6 mg/kg/day in 3 divided doses

Adolescents: Initial: 25-50 mg/day; increase to 100-150 mg/day in divided doses

Adults: Initial: 150 mg/day in 3 divided doses (may ↑ by 50 mg/day every 3-7 days); maximum: 600 mg/day

Reference Range Therapeutic: 0.5-2.5 μg/mL (SI: 1-6 μmol/L); potentially toxic: >2.5 μg/mL (SI: >6 μmol/L); toxic: >4 μg/mL (SI: 10 μmol/L)

Nursing Implications Dosing after meals may ↓ lightheadedness and postural hypotension

Dosage Forms Tablet: 50 mg, 100 mg, 150 mg, 300 mg

Trecator®-SC *see* Ethionamide *on page 235*

Trendar® [OTC] *see* Ibuprofen *on page 300*

Tretinoin (tret' i noyn)

Brand Names Retin-A™

Synonyms Retinoic Acid; *trans*-Retinoic Acid; Vitamin A Acid

Therapeutic Category Acne Product; Retinoic Acid Derivative; Vitamin, Topical

Use Treatment of acne vulgaris, photodamaged skin, and some skin cancers

Pregnancy Risk Factor C

Contraindications Hypersensitivity to tretinoin or any component; sunburn

Warnings Avoid contact with abraded skin, mucous membranes, eyes, mouth, angles of the nose; avoid excessive exposure to sunlight or sunlamps

Precautions Use with caution in patients with eczema

Adverse Reactions

Cardiovascular: Edema

Dermatologic: Excessive dryness, erythema, scaling of the skin, hyperpigmentation or hypopigmentation, photosensitivity, initial acne flare-up

Local: Stinging, blistering

Drug Interactions Sulfur, benzoyl peroxide, salicylic acid, and resorcinol potentiate adverse reactions seen with tretinoin

Mechanism of Action Keratinocytes in the sebaceous follicle become less adherent which allows for easy removal; inhibits microcomedone formation and eliminates lesions already present

Pharmacokinetics

Absorption: Topical: Minimum absorption

Metabolism: Occurs in the liver

Elimination: Excreted in the bile and urine

Usual Dosage Children >12 years and Adults: Topical: Begin therapy with a weaker formulation of tretinoin (0.025% cream or 0.01% gel) and increase the concentration as tolerated; apply once daily before retiring; if stinging or irritation develop, decrease frequency of application

Patient Information Avoid hydration of skin immediately before application; minimize exposure to sunlight; use of a sunscreen is recommended; avoid washing face more frequently than 2-3 times/day; avoid using topical preparations with high alcoholic content during treatment period

Additional Information Therapeutic effects seen after 2-3 weeks; optimum results may require 3-5 months of continuous therapy

Dosage Forms

Cream: 0.025% (20 g, 45 g); 0.05% (20 g, 45 g); 0.1% (20 g, 45 g)
Gel, topical: 0.01% (15 g, 45 g); 0.025% (15 g, 45 g)
Liquid, topical: 0.05% (28 mL)

References

Winston MH, Shalita AR, "Acne Vulgaris, Pathogenesis and Treatment," *Pediatr Clin North Am*, 1991, 38(4):889-903.

Triacetyloleandomycin *see* Troleandomycin *on page 587*

Triam-A® *see* Triamcinolone *on this page*

Triamcinolone (trye am sin' oh lone)

Related Information

Topical Steroids Comparison Chart *on page 728*

Brand Names Amcort®; Aristocort® Forte; Aristocort® Intralesional Suspension; Aristocort® Tablet; Aristospan®; Azmacort™; Cenocort®; Cenocort® Forte; Kenacort® Syrup; Kenacort® Tablet; Kenalog® Injection; Tac™-3; Triam-A®; Triamolone®; Tri-Kort®; Trilog®; Trilone®; Trisoject®

Synonyms Triamcinolone Acetonide, Aerosol; Triamcinolone Acetonide, Parenteral; Triamcinolone Diacetate, Oral; Triamcinolone Diacetate, Parenteral; Triamcinolone Hexacetonide; Triamcinolone, Oral

Therapeutic Category Anti-inflammatory Agent; Corticosteroid, Inhalant; Corticosteroid, Systemic; Corticosteroid, Topical; Glucocorticoid

Use Severe inflammation or immunosuppression; nasal spray for symptoms of seasonal and perennial allergic rhinitis

Pregnancy Risk Factor C

Contraindications Known hypersensitivity to triamcinolone; systemic fungal infections; serious infections, except septic shock or tuberculous meningitis; primary treatment of asthma

Warnings Fatalities have occurred due to adrenal insufficiency in asthmatic patients during and after transfer from systemic corticosteroids to aerosol steroids; several months may be required for recovery from this syndrome; during this period, aerosol steroids do **not** provide the increased systemic steroid requirement needed to treat patients having trauma, surgery or infections

Adverse Reactions

Cardiovascular: Facial edema
Central nervous system: Fatigue
Dermatologic: Itching, hypertrichosis, skin atrophy, hyperpigmentation, hypopigmentation, acne
Gastrointestinal: Oral candidiasis, dry throat, dry mouth, peptic ulcer
Local: Burning, sterile abscesses
Musculoskeletal: Osteoporosis
Ocular: Cataracts
Respiratory: Hoarseness, wheezing, cough

Drug Interactions Barbiturates, phenytoin, rifampin ↑ metabolism of triamcinolone; salicylates; vaccines

Mechanism of Action Decreases inflammation by suppression of migration of polymorphonuclear leukocytes and reversal of increased capillary permeability; suppresses the immune system by reducing activity and volume of the lymphatic system

Pharmacokinetics Peak serum levels: I.M.: Within 8-10 hours

Usual Dosage

Children: 6-12 years:

I.M. (as acetonide or hexacetonide): 0.03-0.2 mg/kg at 1- to 7-day intervals
Inhalation: 1-2 inhalations 3-4 times/day, not to exceed 12 inhalations/day
Intra-articular, intrabursal, or tendon-sheath injection: 2.5-15 mg, repeated as needed

(Continued)

Triamcinolone *(Continued)*

Children and Adults: Topical: Apply a thin film 2-3 times/day

Children >12 years and Adults:

Oral inhalation: 2 inhalations 3-4 times/day, not to exceed 16 inhalations/day

Intranasal: 2 sprays in each nostril once daily; may increase after 4-7 days up to 4 sprays once daily or 1 spray 4 times/day in each nostril

Oral: 4-100 mg/day

Intra-articular, intrasynovial, intralesional (as diacetate or acetonide): 2.5-40 mg, dose may be repeated when signs and symptoms recur

Intra-articular (as hexacetonide): 2-20 mg every 3-4 weeks

Intralesional, sublesional (as diacetate or acetonide): Up to 1 mg per injection site and may be repeated 1 or more times weekly; multiple sites may be injected if they are 1 cm or more apart, not to exceed 30 mg

Nursing Implications Avoid topical application on face; avoid S.C. use; for topical use do not occlude area unless directed; rinse mouth and throat after oral inhalation use to prevent candidiasis

Dosage Forms

Aerosol:

Oral inhalation: 100 μg/metered spray (2 oz)

Topical, as acetonide: 0.2 mg/2 second spray (23 g, 63 g)

Cream, as acetonide: 0.025% (15 g, 60 g, 80 g, 240 g, 454 g); 0.1% (15 g, 30 g, 60 g, 80 g, 90 g, 120 g, 240 g; 0.5% (15 g, 20 g, 30 g, 240 g)

Injection, as acetonide: 10 mg/mL (5 mL); 40 mg/mL (1 mL, 5 mL, 10 mL)

Injection, as diacetate: 25 mg/mL (5 mL); 40 mg/mL (1 mL, 5 mL, 10 mL)

Injection, as hexacetonide: 5 mg/mL (5 mL); 20 mg/mL 1 mL, 5 mL)

Lotion, as acetonide: 0.025% (60 mL); 0.1% (15 mL, 60 mL)

Ointment:

Oral: 0.1% (5 g)

Topical, as acetonide: 0.025% (15 g, 30 g, 60 g, 80 g, 120 g, 454 g); 0.1% (15 g, 30 g, 60 g, 80 g, 120 g, 240 g, 454 g); 0.5% (15 g, 20 g, 30 g, 240 g)

Syrup: 2 mg/5 mL (120 mL); 4 mg/5 mL (120 mL)

Tablet: 1 mg, 2 mg, 4 mg, 8 mg

Triamcinolone Acetonide, Aerosol *see* Triamcinolone *on previous page*

Triamcinolone Acetonide, Parenteral *see* Triamcinolone *on previous page*

Triamcinolone Diacetate, Oral *see* Triamcinolone *on previous page*

Triamcinolone Diacetate, Parenteral *see* Triamcinolone *on previous page*

Triamcinolone Hexacetonide *see* Triamcinolone *on previous page*

Triamcinolone, Oral *see* Triamcinolone *on previous page*

Triamolone® *see* Triamcinolone *on previous page*

Triamterene (trye am' ter een)

Brand Names Dyrenium®

Therapeutic Category Antihypertensive; Diuretic, Potassium Sparing

Use Used alone or in combination with other diuretics to treat edema and hypertension; decreases potassium excretion caused by kaliuretic diuretics

Pregnancy Risk Factor D

Contraindications Hypersensitivity to triamterene or any component; severe renal or hepatic impairment, hyperkalemia

Warnings Do not give triamterene to patients on other potassium-sparing diuretics; see Drug Interactions

Precautions Use with caution in patients with impaired hepatic or renal function, history of renal calculi, diabetes

Adverse Reactions

Cardiovascular: Hypotension,

Central nervous system: Dizziness, weakness, headache,

Endocrine & metabolic: Hyperkalemia, hyponatremia, hypomagnesemia, hyperchloremia, hyperuricemia, metabolic acidosis

Dermatologic: Photosensitivity
Gastrointestinal: Nausea, vomiting, diarrhea, dry mouth
Hematologic: Blood dyscrasias
Hepatic: Abnormal liver function
Musculoskeletal: Muscle cramps
Renal & genitourinary: Slight alkalinization of urine, prerenal azotemia, nephrolithiasis (rarely)
Miscellaneous: Allergic reactions have been reported

Drug Interactions Increased risk of hyperkalemia if given together with other potassium-sparing diuretics (ie, spironolactone); may increase risk of hyperkalemia with angiotensin-converting enzyme (ACE) inhibitor, (ie, captopril, enalapril); concomitant administration of triamterene and indomethacin may increase nephrotoxicity; increased risk of hyperkalemia with potassium-containing preparations; may increase lithium toxicity by decreasing lithium clearance; may increase amantadine toxicity possibly by decreasing its renal excretion

Mechanism of Action Competes with aldosterone for receptor sites in the distal renal tubules, increasing sodium, chloride and water excretion while conserving potassium and hydrogen ions

Pharmacodynamics
Onset of action: Diuresis occurs within 2-4 hours
Duration: 7-9 hours
Note: Maximum therapeutic effect may not occur until after several days of therapy

Pharmacokinetics
Absorption: Oral: Unreliably absorbed
Half-life: 100-150 minutes
Metabolic and excretory pathways have not been fully determined

Usual Dosage Oral:
Children: 2-4 mg/kg/day in 1-2 divided doses; maximum: 6 mg/kg/day and not to exceed 300 mg/day
Adults: 100-300 mg/day in 1-2 divided doses; maximum dose: 300 mg/day

Monitoring Parameters Electrolytes (sodium, potassium, magnesium, HCO_3, chloride), CBC, BUN, creatinine

Test Interactions Interferes with fluorometric assay of quinidine

Patient Information Take with food to avoid GI upset

Additional Information Abrupt discontinuation of therapy may result in rebound kaliuresis; taper off gradually

Dosage Forms Capsule: 50 mg, 100 mg

Triazolam (trye ay' zoe lam)

Related Information
Overdose and Toxicology Information *on page 696-700*

Brand Names Halcion®

Therapeutic Category Benzodiazepine; Hypnotic

Use Short-term treatment of insomnia

Restrictions C-IV

Pregnancy Risk Factor X

Contraindications Hypersensitivity to triazolam, or any component, cross-sensitivity with other benzodiazepines may occur; severe uncontrolled pain; pre-existing CNS depression; narrow-angle glaucoma; not to be used in pregnancy or lactation

Warnings Abrupt discontinuance may precipitate withdrawal or rebound insomnia

Adverse Reactions
Central nervous system: Drowsiness, ataxia, anterograde amnesia, confusion, bizarre behavior, agitation, dizziness, hallucinations, nightmares, headache
Gastrointestinal: Dry mouth, nausea, vomiting
Hepatic: Cholestatic jaundice
Miscellaneous: Physical and psychological dependence

Drug Interactions CNS depressants may ↑ CNS adverse effects; cimetidine may ↓ and enzyme inducers may ↑ the metabolism of triazolam

Mechanism of Action Depresses all levels of the CNS, including the limbic and reticular formation, probably through the increased action of gamma-

(Continued)

Triazolam *(Continued)*

aminobutyric acid (GABA), which is a major inhibitory neurotransmitter in the brain

Pharmacodynamics Hypnotic effects:

Onset: Within 15-30 minutes

Duration: 6-7 hours

Pharmacokinetics

Distribution: V_d: 0.8-1.8 L/kg

Protein binding: 89%

Metabolism: Extensive in the liver

Half-life: 1.7-5 hours

Elimination: Excreted in the urine as unchanged drug and metabolites

Usual Dosage Oral:

Children <18 years: Dosage not established; investigational doses of 0.02 mg/kg given as an elixir have been used in children (n=20) for sedation prior to dental procedures; further studies are needed before this dose can be recommended

Adults: 0.125-0.25 mg at bedtime

Additional Information Onset of action is rapid, patient should be in bed when taking medication

Dosage Forms Tablet: 0.125 mg, 0.25 mg

References

Meyer ML, Mourino AP, and Farrington FH, "Comparison of Triazolam to a Chloral Hydrate/Hydroxyzine Combination in the Sedation of Pediatric Dental Patients," *Pediatr Dent*, 1990, 12(5):283-7.

Triban® *see* Trimethobenzamide Hydrochloride *on page 585*

Tribavirin *see* Ribavirin *on page 511*

Trichloroacetaldehyde Monohydrate *see* Chloral Hydrate *on page 122*

Tridil® *see* Nitroglycerin *on page 415*

Triethanolamine Polypeptide Oleate-Condensate

Brand Names Cerumenex®

Therapeutic Category Otic Agent, Ear Wax Emulsifier

Use Removal of cerumen

Pregnancy Risk Factor C

Contraindications Perforated tympanic membrane or otitis media; hypersensitivity to product or any component

Warnings Discontinue if sensitization or irritation occurs

Precautions Avoid undue exposure to skin during administration and the flushing out of ear canal; exposure of ear canal to otic solution should be limited to 15-30 minutes

Adverse Reactions Local: Localized dermatitis, mild erythema and pruritus, severe eczematoid reactions involving the external ear and periauricular tissue

Mechanism of Action Emulsifies and disperses accumulated cerumen for easier removal

Pharmacodynamics Onset of effect: Produces slight disintegration of very hard ear wax by 24 hours

Usual Dosage Children and Adults: Otic: Fill ear canal, insert cotton plug; allow to remain 15-30 minutes; flush ear with lukewarm water as a single treatment; if a second application is needed for unusually hard impactions, repeat the procedure

Monitoring Parameters Evaluate hearing before and after instillation of medication

Patient Information For external use in the ear only; warm to body temperature before using to improve effect

Nursing Implications Avoid undue exposure of the drug to the periaural skin

Dosage Forms Solution, otic: 6 mL, 12 mL

References

Mehta AK, "An *In Vitro* Comparison of the Disintegration of Human Ear Wax by Five Cerumenolytics Commonly Used in General Practice," *Br J Clin Pract*, 1985, 39(5):200-3.

Triethylenethiophosphoramide *see* Thiotepa *on page 563*

Trifed® [OTC] *see* Triprolidine and Pseudoephedrine *on page 586*

Trifluorothymidine *see* Trifluridine *on this page*

Trifluridine (trye flure' i deen)

Brand Names Viroptic®

Synonyms F_3T; Trifluorothymidine

Therapeutic Category Antiviral Agent, Ophthalmic

Use Treatment of primary keratoconjunctivitis and recurrent epithelial keratitis caused by herpes simplex virus types I and II

Pregnancy Risk Factor C

Contraindications Known hypersensitivity to trifluridine

Adverse Reactions

Local: Burning, stinging

Ocular: Palpebral edema, epithelial keratopathy, keratitis, stromal edema, increased intraocular pressure, hyperemia

Miscellaneous: Hypersensitivity reactions

Stability Store in refrigerator; storage at room temperature may result in a solution with altered pH which could result in ocular discomfort upon administration and/or decreased potency

Mechanism of Action Interferes with viral replication by incorporating into viral DNA in place of thymidine, inhibiting thymidylate synthetase resulting in the formation of defective proteins

Pharmacodynamics Onset of action: Response to treatment occurs within 2-7 days; epithelial healing is complete in 1-2 weeks

Pharmacokinetics Absorption: Ophthalmic: Systemic absorption is negligible, while corneal penetration is adequate

Usual Dosage Children and Adults: Ophthalmic: 1 drop into affected eye every 2 hours while awake, to a maximum of 9 drops/day, until re-epithelialization of corneal ulcer occurs; then use 1 drop every 4 hours for another 7 days; do **not** exceed 21 days of treatment

Monitoring Parameters Ophthalmologic exam (test for corneal staining with fluorescein or rose bengal)

Dosage Forms Solution, ophthalmic: 1% (7.5 mL)

Trihexy® *see* Trihexyphenidyl Hydrochloride *on this page*

Trihexyphenidyl Hydrochloride (trye hex ee fen' i dill)

Related Information

Overdose and Toxicology Information *on page 696-700*

Brand Names Artane®; Trihexy®

Synonyms Benzhexol Hydrochloride

Therapeutic Category Anticholinergic Agent; Antiparkinson Agent

Use Adjunctive treatment of Parkinson's disease; also used in treatment of drug-induced extrapyramidal effects and acute dystonic reactions

Pregnancy Risk Factor C

Contraindications Hypersensitivity to trihexyphenidyl or any component; children younger than 3 years of age; patients with narrow-angle glaucoma, GI or GU obstruction

Precautions May impair ability to perform hazardous duties requiring mental alertness or physical coordination; use with caution in patients with hyperthyroidism, renal or hepatic dysfunction, hypertension, hiatal hernia, peptic ulcer, esophageal reflux

Adverse Reactions

Cardiovascular: Tachycardia

Central nervous system: Dizziness, nervousness, drowsiness, weakness, agitation, delirium, headache

Dermatologic: Rash

Gastrointestinal: Dryness of mouth, nausea, constipation

Ocular: Blurred vision, mydriasis, increased intraocular tension

Renal & genitourinary: Urinary hesitancy or retention

Drug Interactions Amantadine, anticholinergics, tricyclic antidepressants, MAO inhibitors

(Continued)

Trihexyphenidyl Hydrochloride *(Continued)*

Mechanism of Action Presumed to act by blocking excess acetylcholine at cerebral synapses; many of its effects are due to its pharmacologic similarities with atropine

Pharmacodynamics

Onset of effect: 1 hour
Peak effect: 2-3 hours
Duration: 6-12 hours

Pharmacokinetics

Metabolism: Metabolic fate undetermined
Elimination: Some urinary excretion

Usual Dosage Adults: Oral: Extrapyramidal: 5-15 mg/day in 3-4 divided doses

Monitoring Parameters Intraocular pressure monitoring (baseline and at regular intervals)

Dosage Forms

Capsule, sustained release: 5 mg
Elixir: 2 mg/5 mL (480 mL)
Tablet: 2 mg, 5 mg

Tri-Kort® *see* Triamcinolone *on page 579*

Trilisate® *see* Choline Magnesium Trisalicylate *on page 133*

Trilog® *see* Triamcinolone *on page 579*

Trilone® *see* Triamcinolone *on page 579*

Trimazide® *see* Trimethobenzamide Hydrochloride *on next page*

Trimetaphan Camsylate *see* Trimethaphan Camsylate *on this page*

Trimethaphan Camphorsulfonate *see* Trimethaphan Camsylate *on this page*

Trimethaphan Camsylate (trye meth' a fan)

Brand Names Arfonad®

Synonyms Trimetaphan Camsylate; Trimethaphan Camphorsulfonate

Therapeutic Category Adrenergic Blocking Agent; Anticholinergic Agent; Antihypertensive; Ganglionic Blocking Agent

Use Hypertensive emergencies; controlled hypotension during surgery

Pregnancy Risk Factor D

Contraindications Hypersensitivity to trimethaphan camsylate or any component; hypovolemia or shock; anemia; respiratory insufficiency

Precautions Use with caution in patients with allergies; cardiac, hepatic, or renal dysfunction; diabetes mellitus, Addison's disease, or glaucoma

Adverse Reactions

Cardiovascular: Hypotension (especially orthostatic), tachycardia (especially in children and young adults)
Central nervous system: Restlessness, weakness
Dermatologic: Itching, urticaria
Endocrine & metabolic: With prolonged use (>48-72 hours) sodium and water retention
Gastrointestinal: Anorexia, nausea, vomiting, dry mouth, adynamic ileus
Ocular: Mydriasis, cycloplegia
Renal & genitourinary: Urinary retention
Respiratory: Apnea, respiratory arrest (especially with doses >6 mg/minute)

Drug Interactions Anesthetics, procainamide, diuretics and other hypotensive agents may ↑ hypotensive effects of trimethaphan; effects of tubocurarine and succinylcholine may be prolonged by trimethaphan

Stability Solution should be freshly prepared and any unused portion discarded

Mechanism of Action Blocks transmission in both adrenergic and cholinergic ganglia by blocking stimulation from presynaptic receptors to postsynaptic receptors mediated by acetylcholine; possesses direct peripheral vasodilatory activity and is a weak histamine releaser

Pharmacodynamics

Onset of action: I.V.: Immediate

Peak effects: 5 minutes
Duration: 10-30 minutes

Pharmacokinetics
Metabolism: Metabolized primarily by postganglionic pseudocholinesterase
Elimination: Urinary excretion

Usual Dosage I.V.:
Children: 50-150 μg/kg/minute

Adults: Initial: 0.5-2 mg/minute; titrate to effect; usual dose: 0.3-6 mg/minute

Administration Must be diluted; usually mixed as 1 mg/mL concentration in 5% dextrose

Monitoring Parameters Blood pressure and heart rate continuously

Dosage Forms Injection: 50 mg/mL (10 mL)

Trimethobenzamide Hydrochloride

(trye meth oh ben' za mide)

Related Information
Compatibility of Medications Mixed in a Syringe *on page 717*

Brand Names Arrestin®; Tebamide®; T-Gen®; Ticon®; Tigan®; Tiject®; Triban®; Trimazide®

Therapeutic Category Antiemetic

Use Control of nausea and vomiting (especially for long term antiemetic therapy)

Pregnancy Risk Factor C

Contraindications Hypersensitivity to trimethobenzamide or any component or benzocaine (contained in suppository)

Precautions Use in patients with acute vomiting should be **avoided**; may mask emesis due to Reye's syndrome or mimic CNS effects of Reye's syndrome in patients with emesis of other etiologies; may impair ability to perform hazardous duties requiring mental alertness or physical coordination

Adverse Reactions
Cardiovascular: Hypotension (especially after I.M. use)
Central nervous system: Drowsiness, sedation, extrapyramidal symptoms, dizziness, seizures
Gastrointestinal: Diarrhea
Hematologic: Blood dyscrasias
Local: Pain, stinging, burning at I.M. injection site
Ocular: Blurred vision
Miscellaneous: Hypersensitivity skin reactions

Mechanism of Action Acts centrally to inhibit stimulation of the medullary chemoreceptor trigger zone

Pharmacodynamics
Onset of action:
Oral: 10-40 minutes
I.M.: 15-35 minutes
Duration:
Oral: 3-4 hours
I.M.: 2-3 hours

Pharmacokinetics
Bioavailability: Oral dose is ~60% of I.M. dose
Metabolism: Not well determined
Elimination: 20% is excreted unchanged in urine in 24 hours

Usual Dosage Rectal use: Contraindicated in neonates and premature infants; not for I.V. use
Children:
Oral, rectal: 15-20 mg/kg/day or 400-500 mg/m^2/day divided into 3-4 doses
I.M.: Not recommended

Adults:
Oral: 250 mg 3-4 times/day
I.M., rectal: 200 mg 3-4 times/day

Additional Information Note: Less effective than phenothiazines but may be associated with fewer side effects

Dosage Forms
Capsule: 100 mg, 250 mg
Injection: 100 mg/mL (2 mL, 20 mL)
Suppository, rectal: 100 mg, 200 mg

Trimethoprim and Sulfamethoxazole *see* Co-trimoxazole *on page 156*

Trimox® *see* Amoxicillin *on page 44*

Triofed® [OTC] *see* Triprolidine and Pseudoephedrine *on this page*

Triple Antibiotic® *see* Neomycin, Polymyxin B, and Bacitracin *on page 407*

Triposed® [OTC] *see* Triprolidine and Pseudoephedrine *on this page*

Triprolidine and Pseudoephedrine (trye proe' li deen)

Related Information

OTC Cold Preparations, Pediatric *on page 723-726*

Overdose and Toxicology Information *on page 696-700*

Brand Names Actagen® [OTC]; Actifed® [OTC]; Allerfrin® [OTC]; Allerphed [OTC]; Aprodine® [OTC]; Cenafed® Plus [OTC]; Genac® [OTC]; Trifed® [OTC]; Triofed® [OTC]; Triposed® [OTC]

Synonyms Pseudoephedrine and Triprolidine

Therapeutic Category Antihistamine; Sympathomimetic

Use Temporary relief of nasal congestion, running nose, sneezing, itching of nose or throat and itchy, watery eyes due to common cold, hay fever or other upper respiratory allergies

Pregnancy Risk Factor C

Contraindications Known hypersensitivity to triprolidine or pseudoephedrine; severe hypertension or coronary artery disease; MAO inhibitor therapy, GI or GU obstruction, narrow-angle glaucoma

Warnings Not recommended for use in children <4 months of age; may impair ability to perform hazardous activities requiring mental alertness or physical coordination

Precautions Use with caution in patients with mild to moderate high blood pressure, heart disease, diabetes, asthma, thyroid disease, or prostatic hypertrophy

Adverse Reactions

Cardiovascular: Hypertension, tachycardia

Central nervous system: Sedation, CNS stimulation, headache

Gastrointestinal: Nausea, vomiting, dry mouth, anorexia

Drug Interactions MAO inhibitors, beta blocking agents, other sympathomimetics, methyldopa, reserpine, alpha blocking agents, CNS depressants

Usual Dosage Oral:

Children: May dose according to **pseudoephedrine** component: 4 mg/kg/day in divided doses 3-4 times/day **or**

- 4 months to 2 years: 1.25 mL 3-4 times/day
- 2-4 years: 2.5 mL 3-4 times/day
- 4-6 years: 3.75 mL 3-4 times/day
- 6-12 years: 5 mL or ½ tablet 3-4 times/day

Children >12 years and Adults: 10 mL or 1 tablet 3-4 times/day **or** 1 extended release capsule every 12 hours

Additional Information Do not crush or chew sustained release products

Dosage Forms

Capsule: Triprolidine hydrochloride 2.5 mg and pseudoephedrine hydrochloride 60 mg

Capsule, extended release: Triprolidine hydrochloride 5 mg and pseudoephedrine hydrochloride 120 mg

Syrup: Triprolidine hydrochloride 1.25 mg and pseudoephedrine hydrochloride 30 mg per 5 mL

Tablet: Triprolidine hydrochloride 2.5 mg and pseudoephedrine hydrochloride 60 mg

TripTone® Caplets® [OTC] *see* Dimenhydrinate *on page 193*

Tris Buffer *see* Tromethamine *on next page*

Tris(hydroxymethyl)aminomethane *see* Tromethamine *on next page*

Trisoject® *see* Triamcinolone *on page 579*

Troleandomycin (troe lee an doe mye' sin)

Brand Names Tao®

Synonyms Triacetyloleandomycin

Therapeutic Category Antibiotic, Macrolide

Use Adjunct in the treatment of corticosteroid-dependent asthma due to its steroid sparing properties; obsolete antibiotic with spectrum of activity similar to erythromycin

Pregnancy Risk Factor C

Contraindications Hypersensitivity to troleandomycin or any component

Warnings Cholestatic hepatitis has been reported in patients who have received troleandomycin for 2 weeks or longer and in cases where repeated courses were administered

Precautions Use with caution in patients with impaired hepatic function

Adverse Reactions

Central nervous system: Fever

Dermatologic: Urticaria, rash

Gastrointestinal: Abdominal cramping, nausea, vomiting, diarrhea, rectal burning, esophagitis

Hepatic: Cholestatic hepatitis, jaundice

Drug Interactions Theophylline (↓ theophylline clearance since Tao® binds to cytochrome P-450 reducing its oxidizing activity); interferes with metabolism of ergotamine and carbamazepine potentiating their action; methylprednisolone

Mechanism of Action Decreases methylprednisolone clearance from a linear first order decline to a nonlinear decline in plasma concentration; Tao® also has an undefined action independent of its effects on steroid elimination

Pharmacokinetics

Peak serum concentrations: Oral: Within 2 hours

Elimination: 10% to 25% excreted in urine as active drug; excreted in feces via bile

Usual Dosage Oral:

Children: 25-40 mg/kg/day divided every 6 hours

Adjunct in corticosteroid-dependent asthma: 14 mg/kg/day in divided doses every 6-12 hours not to exceed 250 mg every 6 hours; dose is tapered to once daily then alternate day dosing

Adults: 250-500 mg 4 times/day

Monitoring Parameters Hepatic function tests

Dosage Forms Capsule: 250 mg

References

Brenner AM and Szefler SJ, "Troleandomycin in the Treatment of Severe Asthma," *Immunol Allergy Clin North Am*, 1991, 11(1):91-102.

Spector SL, Katz FH, and Farr RS, "Troleandomycin: Effectiveness in Steroid-Dependent Asthma and Bronchitis," *J Allergy Clin Immunol*, 1974, 54(6):367-79.

Tromethamine (troe meth' a meen)

Brand Names Tham®; Tham-E®

Synonyms Tris Buffer; Tris(hydroxymethyl)aminomethane

Therapeutic Category Alkalinizing Agent, Parenteral

Use Correction of metabolic acidosis associated with cardiac bypass surgery or cardiac arrest; to correct excess acidity of stored blood that is preserved with acid citrate dextrose (ACD); to prime the pump-oxygenator during cardiac bypass surgery; indicated in severe metabolic acidosis in patients in whom sodium or carbon dioxide elimination is restricted [eg, infants needing alkalinization after receiving maximum sodium bicarbonate (8-10 mEq/kg/24 hours)]

Pregnancy Risk Factor C

Contraindications Uremia or anuria; chronic respiratory acidosis

Precautions Reduce dose and monitor pH carefully in renal impairment

Adverse Reactions

Cardiovascular: Venospasm

Endocrine & metabolic: Hyperosmolality of serum, hyperkalemia, hypoglycemia

(Continued)

Tromethamine *(Continued)*

Hepatic: Liver cell destruction from direct contact with THAM®
Local: Tissue irritation, necrosis with extravasation
Respiratory: Respiratory depression, apnea

Mechanism of Action Proton acceptor, which combines with hydrogen ions to form bicarbonate and buffer

Pharmacokinetics 30% of dose is not ionized; rapidly eliminated by kidneys

Usual Dosage Dose depends on buffer base deficit; when deficit is known: tromethamine mL of 0.3 M solution = body weight (kg) x base deficit (mEq/L); when base deficit is not known: 3.5-6 mL/kg/dose I.V. (1-2 mEq/kg/dose)

Metabolic acidosis with cardiac arrest: I.V.: 3.5-6 mL/kg (1-2 mEq/kg/dose) into large peripheral vein; maximum: 500 mg/kg/dose

Excess acidity of acid citrate dextrose priming blood: 14-70 mL of 0.3 molar solution added to each 500 mL of blood

Administration Maximum concentration: 0.3 molar; infuse slowly over at least 1 hour (Tham-E® requires the reconstitution with 1 L sterile water before use)

Monitoring Parameters Serum electrolytes, arterial blood gases, serum pH, blood sugar, EKG monitoring, renal function tests

Additional Information 1 mM = 120 mg = 3.3 mL = 1 mEq of THAM®

Dosage Forms Injection:

Tham®: 18 g [0.3 molar] (500 mL)
Tham-E®: 36 g with sodium 30 mEq, potassium 5 mEq, and chloride 35 mEq (1000 mL)

Tropicacyl® *see* Tropicamide *on this page*

Tropicamide (troe pik' a mide)

Brand Names I-Picamide®; Mydriacyl®; Tropicacyl®

Synonyms Bistropamide

Therapeutic Category Ophthalmic Agent, Mydriatic

Use Short-acting mydriatic used in diagnostic procedures; as well as preoperatively and postoperatively; treatment of some cases of acute iritis, iridocyclitis, and keratitis

Pregnancy Risk Factor C

Contraindications Glaucoma, hypersensitivity to tropicamide or any component

Warnings Tropicamide may cause an increase in intraocular pressure

Precautions Use with caution in infants and children since tropicamide may cause potentially dangerous CNS disturbances and psychotic reactions

Adverse Reactions

Cardiovascular: Tachycardia
Central nervous system: Parasympathetic stimulation, drowsiness, headache, behavioral disturbances, psychotic reactions
Gastrointestinal: Dryness of the mouth
Local: Transient stinging
Ocular: Blurred vision, photophobia, increased intraocular pressure, follicular conjunctivitis
Miscellaneous: Allergic reactions

Stability Store at room temperature

Mechanism of Action Prevents the sphincter muscle of the iris and the muscle of the ciliary body from responding to cholinergic stimulation

Pharmacodynamics

Maximum mydriatic effect: ~20-40 minutes
Duration: ~6-7 hours
Maximum cycloplegic effect: Within 30 minutes
Duration: <6 hours

Usual Dosage Children and Adults: Ophthalmic:

Cycloplegia: 1-2 drops (1%); may repeat in 5 minutes. The exam must be performed within 30 minutes after the repeat dose; if the patient is not examined within 20-30 minutes, instill an additional drop. Concentrations <1% are inadequate for producing satisfactory cycloplegia.

Mydriasis: 1-2 drops (0.5%) 15-20 minutes before exam; may repeat every 30 minutes as needed

Dosage Forms Solution, ophthalmic: 0.5% (2 mL, 15 mL); 1% (2 mL, 3 mL, 15 mL)

References

Caputo AR and Schnitzer RE, "Systemic Response to Mydriatic Eyedrops in Neonates: Mydriatics in Neonates," *J Pediatr Ophthalmol Strabismus*, 1978, 15:109-22.

Truphylline® *see* Aminophylline *on page 37*

TSPA *see* Thiotepa *on page 563*

T-Stat® *see* Erythromycin *on page 226*

Tubocurarine Chloride (too boe kyoor ar' een)

Synonyms *d*-Tubocurarine Chloride

Therapeutic Category Neuromuscular Blocker Agent, Nondepolarizing

Use Adjunct to anesthesia to induce skeletal muscle relaxation

Pregnancy Risk Factor C

Contraindications Hypersensitivity to tubocurarine or any component

Warnings Ventilation must be supported during neuromuscular blockade; some commercially available products may contain sulfites

Precautions Use with caution in patients with renal impairment, respiratory depression, impaired hepatic or endocrine function

Adverse Reactions

Cardiovascular: Cardiac arrhythmias, hypotension, tachycardia or bradycardia

Gastrointestinal: Increased salivation, decreased GI motility

Respiratory: Bronchospasm

Miscellaneous: Allergic reactions

Drug Interactions Aminoglycosides, clindamycin, quinidine, magnesium sulfate, verapamil, ketamine, furosemide

Mechanism of Action Nondepolarizing neuromuscular blocking agent which blocks acetylcholine from binding to receptors on motor endplate thus inhibiting depolarization; also has histamine-releasing and ganglionic blocking properties

Pharmacodynamics

Onset of effect:

- I.M.: Unpredictable, 10-25 minutes
- I.V.: 2-5 minutes

Duration: 20-30 minutes

Pharmacokinetics Elimination: ~33% to 75% of a parenteral dose is excreted unchanged in urine in 24 hours; about 11% excreted in bile through a specific organic cation secretion mechanism

Usual Dosage I.V.:

Neonates <1 month: 0.3 mg/kg as a single dose; maintenance: 0.1 mg/kg/dose as needed to maintain paralysis

Children: 0.2-0.5 mg/kg as a single dose; maintenance: 0.04-0.1 mg/kg/dose as needed to maintain paralysis

Adults: 6-9 mg as a single dose followed by maintenance of 3-4.5 mg as needed to maintain paralysis

Administration May infuse direct I.V. without further dilution over a period of 1-1½ minutes

Monitoring Parameters Respiratory status, heart rate, blood pressure, mechanical ventilator status

Dosage Forms Injection: 3 mg/mL [3 units/mL] (5 mL, 10 mL, 20 mL)

Tums® [OTC] *see* Antacid Preparations *on page 53*

Tums® [OTC] *see* Calcium Carbonate *on page 94*

Tusstat® *see* Diphenhydramine Hydrochloride *on page 195*

Twilite® [OTC] *see* Diphenhydramine Hydrochloride *on page 195*

Tylenol® [OTC] *see* Acetaminophen *on page 16*

Tylenol® With Codeine *see* Acetaminophen and Codeine Phosphate *on page 17*

Tylox® *see* Oxycodone Hydrochloride and Acetaminophen *on page 427*

Ucephan® *see* Sodium Phenylacetate and Sodium Benzoate *on page 529*

U-Cort™ *see* Hydrocortisone *on page 293*

Ultralente® Iletin® I *see* Insulin Preparations *on page 311*

Unasyn® *see* Ampicillin and Sulbactam *on page 50*

Undecylenic Acid and Derivatives (un de sill enn' ik)

Brand Names Caldesene® [OTC]; Cruex® [OTC]; Merlenate® [OTC]; Pedi-Dri; Pedi-Pro [OTC]; Quinsana® Plus [OTC]; Undoguent® [OTC]

Synonyms Calcium Undecylenate; Zinc Undecylenate

Therapeutic Category Antifungal Agent, Topical

Use Treatment of athlete's foot (tinea pedis), ringworm (except nails and scalp), prickly heat, jock itch (tinea cruris), diaper rash and other minor skin irritations due to superficial dermatophytes

Contraindications Fungal infections of the scalp or nails

Warnings Do not apply to blistered, raw, or oozing areas of skin or over deep wounds or puncture wounds

Adverse Reactions

Dermatologic: Rash

Local: Skin irritation, stinging, sensitization

Pharmacodynamics Onset of action: Improvement in erythema and pruritus may be seen within one week after initiation of therapy

Usual Dosage Children and Adults: Topical: Apply as needed twice daily after cleansing the affected area for 2-4 weeks

Monitoring Parameters Resolution of skin infection

Patient Information For external use only; avoid contact with the eye; do not inhale the powder

Nursing Implications Clean and dry the affected area before topical application

Additional Information Ointment should be applied at night, the powder may be applied during the day or used alone when a drying effect is needed

Dosage Forms

Cream: Total undecylenate 20% (15 g, 82.5 g)

Foam, topical: Undecylenic acid 10% (42.5 g)

Liquid, topical: Undecylenic acid 10% (42.5 g)

Ointment, topical: Total undecylenate 22% (30 g, 60 g, 454 g); total undecylenate 25% (60 g, 454 g)

Powder, topical: Calcium undecylenate 10% (45 g, 60 g, 120 g); total undecylenate 22% (45 g, 54 g, 81 g, 90 g, 105 g, 165 g, 454 g)

Undoguent® [OTC] *see* Undecylenic Acid and Derivatives *on this page*

Unguentine® [OTC] *see* Benzocaine *on page 77*

Unipen® *see* Nafcillin Sodium *on page 400*

Uniphyl® *see* Theophylline *on page 554*

Uni Tussin® [OTC] *see* Guaifenesin *on page 278*

Urea Peroxide *see* Carbamide Peroxide *on page 103*

Urecholine® *see* Bethanechol Chloride *on page 82*

Urex® *see* Methenamine *on page 369*

Urised® *see* Methenamine *on page 369*

Urobak® *see* Sulfamethoxazole *on page 542*

Urodine® *see* Phenazopyridine Hydrochloride *on page 449*

Urokinase (yoor oh kin' ase)

Brand Names Abbokinase®

Therapeutic Category Thrombolytic Agent

Use Thrombolytic agent used in treatment of recent severe or massive deep vein thrombosis, pulmonary emboli, and occluded arteriovenous cannulas

Pregnancy Risk Factor B

Contraindications Hypersensitivity to urokinase or any component; internal bleeding; CVA (within two months); brain carcinoma, bacterial endocarditis, anticoagulant therapy, surgery or trauma within past 10 days

Warnings Stop urokinase administration if any signs of bleeding occur

Precautions Use with caution in patients with severe hypertension, recent lumbar puncture, patient receiving I.M. administration of medications. If indicated, febrile patients should receive antibiotics for at least 24 hours prior to urokinase therapy; obtain an echocardiogram in febrile patients prior to therapy to rule out intracardiac vegetations; pretreatment lab studies should include: platelet count, PT/PTT, fibrinogen, fibrin degradation products, plasminogen, antithrombin III, protein S, protein C

Adverse Reactions

Central nervous system: Fever
Dermatologic: Rash
Hematologic: Internal bleeding
Local: Bleeding, hematoma at I.M. or L.P. sites
Respiratory: Bronchospasm
Miscellaneous: Allergic reactions

Drug Interactions Anticoagulants, aspirin

Stability Store in refrigerator; reconstitute by gently rolling and tilting, **do not shake**; does not contain preservative; the 5000 unit vial should be reconstituted just prior to use; discard unused portion; a reconstituted 250,000 unit vial is stable for 24 hours under refrigeration

Mechanism of Action Promotes thrombolysis by directly activating plasminogen to plasmin, which degrades fibrin, fibrinogen, and other procoagulant plasma proteins

Pharmacodynamics

Onset of action: I.V.: Fibrinolysis occurs rapidly
Duration: 4 or more hours

Pharmacokinetics

Half-life: 10-20 minutes
Elimination: Cleared by the liver with a small amount excreted in the urine and the bile

Usual Dosage

Infants, Children, and Adults:

- Arterial or venous thrombosis or pulmonary emboli: I.V.: Loading: 4400 units/kg over 10 minutes, then 4400 units/kg/hour for 12-72 hours; continuous infusion doses of 4000-10,000 units/kg/hour have been used; titrate urokinase dose to bring level of plasma fibrinogen to 75% of fibrinogen measured after FFP infusion; reassess clot size every 12-24 hours
- Occluded I.V. catheters:
  - 5000 units/mL concentration; (use only Abbokinase® Open Cath), volume to instill into catheter is equal to the volume of the catheter; administer in each lumen over 1-2 minutes, leave in lumen for 1-4 hours, then aspirate out of catheter, flush catheter with saline; may repeat with 10,000 units in each lumen if 5000 units fails to clear the catheter; **do not infuse into the patient**
  - Continuous I.V. infusion: 200 units/kg/hour in each lumen for 12-48 hours at a rate of at least 20 mL/hour
  - Dialysis patients: 5000 units is administered in each lumen over 1-2 minutes; leave urokinase in lumen for 1-2 days, then aspirate out of lumen

Adults: Myocardial infarction: Intracoronary: 6000 units/minute up to 2 hours

Administration I.V. infusion: Usual concentration: 1250-1500 units/mL; maximum concentration not yet defined

Monitoring Parameters CBC, reticulocyte, platelet count; fibrinogen, plasminogen, FDP, D-dimer, PT, PTT, ATIII, protein C, U/A, ACT

Nursing Implications Use 0.22 or 0.45 micron filter during I.V. systemic therapy

Additional Information Abbokinase® Open Cath 5000 unit product is **not** for systemic administration; it must be aspirated out of the catheter

Dosage Forms

Powder for injection: 250,000 units (5 mL)
Powder for injection, catheter clear: 5000 units (1 mL)

References

Bagnall HA, Gomperts E, and Atkinson JB, "Continuous Infusion of Low-Dose Urokinase in the Treatment of Central Venous Catheter Thrombosis in Infants and Children," *Pediatrics*, 1989, 83(6):963-6.

Urolene Blue® *see* Methylene Blue *on page 377*

Uroplus® DS *see* Co-trimoxazole *on page 156*

Uroplus® SS *see* Co-trimoxazole *on page 156*

Uticort® *see* Betamethasone *on page 81*

Valergen® *see* Estradiol *on page 231*

Valisone® *see* Betamethasone *on page 81*

Valium® *see* Diazepam *on page 182*

Valproic Acid and Derivatives (val proe' ik)

Related Information

Blood Level Sampling Time Guidelines *on page 694-695*

Brand Names Depakene®; Depakote®

Synonyms Dipropylacetic Acid; Divalproex Sodium; DPA; 2-Propylpentanoic Acid; 2-Propylvaleric Acid

Therapeutic Category Anticonvulsant

Use Management of simple and complex absence seizures; mixed seizure types; myoclonic and generalized tonic-clonic (grand mal) seizures; may be effective in partial seizures and infantile spasms

Pregnancy Risk Factor D

Contraindications Hypersensitivity to valproic acid or derivatives or any component; hepatic dysfunction

Warnings Hepatic failure resulting in fatalities has occurred in patients; children <2 years of age, especially those on polytherapy are at considerable risk; monitor patients closely for appearance of malaise, loss of seizure control, weakness, facial edema, anorexia, jaundice and vomiting; hepatotoxicity has been reported after 3 days to 6 months of therapy

Adverse Reactions

Central nervous system: Drowsiness, ataxia, tremor, irritability, confusion, restlessness, hyperactivity, malaise, headache

Dermatologic: Alopecia, erythema multiforme

Endocrine & metabolic: Hyperammonemia, weight gain

Gastrointestinal: Nausea, vomiting, diarrhea, pancreatitis

Hematologic: Thrombocytopenia, prolongation of bleeding time

Hepatic: Transient increased liver enzymes, liver failure (can be fatal)

Drug Interactions Valproic acid may displace phenytoin and diazepam from protein binding sites. Aspirin may displace valproic acid from protein binding sites which may result in toxicity. Valproic acid may significantly increase phenobarbital serum concentrations in patients receiving phenobarbital or primidone. Valproic acid may inhibit the metabolism of phenytoin. Phenobarbital, primidone, phenytoin, and carbamazepine may ↓ serum levels of valproic acid

Mechanism of Action Causes increased availability of gamma-aminobutyric acid (GABA), an inhibitory neurotransmitter, to brain neurons or may enhance the action of GABA or mimic its action at postsynaptic receptor sites

Pharmacokinetics

Protein binding: 80% to 90% (dose dependent)

Metabolism: Extensive in liver

Half-life:

- Newborns 1st week of life: 40-45 hours
- Children 2-14 years: Mean: 9 hours; range: 3.5-20 hours
- Adults: 8-17 hours
- Increased half-life in patients with liver disease

Peak serum levels: Oral: 1-4 hours; divalproex (enteric coated): 3-5 hours

Elimination: 2% to 3% excreted unchanged in urine; faster clearance in children who receive other antiepileptic drugs and those who are younger; age and polytherapy explain 80% of interpatient variability in total clearance

Usual Dosage Children and Adults:

Oral: Initial: 10-15 mg/kg/day in 1-3 divided doses; increase by 5-10 mg/kg/day at weekly intervals until therapeutic levels are achieved; maintenance: 30-60 mg/kg/day in 2-3 divided doses

Children receiving more than 1 anticonvulsant (ie, polytherapy) may require doses up to 100 mg/kg/day in 3-4 divided doses

Rectal: Dilute syrup 1:1 with water for use as a retention enema; loading dose: 17-20 mg/kg one time; maintenance: 10-15 mg/kg/dose every 8 hours

Monitoring Parameters Liver enzymes, CBC with platelets, serum concentrations

Reference Range Therapeutic: 50-100 μg/mL (SI: 350-690 μmol/L); Toxic: >100-150 μg/mL (SI: >690-1040 μmol/L). Seizure control may improve at levels over 100 μg/mL (SI: 690 μmol/L), but toxicity may occur

Test Interactions False-positive result for urine ketones

Nursing Implications Instruct patients/parents to report signs or symptoms of hepatotoxicity; administer with food or milk; do not chew, break or crush the tablet or capsule; do not administer with carbonated drinks; GI side effects of divalproex may be less than valproic acid

Dosage Forms

Capsule, sprinkle, as divalproex sodium (Depakote® Sprinkle®): 125 mg

Capsule, as valproic acid (Depakene®): 250 mg

Syrup, as sodium valproate (Depakene®): 250 mg/5mL (5 mL, 50 mL, 480 mL)

Tablet, delayed release, as divalproex sodium (Depakote®): 125 mg, 250 mg, 500 mg

References

Cloyd JC, Fischer JH, Kriel RL, et al, "Valproic Acid Pharmacokinetics in Children. IV. Effects of Age and Antiepileptic Drugs on Protein Binding and Intrinsic Clearance," *Clin Pharmacol Ther*, 1993, 53(1):22-9.

Cloyd JC, Kriel RL, Fischer JH, et al, "Pharmacokinetics of Valproic Acid in Children: I. Multiple Antiepileptic Drug Therapy," *Neurology*, 1983, 33(2):185-91.

Dreifuss FE, Santilli N, Langer DH, et al, "Valproic Acid Hepatic Fatalities: A Retrospective Review," *Neurology*, 1987, 37(3):379-85.

Valrelease® *see* Diazepam *on page 182*

Vancenase® *see* Beclomethasone Dipropionate *on page 75*

Vancenase® AQ *see* Beclomethasone Dipropionate *on page 75*

Vanceril® *see* Beclomethasone Dipropionate *on page 75*

Vancocin® *see* Vancomycin Hydrochloride *on this page*

Vancoled® *see* Vancomycin Hydrochloride *on this page*

Vancomycin Hydrochloride (van koe mye' sin)

Related Information

Blood Level Sampling Time Guidelines *on page 694-695*

Endocarditis Prophylaxis *on page 659*

Medications Compatible With PN Solutions *on page 649-650*

Brand Names Lyphocin®; Vancocin®; Vancoled®

Therapeutic Category Antibiotic, Miscellaneous

Use Used in the treatment of patients with the following infections or conditions: treatment of infections due to documented or suspected methicillin-resistant *S. aureus* or beta-lactam resistant coagulase negative *Staphylococcus*; treatment of serious or life-threatening infections (ie, endocarditis, meningitis, osteomyelitis) due to documented or suspected staphylococcal or streptococcal infections in patients who are allergic to penicillins and/or cephalosporins; empiric therapy of infections associated with central lines, VP shunts, hemodialysis shunts, vascular grafts, prosthetic heart valves; treatment of febrile granulocytopenic patient who has not responded after 48 hours to antibiotic treatment directed at gram-negative rod infections; used orally for staphylococcal enterocolitis or for antibiotic-associated pseudomembranous colitis produced by *C. difficile*

Pregnancy Risk Factor C

Contraindications Hypersensitivity to vancomycin or any component; avoid in patients with previous hearing loss

Precautions Use with caution in patients with renal impairment or those receiving other nephrotoxic or ototoxic drugs; dosage modification required in patients with impaired renal function

Adverse Reactions Rapid infusion associated with red neck or red man syndrome: Erythema multiforme-like reaction with intense pruritus, tachycardia, hypotension, rash involving face, neck, upper trunk, back and upper arms

(Continued)

Vancomycin Hydrochloride *(Continued)*

Cardiovascular: Cardiac arrest
Central nervous system: Fever, chills
Dermatologic: Red neck or red man syndrome, urticaria, macular skin rash
Gastrointestinal: Nausea
Hematologic: Neutropenia, eosinophilia
Local: Phlebitis
Musculoskeletal: Lower back pain
Otic: Ototoxicity associated with prolonged serum concentration >40 μg/mL
Renal & genitourinary: Nephrotoxicity (higher incidence with trough concentrations >10 μg/mL)
Miscellaneous: Hypersensitivity reactions

Drug Interactions Anesthetic agents (erythema, hypotension, hypothermia, and facial flushing); concurrent ototoxic or nephrotoxic drugs

Stability After the oral or parenteral solution is reconstituted, it should be refrigerated and used within 2 weeks; incompatible with heparin, phenobarbital

Mechanism of Action Inhibits bacterial cell wall synthesis; blocks glycopeptide polymerization of the phosphodisaccharide-pentapeptide complex in the second stage of cell wall synthesis by binding tightly to D-alanyl-D-alanine portion of cell wall precursor

Pharmacokinetics

Absorption:
- Oral: Poor
- I.M.: Erratic
- Intraperitoneal administration can result in 38% systemic absorption

Distribution: Widely distributed in body tissues and fluids except for poor penetration into CSF

Protein binding: 10%

Half-life, biphasic:
- Terminal:
  - Newborns: 6-10 hours
  - 3 months to 4 years: 4 hours
  - >3 years: 2.2-3 hours
  - Adults: 5-8 hours, half-life prolonged significantly with reduced renal function

Elimination: Primarily via glomerular filtration; excreted as unchanged drug in the urine (80% to 90%); oral doses are excreted primarily in the feces

Not dialyzable (0% to 5%)

Usual Dosage Initial dosage recommendation: I.V.:

Neonates:
- Postnatal age ≤7 days:
  - <1200 g: 15 mg/kg/day given every 24 hours
  - 1200-2000 g: 15 mg/kg/dose every 12-18 hours
  - >2000 g: 30 mg/kg/day divided every 12 hours
- Postnatal age >7 days:
  - <1200 g: 15 mg/kg/day given every 24 hours
  - 1200-2000 g: 15 mg/kg/dose every 8-12 hours
  - >2000 g: 45 mg/kg/day divided every 8 hours

Infants >1 month and Children: 40 mg/kg/day in divided doses every 6 hours

Infants >1 month and Children with staphylococcal central nervous system infection: 60 mg/kg/day in divided doses every 6 hours; maximum: 1 g/dose

Adults: With normal renal function: 0.5 g every 6 hours or 1 g every 12 hours

Dosing interval in renal impairment:
- Cl_{cr} >90 mL/minute: Administer every 6 hours
- Cl_{cr} 70-89 mL/minute: Administer every 8 hours
- Cl_{cr} 46-69 mL/minute: Administer every 12 hours
- Cl_{cr} 30-45 mL/minute: Administer every 18 hours
- Cl_{cr} 15-29 mL/minute: Administer every 24 hours

Renal dysfunction, end stage renal disease, or on dialysis: 10-20 mg/kg; subsequent dosages and frequency of administration are best determined by measurement of serum levels and assessment of renal insufficiency

Intrathecal/intraventricular:
Neonates: 5-10 mg/day
Children: 5-20 mg/day
Adults: 20 mg/day

Oral:
Children: 40-50 mg/kg/day in divided doses every 6-8 hours; not to exceed 2 g/day
Adults: 0.5-2 g/day in divided doses every 6-8 hours

Administration Administer vancomycin by I.V. intermittent infusion over 60 minutes at a final concentration not to exceed 5 mg/mL; red man or red neck syndrome usually develops during a rapid infusion of vancomycin or with doses ≥15-20 mg/kg/hour; reaction usually dissipates in 30-60 minutes

Monitoring Parameters Periodic renal function tests, urinalysis, serum vancomycin concentrations, WBC, audiogram

Reference Range Peak: 25-40 μg/mL; Trough: 5-10 μg/mL

Patient Information Report pain at infusion site; dizziness, fullness or ringing in ears with I.V. use

Nursing Implications Do not administer I.M.; peak levels are drawn 1 hour after the completion of a 1-hour infusion; troughs are obtained just before the next dose; if a maculopapular rash appears on face, neck, trunk, and upper extremities, slow the infusion rate to over 1½ to 2 hours and increase the dilution volume; administration of antihistamines just before the infusion may also prevent or minimize this reaction

Dosage Forms

Capsule: 125 mg, 250 mg
Powder for oral solution: 1 g, 10 g
Powder for injection: 500 mg, 1 g, 2 g, 5 g, 10 g

References

American Academy of Pediatrics Committee on Infectious Diseases, "Treatment of Bacterial Meningitis," *Pediatrics*, 1988, 81(6):904-7.

Leonard MB, Koren G, Stevenson DK, et al, "Vancomycin Pharmacokinetics in Very Low Birth Weight Neonates," *Pediatr Infect Dis J*, 1989, 8(5):282-6.

Matzke GR, Zhanel GG, and Guay DRP, "Clinical Pharmacokinetics of Vancomycin," *Clin Pharmacokinet*, 1986, 11(4):257-82.

Rybak MJ, Albrecht LM, Boike SC, et al, "Nephrotoxicity of Vancomycin, Alone and With an Aminoglycoside," *J Antimicrob Chemother*, 1990, 25(4):679-87.

Vanoxide® [OTC] *see* Benzoyl Peroxide *on page 78*

Vantin® *see* Cefpodoxime Proxetil *on page 115*

Vaponefrin® *see* Epinephrine *on page 220*

Varicella-Zoster Immune Globulin (Human) *see* Immunization Guidelines *on page 660-667*

VasoClear® [OTC] *see* Naphazoline Hydrochloride *on page 403*

Vasocon Regular® *see* Naphazoline Hydrochloride *on page 403*

Vasopressin (vay soe press' in)

Brand Names Pitressin®

Synonyms ADH; Antidiuretic Hormone; 8-Arginine Vasopressin; Vasopressin Tannate

Therapeutic Category Antidiuretic Hormone Analog; Hormone, Posterior Pituitary

Use Treatment of diabetes insipidus; prevention and treatment of postoperative abdominal distention; differential diagnosis of diabetes insipidus; adjunct in the treatment of acute massive hemorrhage of GI tract or esophageal varices

Pregnancy Risk Factor B

Contraindications Hypersensitivity to vasopressin or any component; chronic nephritis with nitrogen retention

Precautions Use with caution in patients with seizure disorders, migraine, asthma, vascular disease, renal disease, cardiac disease, goiter with cardiac complications, arteriosclerosis

(Continued)

Vasopressin *(Continued)*

Adverse Reactions

Cardiovascular: Sweating, circumoral pallor; with high doses: hypertension, bradycardia, arrhythmias, venous thrombosis, vasoconstriction, angina, heart block

Central nervous system: Tremor, vertigo, fever, headache

Dermatologic: Urticaria

Endocrine & metabolic: Water intoxication

Gastrointestinal: Abdominal cramps, nausea, vomiting, flatus, diarrhea

Respiratory: Wheezing

Drug Interactions

Decreased antidiuretic activity: Lithium, demeclocycline, large doses of epinephrine, heparin (therapeutic doses), alcohol

Increased antidiuretic activity: Chlorpropamide, carbamazepine, tricyclic antidepressants, clofibrate, fludrocortisone

Mechanism of Action Increases cyclic adenosine monophosphate (cAMP) which increases water permeability at the distal convoluted tubule and collecting duct resulting in decreased urine volume and increased urine osmolality; causes peristalsis by directly stimulating the smooth muscle in the GI tract (in doses greater than those required for its antidiuretic action); causes vasoconstriction (primarily of capillaries and small arterioles)

Pharmacodynamics Duration of action: I.M., S.C.: 2-8 hours

Pharmacokinetics Destroyed by trypsin in GI tract, must be administered parenterally

Half-life: 10-20 minutes

Metabolism: Most of dose is rapidly metabolized in liver and kidney

Usual Dosage

Diabetes insipidus:

- I.M., S.C.: (Highly variable dosage; titrated based upon serum and urine sodium and osmolality in addition to fluid balance and urine output)
  - Children: 2.5-10 units 2-4 times/day
  - Adults: 5-10 units 2-4 times/day as needed (range: 5-60 units/day)
- Continuous infusion: Children and Adults: Initial: 0.5 milliunit/kg/hour (0.0005 unit/kg/hour); double dosage as needed every 30 minutes to a maximum of 10 milliunit/kg/hour

Abdominal distention: Adults: I.M.: 5 units initially, then repeated every 3-4 hours; dosage may be increased to 10 units if necessary

GI hemorrhage: I.V. continuous infusion (may also be infused directly into the superior mesenteric artery):

- Children: 0.01 units/kg/minute; continue at same dosage (if bleeding stops) for 12 hours, then taper off over 24-48 hours
- Adults: Initial: I.V.: 0.2-0.4 unit/minute, then titrate dose as needed; if bleeding stops, continue at same dose for 12 hours, taper off over 24-48 hours

Administration Dilute in normal saline or 5% dextrose to a final concentration of 0.1-1 unit/mL; see Usual Dosage for rate of infusion

Monitoring Parameters Fluid I & O, urine specific gravity, urine and serum osmolality, serum and urine sodium

Dosage Forms Injection, aqueous: 20 pressor units/mL (0.5 mL, 1 mL)

References

Tuggle DW, Bennett KG, Scott J, et al, "Intravenous Vasopressin and Gastrointestinal Hemorrhage in Children," *J Ped Surg,* 1988, 23:627-9.

Vasopressin Tannate *see* Vasopressin *on previous page*

Vasotec® *see* Enalapril/Enalaprilat *on page 219*

V-Cillin K® *see* Penicillin V Potassium *on page 442*

VCR *see* Vincristine Sulfate *on page 602*

Vecuronium Bromide (ve kyoo' roe ni um)

Brand Names Norcuron®

Synonyms ORG NC 45

Therapeutic Category Neuromuscular Blocker Agent, Nondepolarizing

Use Adjunct to anesthesia, to facilitate endotracheal intubation, and provide skeletal muscle relaxation during surgery or mechanical ventilation

Pregnancy Risk Factor C

Contraindications Known hypersensitivity to vecuronium

Warnings Ventilation must be supported during neuromuscular blockade; use only by individuals who are experienced in the maintenance of an adequate airway and respiratory support

Precautions Use with caution in patients with hepatic impairment, neuromuscular disease

Adverse Reactions

Dermatologic: Urticaria

Musculoskeletal: Skeletal muscle weakness

Respiratory: Respiratory insufficiency, bronchospasm, apnea

Drug Interactions Aminoglycosides, clindamycin, metronidazole, tetracyclines, polymyxins, piperacillin, mezlocillin, quinidine, magnesium sulfate (high dose), verapamil, enflurane, isoflurane

Stability Stable for 5 days at room temperature when reconstituted with bacteriostatic water; stable for 24 hours at room temperature when reconstituted with preservative free sterile water (avoid preservatives in neonates); do not mix with alkaline drugs; compatible with dextrose, normal saline, or lactated Ringer's

Mechanism of Action Nondepolarizing neuromuscular blocker which blocks acetylcholine from binding to receptors on motor endplate thus inhibiting depolarization

Pharmacodynamics

Onset of effects: After a single I.V. dose, neuromuscular blockade occurs within 1-3 minutes

Duration of effect (dose dependent): 30-40 minutes

Pharmacokinetics Elimination: Vecuronium bromide and its metabolite(s) appear to be excreted principally in feces via biliary elimination; the drug and its metabolite(s) are also excreted in urine; the rate of elimination is appreciably reduced with hepatic dysfunction but not with renal dysfunction

Usual Dosage I.V.:

Infants >7 weeks to 1 year: Initial: 0.08-0.1 mg/kg/dose; maintenance: 0.05-0.1 mg/kg/every hour as needed

Children >1 year and Adults: Initial: 0.08-0.1 mg/kg/dose; maintenance: 0.05-0.1 mg/kg/every hour as needed; may be administered as a continuous infusion at 0.1 mg/kg/hour

Note: Young children (1-9 years) may require slightly higher initial doses and slightly more frequent supplementation

Administration Dilute vial to a maximum concentration of 2 mg/mL and give by rapid direct injection; for continuous infusion, dilute to a maximum concentration of 1 mg/mL

Monitoring Parameters Assisted ventilation status, heart rate, blood pressure

Nursing Implications Does not alter the patient's state of consciousness; addition of sedation and analgesia are recommended

Additional Information Produces minimal, if any, histamine release

Dosage Forms Powder for injection: 10 mg (5 mL, 10 mL)

Veetids® *see* Penicillin V Potassium *on page 442*

Velban® *see* Vinblastine Sulfate *on page 601*

Velosulin® *see* Insulin Preparations *on page 311*

Velsar® *see* Vinblastine Sulfate *on page 601*

Veltane® *see* Brompheniramine Maleate *on page 88*

Venoglobulin®-I *see* Immune Globulin, Intravenous *on page 307*

Ventolin® *see* Albuterol *on page 26*

VePesid® *see* Etoposide *on page 237*

Verapamil Hydrochloride (ver ap' a mill)

Brand Names Calan®; Isoptin®; Verelan®

Synonyms Iproveratril Hydrochloride

Therapeutic Category Antianginal Agent; Antiarrhythmic Agent, Class IV; Antihypertensive; Calcium Channel Blocker

Use Angina, hypertension; I.V. for supraventricular tachyarrhythmias (PSVT, atrial fibrillation, atrial flutter)

(Continued)

Verapamil Hydrochloride *(Continued)*

Pregnancy Risk Factor C

Contraindications Sinus bradycardia; advanced heart block; ventricular tachycardia; cardiogenic shock; hypersensitivity to verapamil or any component; atrial fibrillation or flutter associated with accessory conduction pathways

Warnings Avoid I.V. use in neonates and young infants due to severe apnea, bradycardia, hypotensive reactions, and cardiac arrest; monitor EKG and blood pressure closely in patients receiving I.V. therapy, have I.V. calcium chloride 10 mg/kg available at bedside to treat hypotension

Precautions Sick-sinus syndrome, severe left ventricular dysfunction, hepatic or renal impairment, hypertrophic cardiomyopathy (especially obstructive), concomitant therapy with beta blockers or digoxin

Adverse Reactions

Cardiovascular: Hypotension, bradycardia, 1st, 2nd, or 3rd degree A-V block, worsening heart failure

Central nervous system: Dizziness, fatigue, seizures (occasionally with I.V. use), headache

Gastrointestinal: Constipation, nausea, abdominal discomfort

Hepatic: Increase in hepatic enzymes

Respiratory: May precipitate insufficiency of respiratory muscle function in Duchenne muscular dystrophy

Drug Interactions ↑ cardiovascular adverse effects with beta-adrenergic blocking agents, digoxin, quinidine, and disopyramide. Verapamil may increase serum concentrations of digoxin, quinidine, carbamazepine, and cyclosporine necessitating a decrease in dosage. Phenobarbital and rifampin may ↓ verapamil serum concentrations by ↑ hepatic metabolism. Avoid combination with disopyramide, discontinue disopyramide 48 hours before starting therapy, do not restart until 24 hours after verapamil has been discontinued.

Stability Store injection at room temperature; protect from heat and from freezing; use only clear solutions; compatible in solutions of pH of 3-6, but may precipitate in solutions having a pH of ≥6

Mechanism of Action Inhibits calcium ion from entering the "slow channels" or select voltage-sensitive areas of vascular smooth muscle and myocardium during depolarization; produces a relaxation of coronary vascular smooth muscle and coronary vasodilation; increases myocardial oxygen delivery in patients with vasospastic angina

Pharmacodynamics

Peak effects:
- Oral (nonsustained tablets): 2 hours
- I.V.: 1-5 minutes

Duration:
- Oral: 6-8 hours
- I.V.: 10-20 minutes

Pharmacokinetics

Protein binding: 90%

Metabolism: Metabolized in the liver, extensive first pass effect

Bioavailability: Oral: 20% to 30%

Half-life:
- Infants: 4.4-6.9 hours
- Adults (single dose): 2-8 hours, increased up to 12 hours with multiple dosing
- Increased half-life with hepatic cirrhosis

Elimination: 70% of a dose excreted in the urine (3% to 4% as unchanged drug), and 16% in the feces

Usual Dosage

Children: I.V.:
- <1 year: Not indicated
- 1-16 years: 0.1-0.3 mg/kg/dose over 2-3 minutes; maximum: 5 mg/dose; may repeat dose once in 30 minutes if adequate response not achieved; maximum for second dose: 10 mg/dose

Children: Oral (dose not well established):

4-8 mg/kg/day in 3 divided doses

or

1-5 years: 40-80 mg every 8 hours

>5 years: 80 mg every 6-8 hours

Adults:

Oral: 240-480 mg/24 hours divided 3-4 times/day

I.V. (1992 ACLS guidelines): PSVT (narrow complex, unresponsive to vagal maneuvers and adenosine): 2.5-5 mg; if no response in 15-30 minutes and no adverse effects seen, give 5-10 mg every 15-30 minutes to a maximum total dose of 20 mg

I.V.: 5-10 mg (0.075-0.15 mg/kg); may repeat 10 mg (0.15 mg/kg) 15-30 minutes after the initial dose if needed and if patient tolerated initial dose

I.V. continuous infusion (investigational): 0.005 mg/kg/minute

Children and Adults: Dosing adjustment in renal impairment: Cl_{cr} <10 mL/minute: Administer at 50% to 75% of normal dose

Administration Infuse I.V. dose over 2-3 minutes; infuse I.V. over 3-4 minutes if blood pressure is in the lower range of normal; I.V. push: Maximum concentration: 2.5 mg/mL

Monitoring Parameters EKG, blood pressure, heart rate

Nursing Implications Do not crush sustained release products

Additional Information I.V. administration, hypertrophic cardiomyopathy, sick sinus syndrome, moderate to severe congestive heart failure, concomitant therapy with beta blockers or digoxin can all increase incidence of adverse effects. Extended release products should be dosed 1-2 times/day.

Dosage Forms

Capsule, sustained release: 120 mg, 180 mg, 240 mg

Injection: 2.5 mg/mL (2 mL, 4 mL)

Tablet: 40 mg, 80 mg, 120 mg

Tablet, sustained release: 120 mg, 180 mg, 240 mg

References

Emergency Cardiac Care Committee and Subcommittees, American Heart Association, "Guidelines for Cardiopulmonary Resuscitation and Emergency Cardiac Care, III: Adult Advanced Cardiac Life Support" and "VI: Pediatric Advanced Life Support," *JAMA*, 1992, 268(16):2199-241 and 2262-75.

Sapire DW, O'Riordan AC, and Black IF, "Safety and Efficacy of Short- and Long-Term Verapamil Therapy in Children With Tachycardia," *Am J Cardiol*, 1981, 48(6):1091-7.

Shakibi JG, "Arrhythmias in Infants and Children," *Pediatrician*, 1981, 10(1-3):117-22.

Verelan® *see* Verapamil Hydrochloride *on page 597*

Vergon® [OTC] *see* Meclizine Hydrochloride *on page 358*

Vermox® *see* Mebendazole *on page 356*

Versed® *see* Midazolam Hydrochloride *on page 388*

Vertab® [OTC] *see* Dimenhydrinate *on page 193*

V-Gan® *see* Promethazine Hydrochloride *on page 488*

Vibramycin® *see* Doxycycline *on page 210*

Vibra-Tabs® *see* Doxycycline *on page 210*

Vicks® Sinex® Long-Acting Nasal Solution [OTC] *see* Oxymetazoline Hydrochloride *on page 429*

Vicks® Sinex® Nasal Solution [OTC] *see* Phenylephrine Hydrochloride *on page 453*

Vicodin® *see* Hydrocodone and Acetaminophen *on page 292*

Vidarabine (vye dare' a been)

Brand Names Vira-A®

Synonyms Adenine Arabinoside; Ara-A; Arabin of Uranosyladenine

Therapeutic Category Antiviral Agent, Ophthalmic; Antiviral Agent, Parenteral

Use Treatment of acute keratoconjunctivitis and epithelial keratitis due to herpes simplex virus; herpes simplex encephalitis; neonatal herpes simplex virus infections; disseminated varicella zoster in immunosuppressed patients

(Continued)

Vidarabine *(Continued)*

Pregnancy Risk Factor C

Contraindications Hypersensitivity to vidarabine or any component

Warnings Vidarabine is potentially mutagenic, teratogenic, and oncogenic

Precautions Vidarabine must be administered slow I.V. to neonates; administration requires dilution in large fluid volumes; use with caution in patients at risk of fluid overload (cerebral edema); and in patients with impaired renal or hepatic function; reduce dosage in patients with severe renal insufficiency

Adverse Reactions

Central nervous system: Weakness, ataxia, disorientation, depression, agitation, tremors
Dermatologic: Rash
Endocrine & metabolic: Hypokalemia, SIADH
Gastrointestinal: Anorexia, nausea, vomiting, diarrhea, weight loss
Hematologic: Decreased WBC and platelets
Hepatic: Increase in AST and total bilirubin
Local: Burning, lacrimation, pain, thrombophlebitis
Musculoskeletal: Myoclonus
Ocular: Keratitis, photophobia, foreign body sensation, uveitis, stromal edema, blurred vision

Drug Interactions Allopurinol (may ↑ vidarabine levels)

Stability Solutions should not be refrigerated

Mechanism of Action Inhibits viral DNA synthesis by blocking DNA polymerase

Pharmacokinetics

Absorption: Oral, I.M., S.C.: Poor
Distribution: Crosses into the CNS
Protein binding:
- Vidarabine: 20% to 30%
- Ara-hypoxanthine: 0% to 3%

Half-life:
- Infants: 2.4-3.1 hours
- Children: 2.8 hours
- Adults: 1.5 hours
- Ara-hypoxanthine: 3.3 hours with normal renal function

Elimination: Following administration, rapidly deaminated to ara-hypoxanthine (active) and excreted in the urine as unchanged drug (1% to 3%) and the active metabolite (40% to 53%)

Usual Dosage

Neonates: I.V.: Herpes simplex infection: 15-30 mg/kg/day once daily as an 18- to 24-hour infusion

Children and Adults:
- I.V.:
  - Herpes simplex encephalitis: 15 mg/kg/day once daily as a 12-hour or longer infusion for 10 days
  - Herpes zoster, varicella zoster infection: 10 mg/kg/day once daily as a 12-hour or longer infusion for 5-7 days
- Dosing adjustment in renal impairment: Cl_{cr} <10 mL/minute: Reduce dose by 25%
- Ophthalmic: Keratoconjunctivitis: ½" of ointment in lower conjunctival sac 5 times/day every 3 hours while awake until complete re-epithelialization has occurred, then twice daily for an additional 7 days

Administration Administer by I.V. infusion over 12 to 24 hours; vidarabine must be filtered with a 0.45 micron or smaller pore size inline filter; administer at a final concentration not to exceed 0.45 mg/mL to prevent precipitation. However, concentrations up to 0.7 mg/mL have been administered to fluid restricted patients.

Monitoring Parameters CBC with platelet count, renal function tests, liver function tests, hemoglobin, and hematocrit

Nursing Implications Rapid infusion may result in nausea and vomiting

Dosage Forms

Injection, suspension: 200 mg/mL [base 187.4 mg] (5 mL)
Ointment, ophthalmic, as monohydrate: 3% [base 2.8%] (3.5 g)

References

Whitley R, Arvin A, Prober C, et al, "A Controlled Trial Comparing Vidarabine

With Acyclovir in Neonatal Herpes Simplex Virus Infection. Infectious Diseases Collaborative Antiviral Study Group," *N Engl J Med*, 1991, 324(7):444-9.

Videx® *see* Didanosine *on page 188*

Vinblastine Sulfate (vin blas' teen)

Related Information

Emetogenic Potential of Single Chemotherapeutic Agents *on page 655*

Extravasation Treatment *on page 640*

Brand Names Alkaban-AQ®; Velban®; Velsar®

Synonyms Vincaleukoblastine; VLB

Therapeutic Category Antineoplastic Agent

Use Palliative treatment of Hodgkin's disease; advanced testicular germinal-cell cancers; non-Hodgkin's lymphoma, histiocytosis, and choriocarcinoma

Pregnancy Risk Factor D

Contraindications In patients with severe leukopenia

Warnings The US Food and Drug Administration (FDA) currently recommends that procedures for proper handling and disposal of antineoplastic agents be considered. For I.V. use only. **Intrathecal administration may result in death**.

Precautions Avoid extravasation; dosage modification required in patients with impaired liver function or neurotoxicity; dosage should be reduced in patients with recent exposure to radiation therapy or chemotherapy

Adverse Reactions

Cardiovascular: Tachycardia, orthostatic hypotension

Central nervous system: Paresthesias, peripheral neuropathy, depression, malaise, seizures, headache

Dermatologic: Rashes, mild alopecia, photosensitivity

Endocrine & metabolic: Hyperuricemia

Gastrointestinal: Nausea, hemorrhagic enterocolitis, vomiting, constipation, abdominal pain, paralytic ileus, stomatitis

Hematologic: Bone marrow depression

Local: Severe tissue burn if infiltrated

Musculoskeletal: Jaw pain, muscle pain

Renal & genitourinary: Urinary retention

Drug Interactions Concomitant administration with mitomycin has resulted in severe bronchospasm and shortness of breath

Stability Store in refrigerator; reconstituted solution is stable for 30 days when refrigerated and protected from light

Mechanism of Action Binds to microtubular protein of the mitotic spindle causing metaphase arrest

Pharmacokinetics

Distribution: Poor penetration into CSF; rapidly distributed into body tissues

Protein binding: 99%

Metabolism: Extensively metabolized in the liver to a more active metabolite

Half-life, terminal: 24 hours

Elimination: Biliary excretion (95%)

Usual Dosage Vinblastine can be given at intervals of every 7 days or greater and only after leukocyte count has returned to at least 4000/mm^3; maintenance therapy should be titrated according to leukocyte count.

I.V. (refer to individual protocols):

Children: 2.5-12.5 mg/m^2/day every 7-10 days

Hodgkin's disease, histiocytosis: 3.5-6 mg/m^2/day once weekly for 3-6 weeks

Adults: 3.7-18.5 mg/m^2/day every 7-10 days or 1.4-1.8 mg/m^2/day for 5 days given as an I.V. continuous infusion or 0.1-0.5 mg/kg/day once weekly

Children and Adults: Dosing adjustment in hepatic impairment: Direct serum bilirubin concentration >3 mg/dL: Reduce dose 50%

Administration May be administered IVP or into a free flowing I.V. over a 1-minute period at a concentration for administration of 1 mg/mL

Monitoring Parameters CBC with differential and platelet count, serum uric acid, hepatic function tests

(Continued)

Vinblastine Sulfate *(Continued)*

Patient Information Report to physician any fever, sore throat, bleeding, or bruising; avoid contact with the eyes since the drug is very irritating and corneal ulceration may result

Nursing Implications Maintain adequate hydration. Allopurinol may be given to prevent uric acid nephropathy; vinblastine is a tissue irritant and can cause sloughing upon extravasation; care should be taken to avoid extravasation. If extravasation occurs, hyaluronidase and a warm pack can be used for treatment.

Additional Information Myelosuppressive effects:

Onset (days): 4-7
Nadir (days): 10
Recovery (days): 17

Dosage Forms

Injection: 1 mg/mL (10 mL)
Powder for injection: 10 mg

References

Balis FM, Holcenberg JS and Bleyer WA, "Clinical Pharmacokinetics of Commonly Used Anticancer Drugs," *Clin Pharmacokinet*, 1983, 8(3):202-32.

Crom WR, Glynn-Barnhart AM, Rodman JH, et al, "Pharmacokinetics of Anticancer Drugs in Children," *Clin Pharmacokinet*, 1987, 12(3):168-213.

Tannock I, Ehrlichman C, Perrault D, et al, "Failure of 5-Day Vinblastine Infusion in the Treatment of Patients With Advanced Refractory Breast Cancer," *Cancer Treat Rep*, 1982, 66(9):1783-4.

Yap HY, Blumenschein GR, Keating MJ, et al, "Vinblastine Given as a Continuous 5-Day Infusion in the Treatment of Refractory Breast Cancer," *Cancer Treat Rep*, 1980, 64(2-3):279-83.

Vincaleukoblastine *see* Vinblastine Sulfate *on previous page*

Vincasar® PFS *see* Vincristine Sulfate *on this page*

Vincristine Sulfate (vin kris' teen)

Related Information

Emetogenic Potential of Single Chemotherapeutic Agents *on page 655*

Extravasation Treatment *on page 640*

Brand Names Oncovin®; Vincasar® PFS

Synonyms LCR; Leurocristine; VCR

Therapeutic Category Antineoplastic Agent

Use Treatment of leukemias, Hodgkin's disease, neuroblastoma, malignant lymphomas, Wilms' tumor, and rhabdomyosarcoma

Pregnancy Risk Factor D

Contraindications Hypersensitivity to vincristine or any component; patients with demyelinating form of Charcot-Marie-Tooth syndrome

Warnings The US Food and Drug Administration (FDA) currently recommends that procedures for proper handling and disposal of antineoplastic agents be considered. For I.V. use only; **intrathecal administration may result in death**

Precautions Dosage modification required in patients with impaired hepatic function, patients receiving other neurotoxic drugs, or patients with preexisting neuromuscular disease; avoid extravasation

Adverse Reactions

Cardiovascular: Orthostatic hypotension

Central nervous system: Neurotoxicity, numbness, weakness, seizures, CNS depression, cranial nerve paralysis

Dermatologic: Alopecia, rash

Endocrine & metabolic: Hyperuricemia, SIADH

Gastrointestinal: Constipation, paralytic ileus, nausea, vomiting, diarrhea, stomatitis

Local: Pain, cellulitis and tissue necrosis if infiltrated, phlebitis

Musculoskeletal: Jaw pain, leg pain, myalgias, cramping, motor difficulties

Respiratory: Dyspnea

Drug Interactions Asparaginase may ↓ vincristine clearance; acute pulmonary reactions may occur with concomitant use of mitomycin C

Stability Store in refrigerator; injectable solution is stable for 1 month at room temperature

Mechanism of Action Binds to microtubular protein of the mitotic spindle causing metaphase arrest

Pharmacokinetics

Distribution: Poor penetration into the CSF

Protein binding: 75%

Metabolism: Extensively metabolized in the liver

Half-life, terminal: 24 hours

Elimination: Excreted primarily in the bile (~80%)

Usual Dosage I.V. (refer to individual protocols):

Children ≤10 kg or BSA <1 m^2: Initial therapy: 0.05 mg/kg once weekly then titrate dose; maximum single dose: 2 mg

Children: 1-2 mg/m^2/week for 3-6 weeks; maximum single dose: 2 mg

Adults: 0.4-1.4 mg/m^2 up to 2 mg; may repeat every week

Children and Adults: Dosing adjustment in hepatic impairment: Direct serum bilirubin concentration >3 mg/dL: Dosage reduction of 50% is recommended

Administration Vincristine is administered IVP or into a free flowing I.V. over a period of 1 minute at a concentration for administration of 1 mg/mL

Monitoring Parameters Serum electrolytes (sodium), hepatic function tests, neurologic examination, CBC, hemoglobin, serum uric acid

Patient Information Stool softener should be used for constipation prophylaxis; report to physician any fever, sore throat, bleeding, bruising, or shortness of breath

Nursing Implications Maintain adequate hydration. Allopurinol may be given to prevent uric acid nephropathy; vincristine is a tissue irritant; care should be taken to avoid extravasation. If extravasation occurs, hyaluronidase and a warm pack can be used for treatment. Avoid contact with the eye since vincristine is very irritating.

Dosage Forms Injection: 1 mg/mL (1 mL, 2 mL, 5 mL)

References

Crom WR, Glynn-Barnhart AM, Rodman JH, et al, "Pharmacokinetics of Anticancer Drugs in Children," *Clin Pharmacokinet*, 1987, 12(3):168-213.

Vioform® [OTC] *see* Iodochlorhydroxyquin *on page 318*

Viokase® *see* Pancrelipase *on page 431*

Viosterol *see* Ergocalciferol *on page 224*

Vira-A® *see* Vidarabine *on page 599*

Virazole® *see* Ribavirin *on page 511*

Viroptic® *see* Trifluridine *on page 583*

Vistaril® *see* Hydroxyzine *on page 298*

Vistazine® *see* Hydroxyzine *on page 298*

Vita-C® [OTC] *see* Ascorbic Acid *on page 59*

Vitacarn® *see* Levocarnitine *on page 338*

Vitamin A (vye' ta min)

Brand Names Aquasol A® [OTC]

Synonyms Oleovitamin A

Therapeutic Category Vitamin, Fat Soluble

Use Treatment and prevention of vitamin A deficiency; supplementation in patients with measles

Pregnancy Risk Factor A (X if dose exceeds RDA recommendation)

Contraindications Hypervitaminosis A, hypersensitivity to vitamin A or any component

Warnings Patients receiving >25,000 units/day should be closely monitored for toxicity

Adverse Reactions Seen only with doses exceeding physiologic replacement

Central nervous system: Irritability, drowsiness, vertigo, delirium, headache, coma, increased intracranial pressure

(Continued)

Vitamin A *(Continued)*

Dermatologic: Erythema, peeling skin
Gastrointestinal: Vomiting, diarrhea
Ocular: Visual disturbances, papilledema

Drug Interactions Cholestyramine decreases absorption of vitamin A; neomycin and mineral oil may also interfere with vitamin A absorption; retinoids may have additive adverse effects, warfarin

Stability Protect injectable preparation from light

Mechanism of Action Needed for bone development, growth, visual adaptation to darkness, testicular and ovarian function, and as a cofactor in many biochemical processes

Pharmacokinetics

Absorption: Vitamin A in dosages **not** exceeding physiologic replacement is well absorbed after oral administration; water miscible preparations are absorbed more rapidly than oil preparations; large oral doses, conditions of fat malabsorption, low protein intake, or hepatic or pancreatic disease reduces oral absorption

Metabolism: Conjugated with glucuronide, undergoes enterohepatic circulation

Elimination: Excreted in feces via biliary elimination

Usual Dosage

Vitamin A supplementation in measles (recommendation of the World Health Organization): Children: Oral: Give as a single dose; repeat the next day and at 4 weeks for children with ophthalmologic evidence of vitamin A deficiency:

6 months to 1 year: 100,000 units
>1 year: 200,000 units

Note: Use of vitamin A in measles is recommended only for patients 6 months to 2 years of age hospitalized with measles and its complications **or** patients >6 months of age who have any of the following risk factors and who are not already receiving vitamin A: immunodeficiency, ophthalmologic evidence of vitamin A deficiency including night blindness, Bitot's spots or evidence of xeropthalmia, impaired intestinal absorption, moderate to severe malnutrition including that associated with eating disorders, or recent immigration from areas where high mortality rates from measles have been observed

Note: Monitor patients closely; dosages of >25,000 units/kg have been associated with toxicity

Vitamin A deficiency (varying recommendations available):

Severe deficiency with xerophthalmia:

Children 1-8 years: Oral: 5000 units/kg/day for 5 days or until recovery occurs; I.M.: 5000-15,000 units/day for 10 days

Children >8 years and Adults: Oral: 500,000 units/day for 3 days, then 50,000 units/day for 14 days; then 10,000-20,000 units/day for 2 months; I.M.: 50,000-100,000 units/day for 3 days; then 50,000 units/day for 14 days

Deficiency (without corneal changes):

Infants and Children: Initial: 100,000 units I.M. dosage once followed by oral intermittent therapy: Infants: 50,000 units once; <1 year: 100,000 units every 4-6 months; 1-8 years: 200,000 units every 4-6 months

Children >8 years and Adults: Oral: 100,000 units/day for 3 days followed by 50,000 units/day for 14 days

Prophylactic therapy for children at risk for developing deficiency: Oral given every 4-6 months:

Infants ≤1 year: 100,000 units
Children >1 year: 200,000 units

Malabsorption syndrome (prophylaxis): Children >8 years and Adults: Oral: 10,000-50,000 units/day of water miscible product

Daily dietary supplement: Oral:

Infants up to 6 months: 1500 units
Children:
6 months to 3 years: 1500-2000 units
4-6 years: 2500 units
7-10 years: 3300-3500 units

Children >10 years and Adults: 4000-5000 units

RDA:

<1 year: 375 μg*
1-3 years: 400 μg*
4-6 years: 500 μg*
7-10 years: 700 μg*
>10 years:
Females: 800 μg*
Males: 1000 μg*

*μg retinol equivalent (0.3 μg retinol = 1 unit vitamin A)

Dosage Forms

Capsule: 10,000 units, 25,000 units, 50,000 units
Drops, oral (water miscible): 5000 units/0.1 mL (30 mL)
Injection: 50,000 units/mL (2 mL)

References

Committee on Infectious Diseases, "Vitamin A in the Treatment of Measles," *Pediatrics*, 1993, 91(5):1014-5.

DeMaeyer EM, "The WHO Programme of Prevention and Control of Vitamin A Deficiency, Xerophthalmia, and Nutritional Blindness," *Nutr Health*, 1986, 4(2):105-12.

Hussey GD and Klein M, "A Randomized, Controlled Trial of Vitamin A in Children With Severe Measles," *N Engl J Med*, 1990, 323(3):160-4.

Vitamin A Acid *see* Tretinoin *on page 578*

Vitamin B_1 *see* Thiamine Hydrochloride *on page 559*

Vitamin B_2 *see* Riboflavin *on page 512*

Vitamin B_3 *see* Niacin *on page 411*

Vitamin B_6 *see* Pyridoxine Hydrochloride *on page 501*

Vitamin B_{12} *see* Cyanocobalamin *on page 160*

Vitamin C *see* Ascorbic Acid *on page 59*

Vitamin D_2 *see* Ergocalciferol *on page 224*

Vitamin E

Brand Names Aquasol E® [OTC]; Vitec® [OTC]

Synonyms *d*-Alpha Tocopherol; *dl*-Alpha Tocopherol

Therapeutic Category Vitamin, Fat Soluble; Vitamin, Topical

Use Prevention and treatment of vitamin E deficiency

Pregnancy Risk Factor A (C if dose exceeds RDA recommendation)

Warnings Necrotizing enterocolitis has been associated with oral administration of large dosages (eg, >200 units/day) of a hyperosmolar vitamin E preparation in low birth weight infants

Adverse Reactions

Central nervous system: Weakness, headache
Dermatologic: Rash
Endocrine & metabolic: Gonadal dysfunction; decreased serum thyroxine and tri-iodothyronine
Gastrointestinal: Nausea, diarrhea, intestinal cramps
Ocular: Blurred vision
Renal & genitourinary: Creatinuria and increased serum creatinine kinase; increased urinary estrogens and androgens
Hepatic: Increased cholesterol and triglycerides

Drug Interactions Iron, mineral oil, warfarin

Mechanism of Action Antioxidant which prevents oxidation of vitamin A and C; protects polyunsaturated fatty acids in membranes from attack by free radicals and protects red blood cells against hemolysis by oxidizing agents

Pharmacokinetics

Absorption: Oral: Depends upon the presence of bile; absorption is reduced in conditions of malabsorption, in low birth weight premature infants, and as dosage increases; water miscible preparations are better absorbed than oil preparations
Metabolism: Metabolized in liver to glucuronides
Elimination: Excreted primarily in the bile

(Continued)

Vitamin E *(Continued)*

Usual Dosage One unit of vitamin E = 1 mg *dl*-alpha-tocopherol acetate.

Oral:

Vitamin E deficiency:

Neonates, premature, low birthweight: 25-50 units/day results in normal levels within 1 week

Children (with malabsorption syndrome): 1 unit/kg/day of water miscible vitamin E (to raise plasma tocopherol concentrations to the normal range within 2 months and to maintain normal plasma concentrations)

Adults: 60-75 units/day

Prevention of vitamin E deficiency:

Neonates:

Low birthweight: 5 units/day

Full term: 5 units/L of formula ingested

Adults: 30 units/day

Prevention of retinopathy of prematurity or BPD secondary to O_2 therapy: (American Academy of Pediatrics considers this use investigational and routine use is not recommended):

Retinopathy prophylaxis: 15-30 units/kg/day to maintain plasma levels between 1.5-2 μg/mL (may need as high as 100 units/kg/day)

Cystic fibrosis, beta-thalassemia, sickle cell anemia may require higher daily maintenance doses:

Cystic fibrosis: 100-400 units/day

Beta-thalassemia: 750 units/day

Sickle cell: 450 units/day

Recommended daily allowance:

Premature infants ≤3 months: 17 mg (25 units)

Infants:

≤6 months: 3 mg (4.5 units)

6-12 months: 4 mg (6 units)

Children:

1-3 years: 6 mg (9 units)

4-10 years: 7 mg (10.5 units)

Children >11 years and Adults:

Females: 8 mg (12 units)

Males: 10 mg (15 units)

Topical: Apply a thin layer over affected area

Monitoring Parameters Plasma tocopherol concentrations (normal range: 6-14 μg/mL)

Dosage Forms

Capsule: 100 units, 200 units, 400 units, 500 units, 600 units, 1000 units

Capsule, water miscible: 73.5 mg, 147 mg, 165 mg, 330 mg, 400 units

Cream: 50 mg/g (15 g, 30 g, 60 g, 75 g, 120 g, 454 g)

Drops, oral: 50 mg/mL

Liquid, topical: 10 mL, 15 mL, 30 mL, 60 mL

Oil: 15 mL, 30 mL, 60 mL

Ointment, topical: 30 mg/g (45 g, 60 g)

Tablet: 200 units, 400 units

References

American Academy of Pediatrics Committee on Fetus and Newborn, "Vitamin E and the Prevention of Retinopathy of Prematurity," *Pediatrics*, 1985, 76(2):315-6.

Vitamin G *see* Riboflavin *on page 512*

Vitamin K_1 *see* Phytonadione *on page 458*

Vitec® [OTC] *see* Vitamin E *on previous page*

V-Lax® [OTC] *see* Psyllium *on page 498*

VLB *see* Vinblastine Sulfate *on page 601*

Voltaren® *see* Diclofenac Sodium *on page 185*

VP-16 *see* Etoposide *on page 237*

VP-16-213 *see* Etoposide *on page 237*

Warfarin Sodium (war' far in)

Related Information

Overdose and Toxicology Information *on page 696-700*

Brand Names Coumadin®; Panwarfin®; Sofarin®

Therapeutic Category Anticoagulant

Use Prophylaxis and treatment of thromboembolic disorders

Pregnancy Risk Factor D

Contraindications Hypersensitivity to warfarin or any component; severe liver or kidney disease; open wounds; uncontrolled bleeding; GI ulcers; neurosurgical procedures; malignant hypertension

Warnings Concomitant use with vitamin K may decrease anticoagulant effect; monitor carefully; concomitant use with ethacrynic acid, indomethacin, NSAIDs, phenylbutazone, or aspirin increases warfarin's anticoagulant effect and may cause severe GI irritation

Precautions Do not switch brands once desired therapeutic response has been achieved; use with caution in patients with active tuberculosis or diabetes

Adverse Reactions

Central nervous system: Fever
Dermatologic: Skin lesions, skin necrosis
Gastrointestinal: Anorexia, nausea, vomiting, diarrhea
Hematologic: Hemorrhage
Respiratory: Hemoptysis

Drug Interactions Alcohol, amiodarone, anabolic steroids, barbiturates, chloral hydrate, chloramphenicol, cholestyramine, cimetidine, clofibrate, disulfiram, ketoconazole, metronidazole, phenylbutazone, phenytoin, salicylates, streptokinase, sucralfate, sulfonamides, urokinase

Stability Protect from light

Mechanism of Action Interferes with hepatic synthesis of vitamin K-dependent coagulation factors (II, VII, IX, X)

Pharmacodynamics Anticoagulation effects:

Onset of action: Within 36-72 hours
Peak effect: Within 5-7 days

Pharmacokinetics

Absorption: Oral: Rapid
Metabolism: Metabolized in the liver
Half-life: 42 hours, highly variable among individuals

Usual Dosage Oral:

Infants and Children: 0.1 mg/kg/day with a range of 0.05-0.34 mg/kg/day; infants <12 months of age may require doses near the high end of this range; adjust dose to achieve the desired PT; consistent anticoagulation may be difficult to maintain in children <5 years of age

Adults: 5-15 mg/day for 2-5 days, then adjust dose according to results of prothrombin time; usual maintenance dose ranges from 2-10 mg/day

Monitoring Parameters Prothrombin, hematocrit, signs and symptoms of bleeding

Reference Range Therapeutic: 2-5 μg/mL (SI: 6.5-16.2 μmol/L); prothrombin time: should be $1\frac{1}{2}$ to 2 times the control or INR should be ↑ 2-3 times based upon indication

Nursing Implications Be aware of drug interactions and foods that contain vitamin K which can alter anticoagulant effects

Dosage Forms Tablet: 1 mg, 2 mg, 2.5 mg, 5 mg, 7.5 mg, 10 mg

4-Way® Long Acting Nasal Solution [OTC] *see* Oxymetazoline Hydrochloride *on page 429*

Wehamine® *see* Dimenhydrinate *on page 193*

Wellcovorin® *see* Leucovorin Calcium *on page 335*

Westcort® *see* Hydrocortisone *on page 293*

White Mineral Oil *see* Mineral Oil *on page 390*

Wigraine® *see* Ergotamine *on page 225*

Wyamycin® *see* Erythromycin *on page 226*

Wycillin® *see* Penicillin G Procaine *on page 441*

Wydase® *see* Hyaluronidase *on page 289*

Wygesic® *see* Propoxyphene and Acetaminophen *on page 492*

Wymox® *see* Amoxicillin *on page 44*

Xanax® *see* Alprazolam *on page 31*

Xerac™ BP [OTC] *see* Benzoyl Peroxide *on page 78*

X-Prep® Liquid [OTC] *see* Senna *on page 522*

Xylocaine® *see* Lidocaine Hydrochloride *on page 342*

Xylocaine® With Epinephrine *see* Lidocaine and Epinephrine *on page 340*

Yellow Fever Vaccine *see* Immunization Guidelines *on page 660-667*

Yodoxin® *see* Iodoquinol *on page 318*

Zantac® *see* Ranitidine Hydrochloride *on page 508*

Zarontin® *see* Ethosuximide *on page 235*

Zaroxolyn® *see* Metolazone *on page 382*

Zartan® *see* Cephalexin Monohydrate *on page 120*

Zeasorb-AF® [OTC] *see* Tolnaftate *on page 573*

Zeroxin® *see* Benzoyl Peroxide *on page 78*

Zetar® [OTC] *see* Coal Tar *on page 147*

Zetran® *see* Diazepam *on page 182*

Zidovudine (zye doe' vue deen)

Brand Names Retrovir®

Synonyms Azidothymidine; AZT; Compound S

Therapeutic Category Antiviral Agent, Oral; Antiviral Agent, Parenteral

Use Management of patients with HIV infections who have had at least one episode of *Pneumocystis carinii* pneumonia or who have CD4 cell counts of $\leq$500/mm^3; patients who have HIV related symptoms or who are asymptomatic with abnormal laboratory values indicating HIV related immunosuppression

Pregnancy Risk Factor C

Contraindications Life-threatening hypersensitivity to zidovudine or any component

Warnings Associated with hematologic toxicity including granulocytopenia and severe anemia requiring transfusions; zidovudine has been shown to be carcinogenic in rats and mice

Precautions Use with caution in patients with bone marrow compromise or in patients with impaired renal or hepatic function; reduce dosage or interrupt therapy in patients with anemia and/or granulocytopenia and myopathy

Adverse Reactions

Central nervous system: Malaise, dizziness, asthenia, manic syndrome, seizures, confusion tremor, fever, severe headache, insomnia

Dermatologic: Rash, pigmentation of nails (blue)

Gastrointestinal: Nausea, diarrhea, vomiting

Hematologic: Granulocytopenia, thrombocytopenia, leukopenia, anemia

Hepatic: Cholestatic hepatitis

Musculoskeletal: Myalgia

Drug Interactions Acyclovir, ganciclovir; coadministration with drugs that inhibit glucuronidation (acetaminophen, cimetidine, indomethacin, lorazepam, probenecid, aspirin) may ↑ toxicity of zidovudine

Mechanism of Action Zidovudine is a thymidine analog which interferes with the HIV viral RNA dependent DNA polymerase resulting in inhibition of viral replication

Pharmacokinetics

Absorption: Oral: Well absorbed (66% to 70%)

Distribution: Significant penetration into the CSF; crosses the placenta

Protein binding: 25% to 38%

Metabolism: Extensive first-pass metabolism; metabolized in the liver via glucuronidation to inactive metabolites

Half-life, terminal: 60 minutes

Peak serum levels: Within 30-90 minutes

Elimination: Urinary excretion (63% to 95%)

Oral: 72% to 74% of the drug is excreted in the urine as metabolites and 14% to 18% as unchanged drug

I.V.: 45% to 60% is excreted in the urine as metabolites and 18% to 29% as unchanged drug

Usual Dosage

Children 3 months to 12 years:

Oral: 90-180 mg/m^2/dose every 6 hours; maximum: 200 mg every 6 hours

I.V. continuous infusion: 0.5-1.8 mg/kg/hour

I.V. intermittent infusion: 100 mg/m^2/dose every 6 hours

Adults:

Oral:

Asymptomatic infection: 100 mg every 4 hours while awake (500 mg/day)

Symptomatic HIV infection: Initial: 200 mg every 4 hours (1200 mg/day), then after one month, 100 mg every 4 hours (600 mg/day)

I.V.: 1-2 mg/kg/dose every 4 hours

Administration Infuse I.V. zidovudine over 1 hour at a final concentration not to exceed 4 mg/mL in D_5W

Monitoring Parameters CBC with differential, hemoglobin, MCV, reticulocyte count, serum creatine kinase, CD4 cell count

Patient Information Take 30 minutes before or 1 hour after a meal with a glass of water; take zidovudine exactly as prescribed and administration every 4 hours means dosing around the clock

Nursing Implications Do not administer I.M.; do not administer I.V. push or by rapid infusion

Dosage Forms

Capsule: 100 mg

Injection: 10 mg/mL (20 mL)

Syrup (strawberry flavor): 50 mg/5 mL (240 mL)

References

Fischl MA, Richman DD, Hansen N, et al, "The Safety and Efficacy of Zidovudine (AZT) in the Treatment of Subjects With Mildly Symptomatic Human Immunodeficiency Virus Type 1 (HIV) Infection. A Double-Blind, Placebo-Controlled Trial. The AIDS Clinical Trials Group," *Ann Intern Med*, 1990, 112(10):727-37.

Mueller BU, Jacobsen F, Butler KM, et al, "Combination Treatment With Azidothymidine and Granulocyte Colony-Stimulating Factor in Children With Human Immunodeficiency Virus Infection," *J Pediatr*, 1992, 121(5 Pt 1):797-802.

Volberding PA, Lagakos SW, Koch MA, et al, "Zidovudine in Asymptomatic Human Immunodeficiency Virus Infection. A Controlled Trial in Persons With Fewer Than 500 CD4-Positive Cells per Cubic Millimeter. The AIDS Clinical Trials Group of the National Institute of Allergy and Infectious Diseases," *N Engl J Med*, 1990, 322(14):941-9.

Zinacef® *see* Cefuroxime *on page 118*

Zinc *see* Trace Metals *on page 574*

Zinca-Pak® *see* Trace Metals *on page 574*

Zinc Oxide

Synonyms Lassar's Zinc Paste

Therapeutic Category Topical Skin Product

Use Protective coating for mild skin irritations and abrasions; soothing and protective ointment to promote healing of chapped skin, diaper rash

Contraindications Hypersensitivity to any component

Stability Avoid prolonged storage at temperatures >30°C

Mechanism of Action Mild astringent with weak antiseptic properties

Usual Dosage Infants, Children, and Adults: Topical: Apply several times daily to affected area

Patient Information Paste is easily removed with mineral oil; for external use only; do not use in the eyes

Dosage Forms

Ointment, topical: 20% (30 g, 60 g, 454 g)

Paste, topical: 25% (in white petrolatum)

Zinc Undecylenate *see* Undecylenic Acid and Derivatives *on page 590*

Zithromax™ *see* Azithromycin *on page 70*

Zofran® *see* Ondansetron *on page 423*

Zolicef® *see* Cefazolin Sodium *on page 110*

ZORprin® *see* Aspirin *on page 61*

Zostrix® [OTC] *see* Capsaicin *on page 99*

Zostrix-HP® [OTC] *see* Capsaicin *on page 99*

Zovirax® *see* Acyclovir *on page 21*

Zydone® *see* Hydrocodone and Acetaminophen *on page 292*

Zyloprim® *see* Allopurinol *on page 30*

Zymase® *see* Pancrelipase *on page 431*

APPENDIX

HOTLINE PHONE NUMBERS

Car Seats	1-800-227-7233 (1-800-CAR-SAFE)
CDC Disease Information	1-404-639-1610
CDC Tuberculosis Section	1-404-639-2530
DSS 51-A	1-800-792-5200
Parental Stress	1-800-632-8188
WIC	1-800-942-1007 (1-800-WIC-1007)

CPR PEDIATRIC DRUG DOSAGES

Drug	Dose
Albumin 5%	5-10 mL/kg, may repeat in 15 minutes
Atropine 0.1 mg/mL	0.02 mg/kg every 5 minutes (minimum dose = 0.1 mg) Maximum single dose: Child: 0.5 mg, Adolescent: 1 mg Total maximum dose: Child: 1 mg, Adolescent: 2 mg May be administered via endotracheal tube. Dilute to 1-2 mL with normal saline prior to endotracheal administration.
Bretylium 50 mg/mL	1st dose: 5 mg/kg 2nd dose: 10 mg/kg every 15-30 minutes Maximum total dose: 30 mg/kg
Calcium chloride 100 mg/mL	0.2 mL/kg/dose every 10 minutes Role in resuscitation questionable, use only when hyperkalemia, hypermagnesemia, hypocalcemia, or calcium channel blocker toxicity is present
Dextrose 50% 0.5 g/mL	0.5 g/kg or (2 mL/kg of dextrose 25%) Dilute to a 25% solution before administration
Epinephrine injection 1:10,000 = 0.1 mg/mL 1:1000 = 1 mg/mL	Neonates: 0.01-0.03 mg/kg (0.1-0.3 mL/kg of **1:10,000** solution) every 3-5 minutes Consider 0.1-0.2 mg/kg by E.T. if no I.V. access and neonate did not respond to standard doses. Pediatric: **Bradycardia**: I.O., I.V.: 0.01 mg/kg (0.1 mL/kg of **1:10,000** solution) every 3-5 minutes E.T.: 0.1 mg/kg (0.1 mL/kg of **1:1000** solution) every 3-5 minutes **Asystolic or pulseless arrest**: Initial dose: I.O., I.V. 0.01 mg/kg (0.1 mL/kg of **1:10,000** solution) E.T.: 0.1 mg/kg (0.1 mL/kg of **1:1000** solution); doses as high as 0.2 mg/kg may be effective Subsequent doses: E.T., I.O., I.V.: 0.1 mg/kg (0.1 mL/kg of **1:1000** solution); doses as high as 0.2 mg/kg may be effective
Lidocaine 10 mg/mL	1 mg/kg loading dose, may repeat to a total dose not >3 mg/kg May be administered via endotracheal tube. Dilute to 1-2 mL with normal saline prior to endotracheal administration. I.V. infusion: 20-50 μg/kg/minute
Naloxone 0.4 mg/mL 1 mg/mL	Birth to 5 y or 20 kg: 0.1 mg/kg/dose >5 y or 20 kg: 2 mg/dose May repeat doses every 2-3 minutes May be administered via endotracheal tube. Dilute to 1-2 mL with normal saline prior to endotracheal administration.
Sodium bicarbonate 1 mEq/mL 0.5 mEq/mL	1 mEq/kg as a single dose, may repeat with 0.5 mEq/kg or calculate mEq = 0.3 x kg x base deficit; infuse slowly and only if ventilation is adequate Use only the 0.5 mEq/mL solution for neonates or dilute 1 mEq/mL solution 1:1 with sterile water for injection. $NaHCO_3$ should be used based on documented metabolic acidosis. Routine use in cardiac arrest is not recommended.

EMERGENCY PEDIATRIC DRIP CALCULATIONS

Drips

Drug	Dose	Calculation*	Rate & Dose
Dobutamine	5-20 μg/kg/min	6 x body wt (kg) is the mg added to make 100 mL	1 mL/h = 1 μg/kg/min
Dopamine	2-20 μg/kg/min	6 x body wt (kg) is the mg added to make 100 mL	1 mL/h = 1 μg/kg/min
Epinephrine	0.1-1 μg/kg/min	0.6 x body wt (kg) is the mg added to make 100 mL	1 mL/h = 0.1 μg/kg/min
Isoproterenol	0.1-1 μg/kg/min	0.6 x body wt (kg) is the mg added to make 100 mL	1 mL/h = 0.1 μg/kg/min
Lidocaine	20-50 μg/kg/min	120 mg in 100 mL of D_5W	1 mL/kg/h = 20 μg/kg/min

*Note: Patients ≥40 kg and those requiring fluid restriction may need more concentrated solutions in order to deliver less fluid per hour. In those cases, or as an alternative to the listed calculations above use the following equation:

$$\text{Rate (mL/h)} = \frac{\text{Dose } (\mu\text{g/kg/min}) \times \text{weight (kg)} \times 60 \text{ min/h}}{\text{concentration } (\mu\text{g/mL})}$$

Defibrillation/Cardioversion

	Indication/Remarks	Dose*
Pediatrics		
Defibrillation	V-fib or pulseless V-tach	2 joules/kg then repeat with 4 joules/kg thereafter
Synchronized cardioversion	May increase stepwise if needed	0.5 joules/kg
Adults		
Defibrillation	V-fib or pulseless V-tach or polymorphic V-tach	200 joules, then 200-300 joules, then 360 joules
Synchronized cardioversion		Initial**
	Atrial fibrillation	100 joules
	Atrial flutter	50 joules
	PSVT	50 joules
	monomorphic V-tach	100 joules

*1 joule = 1 watt • second.

**Increase stepwise if initial fails.

PEDIATRIC ALS ALGORITHM BRADYCARDIA

Fig. 1: Pediatric bradycardia decision tree. ABCs indicates airway, breathing, and circulation; ALS, advanced life support; ET, endotracheal; IO, intraosseous; and IV, intravenous.

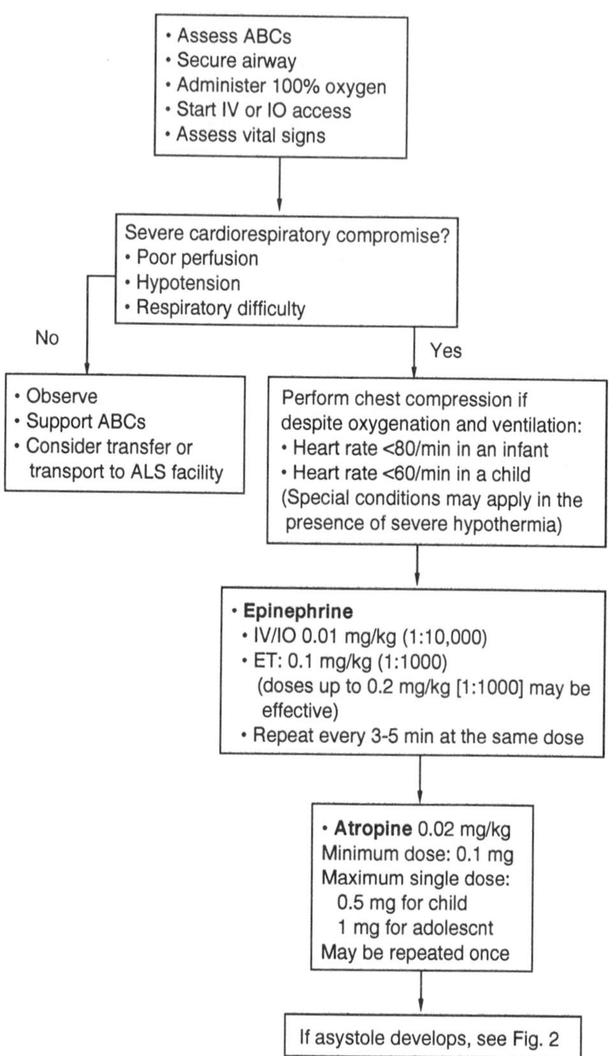

Used with permission: Emergency Cardiac Care Committee and Subcommittees, American Heart Association, "Guidelines for Cardiopulmonary Resuscitation and Emergency Care, IV: Pediatric Advanced Life Support," *JAMA*, 1992: 268:2262-75.

PEDIATRIC ALS ALGORITHM
ASYSTOLE AND PULSELESS ARREST

Fig. 2: Pediatric asystole and pulseless arrest decision tree. CPR indicates cardiopulmonary resuscitation; ET, endotracheal; IO, intraosseous; and IV, intravenous.

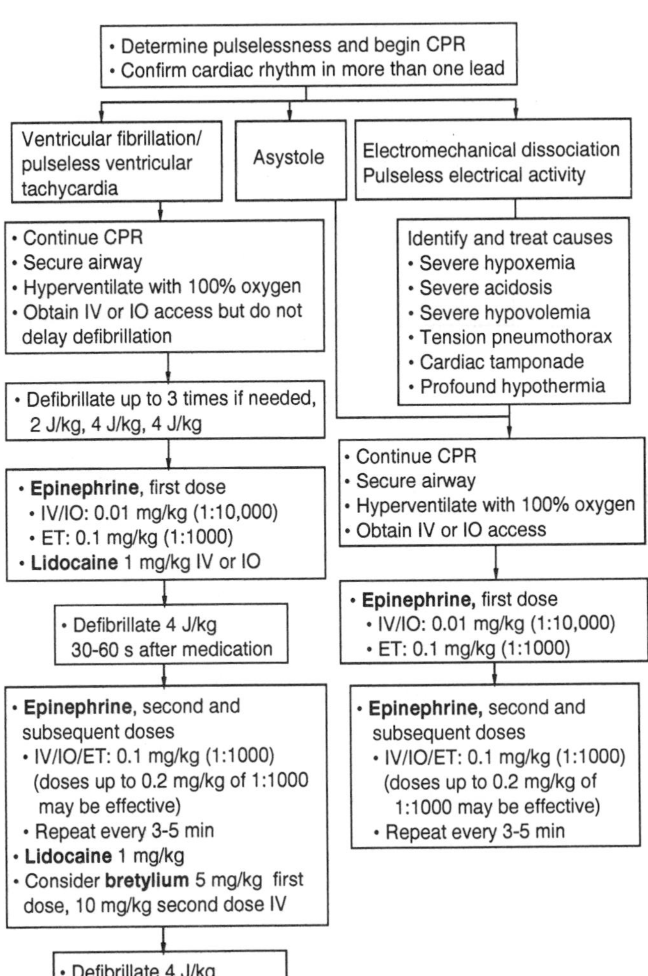

Used with permission: Emergency Cardiac Care Committee and Subcommittees, American Heart Association, "Guidelines for Cardiopulmonary Resuscitation and Emergency Care, IV: Pediatric Advanced Life Support," *JAMA*, 1992: 268:2262-75.

ADULT ACLS ALGORITHM
EMERGENCY CARDIAC CARE

Fig. 1: Universal algorithm for adult emergency cardiac care (ECC)

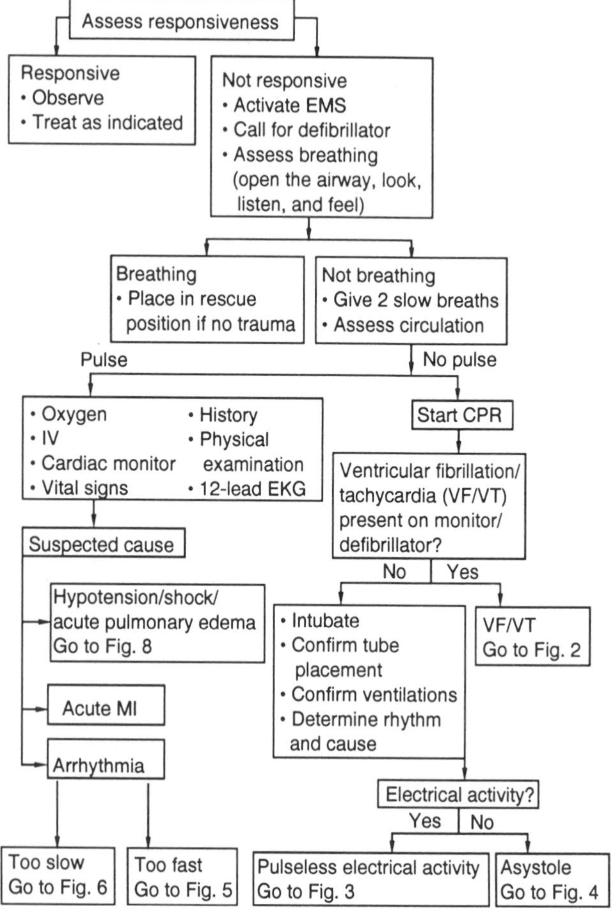

Used with permission: Emergency Cardiac Care Committee and Subcommittees, American Heart Association, "Guidelines for Cardiopulmonary Resuscitation and Emergency Care, III: Adult Advanced Cardiac Life Support," *JAMA*, 1992: 268:2199-2241.

ADULT ACLS ALGORITHM
V. FIB AND PULSELESS V. TACH

Fig. 2: Adult algorithm for ventricular fibrillation and pulseless ventricular tachycardia (VF/VT)

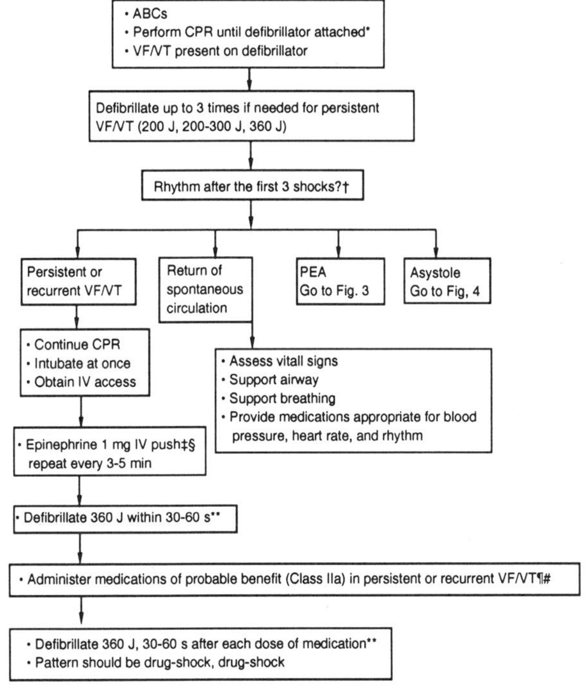

Class I: Definitely helpful
Class IIa: Acceptable, probably helpful
Class IIb: Acceptable, possibly helpful
Class III: Not indicated, may be harmful

*Precordial thump is a Class IIb action in witnessed arrest, no pulse, and no defibrillator immediately available.

†Hypothermic cardiac arrest is treated differently after this point.

‡The recommended dose of **epinephrine** is 1 mg IV push every 3-5 min. If this aproach fails, several Class IIb dosing regimens can be considered:
- Intermediate: **Epinephrine** 2-5 mg IV push, every 3-5 min
- Escalating: **Epinephrine** 1 mg-3 mg-5 mg IV push (3 min apart)
- High: **Epinephrine:** 0.1 mg/kg IV push, every 3-5 min

§**Sodium bicarbonate** (1 mEq/kg) is Class I if patient has known pre-existing hyperkalemia

**Multiple sequenced shocks (200J, 200-300 J, 360 J) are acceptable here (Class I), especially when medications are delayed

¶ •Lidocaine 1.5 mg/kg IV push. Repeat in 3-5 min to total loading dose of 3 mg/kg; then use
- **Bretylium** 5 mg/kg IV push. Repeat in 5 min at 10 mg/kg
- **Magnesium sulfate** 1-2 g IV in torsade de pointes or suspected hypomagnesemic state or severe refractory VF
- **Procainamide** 30 mg/min in refractory VF (maximum total: 17 mg/kg)

•**Sodium bicarbonate** (1 mEq/kg IV):

Class IIa
- If known pre-existing bicarbonate-responsive acidosis
- If overdose with tricyclic antidepressants
- To alkalinize the urine in drug overdoses

Class IIb
- If intubated and continued long arrest interval
- Upon reutrn of spontaneous circulation after long arrest interval

Class III
- Hypoxic lactic acidosis

Used with permission: Emergency Cardiac Care Committee and Subcommittees, American Heart Association, "Guidelines for Cardiopulmonary Resuscitation and Emergency Care, III: Adult Advanced Cardiac Life Support," *JAMA*, 1992: 268:2199-2241.

ADULT ACLS ALGORITHM PULSELESS ELECTRICAL ACTIVITY

Fig. 3: Adult algorithm for pulseless electrical activity (PEA) (electromechanical dissociation [EMD]).

PEA includes
- Electromechanical dissociation (EMD)
- Pseudo-EMD
- Idioventricular rhythms
- Ventricular escape rhythms
- Bradyasystolic rhythms
- Postdefibrillation idioventricular rhythms

- Continue CPR
- Intubate at once
- Obtain IV access
- Assess blood flow using Doppler ultrasound

↓

Consider possible causes
(Parentheses = possible therapies and treatments)
- Hypovolemia (volume infusion)
- Hypoxia (ventilation)
- Cardiac tamponade (pericardiocentesis)
- Tension pneumothorax (needle decompression)
- Hypothermia
- Massive pulmonary embolism (surgery, **thrombolytics**)
- Drug overdoses such as tricyclics, digitalis, beta blockers, calcium channel blockers
- Hyperkalemia*
- Acidosis†
- Massive acute myocardial infarction

↓

Epinephrine 1 mg IV push *‡ repeat every 3-5 min

↓

- If absolute bradycardia (<60 beats/min) or relative bradycardia, give **atropine** 1 mg IV
- Repeat every 3-5 min up to a total of 0.04 mg/kg§

Class I: Definitely helpful
Class IIa: Acceptable, probably helpful
Class IIb: Acceptable, possibly helpful
Class III: Not indicated, may be harmful

***Sodium bicarbonate** 1 mEq/kg is Class I if patient has known pre-existing hyperkalemia

†**Sodium bicarbonate** 1 mEq/kg:

Class IIa
- If known pre-existing bicarbonate-responsive acidosis
- If overdose with tricyclic antidepressants
- To alkalinize the urine in drug overdoses

Class IIb
- If intubated and long arrest interval
- Upon return of spontaneous circulation after long arrest interval

Class III
- Hypoxic lactic acidosis

‡The recommended dose of **epinephrine** is 1 mg IV push every 3-5 min. If this aproach fails, several Class IIb dosing regimens can be considered.
- Intermediate: **Epinephrine** 2-5 mg IV push, every 3-5 min
- Escalating: **Epinephrine** 1 mg-3 mg-5 mg IV push (3 min apart)
- High: **Epinephrine** 0.1 mg/kg IV push every 3-5 min

§Shorter atropine dosing intervals are possibly helpful in cardiac arrest (Class IIb)

ADULT ACLS ALGORITHM ASYSTOLE

Fig. 4: Adult asystole treatment algorithm.

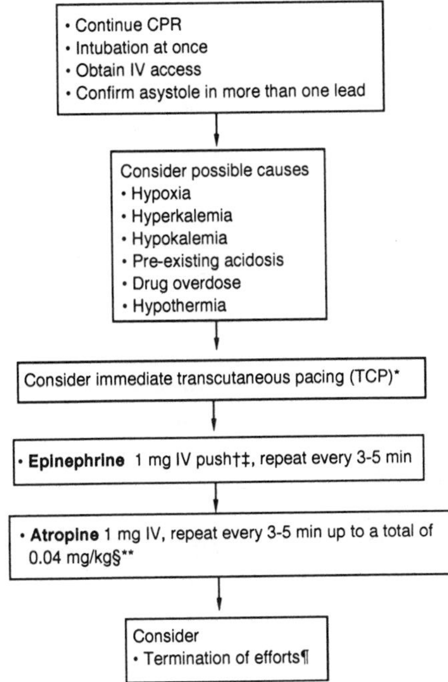

Class I: Definitely helpful
Class IIa: Acceptable, probably helpful
Class IIb: Acceptable, possibly helpful
Class III: Not indicated, may be harmful

* TCP is a Class IIb intervention. Lack of success may be due to delays in pacing. To be effective , TCP must be performed early, simultaneously with drugs. Evidence does not support routine use of TCP for asystole.

†The recommended dose of **epinephrine** is 1 mg IV push every 3-5 min. If this approach fails, several Class IIb dosing regimens can be considered:

- Intermediate: **Epinephrine** 2-5 mg IV push every 3-5 min
- Escalating: **Epinephrine** 1 mg-3 mg-5 mg IV push (3 min apart)
- High: **Epinephrine** 0.1 mg/kg IV push, every 3-5 min

‡**Sodium bicarbonate** 1 mEq/kg is Class I if patient has known pre-existing hyperkalemia.

§Shorter **atropine** dosing intervals are Class IIb in asystolic arrest.

****Sodium bicarbonate** 1 mEq/kg:

Class IIa
- If known pre-existing bicarbonate-responsive acidosis
- If overdose with tricyclic antidepressants
- To alkalinize the urine in drug overdoses

Class IIb
- If intubated and continued long arrest interval
- Upon return of spontaneous circulation after long arrest interval

Class III
- Hypoxic lactic acidosis

¶If patient remains in asystole or other agonal rhythms after successful intubation and initial medications and no reversible causes are identified, consider termination of resuscitative efforts by a physician. Consider interval since arrest.

Used with permission: Emergency Cardiac Care Committee and Subcommittees, American Heart Association, "Guidelines for Cardiopulmonary Resuscitation and Emergency Care, III: Adult Advanced Cardiac Life Support," *JAMA*, 1992: 268:2199-2241.

ADULT ACLS ALGORITHM TACHYCARDIA

Fig. 5: Adult tachycardia algorithm.

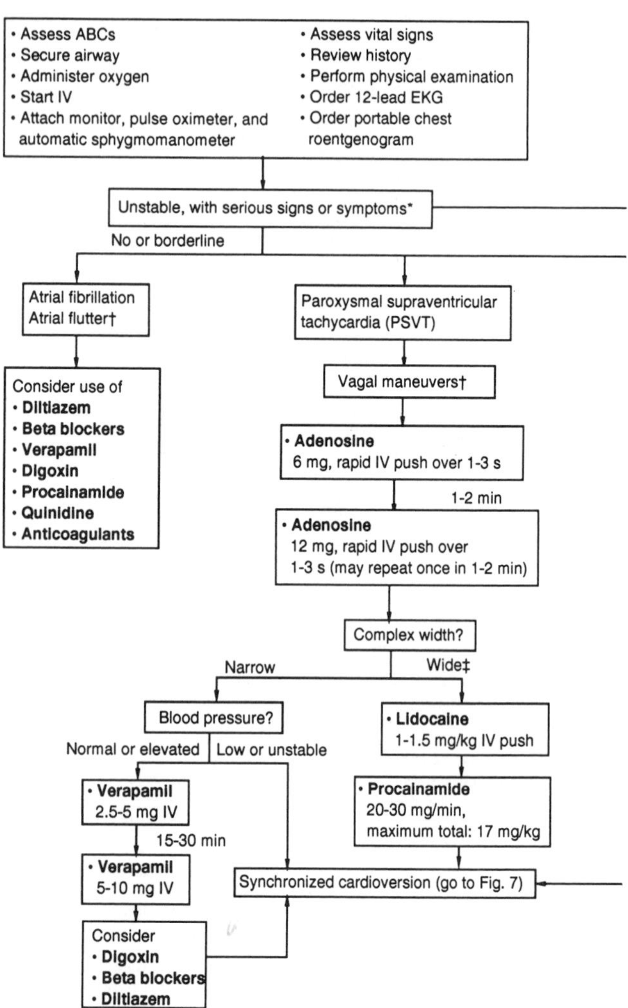

Used with permission: Emergency Cardiac Care Committee and Subcommittees, American Heart Association, "Guidelines for Cardiopulmonary Resuscitation and Emergency Care, III: Adult Advanced Cardiac Life Support," *JAMA*, 1992: 268:2199-2241.

ADULT ACLS ALGORITHM
TACHYCARDIA

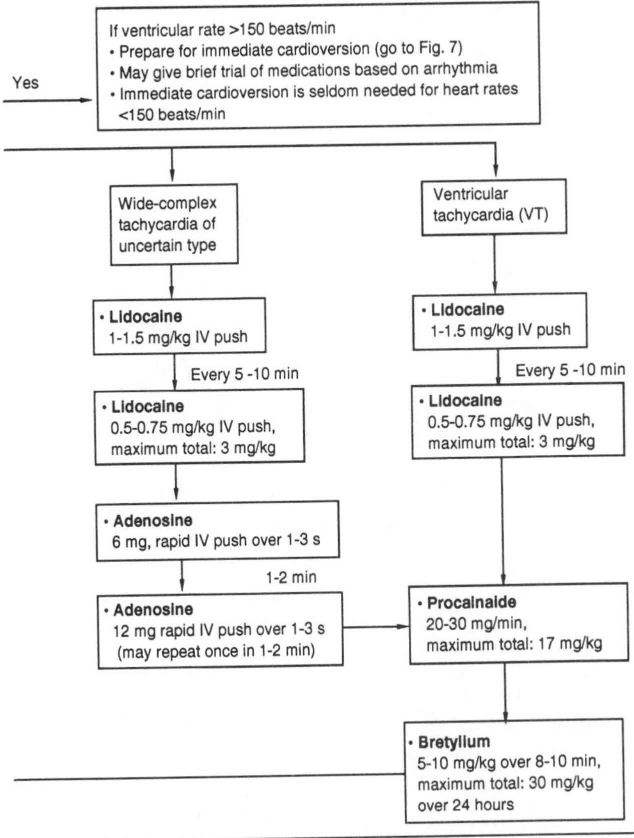

* Unstable condition must be related to the tachycardia. Signs and symptoms may include chest pain, shortness of breath, decreased level of consciousness, low blood pressure (BP), shock, pulmonary congestion, congestive heart failure, acute myocardial infarction.

† Carotid sinus pressure is contraindicated in patients with carotid bruits; avoid ice water immersion in patients with ischemic heart disease.

‡ If the wide-complex tachycardia is known with certainty to be PSVT and BP is normal/elevated, sequence can include **verapamil**.

ADULT ACLS ALGORITHM BRADYCARDIA

Fig. 6: Adult bradycardia algorithm (with the patient not in cardiac arrest).

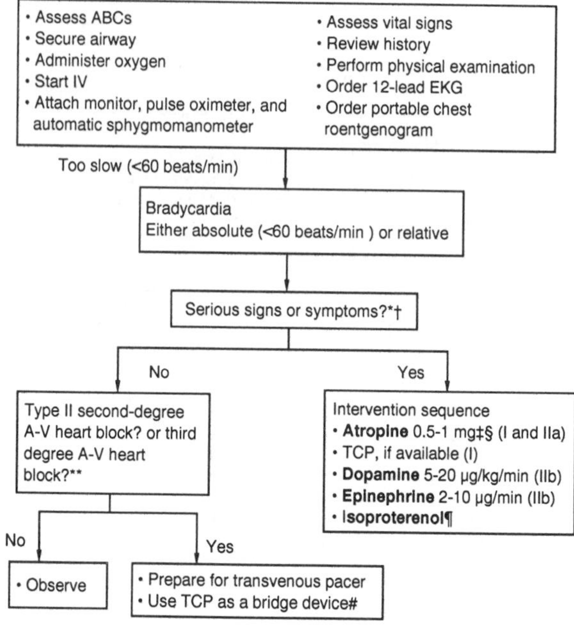

* Serious signs or symptoms must be related to the slow rate.
Clinical manifestations include:
Symptoms (chest pain, shortness of breath, decreased level of consciousness) and Signs (low BP, shock, pulmonary congestion, CHF, acute MI)

† Do not delay TCP while awaiting IV access or for **atropine** to take effect if patient is symptomatic.

‡ Denervated tranplanted hearts will not respond to **atropine**. Go at once to pacing, **catecholamine** infusion, or both.

§ **Atropine** should be given in repeat doses in 3-5 min up to a total of 0.04 mg/kg. Consider shorter dosing intervals in severe clinical conditions. It has been suggested that atropine should be used with caution in atrioventricular (A-V) block at the His-Purkinje level (type II A-V block and new third-degree block with wide QRS complexes) (Class IIb).

** Never treat third degree heart block plus ventricular escape beats with **lidocaine**.

¶ **Isoproterenol** should be used, if at all, with extreme caution. At low doses it is Class IIb (possibley helpful); at higher doses it is Class III (harmful).

Verify patient tolerance and mechanical capture. Use analgesia and sedation as needed.

Used with permission: Emergency Cardiac Care Committee and Subcommittees, American Heart Association, "Guidelines for Cardiopulmonary Resuscitation and Emergency Care, III: Adult Advanced Cardiac Life Support," *JAMA*, 1992: 268:2199-2241.

ADULT ACLS ALGORITHM ELECTRICAL CONVERSION

Fig. 7: Adult electrical cardioversion algorithm (with the patient not in cardiac arrest).

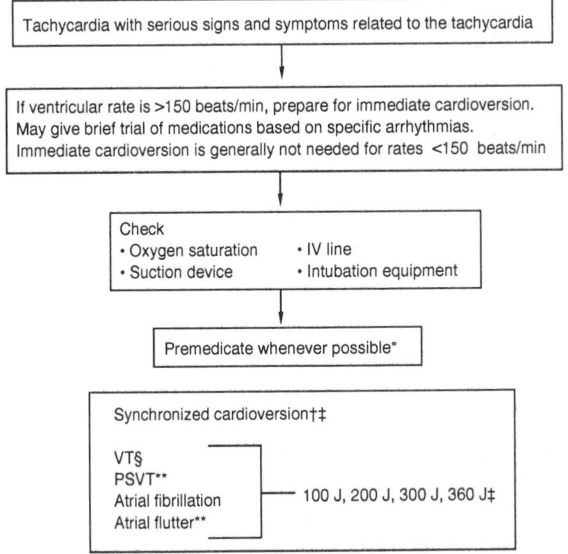

* Effective regimens have included a sedative (eg, **diazepam, midazolam barbiturates, etomidate, ketamine, methohexital**) with or without an analgesic agent (eg, **fentanyl, morphine, meperidine**). Many experts recommend anesthesia if service is readily available.

†Note possible need to resynchronize after each cardioversion.

‡If delays in synchronization occur and clinical conditions are critical, go to immediate unsynchronized shocks

§Treat polymorphic VT (irregular form and rate) like VF: 200 J, 200-300 J, 360 J

**PSVT and atrial flutter often respond to lower energy levels (start with 50 J)

Used with permission: Emergency Cardiac Care Committee and Subcommittees, American Heart Association, "Guidelines for Cardiopulmonary Resuscitation and Emergency Care, III: Adult Advanced Cardiac Life Support," *JAMA*, 1992: 268:2199-2241.

ADULT ACLS ALGORITHM HYPOTENSION, SHOCK

Fig. 8: Adult algorithm for hypotension, shock, and acute pulmonary edema.

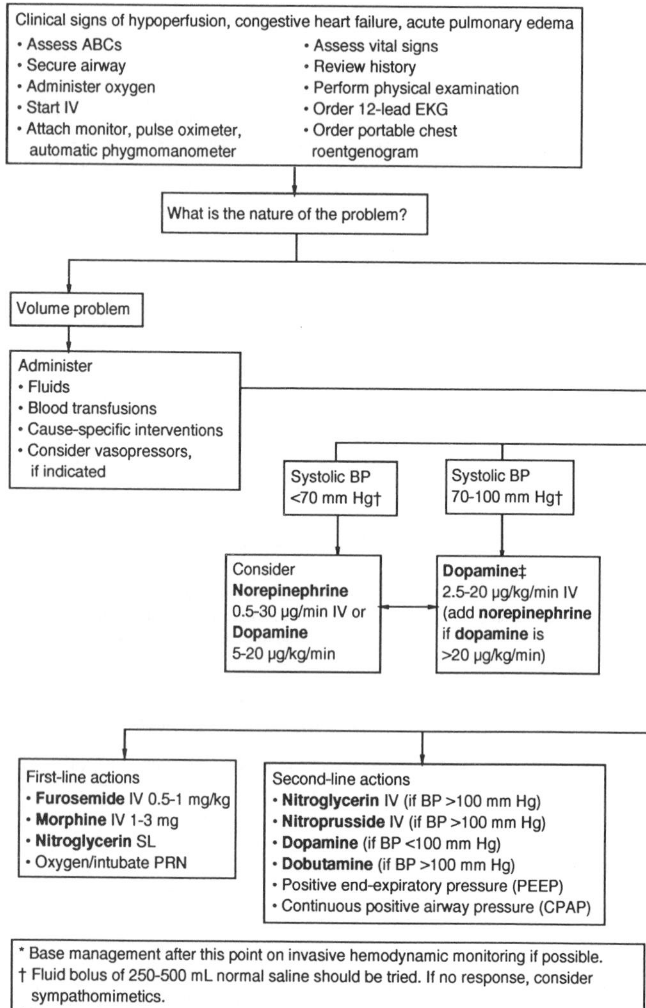

* Base management after this point on invasive hemodynamic monitoring if possible.
† Fluid bolus of 250-500 mL normal saline should be tried. If no response, consider sympathomimetics.
‡ Move to **dopamine** and stop **norepinephrine** when BP improves.
§ Add **dopamine** when BP improves. Avoid **dobutamine** when systolic BP <100 mm Hg.

Used with permission: Emergency Cardiac Care Committee and Subcommittees, American Heart Association, "Guidelines for Cardiopulmonary Resuscitation and Emergency Care, III: Adult Advanced Cardiac Life Support," *JAMA*, 1992: 268:2199-2241.

ADULT ACLS ALGORITHM
HYPOTENSION, SHOCK

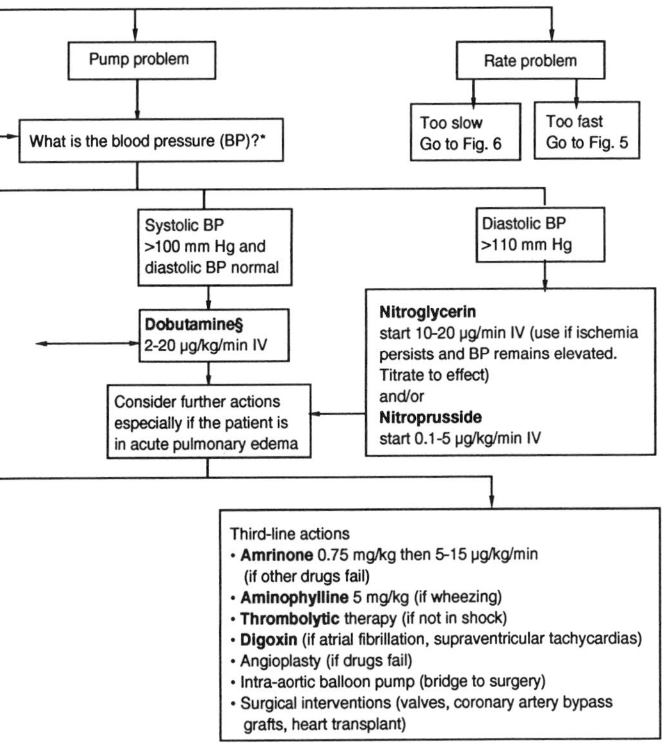

NORMAL HEART RATES

Age	Mean Heart Rate (beats/minute)	Heart Rate Range (2nd – 98th percentile)
<1 d	123	93-154
1-2 d	123	91-159
3-6 d	129	91-166
1-3 wk	148	107-182
1-2 mo	149	121-179
3-5 mo	141	106-186
6-11 mo	134	109-169
1-2 y	119	89-151
3-4 y	108	73-137
5-7 y	100	65-133
8-11 y	91	62-130
12-15 y	85	60-119

Adapted from *The Harriet Lane Handbook*, 12th ed, Greene MG, ed, St Louis, MO: Mosby Yearbook, 1991.

INTERVALS AND SEGMENTS OF AN EKG CYCLE

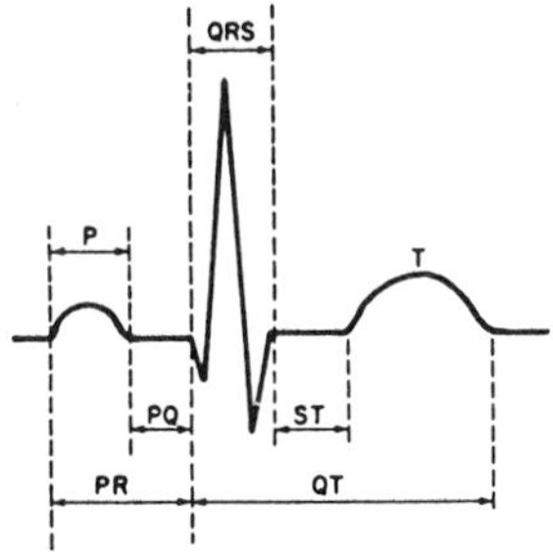

HEXAXIAL REFERENCE SYSTEM

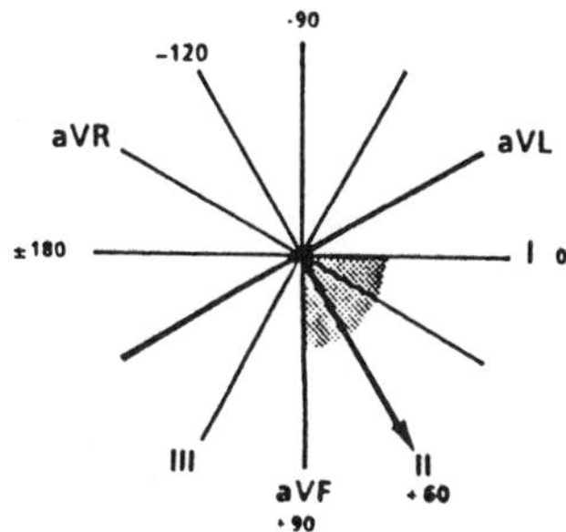

NORMAL QRS AXES (in degrees)

Age	Mean	Range
1 wk – 1 mo	+110	+30 to +180
1–3 mo	+ 70	+10 to +125
3 mo – 3 y	+ 60	+10 to +110
>3 y	+ 60	+20 to +120
Adults	+ 50	– 30 to +105

HYPERTENSION, CLASSIFICATION BY AGE GROUP

Age Group	Significant Hypertension (mm Hg)	Severe Hypertension (mm Hg)
Newborn (7 d)		
systolic BP	≥96	≥106
Newborn (8-30 d)		
systolic BP	≥104	≥110
Infant (<2 y)		
systolic BP	≥112	≥118
diastolic BP	≥74	≥82
Children (3-5 y)		
systolic BP	≥116	≥124
diastolic BP	≥76	≥84
Children (6-9 y)		
systolic BP	≥122	≥130
diastolic BP	≥78	≥86
Children (10-12 y)		
systolic BP	≥126	≥134
diastolic BP	≥82	≥90
Adolescents (13-15 y)		
systolic BP	≥136	≥144
diastolic BP	≥86	≥92
Adolescents (16-18 y)		
systolic BP	≥142	≥150
diastolic BP	≥92	≥98

Adapted from Horan MJ, *Pediatrics*, 1987, 79:1-25.

BLOOD PRESSURE IN PREMATURE INFANTS, NORMAL
(birth weight 600-1750 g)*

	600-999 g		1000-1249 g	
Day	S (± 2SD)	D (± 2SD)	S (± 2SD)	D (± 2SD)
1	37.9 (17.4)	23.2 (10.3)	44 (22.8)	22.5 (13.5)
3	44.9 (15.7)	30.6 (12.3)	48 (15.4)	36.5 (9.6)
7	50 (14.8)	30.4 (12.4)	57 (14)	42.5 (16.5)
14	50.2 (14.8)	37.4 (12)	53 (30)	
28	61 (23.5)	45.8 (27.4)	57 (30)	
	1250-1499 g		**1500-1750 g**	
Day	**S (± 2SD)**	**D (± 2SD)**	**S (± 2SD)**	**D (± 2SD)**
1	48 (18)	27 (12.4)	47 (15.8)	26 (15.6)
3	59 (21.1)	40 (13.7)	51 (18.2)	35 (10)
7	68 (14.8)	40 (11.3)	66 (23)	41 (24)
14	64 (21.2)	36 (24.2)	76 (34.8)	42 (20.3)
28	69 (31.4)	44 (26.2)	73 (5.6)	50 (9.9)

*Blood pressure was obtained by the Dinamap method.

S = systolic; D = diastolic; SD = standard deviation.

Modified from Ingelfinger JR, Powers L, and Epstein MF, "Blood Pressure Norms in Low-Weight Infants: Birth Through Four Weeks", *Pediatr Res*.

BLOOD PRESSURE MEASUREMENTS, AGE-SPECIFIC PERCENTILES

Blood Pressure Measurements: Ages 0-12 Months; Boys

Korotkoff phase IV (K4) used for diastolic BP. Reproduced with permission from Horan MJ, *Pediatrics*, 1987, 79:11-25.

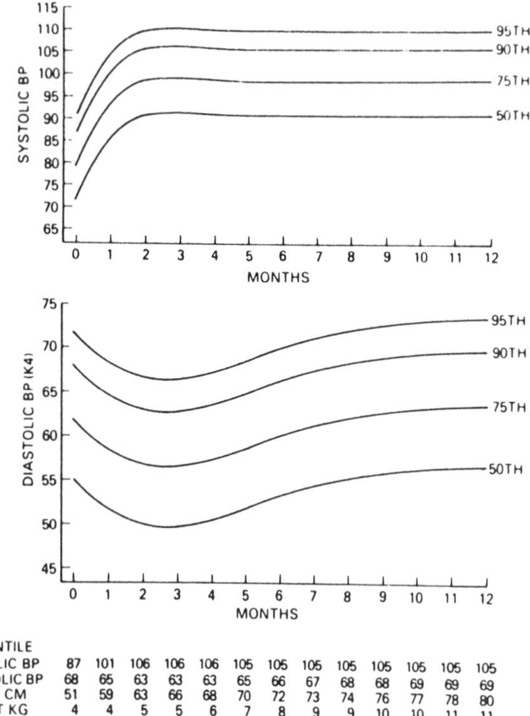

90TH PERCENTILE													
SYSTOLIC BP	87	101	106	106	106	105	105	105	105	105	105	105	105
DIASTOLIC BP	68	65	63	63	63	65	66	67	68	68	69	69	69
HEIGHT CM	51	59	63	66	68	70	72	73	74	76	77	78	80
WEIGHT KG	4	4	5	5	6	7	8	9	9	10	10	11	11

Blood Pressure Measurements: Ages 0-12 Months; Girls

Korotkoff phase IV (K4) used for diastolic BP. Reproduced with permission from Horan MJ, *Pediatrics*, 1987, 79:11-25.

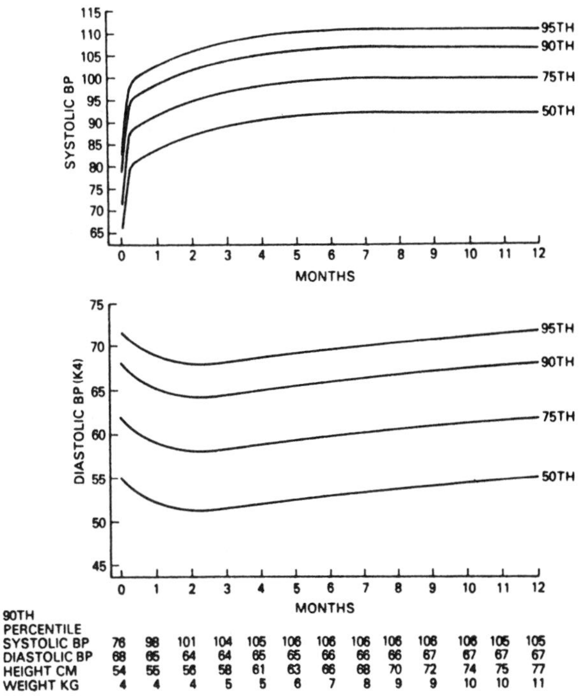

90TH PERCENTILE	0	1	2	3	4	5	6	7	8	9	10	11	12
SYSTOLIC BP	76	98	101	104	105	106	106	106	106	106	106	105	105
DIASTOLIC BP	68	65	64	64	65	65	66	66	66	67	67	67	67
HEIGHT CM	54	55	56	58	61	63	66	68	70	72	74	75	77
WEIGHT KG	4	4	4	5	5	6	7	8	9	9	10	10	11

Blood Pressure Measurements: Ages 1-13 Years; Boys

Korotkoff phase IV (K4) used for diastolic BP. Reproduced with permission from Horan MJ, *Pediatrics*, 1987, 79:11-15.

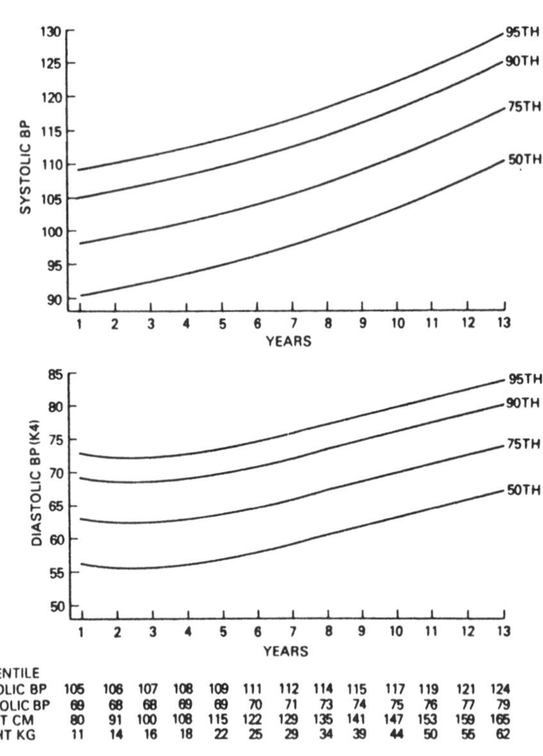

90TH PERCENTILE													
SYSTOLIC BP	105	106	107	108	109	111	112	114	115	117	119	121	124
DIASTOLIC BP	69	68	68	69	69	70	71	73	74	75	76	77	79
HEIGHT CM	80	91	100	108	115	122	129	135	141	147	153	159	165
WEIGHT KG	11	14	16	18	22	25	29	34	39	44	50	56	62

Blood Pressure Measurements: Ages 1-13 Years; Girls

Korotkoff phase IV (K4) used for diastolic BP. Reproduced with permission from Horan MJ, *Pediatrics*, 1987, 79:11-15.

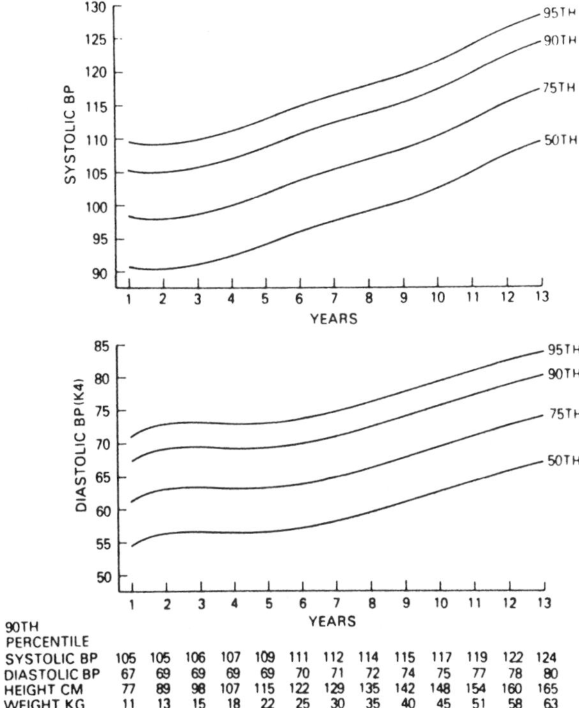

90TH PERCENTILE													
SYSTOLIC BP	105	105	106	107	109	111	112	114	115	117	119	122	124
DIASTOLIC BP	67	69	69	69	69	70	71	72	74	75	77	78	80
HEIGHT CM	77	89	98	107	115	122	129	135	142	148	154	160	165
WEIGHT KG	11	13	15	18	22	25	30	35	40	45	51	58	63

Blood Pressure Measurements: Ages 13-18 Years; Boys

Korotkoff phase IV (K4) used for diastolic BP. Reproduced with permission from Horan MJ, *Pediatrics*, 1987, 79:11-25.

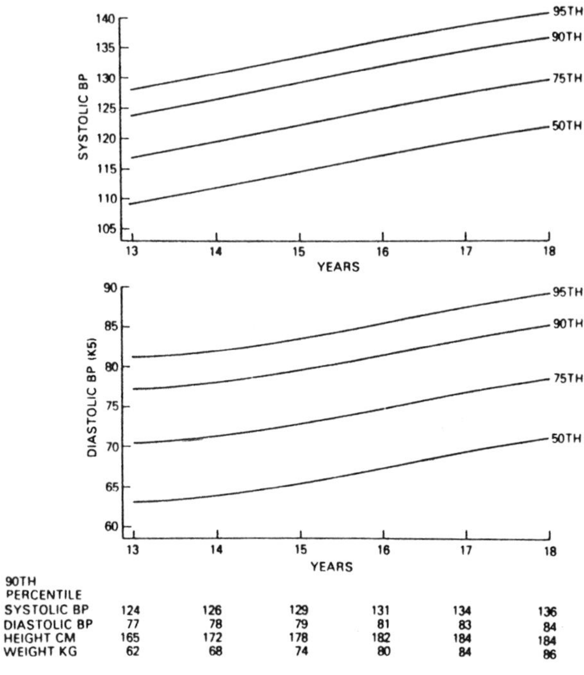

90TH PERCENTILE						
SYSTOLIC BP	124	126	129	131	134	136
DIASTOLIC BP	77	78	79	81	83	84
HEIGHT CM	165	172	178	182	184	184
WEIGHT KG	62	68	74	80	84	86

Blood Pressure Measurements: Ages 13-18 Years; Girls

Korotkoff phase IV (K4) used for diastolic BP. Reproduced with permission from Horan MJ, *Pediatrics*, 1987, 79:11-25.

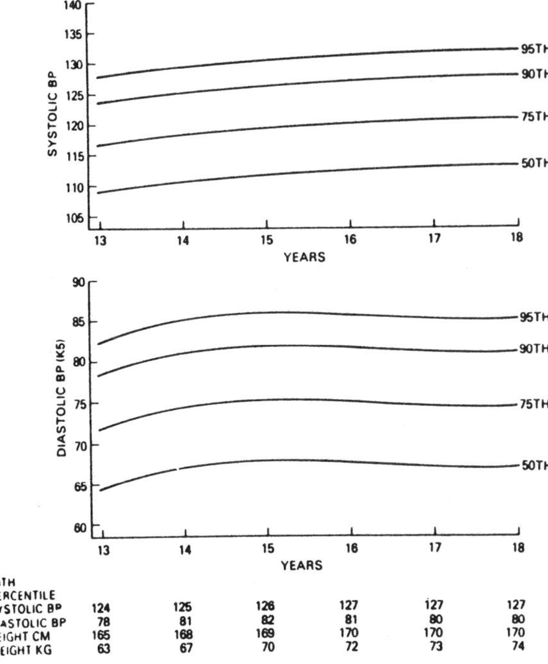

90TH PERCENTILE						
SYSTOLIC BP	124	125	126	127	127	127
DIASTOLIC BP	78	81	82	81	80	80
HEIGHT CM	165	168	169	170	170	170
WEIGHT KG	63	67	70	72	73	74

ANTIHYPERTENSIVE AGENTS BY CLASS

Alpha 2 Agonists
- Clonidine

Alpha 1 Antagonists
- Prazosin

Beta Antagonists
- Atenolol
- Esmolol
- Nadolol
- Propranolol

Mixed Alpha/Beta Antagonists
- Labetalol

Calcium Channel Blockers
- Diltiazem
- Nifedipine
- Verapamil

Angiotensin Converting Enzyme Inhibitors
- Captopril
- Enalapril/Enalaprilat
- Lisinopril

Nitrates
- Isosorbide dinitrate
- Nitroglycerin
- Nitroprusside

Ganglionic Blockers
- Trimethaphan

Diuretics
- Amiloride
- Bumetanide
- Chlorothiazide
- Ethacrynic acid
- Furosemide
- Hydrochlorothiazide
- Mannitol
- Metolazone
- Spironolactone
- Triamterene

Vasodilators (Direct-acting)
- Diazoxide
- Hydralazine
- Minoxidil

POUNDS-KILOGRAMS CONVERSION

1 pound = 0.45359 kilograms
1 kilogram = 2.2 pounds

TEMPERATURE CONVERSION

Celsius to Fahrenheit = (°C x 9/5) + 32 = °F
Fahrenheit to Celsius = (°F - 32) x 5/9 = °C

APOTHECARY-METRIC CONVERSION

Exact Equivalents

1 gram (g)	= 15.43 grains	0.1 mg	= 1/600 gr
1 milliliter (mL)	= 16.23 minims	0.12 mg	= 1/500 gr
1 minim (♍)	= 0.06 milliliter	0.15 mg	= 1/400 gr
1 grain (gr)	= 64.8 milligrams	0.2 mg	= 1/300 gr
1 ounce (℥)	= 31.1 grams	0.3 mg	= 1/200 gr
1 fluid ounce (fl℥)	= 29.57 mL	0.4 mg	= 1/150 gr
1 pint (pt)	= 473.2 mL	0.5 mg	= 1/120 gr
1 ounce (oz)	= 28.35 grams	0.6 mg	= 1/100 gr
1 pound (lb)	= 453.6 grams	0.8 mg	= 1/80 gr
1 kilogram (kg)	= 2.2 pounds	1 mg	= 1/65 gr
1 quart (qt)	= 946.4 mL		

Approximate Equivalents*

Liquids

1 teaspoonful	= 5 mL
1 tablespoonful	= 15 mL

Solids

¼ grain	= 15 mg
½ grain	= 30 mg
1 grain	= 60 mg
1½ grain	= 100 mg
5 grains	= 300 mg
10 grains	= 600 mg

*Use exact equivalents for compounding and calculations requiring a high degree of accuracy.

EXTRAVASATION TREATMENT

Medication Extravasated	Cold/Warm Pack	Antidote
Chemotherapeutic agents		
Anthracyclines Daunorubicin Doxorubicin	Cold	None
Vinca alkaloids Vinblastine Vincristine Vindesine	Warm	Hyaluronidase (Wydase®) 1. Add 1 mL NS to 150 units vial to make 150 units/mL concentration 2. Mix 0.1 mL of above with 0.9 mL NS in 1 mL syringe to make final concentration = 15 units/mL
Alkylating agents Mechlorethamine (Nitrogen mustard)	Cold	Sodium thiosulfate 1/6 molar solution: mix 4 mL of 10% sodium thiosulfate with 6 mL of sterile water
Other vesicant chemotherapeutic agents	Cold	None
Vasopressors		
Dobutamine Dopamine Epinephrine Norepinephrine Phenylephrine	None	Phentolamine (Regitine®) Mix 5 mg with 9 mL of NS Inject a small amount of this dilution into extravasated area. Blanching should reverse immediately. Monitor site. If blanching should recur, additional injections of phentolamine may be needed.
I.V. fluids and other medications		
Nafcillin Calcium	Cold	Hyaluronidase (Wydase®) 1. Add 1 mL NS to 150 units vial to make 150 units/mL concentration 2. Mix 0.1 mL of above with 0.9 mL NS in 1 mL syringe to make final concentration = 15 units/mL

BURN MANAGEMENT

Lund-Browder Chart of Body Surface Area for Estimation of Involvement (in %)

Age — Years

Area	0-1	1-4	4-9	10-15	Adult	Total
Head	19	17	13	10	—	
Neck	2	2	2	2	2	
Trunk	13	13	13	13	13	
Buttock (R/L)	2½	2½	2½	2½	2½	
Genitalia	1	1	1	1	1	
Upper arm (R/L)	4	4	4	4	4	
Lower arm (R/L)	3	3	3	3	3	
Hand (R/L)	2½	2½	2½	2½	2½	
Thigh (R/L)	5½	6½	8½	8½	9½	
Leg (R/L)	5	5	5	6	7	
Foot (R/L)	3½	3½	3½	3½	3½	

Total ______

Parkland Fluid Replacement Formula

A guideline for replacement of deficits and ongoing losses: (Note: For infants, maintenance fluids may need to be added to this): Administer 4 mL/kg/% burn of Ringer's lactate (glucose may be added but beware of stress hyperglycemia) over the first 24 hours; half of this total is given over the first 8 hours **calculated from the time of injury**; the remaining half is given over the next 16 hours. The second 24-hour fluid requirements average 50% to 75% of first day's requirement. Concentrations and rates best determined by monitoring weight, serum electrolytes, urine output, NG losses, etc.

Colloid may be added after 18-24 hours (1 g/kg/day of albumin) to maintain serum albumin >2 g/100 mL.

Potassium is generally withheld for the first 48 hours due to the large amount of potassium that is released from damaged tissues. To manage serum electrolytes, monitor urine electrolytes twice weekly and replace calculated urine losses.

PARENTERAL NUTRITION (PN)

The following information is intended as a brief overview of the use of parenteral nutrition in infants and children.

General Indications for Use

Parenteral nutrition is the provision of required nutrients by the intravenous route to replenish, optimize, or maintain nutritional status.

Specific Indications

Parenteral nutrition of **all** required nutrients (total parenteral nutrition) is indicated in patients for whom it is expected that it would be impossible or dangerous to enterally administer nutrition. Parenteral nutrition in combination with enteral nutrition is indicated in patients who are expected to be unable to meet their nutritional needs by the enteral route alone within 5 days.

1. Patients with an inability to absorb nutrients via the gastrointestinal tract which may include the following: severe diarrhea, short bowel syndrome, developmental anomalies of the GI tract, inflammatory bowel disease, cystic fibrosis, or anatomic or functional loss of GI integrity.
2. Severe malnutrition.
3. Severe catabolic states such as: burns, trauma or sepsis.
4. Patients undergoing high dose chemotherapy, radiation, and bone marrow transplantation.
5. Patients whose clinical condition may necessitate complete bowel rest, eg, necrotizing enterocolitis, pancreatitis, GI fistulas, or recent GI surgery.

Nutritional Assessment

As many as 33% of hospitalized pediatric patients are malnourished and require nutritional therapy. The type of nutritional support indicated depends on the underlying disease, the degree of gastrointestinal function, and the severity of malnutrition. Acutely malnourished patients have an increased risk for serious infection, postoperative complications, and death. Indicators of acute protein-calorie malnutrition include low weight for height, low serum albumin, lymphopenia, decreased body fat folds, and decreased arm muscle area. Nutritional screening may be done by the dietitian. Those patients who are at nutritional risk should receive a complete nutritional assessment.

Nutritional Requirements

Approximate requirements for energy and protein at various ages for normal subjects are listed in Table I at the end of this section. Patients who are severely malnourished or markedly catabolic may require higher levels to achieve catch-up growth or meet increased requirements. Patients who are well-nourished and inactive may require less.

During parenteral nutrition, 10% to 16% of calories should be in the form of amino acids to achieve optimal benefit (approximately 2-3 g/kg/day in infants and 1.5-2.5 g/kg/day ideal body weight in older patients). Exceptions include patients with renal or hepatic failure (where less protein is indicated), or in the treatment of severe trauma, head injury, or sepsis (where more protein may be indicated).

PN ORDERING

Fluid Intake

The patient should be given a total volume of fluid reasonable for his/her age and cardiovascular status. It is generally safe to start with the fluid maintenance level of 1500 mL/m^2/day in children. The fluid requirements in preterm infants are extremely variable due to much greater insensible water losses from radiant warmers and bili-lights. While the standard fluid maintenance of 100 mL/kg/day may be sufficient for term infants, intakes of 150-200 mL/kg/day may be necessary in the very low birth weight infants. Be sure to consider significant fluid intake from medications or other I.V. fluids and enteral diets in planning the fluids available for parenteral nutrition.

Dextrose

For central PN, dextrose is usually begun with a 10% to 12.5% solution or a solution providing dextrose at no more than 5 mg/kg/minute (in neonates and premature infants). The concentration is advanced, if tolerated, by 2.5% to 5% per day (2-2.5 mg/kg/minute increments in neonates and premature infants) to the desired caloric density, usually 20% to 25% dextrose. Fluid restricted patients often need 30% to 35% dextrose to meet their energy needs. For peripheral PN, 5% to 12.5% dextrose is utilized.

Amino Acids

Amino acids may be described as either a "standard" mixture of essential and nonessential amino acids or "specialized" mixtures. Specialized mixtures are intended for use in patients whose physiologic or metabolic needs may not be met with the "standard" amino acid compositions. Examples of specialized solutions include:

TrophAmine®, Aminosyn® PF	Indicated for use in premature infants and young children due to addition of taurine, L-glutamic acid, L-aspartic acid, increased amounts of tyrosine, and reduction in amounts of methionine, phenylalanine, and glycine. Supplementation with a cysteine additive has been recommended.
HepatAmine®	Indicated for treatment in patients with hepatic encephalopathy due to cirrhosis or hepatitis or in patients with liver disease who are intolerant of standard amino acid solutions
NephrAmine®, Aminosyn® RF	Indicated for use in patients with compromised renal function who are intolerant of standard amino acid solutions

Fat Emulsion

There are three roles for intravenous fat in parenteral nutrition:

1. to provide nonprotein calories
2. to provide essential fatty acids and a "balanced" calorie source
3. to provide calories in catabolic patients with limited ability to excrete CO_2

The potential side effects of bolus infusion of fat indicate the need for administration as a slow continuous drip. Neonates are usually started at 0.5-1 g/kg/day and increased to 2-3 g/kg/day as tolerated. Older infants, children and adolescents should receive 0.5-1 g/kg on day 1, 1-2 g/kg on day 2 and each day thereafter. The maximum fat intake is 4 g/kg/day and no more than 60% of the total daily caloric intake. It is given as a continuous drip over 24 hours or no greater than 0.15-0.2 g/kg/hour via a Y-connector with the dextrose-amino acid I.V. line. In patients receiving cyclic PN, the fat emulsion should be given over the duration of the PN infusion. Monitoring triglyceride levels should be drawn **during** lipid infusion. Triglyceride concentration should be checked before the first infusion and daily as the dose is increased. Subsequently, it should be monitored at least weekly. Concentrations should be kept below 150 mg/dL in neonates, below 350 mg/dL in renal patients, and below 250 mg/dL in other patients. Fats should be used cautiously in neonates with hyperbilirubinemia due to displacement of bilirubin from albumin by the free fatty acids. An increase in free bilirubin may increase the risk of kernicterus. Significant displacement occurs when the free fatty acid to serum albumin molar ratio (FFA/SA) >6. For example, infants with a total bilirubin >8-10 mg/dL (assuming an albumin concentration of 2.5-3 g/dL) should not receive more parenteral fat emulsion than required to meet the essential fatty acid requirement of 0.5-1 g/kg/day.

Note: Avoid use of 10% fat emulsion in preterm infants because a greater accumulation of plasma lipids occurs due to the greater phospholipid load of the 10% concentration.

MINERALS, TRACE ELEMENTS, AND VITAMINS

Guideline for Daily Electrolyte Requirements

	Infants-25 kg (mEq/kg)	25-45 kg (mEq/kg)	>45 kg
Sodium	2-6	2-6	60-150 mEq
Potassium	2-5	2-5	60-150 mEq
Calcium gluconate	1-2	1	0.2-0.3 mEq/kg
Magnesium	0.5	0.5	0.35-0.45 mEq/kg
Phosphate	0.5-1 mmol/kg	0.5-1 mmol/kg	7-10 mmol/1000 cal

Vitamins

A pediatric parenteral multivitamin product is indicated for children <11 years of age. Children >11 years of age may receive adult multivitamin formulations.

Trace Mineral Daily Requirements

	Infants	Children
Chromium*	0.2 μg/kg	0.2 μg/kg (max 5 μ)
Copper†	20 μg/kg	20 μg/kg (max 300 μg)
Manganese†,‡	1 μg/kg	1 μg/kg (max 50 μg)
Molybdenum*,§	0.25 μ/kg	0.25 μ/kg (max 5 μg)
Selenium*,§	2 μg/kg	2 μg/kg (max 30 μg)
Zinc	400 μg/kg (preterm) 250 μg/kg (term <3 mo) 100 μ/kg (term >3 mo)	50 μg/kg (max 5 μg)

These are recommended daily trace mineral requirements. Additional supplementation may be indicated in clinical conditions resulting in excessive losses. For example, additional zinc may be needed in situations of excessive gastrointestinal losses.

Developing the PN Goal Regimen

The purpose of this example is to illustrate the thought process in determining what dextrose and amino acid solution and fat emulsion intake would provide the desired daily fluid calorie and protein goals.

1. Calculate the fluid, protein and caloric goals.
   Example:

   Weight = 10 kg
   Fluids = 100 mL/kg/day = 1000 mL
   Calories = 100 cal/kg/day = 1000 cal
   Protein = 2.5 g/kg/day = 25 g

2. If fat emulsion (FE) comprises 40% to 60% of the total daily calories, using the above example: 40% of 1000 cal = 400 cal.

$$\frac{400 \text{ cal}}{2 \text{ cal/mL (20\% FE)}} = 200 \text{ mL}$$

*Omit in patients with renal dysfunction
†Omit in patients with obstructive jaundice
‡Current available commercial products are not in appropriate ratios to maintain this recommendation - doses of up to 10 μg/kg have been used safely.
§Indicated for use in long-term parenteral nutrition patients.

3. To determine the goal dextrose concentration calculate the total daily calories remaining.
Example:

1000 cal	(total daily calories)
− 400 cal	(daily calories from fats)
600 cal	(total daily calories remaining)

4. Determine the concentration of dextrose to achieve the total daily calories remaining.
Example:

$$\frac{600\text{ cal}}{3.5\text{ cal/g}} \times \frac{100}{800\text{ mL*}} = 22\%$$

*Total daily fluids desired minus that from fats.

5. Calculate percent amino acid solution to achieve goal protein intake.
Example:

$$\frac{25\text{ g (total protein)}}{800\text{ mL (total fluid)}} \times 100 = 3.1\%$$

This patient's goal regimen would be: dextrose 22%, amino acid 3.1%, 800 mL/day plus fat emulsion 20% 200 mL/day.

Monitoring Guidelines

Parameter	Frequency: Initial	Frequency: Maintenance
Body weight	Daily	Daily
Height	Weekly	Weekly
Triceps Skin Fold (TSF)/ Mid-arm Circumference (MAC)	PRN	PRN
Cal/pro intakes	Daily	PRN
Intake/output	Every 8 hours	Every 8 hours
Urine glucose	Every 4 hours	Every 8 hours
Urine sp gravity	Every 8 hours	Every 8 hours
Urine protein	Every 8 hours	Every 8 hours
Electrolytes	Daily	1-2 times weekly
Ca, Mg, PO_4	Daily	Weekly
BUN/Cr	Daily	Weekly
Serum glucose	Daily	Weekly
Albumin	Weekly	Weekly
Triglycerides	Daily	Weekly
Transferrin or prealbumin	Weekly	Weekly
Bilirubin, direct	Once	PRN (after a minimum of 2 weeks of PN)
Liver function tests	Once	PRN

Nutritional Guidelines for Pediatric Patients*

Age	kcal/kg/d	Protein g/kg/d
0-1 y	90-120	2.5-3
1-7 y	75-90	1.5-2.5
12 y	60-75	1.5-2.5
12-18 y	30-60	1-1.5

*Kerner JA, *Manual of Pediatric Parenteral Nutrition*, Wiley & Sons, Inc, 1983.

PN cal/mL*

Amino Acid Concentration	Dextrose Concentration						
	5%	10%	15%	20%	25%	30%	35%
1%	0.21	0.38	0.55	0.72	0.89	1.06	1.23
2%	0.25	0.42	0.59	0.76	0.93	1.10	1.27
2.5%	0.27	0.44	0.61	0.78	0.95	1.12	1.29
3%	0.29	0.46	0.63	0.80	0.97	1.14	1.31
4%	0.33	0.50	0.67	0.84	1.01	1.18	1.35
5%	0.37	0.54	0.71	0.88	1.05	1.22	1.39

Dextrose provides 3.4 cal/g.
Amino acids provide 4 cal/g.
Intralipid 10% provides 1.1 cal/mL.
Intralipid 20% provides 2 cal/mL.

*Includes carbohydrate and protein calories

Medications Compatible With PN Solutions (Amino Acid-Dextrose Solution and Fat Emulsion)

To be administered in D_5W or 0.9% sodium chloride via Y-connector to PN line:

Amikacin (not compatible with fat emulsions)
Aminophylline (not compatible with fat emulsions)
Carbenicillin
Cefazolin (Ancef®, Kefzol®, Zolicef®)
Cefotaxime (Claforan®)
Cefoxitin
Ceftazidime (Fortaz®, Tazicef®, Tazidime™)
Ceftriaxone
Cefuroxime (Kefurox®, Zinacef®)
Cephalothin
Cephapirin
Chloramphenicol
Cimetidine (Tagamet®)
Clindamycin (Cleocin Phosphate®)
Cyclophosphamide
Cytarabine
Digoxin (Lanoxin®)
Dobutamine (Dobutrex®)
Dopamine (Dopastat®, Intropin®)
Erythromycin
Foscarnet
Furosemide (Lasix®)
Gentamicin (Garamycin®)*
Heparin
Hydrocortisone sodium succinate (A-hydroCort®, Solu-Cortef®)
Insulin
Isoproterenol
Kanamycin
Lidocaine
Meperidine (Demerol®)
Methicillin (Staphcillin®)
Methylprednisolone sodium succinate (Solu-Medrol®)
Metoclopramide (Reglan®)
Mezlocillin
Miconazole
Morphine sulfate
Nafcillin
Netilmicin
Oxacillin (Prostaphlin®)
Penicillin G
Piperacillin (Pipracil®)
Ranitidine (Zantac®)
Ticarcillin (Ticar®)
Tobramycin (Nebcin®)*
Vancomycin (Vancocin®)*

*Not compatible with amino acid-dextrose solutions containing >0.5 units/mL of heparin.

Reference: Trissel LA, "Handbook on Injectable Drugs," *ASHP*, 7th ed, 1992.

Pharmacologic considerations of mixing medications with PN solutions include:

- Adsorption — bag, bottle, tubing, filter
- Blood levels
- Site of injection/administration
- Flush
- Amino acid-dextrose concentrations
- pH factors
- Temperature
- Additives in solution
- Heparin dose

IDEAL BODY WEIGHT CALCULATION

Adults (18 years and older)

IBW (male) = 50 + (2.3 x height in inches over 5 feet)
IBW (female) = 45.5 + (2.3 x height in inches over 5 feet)

*IBW is in kg.

Children

a. 1-18 years

$$\text{IBW} = \frac{(\text{height}^2 \times 1.65)}{1000}$$

*IBW is in kg.
Height is in cm.

b. 5 feet and taller

IBW (male) = 39 + (2.27 x height in inches over 5 feet)
IBW (female) = 42.2 + (2.27 x height in inches over 5 feet)

*IBW is in kg.

Reference: Traub SL and Johnson CE, "Comparison of Methods of Estimating Creatinine Clearance in Children," *Amer J Hosp Pharm*, 1980, 37:195-201.

BODY SURFACE AREA OF ADULTS AND CHILDREN

Calculating Body Surface Area in Children

In a child of average size, find weight and corresponding surface area on the boxed scale to the left. Or, use the nomogram to the right. Lay a straightedge on the correct height and weight points for the child, then read the intersecting point on the surface area scale.

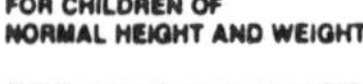

Weight (lb): 90, 80, 70, 60, 50, 40, 30, 20, 15, 10, 9, 8, 7, 6, 5, 4, 3, 2

Surface area (m²): 1.30, 1.20, 1.10, 1.00, .90, .80, .70, .60, .55, .50, .45, .40, .35, .30, .25, .20, .15, .10

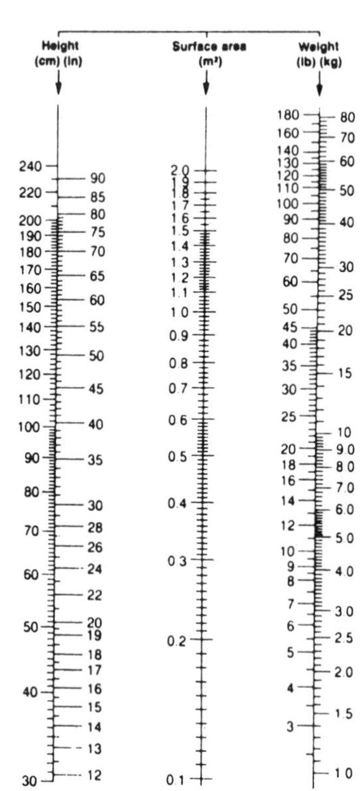

BODY-SURFACE AREA FORMULA
(Adult and Pediatric)

$$\text{BSA (m}^2\text{)} = \sqrt{\frac{\text{Ht (in)} \times \text{Wt (lb)}}{3131}}$$

or, in metric:

$$\text{BSA (m}^2\text{)} = \sqrt{\frac{\text{Ht (cm)} \times \text{Wt (kg)}}{3600}}$$

AVERAGE WEIGHTS AND SURFACE AREAS

Average Weight and Surface Area of Preterm Infants, Term Infants and Children

Age	Average Weight (kg)*	Approximate Surface Area (m^2)
Weeks Gestation		
26	0.9-1	0.1
30	1.3-1.5	0.12
32	1.6-2	0.15
38	2.9-3	0.2
40 (term infant at birth)	3.1-4	0.25
Months		
3	5	0.29
6	7	0.38
9	8	0.42
Year		
1	10	0.49
2	12	0.55
3	15	0.64
4	17	0.74
5	18	0.76
6	20	0.82
7	23	0.90
8	25	0.95
9	28	1.06
10	33	1.18
11	35	1.23
12	40	1.34
Adult	70	1.73

*Weights from age 3 months and over are rounded off to the nearest kilogram.

PHYSICAL DEVELOPMENT

Weight gain
First 6 weeks
20 g/day

Birth weight
regained by day 14
doubles by age 4 mo
triples by age 12 mo
quadruples by age 2 y

Length
increases 50% by age 1 y
doubles by age 4 y
triples by age 13 y

Head circumference
35 cm at birth
44 cm by 6 mo
47 cm by 1 y
1 cm/mo for 1st y
0.3 cm/mo 2nd y

Teeth
1st tooth 6-18 mo
teeth = age (in mo) − 6
(until 30 months)

Tanner Stages of Sexual Development

Stage	Characteristics	Age at onset (mean ± SD)
Genital stages: male		
1	Prepubertal	
2	Scrotum and testes enlarge; skin of scrotum reddens and rugations appear	11.4±1.1 y
3	Penis lengthens; testes enlarge further	12.9±1 y
4	Penis growth continues in length and width; glans develops adult form	13.8±1 y
5	Development completed; adult appearance	14.9±1.1 y
Breast development: female		
1	Prepubertal	
2	Breast buds appear; areolae enlarge	11.2±1.1 y
3	Elevation of breast contour; areolae enlarge	12.2±1.1 y
4	Areolae and papilla form a secondary mound on breast	13.1±1.2 y
5	Adult form	15.3±1.7 y
Menarche		
Pubic hair: both sexes		13.5±1 y
1	Prepubertal, no coarse hair	
2	Longer, silky hair appears at base of penis or along labia	F: 11.7±1.2 y M: 12±1 y
3	Hair coarse, kinky, spreads over pubic bone	F: 12.4±1.1 y M: 13.9±1 y
4	Hair of adult quality but not spread to junction of medial thigh with perineum	F: 13±1 y M: 14.4±1.1 y
5	Spread to medial thigh	F: 14.4±1.1 y M: 15.2±1.1 y
6	"Male escutcheon"	Variable if occurs

Maximum growth rate
Males at 14.1±0.9 y
Females at 12.1±0.9 y

EMETOGENIC POTENTIAL OF SINGLE CHEMOTHERAPEUTIC AGENTS

Class I
Low (<10%)

Chlorambucil
Cyclophosphamide (oral)
Busulfan
Thioguanine (oral)
Thiotepa
Vincristine sulfate

Class II
Moderately Low (10% to 30%)

Bleomycin sulfate
Cytarabine hydrochloride ≤20 mg
Doxorubicin hydrochloride ≤20 mg
Etoposide
Fluorouracil <1000 mg
Methotrexate <100 mg

Class III
Moderate (30% to 60%)

Asparaginase
Azacitidine
Cyclophosphamide <1 g
Doxorubicin <75 mg or >20 mg
Fluorouracil ≥1000 mg
Methotrexate <250 mg or ≥100 mg
Vinblastine sulfate

Class IV
Moderately High (60% to 90%)

Carmustine <200 mg
Cisplatin <75 mg
Cyclophosphamide 1 g
Cytarabine hydrochloride 250 mg - 1 g
Dacarbazine <500 mg
Doxorubicin ≥75 mg
Lomustine <60 mg
Methotrexate ≥250 mg
Mitomycin
Procarbazine hydrochloride

Class V
High (>90%)

Carmustine ≥200 mg
Cisplatin ≥75 mg
Cyclophosphamide >1 g
Cytarabine >1 g
Dacarbazine ≥500 mg
Lomustine ≥60 mg
Mechlorethamine hydrochloride

HEMATOLOGIC ADVERSE EFFECTS OF DRUGS

Drug	Red Cell Aplasia	Thrombo-cytopenia	Neutro-penia	Pancyto-penia	Hemolysis
Acetazolamide		+	+	+	
Allopurinol			+		
Amiodarone	+				
Amphotericin B				+	
Amrinone		++			
Asparaginase		+++	+++	+++	++
Barbiturates		+		+	
Benzocaine					++
Captopril			++		+
Carbamazepine		++	+		
Cephalosporins			+		++
Chloramphenicol		+	++	+++	
Chlordiazepoxide			+	+	
Chloroquine		+			
Chlorothiazides		++			
Chlorpropamide	+	++	+	++	+
Chlortetracycline				+	
Chlorthalidone			+		
Cimetidine		+	++	+	
Codeine		+			
Colchicine				+	
Cyclophosphamide		+++	+++	+++	+
Dapsone					+++
Desipramine		++			
Digitalis		+			
Digitoxin		++			
Erythromycin		+			
Estrogen		+		+	
Ethacrynic acid			+		
Fluorouracil		+++	+++	+++	+
Furosemide		+	+		
Gold salts	+	+++	+++	+++	
Heparin		++		+	
Ibuprofen			+		+
Imipramine			++		
Indomethacin		+	++	+	
Isoniazid		+		+	
Isosorbide dinitrate					+
L-dopa					++
Meperidine		+			
Meprobamate		+	+	+	
Methimazole			++		
Methyldopa		++			+++

(continued)

Drug	Red Cell Aplasia	Thrombo-cytopenia	Neutro-penia	Pancyto-penia	Hemolysis
Methotrexate		+++	+++	+++	++
Methylene blue					+
Metronidazole			+		
Nalidixic acid					+
Naproxen				+	
Nitrofurantoin			++		+
Nitroglycerine		+			
Penicillamine		++	+		
Penicillins		+	++	+	+++
Phenazopyridine					+++
Phenothiazines		+	++	+++	+
Phenylbutazone		+	++	+++	+
Phenytoin		++	++	++	+
Potassium iodide		+			
Prednisone		+			
Primaquine					+++
Procainamide			+		
Procarbazine		+	++	++	+
Propylthiouracil		+	++	+	+
Quinidine		+++	+		
Quinine		+++	+		
Reserpine		+			
Rifampicin		++	+		+++
Spironolactone			+		
Streptomycin		+		+	
Sulfamethoxazole with trimethoprim			+		
Sulfonamides	+	++	++	++	++
Sulindac	+	+	+	+	
Tetracyclines		+			+
Thioridazine			++		
Tolbutamide		++	+	++	
Triamterene					+
Valproate	+				
Vancomycin			+		

+ = rare or single reports.
++ = occasional reports.
+++ = substantial number of reports.

Adapted from D'Arcy PF and Griffin JP, eds, *Iatrogenic Diseases*, New York, NY: Oxford University Press, 1986, 128-30.

METABOLICS OF TUMOR LYSIS, MANAGEMENT

1. **Allopurinol**
   Children: 10 mg/kg/day in 2-3 divided doses **or**
   <6 years: 50 mg P.O. tid
   6-10 years: 100 mg P.O. tid
2. **Hydration**
   3 L/m^2/day
3. **Alkalinization**
   $NaHCO_3$ 150-200 mEq/m^2/day (titrate to keep urine pH 7.5)
4. **Discontinue chemotherapy until metabolically stable**
5. **Monitor:**
   lytes, BUN, creatinine, uric acid, Mg, Ca, P, I & O, BP, neuro exam
6. **Dialyze for:**
   - K >7 mEq/L
   - uric acid >10 mg/dL
   - severe, unmanageable hypertension
   - P >10 mg/dL or rapidly rising
   - symptomatic hypocalcemia, hyponatremia, or hypermagnesemia
   - volume overload

ENDOCARDITIS PROPHYLAXIS*

	Dosage for Adults	Dosage for Children†
DENTAL AND UPPER RESPIRATORY PROCEDURES‡		
Oral§		
Amoxicillin¶	3 g 1 h before procedure and 1.5 g 6 h later	50 mg/kg 1 h before procedure and 25 mg/kg 6 h later
Penicillin allergy:		
Erythromycin	1 g 2 h before procedure and 500 mg 6 h later	20 mg/kg 2 h before procedure and 10 mg/kg 6 h later
Parenteral§,#		
Ampicillin	2 g I.M. or I.V. 30 minutes before procedure	50 mg/kg I.M. or I.V. 30 minutes before procedure
plus Gentamicin	1.5 mg/kg I.M. or I.V. 30 minutes before procedure	2 mg/kg I.M. or I.V. 30 minutes before procedure
Penicillin allergy:		
Vancomycin	1 g I.V. infused **slowly over 1 h** beginning 1 h before procedure	20 mg/kg I.V. infused **slowly over 1 h** beginning 1 h before procedure
GASTROINTESTINAL AND GENITOURINARY PROCEDURES‡		
Oral§		
Amoxicillin	3 g 1 h before procedure and 1.5 g 6 h later	50 mg/kg 1 h before procedure and 25 mg/kg 6 h later
Parenteral§,#		
Ampicillin	2 g I.M. or I.V. 30 minutes before procedure	50 mg/kg I.M. or I.V. 30 minutes before procedure
plus Gentamicin	1.5 mg/kg I.M. or I.V. 30 minutes before procedure	2 mg/kg I.M. or I.V. 30 minutes before procedure
Penicillin allergy:		
Vancomycin	1 g I.V. infused **slowly over 1 h** beginning 1 h before procedure	20 mg/kg I.V. infused **slowly over 1 h** beginning 1 h before procedure
plus Gentamicin	1.5 mg/kg I.M. or I.V. 30 minutes before procedure	2 mg/kg I.M. or I.V. 30 minutes before procedure

*For patients with previous endocarditis, valvular heart disease, prosthetic heart valves, most forms of congenital heart disease (but not uncomplicated secundum atrial septal defect), idiopathic hypertrophic subaortic stenosis, and mitral valve prolapse with regurgitation. Viridans streptococci are the most common cause of endocarditis after dental or upper respiratory procedures; enterococci are the most common cause of endocarditis after gastrointestinal or genitourinary procedures.

†Should not exceed adult dosage.

‡For a review of the risk of bacteremia and endocarditis with various procedures, see D Durack in GL Mandell et al, eds, *Principles and Practice of Infectious Disease*, 3rd ed, New York, NY: Churchill Livingstone, 1990, 716.

§Oral regimens are more convenient and safer. Parenteral regimens are more likely to be effective; they are recommended especially for patients with prosthetic heart valves, those who have had endocarditis previously, or those taking continuous oral penicillin for rheumatic fever prophylaxis.

¶Amoxicillin is recommended because of its excellent bioavailability and good activity against streptococci and enterococci.

#A single dose of parenteral drugs is probably adequate, because bacteremia after most dental and diagnostic procedures is of short duration. An additional dose may be given 8 hours later to patients judged to be at higher risk.

IMMUNIZATION GUIDELINES

Table 1. **Dosage and Administration Guidelines for Vaccines Available in the United States**

Vaccine	Dosage	Route of Administration	Type
DT*	0.5 mL	I.M.	Toxoids
Td*	0.5 mL	I.M.	Toxoids
DTP*	0.5 mL	I.M.	Diphtheria and tetanus toxoids with killed *B. pertussis* organisms
DTaP (Acel-Imune®)‖	0.5 mL	I.M.	Diphtheria and tetanus toxoids with acellular pertussis
DTP-HbOC (Tetramune®)+	0.5 mL	I.M.	Diphtheria and tetanus toxoids with killed *B pertussis* organisms and *Haemophilus* b conjugate (diphtheria CRM_{197} protein conjugate)
Haemophilus B conjugate vaccine	0.5 mL	I.M.	
ProHIBit® (PRP-D), manufactured by Connaught Laboratories	0.5 mL	I.M.	Polysaccharide (diphtheria toxoid conjugate)
HibTITER® (HbOC),† manufactured by Praxis Biologicals	0.5 mL	I.M.	Oligosaccharide (diphtheria CRM_{197} protein conjugate)
PedvaxHIB® (PRP-OMP),‡ manufactured by MSD	0.5 mL	I.M.	Polysaccharide (meningococcal protein conjugate)
Hepatitis B§		I.M. in the anterolateral thigh or in the upper arm; S.C. in individuals at risk of hemorrhage	Yeast recombinant-derived inactivated viral antigen
Infants born to HB_sAg-negative mothers and children <11 y■			
Recombivax HB® (MSD)	2.5 µg (0.25 mL)		
Engerix-B® (SKF)	10 µg (0.5 mL)		
Infants born to HB_sAg-positive mothers (immunization and administration of 0.5 mL hepatitis B immune globulin is recommended for **infants** born to HB_sAg^+ mothers using different administration sites) within 12 hours of birth; administer vaccine at birth; repeat vaccine dose at 1 and 6 months following the initial dose			
Recombivax HB® (MSD)	5 µg (0.5 mL)		
Engerix-B® (SKF)	10 µg (0.5 mL)		
Children 11-19 y			
Recombivax HB® (MSD)	5 µg (0.5 mL)		
Engerix-B® (SKF)	20 µg (1 mL)		
Adults >19 y			
Recombivax HB® (MSD)	10 µg (1 mL)		
Engerix-B® (SKF)	20 µg (1 mL)		

(continued)

Vaccine	Dosage	Route of Administration	Type
Dialysis patients and immunosuppressed patients			
Recombivax HB® (MSD)	<11 y, 20 μg (0.5 mL); ≥11 y, 40 μg (1 mL) using special dialysis formulation		
Engerix-B® (SKF)¶	<11 y, 20 μg (1 mL); ≥11 y, 40 μg (2 mL), give as two 1 mL doses at different sites		
Influenza		I.M. (2 doses 4+ weeks apart in children <9 years of age not previously immunized; only 1 dose needed for annual updates)	Inactivated virus subvirion (split) (contraindicated in patients allergic to chicken eggs)
split virus only in pediatric patients			
6-35 mo	0.25 mL (1 or 2 doses)		
3-8 y	0.5 mL (1 or 2 doses)		
≥9 y	0.5 mL (1 dose)		
Measles	0.5 mL	S.C.	Live virus (contraindicated in patients with anaphylactic allergy to neomycin)

Most areas: Two doses (1st dose at 15 months with MMR; 2nd dose at 4-6 years or 11-12 years, depending on local school entry requirements)

High-risk area: Two doses (1st dose at 12 months with MMR; 2nd dose as above)

Children 6-15 months in epidemic situations: Dose is given at the time of first contact with a health care provider; children <1 year of age should receive single antigen measles vaccine. If vaccinated before 1 year, revaccinate at 15 months with MMR. A 3rd dose is administered at 4-6 years or 11-12 years, depending on local school entry requirements.

Vaccine	Dosage	Route of Administration	Type
Meningococcal	0.5 mL#	S.C.	Polysaccharide
MMR•	0.5 mL	S.C.	Live virus
MR	0.5 mL	S.C.	Live virus
Mumps	0.5 mL	S.C.	Live virus
Pneumococcal polyvalent♦	0.5 mL (≥2 y)	I.M. or S.C. (I.M. preferred)	Polysaccharide
Poliovirus (OPV) trivalent	0.5 mL	Oral	Live virus
Poliovirus (IPV)**·†† trivalent	0.5 mL	S.C.	Inactivated virus
Rabies	1 mL	I.M.‡‡, ID§§	Inactivated virus
Rubella	0.5 mL (≥12 mo)¶¶	S.C.	Live virus
Tetanus (adsorbed)##	0.5 mL	I.M.	Toxoid
Tetanus (fluid)	0.5 mL	I.M., S.C.	Toxoid
Yellow fever	0.5 mL••	S.C.	Live attenuated virus

*DT & DTP for use in children <7 years of age. Td contains same amount of tetanus toxoid as DT & DTP, but a reduced dose of diphtheria toxoid. Td for use in children ≥7 years of age.

‖DTaP (Acel-Imune®) may be used only for the 4th and 5th doses for children >15 months and <7 years of age. The occurrence of fever and local reactions is lower with acellular pertussis vaccine than with whole-cell DTP.

⁺DTP-HbOC may be substituted for DTP and *Haemophilus* B conjugate vaccines which are administered separately, whenever recommended schedules for use of these 2 vaccines coincide. Initiate at 2 months of age for 3 doses (2 months, 4 months, and 6 months), followed by a 4th dose at 15-18 months of age. DTaP and *Haemophilus* B conjugate vaccine may be administered separately as an alternative to DTP-HbOC at 15-18 months of age.

†The conjugate (HbCV) vaccine is preferred over the polysaccharide (HbPV) vaccine. In children with a high risk for *Haemophilus influenzae* type b disease and HbCV is unavailable, an acceptable alternate is to give HbPV at 18 months of age with a 2nd dose at 24 months of age. Children <5 years of age who were previously vaccinated with HbPV between 18-23 months of age should be revaccinated with a single dose of HbCV at least 2 months after the initial dose of HbPV. Either HbCV or HbPV can be administered up to the 5th birthday. However they are generally not recommended for children >5 years of age.

‡PRP-OMP (PedvaxHIB®) manufactured by Merck, Sharp & Dohme is initiated at 2 months of age for 3 doses (2 months, 4 months and 12 months). If initiated at 7-11 months of age, 3 doses are administered (initial 2 doses at 2-month intervals, 3rd dose at 15-18 months of age); initiated at 12-14 months of age, 2 doses are administered at 2- to 3-month intervals between doses; initiated at 15-59 months of age, 1 dose is administered.

§Hepatitis B vaccine can be given at the same time with DTP, HbOC, polio, and/or MMR; administer 3 doses at 0, 1, and 6 months).

■Administer to newborns at 0-2 days of age before hospital discharge; repeat at 1-2 months and 6-18 months following the initial dose. If not vaccinated at birth, administer at 2, 4, and 6-18 months of age.

¶Engerix-B® — an alternate schedule for postexposure prophylaxis or more rapid induction using 4 doses at 0, 1, 2, and 12 months of age is recommended.

#Indicated in children ≥2 years of age at risk in epidemic or highly endemic areas.

•See measles.

♦Indicated for children with sickle cell disease; asplenia; nephrotic syndrome or chronic renal failure; conditions associated with immunosuppression; CSF leaks; HIV infection.

**The primary series consists of 3 doses. The first 2 doses should be administered at an interval of 8 weeks. The 3rd dose should be given at least 6 and preferably 12 months after the 2nd dose. A booster dose of 0.5 mL should be given to all children who have completed the primary series, before entering school. However, if the 3rd dose of the primary series is given on or after the 4th birthday, a 4th dose is not required before entering school. When polio vaccine is given to persons >18 years of age, IPV should be given.

††IPV is indicated for unimmunized or partially immunized patients with compromised immunity; HIV infection; unimmunized adults (>18 years of age) or adults at future risk of exposure to poliomyelitis; household contacts of an immunodeficient individual.

‡‡In infants and small children, I.M. injection can be given into the midlateral aspect of the thigh; in older children and adults, I.M. injection can be given into the deltoid muscle. Repeat doses are given on days 3, 7, 14, and 28 postexposure.

§§For pre-exposure prophylaxis against rabies for high-risk individuals, 1 mL I.M. or 0.1 mL intradermal is administered on days 0, 7, and 21 (or 28). Both I.M. and I.D. dosage forms are available.

¶¶As MMR in a 2-dose schedule.

##Adsorbed preferred to fluid toxoid because of longer lasting immunity.

••≥9 months of age living in or traveling to endemic areas. Contraindicated in infants <4 months of age and in patients who have had an anaphylactic reaction to eggs. Increased risk of encephalitis associated with use of yellow fever vaccine in infants <9 months of age.

Note: For each vaccine, check the manufacturer's package insert for specific product information since preparations may change from time to time.

References:

ACIP, General Recommendations on Immunization, MMWR 1989, 38:205-14, 219-27.

ACIP, Measles Prevention, Recommendations of the Immunization Practices Advisory Committee, MMWR 1989, 38(5-9):1-18.

American Academy of Pediatrics, Report of the Committee on Infectious Diseases (Red Book), 22nd ed, 1991.

American Academy of Pediatrics, Committee on Infectious Diseases, "Acellular Pertussis Vaccines: Recommendations for Use as the Fourth and Fifth Doses," *Pediatrics*, 1992, 90:121-3.

American Academy of Pediatrics, Committee on Infectious Diseases, "Universal Hepatitis B Immunization," *Pediatrics*, 1992, 89:795-800.

Table 2. **Recommended Schedule for Active Immunization of Normal Infants and Children****

Recommended Age	Vaccine(s)	Comments
2 mo	DTP1,* OPV1, HbCV1†	OPV and DTP can be given earlier in areas of high endemicity or during epidemics; DTP-HbOC can be given in place of DTP1 and HbCV1
4 mo	DTP2, OPV2, HbCV2†	6 weeks to 2 months interval desired between OPV doses; DTP-HbOC can be given in place of DTP2 and HbCV2
6 mo	DTP3, HbOC3	An additional dose of OPV is optional in high risk areas; DTP-HbOC can be given in place of DTP3 and HbOC3
12 mo	PRP-OMP	
15 mo	MMR,‡ DTP4,¶ OPV3, HbCV3, or HbCV4§	Completion of primary series of DTP and OPV; DTP-HbOC can be given in place of DTP4 and HbCV
4-6 y	DTP5,¶ OPV4, measles	At or before school entry
11-12 y	MMR	At entry to middle school unless 2nd dose was given at 4-6 years at time of school entry
14-16 y	Td	Repeat every 10 years throughout life

**Please also refer to Hepatitis B Vaccine Guidelines in Table 1.

*DTP may be used up to the 7th birthday. The 1st dose can be given at 6th week of age, and the 2nd and 3rd doses given 4-8 weeks after the preceding dose.

†HbCV — can use either HbOC or PRP-OMP.

‡Can be given at 12 months of age in high-risk areas.

§HbCV — can use either PRP-OMP, PRP-D, or HbOC for children ≥15 months of age.

¶DTaP may be used in place of whole cell DTP only for the 4th and 5th doses for children >15 months and <7 years of age. DTaP can be given at the same time with OPV, IPV, MMR, *Haemophilus influenzae* type b conjugate vaccine, and/or hepatitis B vaccine.

References:

Centers for Disease Control, "Protection Against Viral Hepatitis: Recommendations of the Immunization Practices Advisory Committee (ACIP)," *MMWR*, 1990, 39:11.

American Academy of Pediatrics Committee on Infectious Diseases, "*Haemophilus influenzae* Type B Conjugate Vaccines: Recommendations for Immunization of Infants and Children 2 Months of Age and Older," *Pediatrics*, 1991, 88(1):169-72.

Table 3. **Recommended Immunization Schedule for Infants and Children up to the 7th Birthday Not Immunized at the Recommended Time in Early Infancy**

Timing	Vaccine(s)	Comments
First visit	DTP1, OPV1 MMR* (if child ≥15 months)	DTP, OPV and MMR should be administered simultaneously to children ≥15 months of age
	HbCV†·‡	DTP, OPV, MMR and HbCV may be given simultaneously to children aged 15 months to 5 years at separate sites
2 mo after DTP1, OPV1	DTP2, OPV2 (HbCV)‡	Second HbCV for children whose 1st dose was received when <15 months of age
2 mo after DTP2	DTP3	An additional dose of OPV is optional in high-risk areas
6-12 mo after DTP3	DTP4§ (OPV3)	OPV is given if 3rd dose was not given earlier
4-6 y	DTP5,§ OPV4 (MMR2)	Preferably at or before school entry. OTP5 and OPV4 are not needed if DTP4 and OPV3 were given after the 4th birthday. Local public health regulations may require MMR2 at school entry.
11-12 y	MMR2	MMR2 is given if 2nd dose was not given earlier
14-16 y	Td	Repeat every 10 years throughout life

*Can be given at 12 months of age to children residing in areas at high-risk for measles transmission.

†Only HbOC or PRP-OMP are licensed for use in children <15 months of age.

‡DTP-HbOC may be substituted for DTP and *Haemophilus* B conjugate vaccines which are administered separately, whenever recommended schedules for use of these 2 vaccines coincide. Initiate at 2 months of age for 3 doses (2 months, 4 months, and 6 months), followed by a 4th dose at 15-18 months of age. DTaP and *Haemophilus* B conjugate vaccine may be administered separately as an alternative to DTP-HbOC at 15-18 months.

§DTaP may be used in place of whole cell DTP only for the 4th and 5th doses for children >15 months and <7 years of age.

Table 4. **Recommended Immunization Schedule for Children >7 Years of Age Not Immunized at the Recommended Time in Early Infancy**

Timing	Vaccine(s)	Comments
First visit	Td1, OPV1, MMR, HbCV*	OPV not routinely recommended for persons ≥18 years of age
2 mo after Td1, OPV1	Td2, OPV2	OPV may be given as soon as 6 weeks after OPV1
6-12 mo after Td2, OPV2	Td3, OPV3	OPV3 may be given as soon as 6 weeks after OPV2
10 y after Td3	Td	Repeat every 10 years throughout life
11-12 y	MMR	

*Indicated only in children with a chronic illness associated with increased risk of *Haemophilus influenzae* type B disease.

Table 5. **High-Risk Groups Who Should Receive Hepatitis B Immunization Regardless of Age***

- Hemophiliac patients and other recipients of certain blood products
- Intravenous drug abusers
- Heterosexual persons who have had more than one sex partner in the previous 6 months and/or those with a recent episode of a sexually transmitted disease
- Sexually active homosexual and bisexual males
- Household and sexual contacts of hepatitis B virus (HBV) carriers
- Members of households with adoptees from HBV-endemic, high-risk countries who are hepatitis B surface antigen-positive
- Children and other household contacts in populations of high HBV endemnicity
- Staff and residents of institutions for the developmentally disabled
- Staff of nonresidential day care and school programs for developmentally disabled if attended by known HBV carrier; other attendees in certain circumstances
- Hemodialysis patients
- Health care workers and others with occupational risk
- International travelers who will live for more than 6 months in areas of high HBV endemnicity and who otherwise will be at risk
- Inmates of long-term correctional facilities

*Adapted from Report of the Committee on Infectious Disease, 1991, 246-9.

Table 6. **Guidelines for Spacing Live and Killed Antigen Administration**

Antigen Combinations	Recommended Minimum Interval Between Doses
≥2 killed antigens	None. May be given simultaneously or at any interval between doses.
Killed and live antigens	None. May be given simultaneously or at any interval between doses. (Exception: Concurrent administration of cholera and yellow fever vaccines should be avoided. Separate these vaccines by at least 3 weeks.)
≥2 live antigens	4 weeks minimum interval if not administered simultaneously. (Recent receipt of OPV is not a contraindication to MMR.) Vaccines associated with systemic reactions (cholera and parenteral typhoid or influenza and DTP in young children) should be given on separate occasions.

Table 7. **Passive Immunization Agents — Immune Globulins**

Immune Globulin	Dosage		Route
Hepatitis B (H-BIG®)			I.M.
percutaneous inoculation	0.06 mL/kg/dose (within 24 hours) (5 mL max)		
perinatal	0.5 mL/dose (within 12 hours of birth)		
sexual exposure	0.06 mL/kg/dose (within 14 days of contact) (5 mL max)		
Immune globulin (IG)			I.M.*
hepatitis A prophylaxis	0.02 mL/kg/dose (as soon as possible or within 2 weeks after exposure) (single exposure)		
	0.06 mL/kg/dose (>3 months or continuous exposure) repeat every 4-6 months		
hepatitis B	0.06 mL/kg/dose (H-BIG® should be used)		
hepatitis C	0.06 mL/kg/dose (percutaneous exposure)		
measles†	0.25 mL/kg/dose (max 15 mL/dose) (within 6 days of exposure)		
	0.5 mL/kg/dose (max 15 mL/dose) (immunocompromised children)		
Rabies‡	20 IU/kg/dose (within 3 days)		
Tetanus (serious, contaminated, wounds; <3 previous tetanus vaccine doses)	250-500 units/dose		I.M.
Varicella-zoster§ (VZIG)	Within 48 hours but not later than 96 hours after exposure		I.M.¶
	0-10 kg	125 units = 1 vial	
	10.1-20 kg	250 units = 2 vials	
	20.1-30 kg	375 units = 3 vials	
	30.1-40 kg	500 units = 4 vials	
	>40 kg	625 units = 5 vials	

*Deep I.M. in the gluteal region for large doses only. Deltoid muscle or the anterolateral aspect of the thigh are preferred sites for injection. No greater than 5 mL/site in adults or large children; 1-3 mL/site in small children and infants. Maximum dose: 20 mL at one time.

†IG prophylaxis may not be indicated in a patient who has received IGIV within 3 weeks of exposure.

‡½ of dose used to infiltrate the wound with the remaining ½ of dose given I.M. Rabies immune globulin is not recommended in previously HDCV immunized patients.

§Infants born to women who develop varicella within 5 days before or 48 hours after delivery should receive 125 units I.M. as a single dose.

¶No greater than 2.5 mL of VZIG/one injection site. Doses >2.5 mL should be divided and administered at different sites.

Table 8. **Guidelines for Spacing the Administration of Immune Globulin (IG) Preparations and Vaccines**

Immunobiologic Combinations		Recommended Minimum Interval Between Doses
Simultaneous Administration		
IG and killed antigen		None. May be given simultaneously at different sites or at any time between doses.
IG and live antigen		Should generally not be given simultaneously. If unavoidable to do so, give at different sites and revaccinate or test for seroconversion in 3 months. Example: MMR should not be given to patients who have received immune globulin within the previous 3 months.
Nonsimultaneous Administration		
First	**Second**	
IG	Killed antigen	None
Killed antigen	IG	None
IG	Live antigen	6 weeks, and preferably 3 months
Live antigen	IG	2 weeks

*The live virus vaccines, OPV, and yellow fever are exceptions to these recommendations. Either vaccine may be administered simultaneously or any time before or after IG without significantly decreasing antibody response.

Table 9. **Recommended for Routine Immunization of HIV-Infected Children — United States**

	Known HIV Infection	
Vaccine	**Asymptomatic**	**Symptomatic**
DTP	Yes	Yes
OPV	No	No
IPV	Yes	Yes
MMR	Yes	Yes
HbCV	Yes	Yes
Pneumococcal	Yes	Yes
Influenza	No*	Yes

*Not contraindicated.

IMMUNIZATION SIDE EFFECTS

Vaccine	Side Effect	Incidence/Dose
DPT	Slight fever and irritability (within 2 days of immunization	"Most"
	Pain and swelling at immunization site	1/2
	Continuous crying >3 hours	1/100
	Fever >105°F	1/330
	Unusual, high pitched crying	1/900
	Seizures or episodes of limpness/pallor	1/1750
	Acute encephalopathy (within 3 days of immunization)	1/110,000
	Permanent neurological sequelae*	1/310,000
DT, Td	Pain at immunization site, slight fever	"Not common"
OPV	Paralytic polio in patient immunized	1/8.1 million
	Paralytic polio in close contact of patient immunized	1/5 million
Hib	Swelling and warmth at immunization site	1/100
	Fever >101°F	2/100
	Redness at immunization site	2/100
MMR	Rash or slight fever lasting a few days 1-2 weeks following immunization	1/5
	Rash or lymphadenopathy lasting a few days 1-2 weeks following immunization	1/7
	Arthralgias, joint swelling lasting 2-3 days 1-3 weeks following immunization	1/20 (higher in adults)
	Encephalitis, seizure with fever, nerve deafness	"Very rarely"

**Red Book* (1991, p 355) states "The committee concludes, based on currently available data, that pertussis vaccine has not been proven to be a cause of brain damage. Although the data does not prove that pertussis vaccine will never cause brain damage, it does indicate that such occurrences are exceedingly rare."

Reportable Vaccine Side Effects

Vaccine/Toxoid	Event	Interval From Vaccination
DTP, P, DTP/poliovirus combined	A. Anaphylaxis or anaphylactic shock	24 hours
	B. Encephalopathy (or encephalitis)	7 days
	C. Shock-collapse or hypotonic-hyporesponsive collapse	7 days
	D. Residual seizure disorder	
	E. Any acute complication or sequela (including death) of above events	No limit
	F. See package insert	See package insert
Measles, mumps, and rubella; DT, Td, T toxoid	A. Anaphylaxis or anaphylactic shock	24 hours
	B. Encephalopathy (or encephalitis)	15 days for measles, mumps, and rubella vaccines; 7 days for DT, Td, and toxoids
	C. Residual seizure disorder	
	D. Any acute complication or sequela (including death) of above events	No limit
	E. See package insert	See package insert

(continued)

Vaccine/Toxoid	Event	Interval From Vaccination
Oral poliovirus vaccine	A. Paralytic poliomyelitis	
	– in a nonimmunodeficient recipient	30 days
	– in an immunodeficient recipient	6 months
	– in a vaccine-associated community case	No limit
	B. Any acute complication or sequela (including death) of above events	No limit
	C. See package insert	See package insert
Inactivated poliovirus vaccine	A. Anaphylaxis or anaphylactic shock	24 hours
	B. Any acute complication or sequela (including death) of above events	No limit
	C. See package insert	See package insert

CONTRAINDICATIONS TO IMMUNIZATION

Minor illness is not a contraindication to vaccination, especially if the patient has a minor upper respiratory infection or allergic rhinitis. Delay of immunization should be considered if expected or potential vaccine side effects may accentuate or be accentuated by an underlying illness. Note that fever is not itself a contraindication to vaccination, however, if fever is associated with other signs of serious underlying illness, vaccination should be deferred until the patient has recovered. Moderate or severe illness, with or without fever, is considered a contraindication to DPT administration, as signs and symptoms associated with the underlying illness may be incorrectly attributed to the DPT vaccine.

The following conditions should be evaluated as possible contraindications to vaccination:

Vaccine	Possible Contraindications
DPT (see *Red Book*, p 366-9)	Previous serious reaction to DPT, TD, or dT
	Serious immunosuppressive therapy
	Thimerosal allergy
	Progressive neurological disorder or uncontrolled seizure disorder
	Disorders associated with conditions that predispose to either seizures or neurological deterioration
	Age 7 years or older (dT recommended)
OPV	Immunosuppression
	Immunosuppressive household contacts
	Age 18 years and older (IPV recommended)
	Pregnancy
Hib	Serious thimerosal allergy
	Serious allergic reaction to vaccine containing diphtheria toxoid
	Age 5 years and older
MMR	Serious egg allergy
	Immunosuppression
	Gamma globulin therapy within preceding 3 months
	Serious neomycin or streptomycin allergy
	Pregnancy

Conditions Which Are Not Considered to Be Contraindications to Vaccinations

- Reaction to a previous DTP dose that involved only soreness, redness, or swelling in the area of the vaccination site or temperature of less than 105°F (40.5°C)
- Mild acute illness with low-grade fever or mild diarrheal illness in an otherwise well child
- Current antimicrobial therapy or the convalescent phase of illness
- Prematurity
- Pregnancy of mother or other household contact
- Recent exposure to an infectious disease
- Breast-feeding
- A history of nonspecific allergies or relatives with allergies
- Allergies to penicillin or any other antibiotic, except anaphylactic reactions to neomycin or streptomycin
- Allergies to duck meat or duck feathers
- Family history of convulsions in persons considered for pertussis or measles vaccination
- Family history of sudden infant death syndrome in children considered for DTP vaccination
- Family history of an adverse event, unrelated to immunosuppression, following vaccination

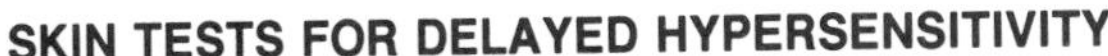

SKIN TESTS FOR DELAYED HYPERSENSITIVITY

Candida 1:100

Dose = 0.1 mL intradermally
(30% of children less than 18 months and 50% older than 18 months respond)
Can be used as a control antigen.

Coccidioidin 1:100

Dose = 0.1 mL intradermally
(apply with PPD **and** a control antigen)
Mercury derivative used as a preservative for spherulin.

Histoplasmin 1:100

Dose = 0.1 mL intradermally
(yeast derived)

Multitest CMI (*Candida,* diphtheria toxoid, tetanus toxoid, *Streptococcus,* old tuberculin, *Trichophyton, Proteus* antigen and negative control)

Press loaded unit into the skin with sufficient pressure to puncture the skin and allow adequate penetration of all points

Mumps 40 cfu per mL

Dose = 0.1 mL intradermally
(contraindicated in patients allergic to eggs, egg products or thimerosal)

Purified Protein Derivative 5 TU (PPD Mantoux Tuberculin)

Dose = 0.1 mL intradermally
A positive immune response is 5 mm or more of induration. Tuberculin positive patients must have an induration of 10 mm or more

Tetanus Toxoid 1:5

Dose = 0.1 mL intradermally
(29% of children less than 2 years and 78% older than 2 years respond if they have received 3 immunizing doses)
Can be used as a control antigen.

Tine Test

Indication: Survey and screen for exposure to tuberculosis (grasp forearm firmly; stretch the skin of the volar surface tightly; apply the tines to the selected site; press for at least one second so that a circular halo impression is left on the skin)

General Information

1. Intradermal skin tests should be injected in the flexor surface of the forearm.
2. A pale wheal 6-10 mm in diameter should form over the needle tip as soon as the injection is administered. If no bleb forms, the injection must be repeated.
3. Space skin tests at least 2 inches apart to prevent reactions from overlapping.
4. Read skin tests for diameter of induration and presence of erythema at 24, 48, and 72 hours. After injection, maximal responses

usually occur at 48 hours. Maximal responses to mumps or coccidioidin may occur at 24 hours.

5. False-negative results may occur in patients with malnutrition, viral infections, febrile illnesses, immunodeficiency disorders, severe disseminated infections, uremia, patients who have received immunosuppressive therapy (steroids, antineoplastic agents), patients who have received a recent live attenuated virus vaccine (MMR, measles) or subdermal injection of the antigen.
6. False-positive results may occur in patients sensitive to ingredients in the skin test solution such as thimerosal; cross sensitivity between similar antigens; or with improper interpretation of skin test.
7. Side effects are pain, blisters, extensive erythema and necrosis at the injection site.

*Emergency equipment and epinephrine should be readily available to treat severe allergic reactions that may occur.

Recommended Interpretation of Skin Test Reactions

	Local Reaction	
Reaction	**After Intradermal Injections of Antigens**	**After Dinitrochlorobenzene**
1+	Erythema >10 mm and/or induration >1-5 mm	Erythema and/or induration covering <½ area of dose site
2+	Induration 6-10 mm	Induration covering >½ area of dose site
3+	Induration 11-20 mm	Vesiculation and induration at dose site or spontaneous flare at days 7-14 at the site
4+	Induration >20 mm	Bulla or ulceration at dose site or spontaneous flare at days 7-14 at the site

References

Ahmed AR and Blose DA, "Delayed-Type Hypersensitivity Skin Testing, A Review," *Arch Dermatol*, 1983, 119:934-45.

Borut TC, Ank BJ, and Gard SE, "Tetanus Toxoid Skin Test in Children: Correlation With *in vitro* Lymphocyte Stimulation and Monocyte Chemotaxis," *J Pediatr*, 1980, 97:567-73.

Corriel RN, Kniker WT, McBryde JL, et al, "Cell-Mediated Immunity in School Children Assessed by Multitest Skin Testing," *Am J Dis Child*, 1985, 139:141-6.

Gordon EG, Krouse HA, Kinney JL, et al, "Delayed Cutaneous Hypersensitivity in Normals: Choice of Antigens and Comparison to *in vitro* Assays of Cell-Mediated Immunity," *J Allergy Clin Immunol*, 1983, 72:487-94.

Sokal JE, "Measurement of Delayed Skin-Test Responses," *N Engl J Med*, 1975, 293:501-2.

NORMAL LABORATORY VALUES FOR CHILDREN

		Normal Values
CHEMISTRY		
Albumin		
	0-1 year	2-4 g/dL
	1 year-adult	3.5-5.5 g/dL
Ammonia		
	Newborn	90-150 μg/dL
	Child	40-120 μg/dL
	Adult	18-54 μg/dL
Amylase		
	Newborn	0-60 units/L
	Adult	30-110 units/L
Bilirubin, conjugated, direct		
	Newborn	<1.5 mg/dL
	1 month-adult	0-0.5 mg/dL
Bilirubin, total		
	0-3 days	2-10 mg/dL
	1 month-adult	0-1.5 mg/dL
Bilirubin, unconjugated, indirect		0.6-10.5 mg/dL
Calcium		
	Newborn	7-12 mg/dL
	0-2 years	8.8-11.2 mg/dL
	2 years-adult	9-11 mg/dL
Calcium, ionized, whole blood		4.4-5.4 mg/dL
Carbon dioxide, total		23-33 mEq/L
Chloride		95-105 mEq/L
Cholesterol		
	Newborn	45-170 mg/dL
	0-1 year	65-175 mg/dL
	1-20 years	120-230 mg/dL
Creatinine		
	0-1 year	≤0.6 mg/dL
	1 year-adult	0.5-1.5 mg/dL
Glucose		
	Newborn	30-90 mg/dL
	0-2 years	60-105 mg/dL
	Child-adult	70-110 mg/dL
Iron		
	Newborn	110-270 μg/dL
	Infant	30-70 μg/dL
	Child	55-120 μg/dL
	Adult	70-180 μg/dL
Iron binding		
	Newborn	59-175 μg/dL
	Infant	100-400 μg/dL
	Adult	250-400 μg/dL
Lactic acid, lactate		2-20 mg/dL
Lead, whole blood		<30 μg/dL
Lipase		
	Child	20-140 units/L
	Adult	0-190 units/L
Magnesium		1.5-2.5 mEq/L
Osmolality, serum		275-296 mOsm/kg
Osmolality, urine		50-1400 mOsm/kg

(continued)

		Normal Values
Phosphorus		
	Newborn	4.2-9 mg/dL
	6 weeks-19 months	3.8-6.7 mg/dL
	18 months-3 years	2.9-5.9 mg/dL
	3-15 years	3.6-5.6 mg/dL
	>15 years	2.5-5 mg/dL
Potassium, plasma		
	Newborn	4.5-7.2 mEq/L
	2 days-3 months	4-6.2 mEq/L
	3 months-1 year	3.7-5.6 mEq/L
	1-16 years	3.5-5 mEq/L
Protein, total		
	0-2 years	4.2-7.4 g/dL
	>2 years	6-8 g/dL
Sodium		136-145 mEq/L
Triglycerides		
	Infant	0-171 mg/dL
	Child	20-130 mg/dL
	Adult	30-200 mg/dL
Urea nitrogen, blood		
	0-2 years	4-15 mg/dL
	2 years - Adult	5-20 mg/dL
Uric acid		
	Male	3-7 mg/dL
	Female	2-6 mg/dL
ENZYMES		
Alanine aminotransferase (ALT) (SGPT)		
	0-2 months	8-78 units/L
	>2 months	8-36 units/L
Alkaline phosphatase (ALKP)		
	Newborn	60-130 units/L
	0-16 years	85-400 units/L
	>16 years	30-115 units/L
Aspartate aminotransferase (AST) (SGOT)		
	Infant	18-74 units/L
	Child	15-46 units/L
	Adult	5-35 units/L
Creatine kinase (CK)		
	Infant	20-200 units/L
	Child	10-90 units/L
	Adult male	0-206 units/L
	Adult female	0-175 units/L
Lactate dehydrogenase (LDH)		
	Newborn	290-501 units/L
	1 month-2 years	110-144 units/L
	>16 years	60-170 units/L

BLOOD GASES

	Arterial	Capillary	Venous
pH	7.35-7.45	7.35-7.45	7.32-7.42
pCO_2 (mm Hg)	35-45	35-45	38-52
pO_2 (mm Hg)	70-100	60-80	24-48
HCO_3 (mEq/L)	19-25	19-25	19-25
TCO_2 (mEq/L)	19-29	19-29	23-33
O_2 saturation (%)	90-95	90-95	40-70
Base excess (mEq/L)	-5 to +5	-5 to +5	-5 to +5

THYROID FUNCTION TESTS

T_4 (thyroxine)

1-7 days	10.1-20.9 μg/dL
8-14 days	9.8-16.6 μg/dL
1 month-1 year	5.5-16 μg/dL
>1 year	4-12 μg/dL

FTI

1-3 days	9.3-26.6
1-4 weeks	7.6-20.8
1-4 months	7.4-17.9
4-12 months	5.1-14.5
1-6 years	5.7-13.3
>6 years	4.8-14

T_3 by RIA

Newborns	100-470 ng/dL
1-5 years	100-260 ng/dL
5-10 years	90-240 ng/dL
10 years-adult	70-210 ng/dL

T_3 uptake 35-45%

TSH

Cord	3-22 μU/mL
1-3 days	<40 μU/mL
3-7 days	<25 μU/mL
>7 days	0-10 μU/mL

HEMATOLOGY VALUES

	Hgb (g/dL)	Hct (%)	MCV (fl)	MCH (pg)	MCHC (%)	RBC (mill/mm^3)	RDW	PLTS (x $10^3/mm^3$)
0-3 days	15-20	45-61	95-115	31-37	29-37	4-5.9	<18	250-450
1-2 weeks	12.5-18.5	39-57	86-110	28-36	28-38	3.6-5.5	<17	250-450
1 month-6 months	10-13	29-42	74-96	25-35	30-36	3.1-4.3	<16.5	300-700
7 months-2 years	10.5-13	33-38	70-84	23-30	31-37	3.7-4.9	<16	250-600
2-5 years	11.5-13	34-39	75-87	24-30	31-37	3.9-5	<15	250-550
5-8 years	11.5-14.5	35-42	77-95	25-33	31-37	4-4.9	<15	250-550
13-18 years	12-15.2	36-47	78-96	25-35	31-37	4.5-5.1	<14.5	150-450
Adult male	13.5-16.5	41-50	80-100	26-34	31-37	4.5-5.5	<14.5	150-450
Adult female	12-15	36-44	80-100	26-34	31-37	4-4.9	<14.5	150-450

WBC and Diff

	WBC (x $10^3/mm^3$)	Segmented Neutrophils	Band Neutrophils	Eosinophils	Basophils	Lymphocytes	Atypical Lymphs	Monocytes	Number of NRBCs
0-3 days	9-35	32-62	10-18	0-2	0-1	19-29	0-8	5-7	0-2
1-2 weeks	5-20	14-34	6-14	0-2	0-1	36-45	0-8	6-10	0
1-6 months	6-17.5	13-33	4-12	0-3	0-1	41-71	0-8	4-7	0
7 months-2 years	6-17	15-35	5-11	0-3	0-1	45-76	0-8	3-6	0
2-5 years	5.5-15.5	23-45	5-11	0-3	0-1	35-65	0-8	3-6	0
5-8 years	5-14.5	32-54	5-11	0-3	0-1	28-48	0-8	3-6	0
13-18 years	4.5-13	34-64	5-11	0-3	0-1	25-45	0-8	3-6	0
Adult	4.5-11	35-66	5-11	0-3	0-1	24-44	0-8	3-6	0

Sedimentation rate, Westergren	Children	0-20 mm/hour
	Adult male	0-15 mm/hour
	Adult female	0-20 mm/hour
Reticulocyte count	Newborn	2-6%
	1-6 months	0-2.8%
	Adult	0.5-1.5%

Sedimentation rate, Wintrobe	Children	0-13 mm/hour
	Adult male	0-10 mm/hour
	Adult female	0-15 mm/hour

CEREBROSPINAL FLUID VALUES, NORMAL

Cell count		% PMNs
Preterm mean	9 (0-25.4 WBC/mm^3)	57%
Term mean	8.2 (0-22.4 WBC/mm^3)	61%
>1 mo	0.7	0

Glucose		
Preterm	24-63 mg/dL	(mean 50)
Term	34-119 mg/dL	(mean 52)
Child	40-80 mg/dL	

CSF glucose/blood glucose (%)	
Preterm	55-105
Term	44-128
Child	50

Lactic acid dehydrogenase: Mean 20 units/mL (range 5-30 units/mL)

Myelin basic protein	<4 ng/mL

Pressure: Initial LP (mm H_2O)	
Newborn	80-110 (<110)
Infant/child	<200 (lateral recumbent position)
Respiratory movements	5-10

Protein		
Preterm	(mean 115)	65-150 mg/dL
Term	(mean 90)	20-170 mg/dL
Children	Ventricular	5-15 mg/dL
	Cisternal	5-25 mg/dL
	Lumbar	5-40 mg/dL

APGAR SCORING SYSTEM

Sign	Score 0	Score 1	Score 2
Heart rate	Absent	Under 100 beats per minute	Over 100 beats per minute
Respiratory effort	Absent	Slow (irregular)	Good crying
Muscle tone	Limp	Some flexion of extremities	Active motion
Reflex irritability	No response	Grimace	Cough or sneeze
Color	Blue, pale	Pink body, blue extremities	All pink

From Apgar V, "A Proposal for a New Method of Evaluation of the Newborn Infant," *Anesth Analg*, 1953, 32:260.

FETAL HEART RATE MONITORING

Normal Heart Rates

Fetal heart rate 120-160 bpm. Isolated accelerations are normal and considered reassuring. Mild (100-120 bpm) and transient bradycardias may be normal. Normal fetal heart rate tracings show beat-to-beat variability of 5-10 bpm (poor-to-beat variability suggests fetal hypoxia).

Abnormal Heart Rates

Bradycardia (FHR <120 bpm): Potential causes include fetal distress, drugs, congenital heart block (associated with maternal SLE, congenital cardiac defects).

Tachycardia (FHR >160 bpm): Potential causes include maternal fever, chorioamnionitis, drugs, fetal dysrhythmias, eg, SVT (with or without fetal CHF).

Decreased Beat-to-Beat Variability

Results from fetal CNS depression;. Potential causes include fetal hypoxia, fetal sleep, fetal immaturity and maternal narcotic/sedative administration.

Fetal Heart Rate Decelerations

Type 1 (early decelerations)

- Seen most commonly in late labor
- Mirror uterine contractions in time of onset, duration and resolution
- Uniform shape
- Usually associated with good beat-to-beat variability
- Heart rate may dip to 60-80 bpm
- Associated with fetal head compression (increases vagal tone)
- Considered benign, and not representative of fetal hypoxia

Type 2 (late decelerations)

- Deceleration 10-30 seconds after onset of uterine contraction
- Heart rate fails to return to baseline after contraction is completed
- Asymmetrical shape (longer deceleration, shorter acceleration)
- Late decelerations of 10-20 bpm may be significant
- Probably associated with fetal CNS and myocardial depression

Type 3 (variable decelerations)

- Heart rate variations do not correlate with uterine contractions
- Variable shape and duration
- Occur occasionally in many normal labors
- Concerning if severe (HR <60 bpm), prolonged (duration >60 seconds), associated with poor beat-to-beat variability, or combined with late decelerations
- Associated with cord compression (including nuchal cord)

Reference

Manual of Neonatal Care, Joint Program in Neonatology, 1991.

CREATININE CLEARANCE ESTIMATING METHODS IN PATIENTS WITH STABLE RENAL FUNCTION

The following formulas provide an acceptable estimate of the patient's creatinine clearance except when:

a. Patient's serum creatinine is changing rapidly (either up or down).
b. Patients are markedly emaciated.

In these situations (a and b above), certain assumptions have to be made:

a. In patients with rapidly rising serum creatinines (ie, >0.5-0.7 mg/dL/day), it is best to assume that the patient's creatinine clearance is probably less than 10 mL/min.
b. In emaciated patients, although their actual creatinine clearance is less than their calculated creatinine clearance (because of decreased creatinine production), it is not possible to predict easily how much less.

Estimation of creatinine clearance using serum creatinine and body length* (to be used when an adequate timed specimen cannot be obtained)

Creatinine clearance = $K \times L/S_{cr}$

where:

K = Constant of proportionality that is age specific

Age	K
Low birth weight ≤1 y	0.33
Full-term ≤1 y	0.45
2-12 y	0.55
13-21 y female	0.55
13-21 y male	0.70

L = Length (cm)

Cr_s = Serum creatinine concentration (mg/dL)

Reference:

Schwartz GJ, Brion LP, and Spitzer A, "The Use of Plasma Creatinine Concentration for Estimating Glomerular Filtration Rate in Infants, Children and Adolescents," *Ped Clin N Amer*, 1987, 34:571-90.

Children 1-18 years (Traub SL, Johnson CE, *Am J Hosp Pharm*, 1980, 37:195-201)

Method 1: Equation:

$$Cl_{cr} = \frac{0.48 \times (\text{height}) \times BSA}{S_{cr} \times 1.73}$$

where

BSA = body surface area in m^2

Cl_{cr} = creatinine clearance in mL/min

S_{cr} = serum creatinine in mg/dL

Height = in cm

*This formula may not provide an accurate estimation of creatinine clearance for children under age 6 months and for patients with severe starvation or muscle wasting.

Method 2: Nomogram:

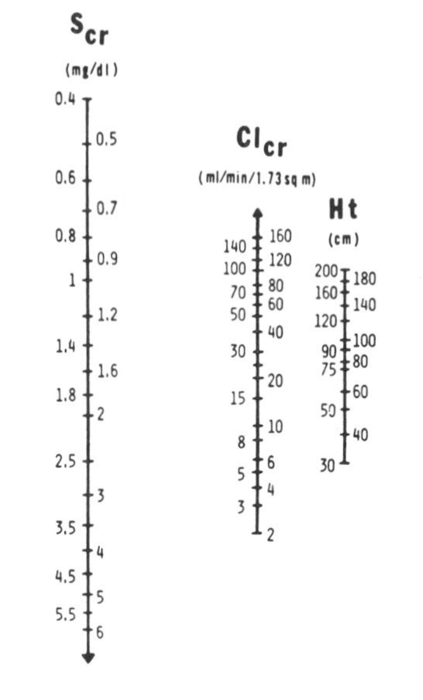

Adults (18 years and older)

Method 1: (Cockroft DW and Gault MH, *Nephron*, 1976, 16:31-41)

Estimated creatinine clearance (Cl_{cr}):
(mL/min)

$$\text{Male} = \frac{(140\text{-age})\ \text{IBW (kg)}}{72 \times \text{serum creatinine}}$$

Female = Estimated Cl_{cr} male x 0.85

Note: The use of the patient's ideal body weight (IBW) is recommended for the above formula except when the patient's actual body weight is less than ideal. Use of the IBW is especially important in obese patients.

Method 2: (Jelliffe RW, *Ann Intern Med*, 1973, 79:604)

Estimated creatinine clearance (Cl_{cr}):
(mL/min/1.73 m^2)

$$\text{Male} = \frac{98\text{-}0.8\ (\text{age-}20)}{\text{serum creatinine}}$$

Female = Estimated Cl_{cr} male x 0.90

RENAL FUNCTION TESTS

Endogenous creatinine clearance vs age (timed collection)

Creatinine clearance (mL/min/1.73 m²) = (Cr_uV/Cr_sT) (1.73/A)

where:

Cr_u = Urine creatinine concentration (mg/dL)
V = Total urine volume collected during sampling period (mL)
Cr_s = Serum creatinine concentration (mg/dL)
T = Duration of sampling period (min) (24 h = 1440 min)
A = Body surface area (m²) (see nomogram page ??)

Age-specific normal values

5-7 d	50.6±5.8 mL/min/1.73 m²
1-2 mo	64.6±5.8 mL/min/1.73 m²
5-8 mo	87.7±11.9 mL/min/1.73 m²
9-12 mo	86.9±8.4 mL/min/1.73 m²
≥18 mo	
male	124±26 mL/min/1.73 m²
female	109±13.5 mL/min/1.73 m²
Adults	
male	105±14 mL/min/1.73 m²
female	95±18 mL/min/1.73 m²

Note: In patients with renal failure (creatinine clearance <25 mL/min), creatinine clearance may be elevated over GFR because of tubular secretion of creatinine.

Serum BUN/Serum Creatinine Ratio

Serum BUN (mg/dL:serum creatinine (mg/dL)

Normal BUN:creatinine ratio is 10-15.

BUN:creatinine ratio >20 suggests prerenal azotemia (also seen with high urea-generation states such as GI bleeding).

BUN:creatinine ratio <5 may be seen with disorders affecting urea biosynthesis such as urea cycle enzyme deficiencies and with hepatitis.

Fractional Sodium Excretion

Fractional sodium secretion (FENa) = Na_uCr_s / Na_sCr_u x 100%

where:

Na_u = Urine sodium (mEq/L)
Na_s = Serum sodium (mEq/L)
Cr_u = Urine creatinine (mg/dL)
Cr_s = Serum creatinine (mg/dL)

FENa <1% suggests prerenal failure
FENa >2% suggest intrinsic renal failure
(for newborns, normal FENa is approximately 2.5%)

Note: Disease states associated with a falsely elevated FENa include severe volume depletion (>10%), early acute tubular necrosis and volume depletion in chronic renal disease. Disorders associated with a lowered FENa include acute glomerulonephritis, hemoglobinuric or myoglobinuric renal failure, nonoliguric acute tubular necrosis and acute urinary tract obstruction. In addition, FENa may be <1% in patients with acute renal failure **and** a second condition predisposing to sodium retention, eg, burns, congestive heart failure, nephrotic syndrome.

Urine Calcium/Urine Creatinine Ratio (spot sample)

Urine calcium (mg/dL): urine creatinine (mg/dL)

Normal values <0.21 (mean values 0.08 males, 0.06 females)

Premature infants show wide variability of calcium: creatinine ratio, and tend to have lower thresholds for calcium loss than older children. Prematures without nephrolithiasis had mean Ca:Cr ratio of 0.75 ± 0.76. Infants with nephrolithiasis had mean Ca:Cr ratio of 1.32 ± 1.03 (Jacinto, et al, *Pediatrics*, vol 81, p 31).

Urine Protein/Urine Creatinine Ratio (spot sample)

P_u/Cr_u	Total Protein Excretion ($mg/m^2/day$)
0.1	80
1	800
10	8000

where:

P_u = Urine protein concentration (mg/dL)
Cr_u = Urine creatinine concentration (mg/dL)

Serum Osmolality

Serum osmolality predicted = 2 x Na (mEq/L) = BUN (mg/dL) / 2.8 + glucose (mg/dL) / 18

High Anion Gap (see Toxicology section)

ACID/BASE ASSESSMENT

Henderson-Hasselbalch Equation

$pH = 6.1 + \log (HCO_3^- \ / (0.03)\ (pCO_2))$

Alveolar Gas Equation

$P_iO_2 = f_iO_2 \times$ (total atmospheric pressure – vapor pressure of H_2O at 37°C)

$= f_iO_2 \times (760 \text{ mm Hg} - 47 \text{ mm Hg})$

$P_AO_2 = P_iO_2 - P_ACO_2 / R$

Alveolar/arterial oxygen gradient = $P_AO_2 - P_aO_2$

Normal ranges:

Children	15-20 mm Hg
Adults	20-25 mm Hg

where:

- P_iO_2 = Oxygen partial pressure of inspired gas (mm Hg) (150 mm Hg in room air at sea level)
- f_iO_2 = Fractional pressure of oxygen in inspired gas (0.21 in room air)
- P_AO_2 = Alveolar oxygen partial pressure
- P_ACO_2 = Alveolar carbon dioxide partial pressure
- P_aO_2 = Arterial oxygen partial pressure
- R = Respiratory exchange quotient (typically 0.8, increases with high carbohydrate diet, decreases with high fat diet)

Acid/Base Disorders

Acute metabolic acidosis (<12 h duration)

$PaCO_2$ expected = $1.5\ (HCO_3^- + 8 \pm 2$

or

expected change in pCO = (1-1.5) x change in HCO_3^-

Acute metabolic alkalosis (<12 h duration)

expected change in pCO_2 = (0.5-1) x change in HCO_3^-

Acute respiratory acidosis (<6 h duration)

expected change in HCO_3^- = 0.1 x pCO_2

Acute respiratory acidosis (>6 h duration)

expected change in HCO_3^- = 0.4 x change in pCO_2

Acute respiratory alkalosis (<6 h duration)

expected change in HCO_3^- = 0.2 x change in pCO_2

Acute respiratory alkalosis (<6 h duration)

expected change in HCO_3^- = 0.5 x change in pCO_2

ACUTE DYSTONIC REACTIONS, MANAGEMENT

1. **Confirm that patient has stable airway and adequate respiratory activity.**
2. Administer **one** of the following:

   Diphenhydramine 0.7-1 mg/kg/dose I.V./P.O. q4-6h or prn

   or

   Hydroxyzine 0.5 mg/kg/dose I.M./P.O. q6h or prn
   (adult dose: 5-25 mg I.M./P.O. q6h)

   or

   Children >3 years: Benztropine 0.02-0.05 mg/kg/dose or maximum of 1-2 mg I.V./P.O. q4-6h or prn (avoid use in children younger than 3 years of age except in cases of extreme emergency)

Agents which predispose patients to acute dystonic reactions, such as phenothiazine neuroleptics or antiemetics, often have long therapeutic half-lives. Anticholinergic administration should therefore be continued for 6-24 hours after discontinuation of phenothiazine therapy.

PREPROCEDURE SEDATIVES IN CHILDREN

Purpose: The following table is a guide to aid the clinician in the selection of the most appropriate sedative to sedate a child for a procedure. One must also consider:

- Not all patients require sedation. It is dependent on the procedure and age of the child.
- When sedation is desired, one must consider the time of onset, the duration of action and the route of administration.
- Each of the following drugs is well absorbed when given by the suggested routes and doses.
- Each drug was assigned an "intensity" based upon the class of drug, dose and route.[1]
  - Conscious sedation: Patient able to maintain airway
  - Deep sedation: May be associated with partial or complete loss of protective reflexes
- Those drugs classified as producing deep sedation require more frequent monitoring postprocedure.
- For painful procedures, an analgesic agent needs to be administered.

References

1. Committee on Drugs, Section on Anesthesiology, "Guidelines for the Elective Use of Conscious Sedation, Deep Sedation and General Anesthesia in Pediatric Patients," *Pediatrics*, 1985, 76(2):317-21.
2. Roelofse JA, van der Bijl P, Stegmann DH, et al, "Preanesthetic Medication With Rectal Midazolam in Children Undergoing Dental Extractions," *J Oral Maxillofac Surg*, 1990, 48(8):791-7.
3. Elman DS and Denson JS, "Preanesthetic Sedation of Children With Intramuscular Methohexital Sodium," *Anesth Analg*, 1965, 44(5):494-8.
4. Miller JR, Grayson M, and Stoelting VK, "Sedation With Intramuscular Methohexital Sodium," *Am J Ophthalmol*, 1966, 62(1):38-43.
5. Burtles R and Astley B, "Lorazepam in Children," *Br J Anaesth*, 1983, 55:275-9.
6. Yager JY and Seshia SS, "Sublingual Lorazepam in Childhood Serial Seizures," *Am J Dis Child*, 1988, 142(9):931-2.
7. "Drug Evaluations," *AMA*, 1980.
8. Burckart GJ, White III TJ, Siegle RL, et al, "Rectal Thiopental Versus an Intramuscular Cocktail for Sedating Children Before Computer Tomography," *Am J Hosp Pharm*, 1980, 37:222-4.
9. Fell D, Gough MB, Northan AA, et al, "Diazepam Premedication in Children," *Anaesthesia*, 1985, 40:12-7.
10. Wilton NC, Leigh J, Rosen DR, et al, "Preanesthetic Sedation of Preschool Children Using Intranasal Midazolam," *Anesthesiology*, 1988, 60(6):972-5.

Preprocedure Sedatives in Children

	Route	Dose (mg/kg)	Onset (min)	Duration (h)	Intensity	Considerations
Chloral hydrate	P.O./P.R.	25–100	30–60	4–8	Conscious sedation	May cause hepatic neoplasms in rats; maximum single dose: 2 g
Diazepam[6,9] (Valium®)	P.O.	0.2–0.4; 90 min prior	60–90	6–8	Conscious sedation	Due to poor absorption and tissue irritation, I.M. route **not** recommended
	I.V.	0.1–0.2	5			Maximum dose I.V.: 10 mg
	P.R.	0.2–0.4	10			May use I.V. solution rectally
"DPT" cocktail[8] (Demerol® Phenergan® Thorazine®)	I.M.	Demerol® 1–2 Phenergan® 0.5–1 Thorazine® 0.5–1	30	2–14	Conscious sedation	May be mixed in single syringe; I.M. only
Fentanyl	P.O./trans-mucosal	15–20 μg/kg	30	30–60 min	Conscious sedation	
	I.M./I.V.	1–3 μg/kg	3–5			
Ketamine	P.O.	6–10; 30 min prior	30–45	10–30 min	Dissociative anesthesia; monitor as if deep sedation	Use only under direct supervision of physicians experienced in administering general anesthetics; has analgesic effects; may use injectable product orally diluted in a beverage of the patient's choice
	I.M.	3–7	7	10–30 min		
	I.V.	0.5–2	1	5–10 min		
Lorazepam[5] (Ativan®)	P.O.	0.05; 90–120 min prior	60	8–12	Conscious sedation	
	Deep I.M.	0.05; 90–120 min prior	30–60	8–12		
	I.V.	0.05; over 5–10 min	15–30	8–12		
Meperidine	P.O.	2–4	15–20	3–4	Conscious sedation	
	I.M.	0.5–2	15–20	3–4		Doses I.M./I.V. >2 mg/kg are considered deep sedation
	I.V.	0.5–2	10	2–3		

(continued)

	Route	Dose (mg/kg)	Onset (min)	Duration (h)	Intensity	Considerations
Methohexital[3,4] (Brevital®)	I.M.	5–10	5	1–1.5	Deep sedation	Maximum concentration for I.M./I.V.: 50 mg/mL; maximum I.M./I.V. dose: 200 mg
	I.V.	0.75–2	1	7–10 min		Greater incidence of adverse effects with I.V. use
	P.R.	20–25	5–10	1–1.5		Shorter duration of action than thiopental; rectal given as a 10% solution in sterile water
Midazolam[2,10] (Versed®)	P.O.	0.2–0.4; 30–45 min prior	30–45	1–2	Conscious sedation	Maximum oral dose: 15 mg
	Deep I.M.	0.08–0.1; 30–60 min prior	15–30	1–2		
	I.V.	0.08–0.15; give over 10–20 min	1–5	1–2		Maximum concentration: 1 mg/mL; maximum I.M./I.V. dose: 10 mg
	P.R.	0.3	20–30	1–2		Dilute injection in 5 mL NS and administer rectally
	Nasal spray	0.2	5–10	1–2		To administer nasally use injectable drug in a 1 or 3 mL syringe
Morphine	P.O.	0.3–0.5	20–30	3–4	Conscious sedation	
	I.M.	0.05–0.2	20–30	3–4		
	I.V.	0.05–0.2	10–15	2–3		
Pentobarbital	P.O./I.M./P.R.	2–6	10–25	1–4	Deep sedation	Maximum I.M./I.V./P.O./P.R. dose: 100 mg
	I.V.	1–3	1	15 min		
Thiopental[7,8] (Pentothal)	I.V.	4–6	0.5–1	5–10 min	Deep sedation	
	P.R.	25; immediately prior to procedure	10	1–5		Variable rectal absorption; may use additional 12.5 mg/kg if necessary; maximum rectal dose: 1–1.5 g

FEBRILE SEIZURES

A febrile seizure is defined as a seizure occurring for no reason other than an elevated temperature. The fever does not have an origin within the CNS. Fever is usually >102°F rectally, but the more rapid the rise in temperature, the more likely a febrile seizure may occur. About 4% of children develop febrile seizures at one time of their life. They usually occur between 3 months and 5 years of age with the majority occurring at 6 months to 3 years of age. There are 3 types of febrile seizures:

1. **Simple** febrile seizures are nonfocal febrile seizures of less than 15 minutes duration. They do not occur in multiples.
2. **Complex** febrile seizures are febrile seizures that are either focal, have a focal component, are longer than 15 minutes in duration or are multiple febrile seizures that occur within 30 minutes.
3. **Febrile status epilepticus** is a febrile seizure that is a generalized tonic clonic seizure lasting longer than 30 minutes.

Note: Febrile seizures should not be confused with a true epileptic seizure associated with a fever or a "seizure with fever." "Seizure with fever" includes seizures associated with acute neurologic illnesses like meningitis and Reye's syndrome.

Long-term prophylaxis with phenobarbital may reduce the risk of subsequent febrile seizures. After the first febrile seizure, long-term prophylaxis should be considered under any of the following:

1. Presence of abnormal neurological development or abnormal neurological exam
2. Febrile seizure was complex in nature:
   duration >15 minutes
   focal febrile seizure
   followed by transient or persistent neurological abnormalities
3. Positive family history of afebrile seizures (epilepsy)

Also consider long-term prophylaxis in certain cases if:

1. the child has multiple febrile seizures
2. the child is <12 months of age

Anticonvulsant prophylaxis is usually continued for 2 years or 1 year after the last seizure, whichever is longer. With the identification of phenobarbital's adverse effects on learning and cognitive function, many physicians will not start long-term phenobarbital prophylaxis after the first febrile seizure unless the patient has more than one of the above risk factors.

Daily administration of phenobarbital and therapeutic phenobarbital serum concentrations of ≥15 μg/mL decrease recurrence rates of febrile seizures. Valproic acid is also effective in preventing recurrences of febrile seizures, but is usually reserved for patients who have significant adverse effects to phenobarbital. Carbamazepine and phenytoin are **not** effective in preventing febrile seizures.

References:

Berg AT, Shinnar S, Hauser WA, et al, "Predictors of Recurrent Febrile Seizures: A Meta-Analytic Review," *Journal of Pediatrics*, 1990, 116:329-37.

NIH Consensus Statement, "Febrile Seizures: A Concensus of Their Significance, Evaluation and Treatment," *Pediatrics*, 1980, 66:1009-12.

ANTICONVULSANTS BY SEIZURE TYPE

Seizure Type	Age	Commonly Used	Alternatives
Primarily generalized tonic-clonic seizures	1-12 mo	Carbamazepine* Phenytoin Phenobarbital	Valproate
	1-6 y	Carbamazepine* Phenytoin Phenobarbital	Valproate
	6-11 y	Carbamazepine	Valproate Phenytoin Phenobarbital
Primarily generalized tonic-clonic seizures with absence or with myoclonic seizures	1 mo - 18 y	Valproate	Phenytoin** Phenobarbital** Carbamazepine**
Absence seizures	Any age	Ethosuximide	Valproate Clonazepam Diamox
Myoclonic seizures	Any age	Valproate Clonazepam	Phenytoin† Phenobarbital†
Tonic and atonic seizures	Any age	Valproate	Phenytoin† Clonazepam Phenobarbital†
Partial seizures	1-12 mo	Phenobarbital	Carbamazepine Phenytoin
	1-6 y	Carbamazepine*	Phenytoin Phenobarbital Valproate†
	6-18 y	Carbamazepine	Phenytoin Phenobarbital Valproate†
Infantile spasms		Corticotropin (ACTH)	Prednisone† Valproate† Clonazepam† Diazepam†

*Not FDA approved for children younger than 6 years of age.

†Not FDA approved for this indication.

**Phenytoin, phenobarbital, carbamazepine will not treat absence seizures. Addition of another anticonvulsant (ie, ethosuximide) would be needed.

COMA SCALES

Glasgow Coma Scale

Activity	Best Response	
Eye opening	Spontaneous	4
	To speech	3
	To pain	2
	None	1
Verbal	Oriented	5
	Confused	4
	Inappropriate words	3
	Nonspecific sounds	2
	None	1
Motor	Follows commands	6
	Localizes pain	5
	Withdraws to pain	4
	Abnormal flexion	3
	Extend	2
	None	1

Modified Coma Scale for Infants

Activity	Best Response	
Eye opening	Spontaneous	4
	To speech	3
	To pain	2
	None	1
Verbal	Coos, babbles	5
	Irritable	4
	Cries to pain	3
	Moans to pain	2
	None	1
Motor	Normal spontaneous movements	6
	Withdraw to touch	5
	Withdraws to pain	4
	Abnormal flexion	3
	Abnormal extension	2
	None	1

References: Jennett B and Teasdale G, *Lancet*, 1977.
James HE, *Pediatr Ann*, 1986, 15:16-22.

NORMAL RESPIRATORY RATES

Hour After Birth	Average Respiratory Rate	Range
1st hour	60 breaths per minute	20-100
2-6 hours	50 breaths per minute	20-80
>6 hours	30-40 per minute	20-60

Age (years)	Mean RR (breaths/minute)
0-2	25-30
3-9	20-25
10-18	16-20

BLOOD LEVEL SAMPLING TIME GUIDELINES

Drug	Infusion Time	Therapeutic Range	When to Draw Levels
Amikacin sulfate			
I.V.	30 min	Peak: 20-30 μg/mL	Peak: 30 min after end of 30 min infusion
		Trough: <10 μg/mL	Trough: Within 30 min before next dose
I.M.			Peak: 1 h after I.M. injection
			Trough: Within 30 min before next dose
Carbamazepine		4-12 μg/mL	Just before next dose
Chloramphenicol			
I.V.	30 min	Peak: 15-25 μg/mL	Peak: 90 min after end of 30 min infusion
			Trough: Just before next dose
P.O.			Peak: 2 h post P.O. dose
Cyclosporine			
I.V./P.O.		BMT 100-200 ng/mL Liver transplant 200-300 ng/mL Renal transplant 100-200 ng/mL	Just before next dose
Digoxin			
I.V./P.O.		Age and disease related: 0.8-2 ng/mL	6 h post dose to just before next dose
Ethosuximide			
P.O.		40-100 μg/mL	Just before next dose
Flucytosine			
P.O.		25-100 μg/mL	Peak: 2 h post dose after at least 4 d of therapy
Gentamicin			
I.V.	30 min	Peak: 4-10 μg/mL	Peak: 30 min after end of 30 min infusion
		Trough: 0.5-2 μg/mL	Trough: Within 30 min before next dose
I.M.			Peak: 1 h after I.M. injection
			Trough: Within 30 min before next dose
Phenobarbital		15-40 μg/mL	Trough: Just before next dose
Phenytoin			
P.O.		10-20 μg/mL	Trough: Just before next dose
Theophylline			
I.V. bolus	30 min	10-20 μg/mL	Peak: 30 min after end of 30 min infusion
Continuous infusion			16-24 h after the start or change in a constant I.V. infusion
P.O. liquid, fast-release tablet (Somophyllin®, Slo-Phyllin® liquid & tablet)			Peak: 1 h post dose
			Trough: Just before next dose
P.O. slow-release (Theo-Dur®, Slo-Phyllin® GC, Slo-bid®)			Peak: 4 h post dose
			Trough: Just before next dose
Tobramycin			
I.V.	30 min	Peak: 4-10 μg/mL	Peak: 30 min after end of 30 min infusion
		Trough: 0.5-2 μg/mL	Trough: Within 30 min before next dose
I.M.			Peak: 1 h post I.M. injection
			Trough: Within 30 min before next dose

(continued)

Drug	Infusion Time	Therapeutic Range	When to Draw Levels
Trimethoprim			
I.V., dose 20 mg/kg	60 min	Peak: 5-10 μg/mL	Peak: 30 min after end of 60 min infusion
I.V., dose 8-10 mg/kg		Peak 1-3 μg/mL	
P.O.			Peak: 1 h post dose
Valproic acid			
P.O.		50-100 μg/mL	Trough: Just before next dose
Vancomycin	60 min	Peak: 25-40 μg/mL	Peak: 20-30 min after end of 60 min infusion*
		Trough: 5-15 μg/mL	Trough: Within 30 min before next dose

*Some institutions may draw vancomycin peak 1 h after 1 h infusion and accept the lower range of therapeutic.

OVERDOSE AND TOXICOLOGY INFORMATION*

Drug or Drug Class	Signs/Symptoms	Treatment/Comments
Acetaminophen	Nausea, vomiting, diaphoresis, delirium, fever, coma, vascular collapse; hepatic necrosis, transient azotemia, renal tubular necrosis	Assess severity of ingestion; for adolescents and adults, doses ≥140 mg/kg are thought to be toxic. Obtain serum concentration ≥4 hours post ingestion and use acetaminophen nomogram to evaluate need for acetylcysteine. Empty stomach with ipecac (if <1 hour post ingestion) or gastric lavage. May administer activated charcoal for one dose, this may decrease absorption of acetylcysteine if given within one hour of acetylcysteine. For unknown ingested quantities and for significant ingestion give acetylcysteine orally (diluted 1:4 with juice or carbonated beverage); initial: 140 mg/kg then give 70 mg/kg every 4 hours for 17 doses.
Alpha-adrenergic blocking agents	Hypotension, drowsiness	Induce emesis, give activated charcoal, additional treatment is symptomatic; use I.V. fluids, dopamine, or ephedrine to treat hypotension. Epinephrine may worsen hypotension due to beta effects.
Aminoglycosides	Ototoxicity, nephrotoxicity, neuromuscular toxicity	Hemodialysis or peritoneal dialysis may be useful in patients with decreased renal function.
Anticholinergics, antihistamines	Coma, hallucinations, delirium, tachycardia, dry skin, urinary retention, dilated pupils	For life-threatening arrhythmias or seizures. Children: I.V., slow: Physostigmine 0.01-0.03 mg/kg/dose up to 0.5 mg/dose over 2-3 minutes, repeat in 5 minutes (maximum total dose is 2 mg). Adolescents and adults: 2 mg/dose physostigmine, may repeat 1-2 mg in 20 minutes and give 1-4 mg slow I.V. over 5-10 minutes if signs and symptoms recur.
Anticholinesterase agents	Nausea, vomiting, diarrhea, miosis, CNS depression, excessive salivation, excessive sweating, muscle weakness	Suction oral secretions, decontaminate skin, atropinize patient; atropine dose must be individualized Infants and children: Initial dose: 0.01-0.02 mg/kg/dose; may need to increase as high as 0.05 mg/kg Adults: Initial atropine dose: 1 mg; may need to increase to 2-5 mg/dose; pralidoxime (2-PAM) may need to be added for severe intoxications.

*As for all overdoses and toxic ingestions, provide airway, breathing, and cardiac support; use appropriate general poisoning management and give general supportive therapy when needed (eg, I.V. fluids, blood pressure support, control seizures, etc). Consult more specific toxicology reference (eg, Poisondex®) for further information.

(continued)

Drug or Drug Class	Signs/Symptoms	Treatment/Comments
Barbiturates	Respiratory depression, circulatory collapse, bradycardia, hypotension, hypothermia, slurred speech, confusion	Repeated oral doses of activated charcoal given every 3-6 hours will increase clearance. Children: 0.5-1 g/kg/dose Adults: 30-60 g Assure GI motility, adequate hydration, and renal function. Urinary alkalinization with I.V. sodium bicarbonate will increase renal elimination of longer acting barbiturates (eg, phenobarbital)
Benzodiazepines	Respiratory depression, apnea, hypoactive reflexes, hypotension, slurred speech, unsteady gait, coma	For comatose patient, use gastric lavage with endotracheal tube in place to prevent aspiration; flumazenil, a benzodiazepine antagonist, can be used to reverse the effects of benzodiazepines. See flumazenil monograph for dose. Action of flumazenil may be shorter than duration of benzodiazepine; repeat doses as needed. Norepinephrine, phenylephrine, or dopamine may be used to treat hypotension; dialysis is of limited value; support blood pressure and respiration.
Beta-adrenergic blockers	Hypotension, bronchospasm, bradycardia, hyperglycemia, or hypoglycemia	Induce emesis, followed by activated charcoal; treat symptomatically; glucagon, atropine, isoproterenol, or cardiac pacing may be needed to treat bradycardia, conduction defects, or hypotension
Carbamazepine	Dizziness, drowsiness, ataxia, involuntary movements, opisthotonos, seizures, nausea, vomiting, agitation, nystagmus, coma, urinary retention, respiratory depression, tachycardia	Use supportive therapy, general poisoning management as needed; use repeated oral doses of activated charcoal given every 3-6 hours to decrease serum concentrations; charcoal hemoperfusion may be needed; treat hypotension with I.V. fluids, dopamine, or norepinephrine, monitor EKG; diazepam may control convulsions but may exacerbate respiratory depression
Cardiac glycosides	Hyperkalemia may develop rapidly and result in life-threatening cardiac arrhythmias, progressive bradyarrhythmias, 2nd or 3rd degree heart block unresponsive to atropine, ventricular fibrillation, asystole	Obtain serum drug level, induce emesis or perform gastric lavage; give activated charcoal to reduce further absorption; atropine may reverse heart block, phenytoin will improve A-V conduction; digoxin immune Fab (digoxin specific antibody fragments) is used in life-threatening cases, each 40 mg of digoxin immune Fab binds with 0.6 mg of digoxin
Heparin	Severe hemorrhage	1 mg of protamine sulfate will neutralize approximately 90 units of heparin sodium (bovine) or 115 units of heparin sodium (porcine) or 100 units of heparin calcium (porcine)

(continued)

Drug or Drug Class	Signs/Symptoms	Treatment/Comments
Hydantoin derivatives	Nausea, vomiting, nystagmus, slurred speech, ataxia, coma	Gastric lavage or emesis; repeated oral doses of activated charcoal may increase clearance of phenytoin. Use 0.5-1 g/kg (30-60 g/dose) activated charcoal every 3-6 hours until nontoxic serum concentration is obtained; assure adequate GI motility, supportive therapy; dialysis may be helpful
Iron	Lethargy, nausea, vomiting, green or tarry stools, hypotension, weak rapid pulse, metabolic acidosis, shock, coma, hepatic necrosis, renal failure, local GI erosions	Induce emesis if awake or lavage with saline solution; give deferoxamine mesylate I.V. at 15 mg/kg/hour in cases of severe poisoning (serum Fe $>$350 μg/mL) and continue chelation therapy for 24 hours after child is excreting normal color urine; urine output should be maintained $>$2 mL/kg/hour to avoid hypovolemic shock
Isoniazid	Nausea, vomiting, blurred vision, CNS depression, intractable seizures, coma, metabolic acidosis	Control seizures with diazepam, give pyridoxine I.V. equal dose to the suspected overdose of isoniazid; lavage after seizure control is reached; force diuresis with I.V. fluids; hemo- or peritoneal dialysis may be beneficial in severe cases
Nonsteroidal anti-inflammatory drugs	Dizziness, abdominal pain, sweating, apnea, nystagmus, cyanosis, hypotension, coma	Induce emesis; give activated charcoal via NG tube; provide symptomatic and supportive care. Forced alkaline diuresis may be helpful for acidic compounds (eg, ibuprofen)
Opiates and morphine analogs	Respiratory depression, miosis, hypothermia, bradycardia, circulatory collapse, pulmonary edema, apnea	Establish airway and adequate ventilation; give naloxone 0.1 mg/kg for children up to 5 years of age or 20 kg; for those $>$5 years or 20 kg give 2 mg naloxone; repeat doses every 2-3 minutes if needed; additional doses may be needed every 20-60 minutes. May need to institute continuous infusion, as duration of action of opiates can be longer than duration of action of naloxone

(continued)

Drug or Drug Class	Signs/Symptoms	Treatment/Comments
Phenothiazines	Deep, unarousable sleep, anticholinergic symptoms, extrapyramidal signs, diaphoresis, rigidity, tachycardia, cardiac dysrhythmias, hypotension, or hypertension	Emesis or gastric lavage; do **not** dialyze; use I.V. benztropine mesylate 0.02-0.05 mg/kg/dose or for adults 1-2 mg/dose slowly over 3-6 minutes for extrapyramidal signs; use loading dose of phenytoin 10-15 mg/kg slow I.V. push for ventricular dysrhythmias; use I.V. fluids and norepinephrine or phenylephrine to treat hypotension; avoid epinephrine which may cause hypotension due to phenothiazine-induced alpha-adrenergic blockade and unopposed epinephrine B_2 action; dantrolene orally 0.5 mg/kg/dose every 12 hours may help with the rigidity
Salicylates	Nausea, vomiting, respiratory alkalosis, hyperthermia, dehydration, hyperapnea, tinnitus, headache, dizziness, metabolic acidosis, coma	Induce emesis or gastric lavage immediately; give charcoal with cathartic via NG tube; correct fluid imbalance by giving D_5LR at 10-20 mL/kg/hour for 1-2 hours, more rapid fluid resuscitation may be needed for patients in shock; use sodium bicarbonate to correct metabolic acidosis and enhance renal elimination by alkalinizing the urine; give supplemental potassium after renal function has been determined to be adequate. Monitor electrolytes; obtain serum salicylate level $\geq$6 hours post ingestion; use poisoning nomogram to assess the significance of the ingestion and the need for more aggressive measures
Tricyclic antidepressants	Agitation, confusion, hallucinations, urinary retention, hypothermia, hypotension, tachycardia	Maintain normal temperature; correct acidosis with Na bicarbonate to increase protein binding and decrease free fraction; correction of acidosis may decrease cardiovascular toxicities; avoid disopyramide, procainamide, and quinidine; lidocaine, phenytoin or propranolol may be necessary; reserve physostigmine for refractory life-treating anticholinergic toxicities. For life-threatening arrhythmias or seizures; Children: I.V., slow: Physostigmine 0.01-0.03 mg/kg/dose up to 0.5 mg/dose over 2-3 minutes, repeat in 5 minutes (maximum total dose is 2 mg). Adolescents and adults: 2 mg/dose physostigmine, may repeat 1-2 mg in 20 minutes and give 1-4 mg slow I.V. over 5-10 minutes if signs and symptoms recur.

(continued)

Drug or Drug Class	Signs/Symptoms	Treatment/Comments
Warfarin	Internal or external hemorrhage, hematuria	For moderate overdoses, give oral or I.V. phytonadione; for severe hemorrhage, give fresh frozen plasma or whole blood
Xanthine derivatives	Vomiting, abdominal pain, bloody diarrhea, tachycardia, extrasystoles, tachypnea, tonic/clonic seizures	Induce emesis, except in a convulsive patient; give activated charcoal orally; repeated oral doses of activated charcoal may increase clearance; use 0.5-1 g/kg (30-60 g/dose) of activated charcoal every 3-6 hours until nontoxic serum concentrations are obtained. Assure adequate GI motility, supportive therapy; charcoal hemoperfusion can also be effective in decreasing serum concentrations.

ANION GAP

Definition: The difference in concentration between unmeasured cation and anion equivalents in serum.

Anion gap = $Na^+ - Cl^- - HCO_3^-$
(The normal anion gap is 10-14 mEq/L.)

Differential diagnosis of increased anion gap
- Organic anions
  - Lactate (sepsis, hypovolemia, large tumor burden)
  - Pyruvate
  - Uremia
  - Ketoacidosis (β-hydroxybutyrate and acetoacetate)
  - Amino acids and their metabolites
  - Other organic acids (eg, formate from methanol, glycolate from ethylene glycol)
- Inorganic anions
  - Hyperphosphatemia
  - Sulfates
  - Nitrates
- Medications and toxins
  - Penicillins and cephalosporins
  - Salicylates (including aspirin)
  - Cyanide
  - Carbon monoxide

Differential diagnosis of decreased anion gap
- Organic cations
  - Hypergammaglobulinemia
- Inorganic cations
  - Hyperkalemia
  - Hypercalcemia
  - Hypermagnesemia
- Medications and toxins
  - Lithium
- Hypoalbuminemia

OSMOLALITY

Definition: The summed concentrations of all osmotically active solute particles.

Predicted serum osmolality =
$2\ Na^+ + \text{glucose (mg/dL)} / 18 + \text{BUN (mg/dL)} / 2.8$

The normal range of serum osmolality is 285-295 mOsm/L.

Differential diagnosis of increased serum osmolal gap ($>$10 mOsm/L)
- Medications and toxins
  - Alcohols (ethanol, methanol, isopropanol, glycerol, ethylene glycol)
  - Mannitol
  - Paraldehyde

SERUM SALICYLATE INTOXICATION NOMOGRAM

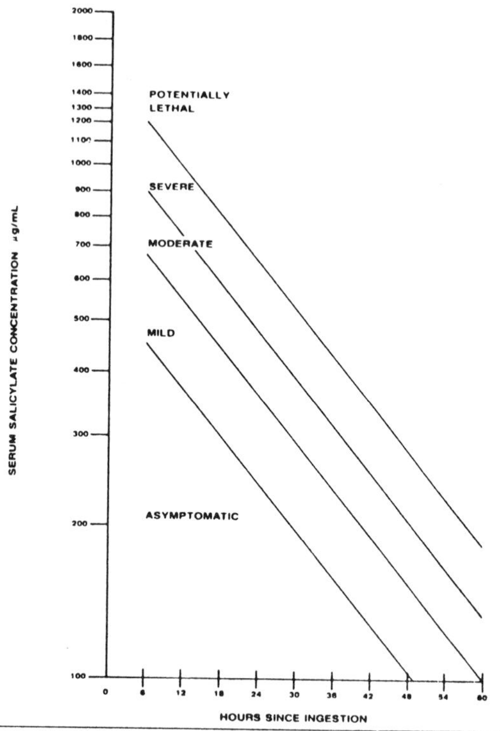

Nomogram relating serum salicylate concentration and estimated severity of intoxication at varying intervals following ingestion of a single toxic dose of salicylate. Modified from Done AK. Salicylate intoxication. Pediatrics. 1960; 26:800–7. © American Academy of Pediatrics 1960.

ACETAMINOPHEN TOXICITY NOMOGRAM

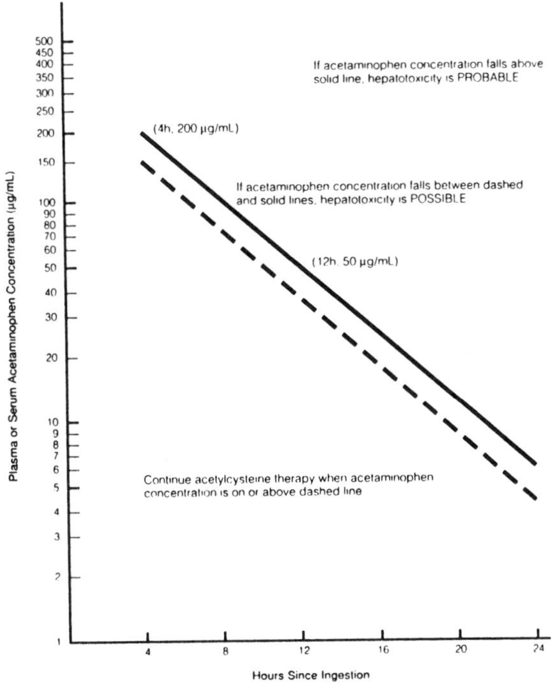

Nomogram relating plasma or serum acetaminophen concentration and probability of hepatotoxicity at varying intervals following ingestion of a single toxic dose of acetaminophen. Modified from Rumack BH, Matthew H. Acetaminophen poisoning and toxicity. Pediatrics. 1975; 55:871-6. © American Academy of Pediatrics 1975.—and from Rumack BH et al. Acetaminophen overdose. Arch Intern Med. 1981; 141:380-5. © American Medical Association.

CONTROLLED SUBSTANCES

Schedule I = C-I

The drugs and other substances in this schedule have no legal medical uses except research. They have a **high** potential for abuse. They include opiates, opium derivatives and hallucinogens.

Schedule II = C-II

The drugs and other substances in this schedule have legal medical uses and a **high** abuse potential which may lead to severe dependence. They include former "Class A" narcotics, amphetamines, barbiturates and other drugs.

Schedule III = C-III

The drugs and other substances in this schedule have legal medical uses and a **lesser** degree of abuse potential which may lead to **moderate** dependence. They include former "Class B" narcotics and other drugs.

Schedule IV = C-IV

The drugs and other substances in this schedule have legal medical uses and **low** abuse potential which may lead to **moderate** dependence. They include barbiturates, benzodiazepines, propoxyphenes and other drugs.

Schedule V = C-V

The drugs and other substances in this schedule have legal medical uses and **low** abuse potential which may lead to **moderate** dependence. They include narcotic cough preparations, diarrhea preparations and other drugs.

Note: These are federal classifications. Your individual state may place a substance into a more restricted category. When this occurs, the more restricted category applies. Consult your state law.

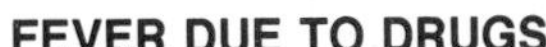

FEVER DUE TO DRUGS

p-Aminosalicylic acid
Amphotericin
Antihistamines
Asparaginase
Barbiturates
Bleomycin
Cephalosporins
Iodides
Methyldopa
Penicillins
Phenolphthalein
Phenytoin
Procainamide
Quinidine
Sulfonamides
Thiouracil

Abstracted from Harrison's *Principles of Internal Medicine*, 11 ed, Braunwald E, ed, New York, NY: McGraw-Hill Book Co, 1987.

DISCOLORATION OF FECES DUE TO DRUGS

Black

Acetazolamide
Alcohols
Alkalies
Aminophylline
Amphetamine
Amphotericin
Antacids
Anticoagulants
Aspirin
Betamethasone
Charcoal
Chloramphenicol
Chlorpropamide
Clindamycin
Corticosteroids
Cortisone
Cyclophosphamide
Cytarabine
Dicumarol
Digitalis
Ethacrynic acid
Ferrous salts
Floxuridine
Fluorouracil
Halothane
Heparin
Hydralazine
Hydrocortisone
Ibuprofen
Indomethacin
Iodine drugs
Iron salts
Levarterenol
Levodopa
Manganese
Melphalan
Methylprednisolone
Methotrexate
Methylene blue
Oxyphenbutazone
Paraldehyde
Phenacetin
Phenolphthalein
Phenylbutazone
Phenylephrine
Phosphorous
Potassium salts
Prednisolone
Procarbazine
Pyrvinium
Reserpine
Salicylates
Sulfonamides
Tetracycline
Theophylline
Thiotepa
Triamcinolone
Warfarin

Blue

Chloramphenicol
Methylene blue

Dark Brown

Dexamethasone

Gray

Colchicine

Green

Indomethacin
Iron
Medroxyprogesterone

Greenish Gray

Oral antibiotics
Oxyphenbutazone
Phenylbutazone

Light Brown

Anticoagulants

Orange-Red

Phenazopyridine
Rifampin

Pink

Anticoagulants
Aspirin
Heparin
Oxyphenbutazone
Phenylbutazone
Salicylates

Red

Anticoagulants
Aspirin
Heparin
Oxyphenbutazone
Phenolphthalein
Phenylbutazone
Pyrvinium
Salicylates
Tetracycline syrup

Red-Brown

Oxyphenbutazone
Phenylbutazone
Rifampin

Tarry

Ergot preparations
Ibuprofen
Salicylates
Warfarin

White/Speckling

Aluminum hydroxide
Antibiotics (oral)
Indocyanine green

Yellow

Senna

Yellow-Green

Senna

Adapted from Drugdex® — Drug Consults, Micromedex, vol 62, Rocky Mountain Drug Consultation Center, Denver, CO: November, 1989.

DISCOLORATION OF URINE DUE TO DRUGS

Black
Cascara
Ferrous salts
Iron dextran
Levodopa
Methocarbamol
Methyldopa
Naphthalene
Phenacetin
Phenols
Quinine
Sulfonamides

Blue
Anthraquinone
Indigo blue
Indigo carmine
Methocarbamol
Methylene blue
Nitrofurans
Resorcinol
Triamterene

Blue-Green
Amitriptyline
Anthraquinone
DeWitt's pills
Doan's® pills
Indigo blue
Indigo carmine
Methylene blue

Brown
Anthraquinone dyes
Cascara
Levodopa
Methocarbamol
Methyldopa
Metronidazole
Nitrofurans
Nitrofurantoin
Phenacetin
Primaquine
Quinine
Rifampin
Senna
Sodium diatrizoate
Sulfonamides

Brown-Black
Quinine

Dark
p-Aminosalicylic acid
Cascara
Levodopa
Metronidazole
Nitrites
Phenacetin
Phenol
Primaquine
Quinine
Resorcinol
Riboflavin
Senna

Green
Anthraquinone
DeWitt's pills
Indigo blue
Indigo carmine
Indomethacin
Methocarbamol
Methylene blue
Nitrofurans
Phenols
Resorcinol
Suprofen

Green-Yellow
DeWitt's pills
Methylene blue

Milky
Phosphates

Orange
Chlorzoxazone
Dihydroergotamine mesylate
Heparin sodium
Phenazopyridine
Rifampin
Sulfasalazine
Warfarin

Orange-Red
Chlorzoxazone
Doxidan
Phenazopyridine
Rifampin

Orange-Yellow
Fluorescein sodium
Rifampin
Sulfasalazine

Pink
Aminopyrine
Anthraquinone dyes
Danthron
Deferoxamine
Merbromin
Phenolphthalein
Phenothiazines
Phenytoin
Salicylates

Red
Anthraquinone
Cascara
Daunorubicin
Dimethylsulfoxide
DMSO
Doxorubicin
Heparin
Ibuprofen
Methyldopa

Red *(cont)*
Oxyphenbutazone
Phenacetin
Phenazopyridine
Phenolphthalein
Phenothiazines
Phensuximide
Phenylbutazone
Phenytoin
Rifampin
Senna

Red-Brown
Cascara
Methyldopa
Oxyphenbutazone
Phenacetin
Phenolphthalein
Phenothiazines
Phenylbutazone
Phenytoin
Quinine

Red-Purple
Chlorzoxazone
Ibuprofen
Phenacetin
Senna

Rust
Cascara
Chloroquine
Metronidazole
Nitrofurantoin
Phenacetin
Riboflavin
Senna
Sulfonamides

Yellow
Nitrofurantoin
Phenacetin
Riboflavin
Sulfasalazine

Yellow-Brown
Cascara
Chloroquine
DeWitt's pills
Methylene blue
Metronidazole
Nitrofurantoin
Primaquine
Quinacrine
Senna
Sulfonamides

Yellow-Pink
Cascara
Senna

Adapted from Drugdex® — Drug Consults, Micromedex, vol 62, Rocky Mountain Drug Consultation Center, Denver, CO: November, 1989.

MILLIEQUIVALENTS FOR SELECTED IONS

Approximate Milliequivalents — Weights of Selected Ions

Salt	mEq/g Salt	Mg Salt/mEq
Calcium carbonate ($CaCO_3$)	20	50
Calcium chloride ($CaCl_2 \bullet 2H_2O$)	14	73
Calcium gluconate (Ca $gluconate_2 \bullet 1H_2O$)	4	224
Calcium lactate (Ca $lactate_2 \bullet 5H_2O$)	6	154
Magnesium sulfate ($MgSO_4$)	16	60
Magnesium sulfate ($MgSO_4 \bullet 7H_2O$)	8	123
Potassium acetate (K acetate)	10	98
Potassium chloride (KCl)	13	75
Potassium citrate (K_3 citrate $\bullet 1H_2O$)	9	108
Potassium iodide (KI)	6	166
Sodium bicarbonate ($NaHCO_3$)	12	84
Sodium chloride (NaCl)	17	58
Sodium citrate (Na_3 citrate $\bullet 2H_2O$)	10	98
Sodium iodide (NaI)	7	150
Sodium lactate (Na lactate)	9	112
Zinc sulfate ($ZnSO_4 \bullet 7H_2O$)	7	144

Valences and Approximate Weights of Selected Ions

Substance	Electrolyte	Valence	Ionic Wt
Calcium	Ca^{++}	2	40
Chloride	Cl^-	1	35.5
Magnesium	Mg^{++}	2	24
Phosphate	PO_4^{---}	3	95*
	HPO_4^{--}	2	96
	$H_2PO_4^-$	1	97
Potassium	K^+	1	39
Sodium	Na^+	1	23
Sulfate	SO_4^{--}	2	96*

*The atomic weight of phosphorus is 31, and of sulfur is 32.

SODIUM CONTENT OF SELECTED MEDICINALS

Name and Dosage Unit*	Sodium mg	Sodium mEq
Antibiotics		
Amikacin sulfate, 1 g	29.9	1.3
Aminosalicylate sodium, 1 g	109	4.7
Ampicillin, suspension 250 mg/5 mL, 5 mL	10	0.4
Ampicillin sodium, 1 g	66.7	3
Azlocillin sodium, 1 g	50	2.2
Carbenicillin disodium 382 mg (tablet)	22	1
Cefazolin sodium, 1 g	47	2
Cefotaxime sodium, 1 g	30.5	2.2
Cefoxitin sodium, 1 g	53	2.3
Ceftriaxone sodium, 1 g	83	3.6
Cefuroxime, 1 g	54.2	2.4
Chloramphenicol sodium succinate, 1 g	51.8	2.3
Dicloxacillin, 250 mg (capsule)	13	0.6
Dicloxacillin, suspension 65 mg/5 mL	27	1.2
Erythromycin ethyl succinate, suspension 200 mg/5 mL	29	1.3
Erythromycin Base Filmtab®, 250 mg	70	3
Methicillin sodium, 1 g	66.7	2.9
Metronidazole, 500 mg I.V.	322	14
Mezlocillin sodium, 1 g	42.6	1.9
Moxalactam sodium, 1 g	88	3.8
Nafcillin sodium, 1 g	66.7	2.9
Nitrofurantoin, suspension 25 mg/5 mL	7	0.3
Penicillin G potassium, 1,000,000 units I.V.	7.6	0.3
Penicillin G sodium, 1,000,000 units I.V.	46	2
Penicillin V potassium, suspension, 250 mg/5 mL	38	1.7
Piperacillin sodium, 1 g	42.6	1.8
Ticarcillin disodium, 1 g	119.6	5.2
Antacids, Liquid (content per 5 mL)		
Amphojel®	<2.3	<0.1
ALternaGEL®	2	0.1
Basaljel®	2.4	0.1
Extra Strength Maalox®-Plus	0.65	~0.05
Gaviscon®	13	0.57
Maalox®	1.3	0.06
Tums E-X™	<4.8	<0.2
Sodium Content of Miscellaneous Medicinals		
Acetazolamide sodium, 500 mg	47.2	2.05
Chlorothiazide sodium, 500 mg	57.5	2
Cisplatin, 10 mg	35.4	1.54
Edetate calcium disodium, 1 g	122	5.3
Fleet® Enema, 4.5 oz	5000†	218
Fleet® Phospho®-Soda, 20 mL	2217	96.4
Hydrocortisone sodium succinate, 1 g	47.5	2.07
Hypaque® M 75%, injection, 20 mL	200	8.7
Hypaque® M 90%, injection, 20 mL	220	9.6
Metamucil® Instant Mix (orange)	6	0.27
Methotrexate sodium, 100 mg vial	20	0.86
Methotrexate sodium, 100 mg vial (low sodium)	15	0.65
Naproxen sodium, 250 mg (tablet)	23	1
Neutra-Phos®, capsule and 75 mL reconstituted solution	164	7.13
Oragrafin® (capsule)	19	0.8
Pentobarbital sodium, 50 mg/mL, 1 mL vial	5	0.2
Phenobarbital sodium, 65 mg, 1 mL vial	6	0.3
Phenytoin sodium, 1 g	88	3.8
Promethazine expectorant, 5 mL	53	2.3
Shohl's solution modified, 1 mL	23	1
Sodium ascorbate, 500 mg acid equivalent	65.3	2.84
Sodium bicarbonate, 50 mL 8.4%	1150	50
Sodium nitroprusside, 50 mg	7.8	0.34
Sodium polystyrene sulfonate, 1 g	94.3‡	4.1
Thiopental sodium, 1 g	86.8	3.8
Valproate sodium, 250 mg/5 mL, 5 mL	23	1

*Product formulations and hence sodium content are subject to change by the manufacturer.

†Average systemic absorption 250-300 mg.

‡Total sodium content. Only about 33% is liberated in clinical use.

SUGAR-FREE LIQUID PHARMACEUTICALS

The following sugar-free liquid preparations are listed by therapeutic category, and alphabetically within each category. Please note that product formulations are subject to change by the manufacturer. Some of these products may contain sorbitol, xylitol, or other sweeteners which may be partially metabolized to provide calories.

Analgesics

Acetaminophen Elixir (various)
APAP/APAP Plus
Aspirin/Buffered Aspirin (Medique®)
Bufferin® A/F Nite Time
Children's Anacin-3® Infants Drops
Children's Myapap® Elixir
Children's Panadol® Drops, Liquid, and Chewable Tablets
Children's Tylenol® Chewable Tablets
Conex® Liquid
Conex® With Codeine Liquid
Dolanex® Elixir
Extra Strength Tylenol® PM
Febrol® and Febrol® EX
I-Prin®
Methadone Hydrochloride Intensol
MS-Aid®
Myapap® Drops
No Drowsiness Tylenol®
Pain-Off®
Paregoric USP (Abbott)
Sep-A-Soothe® II
St Joseph® Aspirin-Free Liquid and Drops
Tempra® Chewable Tablets
Tylenol® Drops

Antacids/Antiflatulents

Alcalak®
Aldroxicon®
Almag® Suspension
Aludrox® Suspension
Aluminum Hydroxide Suspension
Calglycine® Tablets
Camalox® Suspension
Citrocarbonate® Granules
Creamalin® Suspension
Delcid®
Di-Gel® Liquid (mint, lemon & orange flavored)
Digestamic®
Dimacid®
Gaviscon® Liquid
Gelusil® II
Gelusil® Liquid
Gelusil® Liquid Flavor Pack
Gelusil-M® Liquid
Kolantyl® Gel
Maalox® Plus Suspension
Maalox® Suspension
Maalox® Therapeutic Concentrate
Magnatril® Suspension

Magnesia and Alumina Oral Suspension USP (Abbott, Phillips Roxane)
Mallamint® Chewable Tablets
Marblen® Suspension and Tablets
Medi-Seltzer®/Plus
Milk of Bismuth
Milk of Magnesia USP
Mylanta® Liquid
Mylanta®-II Liquid
Mylicon® Drops
Nephrox® Suspension
Nutrajel®
Nutramag®
Pepto-Bismol® Liquid and Tablets
Phosphaljel® Suspension
Riopan Plus®
Riopan® Suspension
Silain-Gel® Liquid
Trisogel®
Titralac® Liquid
Titralac® Plus Liquid
WinGel® Liquid and Tablets

Antiasthmatics

Aerolate® Liquid
Alupent® Syrup
Choledyl® Pediatric Syrup
Droxine®
Elixophyllin® Elixir
Elixophyllin®-GG Liquid
Lanophyllin® Elixir
Lixolin® Liquid
Lufyllin® Elixir
Metaprel® Syrup
Mucomyst®-10
Mucomyst®-20
Mudrane® GG Elixir
Neothylline® Elixir
Neothylline® G
Organidin® Solution
Slo-Phyllin® 80 Syrup
Somophyllin® Oral Liquid
Somophyllin®-DF Oral Liquid
Tedral® Elixir and Suspension
Theolair™ 80 Syrup
Theolixir®
Theon® Syrup
Theo-Organidin® Elixir
Theophylline Elixir (Phillips Roxane)

Antidepressants

Sinequan® Oral Concentrate

Antidiarrheals

Corrective Mixture With Paregoric
Diasorb® Liquid and Tablets
Di-Gon® II

Diotame®
Donnagel®
Infantol® Pink
Kalicon® Suspension
Kaolin Mixture With Pectin NF (Abbott)
Kaolin-Pectin Suspension (Phillips Roxane)
Konsyl® Powder
Lomanate®
Lomotil® Liquid
Paregoric USP (various)
Parepectolin® (various)
Pepto-Bismol®
St Joseph® Antidiarrheal

Antiepileptics

Mysoline® Suspension
Paradione® Solution

Antihistamine-Decongestants

Actifed® With Codeine
Actifed® Syrup
Actidil® Syrup
Bromphen® Elixir
Dimetane® Decongestant Elixir
Dimetapp® Elixir
Hay-Febrol® Liquid
Isoclor® Liquid and Capsules
Naldecon® Pediatric Drops and Syrup
Naldecon® Syrup
Novahistine® Elixir
Phenergan® Fortis Syrup
Phenergan® Syrup
Rondec® DM Drops
Ryna® Liquid
S-T® Forte® Liquid
Tavist® Syrup
Trind® Liquid
Veltap® Elixir
Vistaril® Oral Suspension

Anti-Infectives

Augmentin® Suspension
Furadantin® Oral Suspension
Furoxone® Suspension
Humatin®
Mandelamine® Suspension/Forte®
Minocin® Suspension
Mycifradin® Sulfate Oral Solution
NegGram® Suspension
Proklar® Suspension
Sulfamethoxazole and Trimethoprim Suspension (Biocraft, Beecham, Burroughs Wellcome)
Vibramycin® Syrup

Antiparkinsonism Agents

Artane® Elixir

Antispasmodics

Antrocol® Elixir
Spasmophen® Elixir

Corticosteroids

Decadron® Elixir
Dexamethasone Solution (Roxane)
Dexamethasone Intensol Solution
Pediapred® Oral Liquid

Cough Medicines

Anatuss® With Codeine Syrup
Anatuss® Syrup
Brown Mixture NF (Lannett)
CCP® Caffeine Free
CCP® Cough/Cold Tablets
Cerose-DM®
Chlorgest-HD®
Codagest® Expectorant
Codiclear® DH Syrup
Codimal® DM
Colrex® Compound Elixir
Colrex® Expectorant
Conar® Syrup
Conar® Expectorant Syrup
Conex® Liquid
Conex® With Codeine Syrup
Contac Jr® Liquid
Day-Night Comtrex®
Decoral® Forte®
Dexafed® Cough Syrup
Dimetane®-DC Cough Syrup
Dimetane®-DX Cough Syrup
Entuss® Expectorant Liquid
Fedahist® Expectorant Syrup and Pediatric Drops
Guaificon®-DMS
Histafed® Pediatric Liquid
Hycomine® Syrup and Pediatric Syrup
Lanatuss® Expectorant
Medicon® D
Medi-Synal®
Naldecon-DX® Pediatric Drops and Syrup
Naldecon-DX® Adult Liquid
Non-Drowsy Comtrex®
Noratuss®-II Expectorant and Liquid
Organidin® Solution
Potassium Iodide Solution (various)
Prunicodeine®
Queltuss® Tablets
Robitussin-CF® Liquid
Robitussin® Night Relief Liquid
Rondec®-DM Drops
Rondec®-DM Syrup
Ryna® Liquid
Ryna-C® Liquid
Ryna-CX® Liquid
Scot-Tussin® DM Syrup

Scot-Tussin® Expectorant
Scot-Tussin® DM Cough Chasers
Silexin® Cough Syrup
Sorbutuss®
S-T® Expectorant, SF/D-F
S-T® Forte®, Sugar-Free
Sudodrin®/Sudodrin® Forte®
Terpin® Hydrate With Codeine Elixir (various)
Toclonol® Expectorant
Toclonol® Expectorant With Codeine
Tolu-Sed® Cough Syrup
Tolu-Sed® DM
Tricodene® Liquid
Trind-DM® Liquid
Tuss-Ornade®
Tussar® SF
Tussionex® Extended Release Suspension
Tussi-Organidin® Liquid
Tussirex® Sugar-Free

Dental Preparations and Fluoride Preparations

Cēpacol® Mouthwash
Cēpastat® Mouthwash and Gargle
Chloraseptic® Mouthwash and Gargle
Fluorigard® Mouthrinse
Fluorinse®
Flura-Drops®
Flura-Loz®
Flura® Tablets
Gel-Kam®
Karigel®
Karigel® N
Luride® Drops
Luride® SF Lozi-Tabs
Luride® 0.25 and 0.5 Lozi-Tabs
Luride® Lozi-Tabs
Pediaflor® Drops
Phos-Flur® Rinse/Supplement
Point-Two® Mouthrinse
Prevident® Disclosing Drops
Thera-Flur® Gel and Drops

Diagnostic Agents

Gastrografin®

Dietary Substitutes

Co-Salt®

Iron Preparations/Blood Modifiers

Amicar® Syrup
Beminal® Stress Plus With Iron
Chel-Iron® Drops
Chel-Iron® Liquid
Geritol® Complete Tablets
Geritonic™ Liquid
Hemo-Vite® Liquid

Iberet® Liquid
Iberet®-500 Liquid
Incremin® With Iron Syrup
Kovitonic® Liquid
Niferex®
Nu-Iron® Elixir
Vita-Plus H® Half Strength, Sugar-Free
Vita-Plus H®, Sugar-Free

Laxatives

Agoral® (plain, marshmallow, and raspberry)
Aromatic Cascara Fluidextract USP
Castor Oil
Castor Oil (flavored)
Castor Oil USP
Colace®, Liquid
Cologel®
Disonate™ Liquid
Doxinate® Solution
Emulsoil®
Fiberall® Powder
Haley's MO®
Hydrocil® Instant Powder
Hypaque® Oral Powder
Kondremul®
Kondremul® With Cascara
Kondremul® With Phenolphthalein
Konsyl® Powder
Liqui-Doss®
Magnesium Citrate Solution NF
Metamucil® Instant Mix (lemon-lime or orange)
Metamucil® SF Powder
Milk of Magnesia
Milk of Magnesia/Cascara Suspension
Milk of Magnesia/Mineral Oil Emulsion (various)
Milkinol® Liquid
Mineral Oil (various)
Neoloid® Liquid
Nu-LYTELY®
Phospho-Soda®
Sodium Phosphate & Biphosphate Oral Solution USP (Phillips Roxane)
Zymenol® Emulsion

Potassium Products

Cena-K® Solution
EM-K®-10% Liquid
K-G® Elixir
Kaochlor-Eff® Tablets for Solution
Kaochlor® S-F Solution
Kaon® Elixir (grape and lemon-lime flavor)
Kaon-Cl® 20% Liquid
Kay Ciel® Elixir
Kay Ciel® Powder
Kaylixir®
Klor-Con®/25 Powder
Klor-Con® EF Tablets
Klor-Con® Liquid 20%

Klor-Con® Powder
Klorvess® Effervescent Tablets
Klorvess® Granules
Kolyum® Liquid and Powder
Potachlor® 10% and 20% Liquid
Potasalan® Elixir
Potassine® Liquid
Potassium Chloride Oral Solution USP 5%, 10%, and 20% (various)
Potassium Gluconate Elixir NF
Rum-K® Solution
Tri-K® Liquid
Trikates® Solution

Sedatives-Tranquilizers-Antipsychotics

Butabarbital Sodium Elixir
Butisol Sodium® Elixir
Haldol® Concentrate
Loxitane® C Drops
Mellaril® Concentrate
Serentil® Concentrate
Thorazine® Concentrate

Vitamin Preparations-Nutritionals

Aquasol A® Drops
BioCal® Tablets
Bugs Bunny™ Chewable Tablets
Bugs Bunny™ Plus Iron Chewable Tablets
Bugs Bunny™ With Extra C Chewable Tablets
Bugs Bunny™ Plus Minerals Chewable Tablets
Calciferol™ Drops
Caltrate® 600 Tablets
Ce-Vi-Sol® Drops
Cod Liver Oil (various)
Decagen® Tablets
DHT™ Intensol Solution (Roxane)
Drisdol® in Propylene Glycol
Flintstones™ Complete Chewable Tablets
Flintstones™ With Extra C Chewable Tablets
Flintstones™ Plus Iron Chewable Tablets
Incremin® With Iron Liquid
Kandium® Drops Tablets
Lanoplex® Elixir
Lycolan® Elixir
Oyst-Cal® 500 Tablets
Pediaflor®
PMS® Relief
Poly-Vi-Flor® Drops
Poly-Vi-Flor®/Iron Drops
Poly-Vi-Sol® Drops
Poly-Vi-Sol®/Iron Drops
Posture® Tablets
Spiderman™ Children's Chewable Vitamin Tablets
Spiderman™ Children's Plus Iron Tablets
Theragran® Jr Children's Chewable Tablets
Tri-Vi-Flor® Drops
Tri-Vi-Sol® Drops
Tri-Vi-Sol®/Iron Drops

Vi-Daylin® ADC Drops
Vi-Daylin® ADC/Fluoride Drops
Vi-Daylin® ADC Plus Iron Drops
Vi-Daylin® Drops
Vi-Daylin®/Fluoride Drops
Vi-Daylin® Plus Iron Drops
Vitalize®

Miscellaneous

Altace™ Capsules
Bicitra® Solution
Cibalith-S® Syrup
Colestid® Granules
Dayto® Himbin® Liquid
Digoxin® Elixir (Roxane)
Duvoid®
Glandosane®
Lipomul®
Lithium Citrate Syrup
Nicorette® Chewing Gum
Polycitra®-K Solution
Polycitra®-LC Solution
Tagamet® Liquid

References:

Hill EM, Flaitz CM, and Frost GR, "Sweetener Content of Common Pediatric Oral Liquid Medications," *Am J Hosp Pharm*, 1988, 45:135-42.
Kumar A, Rawlings RD, and Beaman DC, "The Mystery Ingredients: Sweeteners, Flavorings, Dyes, and Preservatives in Analgesic/Antipyretic, Antihistamine/Decongestant, Cough and Cold, Antidiarrheal, and Liquid Theophylline Preparations," *Pediatrics*, 1993, 91:927-33.
"Sugar Free Products," 1992, *Drug Topics Red Book*, 17-8.

COMPATIBILITY OF MEDICATIONS MIXED IN A SYRINGE

	Atropine	Chlorpromazine	Codeine	Diphenhydramine	Droperidol	Fentanyl	Glycopyrrolate	Hydroxyzine	Meperidine	Metoclopramide	Midazolam	Morphine	Pentazocine	Pentobarbital†	Prochlorperazine	Promazine	Promethazine	Trimethobenzamide
Atropine		C	•	C	C	C	C	C	C	C	C	C	C	C	C	C	C	•
Chlorpromazine	C		•	C	C	C	C	C	C	C	C	C	C	X	C	C	C	•
Codeine	•	•		•	•	•	C	C	•	•	•	•	•	X	•	•	•	•
Diphenhydramine	C	C	•		C	C	C	C	C	C	C	C	C	X	C	C	C	•
Droperidol	C	C	•	C		C	C	C	C	C	C	C	C	X	C	C	C	•
Fentanyl	C	C	•	C	C		C	C	C	C	C	C	C	X	C	C	C	•
Glycopyrrolate	C	C	C	C	C	C		C	C	•	C	C	X	X	C	C	C	C
Hydroxyzine	C	C	C	C	C	C	C		C	C	C	C	C	X	C	C	C	•
Meperidine	C	C	•	C	C	C	C	C		C	C	X	C	X	C	C	C	•
Metoclopramide	C	C	•	C	C	C	•	C	C		C	C	C	•	C	C	C	•
Midazolam	C	C	•	C	C	C	C	C	C	C		C	•	X	X	C	C	C
Morphine	C	C	•	C	C	C	C	C	C	C	C		C	X	C*	C	C	•
Pentazocine	C	C	•	C	C	C	C	C	C	C	•	C		X	C	C	C	C
Pentobarbital†	C	X	X	X	X	X	X	X	X	•	X	X	X		X	X	X	•
Prochlorperazine	C	C	•	C	C	C	C	C	C	C	X	C*	C	X		C	C	•
Promazine	C	C	•	C	C	C	C	C	C	C	C	C	C	X	C		C	•
Promethazine	C	C	•	C	C	C	C	C	C	C	C	C	C	X	C	C		•
Trimethobenzamide	•	•	•	•	•	•	C	•	•	•	C	•	C	•	•	•	•	

C = Physically compatible if used within 15 minutes after mixing in a syringe
X = Incompatible
• = No documented information
C* = Potential incompatibility produced by certain manufacturers
† = Compatibility profile is characteristic of most barbiturate salts, such as phenobarbital and secobarbital

The following combinations have been found to be compatible:

atropine / meperidine / promethazine
atropine / meperidine / hydroxyzine
meperidine / promethazine / chlorpromazine

The following drugs should not be mixed with any other drugs in the same syringe:

diazepam, chlordiazepoxide

References:

Forman JK, Sourney PF, "Visual Compatibility of Midazolam Hydrochloride With Common Preoperative Injectable Medications," *Am J Hosp Pharm*, 1987, 44(10):2298-9.

King JC, "Guide to Parenteral Admixtures," St Louis, MO: Cutter Laboratories, 1986.

Parker WA, *Hosp Pharm*, 1984, 19:475-8.

Trissel LA, "Handbook on Injectable Drugs," 5th ed, Bethesda, MD: American Society of Hospital Pharmacists, Inc, 1988.

Stevenson JG, Patriarca C, *Am J Hosp Pharm*, 1985, 42:2651.

ORAL DOSAGES THAT SHOULD NOT BE CRUSHED

There are a variety of reasons for crushing tablets or capsule contents prior to administering to the patient. Patients may have nasogastric tubes which do not permit the administration of tablets or capsules; an oral solution for a particular medication may not be available from the manufacturer or readily prepared by pharmacy; patients may have difficulty swallowing capsules or tablets; or mixing of powdered medication with food or drink may make the drug more palatable.

Generally, medications which should not be crushed fall into one of the following categories:

- **Extended-Release Products**. The formulation of some tablets is specialized as to allow the medication within it to be slowly released into the body. This is sometimes accomplished by centering the drug within the core of the tablet, with a subsequent shedding of multiple layers around the core. Wax melts in the GI tract. Slow-K® is an example of this. Capsules may contain beads which have multiple layers which are slowly dissolved with time.

- **Medications Which Are Irritating to the Stomach**. Tablets which are irritating to the stomach may be enteric coated which delays release of the drug until the time when it reaches the small intestine. Enteric-coated aspirin is an example of this.

- **Foul Tasting Medication**. Some drugs are quite unpleasant in their taste and the manufacturer, to increase their palatability will coat the tablet in a sugar coating. By crushing the tablet, this sugar coating is lost and the patient tastes the unpleasant tasting medication.

- **Sublingual Medication**. Medication intended for use under the tongue should not be crushed. While it appears to be obvious, it is not always easy to determine if a medication is to be used sublingually. Sublingual medications should indicate on the package that they are intended for sublingual use.

- **Effervescent Tablets**. These are tablets which, when dropped into a liquid, quickly dissolve to yield a solution. Many effervescent tablets, when crushed, lose their ability to quickly dissolve.

Recommendations

1. It is not advisable to crush certain medications.
2. Consult individual monographs prior to crushing capsule or tablet.
3. If crushing a tablet or capsule is contraindicated, consult with your pharmacist to determine whether an oral solution exists or can be compounded.

COMPATIBILITIES OF MEDICATIONS WITH SODIUM BICARBONATE

Medications Compatible With Sodium Bicarbonate (when administered via piggyback technique)

acyclovir
amikacin
aminophylline
amphotericin
atropine
bretylium
cefoxitin
chloramphenicol
chlorothiazide
cimetidine
clindamycin
erythromycin lactobionate
famotidine
fentanyl
heparin
heparin/hydrocortisone
hyaluronidase
hydrocortisone
lidocaine
methotrexate
methyldopate
nafcillin
oxacillin
phenobarbital
phenytoin
phytonadione
potassium chloride
prochlorperazine
tolazoline

Medications That Are Incompatible With Sodium Bicarbonate

ampicillin
amrinone
ascorbic acid
calcium chloride
calcium gluconate
carmustine
cefotaxime
ceftazidime
cisplatin
codeine
corticotropin
dobutamine
dopamine
epinephrine
glycopyrrolate
hydromorphone
imipenem/cilastatin
insulin
isoproterenol
labetalol
levorphanol
magnesium sulfate
meperidine
methadone
methylprednisolone
metoclopramide
morphine
norepinephrine
penicillin
pentobarbital
promazine
secobarbital
streptomycin
succinylcholine
tetracycline
thiopental
vancomycin
verapamil

References:

Trissell LA, *Handbook on Injectable Drugs*, 6th ed, Washington, DC: American Society of Hospital Pharmacists, 1990.

Young TE and Mangum OB, *Neofax, a Manual of Drugs Used in Neonatal Care*, 4th ed, Columbus, OH: Ross Laboratories, 1991.

MULTIVITAMIN PRODUCTS AVAILABLE

Product	Content Given Per	A IU	D IU	E IU	C mg	FA mg	B_1 mg	B_2 mg	B_3 mg	B_6 mg	B_{12} μg	Fluoride mg	Other
Drops													
Poly-Vi-Sol®	1 mL	1500	400	5	35		0.5	0.6	8	0.4	2		
Tri-Vit (Tri-Vi-Sol®) (sugar free)	1 mL	1500	400		35								
Tri-Vit w/fluoride 0.25 mg (Tri-Vi-Flor® 0.25 mg)	1 mL	1500	400		35							0.25	
Liquid													
B Complex	10 mL	5000	400	10	50		2.25	2.6	30	3	9		
Tablets													
Nephrovite (Nephrocaps®)	1 tablet				100	1	1.5	1.7	20	10	6		5 mg pantothenic acid 150 μg biotin
Capsule													
B Complex	1 capsule	5000	400	10	50		2.5	2.5	20	0.5	2		15 mg pantothenic acid

NARCOTIC ANALGESICS COMPARISON CHART

Drug	Dosage Form	Onset (min)	Duration (h)	Equianalgesic I.M. Dose (mg)	Equianalgesic P.O. Dose (mg)	Parenteral Oral Ratio	Partial Antagonist
Alfentanil hydrochloride	Inj: 500 μg/mL 5 mL amp	Immediate (I.V.)	ND	ND	—	—	No
Codeine	Inj: 30 mg/mL as phosphate Tab: 15 mg, 30 mg as sulfate, 60 mg as phosphate	10-30 (I.M.)	4-6 (I.M.)	120	200	1/2-2/3	No
Fentanyl citrate (Sublimaze®)	Inj: 50 μg/mL 2 mL, 10 mL amp	7-8 (I.M.)	1-2 (I.M.) 0.5-1 (I.V.)	0.1-0.2	—	—	No
Hydrocodone and acetaminophen	Tab: 5 mg hydrocodone + 500 mg acetaminophen (Vicodin®)	ND	4-6 (P.O.)	—	ND	ND	No
Hydromorphone hydrochloride (Dilaudid®)	Inj: 2 mg/mL amp Tab: 2 mg	15-30 (I.M.)	4-5 (I.M.)	1.5	7.5	1/5	No
Meperidine hydrochloride (Demerol®)	Inj: 25 mg/0.5 mL, 50 mg/mL, 100 mg/mL amp Syrup: 10 mg/mL Tab: 50 mg	10-45 (I.M.)	2-4 (I.M.)	75-100	300	1/3-1/2	No
Methadone hydrochloride (Dolophine®)	Inj: 10 mg/mL amp Solution: 1 mg/mL Tab: 5 mg, 10 mg	30-60 (I.M.)	4-6 (I.M.) Duration increase with repeated use due to cumulative effects	10	20	1/2	No

(continued)

Drug	Dosage Form	Onset (min)	Duration (h)	Equianalgesic I.M. Dose (mg)	Equianalgesic P.O. Dose (mg)	Parenteral Oral Ratio	Partial Antagonist
Morphine sulfate	Inj: 10 mg/mL, 15 mg/mL amp, 2 mg/mL Carbuject®, 1 mg/mL 30 mL PCA syringe Inj: Preservative free 1 mg/mL 10 mL vial, 5 mg/10 mL amp (Duramorph® PF) Solution: 10 mg/5 mL, 20 mg/5 mL Tab (soluble): 10 mg, 30 mg Tab (controlled release): 30 mg MS Contin®	15-60 (epidural or I.T.) 15-30 (S.C.)	4-5 (I.M.) (S.C.)	10	60	1/6 Ratio decreases to 1/1.5-2.5 upon chronic dosing	No
Oxycodone hydrochloride and acetaminophen (P.O.) (Percodan®, Tylox®)	Cap: Oxycodone 5 mg + acetaminophen 500 mg Tab: Oxycodone (~5 mg) + acetaminophen 325 mg	15-30 (P.O.)	4-6 (P.O.)	—	30	—	No
Pentazocine (Talwin® NX)	Tab: 50 mg with 0.5 mg naloxone (Talwin® NX)	15-30 (P.O.)	3-4 (P.O.)	50	150	1/3	Yes
Propoxyphene and acetaminophen (P.O.) (Darvocet-N® 50 Darvocet-N® 100 Darvon®)	Cap: Propoxyphene HCl (Darvon®) 32 mg, 65 mg Tab: Propoxyphene napsylate 50 mg + acetaminophen 325 mg (Darvocet-N® 50) Propoxyphene napsylate 100 mg + acetaminophen 650 mg (Darvocet-N® 100)	30-60 (P.O.)	4-6 (P.O.)	—	130 — HCl salt 200 — napsylate salt	—	No

ND = no data.

*These values are based on adult studies. Duration may be shorter in children due to faster elimination (in general) compared to adults.

OTC COLD PREPARATIONS, PEDIATRIC

The following samples are representative of the more common OTC cold preparations. For specific dosing recommendations, see individual drug monographs.

Brand Name	Decongestant	Antihistamine	Antitussive	Expectorant	Other
Actifed®	Pseudoephedrine 30 mg/5 mL; 60 mg/tab	Triprolidine (1.25 mg/5 mL; 2.5 mg/tab)	—	—	—
Benadryl® Elixir	—	Diphenhydramine	—	—	14% ETOH
Delsym®	—	—	Dextromethorphan polistirex (30 mg/5 mL)	—	Long-acting (bid)
Dimetapp® Cough/Cold Elixir	Phenylpropanolamine (12.5 mg/5 mL)	Brompheniramine (2 mg/5 mL)	Dextromethorphan HBr (10 mg/5 mL)	—	2.3% ETOH
Dimetapp® Elixir	Phenylpropanolamine (12.5 mg/5 mL)	Brompheniramine	—	—	2.3% ETOH
Dorcol® Children's Cough Syrup	Pseudoephedrine (15 mg/5 mL)	—	Dextromethorphan (5 mg/5 mL)	Guaifenesin (50 mg/5 mL)	—
Neo-Synephrine® 12-Hour Children's Nose Drops	Oxymethazoline 0.025%	—	—	—	Benzalkonium chloride, phenylmercuric acetate 0.002% as preservatives
Neo-Synephrine® Nose Drops/Nasal Spray	Phenylephrine (⅛% for infants; ¼% for children)	—	—	—	Benzalkonium chloride, 0.02% (spray)
PediaCare® Allergy Formula	—	Chlorpheniramine (1 mg/5 mL)	—	—	—

(continued)

Brand Name	Decongestant	Antihistamine	Antitussive	Expectorant	Other
PediaCare® Cough-Cold Formula	Pseudoephedrine (15 mg/5 mL; 7.5 mg/tab)	Chlorpheniramine (1 mg/5 mL; 0.5 mg/tab)	Dextromethorphan HBr (5 mg/5 mL; 2.5 mg/tab)	—	—
PediaCare® Infants' Oral Drops	Pseudoephedrine (7.5 mg/0.8 mL dropper)	—	—	—	—
PediaCare® "Night Rest"	Pseudoephedrine (15 mg/5 mL)	Chlorpheniramine (1 mg/5 mL)	Dextromethorphan HBr (7.5 mg/5 mL)	—	—
Robitussin-CF®	Phenylpropanolamine (12.5 mg/5 mL)	—	Dextromethorphan HBr (10 mg/5 mL)	Guaifenesin (100 mg/5 mL)	4.75% ETOH
Robitussin-DM®	—	—	Dextromethorphan HBr (15 mg/5 mL)	Guaifenesin (100 mg/5 mL)	1.4% ETOH
Robitussin-PE®	Pseudoephedrine (30 mg/5 mL)	—	—	Guaifenesin (100 mg/5 mL)	1.4% ETOH
Robitussin® Pediatric Cough Suppressant	—	—	Dextromethorphan HBr (7.5 mg/5 mL)	—	—
Robitussin® Plain	—	—	—	Guaifenesin (100 mg/5 mL)	3.5% ETOH
Sudafed®	Pseudoephedrine	—	—	—	—
Sudafed® Cough Syrup	Pseudoephedrine (15 mg/5 mL)	—	Dextromethorphan HBr (5 mg/5 mL)	Guaifenesin (100 mg/5 mL)	2.4% ETOH

(continued)

Brand Name	Decongestant	Antihistamine	Antitussive	Expectorant	Other
Sudafed™ Plus	Pseudoephedrine (30 mg/5 mL or tab)	Chlorpheniramine (2 mg/5 mL or tab)	—	—	—
Tessalon™	—	—	Benzonatate	—	No sugar
Triaminic™ Expectorant (yellow)	Phenylpropanolamine (12.5 mg/5 mL)	—	—	Guaifenesin (100 mg/5 mL)	5% ETOH
Triaminic™ Nite Light	Pseudoephedrine (15 mg/5 mL)	Chlorpheniramine (1 mg/5 mL)	Dextromethorphan HBr (7.5 mg/5 mL)	—	—
Triaminic™ Syrup (orange)	Phenylpropanolamine (12.5 mg/5 mL)	Chlorpheniramine (2 mg/5 mL)	—	—	—
Triaminic-DM™ Syrup (dark red)	Phenylpropanolamine (12.5 mg/5 mL)	—	Dextromethorphan HBr (10 mg/5 mL)	—	—
Triaminicol™ Multi-Symptom Relief (red)	Phenylpropanolamine (12.5 mg/5 mL)	Chlorpheniramine (2 mg/5 mL)	Dextromethorphan HBr (10 mg/5 mL)	—	—
Tylenol™ Cold, Children's	Pseudoephedrine (7.5 mg/tab)	Chlorpheniramine (0.5 mg/tab)	—	—	Acetaminophen (80 mg/tab)
Vicks NyQuil™, Children's	Pseudoephedrine (30 mg/15 mL)	Chlorpheniramine (2 mg/15 mL)	Dextromethorphan HBr (15 mg/15 mL) larger (15 mL)	—	Less concentrated recommended dosage

(continued)

Brand Name	Decongestant	Antihistamine	Antitussive	Expectorant	Other
Vicks® Pediatric Formula 44® Cough & Cold	Pseudoephedrine (30 mg/15 mL)	Chlorpheniramine (2 mg/15 mL)	Dextromethorphan HBr	—	—
Vicks® Pediatric Formula 44® Cough & Congestion	Pseudoephedrine (30 mg/15 mL)	—	Dextromethorphan HBr (15 mg/15 mL)	—	—

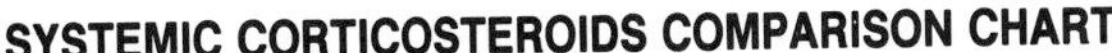

SYSTEMIC CORTICOSTEROIDS COMPARISON CHART

Relative Potencies and Equivalent Doses of Corticosteroids
(Glucocorticoid potency compared to hydrocortisone "mg" for "mg" basis)

Compound	Gluco-corticoid Potency	Mineralo-corticoid Potency	Equivalent Dose (mg)	Duration* of Action
Cortisone (Cortone®) Injection: 50 mg/mL suspension Tablet: 5 mg	0.8	++	25	S
Dexamethasone (Decadron®, Dexone®, Hexadrol®) Elixir: 0.5 mg/5 mL Injection: 4 mg/mL Intensol: 1 mg/mL Tablet: 0.25 mg, 0.5 mg, 0.75 mg, 1 mg, 1.5 mg, 2 mg, 4 mg	25-30	0	0.75	L
Fludrocortisone acetate (Florinef®) Tablet: 0.1 mg	10	+++++		I
Hydrocortisone (Cortef®) Injection: 50 mg/mL Suspension: 10 mg/5 mL Tablet: 5 mg, 10 mg, 20 mg	1.0	++	20	S
Methylprednisolone (Medrol®, Solu-Medrol®, Depo-Medrol®) Injection: 40 mg, 125 mg, 500 mg, 1 g Injection, suspension: 80 mg/mL Tablet: 2 mg, 4 mg, 16 mg, 24 mg	5	0	4	I
Prednisolone (Delta-Cortef®, Prelone® Syrup, Pediapred®) Liquid: 5 mg/5 mL Syrup: 15 mg/5 mL Tablet: 5 mg	4	+	5	I
Prednisone (Deltasone®, Liquid Pred®, Orasone®) Liquid: 5 mg/5 mL Tablet: 1 mg, 2.5 mg, 5 mg, 10 mg, 20 mg, 50 mg	4	+	5	I

* S = Short, 8-12 h biologic activity

I = Intermediate, 12-36 h biologic activity

L = Long, 36-54 h biologic activity

TOPICAL STEROIDS COMPARISON CHART

The following topical steroid preparations are grouped according to relative anti-inflammatory activity. Preparations in each group are approximately equivalent.

Drug	Dosage Form
Lowest Potency	
Hydrocortisone	0.5% cream, ointment
Hydrocortisone	1.0% cream, ointment
Hydrocortisone	2.5% cream, ointment
Hydrocortisone	1.0% solution
Hydrocortisone	1.0% lotion
Low Potency	
Alclometasone Dipropionate (Aclovate®)	0.05% cream, ointment
Desonide (Tridesilon®)	0.05% cream, ointment
Fluocinolone Acetonide	
(Fluonid®)	0.01% solution
(Synalar®)	0.01% cream
Low Intermediate Potency	
Betamethasone Valerate (Valisone®)	0.01% cream
*Flurandrenolide (Cordran®)	0.025% cream, ointment
Hydrocortisone Valerate (Westcort®)	0.2% cream, ointment
Triamcinolone Acetonide (Kenalog®)	0.025% cream, ointment, lotion
High Intermediate Potency	
Betamethasone Valerate (Valisone®)	0.1% cream, ointment, lotion
Desoximetasone (Topicort®)	0.05% gel
*Fluocinolone Acetonide (Synalar®)	0.025% cream, ointment
*Flurandrenolide (Cordran®)	0.05% cream, ointment, lotion
Halcinonide (Halog®)	0.025% cream
Triamcinolone Acetonide (Kenalog®/Aristocort®)	0.1% cream, ointment, lotion
High Potency	
*Amcinonide (Cyclocort®)	0.1% ointment
Betamethasone Dipropionate (Diprosone®)	0.05% cream, ointment, lotion
Desoximetasone (Topicort®)	0.25% cream, ointment
Diflorasone Diacetate (Florone®)	0.05% cream, ointment
Fluocinolone Acetonide (Synalar®-HP)	0.2% cream
Fluocinonide (Lidex®)	0.05% cream, ointment, solution
Halcinonide (Halog®)	0.1% cream, ointment, solution
Triamcinolone Acetonide (Kenalog®/Aristocort®)	0.5% cream, ointment

*Does not contain propylene glycol.

Reference: Cornell RC and Stoughton RB. The use of topical steroids in psoriasis, *Dermatol Clin*, 1984, 2:397-407.

THERAPEUTIC CATEGORY & KEY WORD INDEX

(Continued)

(Continued)

(Continued)

ANTIHYPERTENSIVE *(Continued)*

ANTIHYPOGLYCEMIC AGENT

ANTI-INFLAMMATORY AGENT

ANTILIPEMIC AGENT

ANTIMALARIAL AGENT

ANTIMANIC AGENT

ANTINEOPLASTIC AGENT

ANTIPARASITIC AGENT, TOPICAL

ANTIPARKINSON AGENT

ANTIPLATELET AGENT

ANTIPROTOZOAL

ANTIPSORIATIC AGENT, TOPICAL

ANTIPSYCHOTIC AGENT

ANTIPYRETIC

(Continued)

SEDATIVE *(Continued)*

SEROTONIN ANTAGONIST

SHAMPOOS

SKELETAL MUSCLE RELAXANT, CENTRAL ACTING

SKELETAL MUSCLE RELAXANT, DIRECT ACTING

SKELETAL MUSCLE RELAXANT, LONG ACTING

SOAP

SODIUM SALT

SOMATOSTATIN ANALOG

STOOL SOFTENER

SUGAR FREE

SULFONYLUREA AGENT

SYMPATHOMIMETIC

THROMBOLYTIC AGENT

THYROID PRODUCT

NOTES

NOTES

NOTES

NOTES

NOTES